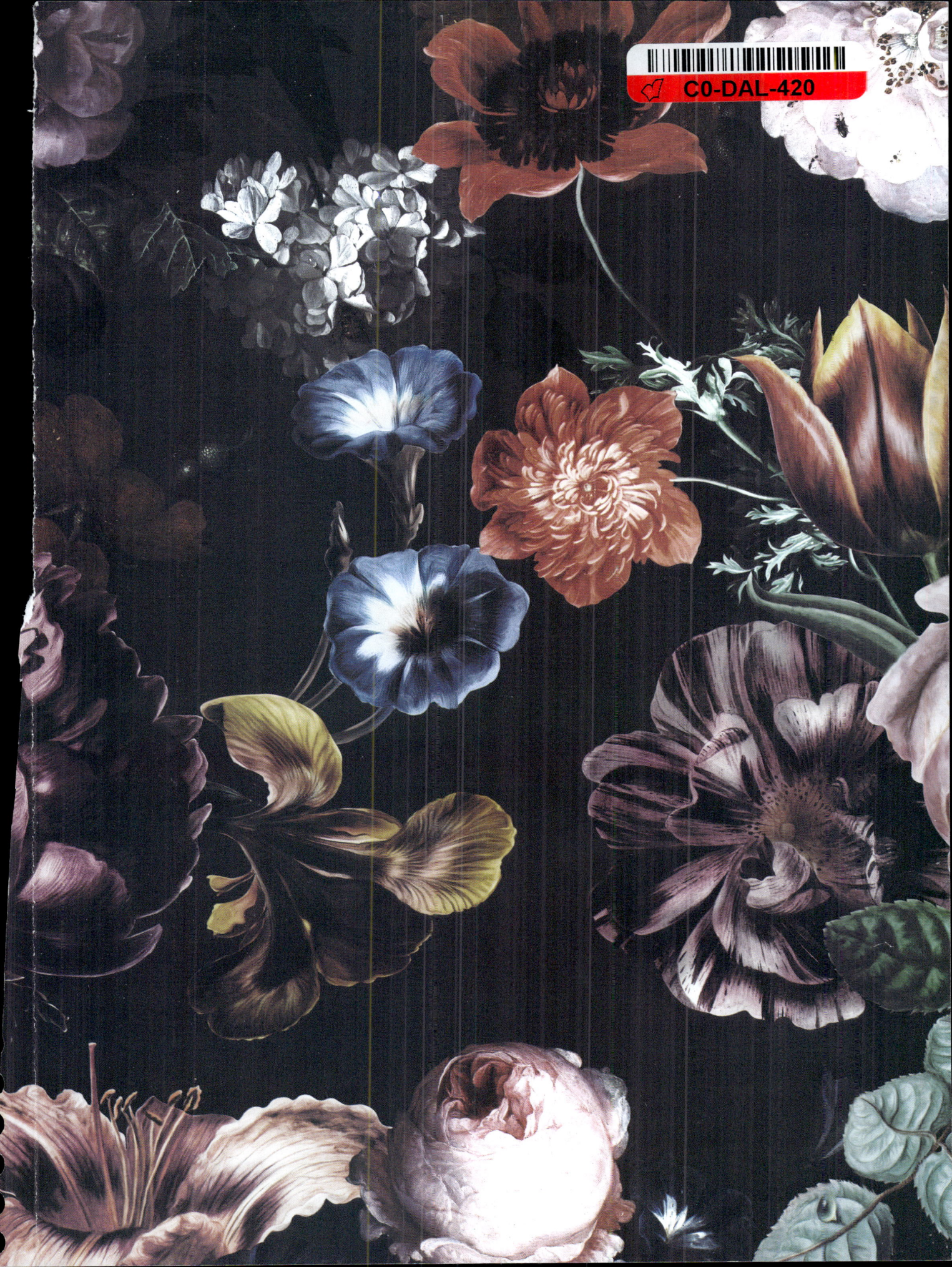

First Edition

Copyright © May 2021   •   Life & Science Publishing

1-800-336-6308   •   www.mylsp.com

ISBN 978-1-953099-04-4

Printed in the USA

All rights reserved. No part of this reference guide may be reproduced or transmitted in any form or by any means, electronic or mechanical, including photocopying, recording, or by any information storage and retrieval system, without permission in writing from the publisher.

Life & Science Publishing is the publisher of this reference guide and is not responsible for its content. The information contained herein is for educational purposes only and as a guideline for your personal use. It should not be used as a substitute for medical counseling with a health care professional. Neither the author nor publisher accepts responsibility for such use.

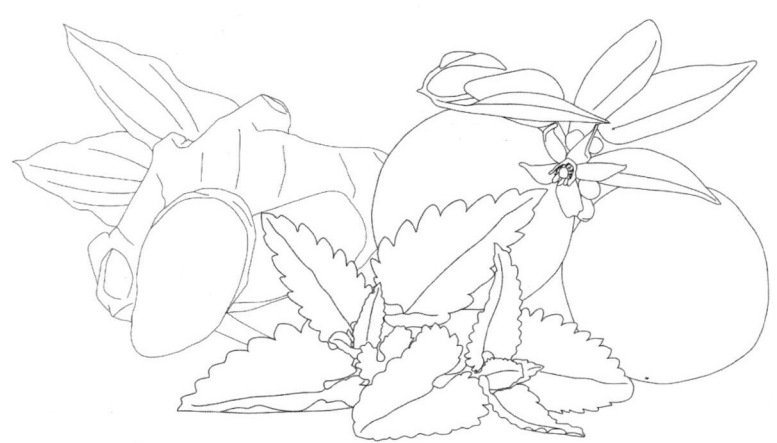

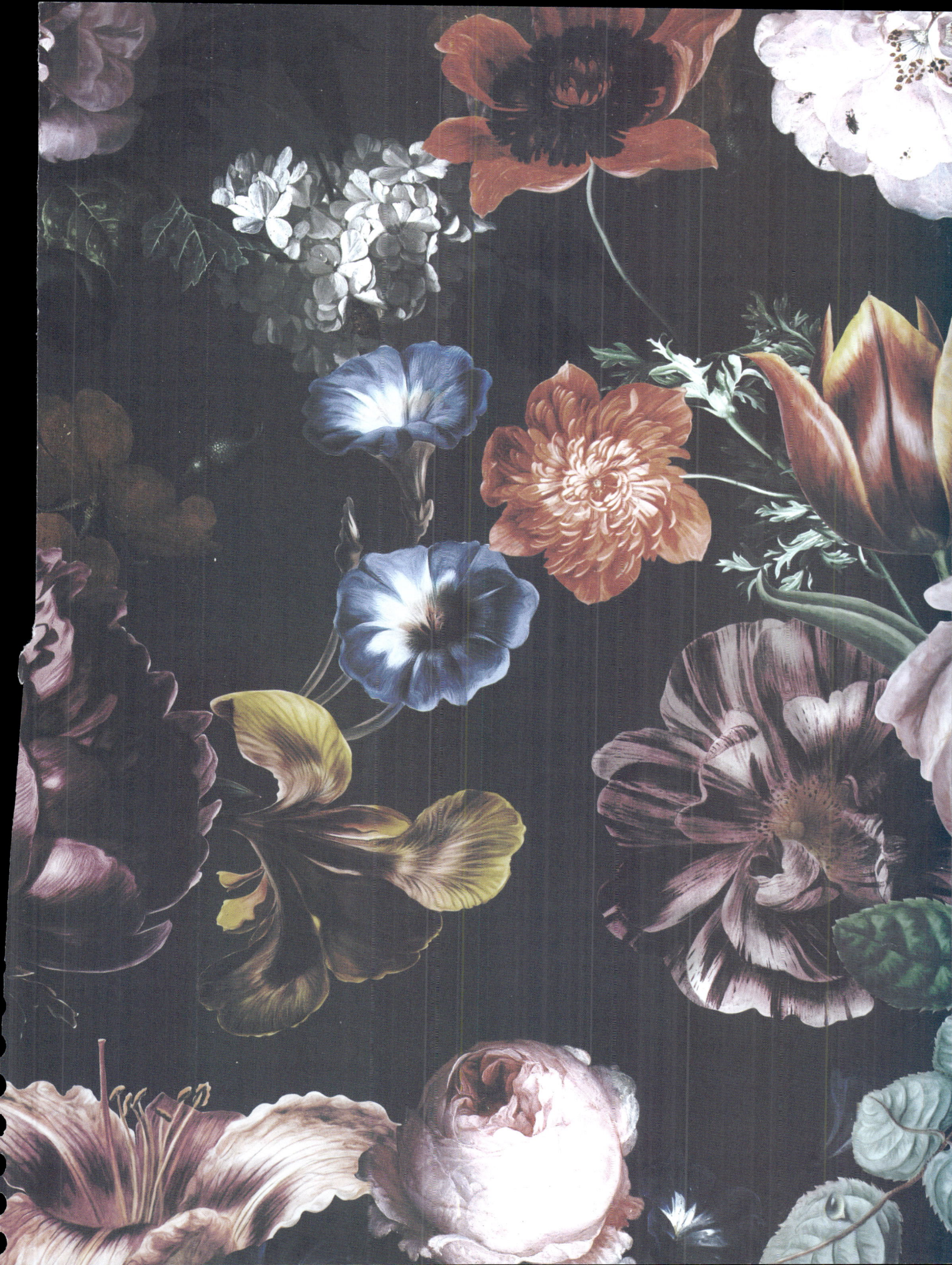

THE HEALTH + WELLNESS MANIFESTO

HEALTH AND WELLNESS ARE SIMPLE, BUT NOT EASY.

They are something we all want. The problem is that they take work -- mental, spiritual, and physical work.

WE BELIEVE THAT WORKING HARD FOR SOMETHING YOU CARE ABOUT IS CALLED "PASSION" NOT "STRESS."

Health and wellness are more than a meal plan and a gym schedule.

They are the mind, body, and soul's pursuit of joy.

WHAT OTHERS THINK ABOUT OUR CHOICE IS NOT OUR CONCERN. OUR BODIES AREN'T UP FOR DEBATE.

Our decisions don't need outside commentary.

APPROVAL ISN'T REQUIRED FOR JOY.

The way we spend our time, money, and energy should be authentic to us and the kind of life we are called to live.

JUST BECAUSE IT'S POPULAR DOESN'T MEAN IT'S GOOD FOR US.

Question everything. Do your own research. Don't take "their" word for it. Never shut up about it.

Our bodies are fearfully and wonderfully made.

We believe that the best health products aren't created in a lab -- they're made in the natural and rich soils of this amazing planet called earth.

WE ARE FEARLESS IN OUR PURSUIT OF TRUTH.

There's nothing we won't do to protect our own and our dreams for the future. There's nothing we can't do when we set our hearts and minds on a goal.

HERE'S TO US!

The wellness warriors, the healer feelers, the health nuts, the tree huggers, the essential oil freaks!

AND HERE'S TO THOSE WHO DON'T KNOW US YET -- THEY'RE ABOUT TO!

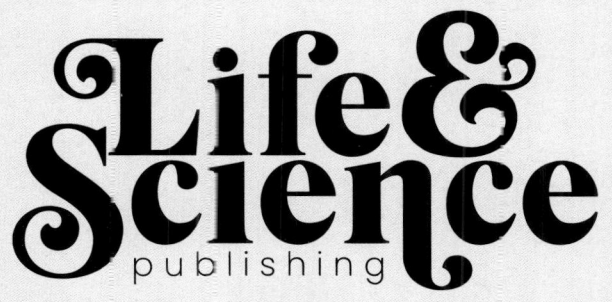

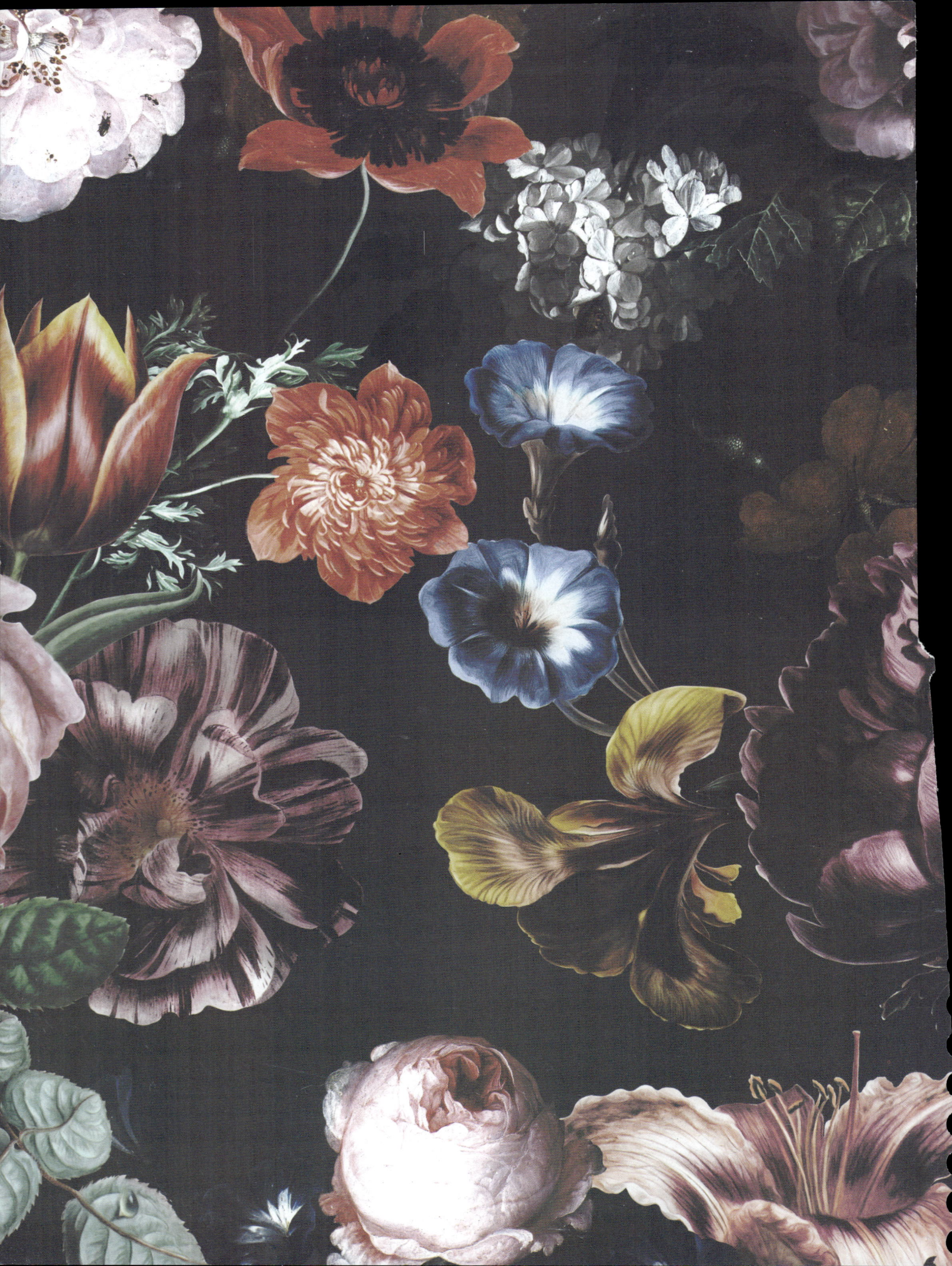

SECTION 1

SECTION 2

SECTION 3

SECTION 4

SECTION 5

SECTION 6

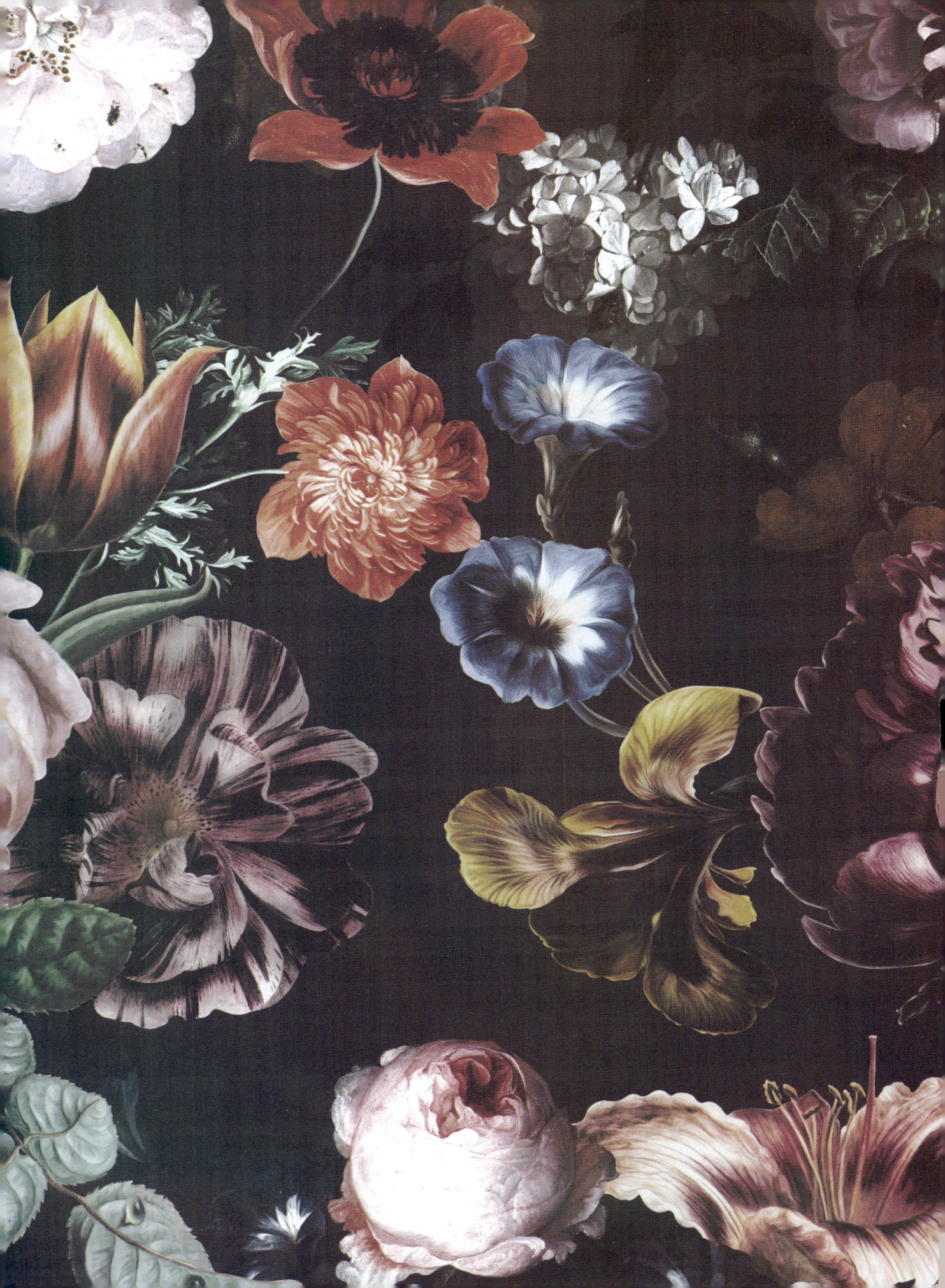

SECTION 1
- CHAPTER 1: WELCOME 1
- CHAPTER 2: ESSENTIAL OIL SINGLES & BLENDS 61

SECTION 2
- CHAPTER 3: NUTRITIONAL PRODUCTS 535
- CHAPTER 4: NINGXIA WOLFBERRY 543
- CHAPTER 5: UNDERSTANDING HORMONE HEALTH 559
- CHAPTER 6: SAFE, NATURAL PERSONAL CARE 571
- CHAPTER 7: HEALTHY CHOICES FOR CHILDREN 615
- CHAPTER 8: CREATING A TOXIN-FREE HOME 623
- CHAPTER 9: ANIMAL CARE WITH ESSENTIAL OILS 629

SECTION 3
- CHAPTER 10: TECHNIQUES FOR ESSENTIAL OIL APPLICATION 647

SECTION 4
- CHAPTER 11: SPIRITUAL, MENTAL & EMOTIONAL SUPPORT . 669
- CHAPTER 12: THE IMPORTANCE OF CLEANSING 681
- CHAPTER 13: BUILDING BLOCKS OF HEALTH 709
- CHAPTER 14: LONGEVITY & VITALITY 727

SECTION 5
- CHAPTER 15: PERSONAL USAGE GUIDE 769

SECTION 6
- APPENDIX & INDEX 933

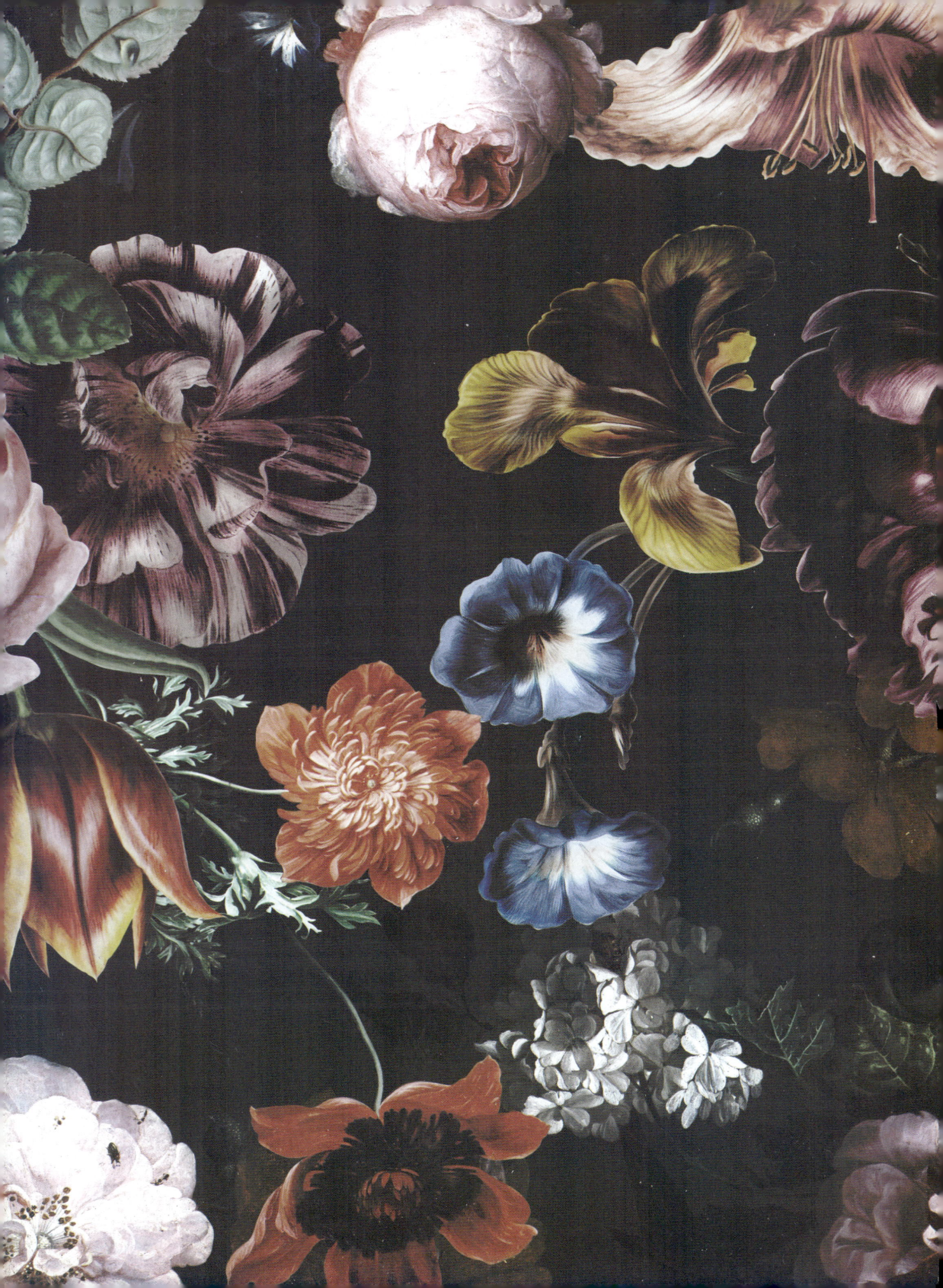

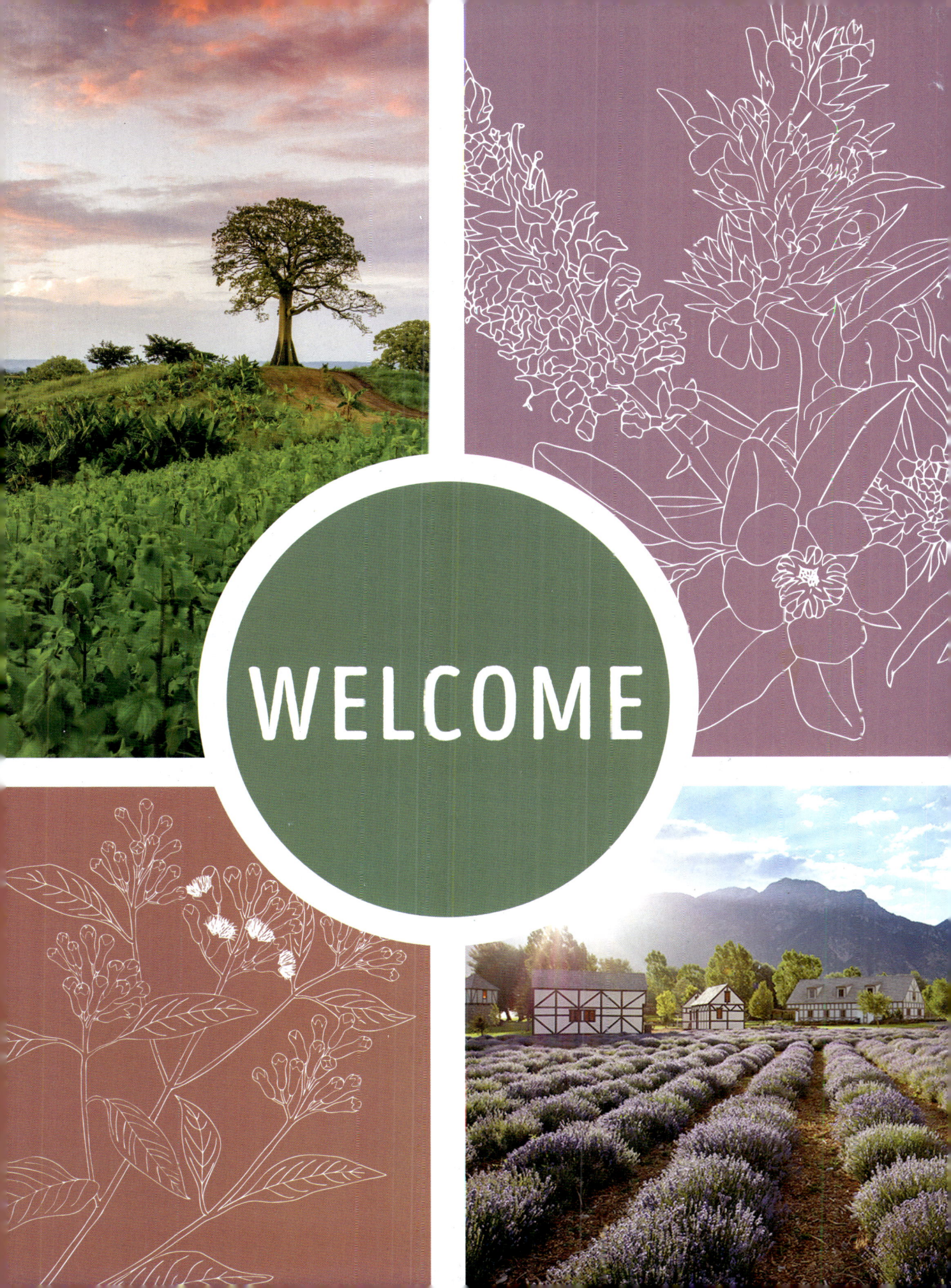

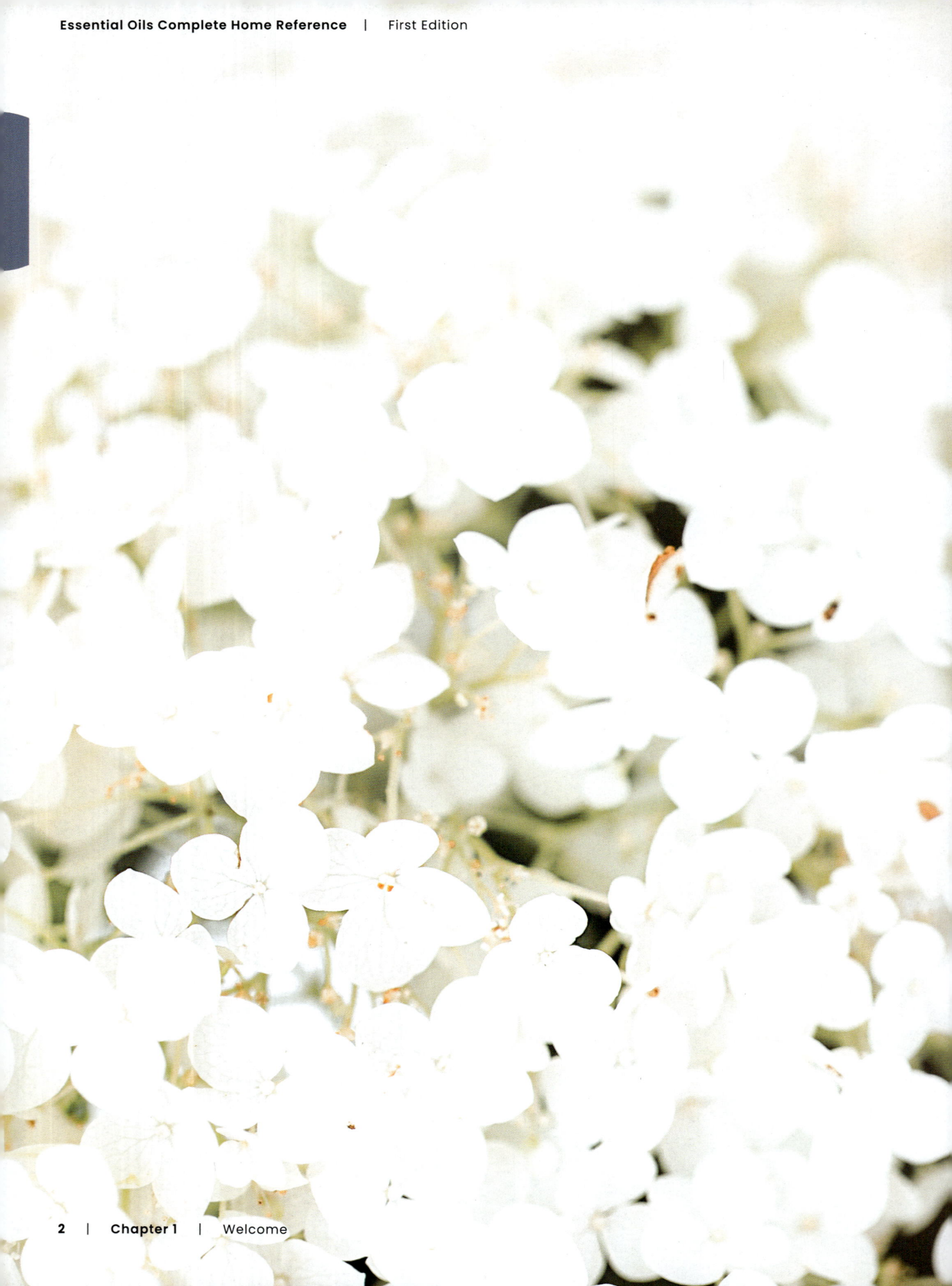

WE'RE GLAD YOU'RE HERE

We're glad you're here. Whether you are a wellness warrior, a healer feeler, a health nut, a tree hugger, an essential oil freak, or just a person who wants to know more about essential oils, you've found the right place. At Life & Science Publishing, we are the science, the tradition, the experience, and the general "go-to" for all things essential oils. If you're looking for the encyclopedia, the "bible" of essential oils, or just a gorgeous coffee table book, then congrats, you've found it.

You may already know this, but it's worth repeating that Young Living essential oils are the top-of-the-line, unmatched, singular standard against which all other oils are—and should be—compared. Each of these gifts, extracted from nature, has been created with a purpose. Each was botanically selected, nurtured, distilled, and sealed in the most ideal way to offer you the maximum health support. It's not so much how these oils smell, but how they make you feel, that truly counts.

If you're like us—and you're a fearless pursuer of truth—it's time to get started. It's time to give your questions what they want, a place to explore the answers.

Whatever challenges you have met that have led you here, we are pleased you agree with us: that the best health products aren't created in a lab, but made in the natural and rich soils of this amazing planet called earth.

Knowledge is power, and this book contains vast amounts of information. We invite you to question everything. We recommend that you do your own research. Don't ever take someone else's word for it. Once you find your truth, never shut up about it, and don't apologize for your hard-earned truth.

The *Essential Oils Complete Home Reference Guide* is the culmination of decades of research. It is our hope that you will use this book often to increase your understanding of the healing power that comes with these incredible oils. We think you will get to know each section like an old friend.

When we have traveled the world as a company, we have met individuals from all walks of life. Although the languages and cultures are different, there is always one thing we find in common: most people are seeking ways to increase health and happiness in their lives.

Millions of people are turning to an expanded view of health, recognizing that our bodies are fearfully and wonderfully made. They are discovering that health and wellness are more than a meal plan and a gym schedule. There's so much more to maintaining a lifelong commitment to health.

We have found that healthy people are happy people. We have witnessed people rejecting the side effects that come from past views of health: that a synthetic pill will fix one thing, yet simultaneously hurt another, and that's somehow okay. There's a reason people are taking a more holistic—or a more complete—approach to health. They are embracing the work it takes to create true health and wellness. They are seeking every possibility, not just one narrow view.

Our purpose in collecting this information and sharing it with you is to help you understand the potential benefits of essential oils and how to use them correctly. Whether you are young or old, able or ailing, a science lover or not, there is a place for you here. We hope this information opens the door to a new level of wellness and happiness for you and the ones you love.

Essential Oils Complete Home Reference | First Edition

WHAT ARE ESSENTIAL OILS?

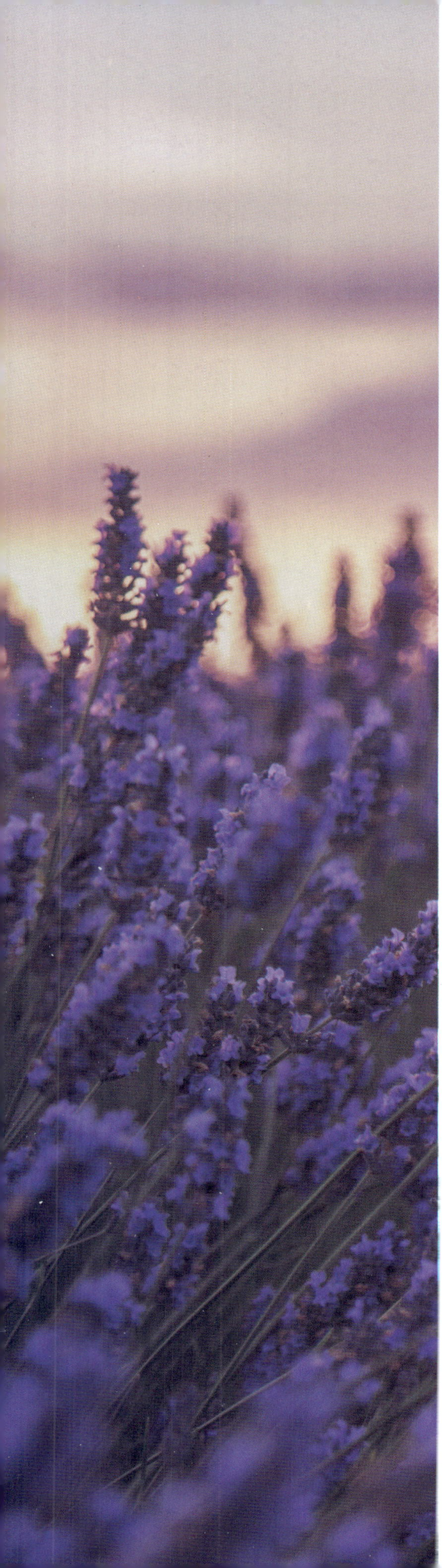

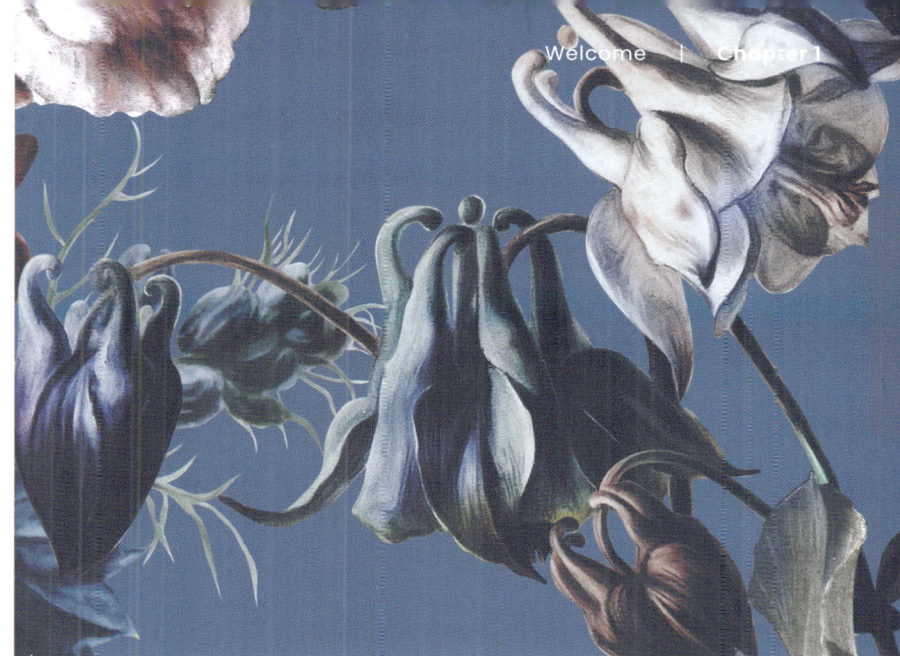

WHAT ARE ESSENTIAL OILS?

Essential oils are nature's volatile aromatic compounds generated within shrubs, flowers, trees, roots, bushes, and seeds. Most extraction is through steam distillation, hydrodistillation, or cold-pressed extraction.

The reason essential oils work, is because of their constituents, which, when in the right ratio, actually create something greater than the sum of the parts. Essential oils are complex. Each may have 100-500 different constituents, and the unique fingerprint is what makes them so effective. No two oils are alike.

Lavender oil, for example, has around 200 different constituents that have been identified so far. Lavender oil has been used for burns, insect bites, headaches, PMS, insomnia, stress, and hair growth. Because essential oils are so diverse and have many natural compounds, each oil can affect more than one tissue or body system. This is why the impact of essential oils on our bodies cannot be easily measured—there are endless possibilities.

Surprisingly, essential oils have a unique ability to penetrate cell membranes and travel throughout the blood and tissues. This is because the lipid-soluble structure of essential oils is very similar to the makeup of our cell membranes, and because the molecules of essential oils are also relatively small, which enhances their ability to penetrate the cells. When you apply them topically to your feet or soft tissue, essential oils can travel throughout your body in a matter of minutes.

WHAT ARE ESSENTIAL OIL GRADES?

WHAT ARE ESSENTIAL OIL GRADES?

There are five grades of essential oils. These grades let you know if what you are using is a pure essential oil from plants, a synthetic copycat, or a partial plant-based product filled with lab-created ingredients, used to increase volume or fragrance.

The grades are as follows:

1. **Naturally Therapeutic ™ Essential Oils:** These are pure, medicinal, steam-distilled essential oils containing therapeutic plant-based compounds.

    Translation: This is the only type of essential oil you want on or in your body.

2. **Natural (Organic) Oils and Certified Oils:** These oils may pass standard tests, and likely won't contain any therapeutic compounds or have a very small percentage of therapeutic compounds. Also, they may not have the ideal ratio of constituents to be effective.

    Translation: Your body deserves the best and this is not it.

3. **Extended or Altered Oils:** These are simply fragrance-grade oils.

    Translation: This is perfume, not medicinal oil.

4. **Synthetic or Nature-Identical Oils:** These oils are chemically created in a laboratory.

    Translation: These have no place near your precious body.

5. **Synthetic Biology:** The new weird laboratory-created synthetic and biological combo. To produce these oils, creative bioengineering combines with some of the nature-identical chemicals. This results in a hybrid that allows some companies to call them "natural" even though they are far from it. This is about using DNA from plant material and then using yeasts, fungi, and enzymes to ferment the chemicals so that they resemble essential oils. These are the Frankensteins of essential oils, and you'll want no part of them, even though they might smell nice.

Pro tip: Often other oil companies copyright a term using misleading labels like: "Certified" or "Therapeutic" or "Organic." Unfortunately, these labels do not necessarily mean it's an actual certification given by an outside quality review board, or that it has met any therapeutic standard. It's just a cleverly worded, copyrighted phrase. It's easy for people to be misled by these tricky labels. Beware of wolves in sheep's clothing!

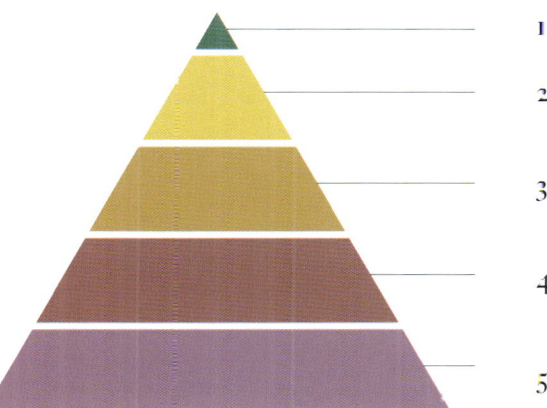

First Edition | Essential Oils Complete Home Reference | 5

NATURALLY THERAPEUTIC ESSENTIAL OILS...

NATURALLY THERAPEUTIC ESSENTIAL OILS...

When you think about the unique abilities of essential oils to help you and your family with personal, holistic health care, it makes sense that you have to use only the purest oils possible. When you look around to choose the best, you have to think about the entire process that goes into producing oils. You want only those that have had careful, natural, sustainable production from the beginning to the end. No matter how costly pure essential oils may be, there can be no substitutes.

Just as chemists can synthetically "copycat" the constituents of a pure essential oil, many essential oil companies today label their oils "therapeutic," even though they buy from anonymous brokers and have no experience in meeting any standards. Young Living was the first to establish guidelines that define what a *Naturally Therapeutic* essential oil is and to create oils that met or exceeded any known medicinal standard.

Synthetic or nature-identical oils are commonplace in the market and can be created cheaply and then sold in places like health food and drug stores or novelty and tourist shops for a very low price. They have no or little *Naturally Therapeutic* effects and may even be harmful. For instance, fragrance-grade lavender may have a harmful effect instead of a healing effect on burned skin.

Extended or altered oils may have an essential oil base but are "enhanced" with certain lab-created constituents to increase volume or fragrance. Due to chemical impurities or an antagonistic balance among oil constituents, these oils may be either ineffective or even cause negative effects.

USDA TO WEAKEN THE PURITY OF THE ORGANIC LABEL?

Plants that produce "natural" and "organic" essential oils may be grown in a natural, chemical-free environment but are not necessarily harvested at the right time or distilled correctly to maximize the *Naturally Therapeutic* potency of the essential oil that is produced. Such oils may be labeled "100% Certified Pure" or "Natural" but may not truly have *Naturally Therapeutic* values, and because of a 2011 decision to allow genetically modified alfalfa to be planted anywhere,[1] the very word "organic" may soon not guarantee freedom from GMO contamination. In the U.S., by 2014, 94% of the planted area of soybeans, 96% of cotton, and 93% of corn were genetically modified varieties.[2] If one GMO plant is approved as organic, the door of impurity has been opened.

SEED TO SEAL®

Young Living Essential Oils is the only company dedicated to the *Naturally Therapeutic* use and application of essential oils that is able to guarantee essential oil quality from seed to seal.

The oils that Young Living provides to consumers are extracted through steam distillation from a wide variety of plants, roots, bushes, trees, and resins and are as powerful and pure as the botanicals from which they are derived.

The life-giving energy of the essential oils that are carefully distilled from nature cannot be duplicated in a sterile laboratory. Synthetic constituents may be similar in structure but have none of the living plant energy that holds the God-given *Naturally Therapeutic* value of the oil that is released from the plant itself.

In *The Living Energy Universe*[3] by Gary Schwartz, PhD, and Linda Russek, PhD, the authors discuss the theory of "systemic memory." They note that the aromatic compounds contained in roses, for example, will have a different systemic memory than the very same aromatic compounds created chemically in a laboratory. "This implication may help explain why aromatherapy and other natural remedies such as herbs work. When the distiller extracts the 'essential' oils from a plant, he or she may be extracting the 'essential' systemic memories that reflect the wholeness of the plants themselves in addition to the unique combination of physical components that the individual plants contain."[3]

This is why Young Living takes so much care to capture the pure energy of the plants and guard the entire Seed to Seal process.

Years of experience have resulted in knowing the optimum species with the most *Naturally Therapeutic* potential and the optimal time and manner to cultivate and harvest them.

Equally important, the freshly produced oil is filtered, and stringent laboratory testing verifies the potency of the oil and desired chemical structure. The oil is then put into glass bottles in Young Living's clean-room facility and shipped.

Young Living's Seed to Seal process guarantees a genuine, pure essential oil that has the highest *Naturally Therapeutic* efficacy. This guarantee includes oils distilled from plants grown on Young Living's own farms and partner farms or sourced from Seed to Seal-certified suppliers. Young Living's essential oils continue to be used worldwide in more clinical and university studies than any other essential oils today.

SEED

Herbs are selected for the proper genus, species, and chemotype. Whether seeking Clove oil from Madagascar, Cistus oil from Spain, or Helichrysum oil from Croatia, Young Living experts constantly travel across the globe to verify plant, cultivation, and extraction quality to ensure absolute integrity of the essential oil.

For example, a huge increase in demand for helichrysum and a similar increase in illegal harvesting from poachers spurred the company to purchase a two-story commercial building in Split, Croatia, and build a new distillery with four 4,000-liter and one 6,000-liter boilers, which began distilling helichrysum from Young Living's Croatian partner farm in June 2015.

CULTIVATION

Young Living's essential oils are extracted from both wildcrafted and cultivated herbs, from established partnerships with growers and distillers all over the world. Some oils come from herbs cultivated in rural areas of countries such as Taiwan,

Australia, Madagascar, Indonesia, and Brazil, harvested by indigenous peoples, who have untold years of experience with the plants and their growing conditions. Other oils come from Young Living farms in Ecuador, France, Canada, Croatia, and the United States, where organic growing practices are adhered to with great care and exactness.

ORGANIC HERB FARMING

The key to producing oils with genuine therapeutic quality starts with the proper cultivation of the herbs in the field.

• Plants should be grown on virgin land uncontaminated by chemical fertilizers, pesticides, fungicides, or herbicides. They should also be grown away from nuclear plants, factories, interstates, highways, and heavily populated cities, if possible.

• Because robust, healthy plants produce higher quality essential oils, the soil should be nourished with enzymes, minerals, and organic mulch. The mineral content of the soil is crucial to the proper development of the plant; soils that lack minerals result in plants that produce inferior oils.

• Land and crops should be watered with deep-well, reservoir, or water-shed water. Mountain stream water is best because of its purity and high mineral content. Municipally treated water or secondary run-off water from residential and commercial areas can introduce undesirable chemical residues into the plant and the essential oil.

• Different varieties of plants produce different qualities of oils. Only those plants that produce the highest quality essential oil should be selected.

• As stewards of the earth, Young Living recognizes that every process, every crop, every fertilizer, and every water source has to be sustainable. Otherwise, the company would only be able to harvest crops of the *Naturally Therapeutic* oils once. They wouldn't be able to produce crops, distillations, and Seed to Seal oils year after year.

HARVESTING

The timing of the harvest is one of the most important factors in the production of *Naturally Therapeutic* oils. If the plants are harvested at the wrong time of the season or even at the incorrect time of day, they may distill into a substandard essential oil. In some instances, changing harvest time by even a few hours can make a huge difference. For example, when Young Living harvests German Chamomile in the morning, they produce oil with far more azulene (a powerful anti-inflammatory compound) than if they were to harvest it in the late afternoon.

Other factors that should be taken into consideration during the harvest include the amount of dew on the leaves, the percentage of the plant that's in bloom, and weather conditions during the two weeks prior to harvest.

To prevent herbs from drying out prior to being distilled, distillation facilities should be located as close to the field as possible. Transporting herbs to distillation facilities hundreds or thousands of miles away heightens the risk of exposure to pollutants, dust, mold, and petrochemical residues.

Young Living continues to expand and develop strategic partnerships with growers and distillers throughout the world.

DISTILLATION

A master distiller must oversee the entire process by harvesting at just the right time for the plant maturity and distilling with the proper temperature, pressure, and time, which varies with different plant material. Young Living often experiments with innovative distillation techniques on its farms to maximize therapeutic potency of the oils. Other oils are distilled traditionally, using techniques that have been passed down through generations from ancestors to descendants today.

STEAM DISTILLATION

Steam distillation is a separation process for materials that are temperature sensitive, like essential oils.

THREE METHODS OF STEAM DISTILLATION:

SIMPLE DISTILLATION: The plant material is loaded into the extraction chamber filled with water, which is heated to soften the plant fiber so that the oil molecules can be released.

As steam begins to rise, the oil molecules are released as vapors, which are carried with the steam into the condenser. The cooling water in the condenser converts the steam to water and the vapors to oil.

The oil and water mixture continues to flow into the separator, where the oil rises to the top of the water so that it can be drained off into containers. Clove and nutmeg are distilled this way.

HYDRODISTILLATION: Oil from resinous material like frankincense and myrrh is extracted through the method of hydrodistillation.

The resin is immersed in boiling water that is in constant motion while steam is injected into the chamber.

The resinous gas is then released into the steam, which carries it to the condenser, where the steam and vapor are gradually cooled to a liquefied form.

The water and oil mixture travels into the separator so that the oil can flow to the top of the water and be poured off into containers.

TRADITIONAL DISTILLATION: Today, the traditional method of steam distillation is still used around the world. This is how Young Living produces Lavender.

Plant material is loaded into the extraction chamber and tightly compacted. As the boiler heats the water, steam is released into the bottom of the chamber and starts to travel upward, saturating the material.

The steam impregnates the plant fiber, causing it to release the oil molecule as a gas from the oil glands of the plant. Then the steam carries the gas to the condenser, where it goes through a phase-change condensation as it passes through the cooling process in the swan neck and liquefies into water and oil.

The water and oil mixture then flows into the separator, where the oil can rise to the top of the water to be poured off into containers.

In each of these processes as the steam rises, it carries the released oil vapor into the condenser, where the water and oil vapor convert to a liquid and flow into the separator so that the oil can rise to the top of the water and be drained off.

THE SCIENCE AND ART OF DISTILLATION

Distillation is as much a science as it is an art. If the pressure or temperature is too high, or if the cooking chambers are constructed from reactive materials, the oil may not be *Naturally Therapeutic*.

Vertical steam distillation offers the greatest potential for protecting the therapeutic benefits and quality of

Welcome | Chapter 1

essential oils. In ancient distillation, low pressure (5 pounds or lower) and low temperature were extremely important to produce the therapeutic benefits. The late Marcel Espieu, who was president of the Lavender Growers Association in Southern France for 20 years, upheld the fact that the best oil quality can be produced only when the pressure is zero pounds during distillation.

Temperature also has a distinct effect. At certain temperatures, the oil fragrance and chemical constituents become altered. High pressures and high temperatures seem to cause harshness in the oil. This even affects the oil pH and the polarity.

For example, *Naturally Therapeutic* Cypress oil from Young Living requires a minimum of 24 hours of distillation at 265°F and 5 pounds of pressure to extract most of the active Naturally Therapeutic constituents. If distillation time is cut by only 2 hours, 18 to 20 constituents will be missing from the resulting oil.

However, most commercial cypress oil is distilled for only 2 hours and 15 minutes! This short distillation time allows the producer to cut costs and produces cheaper oil, since money is saved on the fuel needed to generate the steam. It also causes less wear and tear on equipment. Sadly, it results in oil with little or no *Naturally Therapeutic* value.

In France, lavender produced commercially is often distilled for only 15 to 20 minutes at 155 pounds of pressure with a steam temperature approaching 350°F. Although this high-temperature, high-pressure oil costs less to produce and is easily marketed, it is of poor quality. It retains few, if any, of the therapeutic properties of high-grade lavender distilled at zero pounds of pressure for a minimum of 1 hour and 15 minutes.

In many large commercial operations, distillers introduce chemicals into the steam-distillation process to increase the volume of oil produced. Chemical trucks may even pump solvents directly into the boiler water. This expands oil production by as much as 18 percent. These chemicals inevitably leach into the distilling water and mix

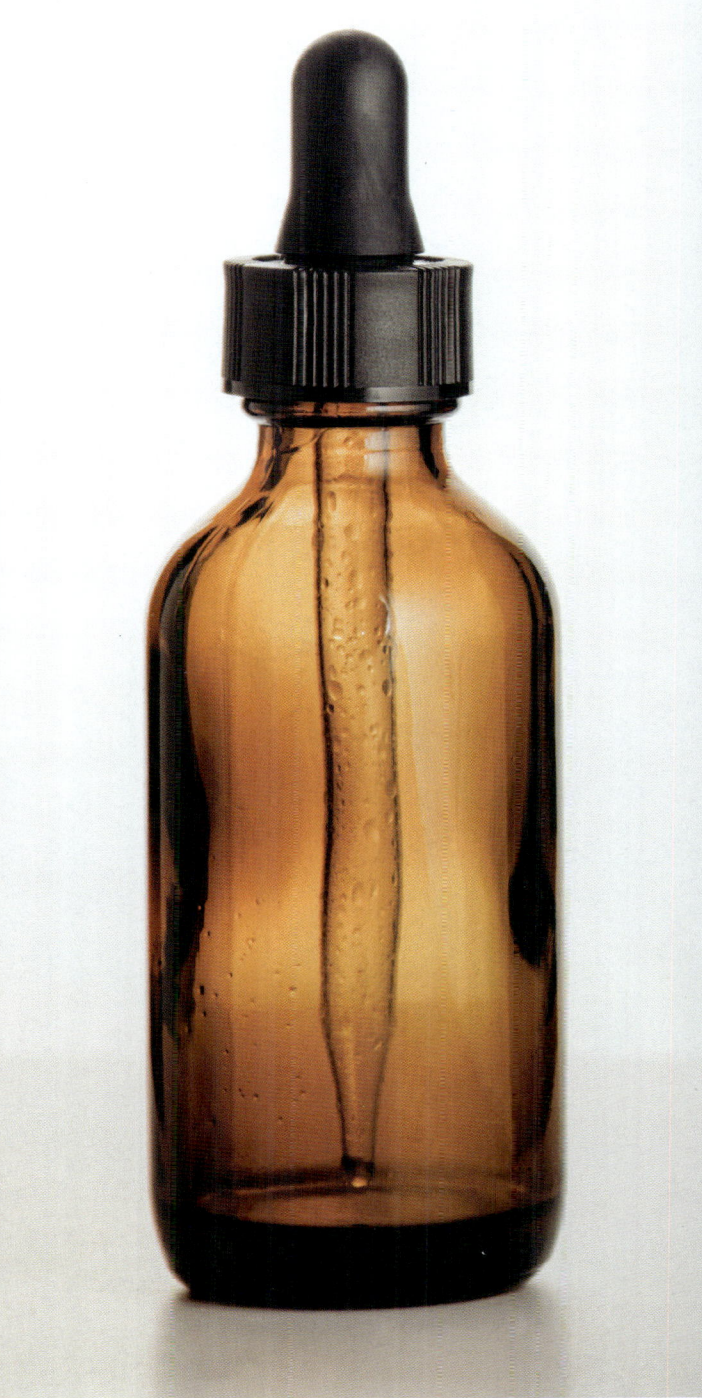

First Edition | Essential Oils Complete Home Reference | 11

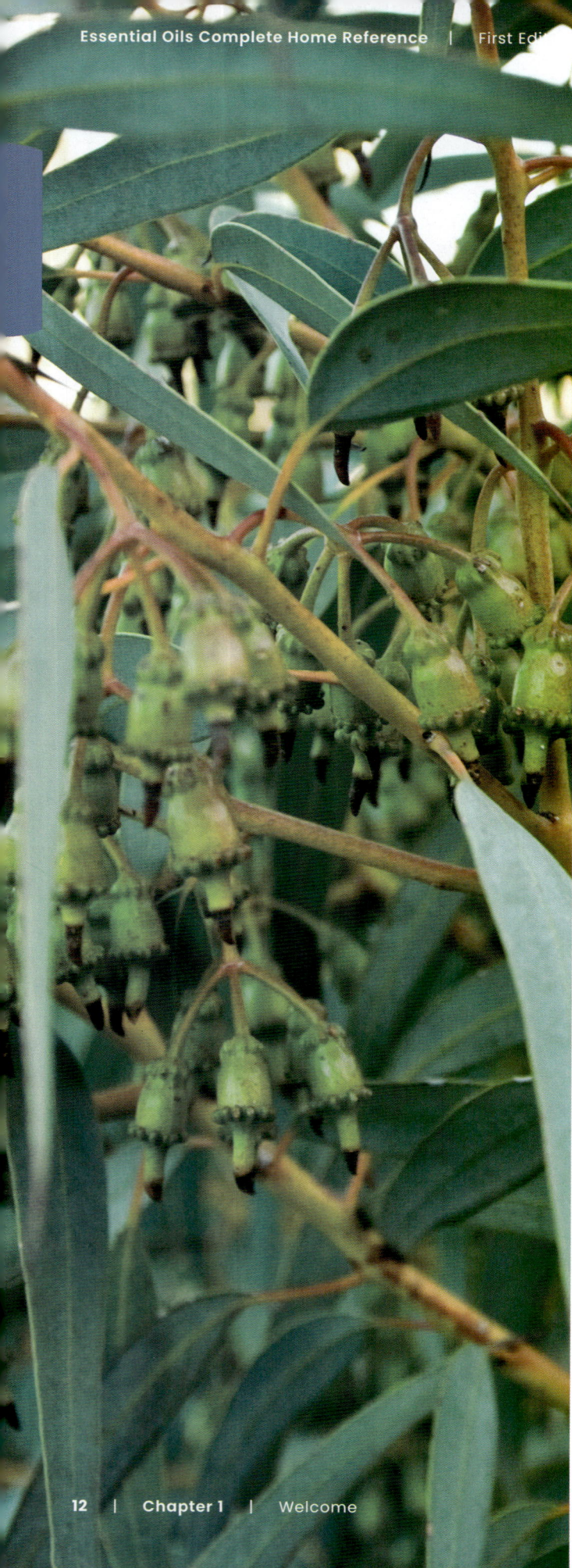

with the essential oil, fracturing the molecular structure of the oil and altering both its fragrance and therapeutic value. These chemicals remain in the oil after it is sold because it is impossible to completely separate them from the oil.

Another way that essential oil producers increase the quantity of the oil extracted is through redistillation. This refers to the repeated distillation of the plant material to maximize the volume of oil by using second, third, and fourth stages of steam distillation. Each successive distillation generates a weaker and less potent essential oil. Such essential oils are also degraded due to prolonged exposure to water and heat used in the redistillation process. Hydrolysis and/or oxidation of the essential oil occurs due to the water and/or heat, and the constituents responsible for its aroma and therapeutic properties begin to chemically break down.

COMBINING TRADITIONAL STEAM DISTILLATION WITH MODERN TECHNOLOGY

Few people appreciate how chemically complex essential oils are. They are rich tapestries of literally hundreds of chemical components, some of which—even in small quantities—contribute important therapeutic benefits. The key to preserving as many as possible of these delicate aromatic constituents is to steam-distill plant material in small batches using low pressure and low heat. This is the traditional method of distillation that has been used for centuries in Europe but is being abandoned in favor of high-volume pressure cookers designed to operate at over 400°F and use over 50 pounds of pressure. More importantly, the cooking chamber where the plants are distilled should be constructed of a nonreactive metal, preferably stainless steel, to reduce the possibility of the essential oil being chemically altered by more reactive metals such as aluminum or copper.

No solvents or synthetic chemicals should be used or added to the water used to generate steam because they might jeopardize the integrity of the essential oil. Even the addition of chemicals to water used in a closed-loop, heat-exchange system of the condenser can be risky, since there is no guarantee that they will be completely isolated from the essential oil. It is unfortunate that many essential oils distilled commercially are processed using boiler water laden with chemicals and descaling agents.

Absolutely no pesticides, herbicides, fungicides, or agricultural chemicals of any kind should be used in the cultivation of herbs earmarked for distillation. These chemicals—even in minute quantities—can react with the essential oil, degrade its purity and quality, and render it therapeutically less effective. During distillation, pesticide residue leaches out of the plant material with the extracted essential oil.

Young Living, the World Leader in Essential Oils and Distillation

During its 28-year history, Young Living Essential Oils has proven again and again to be the world leader in essential oils. With the installation in January 2014 of a true state-of-the-art, large-capacity, computerized distillery at its Highland Flats Tree Farm in Naples, Idaho, the company ushered in a new era in distillation for the production of essential oils, despite many of the challenges.

INNOVATION IN DISTILLERY TECHNOLOGY

If the techie part of the distillation process is exciting you at just the reading of those words, this section is for you. The distilleries in Highland Flats, Idaho, and later in Mona, Utah, are the latest innovation in distillery technology. They run an advanced computer program that monitors the distillation chamber, condenser, separator temperatures and pressures, starting with the steam injection flow into the extraction chamber and following it to the steam exit, monitoring flow temperature levels through the condenser to the separator.

THE FIRST CRITICAL FACTOR is the steam flow volume, which determines the temperature and ability to ramp the steam flow at the precise time to maintain sufficient temperature increase as the oil molecules travel up through the chamber for proper extraction without creating homogenization or reflux that will result in loss of oil, which will compromise the quality. The steam-injection rate and volume are very critical during the entire process.

THE SECOND CRITICAL FACTOR is to make sure the condenser temperature is not too hot or too cold as it descends through 200 12-foot-long tubes to prevent fracturing of the molecules, which could change the chemistry and aroma.

THE THIRD CRITICAL FACTOR is to be sure the temperature of the separator is right because many plants require different separation temperatures. If the temperature is wrong, many of the fine molecules that are important for *Naturally Therapeutic* application are lost, although this is unimportant to the fragrance and food flavoring industry.

With the company's innovative changes, up to 80 percent more of the fine molecules that are lost in normal distilling practices are now being captured.

The computer monitors all systems and makes changes instantly when needed. Manually, the operator may be monitoring, loading, or unloading a chamber and may not be able to make adjustments immediately, which could take several minutes to correct.

Cameras installed inside the swan neck enable the operator to watch the steam as it leaves the plant material carrying the oil into the condenser.

These two automated, state-of-the-art oil-extracting facilities are the most advanced distilling systems for producing essential oils in the world today.

HIGHLAND FLATS TREE FARM, NAPLES, IDAHO

- For the first time, on January 4, 2014, semitrucks were able to drive inside the heated distillery building at the Highland Flats Tree Farm. There the chips were unloaded and then packed into the two 21,000-liter extraction chambers.

- Later in 2014, two more extraction chambers were installed. One was another 21,000-liter chamber for conifer distillation. The other was an 8,500-liter chamber for the distillation of Idaho Tansy, for a total of four extraction chambers.

- The Highland Flats distillery completely eliminated the previous nightly drives of 125 miles in the semitruck pulling two trailers over the treacherous, winding roads covered with snow and ice to the distillery in St. Maries. The workers are safer, the distillation process is infinitely faster, and the oil production is spectacular.

The Highland Flats farm is an amazing place to visit. From distilling, to separating, to decanting/filtering, to

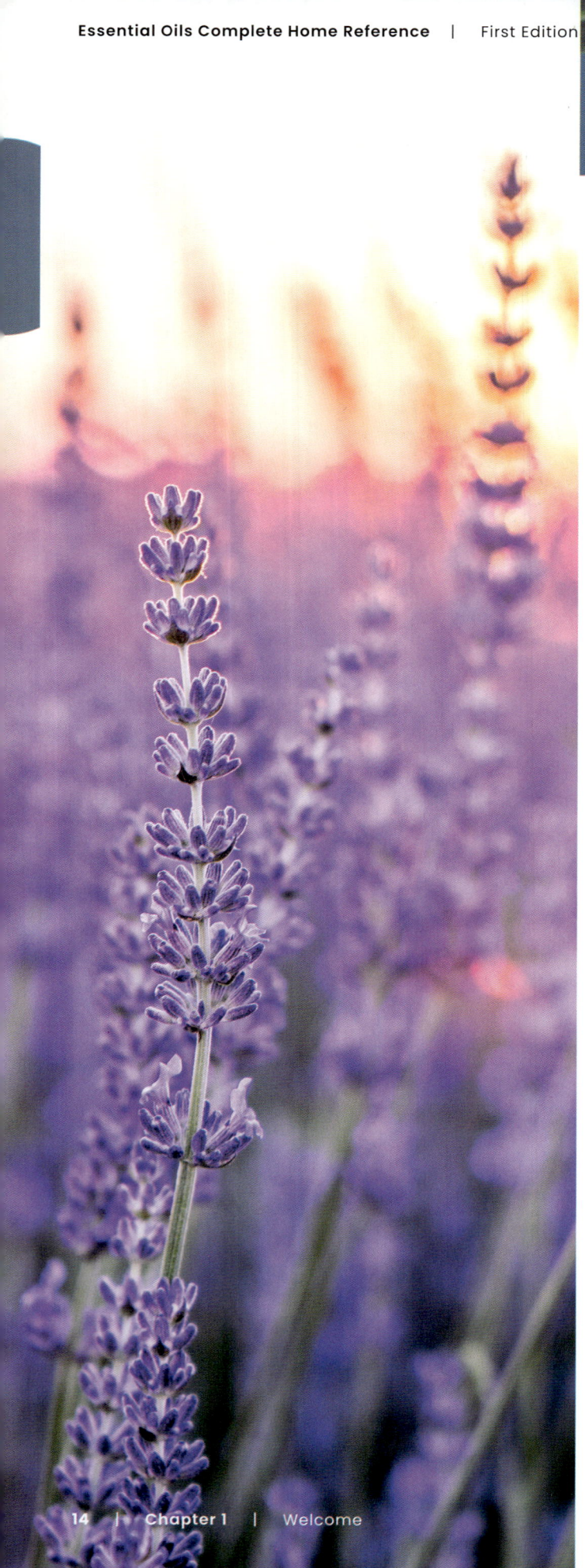

bottling, the oils are transferred from stainless steel to glass containers and never touch hands before they are sealed and packaged for shipping.

TWO NEW DISTILLERIES

After the Highland Flats distillery was finished, two additional distilleries were built, one in Canada and one in Croatia.

NORTHERN LIGHTS FARM, FORT NELSON; BRITISH COLUMBIA, CANADA

In 2014 the company broke ground for a new distillery located 8 miles outside of Fort Nelson in British Columbia, Canada, at Mile 308 on the Alcan Highway, to answer the growing demand for more Black Spruce essential oil.

- The Northern Lights Farm has five extraction chambers: two 12,000-liter, one 20,000-liter, one 10,000-liter, and one 3,500-liter, bringing the total distilling capacity to 57,500 liters. The first distillation of black spruce trees took place on March 9, 2015.

- Between 21 and 42 liters can be extracted from a single distillation. The volume of oil depends on the age of the tree and the branch growth. Older trees with less branch growth and more hard wood naturally produce less oil, and different conifer trees differ in their production. Chips from the entire tree, not just branches, are distilled.

- The new extraction chambers use 30 percent less fuel than the older extraction chambers. The new condenser system reduces the water consumption by 20 percent, and all water in the distillation process is recycled and never leaves the holding reservoir, thus preserving the ecosystem.

- The large, heated truck bay is fully insulated, with heated floors to melt snow and ice and remove the water in the chips for a better and greater distillation.

- Additional crops being considered to be grown and distilled in the future include white fir, a new species of balsam fir, yarrow, German chamomile, goldenrod, ledum, and Canadian fleabane.

SPLIT, CROATIA, FARM

In May 2015 Young Living purchased a two-story commercial building in Split, Croatia, totaling 16,580 square meters, which includes several offices; conference rooms; warehouse space; two large bays for the distillery; an enclosed boiler room; decanting, bottling, and labeling rooms; and a laboratory with a GC instrument for testing the oils.

An amazing accomplishment took place. Distilling of the much-needed Young Living Helichrysum began on June 19, exactly 19 days from when the crew started to assemble everything for the distillery and refit the building, which enabled them to distill during the short 55-day time period allowed by the government for distilling helichrysum.

- The distillery has four 4,000-liter, one 6,000-liter, and four 1,000-liter extraction chambers, bringing the total distilling capacity to 26,000 liters.
- After crops are harvested, they are trucked to the new facility, where the Seed to Seal process continues with distilling, laboratory testing, filtering, and decanting.
- Some of the oil goes to another area of the building, where it is bottled, labeled, and shipped to our European distribution center.
- Bulk oils are shipped to the warehouse in Utah for bottling, additional testing, labeling, and distributing to customers in the U.S. and other countries throughout the world.
- Our new partner farm is growing 78 hectares (192 acres) of helichrysum and contracting with many other farmers who have small acreages of helichrysum.
- Croatia is a country very rich with aromatic plants that will be cultivated at other partner and cooperative farms and are being distilled at Young Living's Split distillery.

Distillery operators say that distilling is both an art and a science. The company has combined research and science with more than 25 years of experience in engineering, designing, building, and operating nine existing distilleries and five partner distilleries in different countries.

All of the distilleries that Young Living built throughout the world on five continents are uncovering great discoveries in modern-day distillation, making them the only company in history to have distilled on such a worldwide scale. Consistency and increased control allow Young Living to further ensure the purity and quality of its world-class products.

The Seed to Seal standard is Young Living's trademark and was developed at the first farm in St. Maries more than 20 years ago. The company then took distilling to a higher level with the new distillery at Highland Flats and the upgrading of the distillery in Mona. Gradually, all of the Young Living distilleries will be upgraded to match the new operation. With the new automation and the most advanced technology available, modernizing the production process will be more efficient and effective than ever.

Young Living has again raised the bar of excellence in the essential oil industry; and with its Seed to Seal process, it is without question the world leader in essential oils.

ESSENTIAL OIL PRODUCTION

Producing pure essential oils is very costly. It often requires several hundred or even thousands of pounds of raw plant material to produce a single pound of essential oil. For example, it can take 2-3 tons of melissa plant material to produce 1 pound of Young Living Melissa oil. This extremely low yield explains why it sells for $9,000 to $15,000 per kilo. It takes 5,000 pounds of rose petals to produce approximately 1 pint of Young Living Rose oil.

It is easy to understand why these oils cost much more than others.

The vast majority of oils throughout the world are produced for the perfume industry, which is interested only in their aromatic qualities. High pressures, high temperatures, and chemical solvents are used in this distillation process to produce greater quantities of oil in a shorter time. To most people, these oils carry a pleasant aroma, but they lack true *Naturally Therapeutic* properties. Many of the important chemical constituents necessary to produce *Naturally Therapeutic* results are either flashed off with the high heat or are not released from the plant material.

TESTING

At Young Living, each essential oil must pass extensive testing to ensure an optimal bioactive profile. Young Living uses its own internal labs, as well as third-party testing from essential oil experts in other countries, to validate the purity and potency of essential oils.

ROUTINE TESTS DONE BY THE QUALITY CONTROL LAB

Each raw oil is sent to our Quality Control lab for identity, composition, purity, and Safety Data Sheet (SDS) testing. This is done by first performing organoleptic testing on qualities such as appearance, color, and odor.

IDENTITY TESTING

Identity testing is done using FTIR, refractive index, optical rotation, and specific gravity.

- **FTIR SPECTROSCOPY:** Fourier transform infrared spectroscopy (FTIR) characterizes an essential oil by its functional components such as ketones, aldehydes, alcohols, etc.

- **REFRACTIVE INDEX:** Measures the bending of light as it passes through the essential oil. It gives an index of refraction for biochemical constituents in the essential oil.

- **OPTICAL ROTATION:** Measures how much polarized light rotates through an essential oil, which indicates the overall chirality of the oil and helps determine if there is adulteration.

- **SPECIFIC GRAVITY:** A measurement that indicates how dense a substance is by comparing it to the density of water.

COMPOSITION TESTING

Composition testing is done by GC and compared to a library containing 400,000+ components based on retention time and peak area. Young Living then uses a proprietary retention index database created by Dr. Hervé Casabianca at CRNS in France via GC-MS and provides firm identification of individual molecules in each essential oil.

- **GAS CHROMATOGRAPHY (GC):** Using polar and nonpolar columns, a GC is able to separate components of an essential oil by the composition of the functional components of the oil.

- **GC/IRMS** (Gas Chromatography, Isotope Ratio, and Mass Spectrometry). This technology identifies ratios of isotopes and determines if those ratios are natural (created by plant metabolism) or synthetic (created in a lab). By this method, the IRMS can identify samples as either natural or synthetic.

PURITY TESTING

Purity is determined by GC, Optical Rotation, ICP-MS, microbiological, and Peroxide Value testing. Using these tests, Young Living ensures that the purity of the essential oil is held to the highest standard.

- **ICP-MS:** Inductively Coupled Plasma-Mass Spectroscopy (ICP-MS) is used to identify heavy metal contaminants that may occur naturally or be man-made. These include, but are not limited to, arsenic, cadmium, lead, and mercury. The ICP-MS is able to detect these heavy metals down to the part-per-billion (ppb) level.

- Microbiological Testing: Each new oil is tested to ensure that no microbial components are present. Although essential oils are not conducive to microbial growth, Young Living tests for the following: aerobic plate count, coliforms, yeast, mold, *Staphylococcus aureus*, *E. coli*, *Salmonella sp.*, and *Pseudomonas aeruginosa*.

- **PEROXIDE VALUE:** The determination of peroxides will give an initial evidence of rancidity in oils. This method is the most widely used to determine if primary oxidation has occurred in the oil.

SAFETY DATA SHEET TESTING

Young Living also provides testing to create Safety Data Sheets (SDS), which include flash point and combustibility.

- **Flash Point:** A test that determines the temperature at which an oil will vaporize and ignite in air.

- **Combustibility:** A test that determines the flammability of an oil.

FINAL PRODUCT TESTING

Once each raw oil is approved by Quality, it is given to Production, where it is bottled. The final product is then sent again to the Quality Control Lab. Oils are then retested in their final packaging using the same tests done on the raw oil. This is done to verify that no contamination or adulteration has occurred in the production process.

SEALING

The final step in Young Living's Seed to Seal process is carefully sealing each bottle of essential oil in Young Living's own clean-room facility and shipping it to customers worldwide.

Seed to Seal and its three pillars—Sourcing, Science, and Standards—are infused into every aspect of Young Living's exacting essential oil production processes.

Literally, from the plant seed that is cropped into the soil to the essential oil sealed in the amber bottle in Young Living's clean room, the Seed to Seal process is carefully supervised from beginning to end to ensure the quality and purity of Young Living's Naturally Therapeutic essential oils.

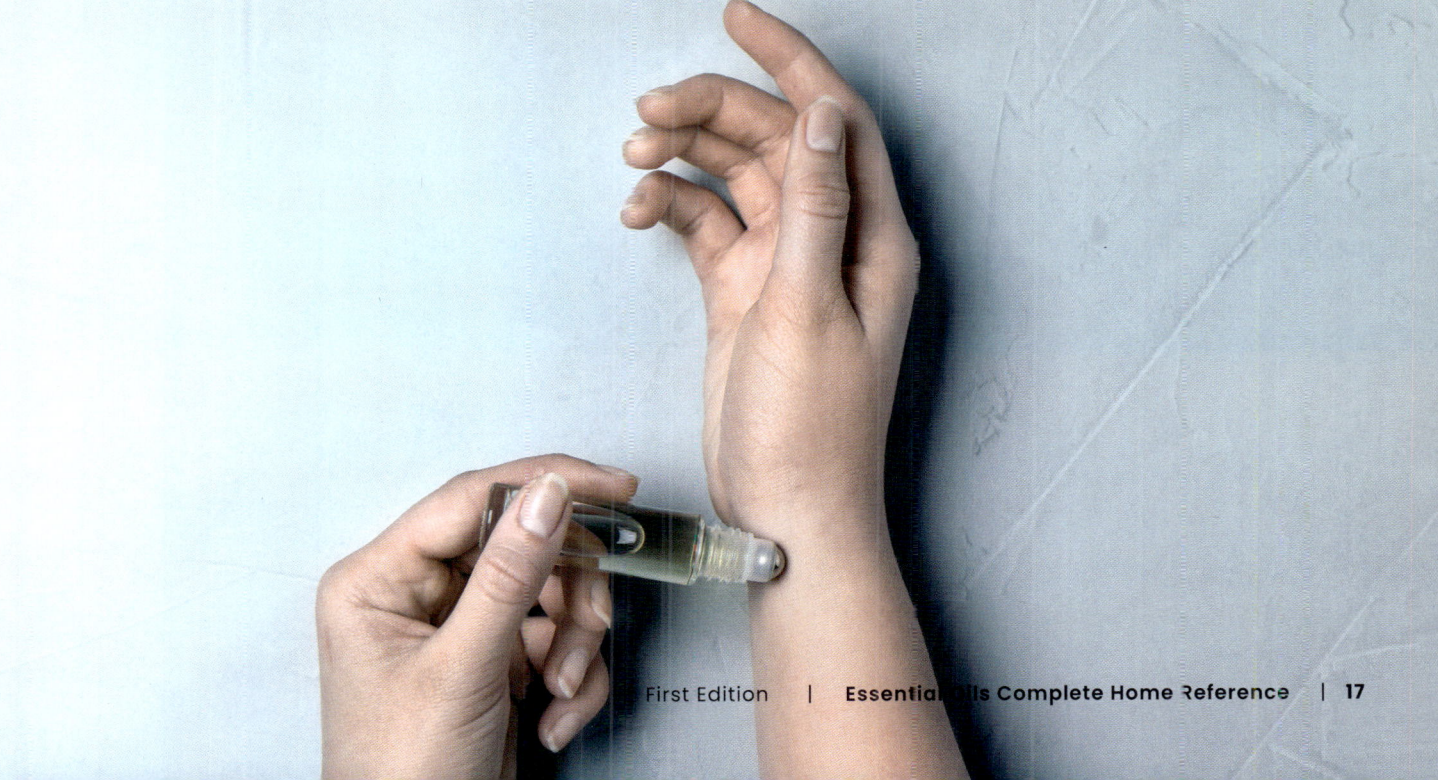

WHY ESSENTIAL OILS?

WHY ESSENTIAL OILS?

Here's some EO history for you that answers the "why" question…

In 1937 the man who coined the term "aromatherapy," Dr. René Maurice Gattefossé, published the first modern book on the discipline of using essential oils therapeutically. In the foreword to his groundbreaking work, Dr. Gattefossé wrote, "Besides their antiseptic and bactericidal properties widely used today (in part thanks to our work), essential oils possess anti-toxic and antiviral properties, have a powerful vitalizing action, an undeniable healing power and extensive therapeutic properties, as we have demonstrated and this work documents." [4]

"From time immemorial," he wrote, "in every country, aromatic plants have always been considered the most effective treatment for the diseases afflicting mankind. In many cases, the essential oil is used, which is evidence that the volatile part is the most effective."

From this humble, modern-day beginning, researchers and scientists from around the world have continued Gattefossé's work. This book continues that tradition in bringing the best research about essential oils to light.

CREATING KILLER MICROBES

The 1940s ushered in the glory days of antibiotics. Dr. Gattefossé would not have believed that nearly seven decades later, resistant bacteria would hurtle medicine back to the pre-antibiotic era.

How deadly are the antibiotic-resistant bacteria? The U.S. Centers for Disease Control and Prevention (CDC) reports that every year in the U.S. at least 2 million people are infected with antibiotic-resistant bacteria, and at least 23,000 people die each year as a direct result of these infections.

These statistics are no longer the worst of the bacterial bad news. From a study published in November 2015, the worst news is that the last-resort antibiotic (colistin) has now been conquered by a bacterial enemy: *Escherichia coli* (also known as E. coli). [5]

Worse news: the mcr-1 gene that confers resistance to colistin found in E. coli has been found together with the gene blaNDM-1, which allows resistance to an important class of antibiotic called carbapenems. This one-two punch found first on a Chinese pig farm has alarmed the media and scientists alike. [6]

The bacterial onslaught of antibiotic resistance started with methicillin-resistant *Staphylococcus aureus* (MRSA), then progressed to bacteria that were *Multidrug* Resistant, quickly expanding to *Extensively* Drug Resistant, and now we are facing Pan Drug Resistant. That's "*pan*" meaning "*all*" (as in pandemic). We now have pan drug-resistant bacteria that are resistant to *all known antibiotics*.

WHAT'S CAUSING ANTIBIOTIC RESISTANCE?

What's a leading cause of antibiotic resistance? Concentrated Animal Feeding Operations (CAFO). Animals raised for food are given *subinhibitory* amounts of antibiotics to increase growth. The subinhibitory amounts kill weaker bacteria but allow the stronger bacteria to become resistant. This is why doctors always tell you to finish an antibiotic because if don't take it all, you are teaching the bacteria how to defeat the antibiotic.

The numbers are shocking: *80 percent* of antibiotics used in the United States are used in livestock farming to increase growth. The last-resort antibiotic, colistin, no longer effective against E. coli (this pan-resistant E. coli strain is now found in China and has spread around the world), was given to food animals in China in horrific numbers. "China alone uses 12,000 tons of colistin in animal farming each year. The U.S. uses 800 tons annually, and another 400 tons is used in Europe to prevent and treat animal diarrhea." Until this practice is stopped, antibiotic resistance will continue to grow. [7]

While in 2006 the European Union banned antibiotics as agricultural growth promoters, by 2013 the only action of the USDA was to issue guidance for "voluntary" plans to phase out the use of medically important antibiotics in livestock for growth purposes.

Antibacterial soaps containing the chemical triclosan were once the popular answer to antibacterial resistance. With overuse, it is not surprising that many virulent strains of bacteria became resistant to triclosan too. *E. coli, Salmonella enterica, Staphylococcus aureus,* and *Mycobacterium tuberculosis* are able to fight triclosan with a cellular mechanism called a "bacterial efflux pump" that discharges the antibacterial agent and keeps it and any other good microbes away from the infected cells.

Thankfully, on September 2, 2016, the FDA issued a final ruling that triclosan (for liquid soaps) and triclocarban (for bar soaps) cannot be marketed because manufacturers failed to prove the ingredients "are both safe for long-term daily use and more effective than plain soap and water in preventing illness and the spread of certain infections."[8]

The superbug C-diff (recently reclassified as Clostridioides difficile) caused 223,900 cases in hospitalized patients and 12,800 deaths in the United States in 2017 according to the 2019 AR Threats Report. *Medical News Today* reported June 27, 2019, that "C-diff does not usually cause problems for people who are otherwise healthy. However, some antibiotics may alter the balance of bacteria in the gut to allow [it] to multiply. It is at this stage that it becomes an infection."

ESSENTIAL OIL COMPLEXITY: A WEAPON AGAINST BACTERIAL RESISTANCE

An infectious disease specialist at Louis Stokes Cleveland V.A. Medical Center and Case Western Reserve University, Dr. Louis B. Rice, warned, "There are strains out there, and they are becoming more and more common, that are resistant to virtually every antibiotic we have." Antibiotics may crumble before these "germs on steroids," but essential oils do not.[9]

The multitude of chemical constituents that make up essential oils present bacteria with a puzzle that cannot be solved. The mosaic of hundreds of chemical constituents simply do not allow for bacterial resistance.

Beginning in the mid-1990s, scientists began to notice the unexpected gift of essential oils against resistant bacteria. A 1995 Australian study found 68 isolates of MRSA were susceptible to tea tree oil.[15] In a study on an essential oil-containing dentifrice on dental plaque microbial composition, researchers observed, "Additionally, there was no evidence of the development of bacterial resistance to the antimicrobial activity of the essential oils or the emergence of opportunistic pathogens."[10]

A study of lemon verbena and lemongrass essential oil against the bacteria that cause ulcers caused the scientists to marvel about the power of lemongrass: "Resistance to lemongrass did not develop even after 10 sequential passages, whereas resistance to clarithromycin developed under the same conditions."[11]

Two antiseptic mouthwashes were compared for their control of plaque and gingivitis. While the chemically based mouthwash can cause brown spots on the teeth and tongue, the essential oil mouthwash was effective with no adverse effects and "no evidence of antimicrobial resistance."[12]

In 2009 essential oils were tested against several common and hospital-acquired bacterial and yeast isolates (six *Staphylococcus* strains, including MRSA; four *Streptococcus* strains; and three Candida strains, including *Candida krusei*). The oils tested were eucalyptus, tea tree, white thyme, lavender, lemon, lemongrass, cinnamon, grapefruit, clove bud, sandalwood, peppermint, Kunzea, and sage. The strongest inhibition was observed with white thyme, lemon, lemongrass, and cinnamon oils, while the other oils showed "considerable efficacy." The control group produced no efficacy. The conclusion: ". . . essential oils represent a cheap and effective antiseptic topical treatment option even for antibiotic-resistant strains [such] as MRSA and antimycotic-resistant Candida species."[12]

Keep an eye on the website of the U. S. National Library of Medicine (PubMed.gov) for research on essential oils against global drug-resistant bacteria.

WORLDWIDE RESEARCH

PubMed.gov [www.ncbi.nlm.nih.gov/pubmed] is the information website for the U.S. National Library of Medicine and the National Institutes of Health. As of July

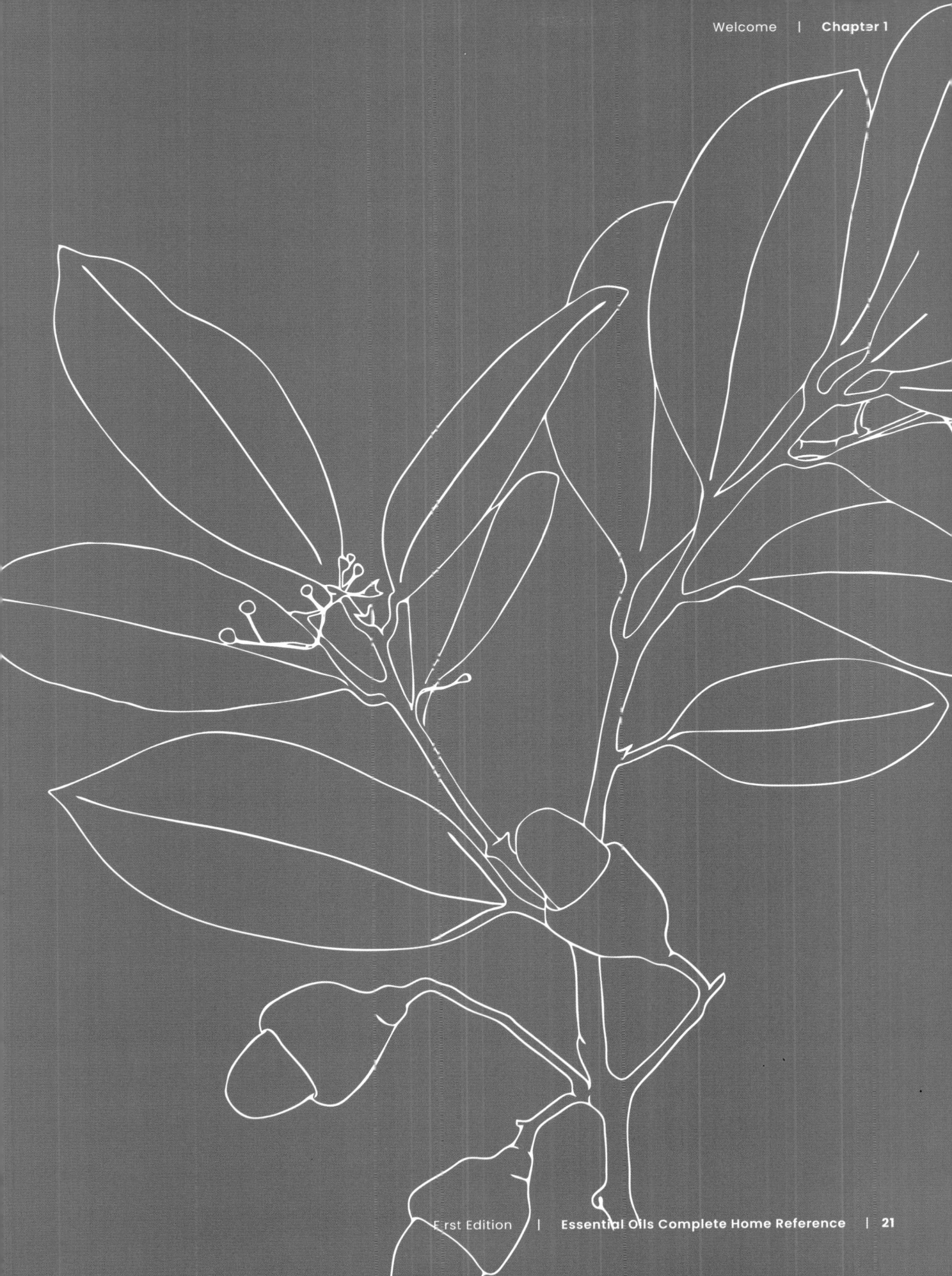

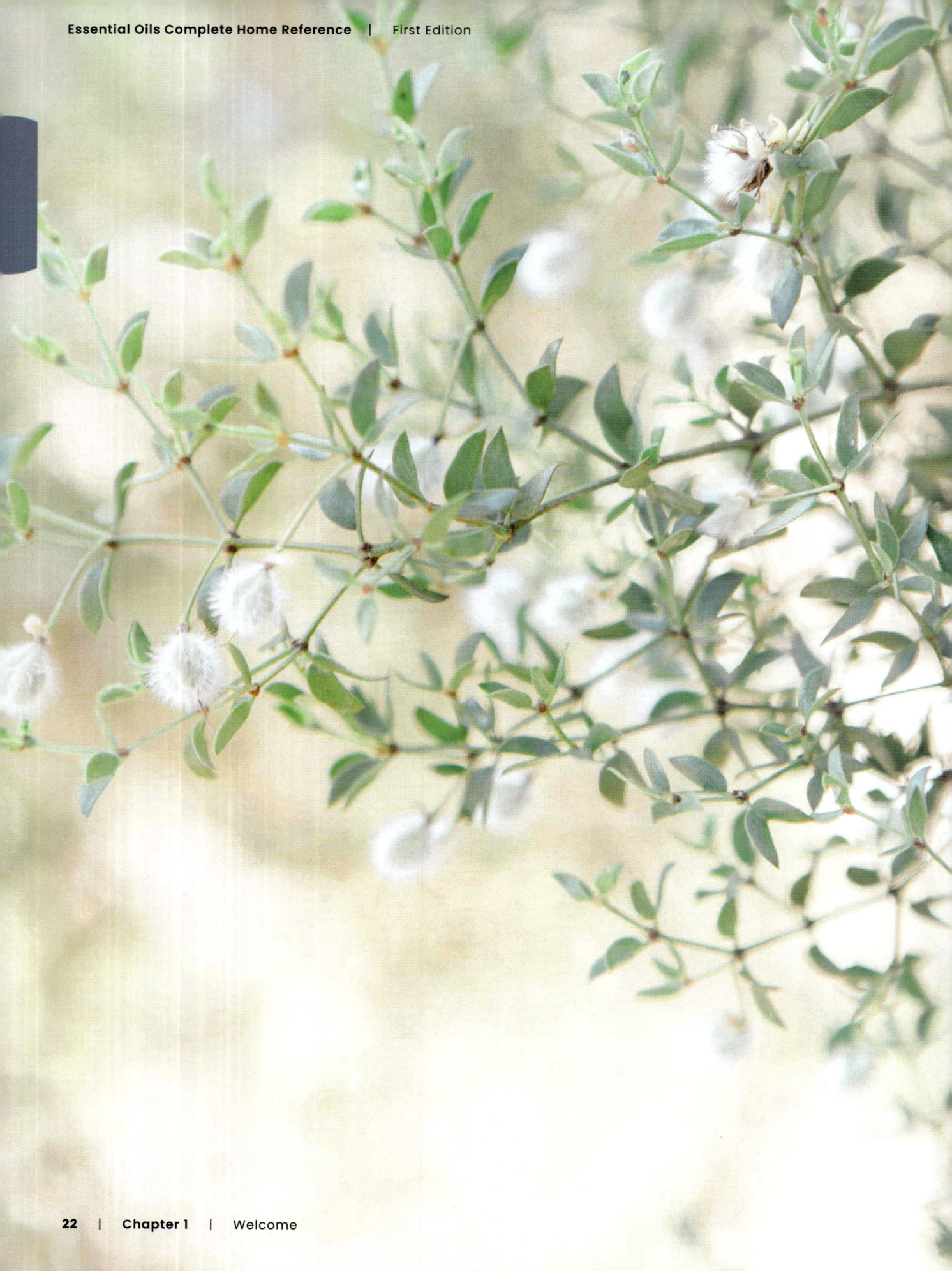

27, 2020, this online library contains more than 30 million citations for biomedical literature from MEDLINE, life science journals, and online books. Essential oils are represented in 178,438 peer-reviewed scientific studies.

Research on essential oils includes a wide array of topics. Italian researchers studied the neuroprotective effects of bergamot. In Iceland, researchers tested basil against otitis media (ear infection). Texas Southern University researchers looked at the antioxidant and free-radical-scavenging power of essential oils. In Germany, a study observed the effects of myrtol (from myrtle), eucalyptus, and orange oil for patients with chronic obstructive pulmonary disease. In Iran, researchers found lavender oil inhalation lowered plasma cortisol levels in patients awaiting open-heart surgery.

We now know it is feasible to wash away *Salmonella enterica* contamination on grape tomatoes with thyme oil, thymol, and carvacrol instead of a chlorine-based washing solution. This 2010 study at the University of Delaware concluded that thymol was the most effective without affecting color or taste of the tomatoes.

Brazilian scientists studied the gastroprotective activity of clove oil, while Iranian researchers discovered the healing advantages of lavender essential oil in healing episiotomies following childbirth. The immune-modifying and antimicrobial effects of eucalyptus oil were studied, and frankincense oil was found to induce tumor cell specific toxicity at the University of Oklahoma by HK Lin, PhD.

Clinical research during the last several decades indicates that essential oils have enormous potential to treat conditions ranging from acne to obesity. The following are just a few examples of the ongoing research in the world of natural solutions for dysfunction and disease. Peppermint (*Mentha piperita*) has been reviewed for its ability to block pain, relieve headaches,[13] combat indigestion,[14] boost mental alertness,[15] induce weight loss,[16] kill lice,[17] and inhibit tumor growth.[18]

Tea Tree (*Melaleuca alternifolia*) has been used to treat acne,[19] kill fungi,[20] and inhibit bacteria growth.[21,22]

Lavender (*Lavandula angustifolia*) fights travel sickness,[23] reduces atherosclerosis,[24] acts as a local anesthetic,[25] has anticonvulsant properties, and initiates human immune response to *Staphylococcus aureus*, responsible for the most important nosocomial (hospital-acquired) infection.[26]

Clove (*Syzygium aromaticum*) has been researched for its action against tooth decay,[27] as well as for its antifungal[28] and anticonvulsant activities.[29]

Rosemary (*Rosmarinus officinalis*) has been shown to enhance alertness,[30] combat fungi such as Candida albicans,[31] and act as an antioxidant.[32]

Orange (*Citrus sinensis*) halts fungus infection[33] and inhibits tumor formation.[34] Limonene, an important component of orange and lemon oil, has demonstrated similar tumor-suppressing effects in studies at Indiana University.[35]

Basil (*Ocimum basilicum*) has been shown to have anticancer properties.[36,37]

Eucalyptus (*Eucalyptus radiata*) contains 1,8-cineole (eucalyptol), which has been studied for reducing inflammation,[38] improving cerebral blood flow,[39] inhibiting Candida growth,[40] and treating bronchitis.[41]

Many other documented benefits of aromatics have been recorded in recent medical literature.[42,43,44,45] Research conducted at two universities was published in 2002 showing that 58 percent of 60 essential oils and 5 essential oil blends showed general cancer inhibition of 50 percent or better.[46] Researchers continue to open new frontiers of study on the health-supporting effects of essential oils.

Whether the topic is mood enhancement, memory, hypertension, Alzheimer's disease, anxiety in a dental office, cancer, or anti-inflammatory action, current medical research on essential oils can be found by searching

TOP QUESTIONS, TOP ANSWERS...

TOP QUESTIONS, TOP ANSWERS

WHAT IS THE PURITY PROCESS FOR YOUNG LIVING ESSENTIAL OILS?

As detailed in previous pages, Young Living's purity process for its essential oils is called Seed to Seal — a five-step process that ensures a quality product that you and your loved ones can trust. Young Living's commitment to authentic ingredients, free of synthetic chemicals, means that you can feel confident that these products are safe and effective. Only Young Living makes this Seed to Seal promise.

Step 1: Seed – Premium seeds and plants become the effective, therapeutic, Young Living Essential Oils. Botanical experts from Young Living in a partnership with university experts are used to verify the plant's essential oil potential.

Step 2: Cultivate – Young Living farms around the world work hard to perfect the best growing and harvesting methods. Experts also visit co-op farms to verify that their cultivation standards match the high expectations Young Living demands. These global farming operations are the continued, sustainable sources for high-quality essential oils.

Step 3: Distill – Young Living is widely recognized in the essential oil industry as an innovator in distillation. Young Living combines ancient and modern techniques to make sure the plant oils remain potent and pure. Young living uses its own proprietary distilling methods depending on the specific oil types. These processes include steam extracting, cold pressing, and resin tapping.

Step 4: Test – To guarantee effectiveness and quality, Young Living tests all oils in its own internal labs. The oils are also tested by third-party labs to ensure consistent potency and excellence. These tests also certify Young Living essential oils meet strict quality international standards and have the ideal amount of pure bio-active plant compounds.

Step 5: Seal – After these rigorous techniques, Young Living completes the Seed to Seal process by carefully bottling and sealing the oils and then distributes them to customers around the world.

Pro tip: Store your oils in a cool, dark place. Although Young Living's oils do not expire, this will ensure an unlimited shelf life and maximize potency. The amber-colored bottle helps maintain the oil's effectiveness.

WHAT DOES ALL THIS INFO ON THE LABEL MEAN?

Young living has designed the labels on their essential oils to be easy to read and understand.

On the Front of the bottle:

Under the Young Living logo, you will find the name of the oil.

Below the oil name you will see "100% pure, Therapeutic-Grade."

This means you can trust that it's the highest quality to use on your loved ones.

Notice it will say, "Essential Oil Single" or "Essential Oil Blend." A "single" means it is from one plant and a "blend" means it is from two or more plants.

The bottom line will tell you the size. Young Living oils come in either 5 ml or 15 ml sizes. There are between 85 to 100 drops in the small bottle, and 250 to 300 drops in the larger size.

On the back of the bottle:

Directions are on the back of the bottle. Not every oil can be used all three ways (topically, aromatically, and internally.) It's important to check the directions to see the usage recommendations. These will provide accurate information on how many drops are safe.

If you ever have an issue with your Young Living oils,

you will find a batch number on the back. Young Living will replace your oil, but they will likely ask for your batch number.

WHERE DOES YOUNG LIVING GET THE PLANTS TO MAKE THESE OILS?

Young Living has farms all over the world, but its main farm is in the small town of Mona Utah, USA. The Young Living Farm has almost 1400 acres of fragrant herbs like Lavender, Melissa, and Tansy. It is the largest herb farm and distillery in the world. Visitors are welcome year-round to tour this beautiful land and facility. The soil here has never been exposed to chemicals or pesticides so it's the perfect foundation to cultivate these plants.

Each farm, no matter the size, no matter the continent, is dedicated to maintaining the highest standards needed to produce quality therapeutic oils. Young Living is also dedicated to sustainably sourcing the plants, protecting the land and natural resources, and providing job opportunities and fair wages to local workers. The amount of time and effort all over the world that goes into growing, processing and providing your family with the best products is incredible. It is done with a sincere purpose.

The Young Living Farm and Distillery in South Africa produces Tea Tree, Eucalyptus, Radiata, Lemon, Orange and Grapefruit essential oils.

In Asia and the Middle East, there are farms in Taiwan, Philippines, Israel, and Oman. These farms produce oils such as: Jojoba, Coconut, Frankincense, Elemi, Jade Lemon, Hong Kuai, and Xiang Mao. The wolfberry used in the NingXia® line of products is also found in this region.

The Farms in Australia grow and distill Blue Cypress and Sandalwood essential oils.

In France, Croatia, Spain and Italy, Young Living's European farms produce products such as Helichrysum, Bergamot, Cistus, Lavender, Frankincense, Myrrh, Sage, and Juniper.

In Ecuador, oils such as Ylang Ylang, Ocotea, Lemongrass, Palo Santo, and Eucalyptus Blue are farmed and distilled.

In North America, Young Living has farms in British Columbia Canada, Mexico, Hawaii, Idaho, and Utah, that bring you the oils Lime, Grapefruit, Black Spruce, Peppermint, Spearmint, Sandalwood, Idaho Blue Spruce, Idaho Balsam Fir, Idaho Grand Fir, Lavender, Melissa, and Goldenrod.

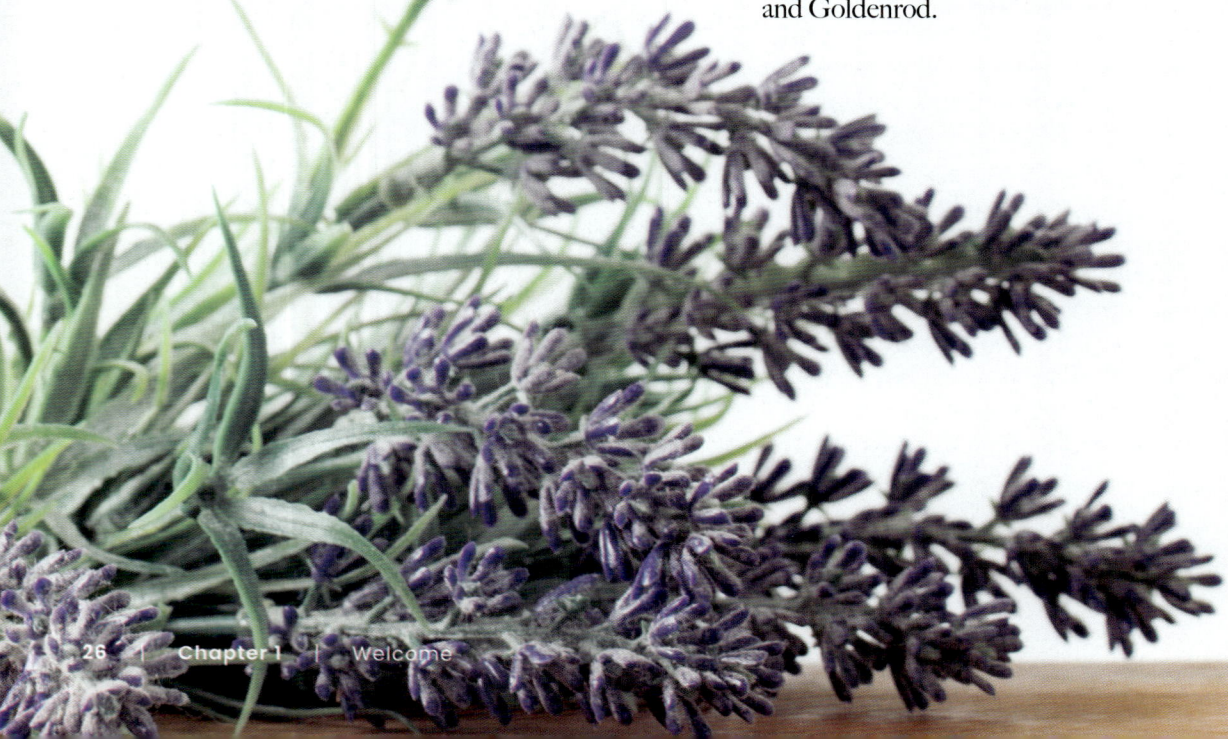

As you explore all of the possibilities with essential oils, you want to make sure you use the highest quality for you and your family. You can feel confident that Young Living Essential Oils focuses on quality—that the oils are not cut with harmful ingredients. Their Seed to Seal® process is followed on every farm they work with throughout the world.

HOW DO ESSENTIAL OILS WORK AROMATICALLY?

Essential oils can have far-reaching benefits both physically and psychologically. The sense of smell is a powerful trigger for the brain. When a molecule is released from a substance, like a flower or coffee, it stimulates our nerve cells located in the nose, called olfactory cells. These cells send the information to the brain, allowing it to identify the smell. But our amazing brains process more than just identifying what the smell is.

Aromatic treatments can have a profound therapeutic effect on our health. Our sense of smell is the only one of our senses that is connected to the limbic system of the brain, which is like the emotional control center. In addition to controlling our emotions, the limbic system also supports functions like behavior, motivation, and long-term memory. This system is connected to the parts of the brain that control heart rate, hormone balance, blood pressure, breathing, and stress.

The emotions we feel—such as joy, fear, anger, frustration, anxiety or sadness—all come from this region of the brain. When you breathe in essential oils, it does more than just smell nice. It produces benefits for your body and mood.

By understanding these facts, it is clear that essential oils will provide numerous health benefits for the household. Using a room diffuser is probably the easiest way to dispense these benefits into the air to improve your health, boost your energy and promote good sleep, among others. By using Young Living Essential Oils, you can have confidence that the oils you are diffusing are toxin free! Not all essential oils are toxin free.

The Essential Oils Complete Home Reference™ Guide and *Essential Oils Field Guide™* will provide valuable education with over 25 years of research on essential oils and how to use them aromatically for health and wellness. You will be an expert in no time! The *Index* and *Personal Usage Guide*® make using essential oils easy. With the use of this guide, creating a healthy lifestyle will become real and the benefits will be noticeable almost immediately.

WHAT ARE THE BEST WAYS TO USE OILS AROMATICALLY?

Aroma. You've heard the word, but what does it really mean?

Breathing in essential oils is a fast and easy way to give you a boost emotionally and physically. Aromatics can stimulate many healing responses in the body. Here are a few ways to use your Young Living Essential Oils aromatically:

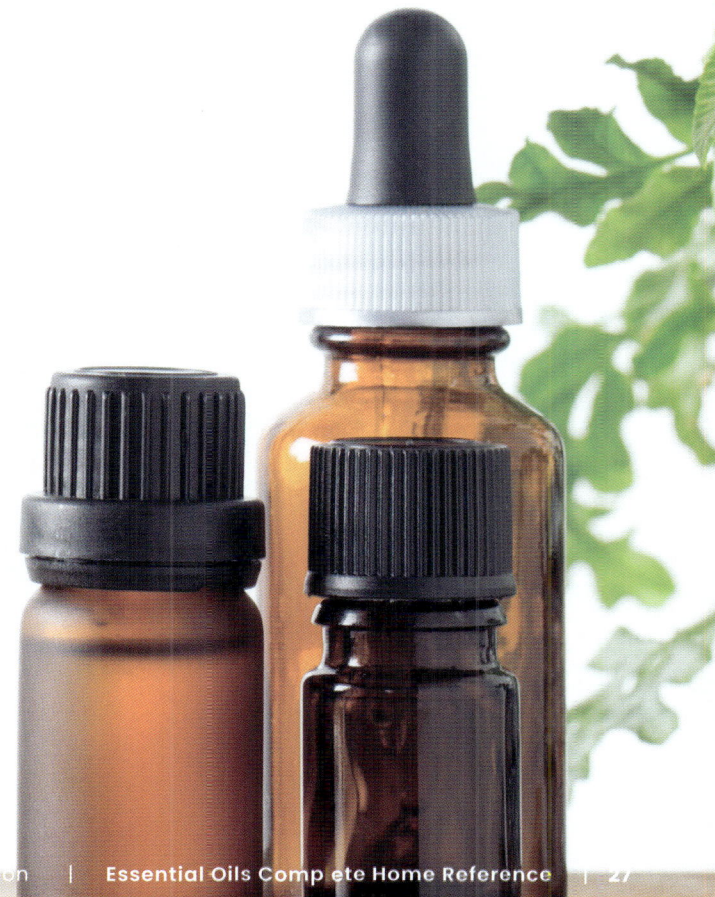

Diffuse: A Young Living ultrasonic, cold-air diffuser is a great way to get the aromatic benefits of essential oils. Simply put drops of oil and water into a diffuser and push the button to start. The diffuser dispenses a micro-fine mist into the air for hours and automatically shuts off. Not only does it make your house smell nice, you and your family get all the health and mood boosting perks with minimum effort. If you change the oil you are using in the diffuser, be sure to empty all the water and clean the small silver disc at the bottom of the diffuser with a cotton swab.

DIY Reed Diffuser: Small vase with a narrow neck. Most of the ones that you can buy will be around 100 ml or 3.5 ounces. Fill it halfway up with a carrier oil such as fractionated coconut oil, V-6™ Vegetable Oil Complex, grapeseed oil, apricot kernel oil, almond oil, or olive oil. Add up to 50 drops of your favorite essential oil, combination of oils or blend. Use more or less, depending on what you personally prefer. Cover the top either using a lid, cork, or your finger. Shake it well. Place fresh rattan reeds and refresh with oils once a week. If you feel the mix isn't giving off enough scent, try adding a teaspoon of 190-proof organic ethyl alcohol to the mix before you shake it up. This will help the oils "lift." Flip the reeds every other day to be sure they are moving the oil. When the sticks are darkened and no longer produce aroma, they are too saturated and should be replaced.

Inhale: Want the easiest method to use essential oils aromatically? You can directly inhale essential oils by putting a few drops into the palms of your hands, rubbing them together, cupping them around your nose to breathe in the benefits! It's a quick and safe pick-me-up! Be sure to avoid touching your eyes or eye area.

Straight from the Bottle: You can get a fast, concentrated effect from essential oils by simply breathing deeply from the bottle. Take off the cap. Place the bottle approximately one-half inch below your nose. Use your finger to close one nostril and inhale deeply. Then switch to the other nostril and repeat.

Breathe Deeply: If you are looking for a more powerful aromatic experience, pour hot water and a few drops of essential oils into a bowl. With a large towel, cover your head and the bowl to create a tent. Breathe in the vapors deep and slow. This is a great technique when you need a little more oomph in your aromatics due to cold, flu, or need a mood boost.

Cotton Inhaler: Cotton inhalers are natural ways to get a concentrated amount of an oil or blend of oils to your limbic system. Place the desired number of drops on an inhaler and place the natural cotton at the base of your nostril. Inhale deeply and enjoy the benefits. These can be washed and re-used or kept as specific inhalers for specific oils.

Cotton Ball: Never underestimate the power of a natural cotton ball. They hold oil, can be quite portable, and may be placed in strategic areas such as air vents, on the floor of a car, gathered in a small burlap bag, or placed in specific spaces around the house. A regular-sized cotton ball can hold up to 5 drops of oil quite easily for natural diffusion.

When it comes to experiencing oils aromatically, remember that the individual experiences and body chemistry is unique to each individual. When you inhale essential oils, no two people will have the same experience. You could have a completely different experience than your friend who's standing right next to you. That's what makes using essential oils so amazing. Your journey to discovering the benefits for you and your family will be endless.

HOW DO I APPLY OILS TOPICALLY?

When you apply essential oils onto your skin, the oils are absorbed through the outer layer of skin (epidermis). They are then absorbed through the second layer of skin (dermis) into the capillaries and into the bloodstream. From there they circulate throughout the body to the parts where they are needed.

You can safely apply oils almost anywhere on the body. For quick and effective absorption, you should apply the oils to the wrists, temples, inner elbow, behind the knee, feet and the back of your neck. These are the areas where the blood vessels are closest to the skin's surface.

One way you can apply oils topically is through massage. Apply a few drops on your skin and start to rub it in. If you have a partner nice enough to massage your back, mix the essential oil with a carrier oil to be able to efficiently cover the large area.

Layering is another technique you can use to get oils to penetrate the skin and maximize each oil's potential. Just as the name implies, layering involves more than one oil. You can begin by rubbing an oil over a specific area until the skin is dry. Then, layer a different oil on top of the first oil. Once the second oil has been absorbed, you can apply a third oil and continue massaging into the skin.

Baths with essential oils and Epsom salts are a heavenly way to use your oils topically. Mix a few drops of oils in with Epsom salts. While you bathe, you absorb the oils through the skin and also aromatically. Homemade essential oil bath salts make a great gift, too!

Pro Tip: After working out, treat sore muscles by layering essential oils on the aching area. A great combo for layering is to begin with Marjoram and massage it gently into the tissue until the area is dry. Next, layer with Peppermint, and massage into the skin until dry. Finally, add Basil as the third layer and rub it in until the skin is dry.

This *Home Reference* can provide you with many more ways to use your oils safely every day. You will love the change in your lifestyle as you incorporate essential oils into daily living.

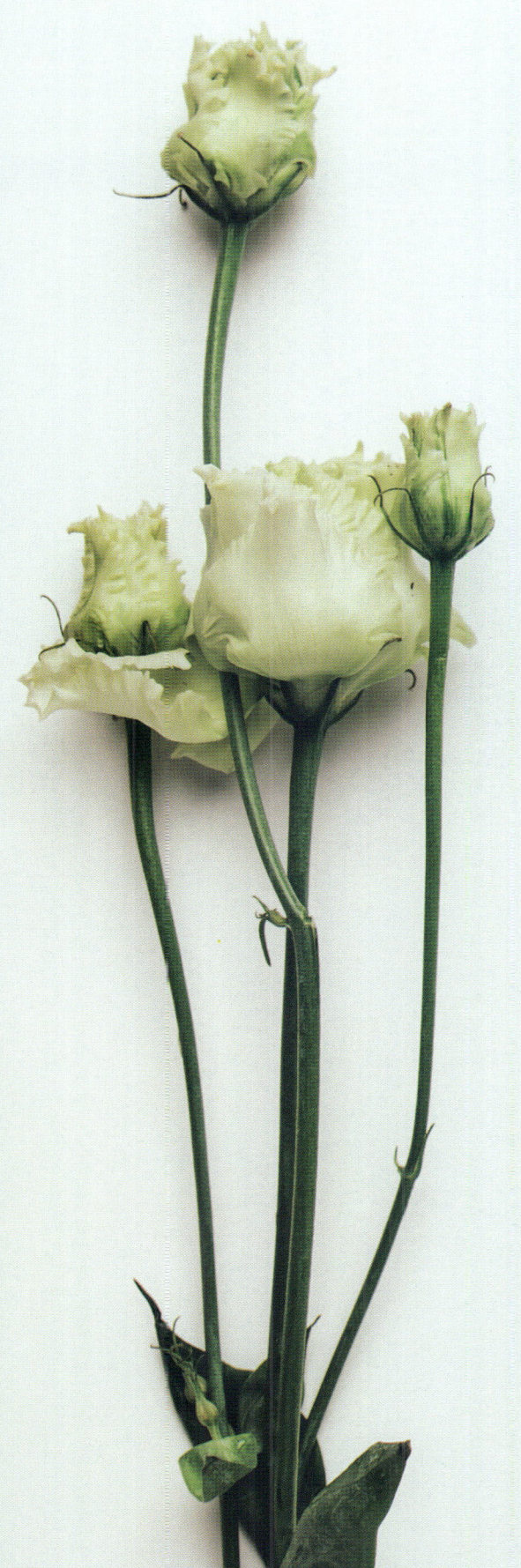

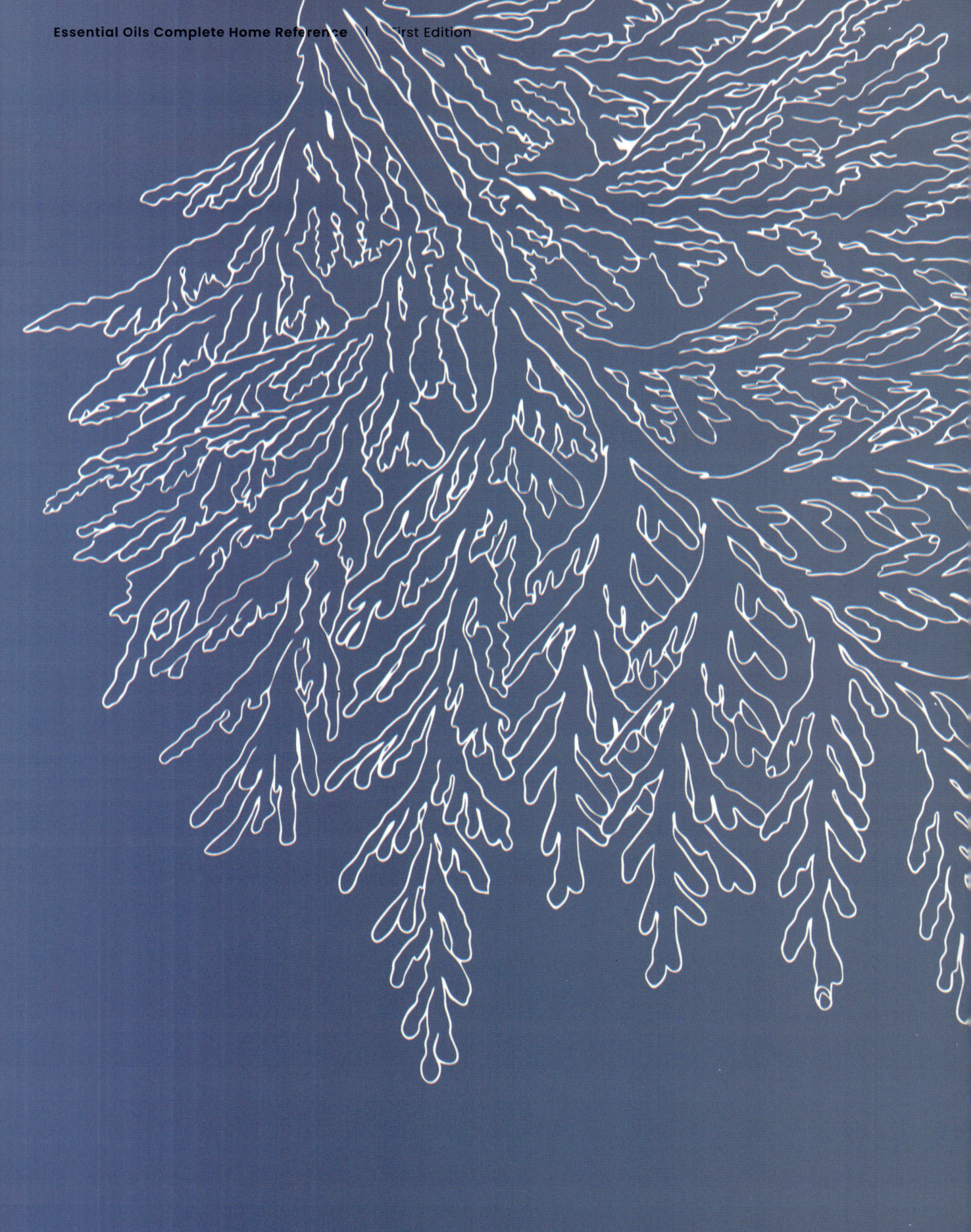

WHAT IS A CARRIER OIL?

A carrier oil is a mild oil used as a base to dilute essential oils. There are many essential oils that are safe to use without diluting them. Some essential oils are so strong, they need to be diluted before putting them directly on the skin. Oregano is an example of an oil that is so potent, you need to pair it with a carrier oil so it doesn't burn or irritate the skin. It's important to exercise caution when trying a new oil because it's possible to have too much of a good thing. Those with sensitive skin who are new to essential oils, or infants and children should almost always start with diluted oil.

Another benefit of diluting your essential oil is that you won't have to use as much of it, making your bottle of oil last longer. On each bottle of Young Living Essential Oils are directions that include how many drops you need for the carrier oil, and how many drops are needed for the essential oil to maximize effectiveness. This takes the guesswork out of it to make it easier on you as you are learning.

Carrier oils can also be used in the layering technique. First, rub the desired essential oil on your skin. Then, layer a carrier oil on top of your essential oil. This will reduce evaporation and allow your essential oil to stay in contact with your skin longer, improving absorption.

Some popular choices for carrier oils are, coconut oil, V-6 Vegetable Oil Complex, jojoba oil, olive oil, grapeseed oil, and almond oil.

Pro tip: Put your contact lenses in before you put your daily essential oils on. It burns! It burns!

WHICH CARRIER OILS ARE NON-COMEDOGENIC?

Young Living puts an incredible amount of effort in its Seed to Seal process to ensure you get the best quality essential oils. It's important that you select a carrier oil that won't jeopardize the amazing benefits of the essential oil. A comedogenic scale measures the likelihood from 0 to 5 of skincare ingredients clogging pores and causing breakouts. The higher the number the more likely it is to clog your pores. Knowing your skin type will help you decide which carrier oil is right for you.

COMEDOGENIC RATINGS

1. Will not clog pores
2. Low
3. Moderately low
4. Fairly high
5. High

In Alphabetical Order:

OILS

Almond Oil - 2
Apricot Kernel Oil - 2
Avocado Oil - 2
Camphor - 2
Castor Oil - 1
Cocoa Butter - 4
Coconut Butter - 4
Coconut Oil - 4
Corn Oil - 3
Cotton Seed Oil - 3
Evening Primrose Oil - 2
Grapeseed Oil - 2
Hazelnut Oil - 2
Hemp seed Oil - 0
Mineral Oil - 0
Mink oil - 3
Olive Oil - 2
Monomethyl Ether - 0
Peanut Oil - 2
Petrolatum - 0
Safflower Oil - 0
Sandalwood Seed Oil - 2
Sesame Oil - 2
Shark Liver Oil - 3
Shea Butter - 0
Soybean Oil - 3
Sunflower Oil - 0
Wheat Germ Oil - 5

WAXES

Beeswax - 2
Candelilla Wax - 1
Carnauba Wax - 0
Ceresin Wax - 0
Emulsifying Wax NF - 2
Jojoba Oil - 2
Lanolin Wax - 1
Sulfated Jojoba Oil - 3

BOTANICALS

Algae Extract - 5
Aloe Vera Gel - 0
Calendula - 1
Carrageenans - 5
Chamomile - 2
Chamomile Extract - 0
Cold-pressed Aloe - 0
Red Algae - 5

VITAMINS AND HERBS

Ascorbic Acid - 0
Black Walnut Extract - 0
Vitamin A - 2
Vitamin E - 2
Panthenol - 0

MINERALS

Algin - 4
Colloidal Sulfur - 3
Flowers of Sulfur - 0
Potassium Chloride - 5
Precipitated Sulfur - 0
Sodium Chloride (salt) - 5
Talc - 1
Zinc Stearate - 0

WHERE ARE THE BEST PLACES TO APPLY ESSENTIAL OILS?

HEADACHES
*Temples
*Top of skull
*Behind ears
*Bridge of nose
*Shoulders
*Back of neck
*Feet

CONGESTION
*Bridge of nose
*Brow bone
*Chest
*Behind ears
*Feet

EARACHES
*Outside of ear
*Behind ear
*Temples
*Along glands
*Feet

COLD AND FLU
*Throat
*Chest
*Wrists
*Behind Ears
*Along glands
*Feet

To get even more tips, check out the "Personal Usage Guide" of this reference book!

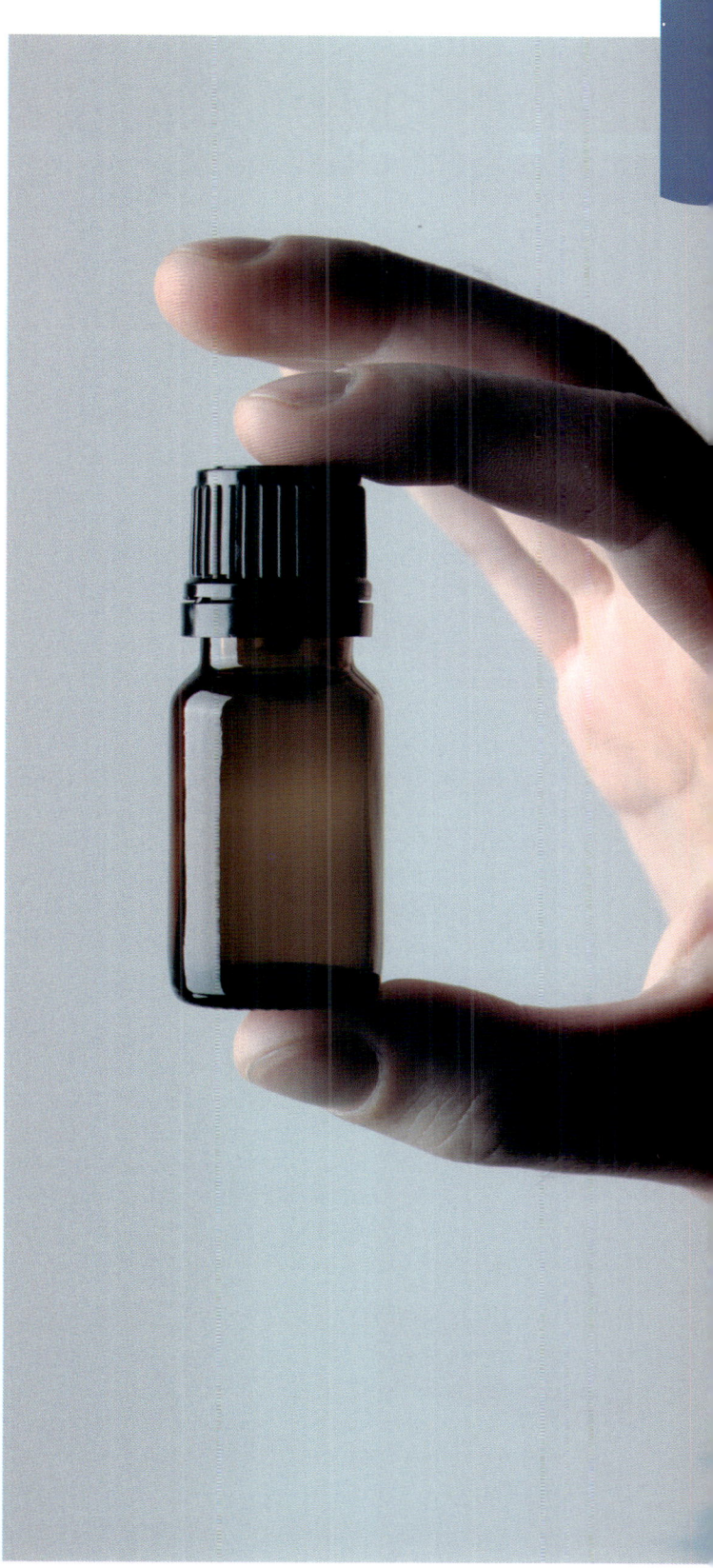

WHAT IS THE VITA FLEX TECHNIQUE?

One simple way to apply oils topically is to the soles and tops of your feet. Did you know there is a signal system within your feet that connects to specific parts of your body? Just as a keyboard connects to send information to a computer, you can send signals to enhance healing and balance from your foot to all other parts of your body, including internal organs. Mind blown over the way everything is connected, right?!

Vita Flex means "Vitality through the reflexes." It can be a powerful aid in revitalizing the body due to its 1500+ electrical reflex points. To learn this method, practice in slow motion on your arm. Take your dominant hand and rest your index, birdie (aka tall man), ring, and pinky fingertips flat on your opposite forearm. Now slowly roll your fingertips upwards so that you are on the actual top part of your fingertips. At this point your hand will be straight up on your arm. Continue rolling your fingertips over until your fingernails are now touching your skin. Continue rolling further until about the mid-digit area before the knuckle. Now release and move lengthwise down the arm and start the rolling motion again. You are looking for medium pressure. Continue with the technique lengthwise down your arm. This is the motion you are looking for, but once you get the hang of it, you can speed it up. Way to go!

You are now ready to try Vita Flex on your feet. First, rub your fingertips in some oil and proceed down the length of the foot. The goal is to cover the entire sole of your foot. Once you have gone down a row of the foot, start back up at the top of the foot and move over a bit to start a new row. This way you can cover the width of the entire foot as well as the length. Repeat this three times. Don't stress if it seems awkward at first. You've got this!

Pro tip: Kids love it when you rub oils on their feet. Try to make it a part of their bedtime routine when you are tucking them in at night. It's a great way to connect with your kiddos, too. After only a few nights of doing this, they will be sure to remind you if you forget! Some bedtime oil favorites are Peace and Calming®, Lavender, Cedarwood, or Valor®.

HOW DO I TAKE ESSENTIAL OILS INTERNALLY?

It is important to use the highest quality essential oils when you are taking them internally. Just as you read the labels on food items in the grocery store, you should always read the label of the oil you are putting in your body. Some oils should not be used internally. Young Living has a dietary line of oils, called "Vitality™" that are safe to ingest. Follow the specific instructions on the bottle of Vitality oils. We encourage you to talk to your medical provider before taking essential oils internally if you plan on taking more than just a few drops daily.

One easy way you can take oils orally is to flavor food and drinks with them. You can add 1 or 2 drops into a glass of ice water, herbal tea, fruit juice, smoothies, rice milk or almond milk. You can also add them to your favorite recipes to enhance the flavor of the food.

Young Living Essential Oils are so pure, you can safely use the Vitality oils along with a carrier oil in an empty vegetable capsule and take it in pill form. Ingesting the plant's therapeutic oils is another way of enhancing your body's health.

If swallowing pills is not your thing, you can put a few drops of Vitality oil under your tongue and hold it there for a few moments to try to let it absorb a bit before swallowing. Once again, use only the Vitality oils in these cases and be sure to follow the dilution instructions. If unsure, start with one drop of essential oil diluted with four drops of olive oil and place under the tongue.

Pro Tip: We all know how healthy it is to drink water, but sometimes it's just boring! Give it a flavor boost to help you chug that H2o. Lemon Vitality™ is a safe choice for beverages, but don't forget to give other citrus fruits a try like Tangerine Vitality™, Orange Vitality™, Grapefruit Vitality™, and Lime Vitality™. It is sure to put some pep in your step! Get creative with flavor combinations like Lemon Vitality™ and Peppermint Vitality™ for a refreshing energy boost!

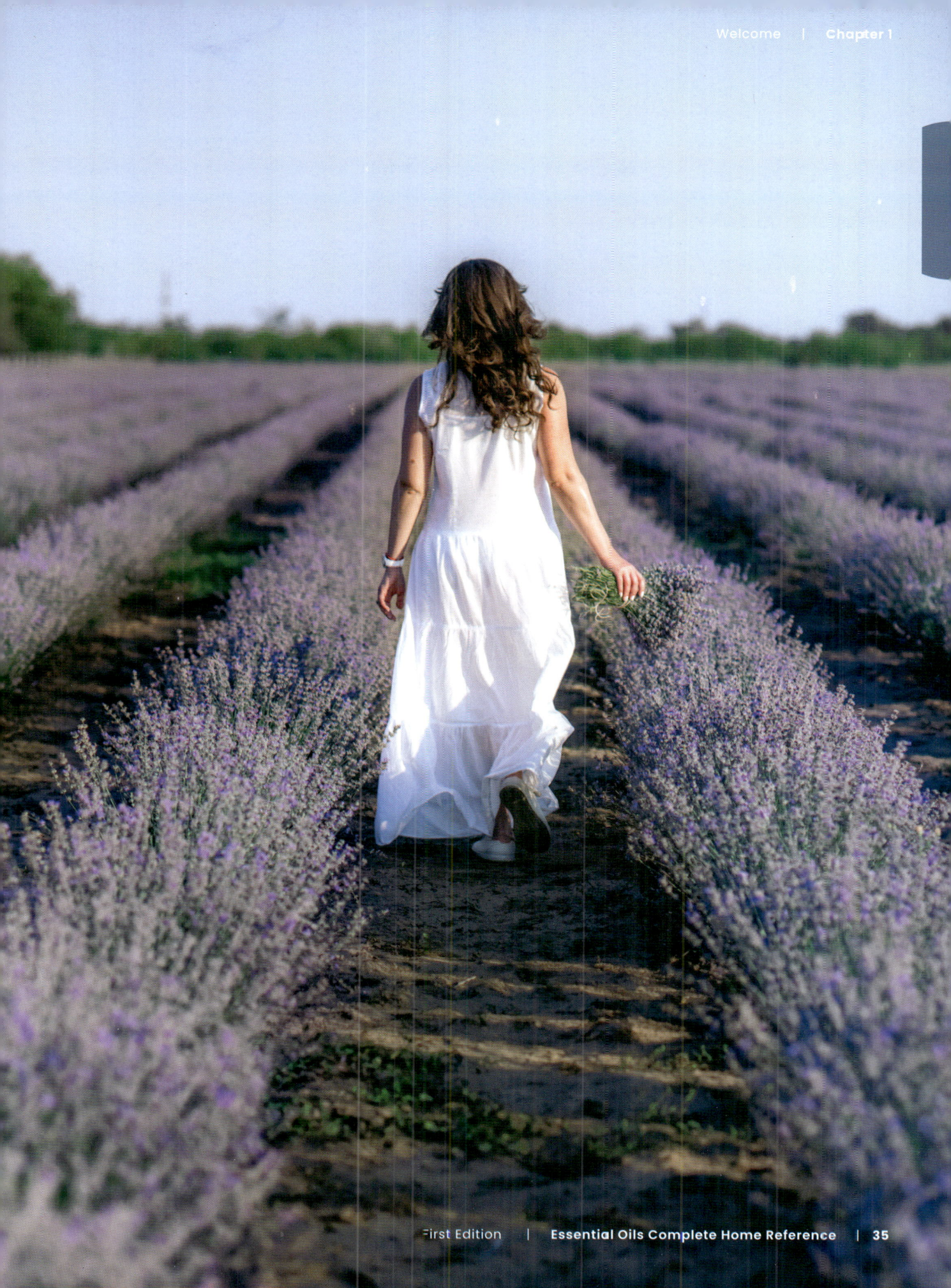

THE ESSENTIAL TOP TWENTY

What do we mean by the "Essential Top Twenty"? This is an alphabetical list of Young Living's Top Twenty Essential Oils and their common uses. This is a way to kickstart your journey with essential oils.

You will want to keep these awesome oil staples on hand for you and your family, always. Use the Personal Usage Guide in the *Essential Oils Complete Home Reference* and the *Essential Oils Field Guide* to get more detail. The detailed *Index* will help you as well.

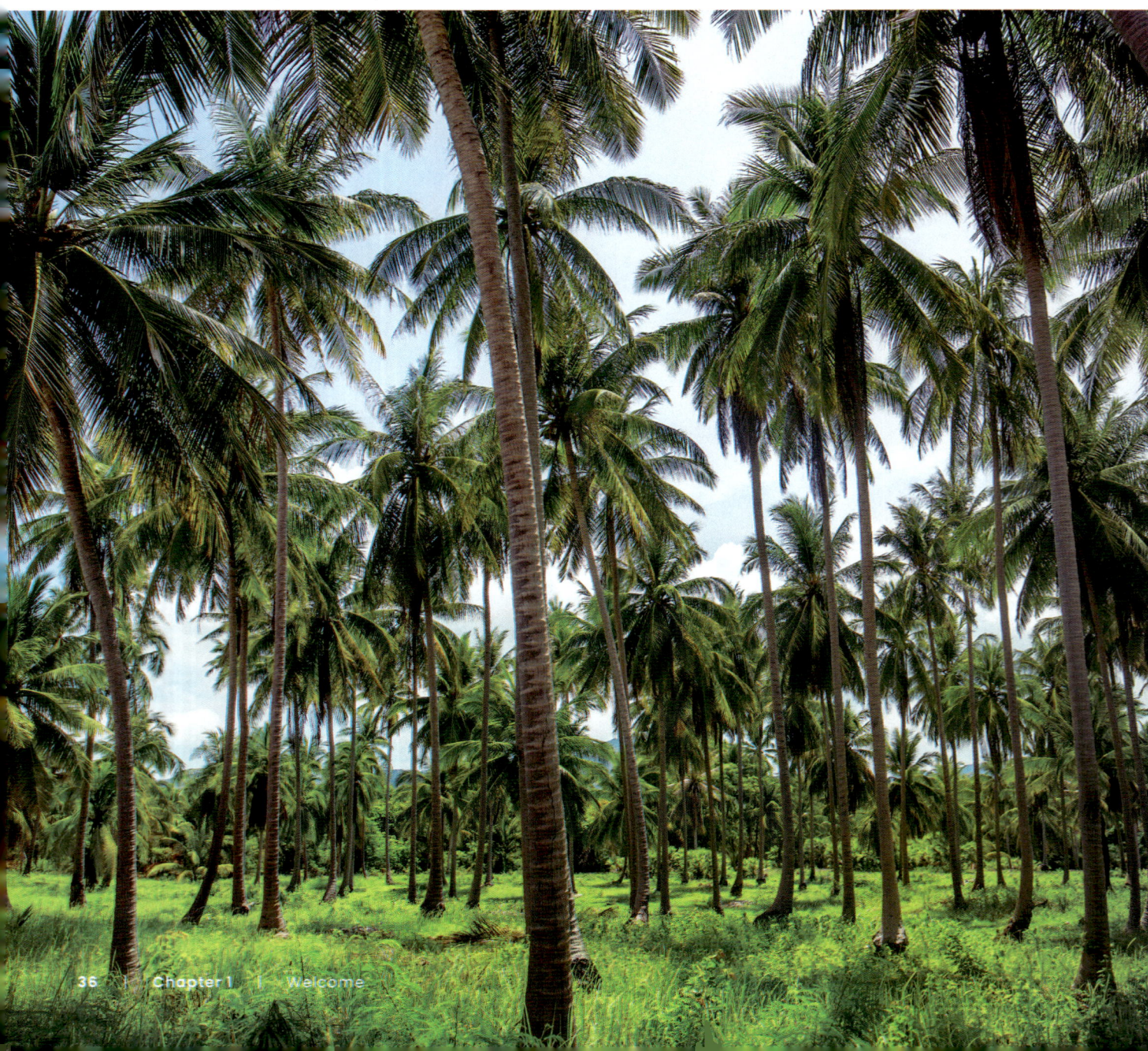

AROMAEASE™
Use to help alleviate symptoms of:

Upset Stomach	Sea Sickness
Low Energy	Tension
Indigestion	Morning Sickness
Stress	Heartburn
Anxiety	

DIGIZE®
Use to help alleviate the symptoms of:

Indigestion	Bloating
Gas	Reflux
Heartburn	Infection
Digestive Problems	Parasites
Upset Stomach	

CEDARWOOD
Use to help alleviate the symptoms of:

Skin Problems	Sleep Issues
Spasms	Immunity Issues
Liver Problems	Inflammation
Restlessness	Antiseptic

FRANKINCENSE
Use to help alleviate the symptoms of:

Scars	Warts
Stretch marks	Swelling
Wrinkles	Stress
Sunspots	Heightened Emotion

CITRUS FRESH™
Use to help alleviate the symptoms of:

Anxiety	Forgetfulness
Brain Fog	Emotional Imbalance
Sadness	Stinky Laundry
Stale Air	Writer's Block

GENTLEBABY™
Use to help alleviate the symptoms of:

Dry Skin	Diaper Rash
Chapped Skin	Fussy Baby
Stretch Marks	Scars
Pregnancy Stress	Wrinkles

COPAIBA
Use to help alleviate the symptoms of:

Stress	Acne
Muscle Pain	Skin Problems
Anxiety	Scrapes
Sagging Skin	Colds
Irritation	Digestion Issues

LAVENDER
Use to help alleviate the symptoms of:

Headaches	Burns
Sunburn	Stress
Fevers	Scrapes
Cramps	Cuts
Dry Skin	Pain
Bacteria	Sleep Issues

LEMON
Use to help alleviate the symptoms of:

- Bloating
- Infection
- Mouth Sores
- Brittle Hair & Nails
- Lethargy
- Household Dirt
- Insect Bites
- Cough

PANAWAY®
Use to help alleviate the symptoms of:

- Bruising
- Warts
- Sciatic Pain
- Stiffness
- Sore Muscles
- Swelling
- Damaged Tissue
- Stress

LEMONGRASS
Use to help alleviate the symptoms of:

- Digestion
- Urinary Tract Issues
- Fluid Retention
- Fungus
- Bacteria
- Circulation Issues
- Varicose Veins
- Swollen Joints
- Stale Air
- Household Dirt

PEACE & CALMING®
Use to help alleviate the symptoms of:

- Nerves
- Anxiety
- Tension
- Hyperactivity
- Sleeplessness
- Moodiness
- Children's Sleep
- Stress

OREGANO
Use to help alleviate the symptoms of:

- Sore Joints
- Fungus
- Parasites
- Digestive Issues
- Infections
- Moles
- Skin Tags
- Immunity Issues
- Inflammation
- Stomach Virus
- Aging

PEPPERMINT
Use to help alleviate the symptoms of:

- Colds
- Congestion
- Fever
- Soreness
- Stress
- Headaches
- Sunburn
- Lethargy
- Gas
- Indigestion
- Constipation

PURIFICATION®
Use to help alleviate the symptoms of:

Insect Bites	Acne
Scrapes	Dirty Air
Cuts	Household Odors
Sore Throat	Bloating
Infections	

TEA TREE
Use to help alleviate the symptoms of:

Acne	Pet Fleas
Insect Bites	Toenail Fungus
Itchy Skin	Mold
Lice Prevention	Stale Laundry

R.C.™
Use to help alleviate the symptoms of:

Breathing Issues	Allergies
Chest Tightness	Colds
Cough	Sore Throat
Congestion	Lung Infections

THIEVES®
Use to help alleviate the symptoms of:

Viruses	Toothaches
Colds	Poison Ivy
Bacteria	Cold Sores
Infection	Cuts
Flu	Household Dirt

STRESS AWAY™
Use to help alleviate the symptoms of:

Anxiety	Sleep Issues
Nervousness	Sadness
Feeling Overwhelmed	Bad Dreams
Stress	

VALOR®
Use to help alleviate the symptoms of:

Sciatic Pain	Bad Dreams
Soreness	Anxiety
Back Problems	Bruising
Attention Issues	Snoring
Stress	Sadness

Essential Oils Complete Home Reference | First Edition

A LITTLE ESSENTIAL OIL CHEMISTRY

A LITTLE ESSENTIAL OIL CHEMISTRY

This section is about to give you more interesting info than all of your high school chemistry lessons combined.

When we talk about the chemistry of essential oils, we're talking about the parts, the constituents. Each of those constituents has to be in perfect harmony to create a *Naturally Therapeutic* essential oil.

Did you ever have that lesson in school, where the teacher brought different batches of cookies for you to taste? She or he would either leave out one important ingredient, like salt, or put a whole bunch of baking soda in another batch so that they tasted awful. The lesson was that the *perfect* cookie has the perfect ingredients in *perfect* combination or *perfect* ratios, cooked at the *perfect* temperature for the *perfect* amount of time to get that *perfect* delectable flavor and texture. It's all about the recipe and the work of the baker.

When it comes to wellness and essential oils, the *perfect* oil comes from the *perfect* plant that was grown in the *perfect* soil under *perfect* sunlit conditions with the *perfect* clean water and rain, harvested at the *perfect* time, with the *perfect* type of equipment, using the *perfect* parts of the plant to be distilled at the *perfect* temperature and *perfect* pressure for the *perfect* length of time. Whew! That's a lot of *perfect*, right? If you don't like the word *perfect*, you may simply switch it out with the word ideal. In other words, nature's ingredients and how we use them will have a huge impact on the end product. And yes, there is a science to that.

Each essential oil may be made up of 200-500 different natural compounds. Each of the natural compounds has to be in the right ratio to affect the outcome. If anything is out of sync, the oil might smell great, but it won't do what it was intended to do—that is, unless it was intended to simply smell great.

Using oils to support health means having the *right* oils with the *right* natural therapeutic compounds (or constituents) in the right ratios that support a particular system of the body. Lavender and Lavandin are two of the best-known examples of this. The camphor in Lavandin can make a burn worse, while pure Lavender (Lavandula angustifolia) is low in camphor and its other constituents can help support wound healing.

BASIC STRUCTURE OF ESSENTIAL OIL CONSTITUENTS

It's good to know a little about the constituents. You can gloss over this science or make it your passion. It's entirely up to you. For those of you who LOVE hard science, take a look at the chemical structure of essential oil constituents.

Aromatic constituents in essential oils (i.e., terpenes, monoterpenes, phenols, aldehydes, etc.) are made up of long chains of carbon and hydrogen atoms, which have a predominantly ring-like structure. Links of carbon atoms form the backbone of these chains, with oxygen, hydrogen, nitrogen, sulfur, and other carbon atoms attached at various points of the chain.

Essential oils have different chemistry than fatty oils (also known as fatty acids). Fatty oils have a simple linear carbon-hydrogen structure. Essential oils have a far more complex ring structure, and contain sulfur and nitrogen atoms that fatty oils do not have.

The terpenoids found in all essential oils are from the same basic building block—a five-carbon molecule known as isoprene. When two isoprene units link together, they create a monoterpene; when three join, they create a sesquiterpene; and so on.

ESSENTIAL OIL CONSTITUENT CATEGORIES

There are 15 categories of essential oil constituents. Following is a list of each category with examples of Young Living oils that have those constituents. When we capitalize the names of common oils, we do so because Young Living's oils are very specific in their constituent percentages. The information below pertains only to Young Living essential oils and has been adapted from *The Chemistry of Essential Oils* by Young Living member David Stewart, PhD,[47] which is highly recommended, and from *L'aromathérapie exactement*[48] by Pierre Franchomme and Daniel Pénoël.

1. Alkanes: Few essential oils contain alkanes, and those that do usually contain less than one percent.

Young Living's Ginger oil contains the alkanes undecane, dodecane, and hexadecane. Their Lemon oil and Ginger oil both contain alkane alcohols. Young Living's Rose oil stands alone as an essential oil that contains 4 to 19 percent alkanes, which may be why this exquisite oil exhibits so many unique characteristics.

2. Phenols: Common phenols found in essential oils are thymol (Thyme and Mountain Savory) and eugenol (Clove, Cinnamon, Basil, and Bay Laurel). Phenol is found in very minute quantities (<1 percent) in Cassia, Cinnamon, and Ylang Ylang. Phenols are believed to be antiseptic and antimicrobial and may boost the immune system in various ways. Some phenols are strong and may cause skin irritation. Always dilute according to label directions.

3. Monoterpenes: This class of constituents is the most common and is found in every essential oil. It is estimated that there are 1,000 different monoterpenes found in essential oils. Monoterpenes contain 10 carbons and are characteristically similar to alkanes. Many oils are composed of mostly monoterpenes, including Grapefruit and Frankincense. They have light fragrances, are supportive, and enhance the therapeutic talents of other constituents. They are commonly the first aroma detected when smelling an essential oil. The monoterpenes α-pinene, d-limonene, l-limonene, sabinene, myrcene, β-phellandrene, camphene, and ocimene are abundant in Pine, Orange, Balsam Fir, Juniper, Frankincense, Ginger, Spruce, and Basil.

4. Sesquiterpenes: As many as 3,000 different sesquiterpenes are found in essential oils. This class of constituents contains fifteen carbons and is characteristically similar to alkanes and monoterpenes. The sesquiterpenes beta-caryophyllene and guaiene are found in Black Pepper, Myrrh, and Patchouli. Oils with high sesquiterpene content include Cedarwood, Patchouli, Ginger, and Myrrh. Many sesquiterpenes are specific to one oil only, and most have light aromas, but not all. Caryophyllene, for example, is one exception because it has a strong, woodsy, spicy aroma and is found in a variety of oils. Sesquiterpenes are soothing to inflamed tissue and can also produce profound effects on emotions and hormonal balance.

5. Other terpenes: Diterpenes (20 carbons) are the heaviest molecules found in distilled essential oils. Jasmine absolute essential oil contains about 14% diterpenes. Therapeutically, diterpenes have some of the same properties as sesquiterpenes and are considered to be expectorants and purgatives.

Triterpenes (30 carbons) and tetraterpenes (40 carbons) are larger molecules than diterpenes and are found mostly in the cold-pressed citrus oils of Orange, Tangerine, Lemon, Grapefruit, and Lime and also in absolutes like Jasmine.

It was once believed that diterpene and triterpene molecules were too large to make it through distillation, but diterpenes like incensole have been documented in essential oils through GC-MS analyses, and triterpenic acids (such as boswellic acids) are detectable in Frankincense essential oil through High Performance Liquid Chromatography (HPLC) testing.

6. Alcohols: The names of these constituents end in –ol. Borneol is found in Lavandin; citronellol is in Rose; linalool is in Ho Wood; α-terpineol and terpinen-4-ol are in Melaleuca; and lavandulol is in Lavender. Alcohols are also found in Eucalyptus and Fennel oils, as well as many more. Alcohols are energizing, cleansing, antiseptic, and antiviral; they have a sweet, floral aroma.

7. Ethers: This constituent form is not as common in essential oils as others like terpenes, alcohols, or ketones. The names of these constituents end in "-ole," "-cin," or "-ether." Examples of ethers are anethole, in Fennel and Anise; estragole, in Tarragon; elemicin, in Elemi; myristicin, in Nutmeg; and eugenol methyl ester found in some Melaleuca species. Ethers are balancing and calming, help release emotions, and have an antidepressant effect.

8. Aldehydes: The names of these constituents end in "–al" or "–aldehyde." Vanillin aldehyde is found in Onycha; trans-cinnamaldehyde, in Cassia and Cinnamon Bark; citral, in Lemon; cuminal, in Cumin; and neral, in Melissa. The aldehyde octanal is in some citrus oils. Decanal is found in Coriander, Lemongrass, and Mandarin oils. Aldehydes are antimicrobial, anti-inflammatory, cooling, and have strong aromas. They can also be calming to the nervous system, emotional stress relievers, and blood-pressure reducers. Oils containing citral and cinnamaldehyde should always be diluted according to label directions.

9. Ketones: A strong, distinctive odor characterizes ketones. Ketones usually end in "-one." Camphor is found in Rosemary; fenchone, in Fennel; jasmone, in Jasmine; piperitone, in Peppermint; β-thujone, in Sage; and α-vetivone, in Vetiver. Ketones are thought to be calming, with decongesting and analgesic benefits; to promote healing (cell regeneration); and to cleanse receptor sites.

10. Carboxylic acids: These constituents are only minor parts of an essential oil, rarely comprising more than 1-2 percent. They are easy to recognize because they always have the word "acid" in their name. Examples are cinnamic acid, in Cinnamon; geranic acid, in Lemongrass; and valerinic acid, in Valerian. Carboxylic acids are stimulating, cleansing, and very reactive with other components.

11. Esters: Wintergreen is an oil composed mainly of esters. The names of esters end in "-ate." Esters usually have a strong, sweet aroma. Linalyl acetate is found in Bergamot; neryl acetate, in Helichrysum; isobutyl angelate, in Roman Chamomile; citronellyl formate, in Geranium; menthyl acetate, in Peppermint; and bornyl acetate, in Pine, Spruce, Juniper, and Fir. To make an ester, a carboxylic acid and an alcohol are combined. Esters are soothing, balancing, antifungal, and stress- and emotion-releasing.

12. Oxides: These are oxygenated hydrocarbons and are usually derived from terpenes, alcohols, or ketones that have been oxidized. Examples are bisabolol oxide, found in German Chamomile; piperitone oxide, in Peppermint; linalool oxide, in Hyssop; rose oxide, in Rose; sclareol oxide, in Clary Sage; and humulene oxide, in Clove. These oxides are in very small quantities, but most oils produce the oxide 1,8-cineole, also known as eucalyptol, in varying amounts. This is more abundantly found in Eucalyptus, Rosemary, and Ginger. Oils with 1,8-cineole are known for decongesting and sinus-clearing benefits.

13. Lactones: This constituent group is characterized by tongue-twisting names like butenolide, cardenolide, and bufadienolide. Celery Seed is an oil with higher amounts of lactones. Lactones, like ketones, are generally decongesting and expectorant. They generally have mild aromas. They seem to have antiseptic, antiparasitic, and anti-inflammatory properties, according to Dr. Daniel Pénoël.

14. Coumarins: Dr. Stewart notes that coumarins are a subgroup of lactones and are found widely in nature. Because there is a similarity to the name of the blood-thinning drug Coumadin®, he explained that coumarins and Coumadin are not similar. One is natural, one synthetic, and they have very different chemical formulas. Coumarins have the fragrance of freshly cut hay or grass. In fact, when you mow your lawn, you are releasing coumarins into the air. They are found in Fleabane, Bitter Orange, Lavandin (in very minute quantities), and Cassia essential oils. Coumarins are powerful and can have strong therapeutic effects, even in small quantities. Coumarins have antispasmodic, antiviral, antibacterial, and antifungal properties.

15. Furanoids: Furanoids, or furans, are lactones or coumarins with names starting with "furano-" or "furo-" or ending with "furan." Most of the essential oils that contain furans are certain expressed citrus oils. Some essential oils with furanoids are photosensitive (i.e., they amplify the effects of the sun) like Angelica, Bergamot, Bitter Orange (neroli), Grapefruit, Lemon, Lime, Petitgrain, and Rue (*Ruta graveolens*). Other oils containing furanoids, like Myrrh and Sweet Orange, are not photosensitive. Myrrh is interesting in that it contains more furanoid components than any other essential oil (up to 27 percent), yet it is not photosensitive. Furanoids can have the benefits of lactones or coumarins.

With this brief explanation of constituent chemistry, Lavender's constituents are categorized as esters (linalyl acetate), alcohols (linalool and terpinen-4-ol), and monoterpenes (cis-β-ocimene and trans-β-ocimene).

Boswellia sacra essential oil constituents are composed of monoterpenes (α-pinene, limonene, sabinene, myrcene, α-thujene, p-cymene), the sesquiterpene β-caryophyllene, and many more components.

Lemon's constituents can be categorized as monoterpenes (limonene, gamma-terpinene, β-pinene, α-pinene, and sabinene), as well as aldehydes, alcohols, esters, sesquiterpenes, tetraterpenes, coumarins, and furocoumarins.

The constituents of peppermint are categorized as alcohols (menthol), ketones (menthone), monoterpenes (1,8-cineole and pulegone), sesquiterpenes (germacrene D), esters (methyl acetate), oxides (1,8 cineol), furanoids (menthofuran), alcohols, sesquiterpenols, furocoumarins, sulphides, and esters (menthyl acetate).

The constituents listed are only a small percentage of the total number of constituents present in each essential oil.

PLANT CHEMOTYPES AND CONSTITUENT VARIABILITY

A single species of plant can have several different chemotypes (biomolecularly unique variants) based on molecular composition. This means that basil *(Ocimum basilicum)* grown in one area might produce an essential oil with different chemistry than a basil grown in another location. The plant's growing environment, such as soil pH and mineral content, can dramatically affect the plant's ultimate chemistry. Different chemotypes of basil are listed below:

- *Ocimum basilicum* CT linalool fenchol (Germany)—antiseptic

- *Ocimum basilicum* CT methyl chavicol (Reunion, Comoro, or Egypt)—anti-inflammatory

- *Ocimum basilicum* CT eugenol (Madagascar)—anti-inflammatory, pain-relieving. Another plant species that occurs in a variety of different chemotypes is rosemary (Rosmarinus officinalis).

- *Rosmarinus officinalis* CT camphor is high in camphor, which serves best as a general stimulant and works synergistically with other oils, such as black pepper (Piper nigrum), and can be a powerful energy stimulant.

- *Rosmarinus officinalis* CT cineole is rich in 1,8-cineole, which is used in other countries for pulmonary congestion and to help with the elimination of toxins from the liver and kidneys. Young Living offers this chemotype of rosemary because of its great value.

- *Rosmarinus officinalis* CT verbenone is high in verbenone and is the most gentle of the rosemary chemotypes. It offers powerful regenerative properties and has outstanding benefits for skin care.

Common thyme *(Thymus vulgaris)* produces several different chemotypes, depending on the conditions of its growth, climate, and altitude. The following are just two chemotypes out of many more.

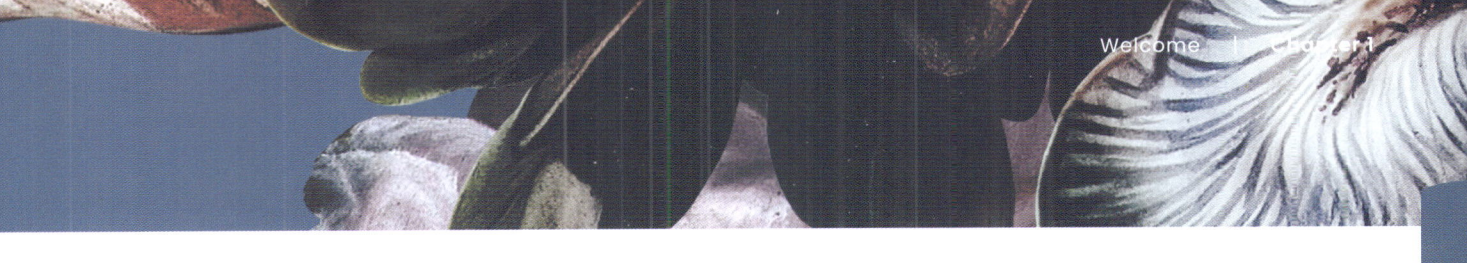

- *Thymus vulgaris* CT thymol is germicidal and anti-inflammatory.

- *Thymus vulgaris* CT linalool is anti-infectious.

One chemotype of thyme will yield an essential oil with high levels of thymol, depending on the time of year it is distilled. The later it is distilled in the growing season (e.g., mid-summer or fall), the more thymol the oil will contain.

Another example of this variability in chemotype is shown in a Turkish study on *Origanum onites*.[3] Researchers found that the altitude at which the plants grew affected the morphology of the plant and amount of volatile oil the plant produced. The plant produced more volatile oil the higher the altitude at which it grew. Even on the same mountainside, wildcrafted plants produced varying levels of oil.

Proper cultivation assures that more variable-specific chemotypes, like *Thymus vulgaris* and *Origanum compactum*, will maintain more consistent levels of constituents and oil produced.

PURITY AND POTENCY OF ESSENTIAL OILS

There are two things that make an oil *Naturally Therapeutic*. They are purity and potency. Nothing affects these qualities more than the constituents. These constituents can be affected by so many things—the part(s) of the plant from which the oil was produced, soil condition, fertilizer (organic or chemical), geographical region, climate, altitude, water purity, harvesting methods, and distillation processes. In other words, where and how the plant is grown really affects the kind of oil that can be extracted.

The key to producing a *Naturally Therapeutic* essential oil is to preserve as many of the delicate aromatic components within the essential oil as possible. Fragile aromatic components are easily destroyed by high temperature and pressure, as well as by contact with certain metals like copper or aluminum. People think of copper as a better conductor of heat, and while that makes it more efficient for cooking, it happens to be a very reactive metal with essential oils. This is why all *Naturally Therapeutic* essential oils should be distilled in stainless steel cooking chambers at low pressure and low temperature.

The plant material should also be free of herbicides and other agrichemicals. These can react with the essential oil during distillation to produce toxic compounds. Because many pesticides are oil-soluble, they can also mix into the essential oil. Who wants to gather a field of poison and put it in an essential oil? Nope.

Even though chemists have successfully recreated the main constituents and fragrances of some essential oils in the laboratory, these synthetic oils lack therapeutic benefits and may even carry risks. Pure essential oils contain hundreds of different constituents, which add important therapeutic properties to the oil, if they're in the right combination. Also, many essential oils have molecules and isomers that can't be manufactured in the lab.

Today approximately three hundred essential oils are distilled or extracted worldwide. Several thousand constituents and aromatic molecules are identified and registered in these essential oils. Ninety-eight percent of essential oil volume produced today is used in the perfume and cosmetic industry. Only about 2% of the production volume is for therapeutic and medicinal purposes.

Young Living requires all distillers who want to sell to Young Living to submit samples to be analyzed to ensure that all the constituents are present at the right percentage to be therapeutic.

You can have pure oils, but if the plants are distilled at the wrong time of day or with incorrect distillation procedures, the constituents that make the oils therapeutic will not be there, and you will not have a *Naturally Therapeutic* profile.

In addition, Young Living requires that the farms and essential oil distillation facilities be subject to site inspection. Of oil samples submitted between May 2007 and October 2011 by distillers wanting to partner with Young Living, over 34 percent did not meet Young Living standards and were rejected. However, currently, by 2020,

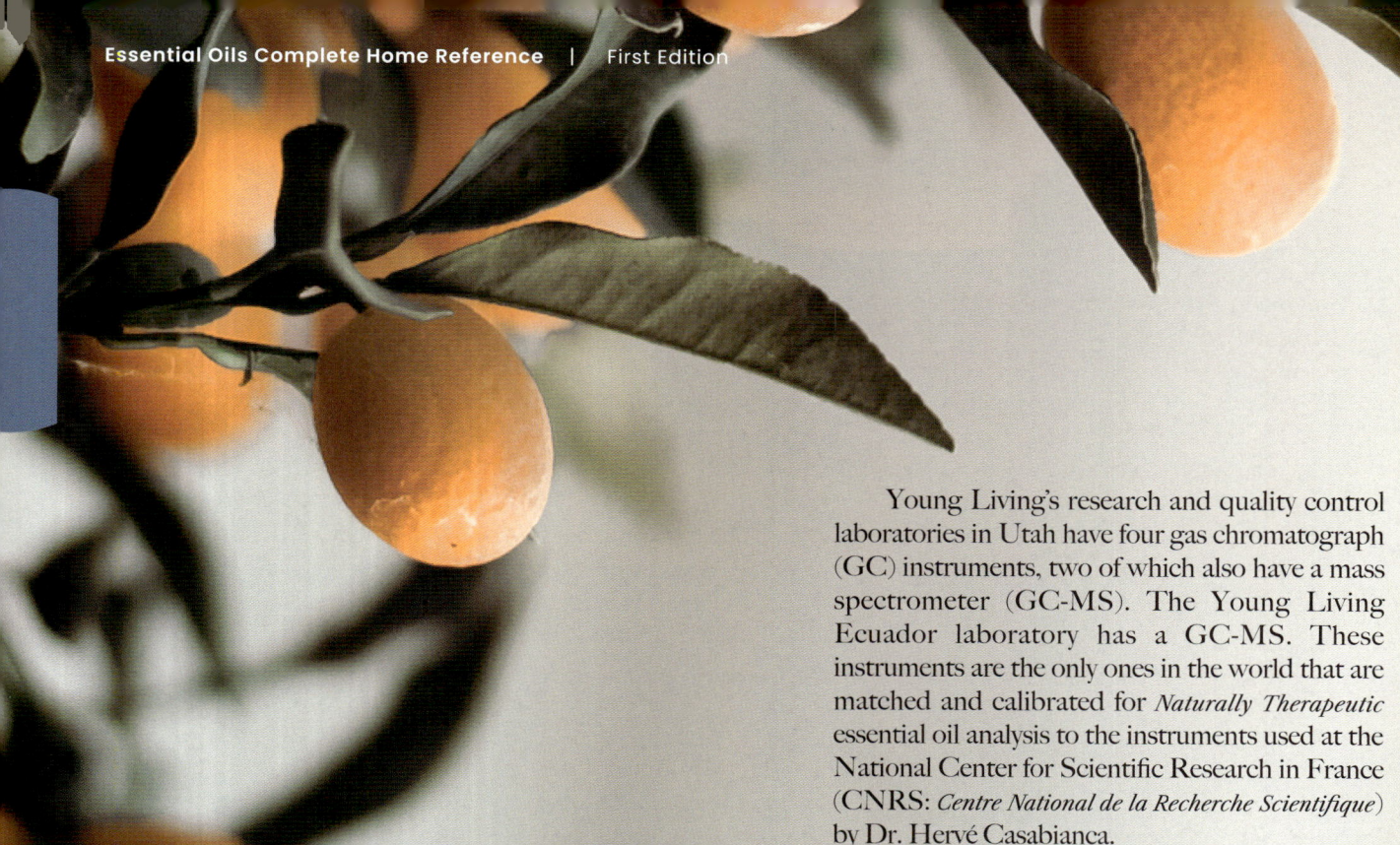

Young Living's research and quality control laboratories in Utah have four gas chromatograph (GC) instruments, two of which also have a mass spectrometer (GC-MS). The Young Living Ecuador laboratory has a GC-MS. These instruments are the only ones in the world that are matched and calibrated for *Naturally Therapeutic* essential oil analysis to the instruments used at the National Center for Scientific Research in France (CNRS: *Centre National de la Recherche Scientifique*) by Dr. Hervé Casabianca.

As a general rule, if one or more marker components in an essential oil falls outside the numbers, the oil does not meet Young Living's *Naturally Therapeutic* essential oil standards. A lavender essential oil produced in one region of France might have a slightly different chemistry than that grown in another region and as a result may not meet the standard. It may have excessive camphor levels (1.0 instead of 0.5), a condition that might be caused by distilling lavender that was too green, or the levels of lavandulol may be too low due to certain weather conditions at the time of harvest.

By comparing the gas chromatograph chemistry profile of a lavender essential oil with the Young Living *Naturally Therapeutic* standard, one may also distinguish true lavender from various species of lavandin (hybrid lavender). Usually, lavandin has high camphor levels, almost no lavandulol, and is easily identified. However, Tasmania produces a lavandin that yields an essential oil with naturally low camphor levels that mimics the composition of true lavender. Only by analyzing the essential oil composition of this Tasmanian lavandin using high-resolution gas chromatography and comparing it with the Young Living *Naturally Therapeutic* standard for genuine lavender can this hybrid lavender be identified.

Young Living has developed such good partnerships with its Seed to Seal suppliers that its rejection numbers are low. Additionally, Young Living rarely accepts samples from suppliers that haven't already qualified.

Because Young Living interacts with the end-users who purchase essential oils, the company is able to monitor human response and determine the actual therapeutic benefits of various oils, and truly compare the constituents of different oils to determine their maximum, health-giving potential. Quality and efficacy are moving, evolving targets. No one understands this more than Young Living.

STANDARDS AND TESTING

YOUNG LIVING STANDARDS

Over the years, Young Living has bought and compiled an essential oil retention index and mass spectral reference library that contains over 400,000 components. Using this research reference library, Young Living developed its own standards to guarantee the highest possible therapeutic potency for its essential oils.

TESTING INSTRUMENTS

In the United States, few companies use the necessary instruments and methods to analyze essential oils properly. Most labs use equipment best suited for synthetic chemicals—not for natural essential oil analysis.

Young Living Essential Oils, LC uses the proper instruments and has made great effort to calibrate Young Living's GC-MS instruments to the column-wall thickness set by Dr. Casabianca, laboratory director of Natural Product Research, at CNRS labs in France. This ensures identification of more components that otherwise might be missed. In addition to operating its analytical instruments with the same calibration as the CNRS laboratories, Young Living is continually expanding its analytical component library in order to perform a more thorough compositional analysis.

GAS CHROMATOGRAPHY AND MASS SPECTROMETRY

Properly analyzing an essential oil by gas chromatography (GC) is a complex thing. The injection mixture, capillary column diameter, column length, and oven temperature must fall within certain parameters. GC is the analytical instrument used to separate the many natural components biogenerated by the aromatic plant that make up the essential oil. The key components of a GC are the injector, capillary GC column, detector, and oven. A small sample of essential oil is injected into the capillary GC column with a syringe. The capillary GC column is slowly heated within the oven to separate the essential oil components. Finally, the separated components exit the GC column, and the percentage of each component is determined by a Flame Ionization Detector (FID).

Using a longer capillary GC column length increases the separation of each of the components in a complex essential oil. Young Living has found that a 50- or 60-meter-long capillary GC column provides the best separation for essential oil components. Shorter 25- or 30-meter columns provide adequate separation of many components, but they are too short to properly analyze the complex mosaic of natural bioconstituents found in an essential oil. A more detailed analysis of an essential oil can be obtained using a 100-meter-long capillary GC column.

Every capillary GC column has an internal polymer coating (stationary phase) that helps separate the essential oil components. The most common stationary phase for essential oil separations is the polydimethylsiloxane phase that generates a separation based on the boiling points of each essential oil component. In addition, using a "wax-based" stationary phase composed of polyethylene oxide, the GC operator can obtain a separation based on both the boiling points and the polarity of each essential oil component. Young Living uses both of these phases simultaneously in one GC to provide two separations from a single injection of essential oil. This process allows for a more certain identification of essential oil components.

Another common analytical instrument for the separation and identification of essential oil components is the GC-MS (gas chromatograph-mass spectrometer). The MS is a special detector attached to the instrument that can identify by name each essential oil component from a library of known essential oil components. The MS identifies the components based on the arrangement of their individual carbon, hydrogen, and oxygen atoms. The GC-MS is used in the first stages of research in order to separate and identify each component of a new essential oil. After the initial research, the GC (with an FID detector) is used for routine quality control to determine percentages of each component in the essential oil.

CHIRAL GC-MS

While GC-MS is an excellent tool to analyze essential oils, it does have limitations. Sometimes it can be difficult to distinguish between natural and synthetic bioconstituents using GC-MS analysis alone. If synthetic linalyl acetate is added to pure lavender, a GC-MS analysis cannot confidently determine whether that constituent is synthetic or natural, only that it is linalyl acetate. Adding a chiral (pronounced "ky-ral") capillary GC column in the GC-MS can help in distinguishing between synthetic and natural components.

Research scientists can use chiral GC-MS to identify whether an essential oil is composed of its natural proportions of chiral components. Some components have what is called "chiral polarity." This means they have left or right versions of the component, called "enantiomers."

To see the perfect example of chirality, bring your hands up, palms facing you. They are mirror images but exact opposites. They are different in that you could not put a right-handed glove on your left hand. The term used to identify rotating to the right is *dextrorotary*, or "*d*," and rotating to the left, *levorotary*, or "*l*." Not all essential oil molecules have chirality, but many do.

A trained scientist can check for adulteration by looking at the ratio between the two chiral enantiomers. Nature tends to favor one over the other. For instance, in the Young Living 2012 study[4] on chiral differences, the Frankincense constituent α-pinene in *Boswellia sacra* is +8.24, while in *Boswellia carterii*, it is -0.68. When adding an unspecified synthetic, you get equal amounts of both enantiomers. It is possible to purify a synthetic mixture down to the individual enantiomers, but this is not seen much because of the expense.

IRMS (Isotope Ratio Mass Spectrometry) takes it to another extreme. This is needed because sometimes people get really clever and adulterate oils to the point that their purity cannot be determined by chirality alone. IRMS measures the isotopic ratios of the individual atoms in oil. By comparing these ratios to both a natural standard and a synthetic one, adulteration can be determined at the atomic level.

Young Living researchers use a polarimeter to identify the optical rotation of molecules. If the "d" or "l" form deviates from what is listed in a chiral library of left and right enantiomers, the sample will be further analyzed with IRMS testing. Adulterated or synthetic-based oil is then rejected.

This complexity is why oils must be analyzed by an analytical chemist specially trained on the interpretation of gas chromatography and mass spectroscopy. The chemist examines the entire essential oil composition to determine its purity, measuring how various components in the oil occur in relation to each other. If some components occur in higher quantities than others, these provide important clues to determine if the oil is adulterated or pure.

Adulteration is such a major concern that each essential oil Young Living offers is tested initially by GC-MS, and every subsequent batch of essential oil is tested using GC-FID by Young Living's trained research and quality control scientists. Batches that do not meet established standards are rejected and returned to the sender.

Adulteration of essential oils has become more and more common as the supply of top-quality essential oils has dwindled, and the demand continues to increase. Adulteration may occur by diluting the essential oil with fatty lipid oils. This is a common practice by some essential oil companies to increase supply and reduce cost. Other methods include adulterating with synthetic components or using a cheaper essential oil to increase volume and maximize profits. These adulterated essential oils will jeopardize the integrity of aromatherapy and essential oil use.

ADULTERATED OILS AND THEIR DANGER

Many lavender crops are dying worldwide. Since the late nineties, the soil has been burning out, the immune systems of the plants are compromised, and viruses are taking them out. There is almost no pure lavender on the open market.

Today, much of the lavender oil sold in America is a hybrid called lavandin, grown and distilled throughout the world. Lavandin is often heated to evaporate the camphor, mixed with synthetic linalyl acetate to improve the fragrance, and then sold as lavender oil. Most consumers don't know the difference and are happy to buy it for $7 to $10 per half ounce in various stores and on the internet. This is one of the reasons why it's important to know about the integrity of the essential oil company or vendor.

Adulterated and mislabeled essential oils may present dangers for consumers. One woman who had heard of the ability of lavender oil to heal burns used "lavender oil" purchased from a local health food store when she spilled boiling water on her arm. But the pain intensified and the

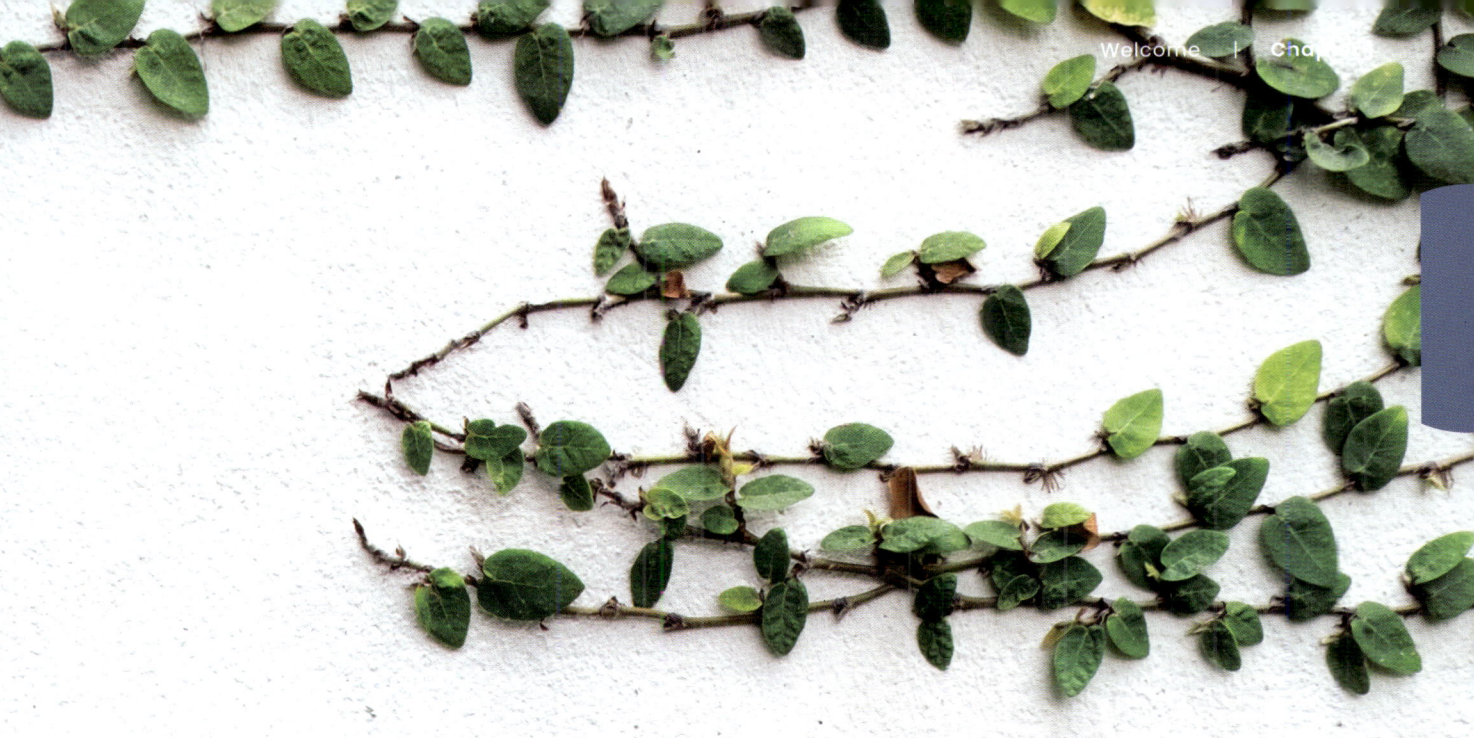

burn worsened, so she later complained that lavender oil was worthless for healing burns. When her "lavender" oil was analyzed, it was found to be lavandin, a hybrid of lavender that is biologically different from pure *Lavandula angustifolia*.

Adulterated oils that are mixed with synthetic extenders can be very detrimental, causing rashes, burns, and skin irritations. Common additives such as propylene glycol, DEP, or DOP (solvents that have no smell and increase the volume) can cause allergic reactions, besides having no therapeutic effects.

Some people assume that because an essential oil is "100 percent pure," it will not burn their skin. This is not true. Some pure essential oils may cause skin irritation if applied undiluted. If some people apply Oregano oil to their skin, it may cause severe reddening. Citrus and spice oils like Orange and Cinnamon may also produce rashes. Even the terpenes in conifer oils like Pine may cause skin irritation on sensitive people.

Some researchers feel that because of their complexity, essential oils do not disturb the body's natural balance or homeostasis: if one constituent exerts too strong an effect, another constituent may block or counteract it. However, synthetic chemicals, like pharmaceuticals, usually have only one action, may disrupt the body's homeostasis, and may cause various adverse side effects.

POWERFUL INFLUENCE OF AROMAS

Human beings can potentially see several million different colors and hear potentially 500,000 tones. Those may seem like large numbers, until you look at modern research on the human sense of smell. Recent research implies that we can smell more than 1 trillion scents. The National Institutes of Health (NIH) funded a study led by Dr. Andreas Keller of Rockefeller University with the results published in *Science* magazine on March 21, 2014.[49] In this study researchers had participants differentiate between multiple sets of fragrance where only one smell was different. Some of the scents had 275 smells contributing to the overall total. Based on the number the participants were able to distinguish, researchers estimated conservatively that humans can potentially smell over 1 trillion smells.

It's no surprise that the fragrance of an essential oil can directly affect everything from your emotional state to your lifespan. Scientists from all walks and specialties are still exploring how aroma/fragrance/smell work. Some have described our sense of smell as working like a lock and key or an odor molecule fitting a specific receptor site.

When you inhale a fragrance, the airborne odor molecules travel up your nostrils to the olfactory epithelium or the center of your olfactory sensation. At the olfactory epithelium, which is only about one square inch of your

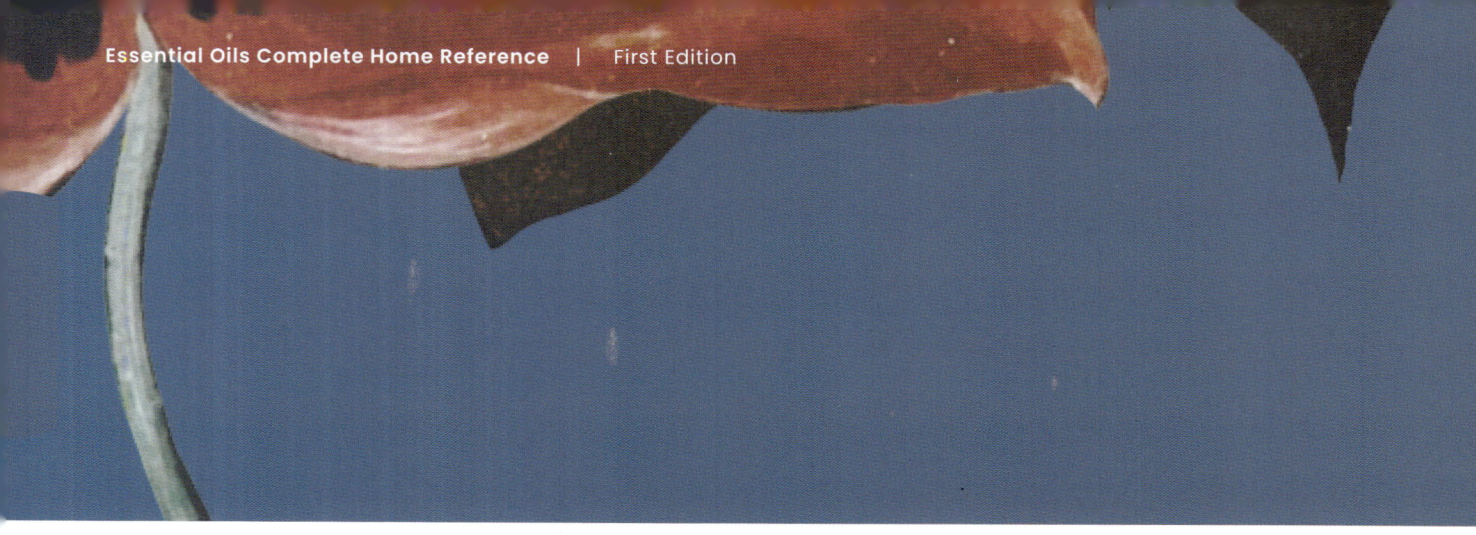

nasal cavity, the scent triggers your olfactory receptor cells and sends an impulse to your olfactory bulb. Each olfactory receptor type sends an impulse to a particular microregion, or glomerulus, of your olfactory bulb. There are around 2,000 glomeruli in your olfactory bulb, which receives the impulses from your olfactory receptors and allows you to perceive many smells. The olfactory bulb then transmits the impulses to other parts of your brain, including the gustatory center (where the sensation of taste is perceived), the amygdala (where emotional memories are stored), and other parts of your limbic system.

Because the limbic system is directly connected to those parts of the brain that control heart rate, blood pressure, breathing, memory, stress levels, and hormone balance, essential oils can have profound physiological and psychological effects.

An article in the December 15, 2006, issue of *Scientific American* raised an interesting question regarding the lock and key theory: "the shape theory doesn't explain why some nearly identically shaped molecules smell vastly different, such as ethanol, which smells like vodka, and ethane thiol (which is the primary scent of rotten eggs)."[50]

An Italian scientist named Luca Turin proposed another theory of smell, called the vibration theory, in a paper published in 1996.[51] He theorizes that rather than the "lock and key" theory of olfaction, it is the vibrational properties of molecules that enable us to distinguish smells. He suggests that the olfactory receptors sense the quantum vibration of each odorants' atoms, which would allow humans to perceive almost limitless numbers of odors, as olfactory receptors are tuned to different frequencies.

While the vibrational theory is still somewhat controversial, Jennifer Brookes, a University College London researcher based at MIT, was lead author on a study that discusses models of receptor selectivity, including those based on shape and other factors like vibrational frequencies.[52] Speaking of Turin's theory, she told the BBC in March 2011, "It's a very interesting idea; there's all sorts of interesting biological physics that implement quantum processes that's cropping up. I believe it's time for the idea to develop and for us to get on with testing it."

A colleague of Brookes, A. P. Horsfield, of Imperial College London, was also interviewed by the BBC about the vibrational theory and said, "There's still lots to understand, but the idea that it cannot possibly be right is no longer tenable really. The theory has to at least be considered respectable at this point."

In February of 2015, writer Christina Agapakis discussed the reasoning of the original proponent of the vibration theory, chemist Malcom Dyson, who proposed the theory in 1928. For Dyson, the idea that molecular vibrations might underlie our sense of smell suggested a tantalizing symmetry with our other senses. The rods and cones in our retinas respond to the vibrating wavelengths of light; the hair cells in our ear activate in response to the frequencies of sound waves vibrating in the air. Is smell also a vibrational sense?[53]

Whatever the mechanism, the sense of smell is the only one of the five senses directly linked to the limbic lobe of the brain, the emotional control center. Anxiety, depression, fear, anger, and joy all emanate from this region. The scent of a special fragrance can evoke memories and emotions before we are even consciously aware of it. When smells are concerned, we react first and think later. All other senses (touch, taste, hearing, and sight) are routed through the thalamus, which acts as the switchboard for the brain,

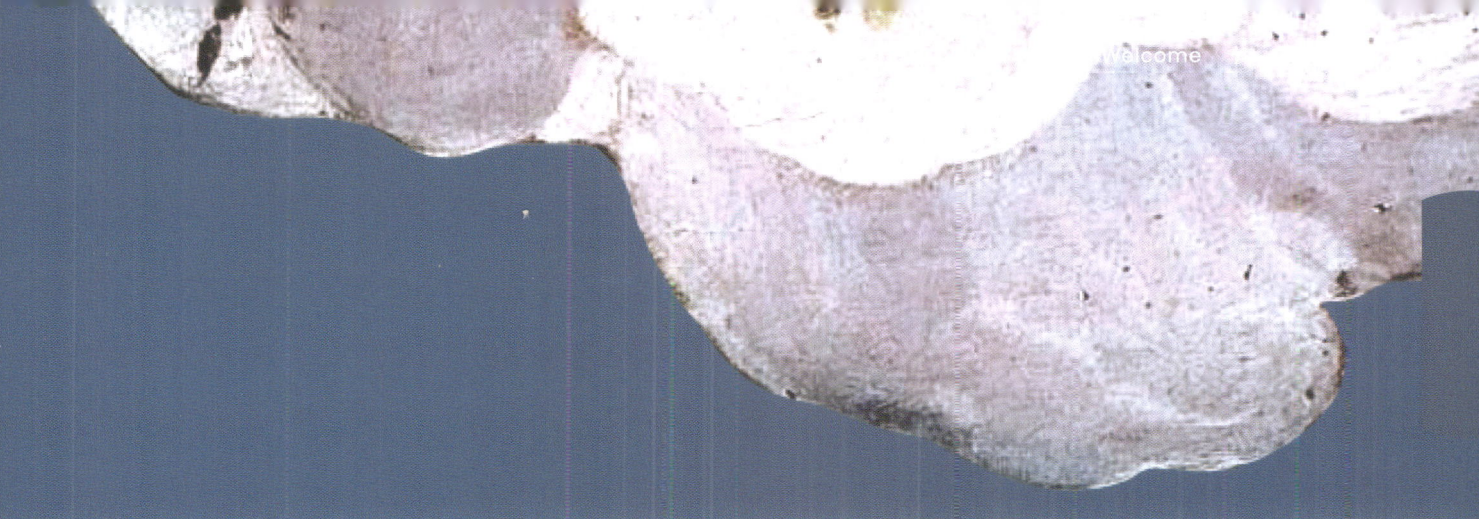

passing stimuli onto the cerebral cortex (the conscious thought center) and other parts of the brain.

The limbic lobe (a group of brain structures that includes the hippocampus and amygdala located below the cerebral cortex) can also directly activate the hypothalamus, which is one of the most important parts of the brain. It controls body temperature, hunger, thirst, fatigue, sleep, and circadian cycles. It acts as our hormonal control center and releases hormones that can affect many functions of the body. The production of growth hormones, sex hormones, thyroid hormones, and neurotransmitters such as serotonin are all governed by the hypothalamus.

Essential oils—through their fragrance and unique molecular structure—can directly stimulate the limbic lobe and the hypothalamus, which is responsive to olfactory stimuli. Not only can the inhalation of essential oils be used to combat stress and emotional trauma, but it can also stimulate the production of hormones from the hypothalamus. This results in increased thyroid hormones (our energy hormone) and growth hormones (our youth and longevity hormone).

Essential oils may also be used to reduce appetite and increase satiety through their ability to stimulate the hypothalamus, which governs our feeling of satiety or fullness following meals. In a large clinical study, Alan Hirsch, MD, used fragrances, including peppermint, to trigger weight loss in a large group of patients (over 3,000 individuals) who had previously been unsuccessful in any type of weight-management program.[54] The amount of weight loss among the subjects directly correlated with the frequency of their use of their aroma inhalers. One group in the study lost an average of 4.7 pounds per month over the course of the six months. Hirsch suggests that by inhaling certain aromas, individuals with good olfaction may have induced and sustained weight loss over a six-month period.

Another double-blind, randomized study by Hirsch documents the ability of aroma to enhance libido and sexual arousal.[55] When thirty-one male volunteers were subjected to the aromas of thirty different essential oils, each one exhibited a marked increase in arousal, based on measurements of brachial penile index and the measurement of both penile and brachial blood pressures. Among the scents that produced the highest increase in penile blood flow was a combination of lavender and pumpkin fragrances. This study shows that fragrances can enhance sexual arousal by stimulating the limbic system, the emotional center of the brain.

People who have undergone nose surgery or suffer olfactory impairment may find it difficult or impossible to completely detect an odor. These people may not derive the full physiological and emotional benefits of essential oils and their fragrances.

Proper stimulation of the olfactory nerves may offer a powerful and entirely new form of therapy that could be used as an adjunct against many forms of illness. Essential oils, through inhalation, may occupy a key position in this relatively unexplored frontier in medicine.

Here's the bottom line: Essential oils should not be dismissed as simple perfumes. Instead, more and more research shows they are complex and have measurable effects on the human body. This helps you understand the complexity and value of each essential oil with its hundreds of different components—and why it's important to give each one our careful study and consideration.

THE MEDICINE OF THE BIBLE...

THE MEDICINE OF THE BIBLE

Ancient civilizations discovered the healing powers of plants from as early as 4500 BC. The Egyptians, Mesopotamians, Greeks, and Romans all used essential oils to purify, heal, invigorate themselves, and to ward off disease.

The Bible contains over 200 references to aromatics, incense, and ointments. Aromatics such as frankincense, myrrh, galbanum, cinnamon, cassia, rosemary, hyssop, and spikenard were used for anointing and healing the sick. In Exodus, the Lord gave the following recipe to Moses for a holy anointing oil:

Myrrh	*"five hundred shekels" (about 1 gallon)*
Cinnamon	*"two hundred and fifty shekels"*
Calamus	*"two hundred and fifty shekels"*
Cassia	*"five hundred shekels"*
Olive Oil	*"an hin" (about 1⅓ gallons)*

Psalm 133:2 speaks of the sweetness of brethren dwelling together in unity: "It is like the precious ointment upon the head, that ran down the beard, even Aaron's beard: that went down to the skirts of his garments." Another scripture that refers to anointing and the overflowing abundance of precious oils is Ecclesiastes 9:8: "Let thy garments be always white; and let thy head lack no ointment."

The Bible also lists an incident where an incense offering by Aaron stopped a plague. Numbers 16:46-50 records that Moses instructed Aaron to take a censer, add burning coals and incense, and "go quickly into the congregation to make an atonement for them: for there is a wrath gone out from the Lord; the plague is begun." The Bible records that Aaron stood between the dead and the living, and the plague was stayed. It is significant that according to the biblical and Talmudic recipes for incense, three varieties of cinnamon were involved. Cinnamon is known to be highly antimicrobial, anti-infectious, and antibacterial. The incense ingredient listed as "stacte" is believed to be a sweet, myrrh-related spice, which would make it anti-infectious and antiviral as well.

The New Testament records that wise men presented the Christ child with frankincense and myrrh. There is another precious aromatic, spikenard, described in the anointing of Jesus in Mark 14:3:

And being in Bethany in the house of Simon the leper, as he sat at meat, there came a woman having an alabaster box of ointment of spikenard very precious; and she brake the box, and poured it on his head.
The anointing of Jesus is also referred to in John 12:3:

Then took Mary a pound of ointment of spikenard, very costly, and anointed the feet of Jesus, and wiped his feet with her hair: and the house was filled with the odour of the ointment.

Following is a list of oils and references in the Bible.

CEDARWOOD

Leviticus 14:51 – "And he shall take the cedar wood, and the hyssop, and the scarlet, and the living bird, and dip them in the blood of the slain bird, and in the running water, and sprinkle the house seven times:"

Leviticus 14:52 – "And he shall cleanse the house with the blood of the bird, and with the running water, and with the living bird, and with the cedar wood, and with the hyssop, and with the scarlet."

Numbers 19:6 – "And the priest shall take cedar wood, and hyssop, and scarlet, and cast it into the midst of the burning of the heifer."

Numbers 24:6 – "As the valleys are they spread forth, as gardens by the river's side, as the trees of lign aloes which the Lord hath planted, *and* as cedar trees beside the waters."

2 Samuel 5:11 – "And Hiram king of Tyre sent messengers to David, and cedar trees, and carpenters, and masons: and they built David an house."

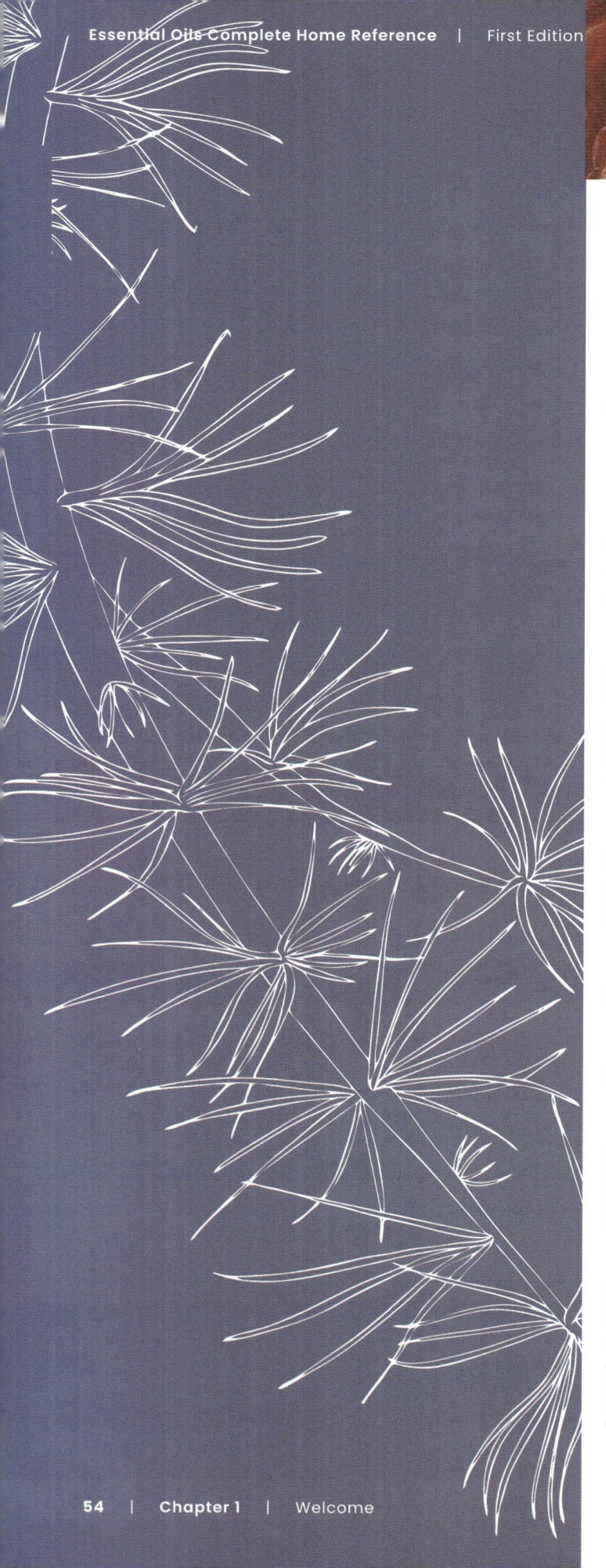

2 Samuel 7:2—"That the king said unto Nathan the prophet, See now, I dwell in an house of cedar, but the ark of God dwelleth within curtains."

2 Samuel 7:7—"In all *the places* wherein I have walked with all the children of Israel spake I a word with any of the tribes of Israel, whom I commanded to feed my people Israel, saying, Why build ye not me an house of cedar?"

1 Kings 4:33—"And he spake of trees, from the cedar tree that *is* in Lebanon even unto the hyssop that springeth out of the wall: he spake also of beasts, and of fowl, and of creeping things, and of fishes."

1 Kings 5:6—"Now therefore command thou that they hew me cedar trees out of Lebanon; and my servants shall be with thy servants: and unto thee will I give hire for thy servants according to all that thou shalt appoint: for thou knowest that *there* is not among us any that can skill to hew timber like unto the Sidonians."

1 Kings 5:8—"And Hiram sent to Solomon, saying, I have considered the things which thou sentest to me for: *and* I will do all thy desire concerning timber of cedar, and concerning timber of fir."

1 Kings 5:10—"So Hiram gave Solomon cedar trees and fir trees *according* to all his desire."

1 Kings 6:9—"So he built the house, and finished it; and covered the house with beams and boards of cedar."

1 Kings 9:11—"(*Now* Hiram the king of Tyre had furnished Solomon with cedar trees and fir trees, and with gold, according to all his desire,) that then king Solomon gave Hiram twenty cities in the land of Galilee."

2 Kings 19:23—"By thy messengers thou hast reproached the Lord, and hast said, With the multitude of my chariots I am come up to the height of the mountains, to the sides of Lebanon, and will cut down the tall cedar trees thereof, *and* the choice fir trees thereof: and I will enter into the lodgings of his borders, *and into* the forest of his Carmel."

1 Chronicles 22:4—"Also cedar trees in abundance: for the Zidonians and they of Tyre brought much cedar wood to David."

2 Chronicles 1:15—"And the king made silver and gold at Jerusalem *as plenteous* as stones, and cedar trees made he as the sycomore trees that are in the vale for abundance."

2 Chronicles 2:8—"Send me also cedar trees, fir trees, and algum trees, out of Lebanon: for I know that thy servants can skill to cut timber in Lebanon; and behold, my servants *shall be* with thy servants. . . ."

2 Chronicles 9:27—"And the king made silver in Jerusalem as stones, and cedar trees made he as the sycomore trees that *are* in the low plains in abundance."

Ezra 3:7—"They gave money also unto the masons, and to the carpenters; and meat, and drink, and oil, unto them of Zidon, and to them of Tyre, to bring cedar trees from Lebanon to the sea of Joppa, according to the grant that they had of Cyrus king of Persia."

Isaiah 41:19—"I will plant in the wilderness the cedar, the shittah tree, and the myrtle, and the oil tree; I will set in the desert the fir tree, *and* the pine, and the box tree together. . . ."

Ezekiel 17:3—"And say, Thus saith the Lord God; A great eagle with great wings, longwinged, full of feathers, which had divers colours, came unto Lebanon, and took the highest branch of the cedar:"

Ezekiel 17:22—"Thus saith the Lord God; I will also take of the highest branch of the high cedar, and will set *it*; I will crop off from the top of his young twigs a tender one, and will plant *it* upon an high mountain and eminent:"

Ezekiel 17:23—"In the mountain of the height of Israel will I plant it: and it shall bring forth boughs, and bear fruit, and be a goodly cedar: and under it shall dwell all fowl of every wing; in the shadow of the branches thereof shall they dwell."

Zechariah 11:2—"Howl, fir tree; for the cedar is fallen; because the mighty are spoiled: howl, O ye oaks of Bashan; for the forest of the vintage is come down."

CINNAMON

Proverbs 7:17—"I have perfumed my bed with myrrh, aloes, and cinnamon."

Song of Solomon 4:14—"Spikenard and saffron; calamus and cinnamon, with all trees of frankincense; myrrh and aloes, with all the chief spices:"

Revelation 18:13—"And cinnamon, and odours, and ointments, and frankincense, and wine, and oil, and fine flour, and wheat, and beasts, and sheep, and horses, and chariots, and slaves, and souls of men."

FIR

1 Kings 6:15—"And he built the walls of the house within with boards of cedar, both the floor of the house, and the walls of the ceiling: and he covered them on the inside with wood, and covered the floor of the house with planks of fir."

1 Kings 6:34—"And the two doors were of fir tree: the two leaves of the one door were folding, and the two leaves of the other door were folding."

1 Kings 9:11—"(Now Hiram the king of Tyre had furnished Solomon with cedar trees and fir trees, and with gold, according to all his desire,) that then king Solomon gave Hiram twenty cities in the land of Galilee."

2 Kings 19:23—"By thy messengers thou hast reproached the Lord, and hast said, With the multitude of my chariots I am come up to the height of the mountains, to the sides of Lebanon, and will cut down the tall cedar trees thereof, and the choice fir trees thereof: and I will enter into the lodgings of his borders, and into the forest of his Carmel."

2 Chronicles 2:8—"Send me also cedar trees, fir trees, and algum trees, out of Lebanon: for I know that thy servants can skill to cut timber in Lebanon; and, behold, my servants shall be with thy servants."

2 Chronicles 3:5—"And the greater house he cieled with fir tree, which he overlaid with fine gold, and set thereon palm trees and chains."

Psalm 104:17—"Where the birds make their nests: as for the stork, the fir trees are her house."

Song of Solomon 1:17—"The beams of our house are cedar, and our rafters of fir."

Isaiah 14:8—"Yea, the fir trees rejoice at thee, and the cedars of Lebanon, saying, Since thou art laid down, no feller is come up against us."

Isaiah 37:24—"By thy servants hast thou reproached the Lord, and hast said, By the multitude of my chariots am I come up to the height of the mountains, to the sides of Lebanon; and I will cut down the tall cedars thereof, and the choice fir trees thereof: and I will enter into the height of his border, and the forest of his Carmel."

Isaiah 41:19—"I will plant in the wilderness the cedar, the shittah tree, and the myrtle, and the oil tree; I will set in the desert the fir tree, and the pine, and the box tree together:"

Isaiah 55:13—"Instead of the thorn shall come up the fir tree, and instead of the brier shall come up the myrtle tree: and it shall be to the Lord for a name, for an everlasting sign that shall not be cut off."

Isaiah 60:13—"The glory of Lebanon shall come unto thee, the fir tree, the pine tree, and the box together, to beautify the place of my sanctuary; and I will make the place of my feet glorious."

Ezekiel 27:5—"They have made all thy ship boards of fir trees of Senir: they have taken cedars from Lebanon to make masts for thee."

Ezekiel 31:8—"The cedars in the garden of God could not hide him: the fir trees were not like his boughs, and the chestnut trees were not like his branches; nor any tree in the garden of God was like unto him in his beauty."

Hosea 14:8—"Ephraim shall say, What have I to do any more with idols? I have heard him, and observed him: I am like a green fir tree. From me is thy fruit found."

Nahum 2:3—"The shield of his mighty men is made red, the valiant men are in scarlet: the chariots shall be with flaming torches in the day of his preparation, and the fir trees shall be terribly shaken."

Zechariah 11:2—"Howl, fir tree; for the cedar is fallen; because the mighty are spoiled: howl, O ye oaks of Bashan; for the forest of the vintage is come down."

FRANKINCENSE

Leviticus 2:15—"And thou shalt put oil upon it, and lay frankincense thereon: it is a meat offering."

Leviticus 2:16—"And the priest shall burn the memorial of it, part of the beaten corn thereof, and part of the oil thereof, with all the frankincense thereof: it is an offering made by fire unto the Lord."

Leviticus 5:11—"But if he be not able to bring two turtledoves, or two young pigeons, then he that sinned shall bring for his offering the tenth part of an ephah of fine flour for a sin offering; he shall put no oil upon it, neither shall he put any frankincense thereon: for it is a sin offering."

Leviticus 6:15—"And he shall take of it his handful, of the flour of the meat offering, and of the oil thereof, and all the frankincense which is upon the meat offering, and shall burn it upon the altar for a sweet savour, even the memorial of it, unto the Lord."

Leviticus 24:7—"And thou shalt put pure frankincense upon each row, that it may be on the bread for a memorial, even an offering made by fire unto the Lord."

Numbers 5:15—"Then shall the man bring his wife unto the priest, and he shall bring her offering for her, the tenth part of an ephah of barley meal; he shall pour no oil upon it, nor put frankincense thereon; for it is an offering of jealousy, an offering of memorial, bringing iniquity to remembrance."

1 Chronicles 9:29—"Some of them also were appointed to oversee the vessels, and all the instruments of the sanctuary, and the fine flour, and the wine, and the oil, and the frankincense, and the spices."

Nehemiah 13:5—"And he had prepared for him a great chamber, where aforetime they laid the meat offerings, the frankincense, and the vessels, and the tithes of the corn, the new wine, and the oil, which was commanded to be given to the Levites, and the singers, and the porters; and the offerings of the priests."

Nehemiah 13:9—"Then I commanded, and they cleansed the chambers: and thither brought I again the vessels of the house of God, with the meat offering and the frankincense."

Song of Solomon 3:6—"Who is this that cometh out of the wilderness like pillars of smoke, perfumed with myrrh and frankincense, with all powders of the merchant?"

Song of Solomon 4:6—"Until the day break, and the shadows flee away, I will get me to the mountain of myrrh, and to the hill of frankincense."

Song of Solomon 4:14—"Spikenard and saffron; calamus and cinnamon, with all trees of frankincense; myrrh and aloes, with all the chief spices:"

Matthew 2:11—"And when they were come into the house, they saw the young child with Mary his mother, and fell down, and worshiped him: and when they had opened their treasures, they presented unto him gifts; gold, and frankincense, and myrrh."

Revelation 18:13—"And cinnamon, and odours, and ointments, and frankincense, and wine, and oil, and fine flour, and wheat, and beasts, and sheep, and horses, and chariots, and slaves, and souls of men."

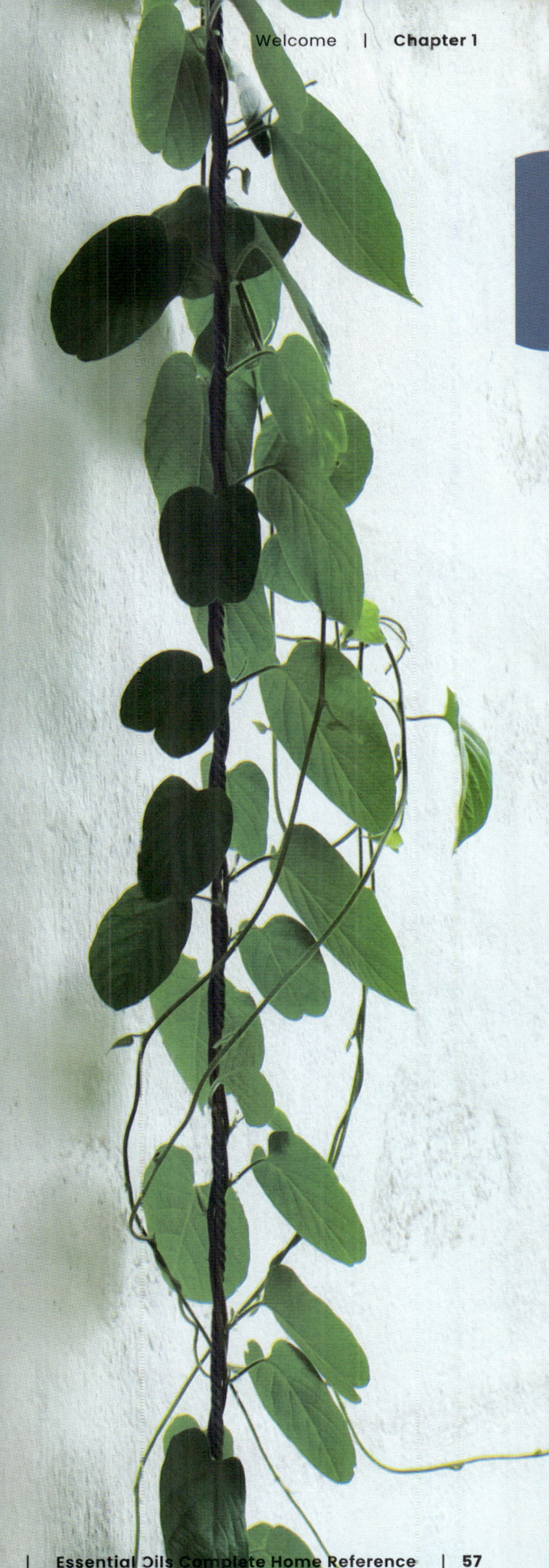

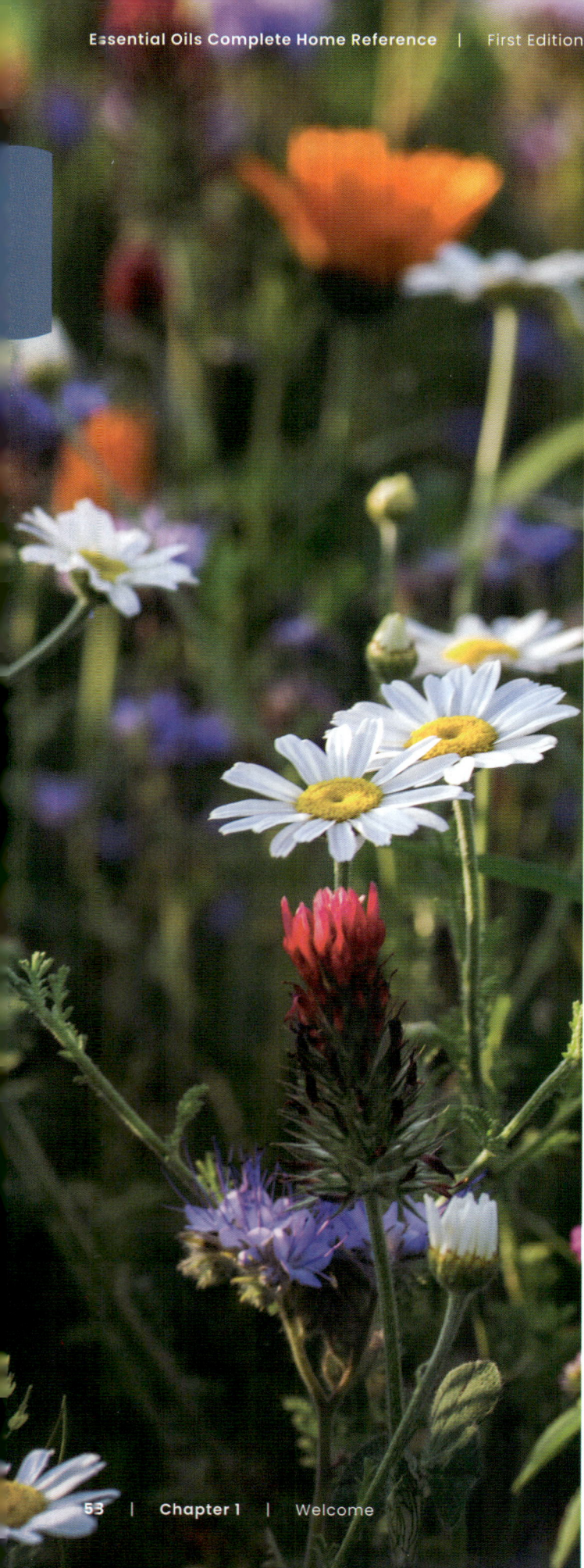

HYSSOP

Leviticus 14:49—"And he shall take to cleanse the house two birds, and cedar wood, and scarlet, and hyssop:"

Leviticus 14:51—"And he shall take the cedar wood, and the hyssop, and the scarlet, and the living bird, and dip them in the blood of the slain bird, and in the running water, and sprinkle the house seven times:"

Leviticus 14:52—"And he shall cleanse the house with the blood of the bird, and with the running water, and with the living bird, and with the cedar wood, and with the hyssop, and with the scarlet:"

Numbers 19:6—"And the priest shall take cedar wood, and hyssop, and scarlet, and cast it into the midst of the burning of the heifer."

Numbers 19:18—"And a clean person shall take hyssop, and dip it in the water, and sprinkle it upon the tent, and upon all the vessels, and upon the persons that were there, and upon him that touched a bone, or one slain, or one dead, or a grave:"

1 Kings 4:33—"And he spake of trees, from the cedar tree that is in Lebanon even unto the hyssop that springeth out of the wall: he spake also of beasts, and of fowl, and of creeping things, and of fishes."

Psalms 51:7—"Purge me with hyssop, and I shall be clean: wash me, and I shall be whiter than snow."

John 19:29—"Now there was set a vessel full of vinegar: and they filled a sponge with vinegar, and put it upon hyssop, and put it to his mouth."

Hebrews 9:19—"For when Moses had spoken every precept to all the people according to the law, he took the blood of calves and of goats, with water, and scarlet wool, and hyssop, and sprinkled both the book, and all the people."

MYRRH

Esther 2:12—"Now when every maid's turn was come to go in to king Ahasuerus, after that she had been twelve months, according to the manner of the women, (for so were the days of their purifications accomplished, to wit, six months with oil of myrrh, and six months with sweet odours, and with other things for the purifying of the women;)"

Psalms 45:8—"All thy garments smell of myrrh, and aloes, and cassia, out of the ivory palaces, whereby they have made thee glad."

Proverbs 7:17—"I have perfumed my bed with myrrh, aloes, and cinnamon."

Song of Solomon 1:13—"A bundle of myrrh is my well-beloved unto me; he shall lie all night betwixt my breasts."

Song of Solomon 3:6—"Who is this that cometh out of the wilderness like pillars of smoke, perfumed with myrrh and frankincense, with all powders of the merchant?"

Song of Solomon 4:6—"Until the day break, and the shadows flee away, I will get me to the mountain of myrrh, and to the hill of frankincense."

Song of Solomon 4:14—"Spikenard and saffron; calamus and cinnamon, with all trees of frankincense; myrrh and aloes, with all the chief spices:"

Song of Solomon 5:1—"I am come into my garden, my sister, my spouse: I have gathered my myrrh with my spice; I have eaten my honeycomb with my honey; I have drunk my wine with my milk: eat, O friends; drink, yea, drink abundantly, O beloved."

Song of Solomon 5:5—"I rose up to open to my beloved; and my hands dropped with myrrh, and my fingers with sweet smelling myrrh, upon the handles of the lock."

Song of Solomon 5:13—"His cheeks are as a bed of spices, as sweet flowers: his lips like lilies, dropping sweet smelling myrrh."

Matthew 2:11—"And when they were come into the house, they saw the young child with Mary his mother, and fell down, and worshiped him: and when they had opened their treasures, they presented unto him gifts; gold, and frankincense, and myrrh."

Mark 15:23—"And they gave him to drink wine mingled with myrrh: but he received it not."

John 19:39—"And there came also Nicodemus, which at the first came to Jesus by night, and brought a mixture of myrrh and aloes, about an hundred pound weight."

MYRTLE

Zechariah 1:8—"I saw by night, and behold a man riding upon a red horse, and he stood among the myrtle trees that were in the bottom; and behind him were there red horses, speckled, and white."
Zechariah 1:10—"And the man that stood among the myrtle trees answered and said, These are they whom the Lord hath sent to walk to and fro through the earth."

Zechariah 1:11—"And they answered the angel of the Lord that stood among the myrtle trees, and said, We have walked to and fro through the earth, and, behold, all the earth sitteth still, and is at rest."

SPIKENARD

Song of Solomon 4:14—"Spikenard and saffron; calamus and cinnamon, with all trees of frankincense; myrrh and aloes, with all chief spices."

Mark 14:3—"And being in Bethany in the house of Simon the leper, as he sat at meat, there came a woman having an alabaster box of ointment of spikenard very precious; and she brake the box, and poured it on his head."

John 12:3—"Then took Mary a pound of ointment of spikenard, very costly, and anointed the feet of Jesus, and wiped his feet with her hair: and the house was filled with the odour of the ointment."

Using essential oils in daily life—spiritual, physical, emotional—is not a new concept. It has been part of the human experience for thousands of years. As time moves on, the rediscovery of these remarkable gifts is becoming more and more widespread. While most people have heard about essential oils, there are still many who have yet to experience how wonderful they are and how they can do wonders in supporting the health of their families.

ENDNOTES

1. The Atlantic [Internet]. Washington: Emerson Collective; c2018. Genetically modified alfalfa officially on the way; 2011 Jan 28 [cited 2018 Dec 4]. Available from: https://www.theatlantic.com/health/archive/2011/01/genetically-modified-alfalfa-officially-on-the-way/70401/.
2. Wikipedia [Internet]. San Francisco: Wikimedia Foundation; [cited 2018 Dec 4]. Available from: https://en.wikipedia.org/wiki/Genetically_modified_crops.
3. Schwartz G, Russek L. The Living Energy Universe. 1st ed. Charlottesville, VA: Hampton Roads Publishing Company; c1999. p. 146.
4. Gattefossé RM. Gattefossé's aromatherapy. 4th ed. Tisserand RB, ed. Essex, England: C.W. Daniel Company Ltd; c1993. p. xii.
5. Liu YY, Wang Y, Walsh TR, Yi LX, Zhang R, Spencer J, Doi Y, Tian G, Dong B, Huang X, Yu LF, Gu D, Ren H, Chen X, Lv L, He D, Zhou H, Liang Z, Liu JH, Shen J. Emergence of plasmid-mediated colistin resistance mechanism MCR-1 in animals and human beings in China: a microbiological and molecular biological study. Lancet Infect Dis. 2016 Feb;16(2):161-8.
6. The Atlantic [Internet]. Washington: Emerson Collective; c2018. Resistance to the antibiotic of last resort is silently spreading. 2017 Jan 12 [cited 2018 Dec 4]. Available from: https://www.theatlantic.com/health/archive/2017/01/colistin-resistance-spread/512705/.
7. Mercola: Take control of your health [Internet]. Chicago: Joseph Mercola, DO; c1997-2018. End of antibiotics grows near as drug-resistant gene with epidemic potential is found in animals, meats, and humans. 2015 Dec 2 [cited 2018 Dec 4]. Available from: http://articles.mercola.com/sites/articles/archive/2015/12/02/antibiotic-resistance-apocalypse.aspx.
8. FDA: U.S. Food & Drug Administration [Internet]. Silver Spring: U.S. Food and Drug Administration; c2018 Dec 4 [cited 2018 Dec 4]. Available from: chttp://www.fda.gov/NewsEvents/Newsroom/PressAnnouncements/ucm517478.htm.
9. 14. Case Western Reserve University Department of Medicine News [Internet]. Cleveland: Case Western Reserve University; c2010 Jul 16 [cited 2018 Dec 4]. Available from: https://cwrumedicine.wordpress.com/2010/02/28/ny-times-id-expert-dr-louis-rice-discusses-rising-threat-of-infections-unfazed-by-antibiotics/.
10. Charles CH, Vincent JW, Borycheski L, Amatnieks Y, Sarina M, Qagish J, Proskin HM. Effect of an essential-oil containing dentifrice on dental plaque microbial composition. Am J Dent. 2000 Sep;13(Spec No):26C-30C.
11. Carson CF, Cookson BD, Farrelly HD, Riley TV. Susceptibility of methicillin-resistant Staphylococcus aureus to the essential oil of Melaleuca alternifolia. J Antimrob Chemother. 1995 Mar;35(3):421-4.
12. Warnke PH, Becker ST, Podschun R, Sivananthan S, Springer IN, Russo PA, Wiltfang J, Fickenscher H, Sherry E. The battle against multi-resistant strains: Renaissance of antimicrobial essential oils as a promising force to fight hospital-acquired infections. J Craniomaxillofac Surg. 2009 Oct;37(7):392-397.
13. Göbel H, Schmidt G, Soyka D. Effect of peppermint and eucalyptus oil preparations on neurophysiological and experimental algesimetric headache parameters. Cephalalgia. 1994 Jun;14(3):228-34; discussion 182.
14. Dalvi SS, Nadkarni PM, Pardesi R, Gupta KC. Effect of peppermint oil on gastric emptying in man: a preliminary study using a radiolabelled solid test meal. Indian J Physiol Pharmacol. 1991 Jul;35(3):212-4.
15. Dember WN, Warm JS, Parasuraman R. Olfactory stimulation and sustained attention. Compendium of Olfactory Research 1982-1994, Kendall/Hunt Publishing Company 1995; 39-46.
16. Hirsch A. A scentsational guide to weight loss. Rockport, MA: Element Books; c1997. 176 p.
17. Veal L. The potential effectiveness of essential oils as a treatment for headlice, Pediculus humanus capitis. Complement Ther Nurs Midwifery. 1996 Aug;2(4):97-101.
18. Russin WA, Hoesly JD, Elson CE, Tanner MA, Gould MN. Inhibition of rat mammary carcinogenesis by monoterpenoids. Carcinogenesis. 1989 Nov;10(11):2161-4.
19. Bassett IB, Pannowitz DL, Barnetson RS. A comparative study of tea-tree oil versus benzoylperoxide in the treatment of acne. Med J Aust. 1990 Oct 15;153(8):455-8.
20. Nenoff P, Haustein UF, Brandt W. Antifungal activity of the essential oil of Melaleuca alternifolia (tea tree oil) against pathogenic fungi in vitro. Skin Pharmacol. 1996;9(6):388-94.
21. Cox SD, Mann CM, Markham JL, Bell HC, Gustafson JE, Warmington JR, Wyllie SG. The mode of antimicrobial action of the essential oil of Melaleuca alternifolia (tea tree oil). J Appl Microbiol. 2000 Jan;88(1):170-5.
22. Carson CF, Riley TV. Antimicrobial activity of the major components of the essential oil of Melaleuca alternifolia. J Appl Bacteriol. 1995 Mar;78(3):264-9.
23. Bradshaw RH, Marchant JN, Meredith MJ, Broom DM. Effects of lavender straw on stress and travel sickness in pigs. J Altern Complement Med. 1998 Fall;4(3):271-5.
24. Nikolaevskiĭ VV, Kononova NS, Pertsovskiĭ AI, Shinkarchuk IF. [Effect of essential oils on the course of experimental atherosclerosis]. Patol Fiziol Eksp Ter 1990 Sep-Oct;5:52-53. Russian.
25. Ghelardini C, Galeotti N, Salvatore G, Mazzanti G. Local anaesthetic activity of the essential oil of Lavandula angustifolia. Planta Med. 1999 Dec;65(8):700-3.
26. Giovannini D, Gismondi A, Basso A, Canuti L, Braglia R, Canini A, Mariani F, Cappelli G. Lavendula angustifolia Mill. essential oil exerts antimicrobial and anti-inflammatory effect in macrophage mediated immune response to Staphylococcus aureus. Immunol Invest. 2016;45(1):11-28.
27. Cai L, Wu CD. Compounds from Syzygium aromaticum possessing growth inhibitory activity against oral pathogens. J Nat Prod. 1996 Oct;59(10):987-90.
28. Fu Y, Zu Y, Chen L, Shi X, Wang Z, Sun S, Efferth T. Antimicrobial activity of clove and rosemary essential oils alone and in combination. Phytother Res. 2007;21(10):989-94.
29. Pourgholami MH, Kamalinejad M, Javadi M, Majzoob S, Sayyah M. Evaluation of the anticonvulsant activity of the essential oil of Eugenia caryophyllata in male mice. J Ethnopharmacol. 1999 Feb;64(2):167-71.
30. Diego MA, Jones NA, Field T, Hernandez-Reif M, Schanberg S, Kuhn C, McAdam V, Galamaga R, Galamaga M. Aromatherapy positively affects mood, EEG patterns of alertness and math computations. Int J Neurosci. 1998 Dec;96(3-4):217-24.
31. Fu Y, Zu Y, Chen L, Shi X, Wang Z, Sun S, Efferth T. Antimicrobial activity of clove and rosemary essential oils alone and in combination. Phytother Res. 2007;21(10):989-94.
32. Lopez-Bote CJ, Gray JI, Gomaa EA, Flegal CJ. Effect of dietary administration of oil extracts from rosemary and sage on lipid oxidation in broiler meat. Br Poult Sci. 1998 May;39(2):235-40.
33. Ramadan W, Mourad B, Ibrahim S, Sonbol F. Oil of bitter orange: new topical antifungal agent. Int J Dermatol. 1996 Jun;35(6):448-9.
34. Alderman GG, Marth EH. Inhibition of growth and aflatoxin production of Aspergillus parasiticus by citrus oils. Z Leb Unters-Forsch. 1976 Apr 28;160(4):353-8.
35. Wattenberg LW, Hanley AB, Barany G, Sparnins VL, Lam LK, Fenwick GR. Inhibition of carcinogenesis by some minor dietary constituents. Princess Takamatsu Symp. 1985; 16:193-203.
36. Crowell PL. Prevention and therapy of cancer by dietary monoterpenes. J Nutr. 1999 Mar;129(3):775S-778S.
37. Aruna K, Sivaramakrishnan VM. Anticarcinogenic effects of the essential oils from cumin, poppy and basil. Phytotherapy Research. 1996 Nov;10(7):577-80.
38. Juergens UR, Dethlefsen U, Steinkamp G, Gillissen A, Repges R, Vetter H. Anti-inflammatory activity of 1.8-cineole (eucalyptol) in bronchial asthma: a double-blind placebo-controlled trial. Respir. Med. 2003; 97(3):250-6.
39. Nasel C, Nasel B, Samec P, Schindler E, Buchbauer G. Functional imaging of effects of fragrances on the human brain after prolonged inhalation. Chem Senses. 1994 Aug;19(4):359-64.
40. Steinmetz M, et al. Transmission and scanning electronmicroscopy study of the action of sage and rosemary essential oils and eucalyptol on Candida albicans. Mycoses. 1988 Jan;31(1):40-51.
41. Ulmer WT, Schött D. Chronic obstructive bronchitis. Effect of Gelomyrtol forte in a placebo-controlled double-blind study. Fortschr Med 1991 Sep;109(27):547-550.
42. Horne D, Holm M, Oberg C, Chao S, Young DG. Antimicrobial effects of essential oils on Streptococcus pneumoniae. Journal of Essential Oil Research. 2001;13(5):387-392.
43. Halliwell B, Gutteridge JM. Free radicals in biology and medicine. 2nd Ed. Oxford: Clarendon Press; c1989. 896 p.
44. Recsan Z, Pagliuca G, Piretti MV, Penzes LG, Youdim KA, Noble RC, Deans SG. Effect of essential oils on the lipids of the retina in the ageing rat: a possible therapeutic use. Journal of Essential Oil Research. 1997;9(1):53-6.
45. Youdim KA, Deans SG. Effect of thyme oil and thymol dietary supplementation on the antioxidant status and fatty acid composition of the ageing rat brain. Br J Nutr. 2000 Jan;83(1):87-93.
46. Stevens N. Natural synergy: essential oils in cancer research [master's thesis]. [Provo (UT), Las Vegas (NV)]: Brigham Young University/University of Nevada Las Vegas; August 2002.
47. Stewart D. The chemistry of essential oils made simple: God's love manifest in molecules. Marble Hill, MO: Care Publications; 2006. 625 p.
48. Franchomme P, Pénoël D. L'aromathérapie exactement. France: Roger Jollois; 31 Août 2003. 446 p.
49. C. Bushdid, M. O. Magnasco, L. B. Vosshall, A. Keller. Humans Can Discriminate More than 1 Trillion Olfactory Stimuli. Science 21 Mar 2014: Vol. 343, Issue 6177, pp. 1370-1372
50. Scientific American [Internet]. New York: Springer Nature; 2018. Is sense of smell powered by quantum vibrations? 2006 Dec 15 [cited 2018 Dec 4]. Available from: https://www.scientificamerican.com/article/is-sense-of-smell-powered/.
51. Turin L. A spectroscopic mechanism for primary olfactory reception. Chem. Senses. 1996. 21(6): 773–91.
52. Brookes JC, Horsfield AP, Stoneham AM. Odour character differences for enantiomers correlate with molecular flexibility J.R. Soc. Interface. 2009 Jan 6;6(3):75-86. doi: 10.1098/rsif.2008.0165.
53. The New Inquiry [Internet]. Brooklyn: The New Inquiry; 2018. Osmic frequencies. 2015 Feb 13 [cited 2018 Dec 4]. Available from: https://thenewinquiry.com/osmic-frequencies/.
54. Hirsch AR, Gomez R. Weight reduction through inhalation of odorants. J. Neurol. Orthop. Med. Surg. 1995;16:28-31.
55. Hirsch AR, Gruss JJ. Human male sexual response to olfactory stimuli. J. Neurol. Orthop. Med. Surg. 1999;19(1):14-19.

Essential Oil Singles & Blends

Common Uses: Almost all oils can be diffused, directly inhaled, and/or applied topically. Many have dietary uses.

Aromatic: Certain oils should be diffused 3 times daily for up to 10, 30, or 60 minutes at a time. Note time recommendations under each oil's listing.

Topical: Apply 2-4 drops on location, temples, neck, or on chakras and/or Vita Flex points (crown of head, forehead, heart, and navel).

- **Neat = Straight, undiluted**

    Dilution usually NOT required; suitable for all but the most sensitive skin. Safe for children over 2 years old.

- **50-50 = Dilute 50-50**

    Dilute 1 part essential oils to 1 part V-6 Vegetable Oil Complex or other pure carrier oil for topical and internal use, especially when used on sensitive areas—face, neck, genital area, underarms, etc.

- **20-80 = Dilute 20-80**

    Dilute 1 part essential oils to 4 parts V-6 Vegetable Oil Complex or other pure carrier oil for topical and internal use, especially when used on sensitive areas—face, neck, genital area, underarms, etc.

- Full-body Massage: Unless otherwise specified on the product label, dilute 1 drop essential oil with 15 drops of V-6 or other pure carrier oil.

Dietary and/or Culinary Use (Vitality™): Vitality essential oils can be diluted, put in a capsule, and taken daily. Note dilution ratios under each oil's listing. Vitality oils can also be added to food for delicious, concentrated flavor. Follow the directions on the product labels.

Note: Found-in List: A list of the products containing each oil can be found in Appendix B.

CAUTIONS

Note which cautions are applicable to which oil under each oil's listing. Not all cautions apply to all oils.

 Keep out of reach of children.

 For external use only.

 Avoid contact with eyes and mucous membranes.

 If you are pregnant, nursing, taking medication, or have a medical condition, consult a health professional prior to use.

 Flammable. Keep away from fire, heat, or sparks. Do not store above room temperature.

 PH = Photosensitizing. Avoid direct sunlight or UV rays (e.g., sunlamps, tanning beds, etc.) for up to 12 hours after applying oil. Sunlight should be avoided for 24 hours after applying some oils, shown as (24).

 May stain some surfaces, skin, or clothing.

 Some oils might cause a stinging, burning sensation, rash, redness, pain, blisters, inflammation, swelling, itching, or darkening of the skin. Test for sensitivity on a small area of skin on the underside of your arm and apply as needed.

These statements have not been evaluated by the Food and Drug Administration. These products are not intended to diagnose, treat, cure, or prevent any disease. Consult individual product labels for safety information.

All Young Living Vitality™ essential oils are Non-GMO Project Verified! To receive this certification, all Vitality oils passed through third-party verification, auditing, and testing.

SINGLE ESSENTIAL OIL APPLICATION CODES

Neat = Straight, undiluted
Dilution usually NOT required; suitable for all but the most sensitive skin. Safe for children over 2 years old.

50-50 = Dilute 50-50
Dilution recommended in equal parts (1 part essential oils to 1 part V-6 Vegetable Oil Complex) for topical and internal use, especially when used on sensitive areas—face, neck, genital area, underarms, etc.

20-80 = Dilute 20-80
Always dilute one part to four parts (1 part essential oils to 4 parts V-6 Vegetable Oil Complex) before applying to the skin or taking internally.

PH = Photosensitizing
Avoid using on skin exposed to direct sunlight or UV rays (e.g., sunlamps, tanning beds, etc.).

Angelica	PH 50-50
Anise	50-50
Australian Ericifolia	50-50
Basil	50-50
Bergamot	PH 50-50
Biblical Sweet Myrrh	50-50
Black Pepper	50-50
Black Spruce	50-50
Black Spruce, Northern Lights	50-50
Blue Cypress	Neat
Blue Spruce, Idaho	Neat
Blue Tansy	Neat
Blue Yarrow	Neat
Calamus	50-50
Camphor (syn. Ho Wood)	Neat
Canadian Fleabane	PH 50-50
Caraway	Neat
Cardamom	50-50
Carrot Seed	Neat
Cassia	PH 20-80
Cedarwood	PH Neat
Celery Seed	50-50
Chamomile, German	Neat
Chamomile, Roman	Neat
Cilantro	50-50
Cinnamon Bark	PH 20-80
Cistus	Neat
Citronella	50-50
Citrus Hystrix	50-50
Clary Sage	PH 50-50
Clove	20-80
Copaiba	Neat
Coriander	50-50
Cumin	PH 20-80
Cypress	Neat
Davana	Neat
Dill	50-50
Dorado Azul	50-50
Douglas Fir	50-50
Elemi	Neat
Eucalyptus Blue	50-50
Eucalyptus Citriodora	50-50
Eucalyptus Globulus	50-50
Eucalyptus Radiata	50-50
Eucalyptus Staigeriana	50-50
Fennel	Neat
Fragonia	Neat
Frankincense	Neat
Frankincense, Frereana	20-80
Frankincense, Sacred	Neat
Geranium	Neat
Ginger	PH 50-50
Goldenrod	50-50
Grand Fir, Idaho	Neat
Grapefruit	PH 50-50
Helichrysum	Neat
Hinoki	50-50
Hong Kuai	20-80
Hyssop	50-50
Ishpingo	20-80
Jade Lemon	PH 50-50
Jasmine	Neat
Juniper	50-50
Kunzea	50-50
Laurus Nobilis	50-50
Lavandin	Neat
Lavender	Neat
Ledum	50-50
Lemon	PH 50-50
Lemongrass	20-80
Lemon Myrtle	50-50
Lemon Verbena	50-50
Lime	PH 50-50
Mandarin	PH 50-50
Manuka	Neat
Marjoram	50-50
Mastrante	50-50
Melaleuca Quinquenervia	50-50
Melissa	Neat
Micromeria	20-80
Mountain Savory	50-50
Myrrh	Neat
Myrtle	50-50
Nerol	iPH Neat
Nutmeg	50-50
Ocotea	20-80
Orange	PH 50-50
Oregano	20-80
Oregano, Ecuadorian	20-80
Palmarosa	Neat
Palo Santo	50-50
Parsley	PH 50-50
Patchouli	PH Neat
Peppermint	20-80
Petitgrain	Neat
Pine	50-50
Plectranthus Oregano	20-80
Ravintsara	50-50
Rose	Neat
Rosemary	20-80
Rue	PH 50-50
Sage	20-80
Sandalwood, Royal Hawaiian	Neat
Sandalwood, Sacred	Neat
Spanish Sage	50-50
Spearmint	50-50
Spikenard	Neat
Tangerine	PH 50-50
Tarragon	50-50
Tea Tree	Neat
Thyme	20-80
Tsuga	50-50
Valerian	Neat
Vanilla	Neat
Vetiver	Neat
Western Red Cedar	50-50
White Fir	Neat
White Lotus	50-50
Wintergreen	PH 20-80
Xiang Mao	Neat
Ylang Ylang	Neat
Yuzu	PH Neat

ESSENTIAL OIL BLEND APPLICATION CODES

Neat = Straight, undiluted
Dilution usually NOT required; suitable for all but the most sensitive skin. Safe for children over 2 years old.

50-50 = Dilute 50-50
Dilution recommended in equal parts (1 part essential oils to 1 part V-6 Vegetable Oil Complex) for topical and internal use, especially when used on sensitive areas—face, neck, genital area, underarms, etc.

20-80 = Dilute 20-80
Always dilute one part to four parts (1 part essential oils to 4 parts V-6 Vegetable Oil Complex) before applying to the skin or taking internally.

PH = Photosensitizing
Avoid using on skin exposed to direct sunlight or UV rays (e.g., sunlamps, tanning beds, etc.).

Blend	Code	Blend	Code	Blend	Code
3 Wise Men™	Neat	Freedom™	PH Neat	M-Grain™	Neat
25 Years Young™	PH Neat	Fulfill Your Destiny™	PH 20-80	Mister™	Neat
Abundance™	PH 50-50	Gary's Light™	PH Neat	Motivation™	50-50
Acceptance™	PH Neat	Gathering™	PH Neat	My Destiny™	PH 20-80
Amoressence™	50-50	Gentle Baby™	PH 50-50	One Heart™	PH 50-50
AromaEase™	50-50	GLF™	PH 50-50	PanAway™	20-80
Aroma Life™	Neat	Gratitude™	Neat	Peace & Calming & R-O™	PH 50-50
Aroma Siez™	50-50	Grounding™	PH 50-50	Peace & Calming II™	PH 50-50
Australian Blue™	PH Neat	Harmony™	PH Neat	Present Time™	PH Neat
Australian Kuranya™	50-50	Higher Unity™	PH 50-50	Purification™	Neat
Awaken™	PH Neat	Highest Potential™	PH Neat	Raven™	PH 50-50
Believe™	Neat	Hope™	Neat	R.C.™	50-50
Brain Power™	PH Neat	Humility™	PH Neat	Reconnect™	PH Neat
Breathe Again™ & Roll-On	Neat	ImmuPower™	PH 20-80	Release™	PH Neat
Build Your Dream™	PH 50-50	Inner Child™	PH 50-50	Relieve It™	50-50
CBD Blends	PH Neat	Inspiration™	PH Neat	RutaVaLa™ & Roll-On	PH 50-50
Celebration™	PH Neat	Into the Future™	PH 20-80	Sacred Angel™	Neat
Chivalry™	PH 50-50	InTouch™	PH Neat	SacredMountain™	PH 50-50
Christmas Spirit™	PH 20-80	Journey On™	PH 20-80	SARA™	PH 20-80
Citrus Fresh™	PH 50-50	Joy®	PH Neat	SclarEssence™	PH 50-50
Clarity™	PH 50-50	JuvaCleanse™	50-50	Sensation™	Neat
Common Sense™	PH 20-80	JuvaFlex™	Neat	Shutran™	PH Neat
Cool Azul™	PH Neat	KidScents® GeneYus™	PH Neat	Slique® Essence	Neat
Deep Relief™ Roll-On	PH Neat	KidScents® KidPower™ & Roll-On	Neat	Stress Away & Roll-On	PH Neat
DiGize™	PH 50-50	KidScents® Owie™ & Roll-On	Neat	Surrender™	PH Neat
Divine Release™	PH Neat	KidScents® SleepyIze™ & Roll-On	Neat	The Gift™	50-50
Dragon Time™	PH 50-50	KidScents® SniffleEase™ & Roll-On	Neat	Thieves & Roll-On	PH 20-80
Dream Catcher™	PH 50-50	KidScents® TummyGize™ & R-O	PH Neat	Tranquil™ Roll-On	PH Neat
Egyptian Gold™	PH 20-80	Lady Sclareol™	PH Neat	Transformation™	PH 50-50
EndoFlex™	50-50	Light the Fire™	PH 20-80	Trauma Life™	50-50
En-R-Gee™	20-80	Live with Passion™	PH 50-50	T.R. Care™	PH Neat
Envision™	PH 50-50	Live Your Passion™	PH 50-50	Treasure of the Season™	50-50
Evergreen Essence™	50-50	Longevity™	PH 20-80	Valor & Roll-On	Neat
Excite™	PH 20-80	Loyalty™	Neat	White Angelica™	PH Neat
Exodus II™	PH 20-80	Magnify Your Purpose™	50-50	White Light™	50-50
Forgiveness™	PH Neat	Melrose™	50-50		

3 WISE MEN™
(Essential Oil Blend)

This blend promotes feelings of reverence and spiritual awareness based on the power of therapeutic-grade essential oils that open the subconscious. It enhances emotional equilibrium as it soothes and uplifts the heart.

MEDICAL PROPERTIES & USES:
Anti-inflammatory, antimicrobial, empowering, calming, disease-inhibitory, nervous system supportive

INGREDIENTS:
Sweet almond oil, Royal Hawaiian Sandalwood, Juniper, Frankincense, Black Spruce, Myrrh

DIRECTIONS:
Aromatic: 6o. Topical: Neat.

CAUTIONS:

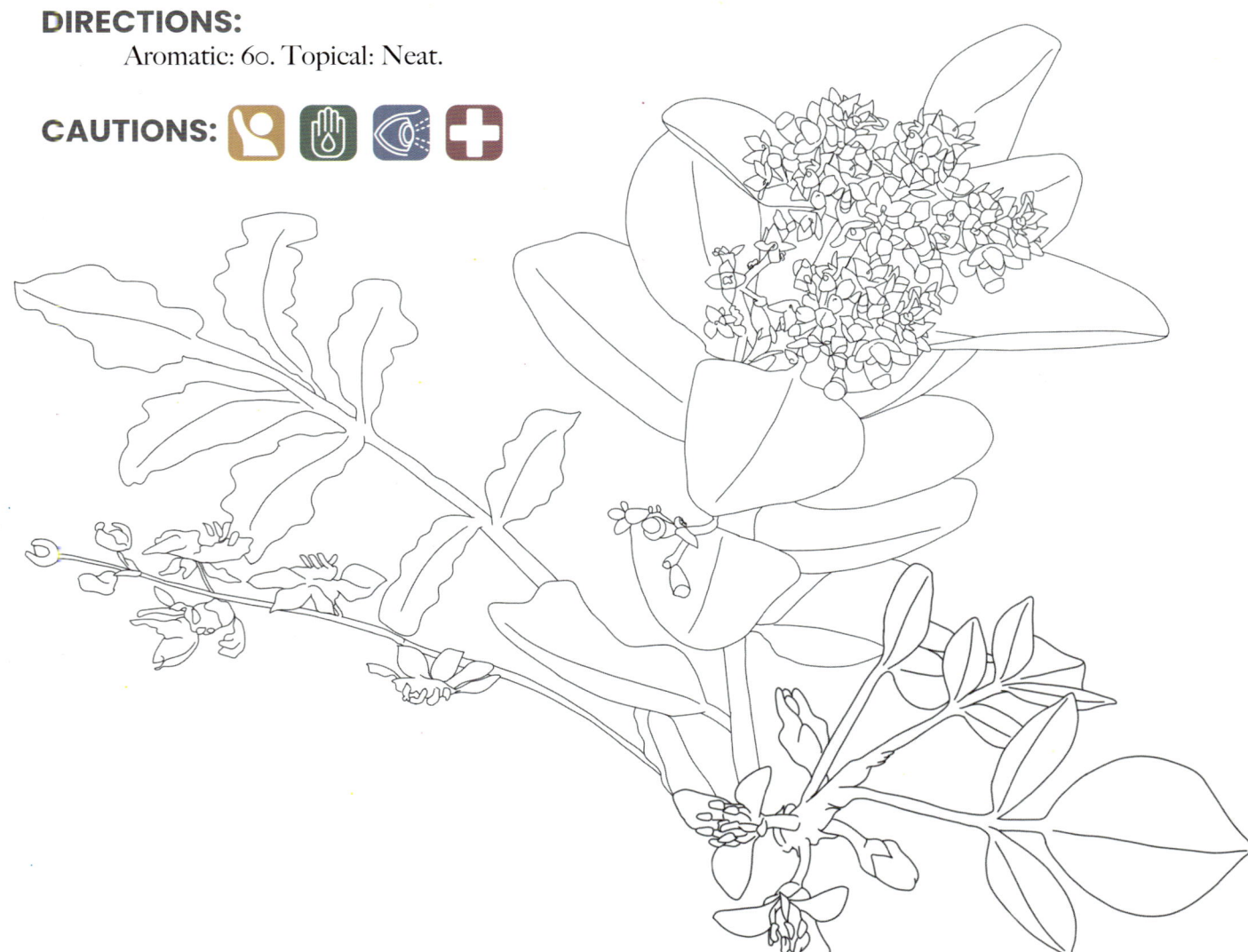

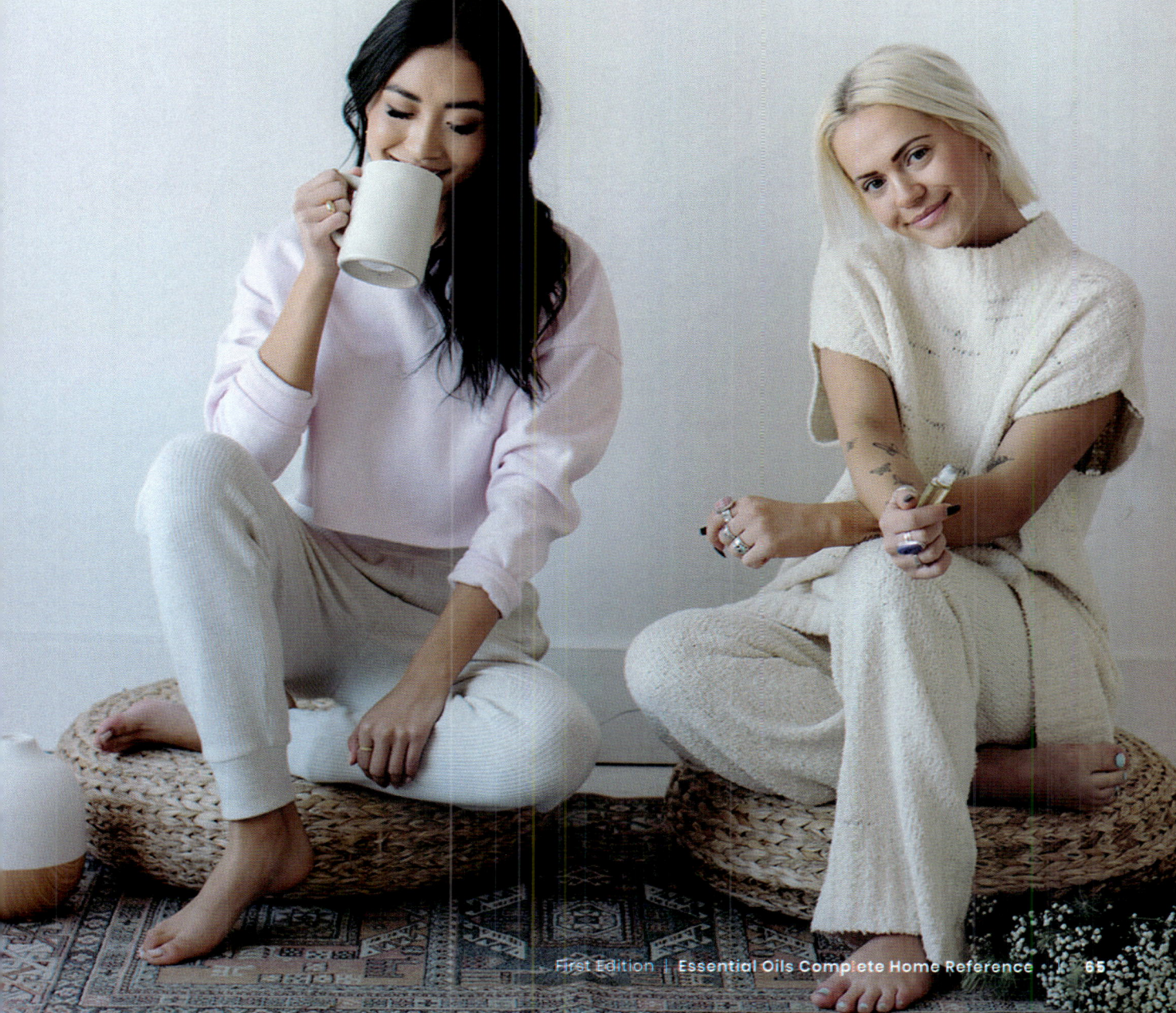

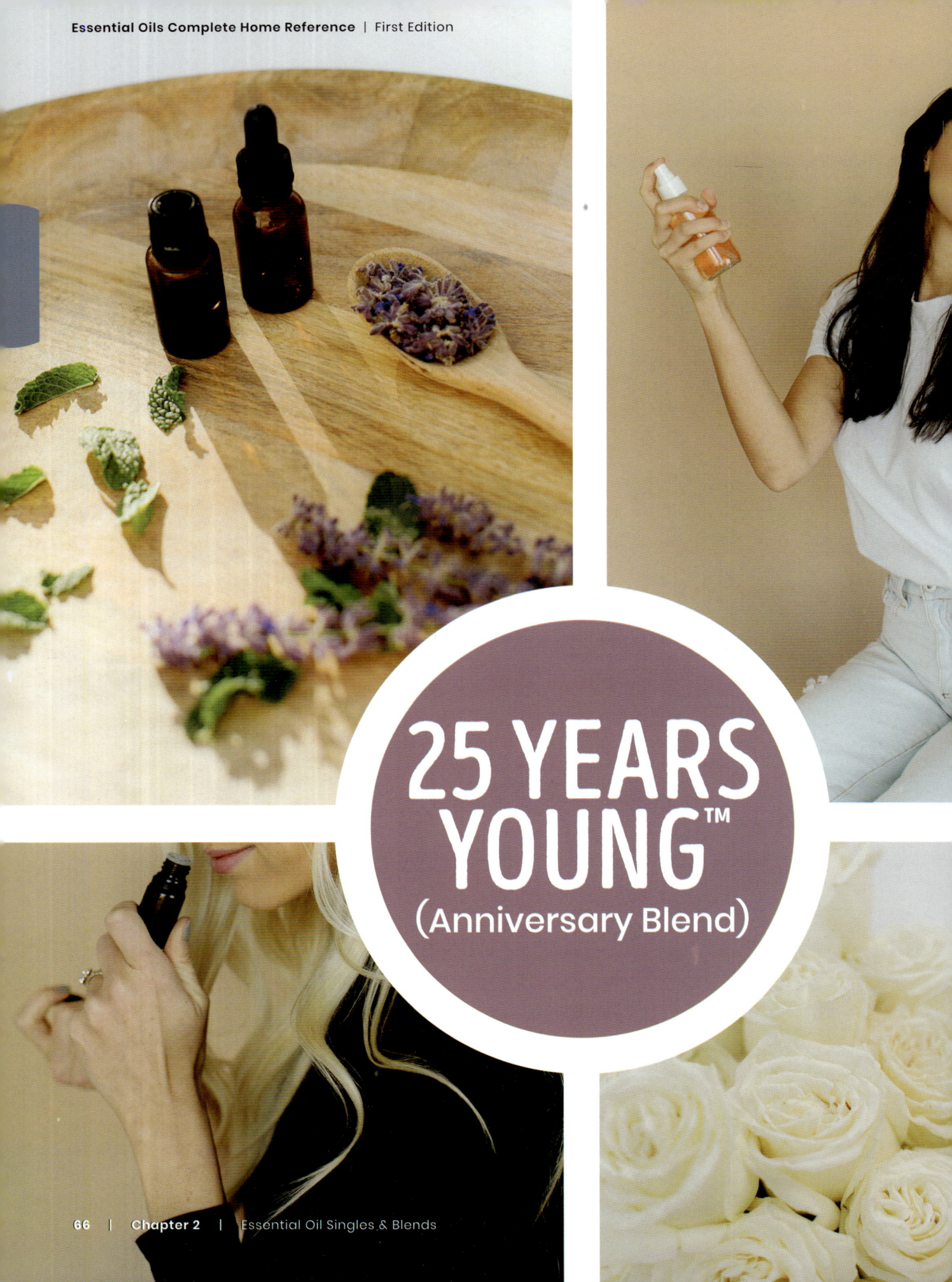

ABOUT 25 YEARS YOUNG:

Formulated exclusively for Young Living's 25th anniversary and the 2019 International Grand Convention, this blend brings together some of the first essential oils produced by Young Living, such as Lavender and Ylang Ylang, as well as some of the world's most sought-after oils, like Sacred Sandalwood, Rose, Frankincense, Myrrh, and Helichrysum. All of these oils combine to promote strong feelings of youthful energy and complexion. When diluted and topically applied, they make for a wonderfully soothing massage.

MEDICAL PROPERTIES & USES:
Antitumoral, antimicrobial, antiviral, anti-inflammatory, emotion supporting, relaxing, neuroprotective, antidepressant, antifungal, antioxidant, insecticidal, sedative

INGREDIENTS:
Sacred Sandalwood, Myrrh, Lavender, Frankincense, Helichrysum, Ylang Ylang, Cedarwood, Rose

DIRECTIONS:
Aromatic: 6o. Topical: Neat.

CAUTIONS:

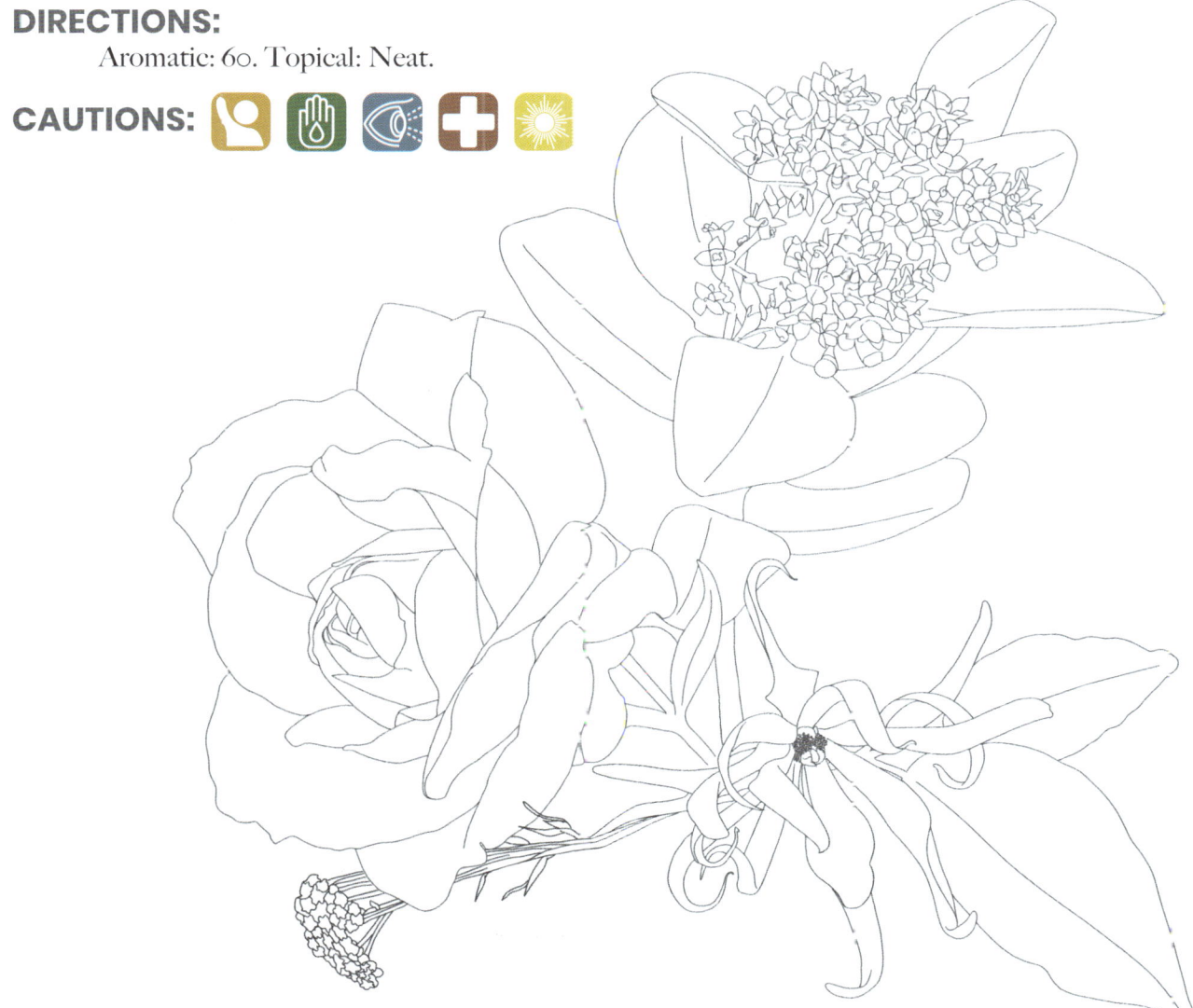

ABUNDANCE™
(Essential Oil Blend)

This blend exemplifies the true power of synergy. Together, all of its component oils are magnified in vibration, creating the law of attraction, the energy and frequency of prosperity and plentitude.

MEDICAL PROPERTIES & USES:
Antiallergy, anti-inflammatory, antimicrobial, antioxidative, emotion supporting, calming, cardiovascular supportive, muscle relaxant/bone or joint preservative, nervous system protective, pain or swelling reducing, respiratory supportive, skin and hair improving

INGREDIENTS:
Orange, Frankincense, Patchouli, Clove, Ginger, Myrrh, Cinnamon Bark, Black Spruce

DIRECTIONS:
Aromatic: 6o. Topical: 50-50. Use Release first to let go of emotions that prevent recipient from receiving abundance. Follow with one or several blends such as Acceptance, Believe, Envision, Into the Future, The Gift, Joy, Magnify Your Purpose, Motivation, or Valor.

CAUTIONS:

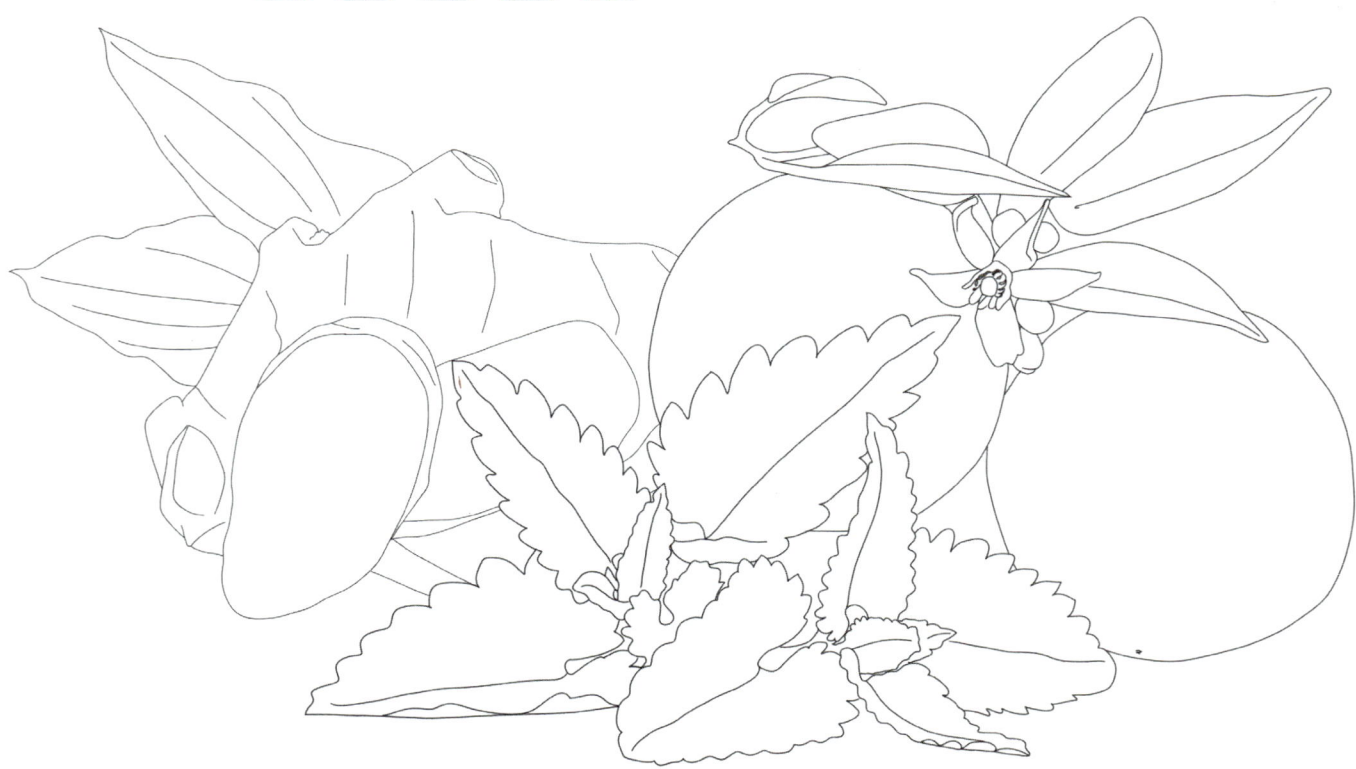

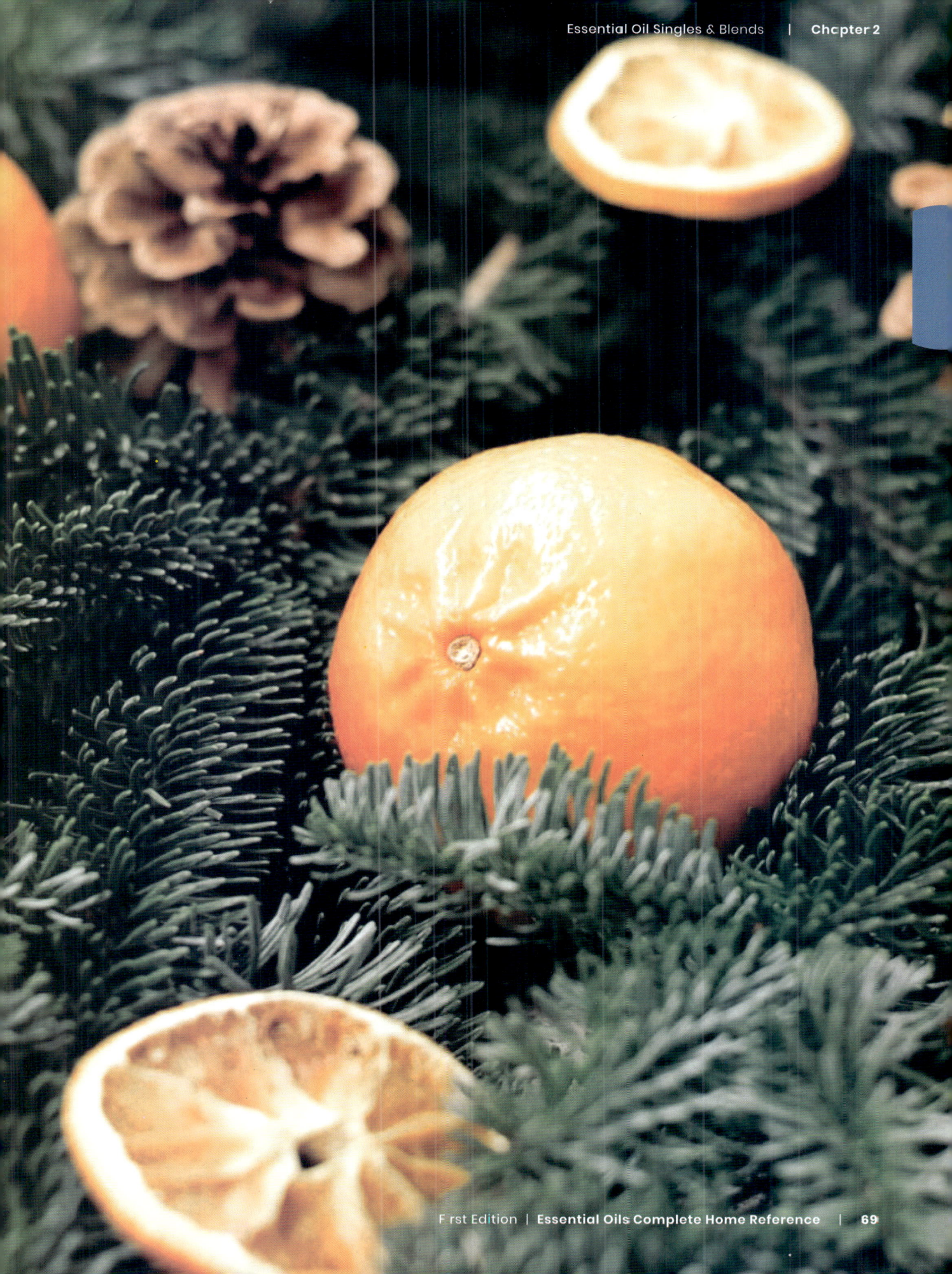

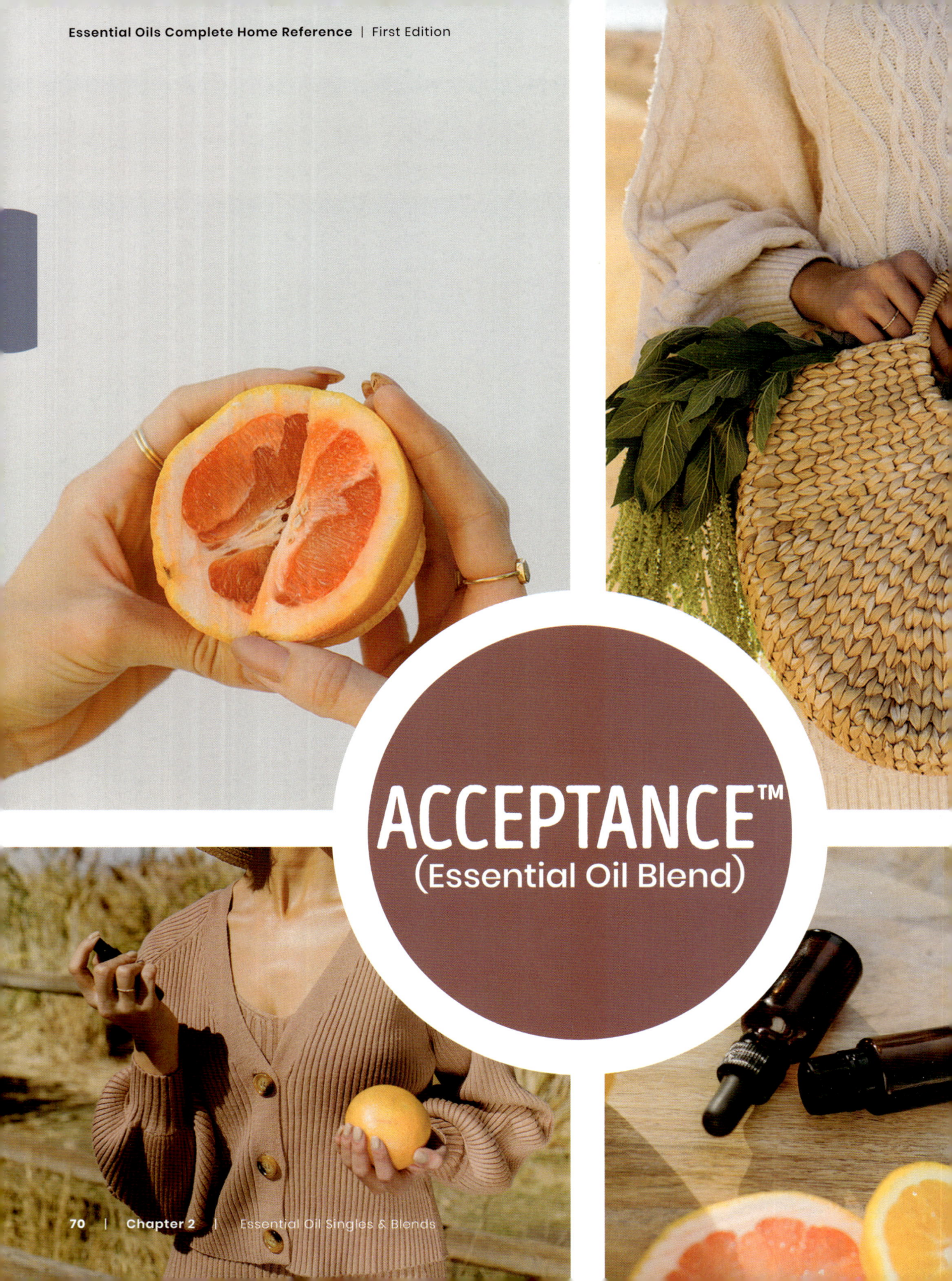

ABOUT ACCEPTANCE:

Acceptance stimulates the mind, compelling us to open and accept new things, people, or relationships in life, allowing one to reach a higher potential. It also helps us to overcome procrastination and denial.

MEDICAL PROPERTIES & USES:

Anti-inflammatory, antimicrobial, antioxidative, emotion supporting, calming, cardiovascular supportive, disease inhibitory, organ protective, pain/swelling reducing, performance enhancing/stimulating, skin and hair improving

INGREDIENTS:

Sweet almond oil, Coriander, Geranium, Bergamot, Frankincense, Royal Hawaiian Sandalwood, Bitter Orange (Neroli), Grapefruit, Tangerine, Spearmint, Lemon, Blue Cypress, Davana, Kaffir Lime, Ocotea, Jasmine, Matricaria (German Chamomile), Ylang Ylang, Blue Tansy, Rose

DIRECTIONS:

Aromatic: 6o. Topical: Neat.

CAUTIONS: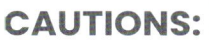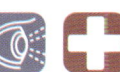

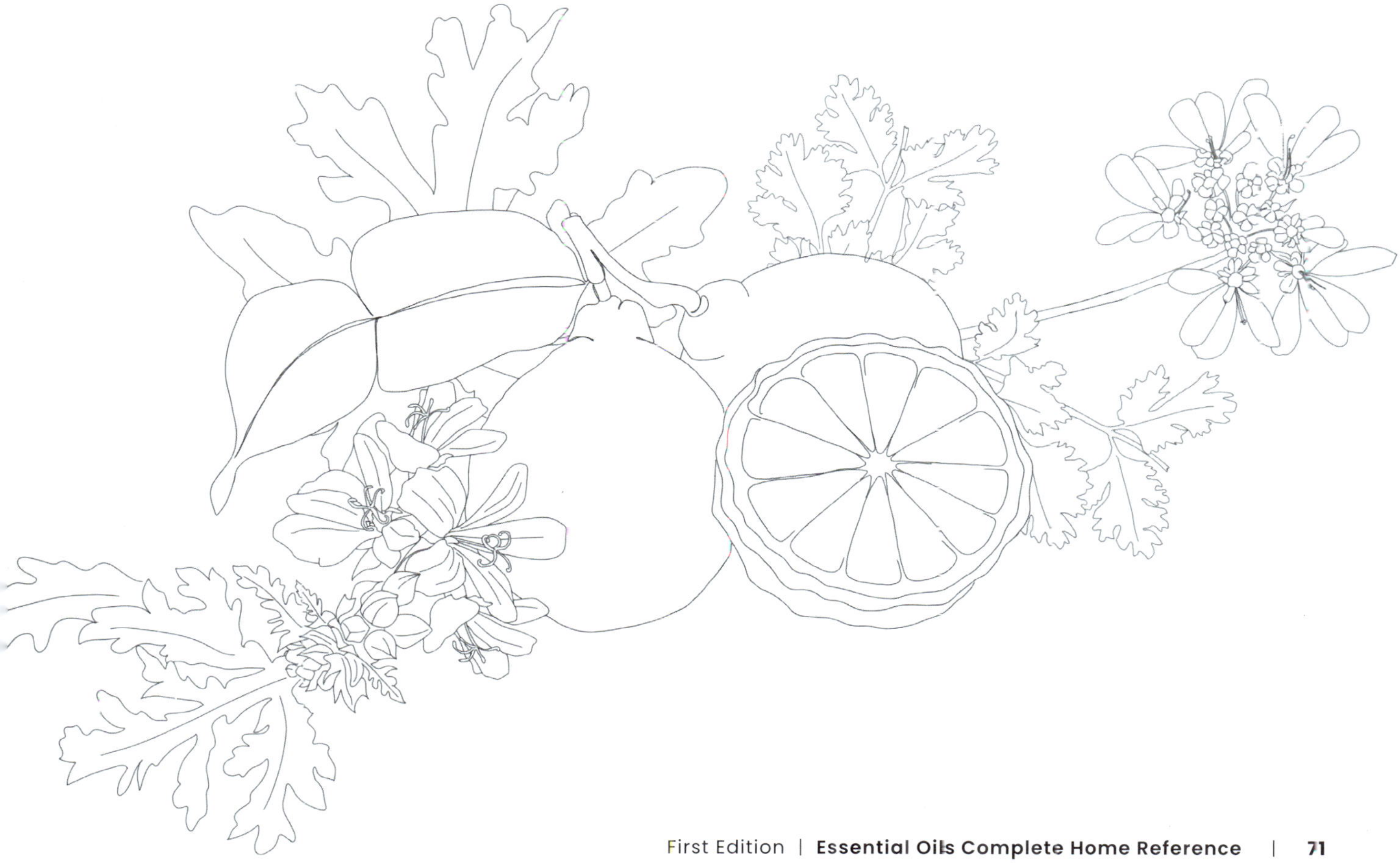

AMORESSENCE™
(Essential Oil Blend)

A limited-edition blend available only at a Young Living Beauty School event, Amoressence is formulated with exotic essential oils that pamper and beautify the skin. It will help you improve and maintain your youthful look and radiant glow.

MEDICAL PROPERTIES & USES:
Skin supporting, anti-inflammatory, antimicrobial, antioxidative, calming, disease inhibitory, pain or swelling reducing, performance-enhancing/stimulating

INGREDIENTS:
Vetiver, Idaho Blue Spruce, Jasmine, Davana, Ocotea, Ylang Ylang, Roman Chamomile, Vanilla, Geranium

DIRECTIONS:
Aromatic: 30. Topical: 50-50. Dilute as needed and apply to desired area.

CAUTIONS:

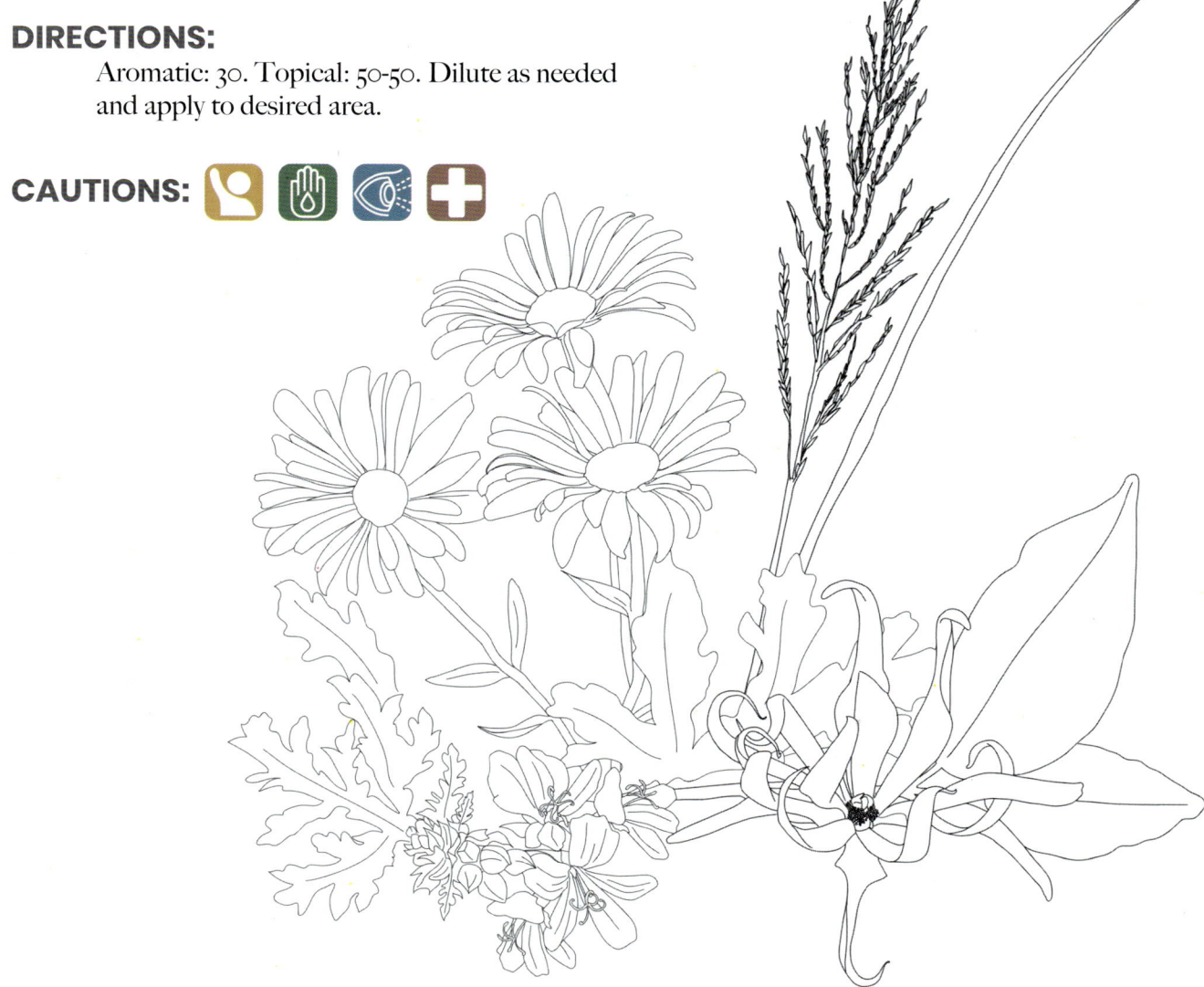

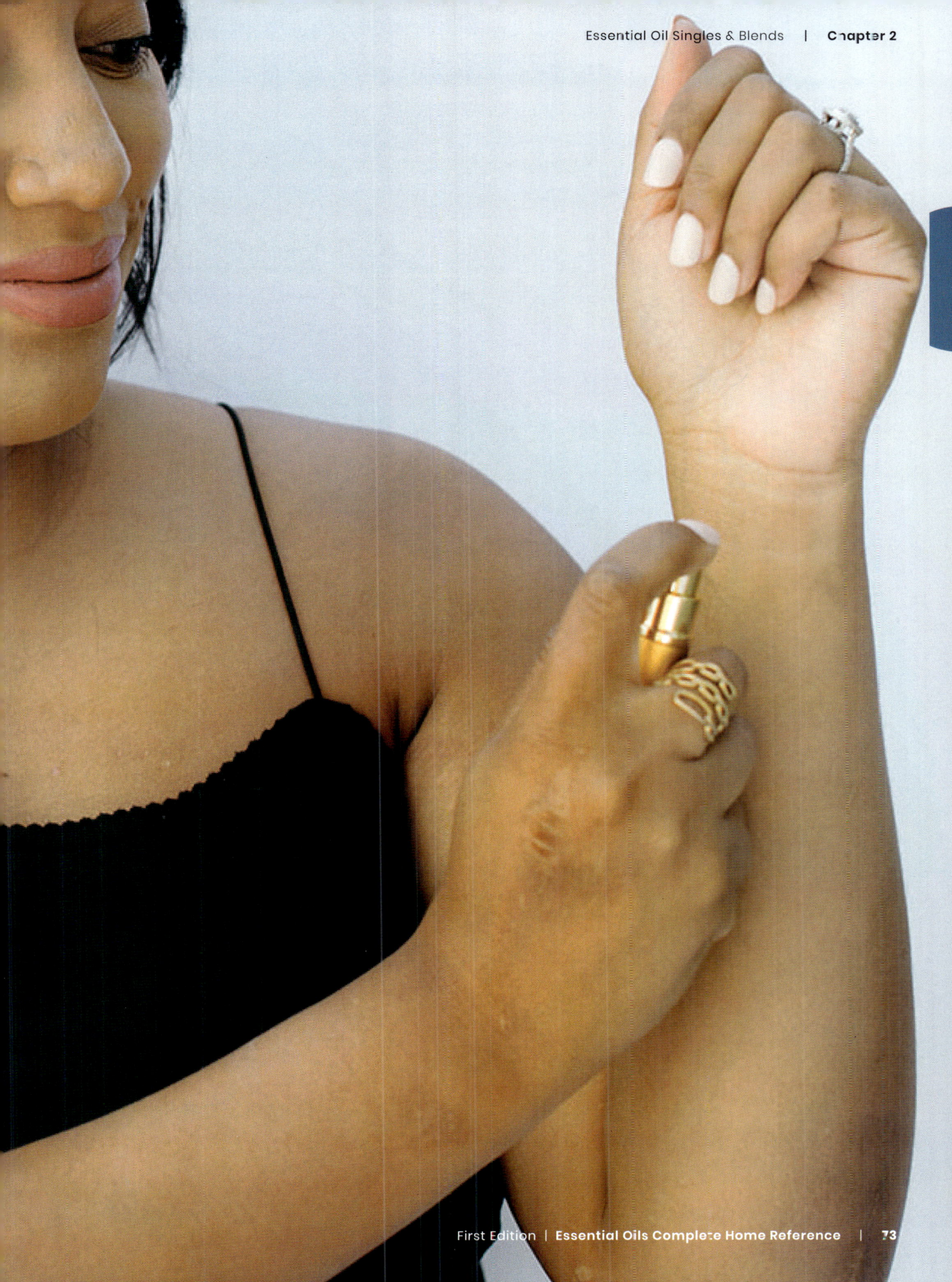

BOTANICAL FAMILY:
Apiaceae

PLANT ORIGIN:
Belgium, Bulgaria, Netherlands

EXTRACTION METHOD:
Steam distilled from root

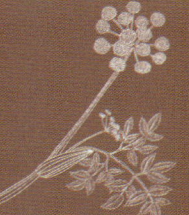

KEY CONSTITUENTS:
Beta-Phellandrene (≤30%), Alpha-Phellandrene (7-28%), Alpha-Pinene (10-27%), Delta-3-Carene (8-15%), Limonene (3-13%), Sabinene (≤12%), Trans-Beta Ocimene (≤7%), Cis-Beta-Ocimene (≤4%)

ANGELICA
(Angelica archangelica)

Known as the "holy spirit root" or the "oil of angels" by the Europeans, angelica's healing powers were so strong that it was believed to be of divine origin. From the time of Paracelsus, it was credited with the ability to protect from the plague. The stems were chewed during the plague of the 1660s to prevent infection. When burned, the seeds and roots were thought to purify the air.

MEDICAL PROPERTIES:
Anticoagulant, relaxant, antispasmodic

USES:
Throat/lung infections, indigestion, menstrual problems/PMS, symptoms of dementia

FRAGRANT INFLUENCE:
Assists in the release of pent-up negative feelings and restores memories to the point of origin before trauma or anger was experienced

DIRECTIONS:
Aromatic: 30. Topical: 50-50.

CAUTIONS:

SELECTED RESEARCH:

Kaur A, Garg S, Shiekh BA, Singh N, Singh P, Bhatti R. InSilico Studies and In Vivo MAOα Inhibitory Activity of Coumarins Isolated from Angelica archangelica Extract: An Approach toward Antidepressant Activity. ACS Omega. 2020 Jun 30; 5(25): 15069-15076. Published online 2020 June 18.

Bhat ZA, Kumar D, Shah MY. Angelica archangelica Linn. is an angel on earth for the treatment of diseases. Int J Nutr Pharmacol Neurol Dis. 2011;1(1):36-50.

Fraternale D, Flamini G, Ricci D. Essential oil composition and antimicrobial activity of Angelica archangelica L. (Apiaceae) roots. J Med Food. 2014 Sep;17(9):1043-7.

Fraternale D, Teodori L, Rudov A, Prattichizzo F, Olivieri F, Guidarelli A, Albertini MC. The in vitro activity of Angelica archangelica L. essential oil on inflammation. J Med Food. 2018 Aug 29.

Kimura T, Hayashida H, Murata M, Takamatsu J. Effect of ferulic acid and Angelica archangelica extract on behavioral and psychological symptoms of dementia in frontotemporal lobar degeneration and dementia with Lewy bodies. Geriatr Gerontol Int. 2011 Jul;11(3):309-14. Epub 2011 Jan 29.

Kumar D, Bhat ZA, Kumar V, Shah MY. Coumarins from Angelica archangelica Linn. and their effects on anxiety-like behavior. Prog Neuropsychopharmacol Biol Psychiatry. 2013 Jan 10;40:180-6. Epub 2012 Aug 29.

Prakash B, Singh P, Goni R, Raina AK, Dubey NK. Efficacy of Angelica archangelica essential oil, phenyl ethyl alcohol and α-terpineol against isolated molds from walnut and their antiaflatoxigenic and antioxidant activity. J Food Sci Technol. 2015 Apr;52(4):2220-8. Epub 2014 Feb 16.

Yeh ML, Liu CF, Huang CL, Huang TC. Hepatoprotective effect of Angelica archangelica in chronically ethanol-treated mice. Pharmacology. 2003 Jun;68(2):70-73. Epub 2003 Apr 25.

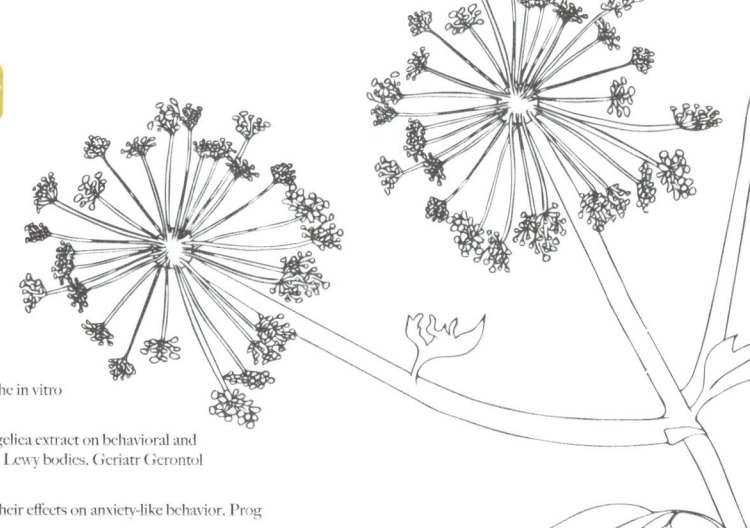

Essential Oil Singles & Blends | **Chapter 2**

Think of it as an angel watching over your sleep...

First Edition | **Essential Oils Complete Home Reference** | 75

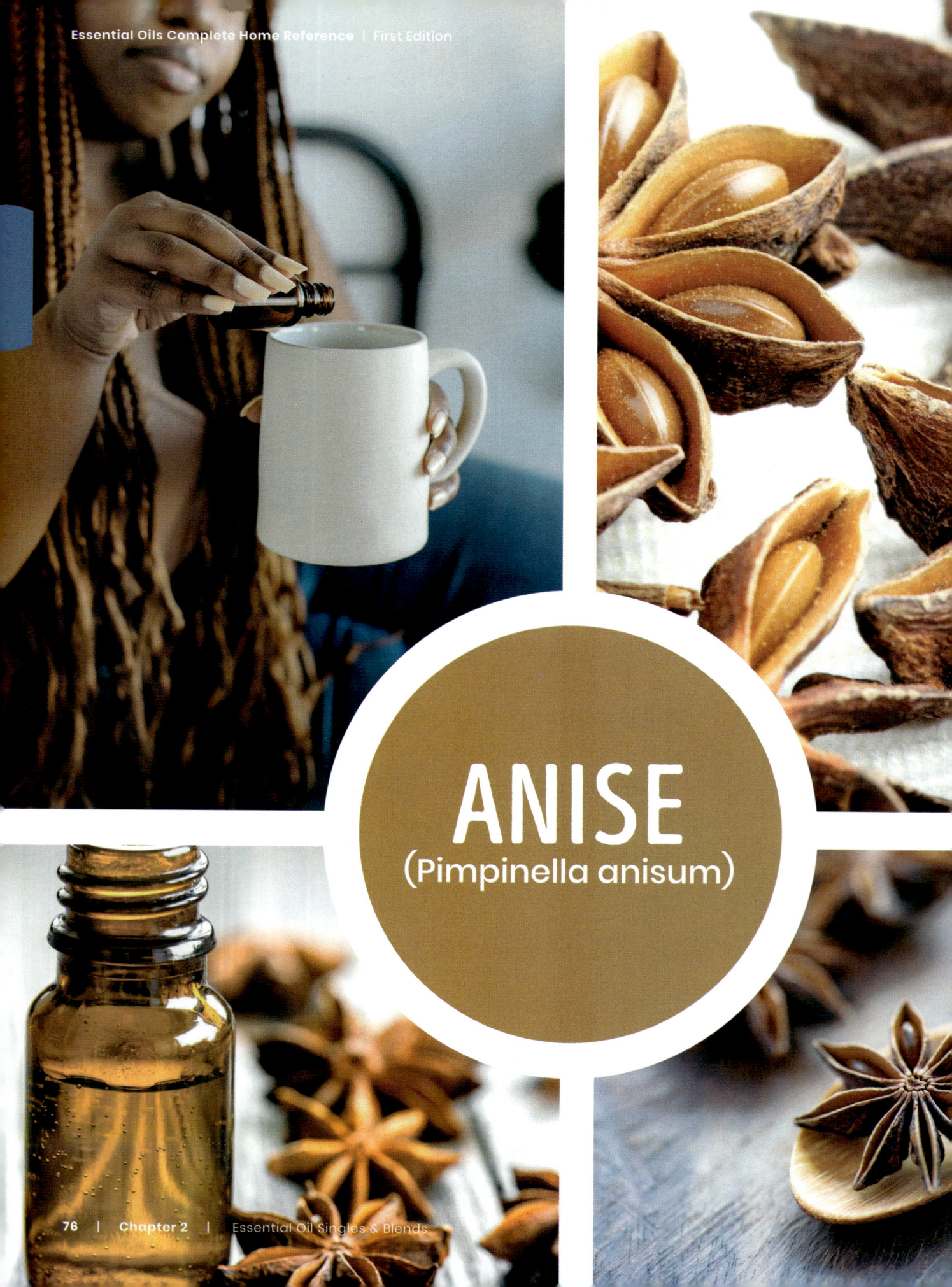

BOTANICAL FAMILY:
Apiaceae

PLANT ORIGIN:
Spain

EXTRACTION METHOD:
Steam distilled from seeds

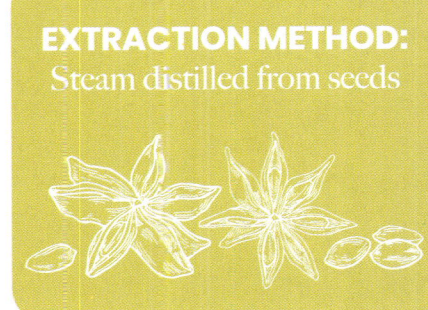

KEY CONSTITUENTS:
Trans-Anethole (88-98%)
Methyl Chavicol (up to 3%)
Gamma-Himachalene (up to 2%)
Anisic Aldehyde (up to 2%)

HISTORICAL DATA:
Listed in Dioscorides' De Materia Medica (AD 78), Europe's first authoritative guide to medicines, which became the standard reference work for herbal treatments for over 1,700 years.

MEDICAL PROPERTIES:
Digestive stimulant, anticoagulant, anesthetic/analgesic, antioxidant, diuretic, antitumoral, anti-inflammatory

USES:
Arthritis/rheumatism, cancer

FRAGRANT INFLUENCE:
Opens emotional blocks and recharges vital energy

DIRECTIONS:
Aromatic: 30. Topical: 50-50.
Dietary: Put in a capsule and take up to 3 times daily or as needed.

CAUTIONS:

SELECTED RESEARCH:
Asadollahpoor A, Abdollahi M, Rahimi R. Pimpinella anisum L. fruit: chemical composition and effect on rat model of nonalcoholic fatty liver disease. J Res Med Sci. 2017 Mar 15;22:37.

Gradinaru AC, Miron A, Trifan A, Spac A, Brebu M, Aprotosoaie AC. Screening of antibacterial effects of anise essential oil alone and in combination with conventional antibiotics against Streptococcus pneumoniae clinical isolates. Rev Med Chir Soc Med Nat Iasi. 2014 Apr-Jun;118(2):537-43.

Jamshidzadeh A, Heidari R, Razmjou M, Karimi F, Moein MR, Farshad O, Akbarizadeh AR, Shayesteh MR. An in vivo and in vitro investigation on hepatoprotective effects of Pimpinella anisum seed essential oil and extracts against carbon tetrachloride-induced toxicity. Iran J Basic Med. 2015 Feb;18(2):205-11.

Koriem KMM, Arbid MS, El-Gendy NF. The protective role of anise oil in oxidative stress and genotoxicity produced in favism. J Diet Suppl. 2016;13(5):505-21. Epub 2016 Jan 8.

Lee JB, Yamagishi C, Hayashi K, Hayashi T. Antiviral and immunostimulating effects of lignan-carbohydrate-protein complexes from Pimpinella anisum. Biosci Biotechnol Biochem. 2011;75(3):459-65. Epub 2011 Mar 11.

Mohammed MJ. Isolation and identification of anethole from Pimpinella anisum L. fruit oil. An antimicrobial study. Journal of Pharmacy Research. 2009 May;2(5):915-919.

Shukla HS, Dubey P, Chaturvedi RV. Antiviral properties of essential oils of Foeniculum vulgare and Pimpinella anisum L. 1989;9(3):277-279.

Tas A. Analgesic effect of Pimpinella anisum L. essential oil extract in mice. Indian Veterinary Journal. 2009;86(2):145-147.

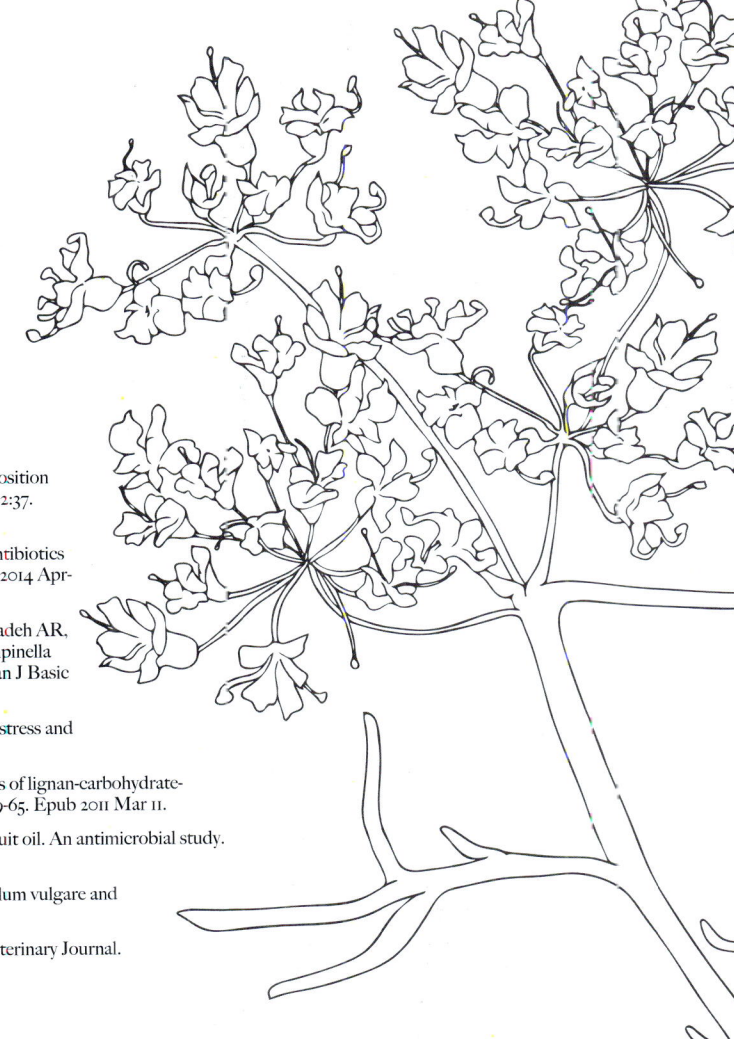

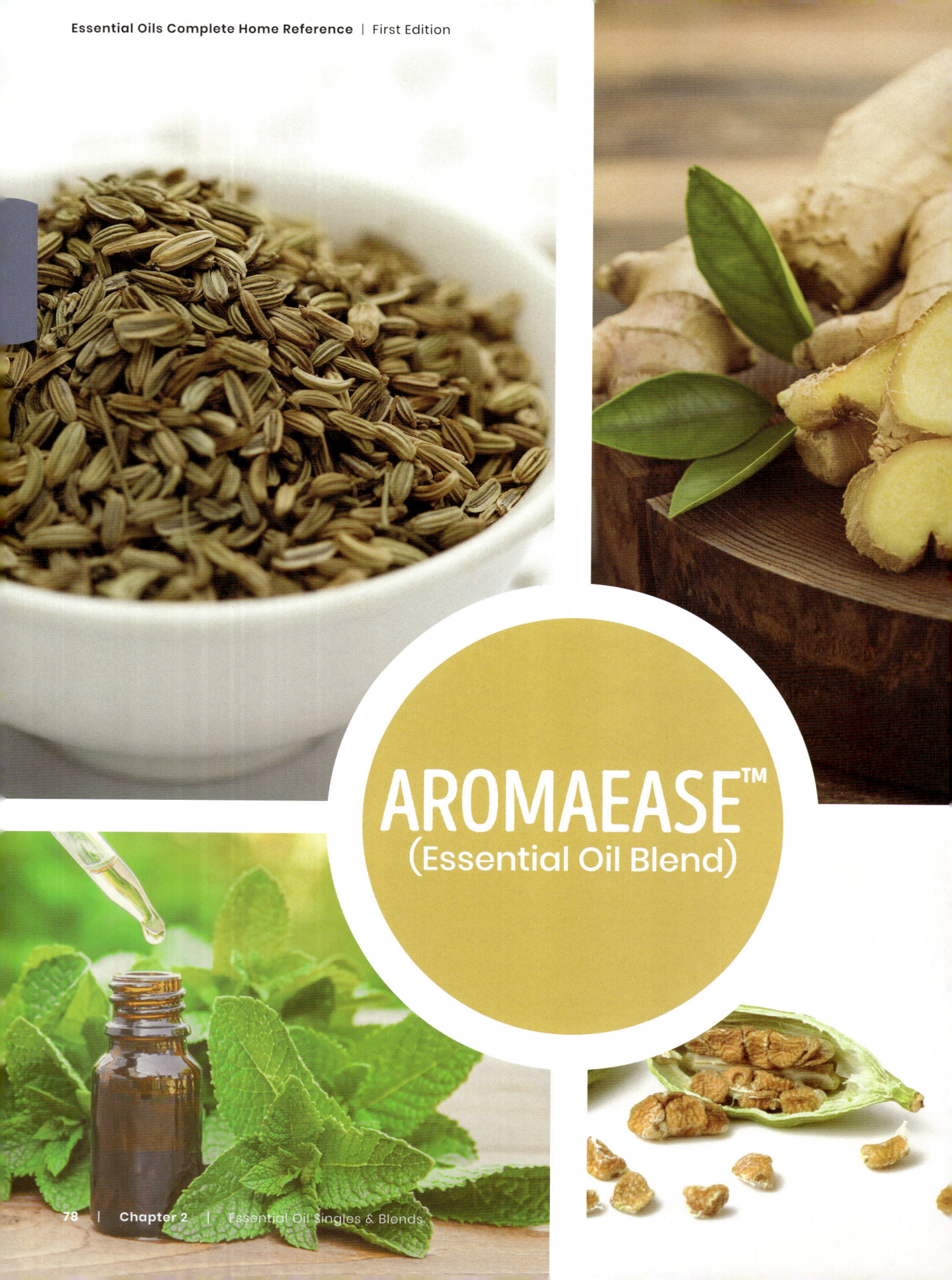

ABOUT AROMAEASE:

This comforting blend has a cool, minty aroma that contains powerful essential oil constituents. Use AromaEase to reduce the effects of nausea and other sensations of digestive discomfort.

MEDICAL PROPERTIES & USES:
Anti-allergy, anti-inflammatory, antimicrobial, antioxidative, calming, digestion/elimination supportive, nausea reducing, pain or swelling reducing, performance enhancing/stimulating

INGREDIENTS:
Peppermint, Spearmint, Ginger, Cardamom, Fennel

DIRECTIONS:
Aromatic: 30. Topical: 50-50.

CAUTIONS:

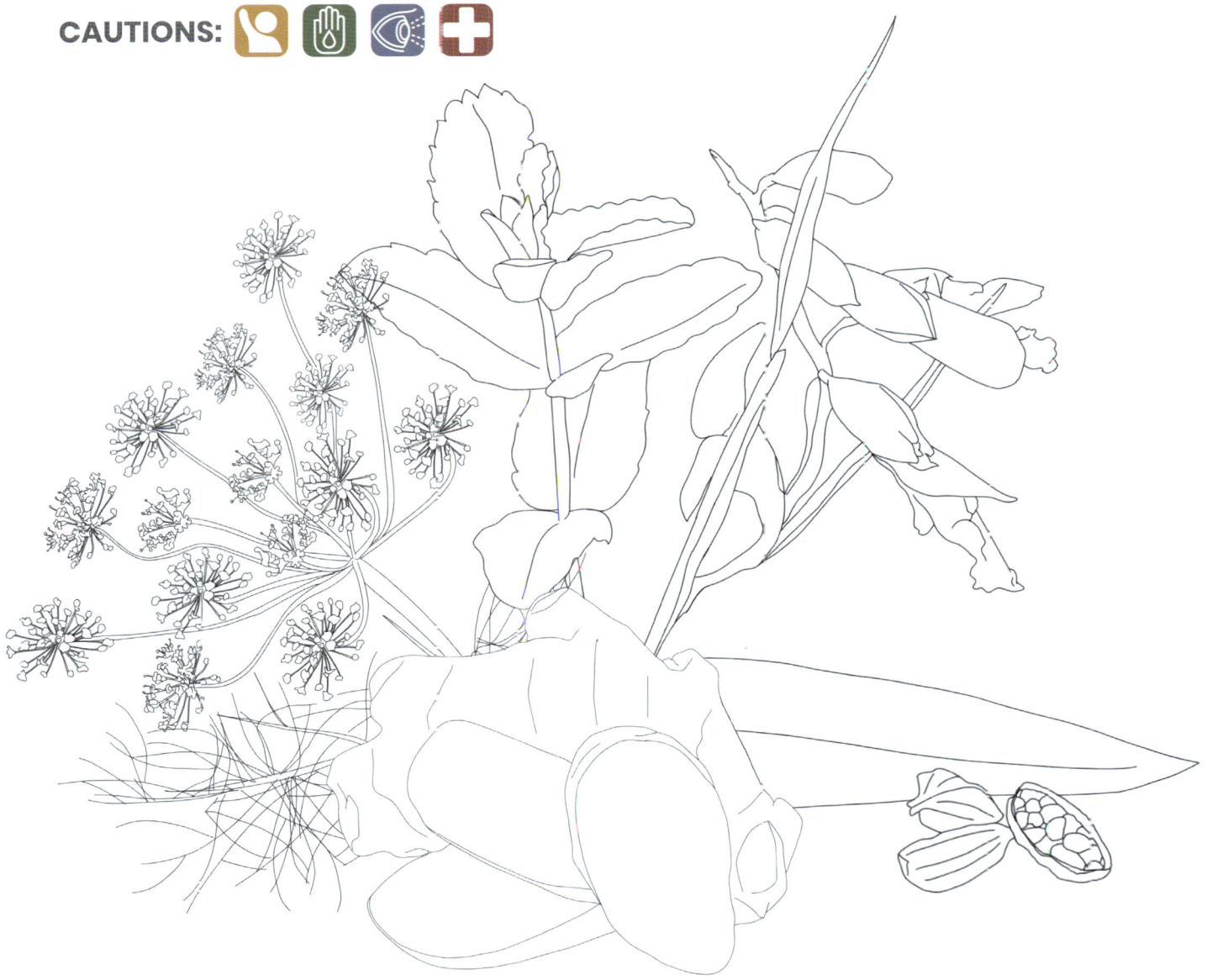

AROMA LIFE™
(Essential Oil Blend)

Aroma Life improves cardiovascular, lymphatic, and circulatory systems, lowers high blood pressure; and reduces stress.

MEDICAL PROPERTIES & USES:
Anti-inflammatory, antimicrobial, antioxidative, calming, digestion or elimination supportive, nausea reducing, cardiovascular system supportive, lymphatic system supportive, disease inhibitory, insecticidal, organ protective, respiratory system supportive

INGREDIENTS:
Sesame seed oil, Cypress, Marjoram, Ylang Ylang, Helichrysum

DIRECTIONS:
Aromatic: 6o. Topical: Neat. Apply 1-2 drops over heart and along spine from first to fourth thoracic vertebrae (which correspond to the cardiopulmonary nerves).

CAUTIONS:

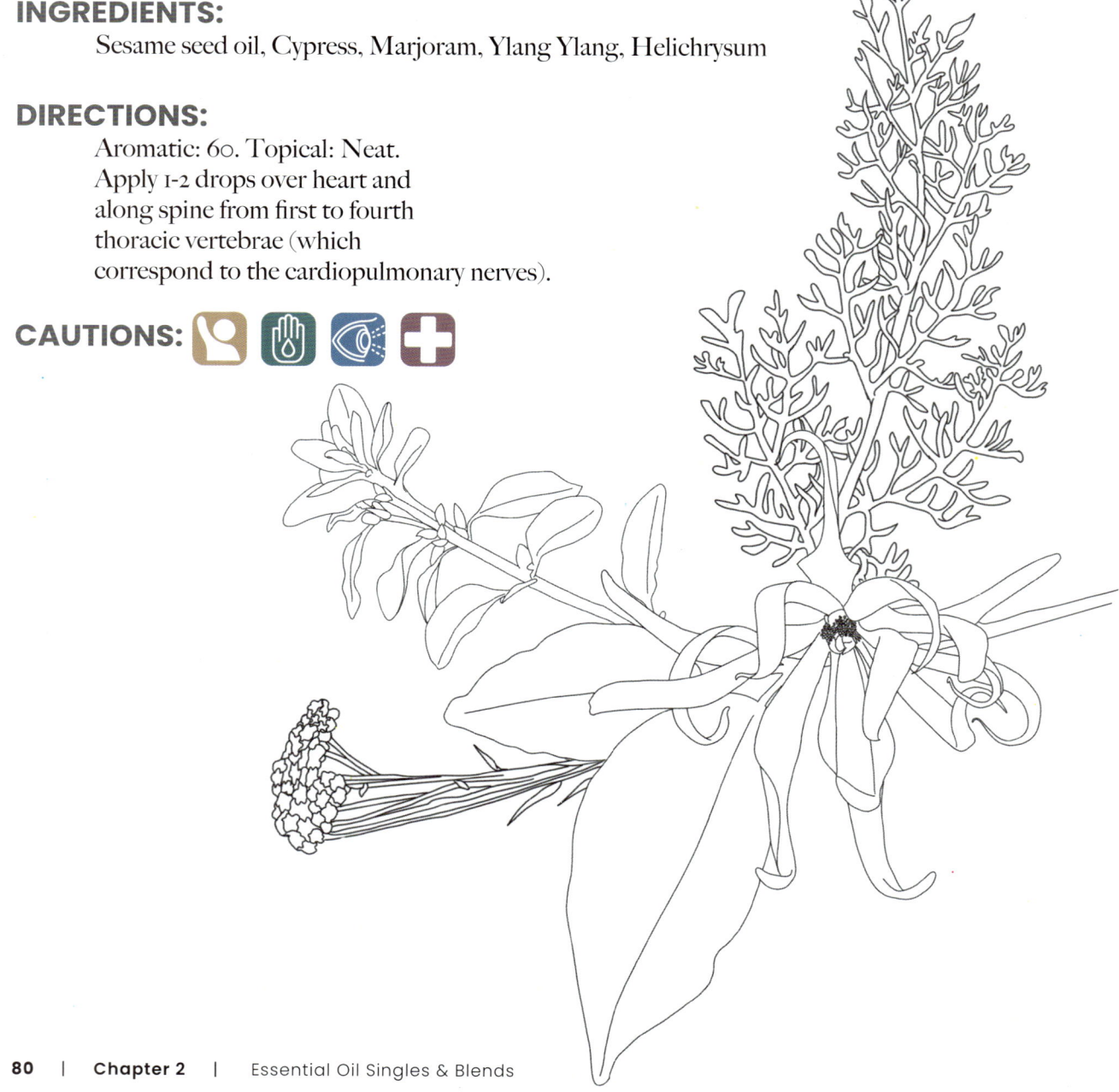

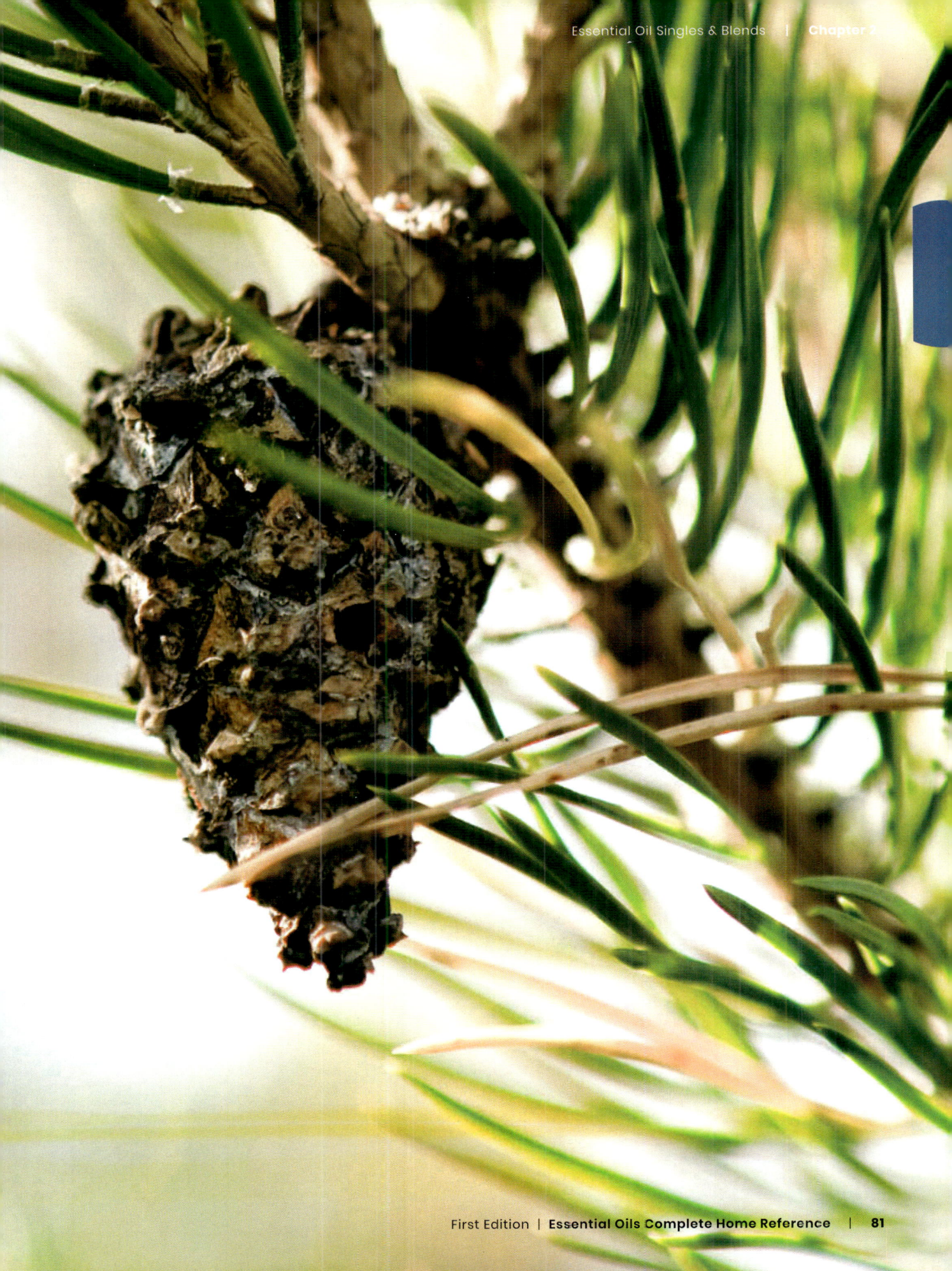

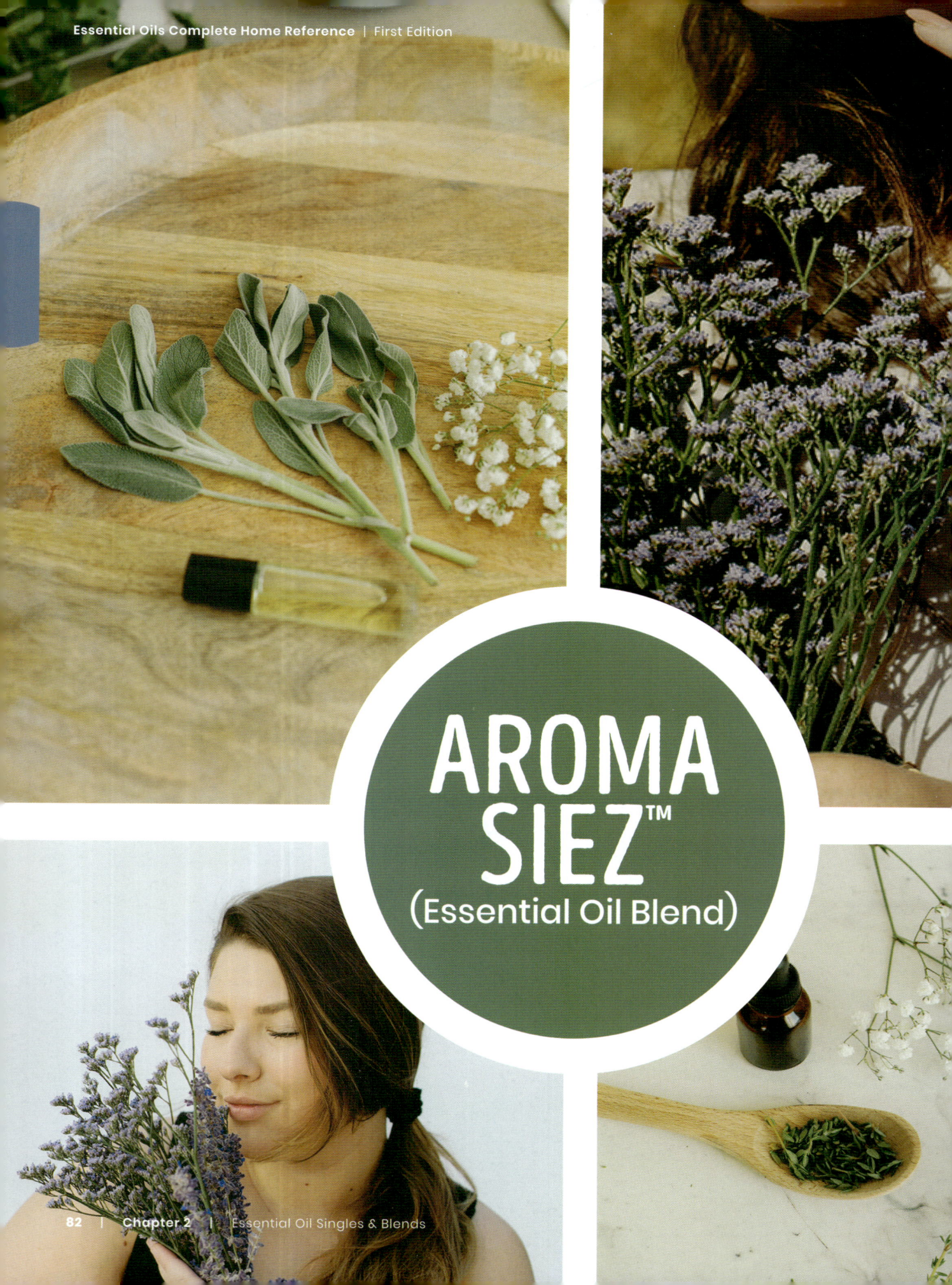

ABOUT AROMA SIEZ:
Aroma Siez is an advanced complex of anti-inflammatory, muscle-relaxing essential oils that promote circulation and relieve headaches and tight, inflamed, aching muscles resulting from injury, fatigue, or stress.

MEDICAL PROPERTIES & USES:
Anti-inflammatory, antimicrobial, calming, digestion or elimination supportive, nausea reducing, organ protective, pain or swelling reducing, muscle relaxing and supportive, performance enhancing/stimulating, circulatory system supportive, skin and hair improving

INGREDIENTS:
Basil, Marjoram, Lavender, Peppermint, Cypress

DIRECTIONS:
Topical: 50-50. Apply on sore muscles, ligaments, locations of poor circulation, or desired location as needed. Use in Raindrop Technique.

CAUTIONS:

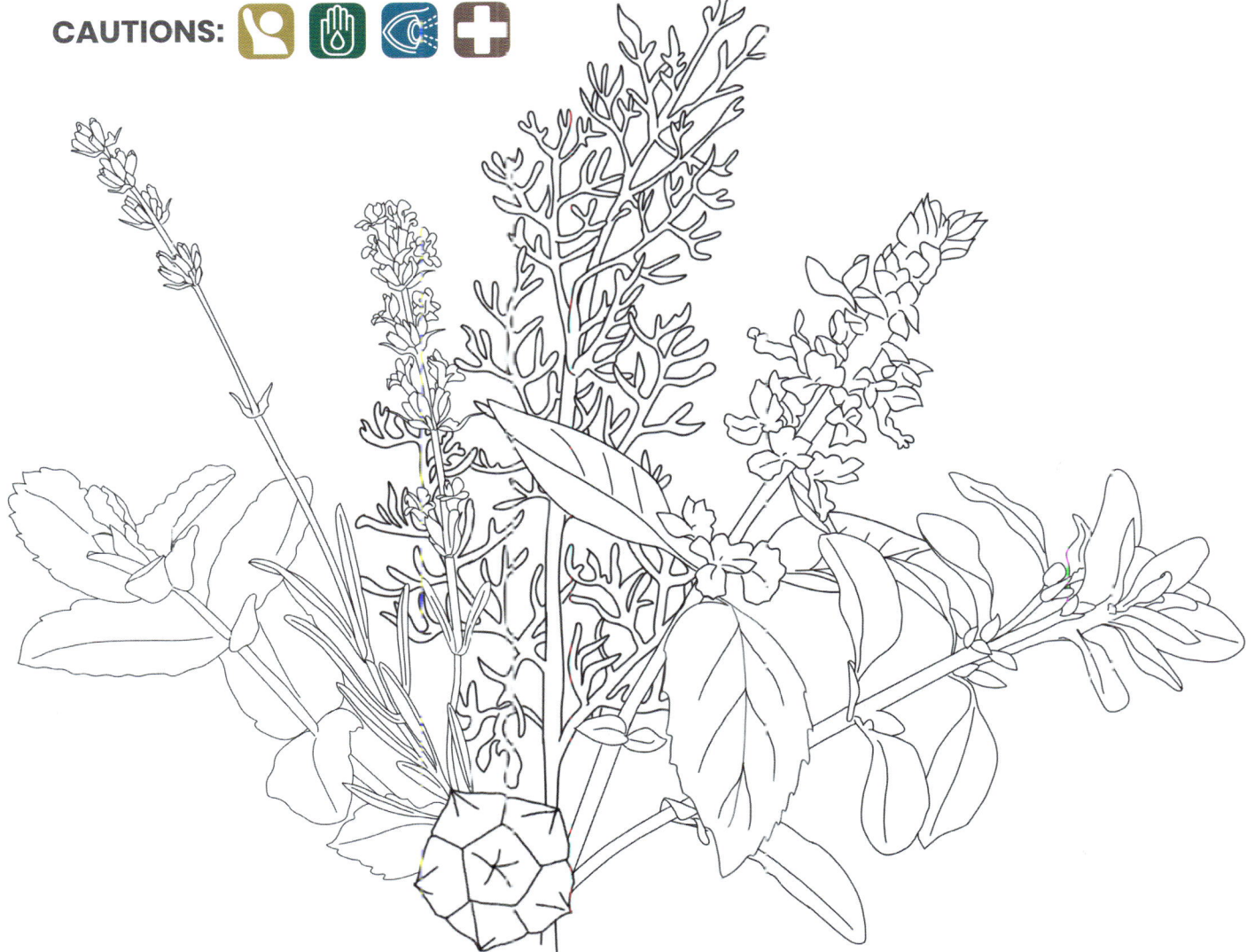

AUSTRALIAN BLUE™
(Essential Oil Blend)

This blend includes a rare Australian aromatic called Blue Cypress, a part of the aboriginal pharmacopoeia for thousands of years. It is distilled from the wood of Callitris intratropica, the northern cypress pine, which has antiviral properties. Its aromatic influence uplifts and inspires while simultaneously grounds and stabilizes.

MEDICAL PROPERTIES & USES:
Anti-inflammatory, antimicrobial, antioxidative, antiviral, calming, cardiovascular supportive, digestion or elimination supportive/nausea reducing, disease inhibitory, insecticidal, organ protective, pain or swelling reducing, skin and hair improving

INGREDIENTS:
Blue Cypress, Ylang Ylang, Cedarwood, White Fir, Geranium, Grapefruit, Tangerine, Spearmint, Davana, Kaffir Lime, Lemon, Ocotea, Jasmine, Matricaria (German Chamomile), Blue Tansy, Rose

DIRECTIONS:
Aromatic: 6o. Topical: Neat.

CAUTIONS:

Essential Oil Singles & Blends | **Chapter 2**

Rare & precious — only from Australia!

BOTANICAL FAMILY:
Myrtaceae

PLANT ORIGIN:
Australia

EXTRACTION METHOD:
Steam distilled from leaves

KEY CONSTITUENTS:
Linalool (30-55%)
Eucalyptol (15-36%)
Alpha-Pinene (3-14%)
Para-Cymene (up to 5%)
Aromadendrene (1-5%)
Limonene (1-5%)
Alpha-Terpineol (2-5%)

AUSTRALIAN ERICIFOLIA
(Melaleuca ericifolia)

The Aboriginal people of Australia used the bark of Melaleuca ericifolia as roofing for their shelters and for blankets and paintings. Oil from the leaves was used for medicine.

MEDICAL PROPERTIES:
Powerful antibacterial, antifungal, antiviral, antiparasitic, anti-inflammatory

USES:
Herpes virus, respiratory/sinus infections, skin irritations, uplifting, improving hair

FRAGRANT INFLUENCE:
Soothing, calming, uplifting

DIRECTIONS:
Aromatic: 6O. Topical: 50-50.

CAUTIONS:

SELECTED RESEARCH:

Abdel Bar FM, Khanfar MA, Elnagar AY, Badria FA, Zaghloul AM, Ahmad KF, Sylvester PW, El Sayed KA. Design and pharmacophore of biaryl methyl eugenol analogs as breast cancer invasion inhibitors. Bioorg Med Chem. 2010 Jan 15;18(2):496-507. Epub 2009 Dec 11.

Abdel Bar FM, Zaghloul AM, Bachawal SV, Sylvester PW, Ahmad KF, El Sayed KA. Antiproliferative triterpenes from Melaleuca ericifolia. J Nat Prod. 2008 Oct;71(10):1787-90. Epub 2008 Oct 1

Abuznait AH, Qosa H, O'Connell ND, Akbarian-Tefaghi J, Sylvester PW, El Sayed KA, Kaddoumi A. Induction of expression and functional activity of P-glycoprotein efflux transporter by bioactive plant natural products. Food Chem Toxicol. 2011 Nov;49(11):2765-72. Epub 2011 Aug 10.

Farag RS, Shalaby AS, El-Baroty GA, Ibrahim NA, Ali MA, Hassan EM. Chemical and biological evaluation of the essential oils of different Melaleuca species. Phytother Res. 2004 Jan;18(1):30-5.

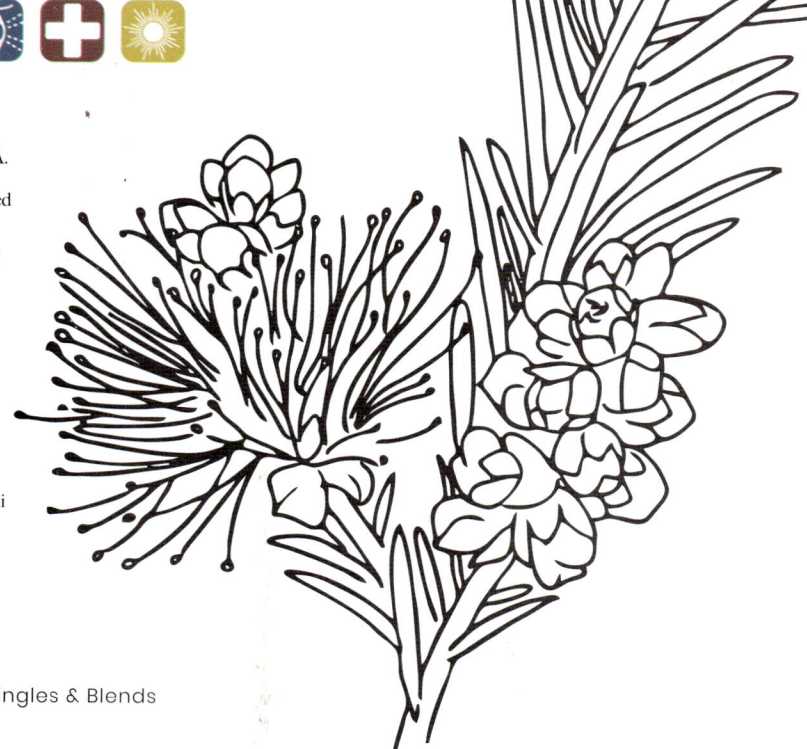

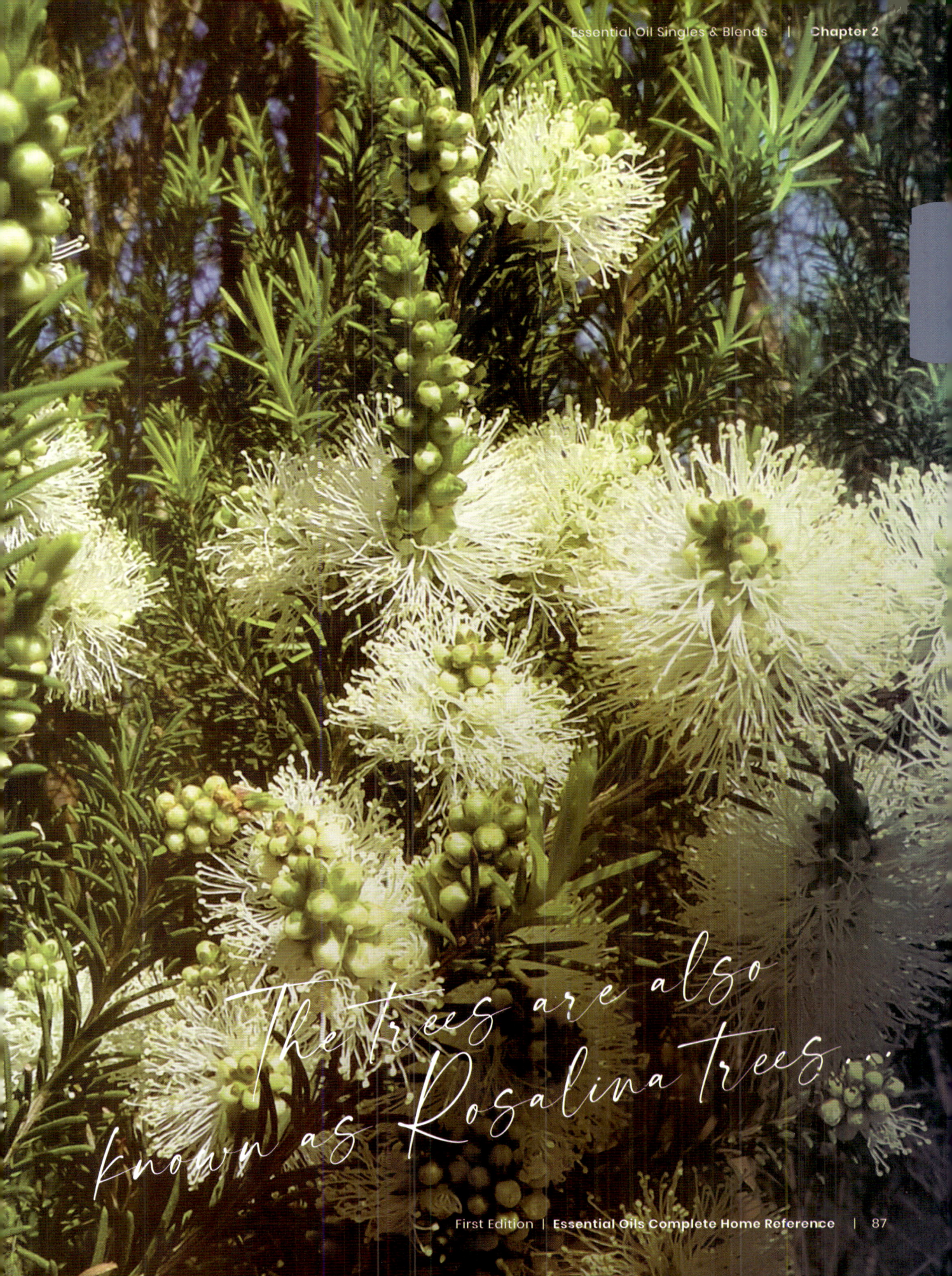

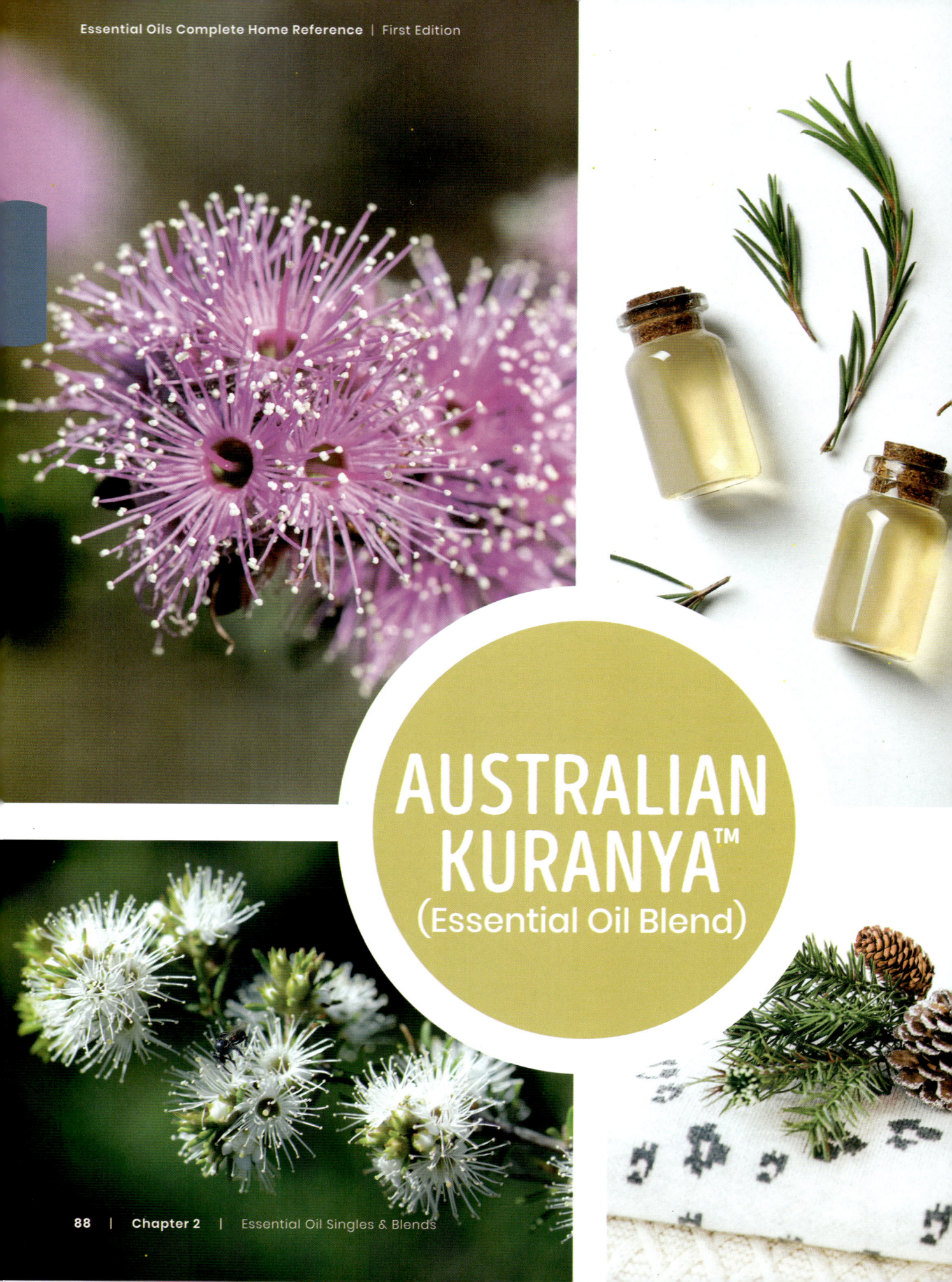

AUSTRALIAN KURANYA™
(Essential Oil Blend)

ABOUT AUSTRALIAN KURANYA:

The legend of a treasure held in a golden pot at the end of the rainbow just came true! Australia is the home to many of the world's most beloved and powerful essential oils. A new blend of essential oils all from Australia is called Kuranya. This is an Australian Aboriginal word meaning "rainbow." Kuranya is truly the treasure at a rainbow's end.

MEDICAL PROPERTIES & USES:

Anti-inflammatory, antimicrobial, antioxidative, calming, cardiovascular supportive, disease inhibitory, insecticidal, muscle relaxant/bone or joint preservative, organ protective, pain or swelling reducing, respiratory system supportive, skin and hair improving

INGREDIENTS:

Lemon Myrtle, Blue Cypress, Kunzea, Sacred Sandalwood, Fennel, Melaleuca Ericifolia, Eucalyptus Radiata, Tea Tree

DIRECTIONS:

Aromatic: 3o. Topical: 5o-5o.

CAUTIONS:

AWAKEN™
(Essential Oil Blend)

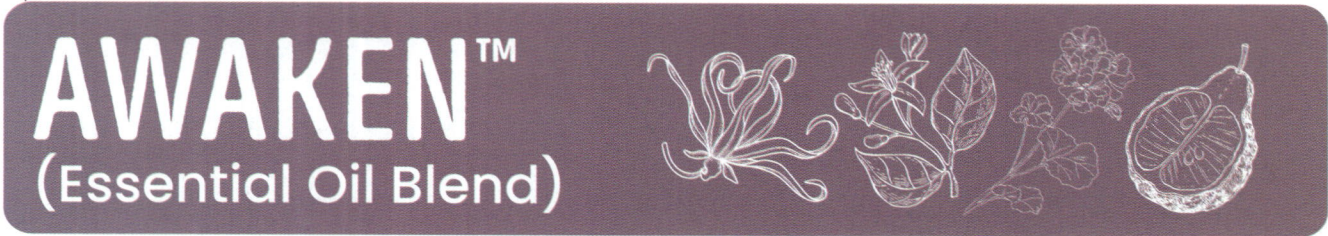

Five specific blends combine to awaken and enhance inner self-awareness that strengthens the desire to reach one's highest potential. It stimulates right brain creativity, amplifying the function of the pineal and pituitary glands in balancing the energy centers of the body and helps us identify our true desires and how best to pursue them.

MEDICAL PROPERTIES & USES:
Anti-inflammatory, antimicrobial, antioxidative, anti-allergy, calming, cardiovascular supportive, digestion or elimination supportive/nausea reducing, disease inhibitory, insecticidal, organ protective, pain or swelling reducing, skin and hair improving

INGREDIENTS:
Caprylic/capric triglyceride (Coconut), Sweet almond oil, Bergamot (Furocoumarin-free), Ylang Ylang, Sesame seed oil, Geranium, Royal Hawaiian Sandalwood, Neroli (Bitter Orange), Tangerine, Lemon, Coriander, Black Pepper, Frankincense, Melissa, Lavender, Jasmine, Roman Chamomile, Lemongrass, Hyssop, Helichrysum, Blue Cypress, Davana, Lime, Rose, German Chamomile, Blue Tansy, Ocotea, Grapefruit, Spearmint

DIRECTIONS:
Aromatic: 6o. Topical: Neat. For clearing allergies, rub over sternum.

CAUTIONS:

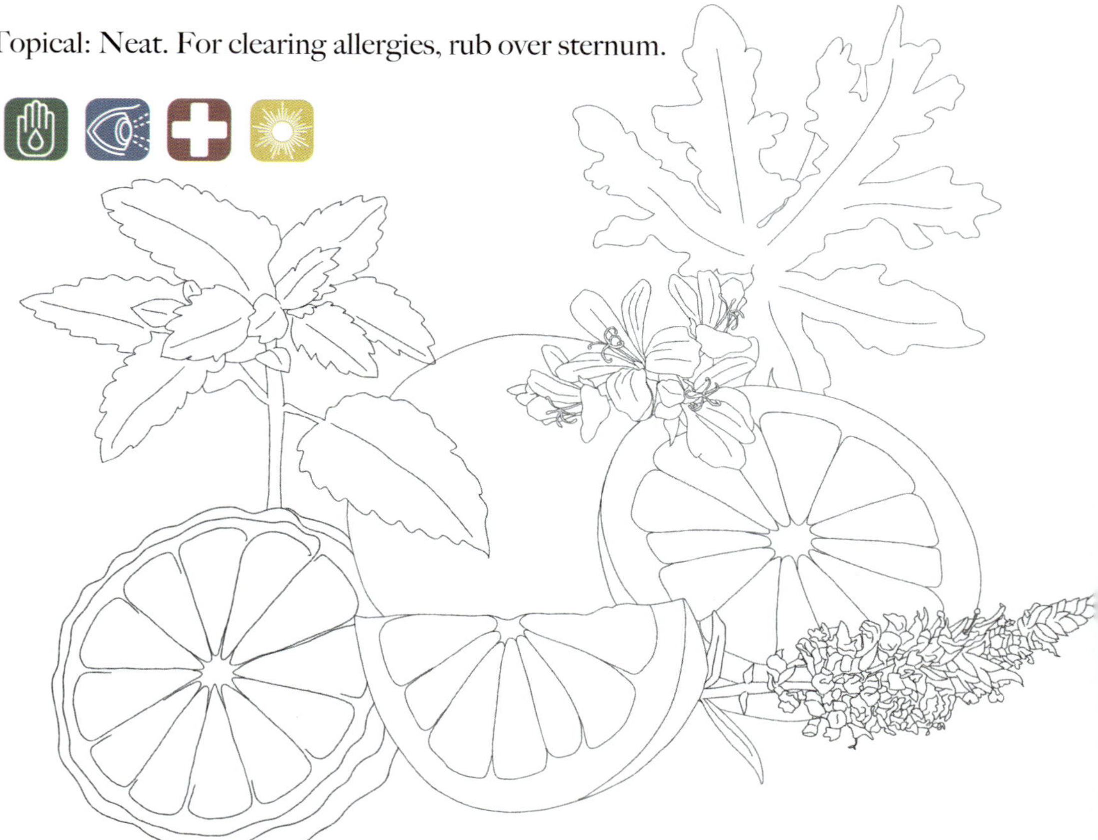

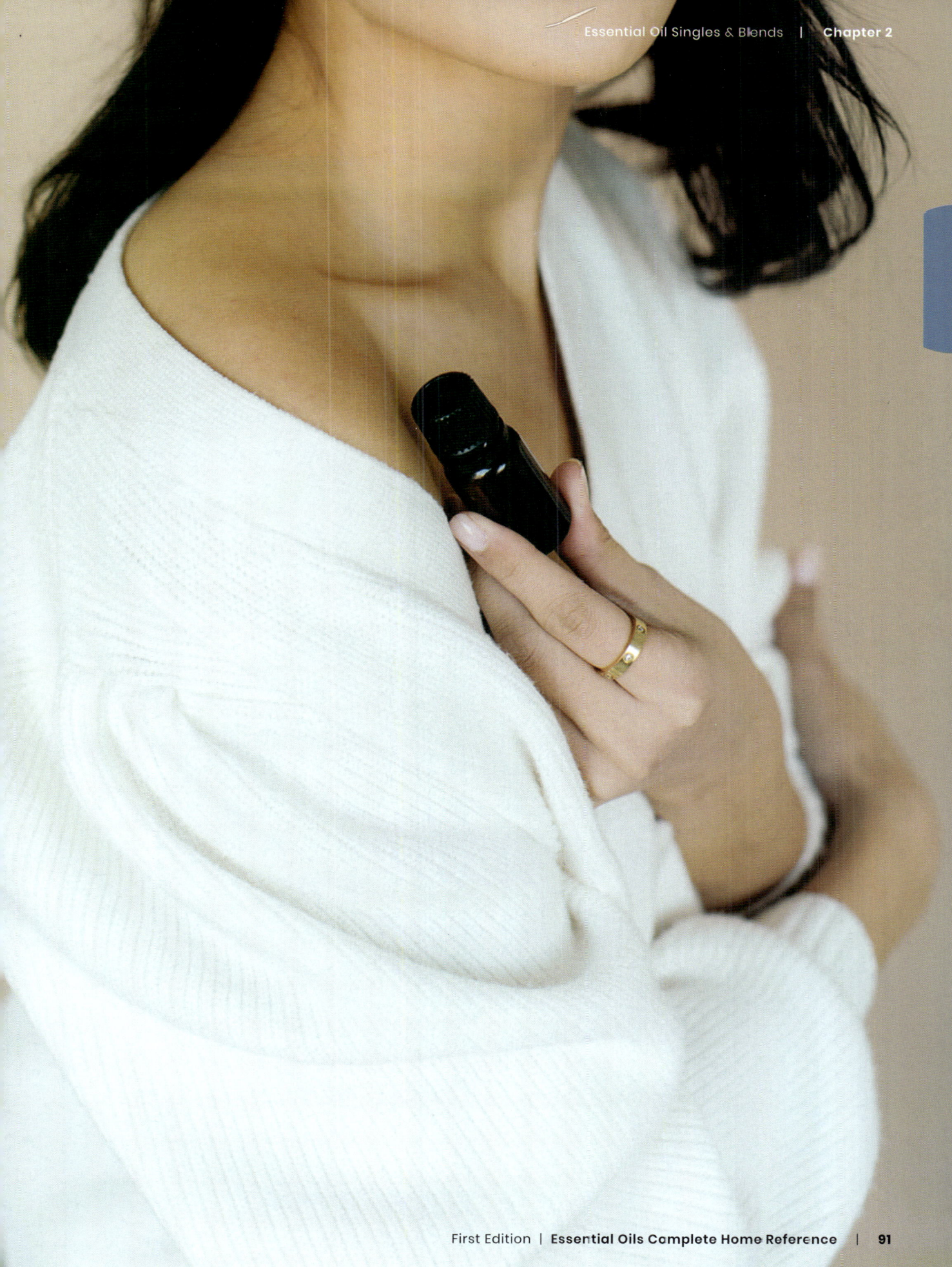

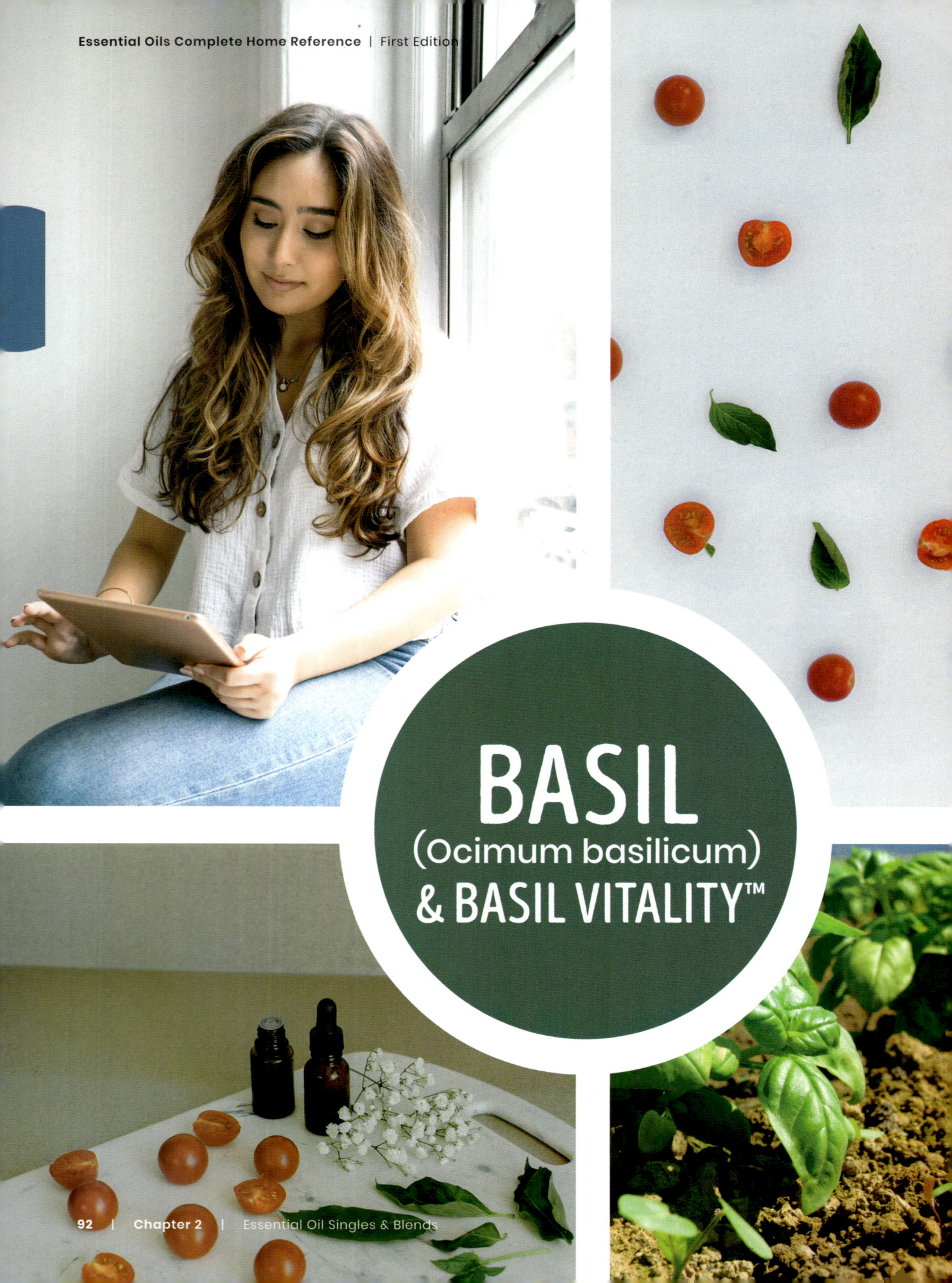

BASIL (Ocimum basilicum) & BASIL VITALITY™

Essential Oil Sigles & Blends | Chapter 2

BOTANICAL FAMILY:
Lamiaceae

PLANT ORIGIN:
Vietnam

EXTRACTION METHOD:
Steam distilled from herb/leaf

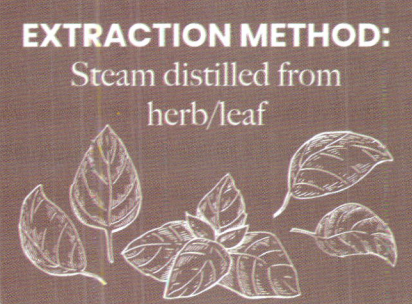

KEY CONSTITUENTS:
Methyl Chavicol (75-88%)
Linalool (up to 5%)
Eucalyptol (1-5%)
Trans-Beta-Ocimene (up to 3%)
Methyl Eugenol (up to 3%)
Camphor (up to 1%)

HISTORICAL DATA:
Used extensively in traditional Asian Indian medicine, basil's name is derived from "basileum," the Greek name for king. In the 16th century, the powdered leaves were inhaled to treat migraines and chest infections. The Hindu people put basil sprigs on the chests of the dead to protect them from evil spirits. Italian women wore basil to attract possible suitors. It was listed in Hildegard's Medicine, a compilation of early German medicines by highly regarded Benedictine herbalist Hildegard of Bingen (1098-1179).

MEDICAL PROPERTIES:
Powerful antispasmodic, antiviral, antibacterial, anti-inflammatory, muscle relaxant

USES:
Migraines, throat/lung infections, insect bites

FRAGRANT INFLUENCE:
Fights mental fatigue

DIRECTIONS:
Aromatic: 30. Topical: 50-50. Apply around ear for earache.
Use in Raindrop Technique. Dietary (Vitality): Dilute 1 drop with 4 drops of carrier oil. Put in a capsule and take 1 daily.

CAUTIONS:

SELECTED RESEARCH:

Hirai M, Ito M. Sedative effects of the essential oil and headspace air of Ocimum basilicum by inhalation in mice. J Nat Med. 2019 Jan;73(1):283-288.

Kavoosi G, Amirghofran Z. Chemical composition, radical scavenging and antioxidant capacity of Ocimum basilicum essential oil. Journal of Essential Oil Research. 2017;29(2):189-199.

Basil (Ocimum basilicum L.) essential oil. Journal of Essential Oil Bearing Plants. 2017 Nov 02;20(6):1557-1569. Epub 2018 Jan 17.

Snoussi M, Dehmani A, Noumi E, Flamini G, Papetti A. Chemical composition and antibiofilm activity of Petroselinum crispum and Ocimum basilicum essential oils against Vibrio spp. strains. Microb Pathog. 2016 Jan;90:13-21. Epub 2015 Nov 16.

Ogaly HA, Eltablawy NA, El-Behairy AM, El-Hindi H, Abd-Elsalam RM. Hepatocyte growth factor mediates the antifibrogenic action of Ocimum basilicum essential oil against CCl4-induced liver fibrosis in rats. Molecules. 2015 Jul 23;20(8):13518-35.

Shirazi MT, Gholami H, Kavoosi G, Rowshan V, Tafsiry A. Chemical composition, antioxidant, antimicrobial and cytotoxic activities of Tagetes minuta and Ocimum basilicum essential oils. Food Sci & Nutr. 2014 Mar;2(2):146-55. Epub 2014 Jan 16.

Siddiqui BS, Bhatti HA, Begum S, Perwaiz S. Evaluation of the antimycobacterium activity of the constituents from Ocimum basilicum against Mycobacterium tuberculosis. J Ethnopharmacol. 2012 Oct 31;144(1):220-2. Epub 2012 Aug 17.

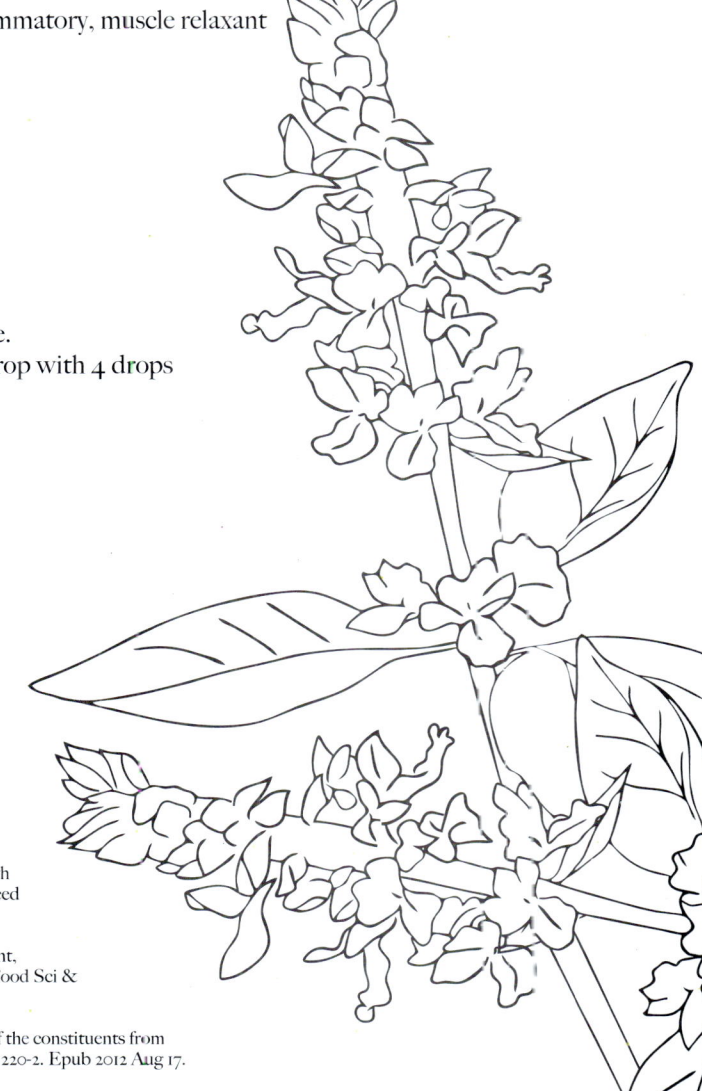

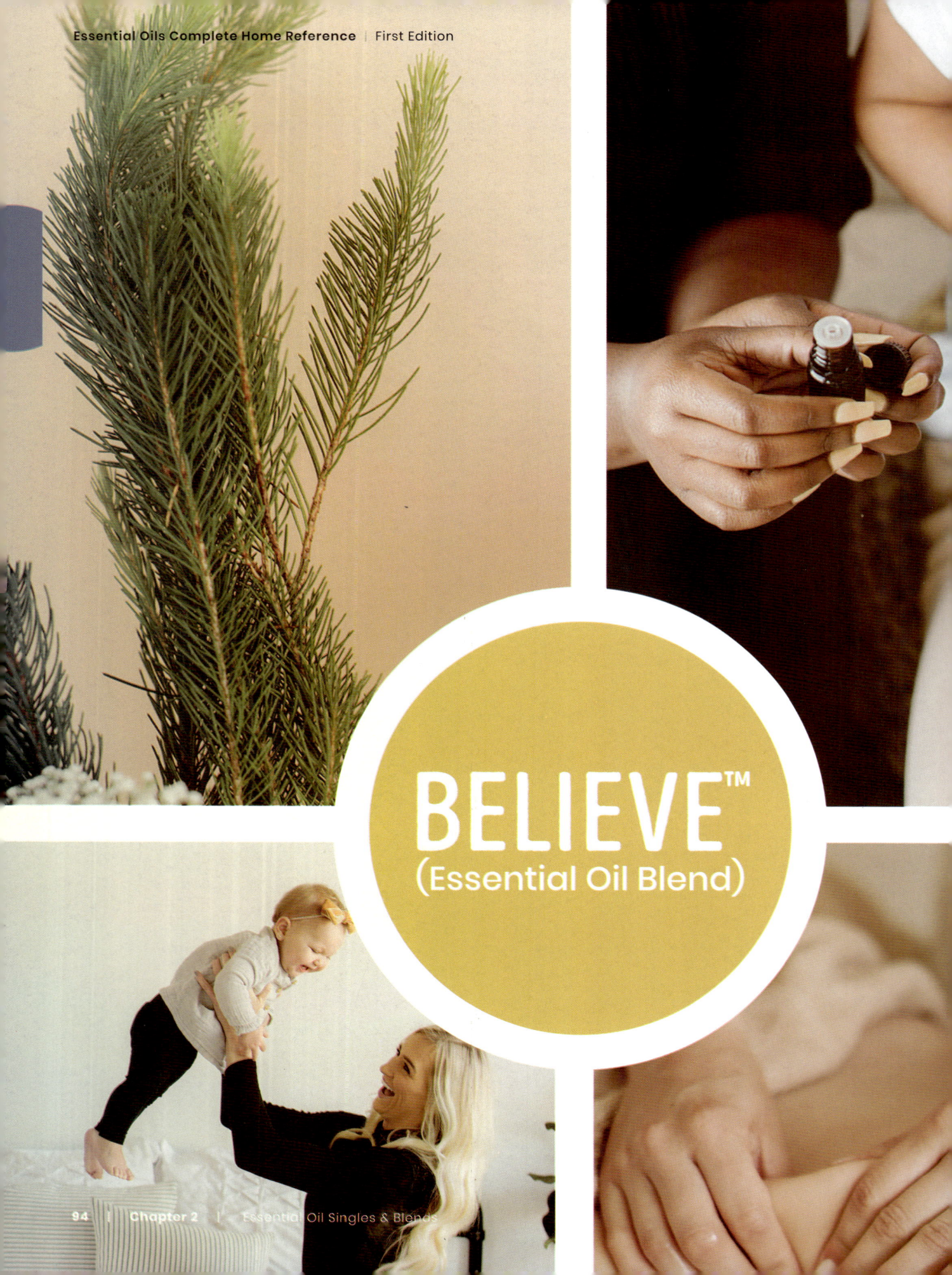

Essential Oils Complete Home Reference | First Edition

BELIEVE™
(Essential Oil Blend)

94 | Chapter 2 | Essential Oil Singles & Blends

ABOUT BELIEVE:

Believe helps release the unlimited potential everyone possesses. It restores feelings of hope, making it possible to more fully experience health, happiness, and vitality.

MEDICAL PROPERTIES & USES:
Anti-inflammatory, antimicrobial, antioxidative, emotion supportive, calming, uplifting, disease inhibitory, insecticidal, organ protective, pain reducing, skin and hair improving

INGREDIENTS:
Idaho Grand Fir, Coriander, Bergamot (Furocoumarin-free), Frankincense, Idaho Blue Spruce, Ylang Ylang, Geranium

DIRECTIONS:
Aromatic: 6o. Topical: Neat.

CAUTIONS:

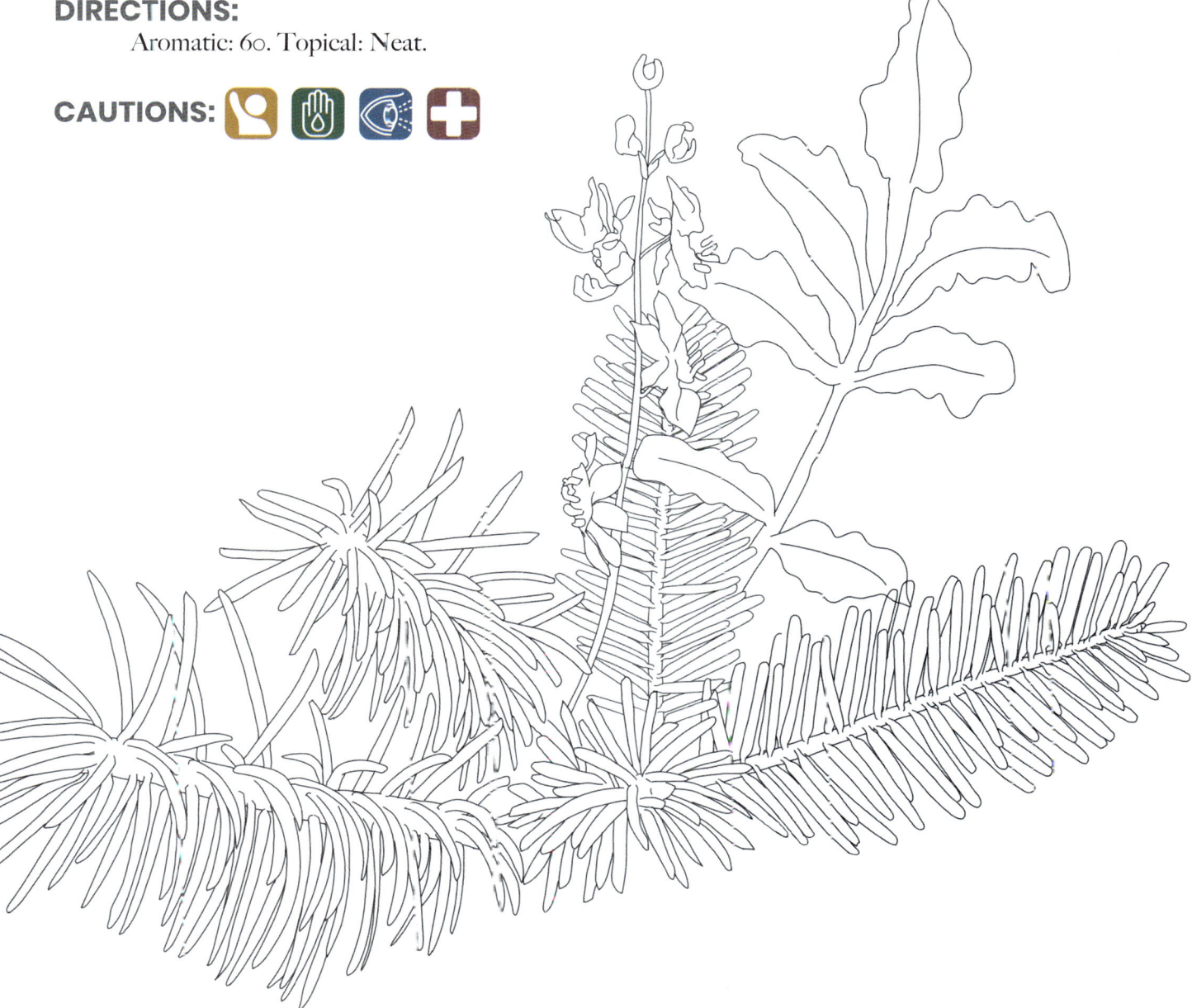

BOTANICAL FAMILY:
Rutaceae

PLANT ORIGIN:
Italy

EXTRACTION METHOD:
Pressed from the peel of the fruit. Furocoumarin-free bergamot oil is specially distilled to minimize the concentration of sun-sensitizing compounds in the oil.

KEY CONSTITUENTS:
Limonene (30-45%), Linalyl Acetate (22-36%), Linalool (3-15%), Gamma-Terpinene (6-10%), Beta-Pinene (5-10%)

BERGAMOT & BERGAMOT VITALITY™
(Citrus aurantium bergamia)

Christopher Columbus is believed to have brought bergamot to Bergamo in Northern Italy from the Canary Islands. A mainstay in traditional Italian medicine, bergamot has been used in the Middle East for hundreds of years for skin conditions associated with an oily complexion. Bergamot is responsible for the distinctive flavor of the renowned Earl Grey Tea and was used in the first genuine eau de cologne.

MEDICAL PROPERTIES:
Calming, antimicrobial, anti-inflammatory, some anticancer efficacy, antinociceptive, neuroprotective, antifungal, antibacterial, hormonal support, antidepressant

USES:
Reduces stress, cleansing and purifying, skin cleansing, may reduce the appearance of blemishes, agitation, depression, anxiety, intestinal parasites, insomnia, viral infections (herpes, cold sores)

FRAGRANT INFLUENCE:
Citrus aroma with a hint of floral, relieves anxiety, mood-lifting qualities

DIRECTIONS:
60. Topical: 50-50. Dietary (Vitality): Dilute 1 drop with a drop of carrier oil. Put in a capsule and take up to 3 times daily.

CAUTIONS:

SELECTED RESEARCH:

Lombardo GE, Cirmi S, Musumeci L, Pergolizzi S, Maugeri A, Russo C, Mannucci C, Calapai G, Navarra M. Mechanisms Underlying the Anti-Inflammatory Activity of Bergamot Essential Oil and Its Antinociceptive Effects. Plants (Basel) 2020 Jun; 9(6): 704.

Parafati M, Lascala A, La Russa D, Mignogna C, Trimboli F, Morittu VM, Riillo C, Macirella R, Mollace V, Brunelli E, Janda E. Bergamot polyphenols boost therapeutic effects of the diet on non-alcoholic steatohepatitis (NASH) induced by "junk food": evidence for anti-inflammatory activity. Nutrients. 2018 Nov 1;10(11).

Han X, Gibson J, Eggett DL, Parker TL. Bergamot (Citrus bergamia) essential oil inhalation improves positive feelings in the waiting room of a mental health treatment center: a pilot study. Phytother Res. 2017 May;31(5):812-816. Epub 2017 Mar 24.

Rombolà L, Amantea D, Russo D, Adornetto A, Berliocchi L, Tridico L, Corasaniti MT, Sakurada S, Sakurada T, Bagetta G, Morrone LA. Rational basis for the use of bergamot essential oil in complementary medicine to treat chronic pain. Mini Rev Med Chem. 2016;16(9):721-8. Toth PP, Patti AM, Nikolic D, Giglio RV, Castellino G, Biancucci T, Geraci F, David S, Montalto G, Rizvi A, Rizzo M. Bergamot reduces plasma lipids, atherogenic small dense LDL, and subclinical atherosclerosis in subjects with moderate hypercholesterolemia: a 6 months prospective study. Front Pharmacol. 2016 Jan 6;6:299. eCollection 2015.

Watanabe E, Kuchta K, Kimura M, Rauwald HW, Kamei T, Imanishi J. Effects of bergamot (Citrus bergamia (Risso) Wright & Arn.) essential oil aromatherapy on mood states, parasympathetic nervous system activity, and salivary cortisol levels in 41 healthy females. Forsch Komplementmed. 2015;22(1):43-9. Epub 2015 Apr 01.

Cosentino M, Luini A, Bombelli R, Corasaniti MT, Bagetta G, Marino F. The essential oil of bergamot stimulates reactive oxygen species production in human polymorphonuclear leukocytes. Phytother Res. 2014 Aug;28(8):1232-9.

Saiyudthong S, Marsden CA. Acute effects of bergamot oil on anxiety-related behaviour and corticosterone level in rats. Phytother Res. 2011 Jun;25(6):858-62. Epub 2010 Nov 23.

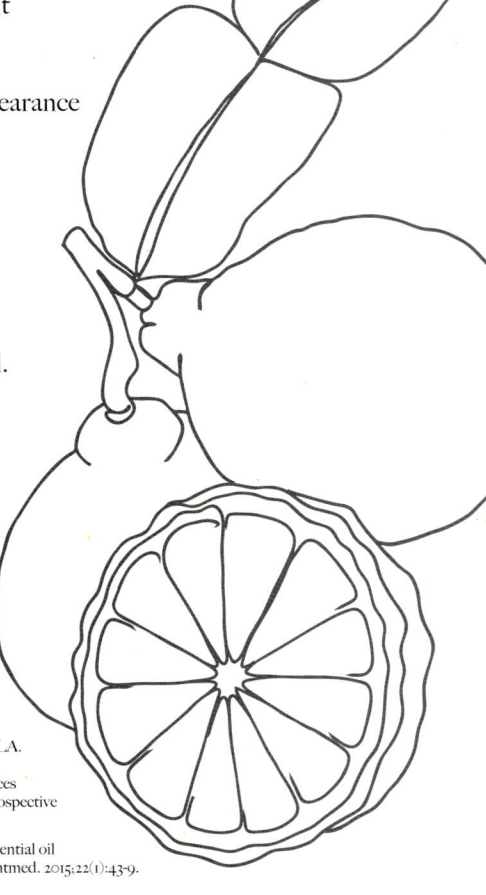

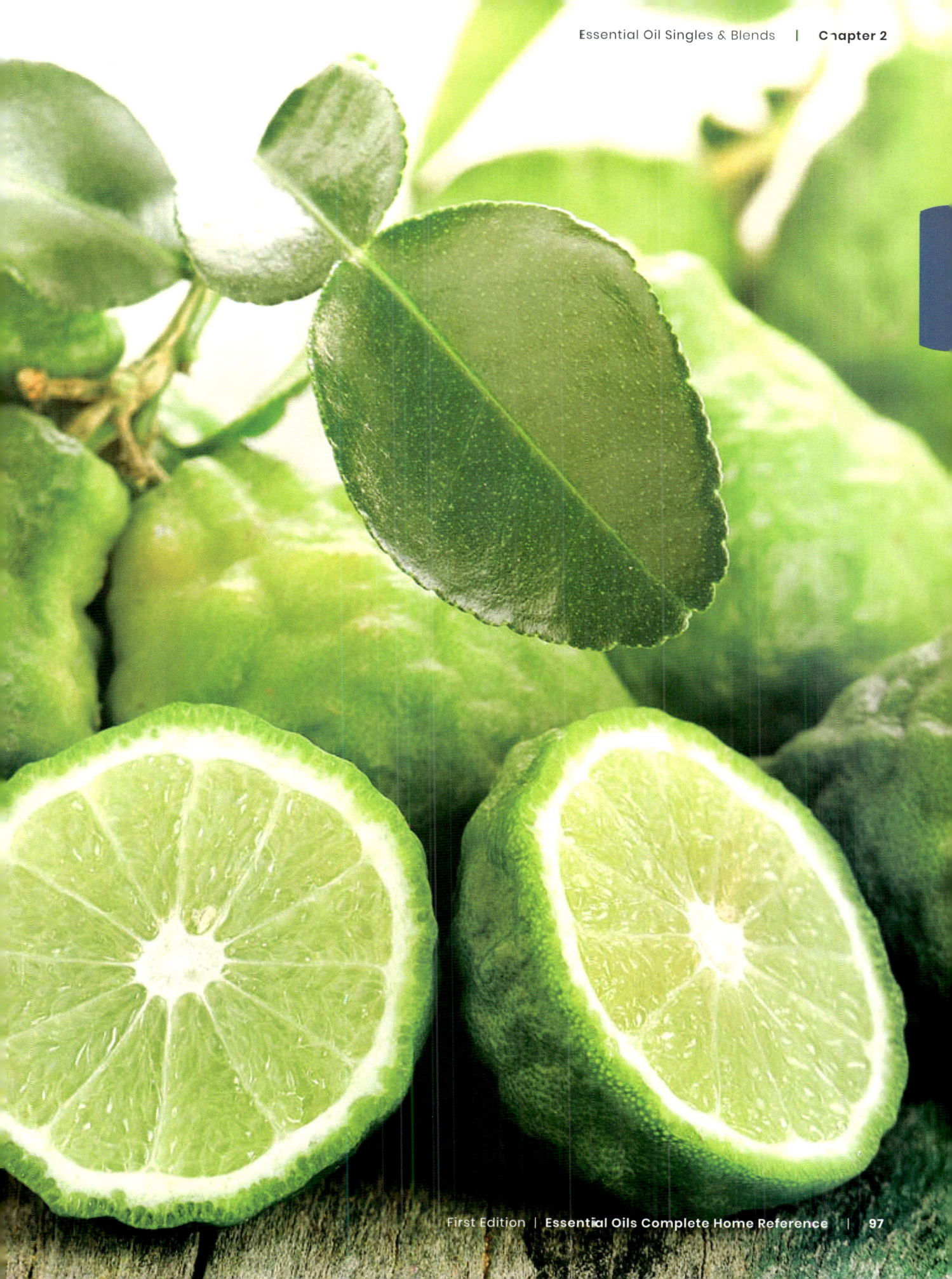

BOTANICAL FAMILY:
Burseraceae

PLANT ORIGIN:
Socotra Island, Yemen

EXTRACTION METHOD:
Steam distilled from resin

KEY CONSTITUENTS:
Trans-Beta-Ocimene (45-65%)
Cis-Alpha-Bisabolene (10-15%)
Alpha-Santalene (12-20%)
Trans-Alpha-Bergamotene (3-8%)
Cis-Alpha-Bergamotene (1-4%)

BIBLICAL SWEET MYRRH
(Commiphora erythraea)

A close cousin to the more well-known Commiphora myrrha, Biblical Sweet Myrrh is also called Opoponax. Used in dozens of perfumes to impart sweet balsamic notes, this myrrh species is found in Chanel's Coco Mademoiselle and Dior's Poison. Biblical Sweet Myrrh comes from myrrh resin gathered on the island of Socotra, off the coast of Yemen, and is distilled at the Young Living Arabian Frankincense Distillery in Muscat, Oman. Like other frankincense species, it is highly anti-inflammatory, antimicrobial, and antioxidative.

MEDICAL PROPERTIES:
Analgesic, antioxidant, anti-inflammatory, antimicrobial, antifungal, antiviral

USES:
Arthritis, digestive problems, nerve/muscle pain, fungal infections

FRAGRANT INFLUENCE:
Promotes spiritual awareness and is uplifting. It contains sesquiterpenes, which stimulate the limbic system of the brain (the center of memory and emotions) and the hypothalamus, pineal, and pituitary glands. The hypothalamus is the master gland of the human body, producing many vital hormones, including thyroid and growth hormone.

DIRECTIONS:
Aromatic: 3o. Topical: 50-50

CAUTIONS:

SELECTED RESEARCH:

Bellezza I, Mierla A, Grottelli S, Marcotullio MC, Messina F, Roscini L, Cardinali G, Curini M, Minelli A. Furanodien-6-one from Commiphora erythraea inhibits the NF-kB signaling and attenuates LPS-induced neuroinflammation. Mol Immunol. 2013 Jul;54(3-4):347-54. Epub 2013 Jan 26.

Cai T, Tiscione D, Cocci A, Puglisi M, Cito G, Malossini G, Palmieri A. Hibiscus extract, vegetable proteases and Commiphora myrrha are useful to prevent symptomatic UTI episode in patients affected by recurrent uncomplicated urinary tract infections. Arch Ital Urol Androl. 2018 Sep 30;90(3):203-207.

Cenci E, Messina F, Rossi E, Epifano F, Marcotullio MC. Antiviral furanosesquiterpenes from Commiphora erythraea. Nat Prod Commun. 2012 Feb;7(2):143-4.

Fraternale D, Sosa S, Ricci D, Genovese S, Messina F, Tomasini S, Montanari F, Marcotullio MC. Anti-inflammatory, antioxidant and antifungal furanosesquiterpenoids isolated from Commiphora erythraea (Ehrenb.) Engl. resin. Fitoterapia. 2011 Jun;82(4):654-61. Epub 2011 Feb 21.

Marcotullio MC, Messina F, Curini M, Macchiarulo A, Cellanetti M, Ricci D, Giamperi L, Bucchini A, Minelli A, Mierla AL, Bellezza I. Protective effects of Commiphora erythraea resin constituents against cellular oxidative damage. Molecules. 2011 Dec 14;16(12):10357-69.

Santoro S, Superchi S, Messina F, Santoro E, Rosati O, Santi C, Marcotullio MC. Agarsenone, a cadinane sesquiterpenoid from Commiphora erythraea. J Nat Prod. 2013 Jul 26;76(7):1254-9. Epub 2013 Jul 11.

Shen T, Li GH, Wang XN, Lou HX. The genus Commiphora: a review of its traditional uses, phytochemistry and pharmacology. J Ethnopharmacol. 2012 Jul 13;142(2):319-30. Epub 2012 May 21.

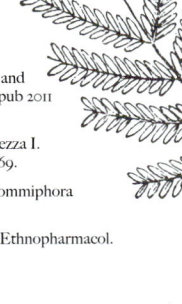

Essential Oil Singles & Blends | **Chapter 2**

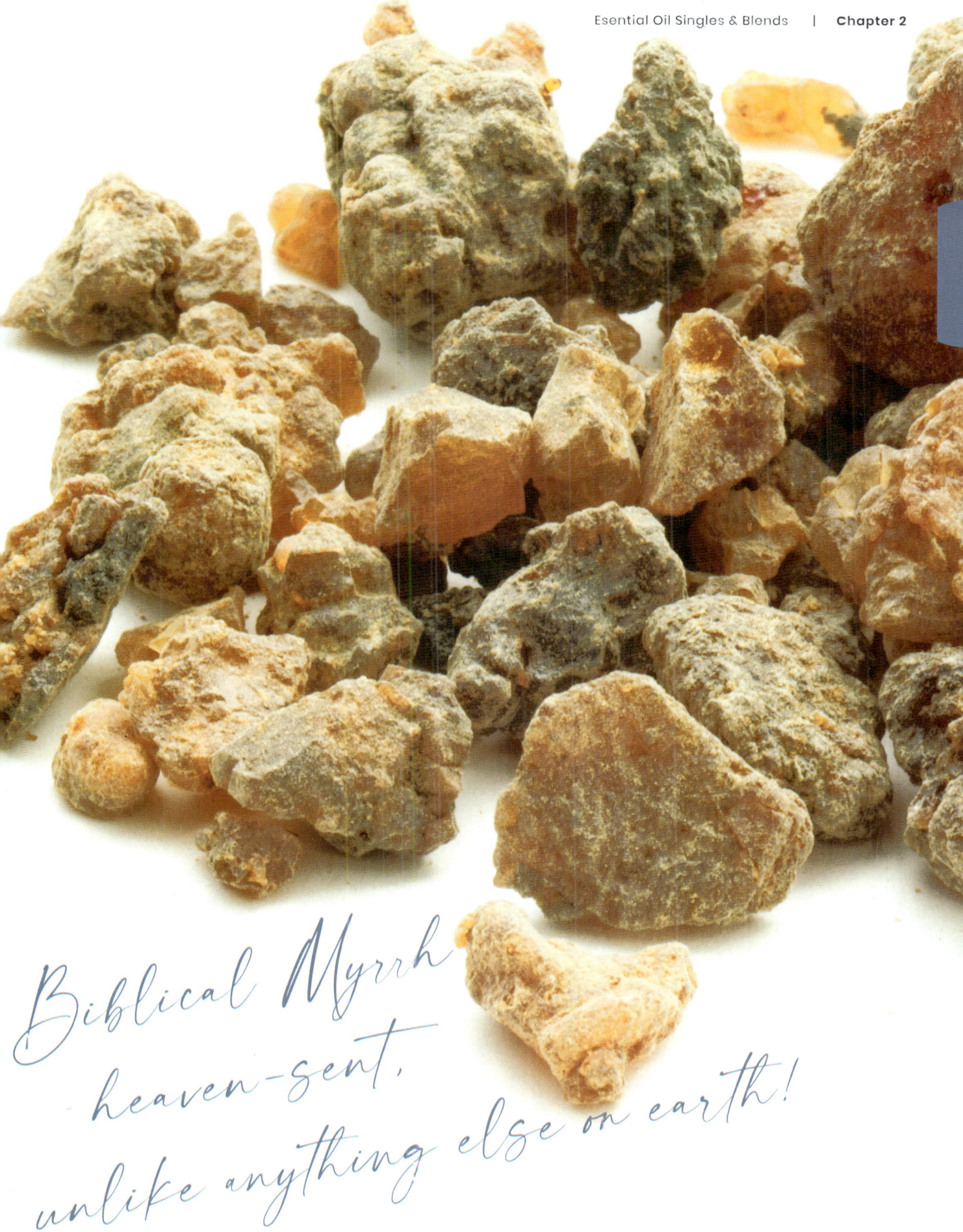

Biblical Myrrh heaven-sent, unlike anything else on earth!

First Edition | **Essential Oils Complete Home Reference** | 99

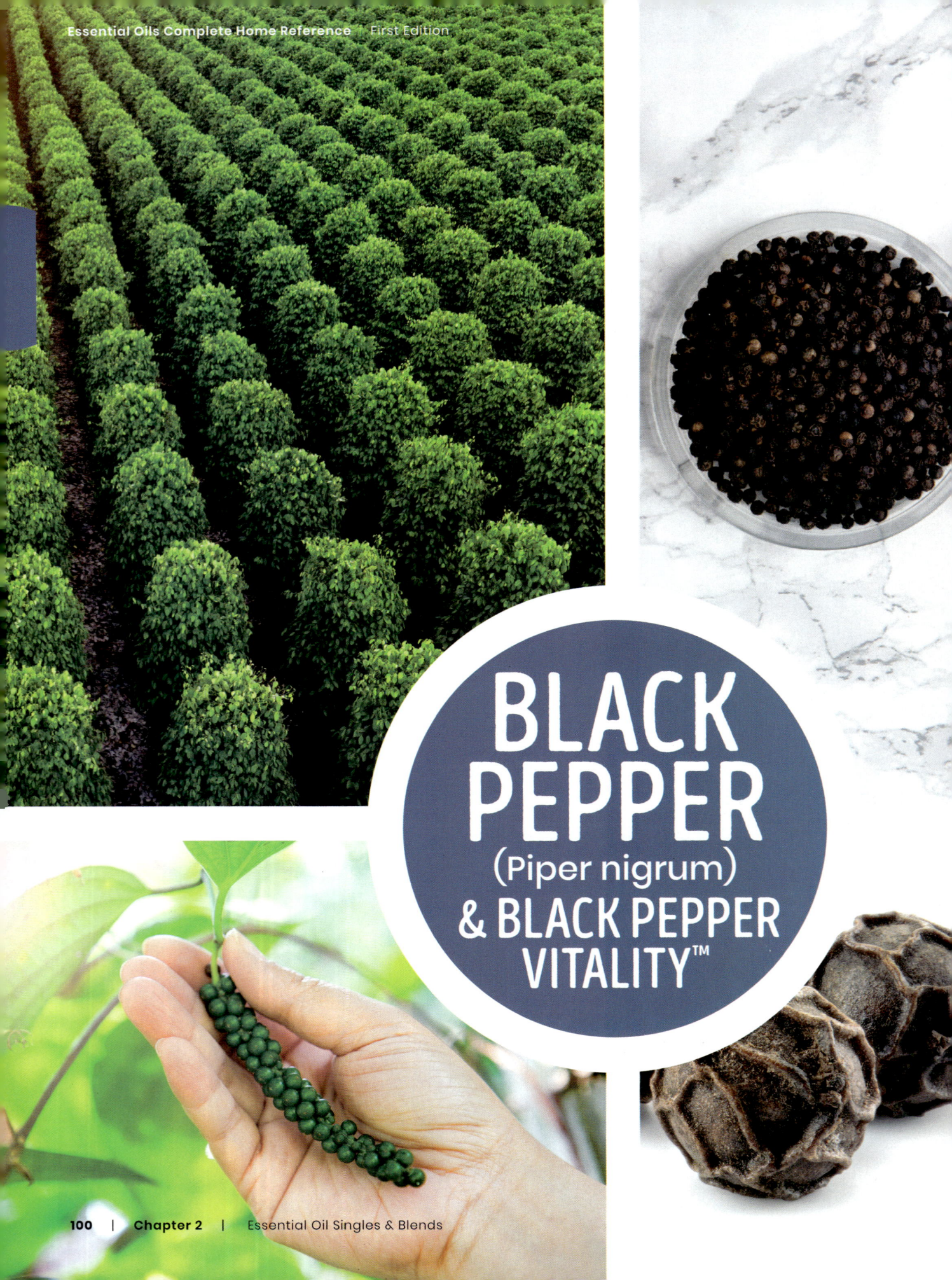

BLACK PEPPER
(Piper nigrum)
& BLACK PEPPER VITALITY™

Essential Oil Singles & Blends | Chapter 2

BOTANICAL FAMILY:
Piperaceae

PLANT ORIGIN:
Indonesia, Madagascar

EXTRACTION METHOD:
Steam distilled from fruit/berries

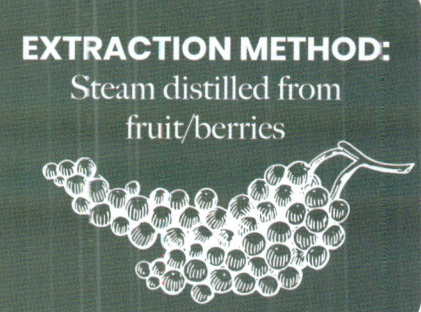

KEY CONSTITUENTS:
Beta-Caryophyllene (10-40%), Alpha-Pinene (2-26%), Limonene (7-25%), Delta-3-Carene (3-20%), Sabinene (up to 17%), Beta-Pinene (up to 15%), Germacrene (up to 7%), Delta-Elemene (up to 5%), Alpha-Copaene (up to 5%), up to Beta-Selinene (up to 5%), Alpha-Selinene (up to 4%)

HISTORICAL DATA:
Black Pepper was used by the Egyptians in mummification, as evidenced by the discovery of black pepper in the nostrils and abdomen of Ramses II. Indian monks ate several black peppercorns a day to give them endurance during their arduous travels. In ancient times, pepper was as valuable as gold or silver. When the barbarian Goth tribes of Europe vanquished Rome in 410 AD, they demanded 3,000 pounds of pepper as well as other valuables as a ransom. Traditional Chinese healers used pepper to treat cholera, malaria, and digestive problems.

MEDICAL PROPERTIES:
Analgesic, antifungal, antimicrobial, insecticidal, antioxidant

USES:
Obesity, arthritis, digestive problems, fatigue, nerve/muscle pain, fungal infections, tobacco cessation

FRAGRANT INFLUENCE:
Stimulating, energizing, and empowering. A 2002 study found that fragrance inhalation of pepper oil induced a 1.7-fold increase in plasma adrenaline concentration (Haze, et al.).

DIRECTIONS:
Aromatic: 30. Topical: 50-50. Dietary (Vitality): Dilute 1 drop with a drop of carrier oil. Put in a capsule and take up to 3 times daily. Use in cooking as desired.

CAUTIONS:

SELECTED RESEARCH:
Leja K, Majcher M, Juzwa W, Czaczyk K, Komosa M. Comparative Evaluation of piper nigrum, Rosmarinus officinalis, Cymbopogon citratus and Junperus communis l. Essential Oils of Different Origin as Functional Antimicrobials in Foods. Foods. 2020 Feb; 9(2): 141. Published online 2020 Jan. 31.

Han X, Beaumont C, Rodriguez D, Bahr T. Black pepper (Piper nigrum) essential oil demonstrates tissue remodeling and metabolism modulating potential in human cells. Phytother Res. 2018 Sept;32(9):1848-1852. Epub 2018 May 18.

Chavarria D, Silva T, Magalhães e Silva D, Remião F, Borges F. Lessons from black pepper: piperine and derivatives thereof. Expert Opin Ther Pat. 2016;26(2):245-64. Epub 2015 Nov 13.

Cordell B, Buckle J. The effects of aromatherapy on nicotine craving on a U.S. campus: a small comparison study. J Altern Complement Med. 2013 Aug;19(8):709-13. Epub 2013 Mar 30.

Haze S, Sakai K, Gozu Y. Effects of fragrance inhalation on sympathetic activity in normal adults. Jpn J Pharmacol. 2002 Nov;90(3):247-53. Epub 2002 Dec 25.

Kapoor IPS, Singh B, Singh G, De Heluani CS, De Lampasona MP, Catalan CAN. Chemistry and in vitro antioxidant activity of volatile oil and oleoresins of black pepper (Piper nigrum). J Agric Food Chem. 2009 Jun 24;57(12):5358-64.

Kristiniak S, Harpel J, Breckenridge DM, Buckle J. Black pepper essential oil to enhance intravenous catheter insertion in patients with poor vein visibility: a controlled study. J Altern Complement Med. 2012 Nov;18(11):1003-7.

Majdalawieh AF, Carr RI. In vitro investigation of the potential immunomodulatory and anti-cancer activities of black pepper (Piper nigrum) and cardamom (Elettaria cardamomum). J Med Food. 2010 Apr;13(2):371-381. Epub 2010 Mar 10.

Morsy NSF, Abd El-Salam EA. Antimicrobial and antiproliferative activites of black pepper (Piper nigrum L.) essential oil and oleoresin. Journal of Essential Oil Bearing Plants. 2017 May 04;20(3):779-790.

Vijayakumar RS, Surya D. Nalini N. Antioxidant efficacy of black pepper (Piper nigrum L.) and piperine in rats with high fat diet induced oxidative stress. Redox Rep:9(2):105-110. Epub 2004 July 03.

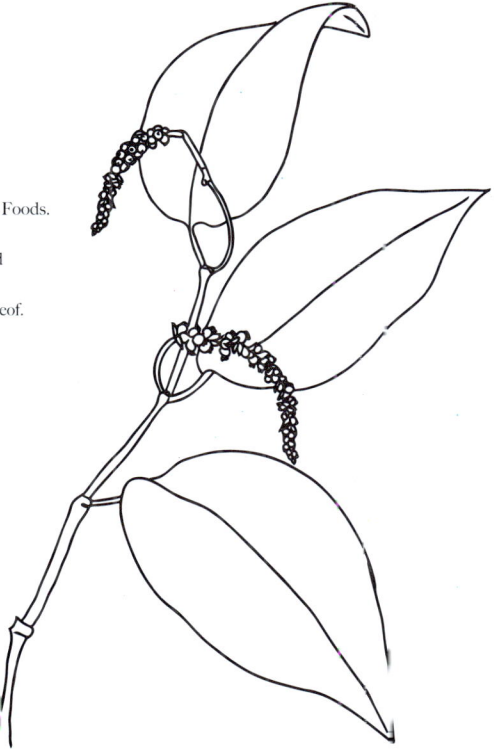

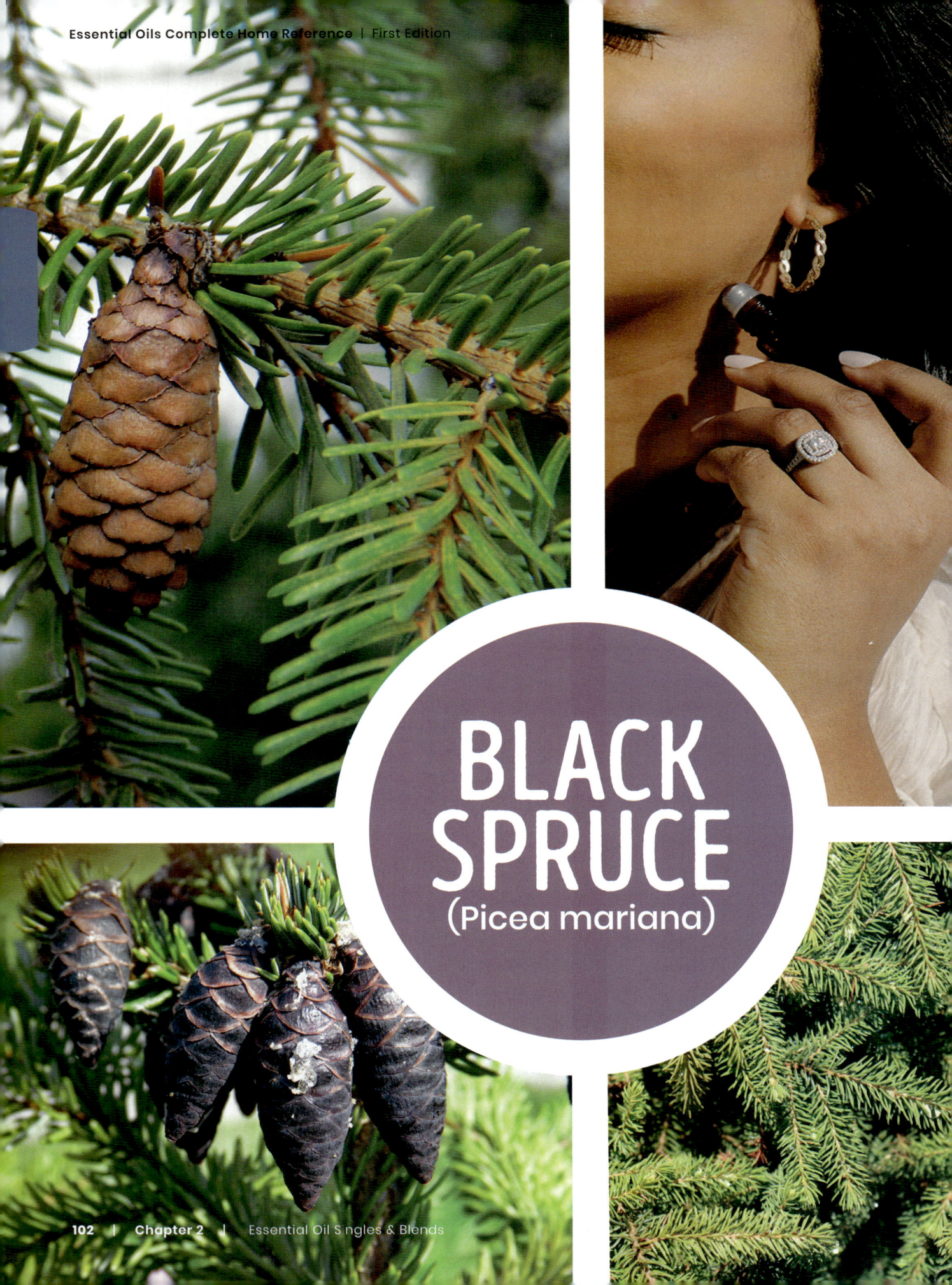

BOTANICAL FAMILY: Pinaceae

PLANT ORIGIN: Canada

EXTRACTION METHOD: Steam distilled from branches, needles, and twigs

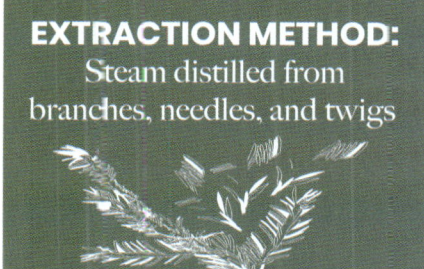

KEY CONSTITUENTS: Bornyl Acetate (13-39%), Camphene (10-28%), Alpha-Pinene (11-21%), Delta-3-Carene (3-13%), Beta-Pinene (up to 11%), Limonene (1-7%), Santene (1-6%), Myrcene (2-6%), Tricyclene (1-4%)

HISTORICAL DATA:
The Lakota Indians used black spruce to strengthen their ability to communicate with the Great Spirit. Traditionally, it was believed to possess the frequency of prosperity.

MEDICAL PROPERTIES:
Antispasmodic, antiparasitic, antiseptic, anti-inflammatory, hormone-like, cortisone-like, immune stimulant, antidiabetic

USES:
Arthritis/rheumatism, fungal infections (candida), sinus/respiratory infections, sciatica/lumbago/diabetes neuropathy symptoms

FRAGRANT INFLUENCE:
Refreshing, woodsy aroma; releases emotional blocks, bringing about a feeling of balance and grounding

DIRECTIONS:
Aromatic: 3o. Topical: 50-50. Dietary: Take as a dietary supplement: 1-10 drops in a capsule or 1-2 drops under the tongue or add to drinking water.

CAUTIONS: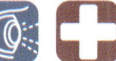

SELECTED RESEARCH:

Downing AD, Eid HM, Tang A, Ahmed F, Harris CS, Haddad PS, Johns T, Arnason JT, Bennett SAL, Cuerrier A. Growth environment and organ specific variation in in-vitro cytoprotective activities of Picea mariana in PC12 cells exposed to glucose toxicity: a plant used for treatment of diabetes symptoms by the Cree of Eeyou Istchee (Quebec, Canada). BMC Complement Altern Med. 2019; 19: 137. Published online 2019 June 18.

Francezon N, Meda NR, Stevanovic T. Optimization of bioactive polyphenols extraction from Picea mariana bark. Molecules. 2017 Dec 1;22(12).

Garcia-Pérez ME, Allaeys I, Rusu D, Pouliot R, Janezic TS, Poubelle PE. Picea mariana polyphenolic extract inhibits phlogogenic mediators produced by TNF-α-activated psoriatic keratinocytes: impact on NF-kB pathway. J Ethnopharmacol. 2014;151(1):265-78. doi: 10.1016/j.jep.2013.10.034. Epub 2013 Nov 6.

Garcia-Pérez ME, Royer M, Herbette G, Desjardins Y, Pouliot R, Stevanovic T. Picea mariana bark: a new source of trans-resveratrol and other bioactive polyphenols. Food Chem. 2012 Dec 1; 135(3):1173-82.

Prunier J, Tessier G, Bousquet J, MacKay J. From genotypes to phenotypes: expression levels of genes encompassing adaptive SNPs in black spruce. Plant Cell Rep. 2015 Dec;34(12):2111-25. Epub 2015 Aug 11.

Tam TW, Liu R, Arnason JT, Krantis A, Staines WA, Haddad PS, Foster BC. Cree antidiabetic plant extracts display mechanism-based inactivation of CYP3A4. Can J Physiol Pharmacol. 2011 Jan;89(1):13-23.

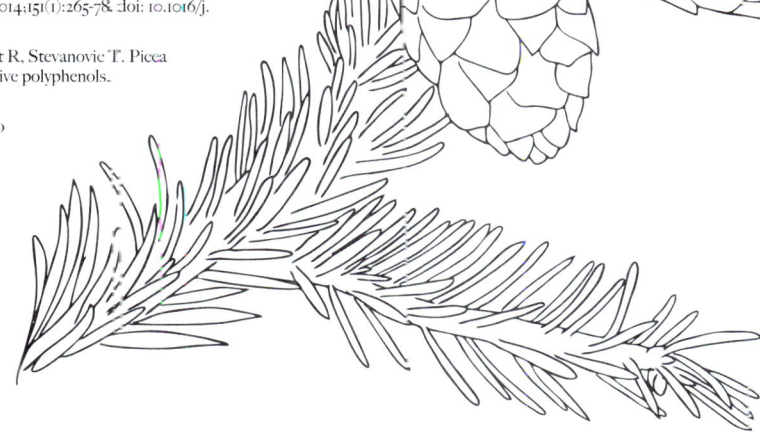

BOTANICAL FAMILY: Pinaceae

PLANT ORIGIN: Canada

EXTRACTION METHOD: Steam distilled from entire tree

KEY CONSTITUENTS: Alpha-Pinene (18-22%), Beta-Pinene (12-18%), Bornyl Acetate (12-17%), Delta-3-Carene (12-13%), Camphene (7-11%), Limonene (1-5%), Myrcene (2-4%), Tricyclene (up to 2%), Santene (up to 2%)

BLACK SPRUCE, NORTHERN LIGHTS
(see also Black Spruce)

The Cree Indians of Quebec, Canada, traditionally used a poultice of Black Spruce inner bark for infections and an infusion of the bark for pain relief. They call Black Spruce "Innatuck." Traditionally, Black Spruce was believed to possess the frequency of prosperity. Northern Lights Black Spruce is made from the entire tree not just branches, needles, and twigs.

MEDICAL PROPERTIES:
Antispasmodic, antiparasitic, antiseptic, anti-inflammatory, hormone-like, cortisone-like, immune stimulant, diabetes neuropathy symptoms

USES:
Arthritis/rheumatism, fungal infections (candida), sinus/respiratory infections, sciatica/lumbago

FRAGRANT INFLUENCE:
Rich, woody, invigorating; releases emotional blocks, bringing about a feeling of balance and grounding

DIRECTIONS:
Aromatic: 30. Topical: 50-50.

CAUTIONS:

SELECTED RESEARCH:

Downing AD, Eid HM, Tang A, Ahmed F, Harris CS, Haddad PS, Johns T, Arnason JT, Bennett SAL, Cuerrier A. Growth environment and organ specific variation in in-vitro cytoprotective activities of Picea mariana in PC12 cells exposed to glucose toxicity: a plant used for treatment of diabetes symptoms by the Cree of Eeyou Istchee (Quebec, Canada). BMC Complement Altern Med. 2019; 19: 137. Published online 2019 June 18.

Garcia-Pérez ME, Allaeys I, Rusu D, Pouliot R, Janezic TS, Poubelle PE. Picea mariana polyphenolic extract inhibits phlogogenic mediators produced by TNF-α-activated psoriatic keratinocytes: impact on NF-kB pathway. J Ethnopharmacol. 2014;151(1):265-78. Epub 2013 Nov 1.

Garcia-Pérez ME, Royer M, Herbette G, Desjardins, Pouliot R, Stevanovic T. Picea mariana bark: a new source of trans-resveratrol and other bioactive polyphenols. Food Chem. 2012 Dec 1; 135(3):1173-82. 2012.05.050. Epub 2012 May 22.

Prunier J, Tessier G, Bousquet J, MacKay J. From genotypes to phenotypes: expression levels of genes encompassing adaptive SNPs in black spruce. Plant Cell Rep. 2015 Dec;34(12):2111-25. Epub 2015 Aug 11.

Tam TW, Liu R, Arnason JT, Krantis A, Staines WA, Haddad PS, Foster BC. Cree antidiabetic plant extracts display mechanism-based inactivation of CYP3A4. Can J Physiol Pharmacol. 2011 Jan;89(1):13-23.

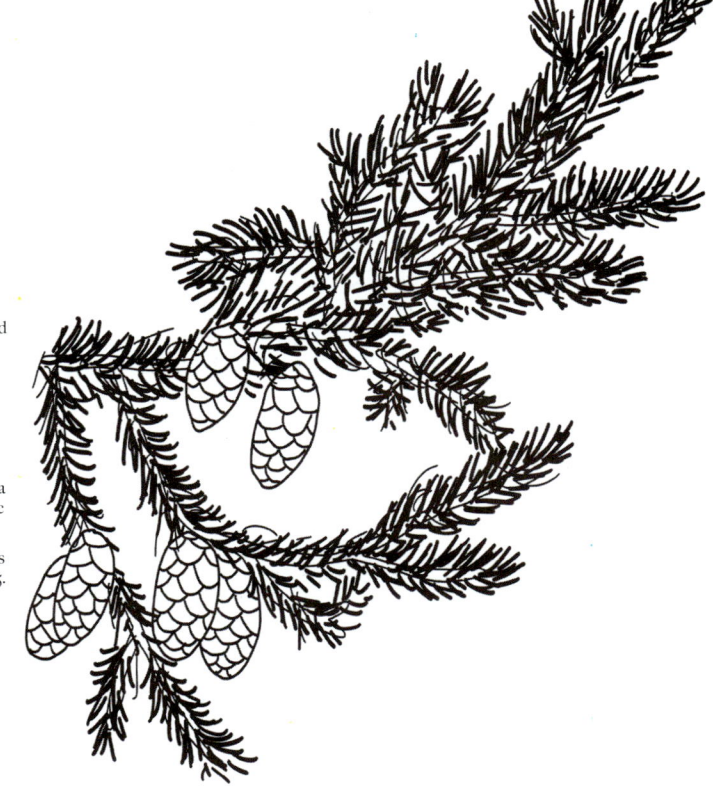

Essential Oil Singles & Blends | **Chapter 2**

Infused with the natural energy of the Northern Lights!

First Edition | **Essential Oils Complete Home Reference** | 105

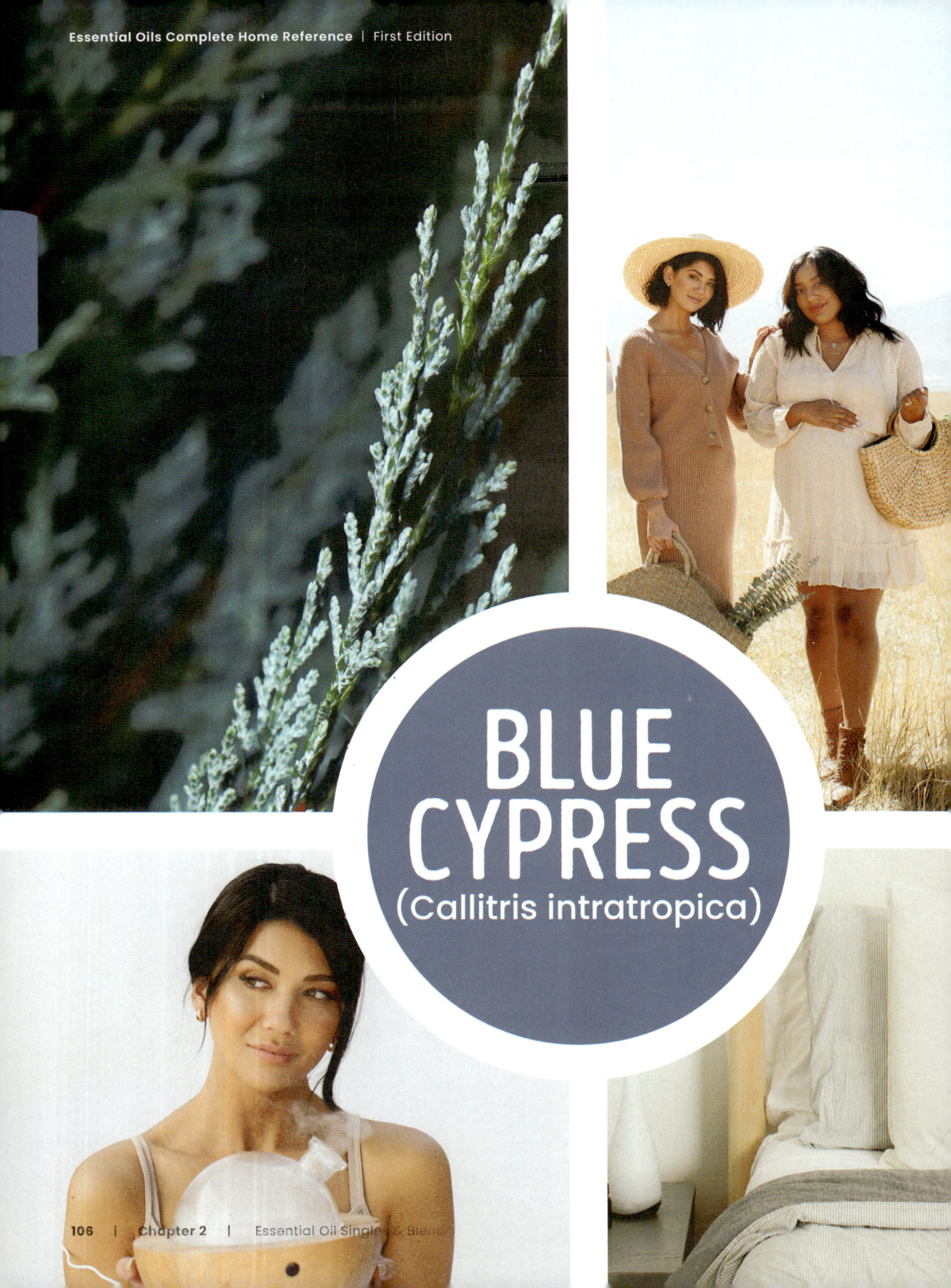

BLUE CYPRESS
(Callitris intratropica)

Single Oils | Chapter 2

BOTANICAL FAMILY:
Cupressaceae

PLANT ORIGIN:
Australia

EXTRACTION METHOD:
Steam distillation from leaves, wood, and bark

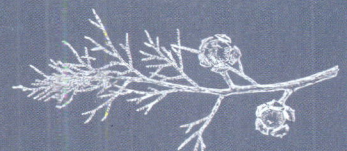

KEY CONSTITUENTS:
Dihydrocolumellarin (1-27%), Guaiol (10-23%), Bulnesol (4-14%), Gamma-Eudesmol (5-13%), Beta-Eudesmol (2-11%), Alpha-Eudesmol (2-10%), Gamma-Costol (2-7%), Beta-Selinene (up to 5%)

HISTORICAL DATA:
In ancient times, blue cypress was used for incense, perfume, and embalming.

MEDICAL PROPERTIES:
Antimicrobial, antioxidative, antitumoral, anti-inflammatory, antiviral

USES:
Skin moisturizing, promotes the appearance of healthy-looking skin, viral infections (herpes simplex, herpes zoster, cold sores, human papilloma virus, genital warts, etc.)

FRAGRANT INFLUENCE:
Good aroma for outdoor activities

DIRECTIONS:
Aromatic: 6o. Topical: Neat.

CAUTIONS:

SELECTED RESEARCH:
Sadgrove NJ, Senbill H, Van Wyk B-E, Greatrex BW. New Labdanes with Antimicrobial and Acaridical Activity: Terpenes of Callitris and Widdringtonia (Cupressaceae). Antibiotics (Basel). 2020 Apr; 9(4): 173. Published online 2020 Apr 11.

Doimo L. Azulenes, costols and γ-lactones from cypress-pines (Callitris columellaris, C. glaucophylla and C. intratropica) distilled oils and methanol extracts. J Essent Oil Res. 2001 Jan 1;13(1):25-9.

Horak S, Koschak A, Stuppner H, Striessnig J. Use-dependent block of voltage-gated Cav2.1 Ca2+ channels by petasins and eudesmol isomers. J Pharmacol Exp Ther. 2009 Jul;330(1):220-6. Epub 2009 Apr 17.

Oyedeji AO, Ekundayo O, Sonwa MM, Fricke C, Konig WA. (-)-Eudesma-1,4(15),11-triene from the essential oil of Callitris intratropica. Phytochemistry. 1998 Jun;48(4):657-60. doi: 10.1016/s0031-9422(98)00158-7.

Wanner J, Jirovetz L, Schmidt E. Callitris intratropica RT Baker & HG Smith as a novel rich source of deoxypodophyllotoxin. Current Bioactive Compounds. 2015 Jun 1;11(2):173-7.

Zhao Q, Bowles EJ, Zhang HY. Antioxidant activities of eleven Australian essential oils. Nat Prod Comm. 2008;3,5:1837-42.

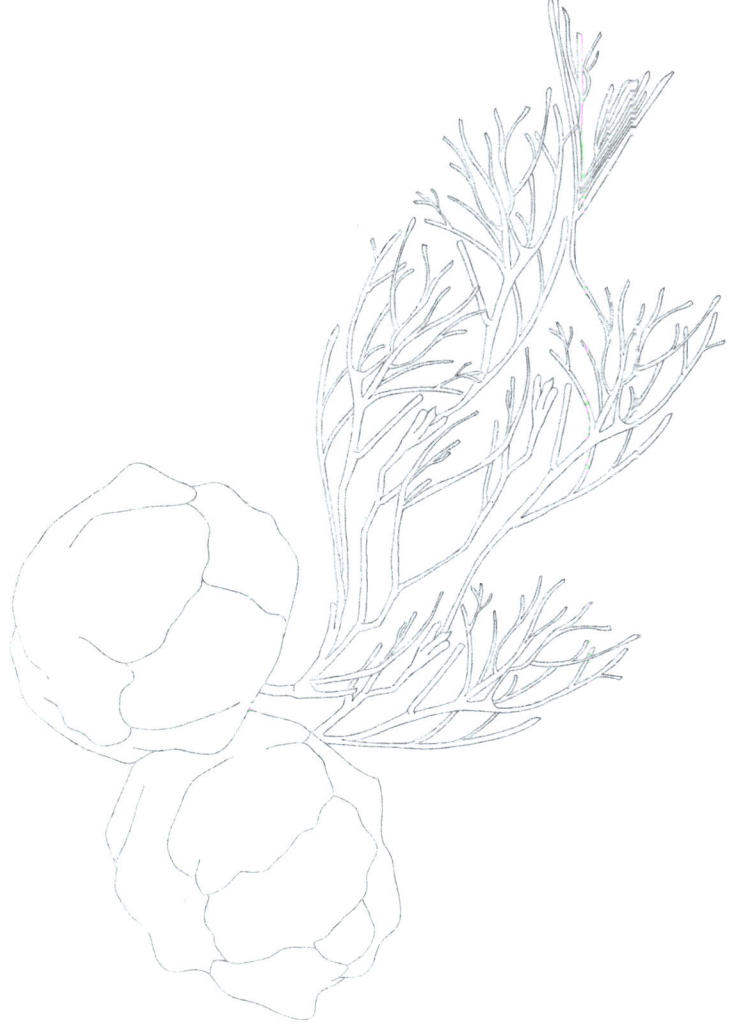

BOTANICAL FAMILY:
Pinaceae

PLANT ORIGIN:
USA, Highland Flats in Naples, Idaho

EXTRACTION METHOD:
Steam distilled from wood/branches/leaves

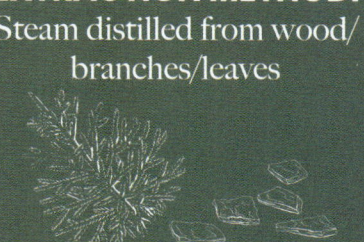

KEY CONSTITUENTS:
Alpha-Pinene (20-47%), Limonene (15-30%), Beta-Pinene (2-17%), Delta-3-Carene (3-11%), Camphene (4-9%), Myrcene (3-7%), Bornyl Acetate (1-6%), Cembrene (up to 2%)

BLUE SPRUCE, IDAHO
(Picea pungens)

Northwestern Native Americans considered the Idaho blue spruce to be a sacred tree and used it for smudging/purification rites. Spruce leaves, inner bark, gum, and twigs have been used historically by Native Americans for a variety of functions. Leaves were used as inhalants, fumigators, and revivers. The inner bark of the spruce was used for lung and throat troubles, inward negative feelings, in a poultice applied to wounds and for cuts and swelling, as a medicinal salt, applied to areas of inflammation, and in an antiscorbutic drink for scurvy and colds. Spruce gum was also used for caulking canoes. Various parts of the tree were also combined and used for stomach troubles, scabs, sores, as a salve for cuts and wounds, and in a tea for scurvy and as a cough remedy.

MEDICAL PROPERTIES:
Antinociceptive (analgesic; reduces sensitivity to pain), antioxidative, antibacterial, antimicrobial, relaxant, possibly anticancerous

USES:
Pain relief, insecticide, expectorant, induces relaxation, nAChR (nicotinic acetylcholine receptor) inhibitor, prevents oxidation of LDL, GABA agonist

FRAGRANT INFLUENCE:
Releases emotional blocks, bringing about a feeling of balance and grounding

DIRECTIONS:
Aromatic: 6o. Topical: Neat.
Dietary: Take 2 drops in a capsule daily as a dietary supplement.

CAUTIONS:

SELECTED RESEARCH:

Pack JA, et al. Physical and emotional effects of Idaho blue spruce. Unpublished Young Living Essential Oils study. 2013.

Leite AM, Lima E. de O, de Souza EL, Diniz M de FFM, Trajano VN, de Medeiros IA. Inhibitory effect of β-pinene, α-pinene and eugenol on the growth of potential infectious endocarditis causing gram-positive bacteria. Brazilian J of Pharmaceut Sci. 2007 Jan/Mar;43(1):121-126.

Matsubara E, Fukagawa M, Okamoto T, Ohnuki K, Shimizu K, Kondo R. (-)-Bornyl acetate induces autonomic relaxation and reduces arousal level after visual display terminal work without any influences of task performance in low-dose condition. Biomed Research. 2011 Apr;32(2):151-7. Epub May 10.

Pacheco A, Lindner AS. Effects of alpha-pinene and trichloroethylene on oxidation potentials of methanotrophic bacteria. Bull Environ Contam Toxicol. 2005 Jan;74(1):133-140. Epub 2005 Mar 17.

Tiwari M, Kakkar P. Plant derived antioxidants—Geraniol and camphene protect rat alveolar macrophages against t-BHP induced oxidative stress. Toxicology in Vitro. 2009 Mar;23(2):295-301. Epub 2008 Jan 13.

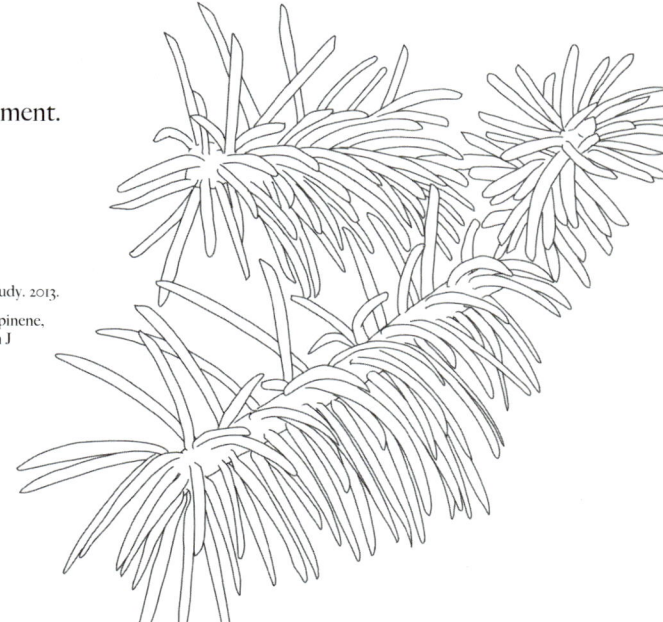

Essential Oil Singles & Blends | Chapter 2

Say hello to an evergreen immune system

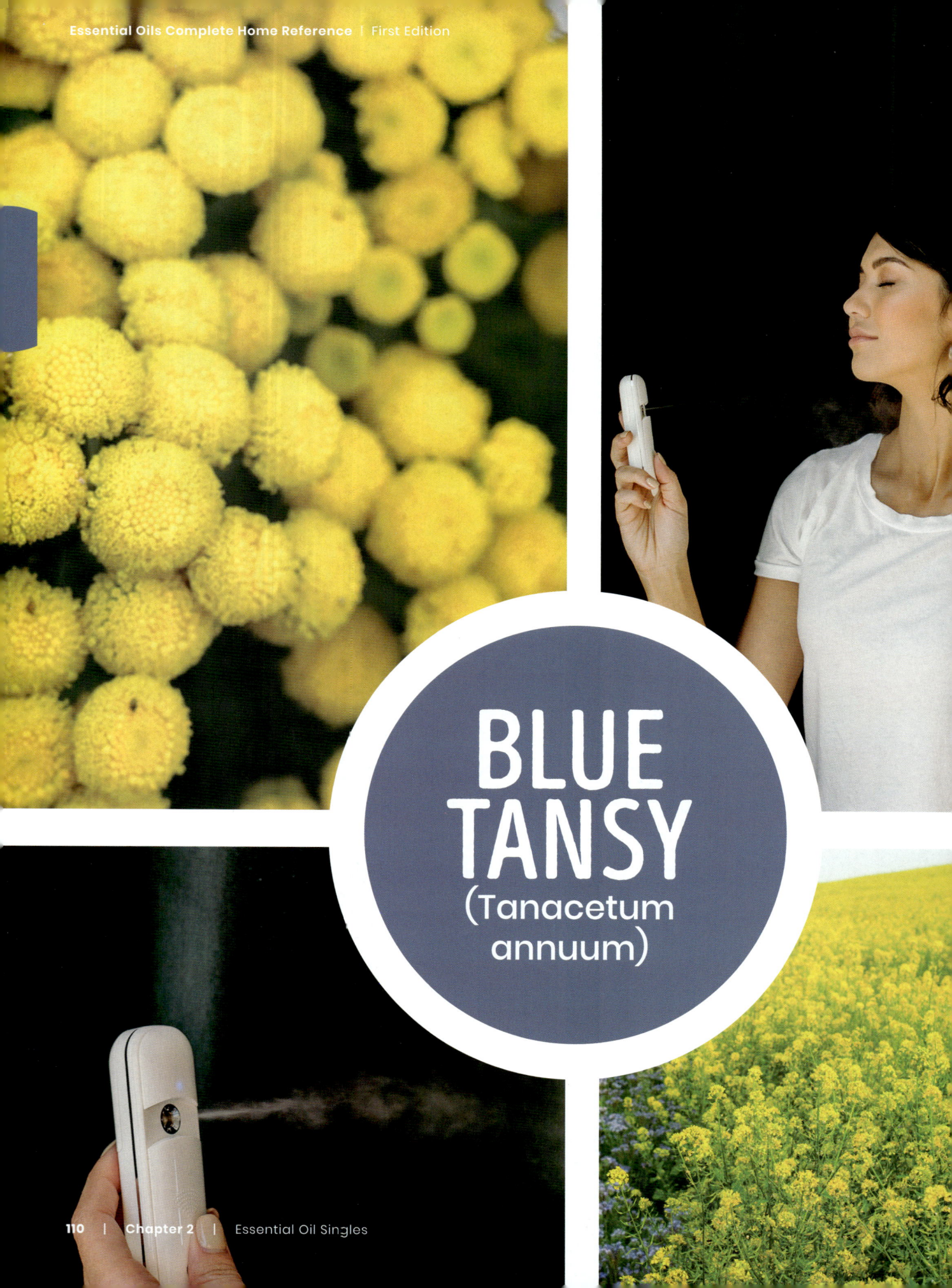

BLUE TANSY
(Tanacetum annuum)

Essential Oil Singles & Blends | **Chapter 2**

BOTANICAL FAMILY:
Compositae

PLANT ORIGIN:
Morocco

EXTRACTION METHOD:
Steam distilled from flowering tops and herbs

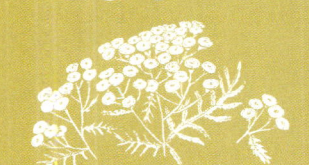

KEY CONSTITUENTS:
Sabinene (8-27%), Camphor (2-17%), Chamazulene (5-15%), Myrcene (1-13%), 3,6-Dihydrochamazulene (3-13%), Beta-Pinene (2-8%), Alpha-Phellandrene (3-8%), Para-Cymene (2-7%)

HISTORICAL DATA:
Moroccan Blue Tansy receives its lovely blue color from the constituent chamazulene.

MEDICAL PROPERTIES:
Antimicrobial anti-inflammatory, analgesic/anesthetic, antifungal, anti-itching, relaxant, hormone-like

USES:
Helps reduce the appearance of blemishes, skin cleansing, mood uplifting

FRAGRANT INFLUENCE:
Sweet, floral fragrance; soothing, relaxing

DIRECTIONS:
Aromatic: 60. Topical: Neat.

CAUTIONS: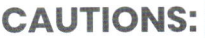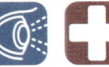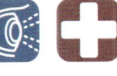
Not intended for use during pregnancy.

SELECTED RESEARCH:
Saleh MA, Clark S, Woodard B, Deolu-Sobogun SA. Antioxidant and free radical scavenging activities of essential oils. Ethn Dis. 2010 Winter;20(1 Suppl 1):S1-78-82. Epub 2010 Jun 4.

Greche H, Hajjaji N, Ismaï-Alaoui M, Mrabet N, Benjilali B. Chemical composition and antifungal properties of the essential oil of Tanacetum annuum. Journal of Essential Oil Research. 2000 Jan/Feb;12(1):122-4.

Barrero AF, Sánchez JF, Altarejos J, Zafra MJ. Homoditerpenes from the essential oil of Tanacetum annuum. Phytochemistry. 1992 May 1; 31(5):1727-30.

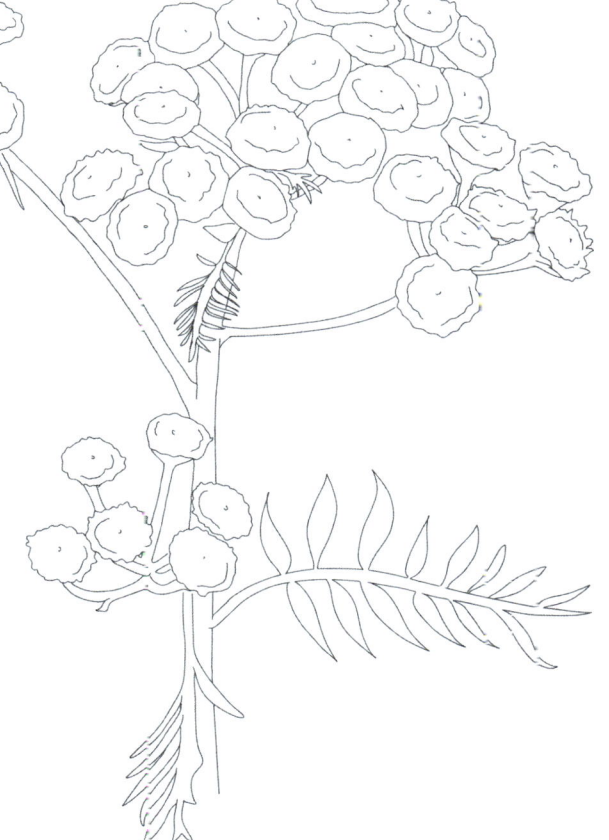

Essential Oils Complete Home Reference | First Edition

BOTANICAL FAMILY: Asteraceae

PLANT ORIGIN: Bulgaria, Canada, USA

EXTRACTION METHOD: Steam distilled from flowering tops

KEY CONSTITUENTS: Germacrene D (4-30%), Sabinene (1-22%), Chamazulene (2-21%), Beta-Pinene (3-18%), Trans-Beta-Caryophyllene (4-15%), Eucalyptol (2-11%), Camphor (up to 8%), Myrcene (up to 7%)

BLUE YARROW
(Achillea millefolium)

The Greek Achilles, hero of the Trojan War, was said to have used the yarrow herb to help cure the injury to his Achilles tendon. Yarrow was considered sacred by the Chinese, who recognized the harmony of the Yin and Yang energies within it. It has been said that the fragrance of yarrow makes possible the meeting of heaven and earth. Yarrow was used by Germanic tribes for the treatment of battle wounds.

MEDICAL PROPERTIES:
Anti-inflammatory, hormone-like, combats scarring, supports prostate

USES:
Prostate problems, menstrual problems/PMS, varicose veins

FRAGRANT INFLUENCE:
Balancing highs and lows, both external and internal, yarrow simultaneously inspires and grounds us. Useful during meditation and supportive to intuitive energies. Reduces confusion and ambivalence.

DIRECTIONS:
Aromatic: 6o. Topical: Neat.

CAUTIONS: Possible drug interaction.

SELECTED RESEARCH:

Rezaei S, Ashkar F, Koohpeyma F, Mahmood M, Gholamalizadeh M, Mazloom Z, Doei S. Hydroalcoholic extract of Achillea millefolium improved blood glucose, liver enzymes and lipid profile compared to metformin in strepozotocin-induced diabetic rats. Lipids Health Dis. 2020; 19:81. Published online 2020 Apr 27.

El-Kalamouni C, Venskutonis PR, Zebib B, Merah O, Raynaud C, Talou T. Antioxidant and antimicrobial activities of the essential oil of Achillea millefolium L. grown in France. Medicines (Basel). 2017 May 19;4(2).

Ayoobi F, Shamsizadeh A, Fatemi I, Vakilian A, Allahtavakoli M, Hassanshahi G, Moghadam-Ahmadi A. Bio-effectiveness of the main flavonoids of Achillea millefolium in the pathophysiology of neurodegenerative disorders-a review. Iran J Basic Med Sci. 2017 Jun;20(6):604-612.

Freysdottir J, Logadottir OT, Omarsdottir SS, Vikingsson A, Hardardottir I. A polysaccharide fraction from Achillea millefolium increases cytokine secretion and reduces activation of Akt, ERK and NF-kB in THP-1 monocytes. Carbohydr Polym. 2016 Jun 5;143:131-8. Epub 2016 Feb Jenabi E, Fereidoony B. Effect of Achillea millefolium on relief of primary dysmenorrhea: a double-blind randomized trial. J Pediatr Adolesc Gynecol. 2015 Oct;28(5):402-4. Epub 2014 Dec 23.

Shahani S, Rostamnezhad M, Ghaffari-Rad V, Ghasemi A, Allahverdi Pourfallah T, Hosseinimehr SJ. Radioprotective effect of Achillea millefolium L. against genotoxicity induced by ionizing radiation in human normal lymphocytes. Dose Response. 2015 Apr 29;13(1):1559325815583761. eCollection 2015 Jan-Mar.

Peng HY, Lin CC, Wang HY, Shih Y, Chou ST. The melanogenesis alteration effects of Achillea millefolium L. essential oil and linalyl acetate: involvement of oxidative stress and the JNK and ERK signaling pathways in melanoma cells. PLoS One. 2014 Apr 17;9(4):e95186. Epub 2014 Apr 20.

Applequist WL, Moerman DE. Yarrow (Achillea millefolium L.): a neglected panacea? A review of ethnobotany, bioactivity, and biomedical research. Economic Botany. 2011 Jun 01;65(2):209-225.

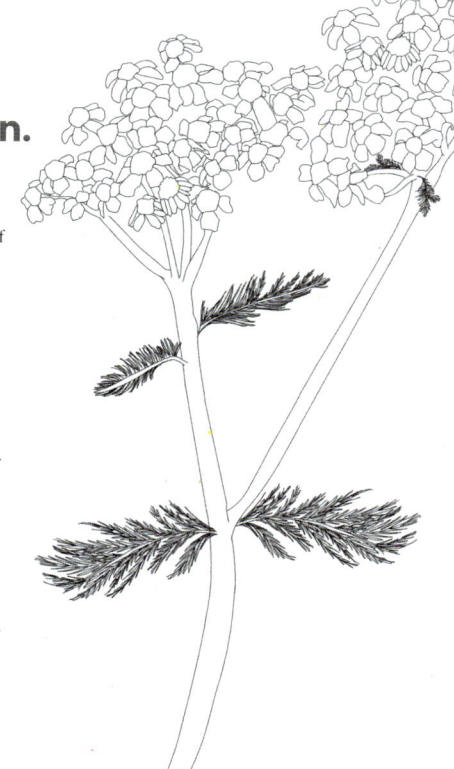

Essential Oil Singles & Blends | Chapter 2

In a field of flowers, be the oil-giving kind!

First Edition | Essential Oils Complete Home Reference | 113

BRAIN POWER™
(Essential Oil Blend)

Brain Power promotes deep concentration and channels physical energy into mental energy. It also increases mental potential and clarity, and long-term use may retard the aging process. Many of the oils in this blend are high in sesquiterpene compounds that increase activity in the pineal, pituitary, and hypothalamus glands and thereby increase output of growth hormone and melatonin. The oils also help dissolve petrochemicals that congest the receptor sites, clearing the "brain fog" that people experience due to exposure to synthetic petrochemicals in food, skin, hair care products, and air.

MEDICAL PROPERTIES & USES:
Anti-inflammatory, antimicrobial, antioxidative, calming, energizing, mental clarity supporting, disease inhibitory, organ protective, skin and hair improving

INGREDIENTS:
Sacred Sandalwood, Cedarwood, Frankincense, Melissa, Blue Cypress, Lavender, Helichrysum

DIRECTIONS:
Aromatic: 6o. Topical: Neat. Also, apply 1 or 2 drops with a finger on insides of cheeks in mouth.

CAUTIONS:

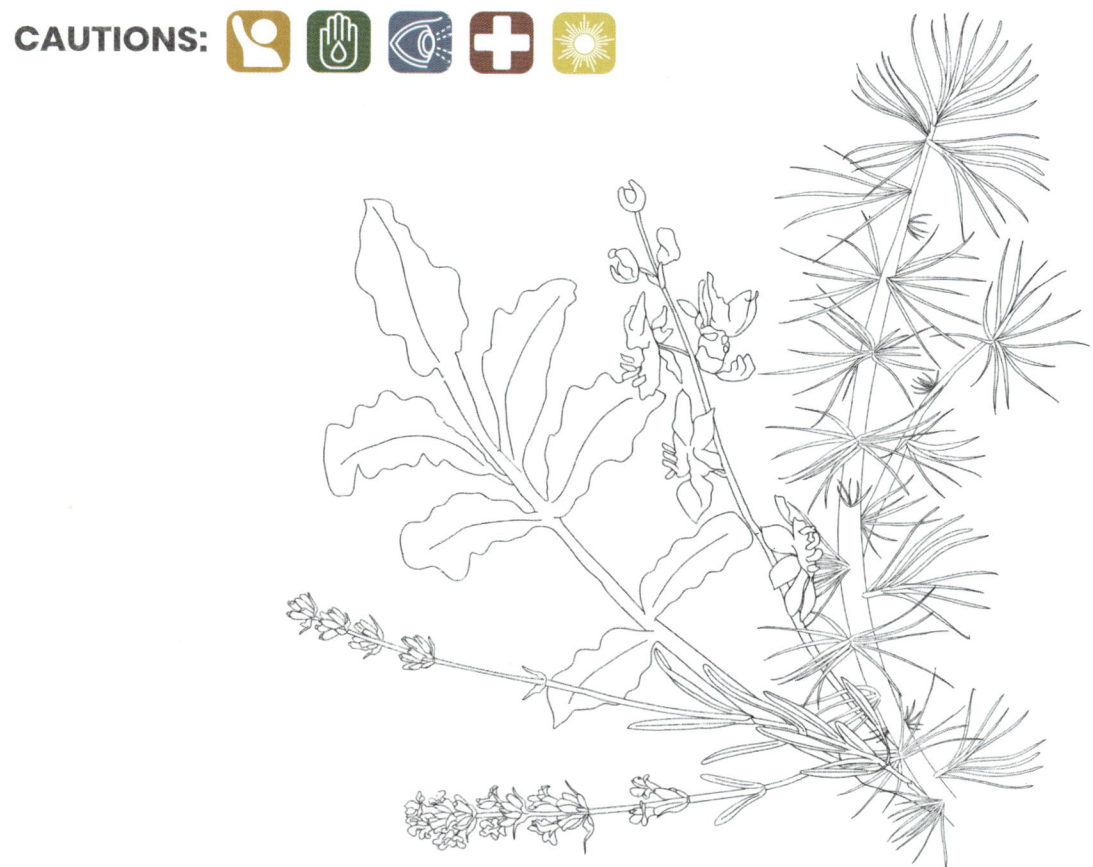

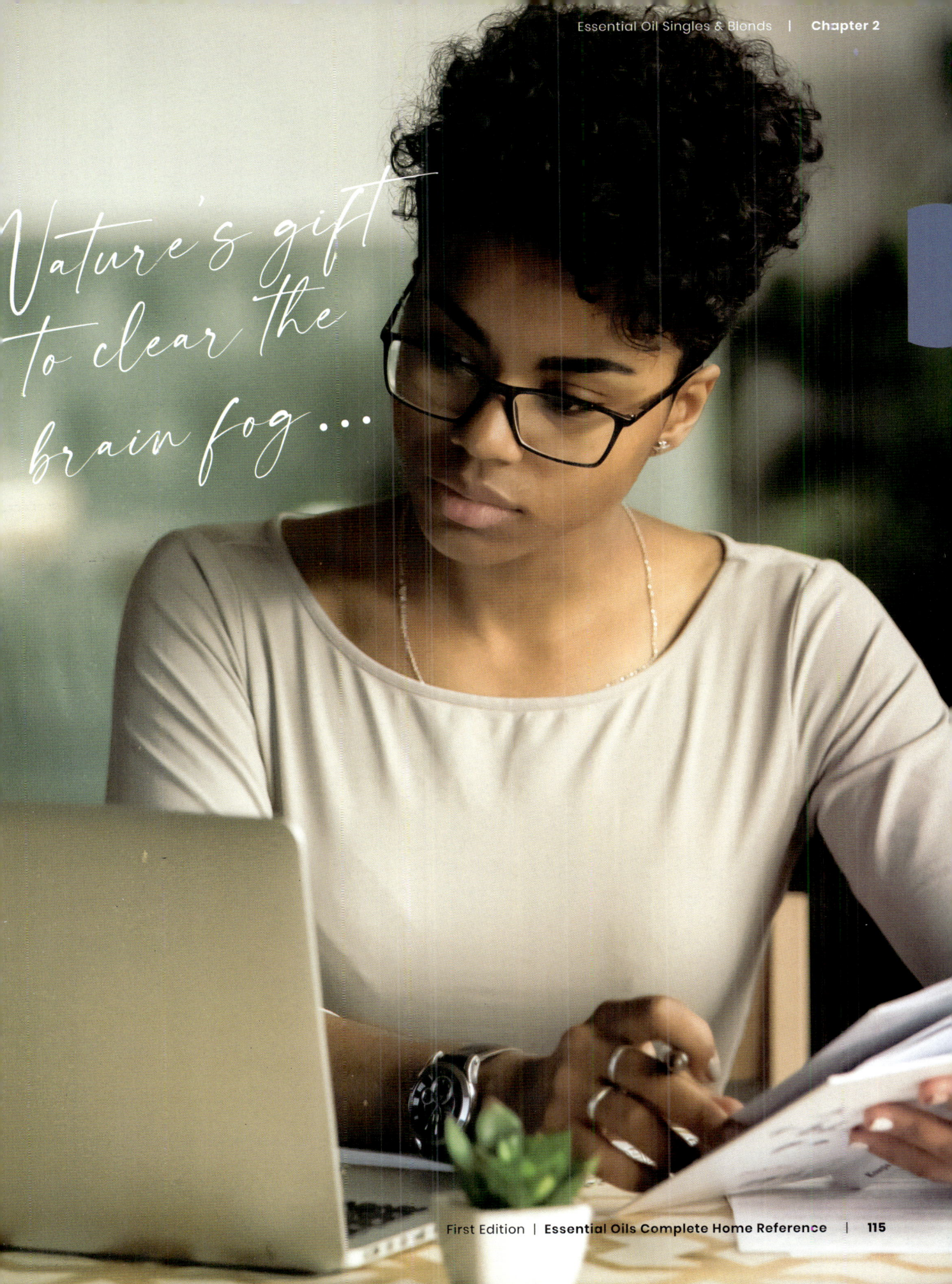

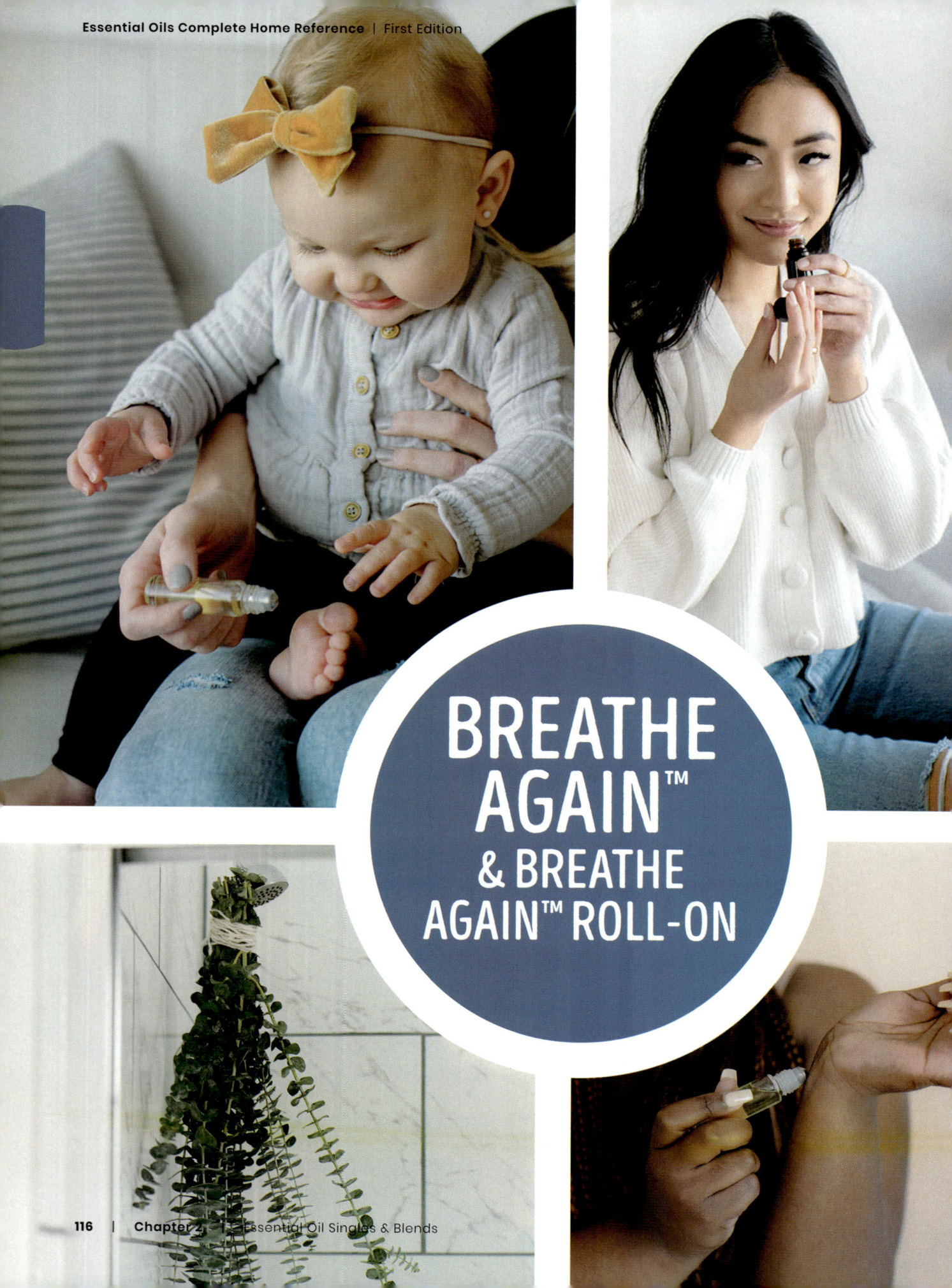

ABOUT BREATHE AGAIN™ & BREATHE AGAIN™ ROLL-ON:

This supercharged version of the R.C. blend is packaged in a convenient dispenser for easy use when air pollution makes it difficult to breathe, or throat and nasal congestion strike. Contains four different eucalyptus oils and five additional essential oils, all known for their ability to relax airways, make breathing easier, and reduce coughing. In addition, these oils have anti-inflammatory characteristics.

MEDICAL PROPERTIES & USES:

Anti-inflammatory, antimicrobial, antioxidative, digestion or elimination supportive/nausea reducing, disease inhibitory, insecticidal, muscle relaxant/bone-joint preservative, pain or swelling reducing, performance enhancing/stimulating, respiratory system supportive

INGREDIENTS:

Caprylic/capric triglyceride, Eucalyptus Staigeriana, Eucalyptus Globulus, Laurus Nobilis (Bay Laurel), Rose Hip seed oil, Peppermint, Eucalyptus Radiata, Copaiba, Blue Cypress, Eucalyptus Blue, Myrtle

DIRECTIONS:

Neat. Apply generously to chest and neck as desired for relief of symptoms related to colds, coughs, or sinus/lung congestion.

CAUTIONS:

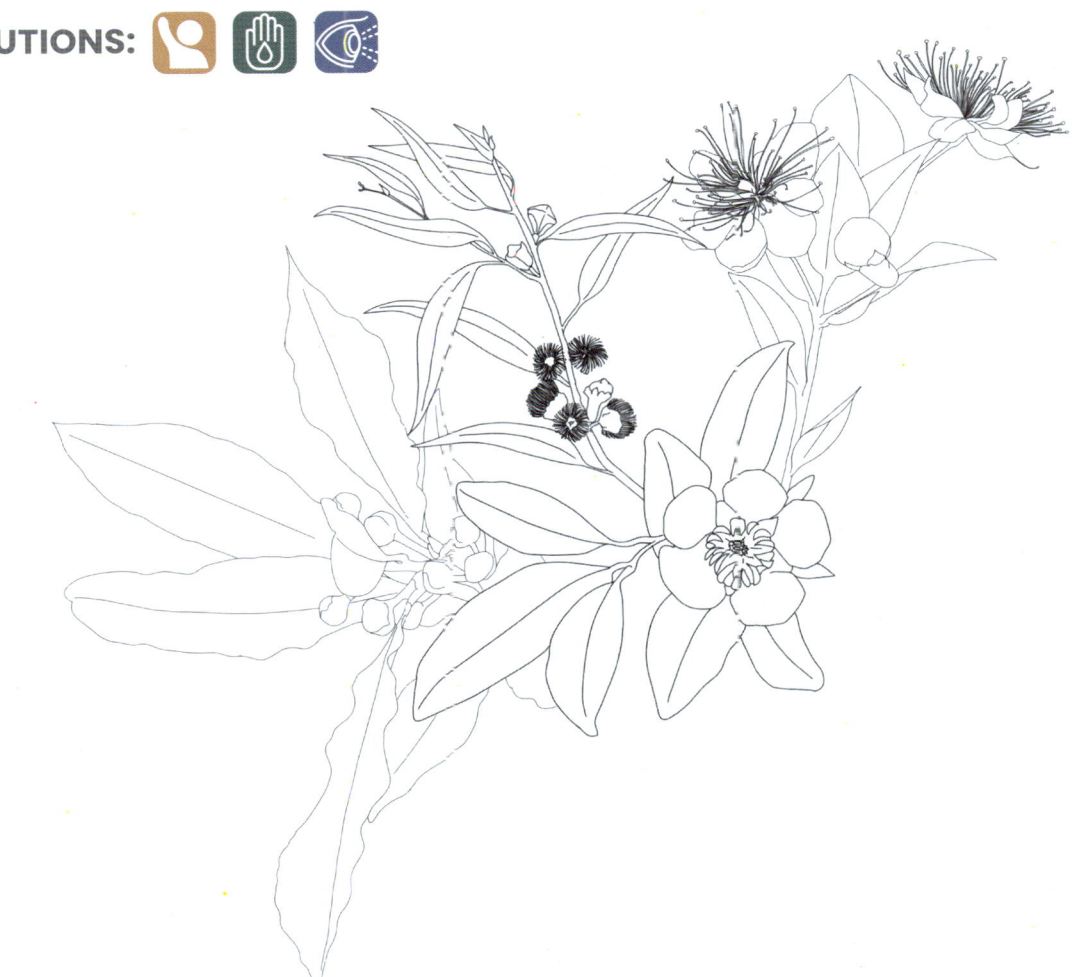

BUILD YOUR DREAM™
(Essential Oil Blend)

A unique blend, Build Your Dream is designed to empower and give clarity to your thoughts and purpose when used aromatically.

MEDICAL PROPERTIES & USES:
Anti-inflammatory, antimicrobial, antioxidative, emotion supportive, disease inhibitory, insecticidal, organ protective, pain or swelling reducing

INGREDIENTS:
Lavender, Ylang Ylang, Blue Cypress, Sacred Frankincense, Hong Kuai, Melissa, Idaho Blue Spruce, Idaho Grand Fir, Royal Hawaiian Sandalwood, Coriander, Tangerine, Black Pepper, Blue Lotus, Bergamot, Frankincense, Anise, Juniper, Citrus Hystrix, Davana, Geranium, Jasmine, Matricaria (German Chamomile), Rose, Blue Tansy, Grapefruit, Spearmint, Lemon, Ocotea

DIRECTIONS:
Aromatic: 60. Topical: 50-50.

CAUTIONS:

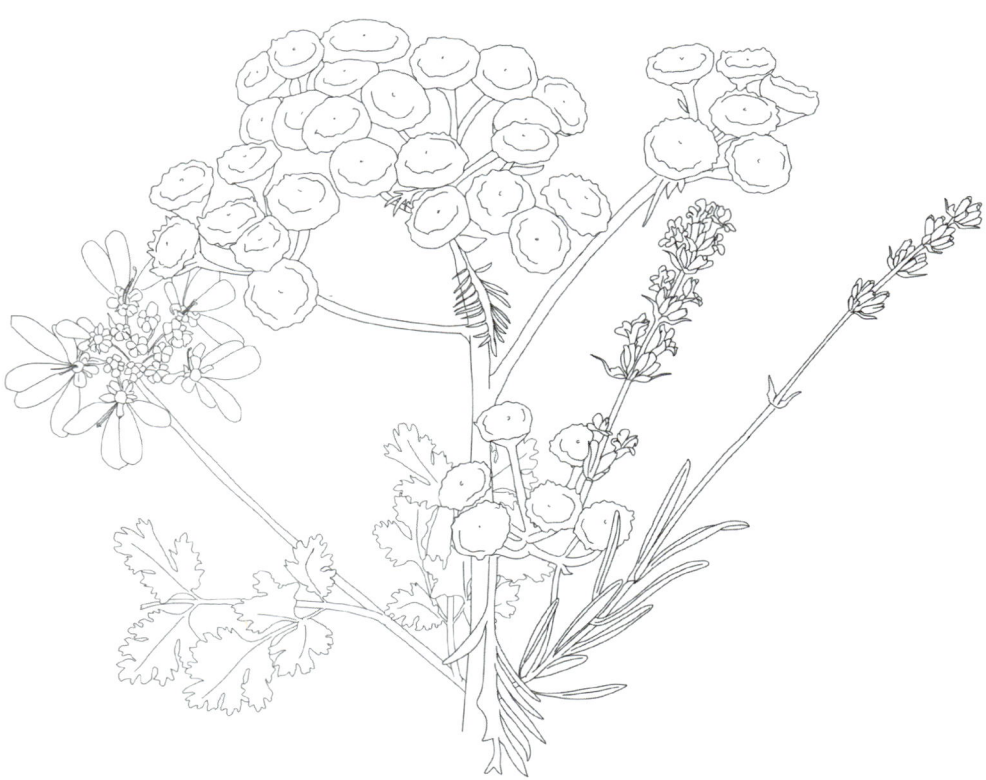

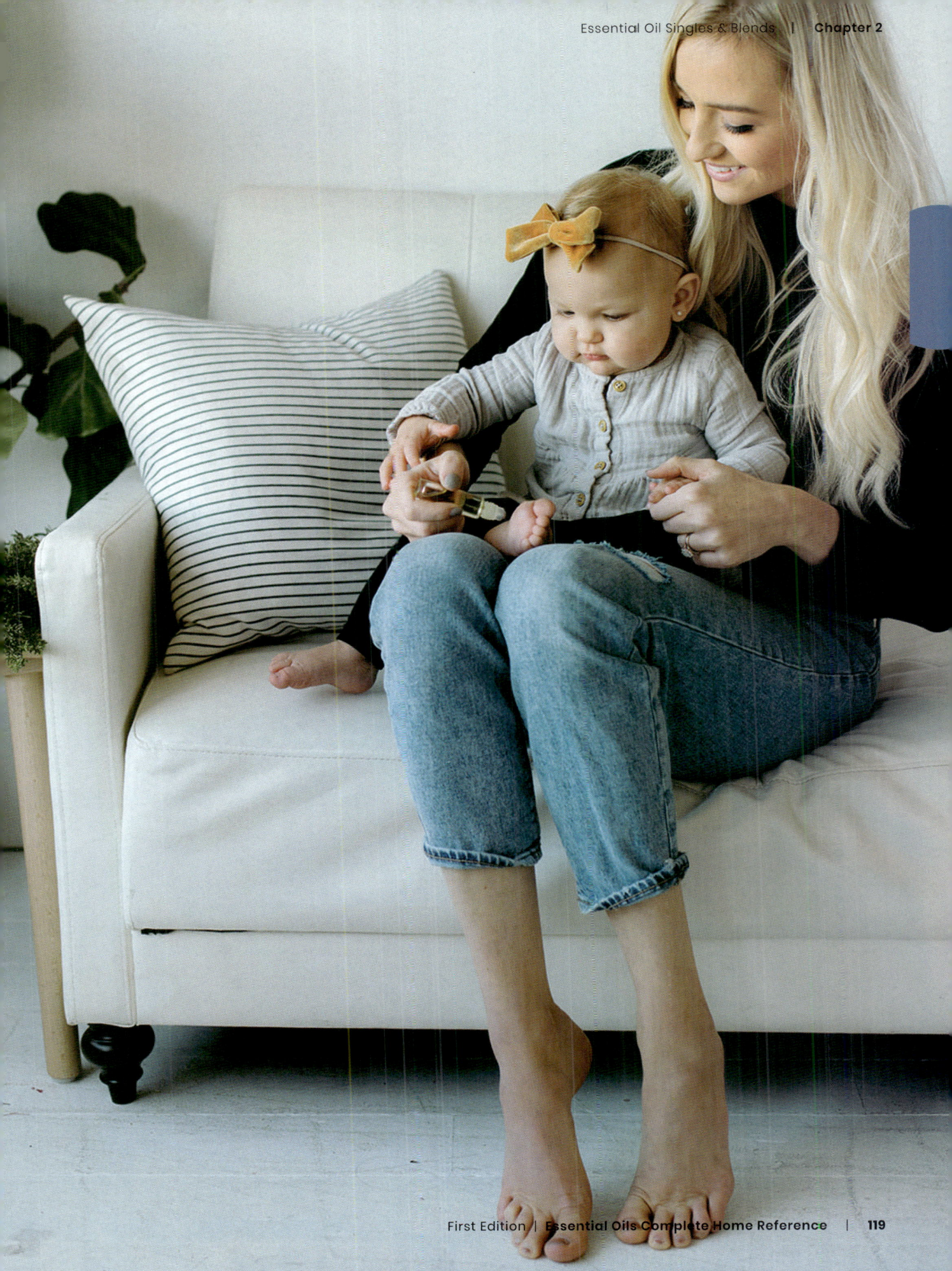

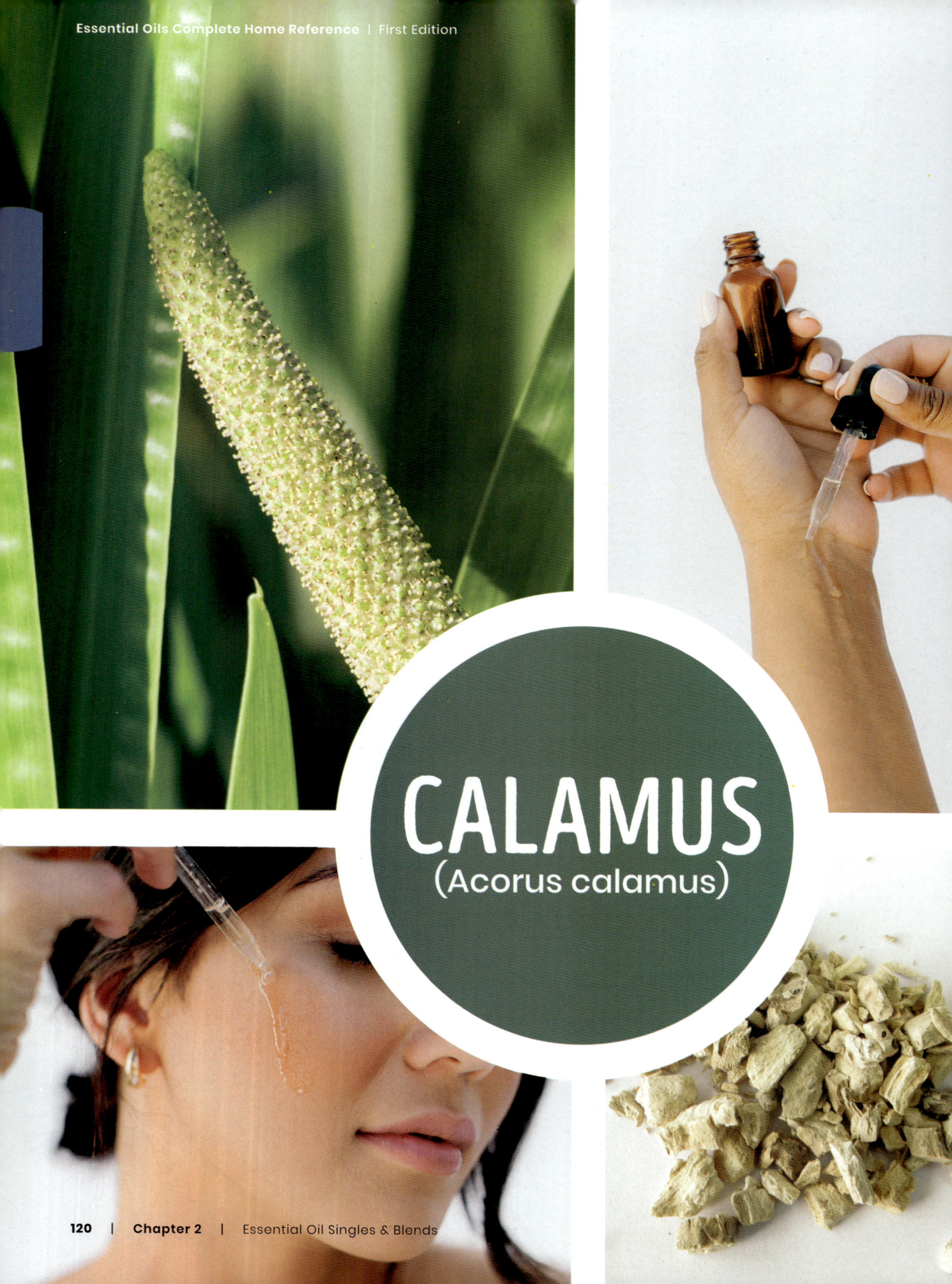

Essential Oil Singles & Blends | Chapter 2

BOTANICAL FAMILY:
Acoraceae

PLANT ORIGIN:
India, Nepal, Brazil

EXTRACTION METHOD:
Steam distilled from roots

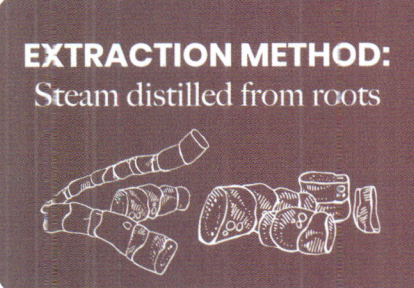

KEY CONSTITUENTS:
Cis Methyl Isoeugenol (6-27%), Acorenone (4-26%), Beta Asarone (6-26%), Shyobunone (1-22%), Preisocalamendiol (up to 12%), Calamuscenone (1-12%), Isoshyobunone (2-8%), Calamendiol (1-5%)

HISTORICAL DATA:
Commonly known as sweet flag, this plant may have been the biblical calamus of Exodus 30:23 used in the holy anointing oil. It seems to have originated in India or Arabia but now is found in many places throughout the world. Native Americans used calamus as a medicine and a stimulant, but low doses are also believed to be calming and to induce sleep. The Penobscot people have a tradition that it saved their people from a serious illness.

MEDICAL PROPERTIES:
Antibacterial, sedative, carminative, expectorant, antispasmodic, bronchodilator, hepatoprotective

USES:
Relaxes spasms, lung infections, agitation, memory boosting

FRAGRANT INFLUENCE:
Believed to induce and promote positive thoughts

DIRECTIONS:
Aromatic: 60. Topical: 50-50.

CAUTIONS:
Large doses can cause mild hallucinations.
Use oil only from the diploid species that does not contain B-asarone.

SELECTED RESEARCH:
Sharma V, Sharma R, Guatam DS, Kuca K, Nepovimova E, Martins N. Role of Vacha (Acorus calamus Linn.) in Neurological and Metabolic Disorders: Evidence from Ethnopharmacology, Phytochemistry, Pharmacology and Clinical Study. J Clin Med. 2020 Apr 19.

Esfandiari E, Ghanadian M, Rashidi B, Mokhtarian A, Vatankhah AM. The effects of Acorus calamus L. in preventing memory loss, anxiety, and oxidative stress on lipopolysaccharide-induced neuroinflammation rat models. Int J Prev Med. 2018 Oct 12;9:85. eCollection 2018.

Haiyaraja N, Khanum F. Amelioration of alcohol-induced hepatotoxicity and oxidative stress in rats by Acorus calamus. J Diet Suppl. 2011 Dec;8(4):331-45. Epub 2011 Sep 26.

Joshi RK Acorus calamus Linn.: phytoconstituents and bactericidal property. World J Microbiol Biotechnol. 2016 Oct;32(10):164. Epub 2016 Aug 25.

Muthuraman A, Singh N. Neuroprotective effect of saponin rich extract of Acorus calamus L. in rat model of chronic constriction injury (CCI) of sciatic nerve-induced neuropathic pain. J Ethnopharmacol. 2012 Aug 1;142(3):723-31. Epub 2012 Jun 15.

Reddy S, Rao G, Shetty B, Hn G. Effects of Acorus calamus rhizome extract on the neuromodulatory system in restraint stress male rats. Turk Neurosurg. 2015;25(3):425-31. Epub Jun 4.

Shah AJ, Gilani AH. Bronchodilatory effect of Acorus calamus (Linn.) is mediated through multiple pathways. J Ethnopharmacol. 2010 Sep 15;131(2):471-7. Epub 2010 Jul 17.

Sharma V, Singh I, Chaudhary P. Acorus calamus (the healing plant): a review on its medicinal potential, micropropagation and conservation. Nat Prod Res. 2014;28(18):1454-66. Epub 2014 May 13.

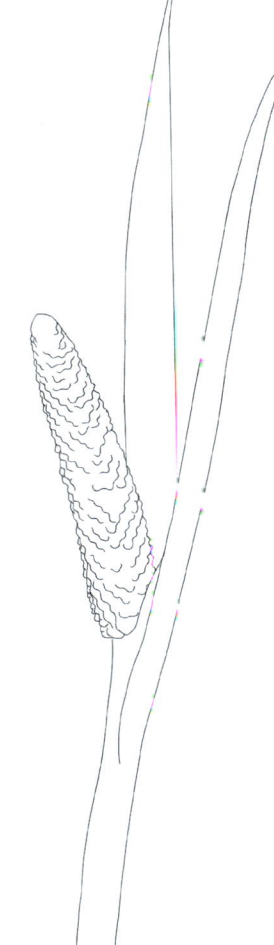

BOTANICAL FAMILY: Lauraceae

PLANT ORIGIN: China

EXTRACTION METHOD: Steam distilled from wood

KEY CONSTITUENTS: Linalool (93-100%)

CAMPHOR (HO WOOD)
(Cinnamomum camphora CT linalool)

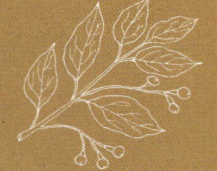

The camphor tree is native to China, Taiwan, Japan, Korea, and Vietnam. It has been introduced into other countries, where geographical influences have changed the tree's chemical makeup or chemotype. There are five commonly accepted chemotypes (cineole, linalool, camphor, isonerolidol, and safrole). Young Living uses the linalool chemotype. Trees in India and Sri Lanka have a high camphor content, while in Madagascar the tree yields a higher 1,8 cineole (eucalyptol) content and is known as ravintsara.

Some essential oil sellers of ho wood state their product is distilled from the wood, bark, or even from resin of the tree; however, the camphor tree is not resinous.

Young Living scientists tested and confirmed their variety of Ho Wood by traveling to China to take actual distillation samples. They learned their chosen oil has high levels of the constituent linalool and is distilled from the tree's branches and leaves. Young Living's Ho Wood essential oil is distilled in China under the direction of YL's Taiwan partner farm specialists.

A Nepali ho wood essential oil was found to be toxic to human breast cancer cells, while ho wood linalool chemotype was found to be a chemopreventive agent.

MEDICAL PROPERTIES:
Anticoagulant, relaxant, antispasmodic

USES:
Throat/lung infections, indigestion, menstrual problems/PMS, symptoms of dementia

FRAGRANT INFLUENCE:
Assists in the release of pent-up negative feelings and restores memories to the point of origin before trauma or anger was experienced

DIRECTIONS:
Aromatic: 30. Topical: 50-50.

CAUTIONS: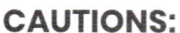

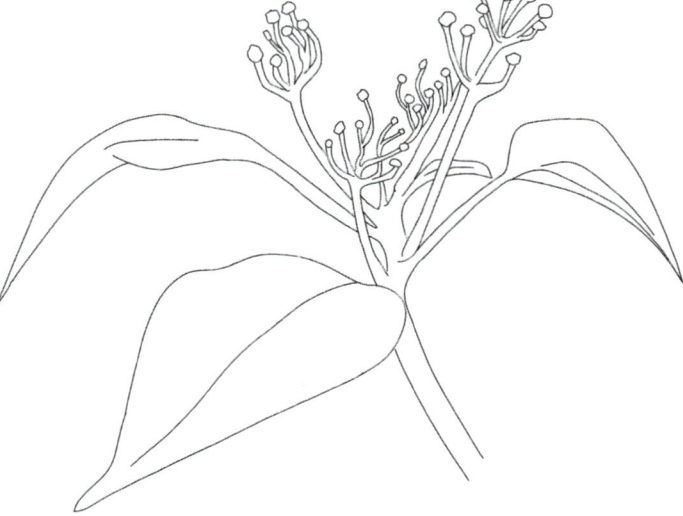

SELECTED RESEARCH:

Kang N-J, Han S-C, Yoon S-H, Sim J-Y, Maeng Y-H, Yoo E-S. Cinnamomum camphora Leaves Alleviate Skin Inflammatory Responses In Vitro and In Vivo. Toxicol Res. 2019 Jul; 35(3): 279-285.

Wang W, Li D, Huang X, Yang H, Qiu Z, Zou L, Liang Q, Shi Y, Wu Y, Wu S, yang C, Li Y. Study on Antibacterial and Quorum-Sensing Inhibition Activities of Cinnamomum camphora Leaf Essential Oil. Molecules. 2019 Oct; 24(20): 3792

Suleiman WB. In vitro estimation of superfluid critical extracts of some plants for their antimicrobial potential, phytochemistry, and GC-MS analyses. Am Clin Microbial Antimicrobial. 2020; 19:29.

Wang W, Li D, Huang X, Yang H, Qiu Z, Zou L, Liang Q, Shi Y, Wu Y. Study on Antibacterial and Quorum-Sensing Inhibition Activities of Cinnamomum camphora Leaf Essential Oil. Moleculews. 2019 Oct; 24(20):3792.

Skariyachan S, Pachiappan A, Joy J, Bhaduri R, Aier I, Vasist KS. Investigating the therapeutic potential of herbal leads against drug resistant Listeria monocytogenes by computational virtual screening and in vitro assays. J Biomol Struct Dyn. 2015;33(12):2682-94. Epub 2015 Feb 11.

Marasini BP, Baral P, Aryal P, Ghimire KR, Neupane S, Dahal N, Singh A, Ghimire L, Shrestha K. Evaluation of antibacterial activity of some traditionally used medicinal plants against human pathogenic bacteria. Biomed Res Int. 2015;2015:265425. Epub 2015 Feb 9.

Lee HJ, Hyun EA, Yoon WJ, Kim BH, Rhee MH, Kang HK, Cho JY, Yoo ES. In vitro anti-inflammatory and anti-oxidant effects of Cinnamomum camphora extracts. J Ethnopharmacol. 2006 Jan 16;103(2):208-16. Epub 2005 Sep 22.

Satyal P, Paudel P, Poudel A, Dosoky NS, Pokharel KK, Setzer WN. Bioactivities and compositional analyses of Cinnamomum essential oils from Nepal: C. camphora, C. tamala, and C. glaucescens. Nat Prod Commun 2013 Dec;8(12):1777-84. Epub 2014 Feb 22.

Shen T, Chen XM, Harder B, Long M, Wang XN, Lou HX, Wondrak GT, Ren DM, Zhang DD. Plant extracts of the family Lauraceae: a potential resource for chemopreventive agents that activate the nuclear factor-erythoid 2-related factor 2/antioxidant response element pathway. Planta Med. 2014 Mar;80(5):426-34. Epub 2014 Mar.

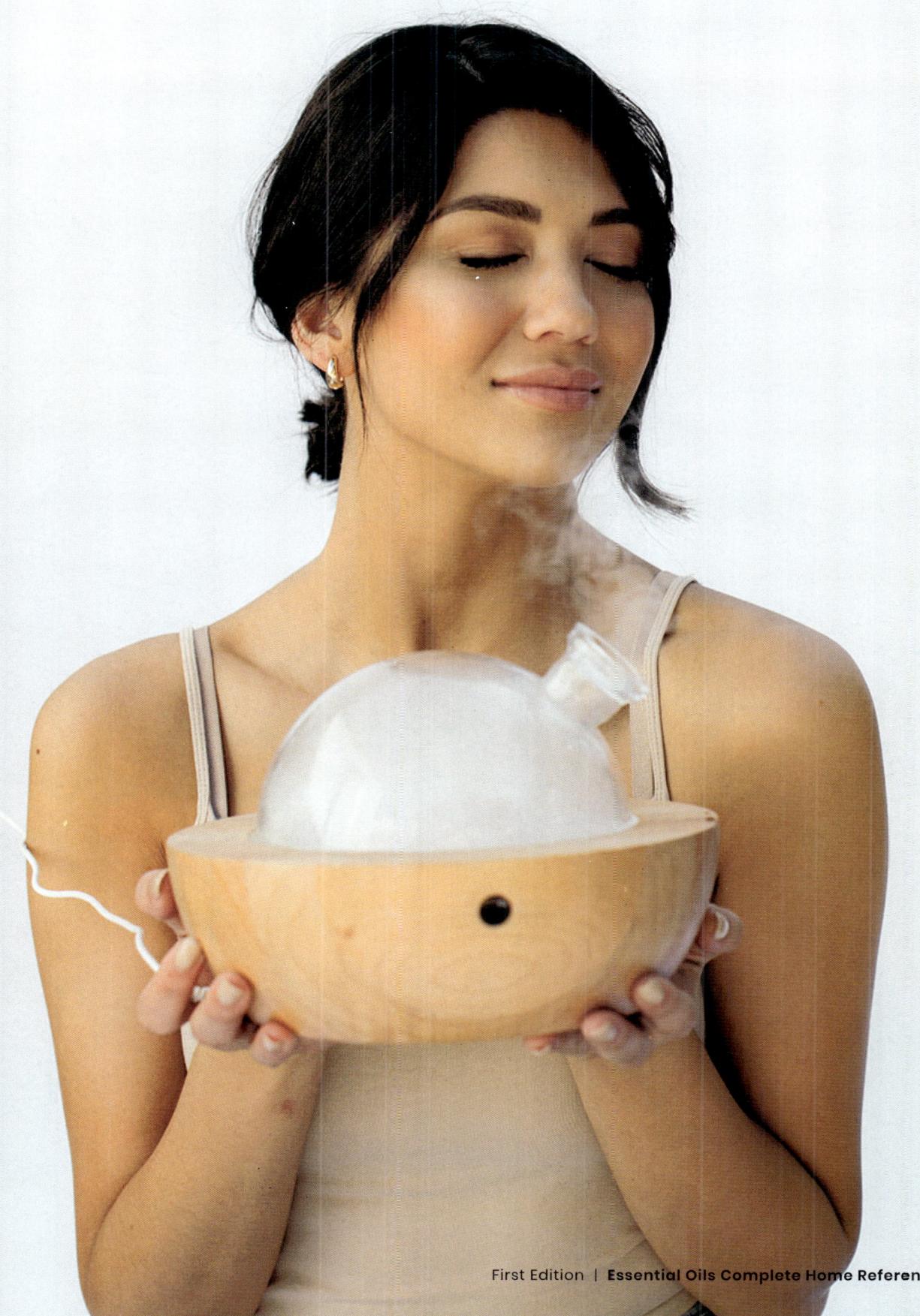

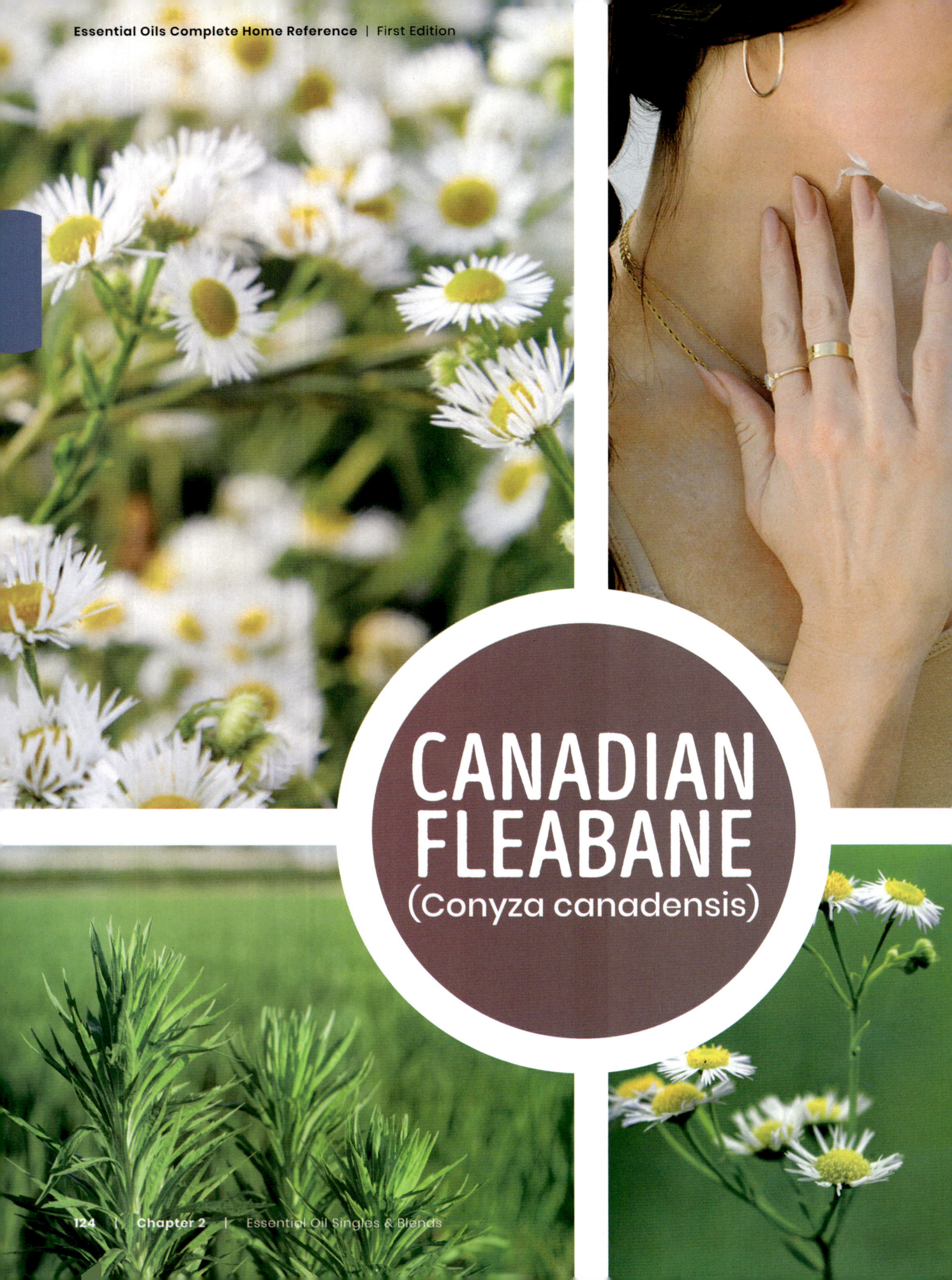

CANADIAN FLEABANE
(Conyza canadensis)

BOTANICAL FAMILY:	EXTRACTION METHOD:	KEY CONSTITUENTS:
Asteraceae	Steam distilled from leaves	Limonene (60-75%), Cis-Matricaria Ester (up to 17%), Gamma-Curcumene (up to 10%), Germacrene D (up to 10%), Trans-Alpha-Bergamotene (1-9%), Trans-Beta-Ocimene (up to 8%), Myrcene (1-3%)
PLANT ORIGIN: Canada, USA		

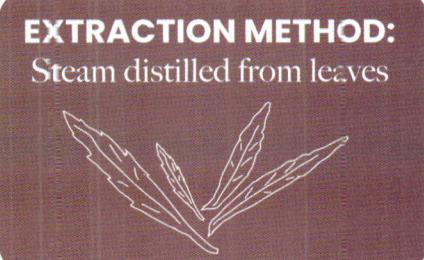

HISTORICAL DATA:
When bothered by rhinitis, the Zuni people inserted the crushed flowers of conyza in their nostrils for the relief of a good sneeze.

MEDICAL PROPERTIES:
Stimulates liver and pancreas, antiaging (stimulates growth hormone), antirheumatic, antispasmodic, vasodilating, antifungal, antimicrobial, antihypertensive

USES:
Hepatitis, Bronchitis, accelerated aging, high blood pressure, bleeding hemorrhoids, diarrhea, inflammation of the throat, joint pain

FRAGRANT INFLUENCE:
Earthy, carrot-like herbal aroma

DIRECTIONS:
Aromatic: 3o. Topical: 50-50. Dietary: Take as a dietary supplement: 1-10 drops in a capsule or 1-2 drops under the tongue or add to drinking water.

CAUTIONS: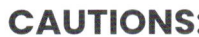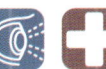

SELECTED RESEARCH:

Suleiman WB. In vitro estimation of superfluid critical exctracts of some plants for their antimicrobial potential, phytochemistry, and GC-MS analyses. Ann Clin Microbiol Antimicrob. 2020; 19:29.

Liu K, Qin YH, Yu JY, Ma H, Song XL. 3-β-Erythrodiol isolated from Conyza canadensis inhibits MKN-45 human gastric cancer cell proliferation by inducing apoptosis, cell cycle arrest, DNA fragmentation, ROS generation and reduces tumor weight and volume in mouse xenograft model. Oncol Rep. 2016 Apr;35(4):2328-38. Epub 2016 Feb 3.

Banday JA, Faroog S, Qurishi MA, Koul S, Razdan TK. Conyzagenin-A and B, two new epimeric lanostane triterpenoids from Conyza canadensis. Nat Prod Res. 2013 27(11):975-81. Epub 2012 Jul 11.

Shakirullah M, Ahmad H, Shah MR, Ahmad I, Ishaq M, Khan N, Badshah A, Khan I. Antimicrobial activities of Conyzolide and Conysoflavone from Conyza Canacensis. J Enzyme Inhib Med Chem. 2011 Aug;26(4):468-71. Epub 2010 Nov 9.

Veres K, Csupor-Löffler B, Lázár A, Hohmann J. Antifungal activity and composition of essential oils of Conyza canadensis herbs and roots. Scientific World Journal. 2012;2012:489646. Epub 2012 Oct 11.

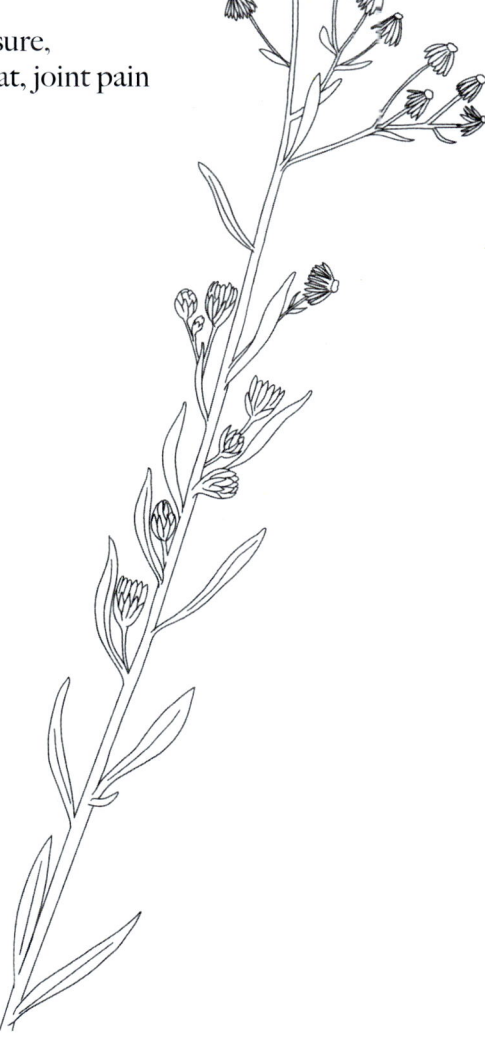

BOTANICAL FAMILY: Apiaceae

PLANT ORIGIN: Finland

EXTRACTION METHOD: Steam distilled from ripe fruit

KEY CONSTITUENTS: Carvone (49-68%), Limonene (33-48%)

CARAWAY & CARAWAY VITALITY™
(Carum carvi)

Caraway was used during the Renaissance era for treating epilepsy, along with a variety of other essential oils. Fossilized caraway seeds have been discovered among debris of the Neolithic dwellers of the Swiss lakes. Caraway is thought to have been cultivated and consumed in Europe longer than any other spice and is a frequent flavoring in European cooking. Dioscorides (c. 40-90 AD) describes karos (caraway) as a "well-known little seed". It is urinary, warming, good for the stomach, pleasant to the mouth and digestive." Both the seed and the essential oil have long been valued for their carminative and stomachic properties. Caraway seed essential oil is employed medicinally in laxative and carminative preparations, including gripe water.

MEDICAL PROPERTIES:
Antibacterial, anti-inflammatory, antioxidant, digestion or elimination supportive, nausea reducing, insecticidal

USES:
Digestive discomfort and support, immune system support, weight management support, insect repellent, breath freshener

FRAGRANT INFLUENCE:
Warm, nutty, bittersweet, slightly spicy-anisic odor, with subtle minty top note and a woody dry-out.

DIRECTIONS:
Neat. In case of sensitivity, dilute 3 drops in 10 ml of V-6. Dietary (Vitality): 50:50. Put in a capsule and take up to 3 times daily.

CAUTIONS: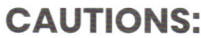

SELECTED RESEARCH:

Yousefi SS, Sadeghpour O, Hamzehgardeshi Z, Sohrabvand F. The effects of Carum Carvi (Bunium Persicum Boiss) on Early Return of Bowel Motility After Caesarean Section: Double-Blind, Randomized, Placebo-Controlled Trial. J Family Reprod Health. 2019 Mar; 13(1): 35-41.

Adebayo SA, Ondua M, Shai LJ, Lebelo SL. Inhibition of nitric oxide production and free radical scavenging activities of four South African medicinal plants. J Inflamm Res. 2019; 12: 195-203.

Mahboubi M. Caraway as important medicinal plants in management of diseases. Nat Prod Bioprospect. 2019 Jan;9(1):1-11. Epub 2018 Oct 29.

Whiley H, Gaskin S, Schroder T, Ross K. Antifungal properties of essential oils for improvement of indoor air quality: a review. Rev Environ Health. 2018 Mar 28;33(1):63-76.

Showraki A, Emamghoreishi M, Oftadegan S. Anticonvulsant effect of the aqueous extract and essential oil of Carum carvi L. seeds in a pentylenetetrazol model of seizure in mice. Iran J Med Sci. 2016 May;41(3):200-8.

Trifan A, Aprotosoaie AC, Cioancă O, Hăcianu M, Jităreanu A, Gille E, Miron A. Antioxidant activity of essential oil from carum carvi L. cultivated in north-eastern Romania. Rev Med Chir Soc Med Nat Iasi. 2016 Jul-Sep;120(3):732-6.

Keshavarz A, Minaiyan M, Ghannadi A, Mahzouni P. Effects of Carum carvi L. (Caraway) extract and essential oil on TNBS-induced colitis in rats. Res Pharm Sci. 2013 Jan;8(1):1-8.

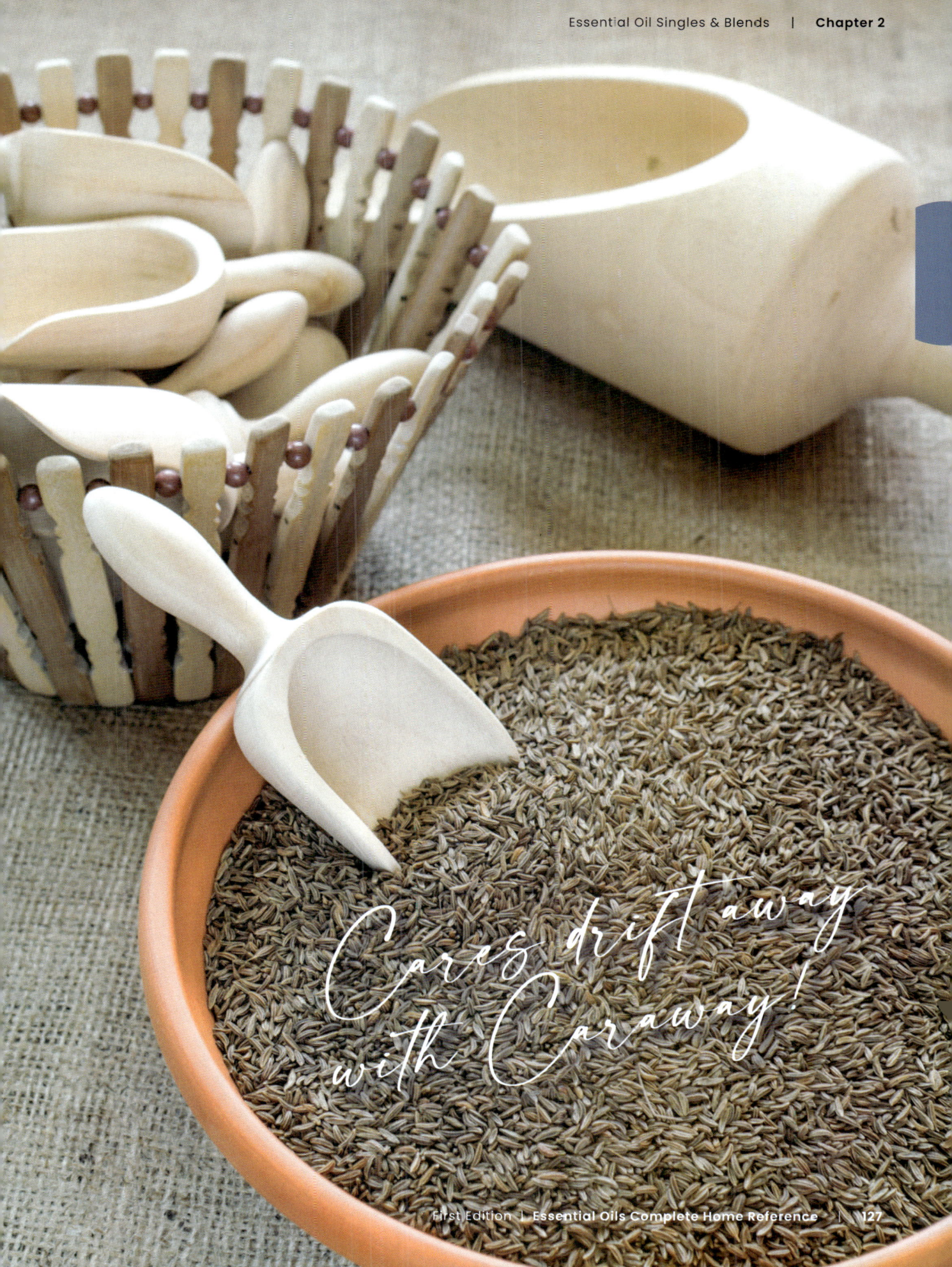

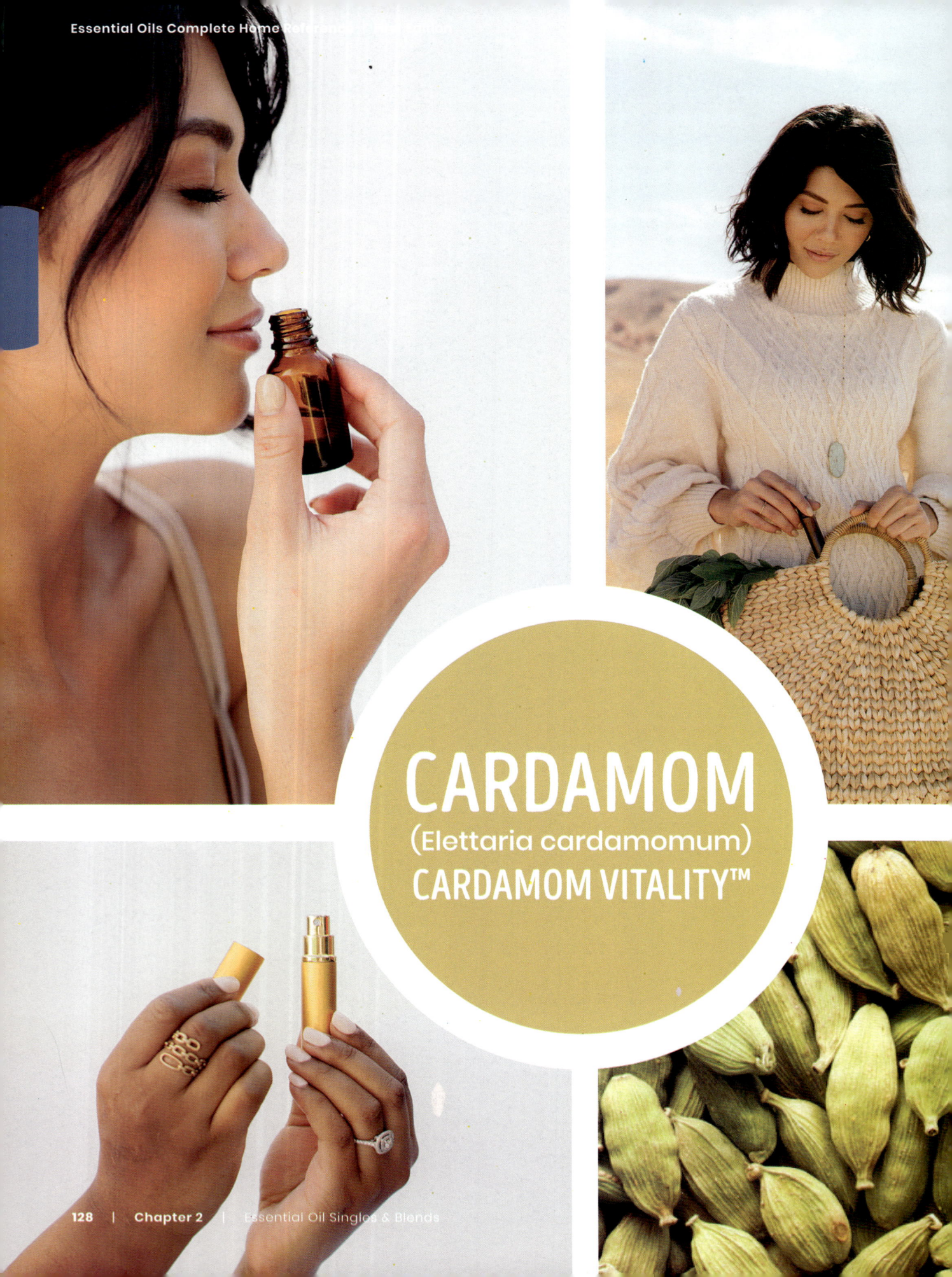

CARDAMOM
(Elettaria cardamomum)
CARDAMOM VITALITY™

Essential Oil Singles & Blends | **Chapter 2**

BOTANICAL FAMILY:
Zingiberaceae

PLANT ORIGIN:
Guatemala

EXTRACTION METHOD:
Steam distilled from seeds

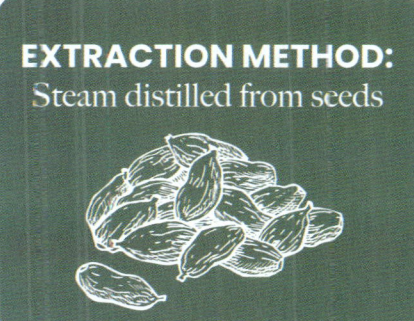

KEY CONSTITUENTS:
Terpinyl Acetate (32-50%),
Eucalyptol (22-42%),
Linalyl Acetate (4-7%),
Sabinene (2-6%),
Linalool (3-6%)

HISTORICAL DATA:
Called "Grains of Paradise" since the Middle Ages, it has been used medicinally by Indian healers for millennia. One of the most prized spices in ancient Greece and Rome, cardamom was cultivated by the king of Babylon around the 7th century BC.
It is mentioned in one of the oldest known medical records, the Ebers Papyrus (dating from 16th century BC), an ancient Egyptian list of 877 prescriptions and recipes.

MEDICAL PROPERTIES:
Antispasmodic (neuromuscular), expectorant, antiparasitic (worms), antioxidant, antimicrobial

USES:
Supports digestion and overall wellness, lung/sinus infection, indigestion, senility, headaches, aphrodisiac, cosmetics

FRAGRANT INFLUENCE:
Uplifting, refreshing, and invigorating; encourages mental clarity

DIRECTIONS:
Aromatic: 30. Topical: 50-50. Dietary (Vitality): Dilute 1 drop essential oil with 1 drop V-6 or other pure carrier oil. Put in a capsule and take up to 3 times daily as a dietary supplement.

CAUTIONS:

SELECTED RESEARCH:

da Fonsêca DV, Filho C daSMB, Lima TC, de Almeida RN, de Sousa DP. Anticonvulsant Essential Oils and Their Relationship with Oxidative Stress in Epilepsy. Biomolecules. Dec 9(12): 835. Published online 2019 Dec 6.

Gomaa AA, Makboul RM, El-Mokhtar MA, Abdel-Rahman EA, Ahmed IA, Nicola MA. Terpenoid-rich Elettaria cardamomum extract prevents Alzheimer-like alterations induced in diabetic rats via inhibition of GSK3β activity, oxidative stress and pro-inflammatory cytokines. Cytokine. 2019 Jan;113:405-416. Epub 2018 Oct 24.

Masoumi-Ardakani Y, Mahmoudvand H, Mirzaei A, Esmaeilpour K, Ghazvini H, Khalifeh S, Sepehri G. The effect of Elettaria cardamomum extract on anxiety-like behavior in a rat model of post-traumatic stress disorder. Biomed Pharmacother. 2017 Mar;87:489-95. Epub 2017 Jan 7.

Nagashree S, Archana KK, Srinivas P, Srinivasan K, Sowbhagya HB. Anti-hypercholesterolemic influence of the spice cardamom (Elettaria cardamomum) in experimental rats. J Sci Food Agric. 2017 Aug;97(10):3204-3210. Epub 2017 Jan 23.

Kumari S, Dutta A. Histological and ultrastructural studies on the toxic effect of pan masala and amelioration by Elettaria cardamomum. Chin J Nat Med. 2014 Mar;12(3):199-203.

Nitasha Bhat GM, Nayak N, Vinodraj K, Chandralekha N, Mathai P, Cherian C. Comparison of the efficacy of cardamom (Elettaria cardamomum) with pioglitazone on dexamethasone-induced hepatic steatosis, dyslipidemia, and hyperglycemia in albino rats. J Adv Pharm Technol Res. 2015 Jul-Sep;6(3):136-40. Epub Sep 1.

Qiblawi S, Al-Hazimi A, Al-Mogbel M, Hossain A, Bagchi D. Chemopreventive effects of cardamom (Elettaria cardamomum L.) on chemically induced skin carcinogenesis in Swiss albino mice. J Med Food. 2012 Jun;15(6):576-80. Epub 2012 Mar 9.

Singh G, Kiran Shashi, Marimuthu P, Isidorov V, Vinogorova V. Antioxidant and antimicrobial activities of essential oil and various oleoresins of Elettaria cardamomum (seeds and pods). J Sci Food Agric. 2008 Jan;88(2):280-9.

Essential Oils Complete Home Reference | First Edition

BOTANICAL FAMILY: Apiaceae

PLANT ORIGIN: France

EXTRACTION METHOD: Steam distilled from seeds

KEY CONSTITUENTS: Carotol (25-49%), Alpha-Pinene (2-18%), Sabinene (1-16%), Beta-Caryophyllene (3-10%), Beta-Bisabolene (up to 7%), Caryophyllene Oxide (up to 6%), Daucol (up to 2%)

CARROT SEED & CARROT SEED VITALITY™
(Daucus carota sativa)

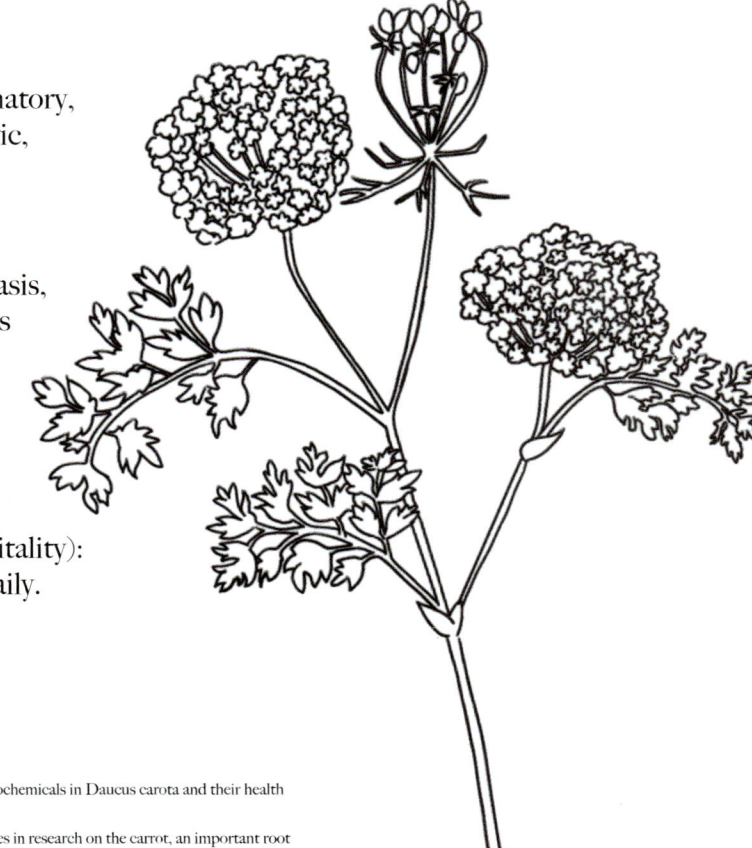

Carrot seed oil is traditionally used for kidney and digestive disorders and to relieve liver congestion.

MEDICAL PROPERTIES:
Antiparasitic, antibacterial, anti-inflammatory, antiseptic, antioxidant, purgative, diuretic, vasodilatory, antifungal

USES:
Skin conditions (eczema, oily skin, psoriasis, wrinkles), water retention, liver problems

FRAGRANT INFLUENCE:
Woody, earthy, sweet smell

DIRECTIONS:
Aromatic: 3O. Topical: Neat. Dietary (Vitality): Put 4 drops in a capsule. Take 3 times daily.

CAUTIONS:

SELECTED RESEARCH:

Ahmad T, Cawood M, Iqbal Q, Ariño A, Batool A, Tariq RMS, Azam M, Akhtar S. Phytochemicals in Daucus carota and their health benefits—Review Article. Foods. 2019 Sep 19.

Que F, Hou X-L, Wang G-L, Xu Z-S, Tan G-F, Wang Y-H, Khadr A, Xiong A-S. Advances in research on the carrot, an important root vegetable in the Apiaceae family. Hortic Res. 2019; 6:69. Published online 2019 Jun 1.

Afzal M, Kazmi I, Kaur R, Ahmad A, Pravez M, Anwar F. Comparison of protective and curative potential of Daucus carota root extract on renal ischemia reperfusion injury in rats. Pharm Biol. 2013 Jul;51(7):856-62. Epub 2013 Apr 29.

Alves-Silva JM, Zuzarte M, Gonçalves MJ, Cavaleiro C, Cruz MT, Cardoso SM, Salgueiro L. New claims for wild carrot (Daucus carota subsp. carota) essential oil. Evid Based Complement Alternat Med. 2016;2016:9045196. Epub 2016 Feb 14.

Rokbeni N, M'rabet Y, Dziri S, Chaabane H, Jemli M, Fernandez X, Boulila A. Variation of the chemical composition and antimicrobial activity of the essential oils of natural populations of Tunisian Daucus carota L. (Apiaceae). Chem & Biodivers. 2013 Dec;10(12):2278-90.

Shebaby WN, Daher CF, El-Sibai M, Bodman-Smith K, Mansour A, Karam MC, Mroueh M. Antioxidant and hepatoprotective activities of the oil fractions from wild carrot (Daucus carota ssp. carota). Pharm Biol. 2015 Sep;53(9):1258-94. Epub 2015 Apr 9.

Zgheib P, Daher CF, Mroueh M, Nasrallah A, Taleb RI, El-Sibai M. Daucus carota pentane/diethyl ether fraction inhibits motility and reduces invasion of cancer cells. Chemotherapy. 2014;60(5-6):302-9. Epub 2015 Jun 13.

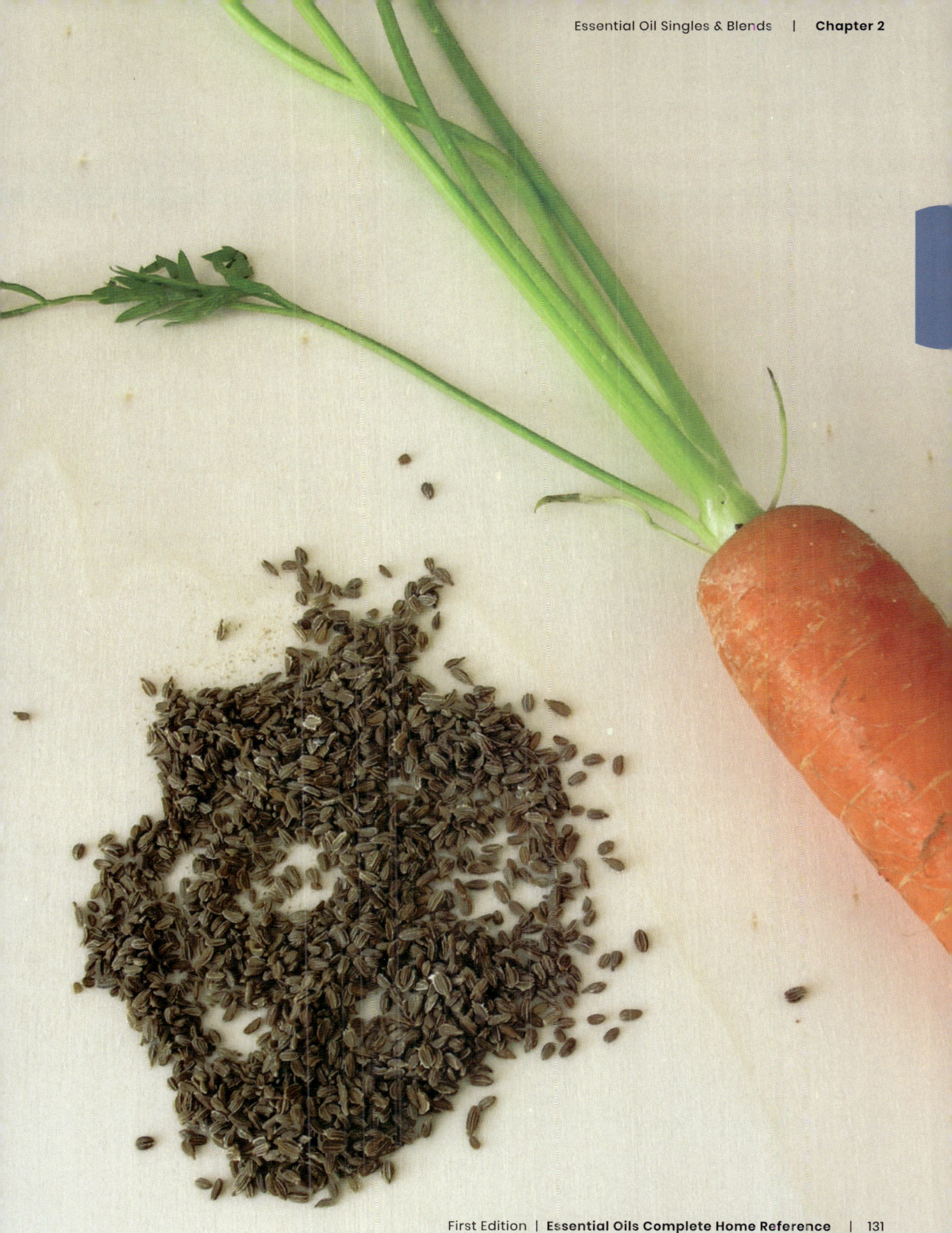

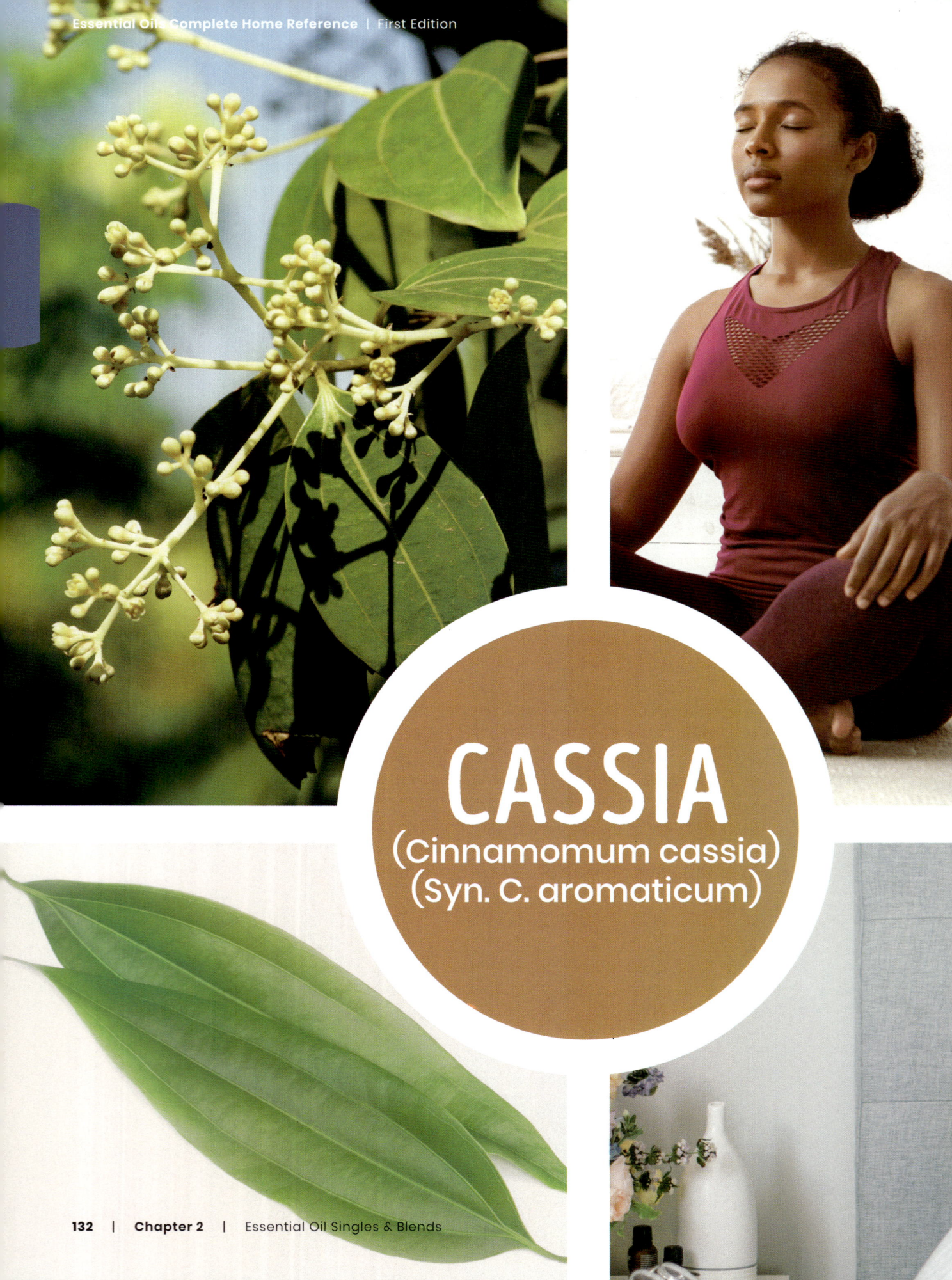

CASSIA
(Cinnamomum cassia)
(Syn. C. aromaticum)

Essential Oil Singles & Blends | Chapter 2

BOTANICAL FAMILY:
Lamiaceae

PLANT ORIGIN:
Vietnam

EXTRACTION METHOD:
Steam distilled from herb/leaf

KEY CONSTITUENTS:
Methyl Chavicol (75-88%)
Linalool (up to 5%)
Eucalyptol (1-5%)
Trans-Beta-Ocimene (up to 3%),
Methyl Eugenol (up to 3%),
Camphor (up to 1%)

HISTORICAL DATA:
Cassia is rich in biblical history and is mentioned in one of the oldest known medical records, the Ebers Papyrus (dating from 16th century BC), an ancient Egyptian list of 877 prescriptions and recipes. It is mentioned as a holy anointing oil in the Old Testament. It is also listed as one of the 50 fundamental herbs of Chinese tradition.

Note: While its aroma is similar to cinnamon, cassia is chemically and physically quite different.

MEDICAL PROPERTIES:
Anti-inflammatory (COX-2 inhibitor), antifungal, antibacterial, antiviral, antiparasitical, anticoagulant

USES:
Cataracts, fungal infections (ringworm, candida), atherosclerosis, anxiolytic, diabetes, arteriosclerosis, uplifting, comforting, centering, self-awareness, grounding and balancing aroma that inspires emotional release, purifies air of odors

FRAGRANT INFLUENCE:
Similar to cinnamon, but a little hotter and more pungent

DIRECTIONS:
Aromatic: 30. Topical: 20-80. Dietary: Dilute 1 drop essential oil with 4 drops V-6 or other pure carrier oil. Put in a capsule and take 1 daily or as directed by a health care professional.

CAUTIONS:

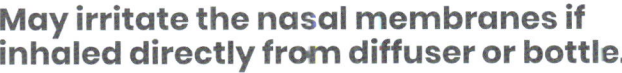

May irritate the nasal membranes if inhaled directly from diffuser or bottle.

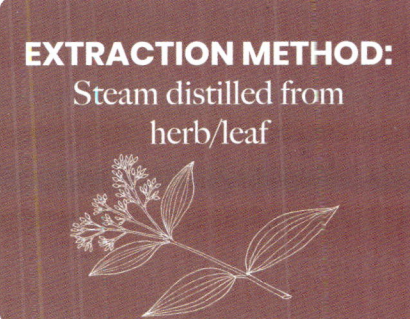

SELECTED RESEARCH:

Afrin F, Chouhan G, Islamuddin M, Want MY, Ozbak HA, Hemeg HA. Cinnamomum cassia exhibits antileishmanial activity against Leishmania donovani infection in vitro and in vivo. PLoS Negl Trop Dis. 2019 May; 13(5): e0007227. Published online 2019 May 9.

Lee EJ, Chung TW, Lee JH, Kim BS, Kim EY, Lee SO, Ha KT. Water-extracted branch of Cinnamomum cassia promotes lung cancer cell apoptosis by inhibiting pyruvate dehydrogenase kinase activity. J Pharmacol Sci. 2018 Oct;138(2):146-154. doi: 10.1016/j.jphs.2018.10.005. Epub 2018 Oct 18.

Chang WL, Cheng FC, Wang SP, Chou ST, Shih Y. Cinnamomum cassia essential oil and its major constituent cinnamaldehyde induced cell cycle arrest and apoptosis in human oral squamous cell carcinoma HSC-3 cells. Environ Toxicol. 2017 Feb;32(2):456-68.

Hoehn AN, Stockert AL. The effects of Cinnamomum cassia on blood glucose values are greater than those of dietary changes alone. Nutr Metab Insights. 2012 Dec 13;5:77-83. Epub 2012 Jan 1.

Luo Q, Wang SM, Lu Q, Luo J, Cheng YX. Identification of compounds from the water soluble extract of Cinnamomum cassia barks and their inhibitory effects against high-glucose-induced mesangial cells. Molecules. 2013 Sep 5;18(9):10930-43.

Sun L, Zong SB, Li JC, Lv YZ, Liu LN, Wang ZZ, Zhou J, Cao L, Kou JP, Xiao W. The essential oil from the twigs of Cinnamomum cassia Presl alleviates pain and inflammation in mice. J. Ethnopharmacol. 2016 Oct 22;194:904-912. Epub 2016 Nov 5.

Trinh NT, Dumas E, Thanh ML, Degraeve P, Amara CB, Gharsallaoui A, Oulahal N. Effect of a Vietnamese Cinnamomum cassia essential oil and its major component trans-cinnamaldehyde on the cell viability, membrane integrity, membrane fluidity, and proton motive force of Listeria innocua. Can J Microbiol. 2015 Apr;61(4):263-71. Epub 2015 Jan 13.

Yu C, Liu SL, Qi MH, Zou X. Cinnamaldehyde/chemotherapeutic agents interaction and drug-metabolizing genes in colorectal cancer. Mol Med Rep. 2014 Feb;9(2):669-76. Epub 2013 Nov 26.

First Edition | Essential Oils Complete Home Reference

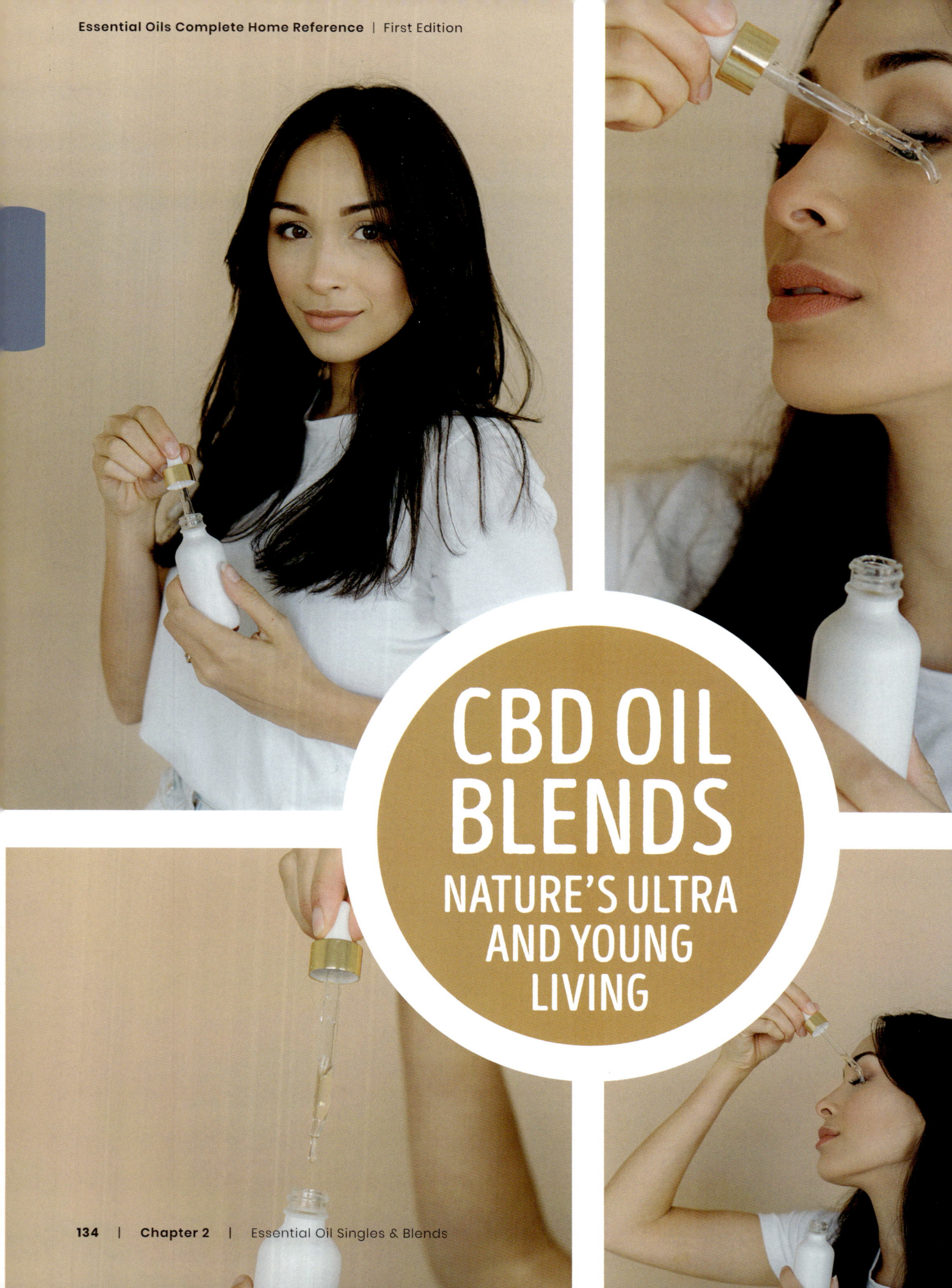

Essential Oils Complete Home Reference | First Edition

CBD OIL BLENDS
NATURE'S ULTRA AND YOUNG LIVING

134 | Chapter 2 | Essential Oil Singles & Blends

ABOUT CBD OIL BLENDS™:

These Smart Spectrum CBD products are made from a combination of CBD (cannabidiol) isolate, which is one of the primary cannabinoids found in the hemp plant, and Young Living's pure, therapeutic-grade essential oils. These CBD products are Young Living Seed to Seal certified. No high-inducing THC is present, but the isolate-and-essential-oil combination provides a variety of benefits, depending on the product used.

While both plants are from the same Cannabis plant family, hemp is completely different from marijuana in its function, cultivation, and application. CBD will not get you high; it does not have euphoric side effects. Cannabinoids interact with your body's endocannabinoid system receptors, which are found in places such as your brain, connective tissues, immune cells, organs, and glands. They help regulate critical processes throughout your body, including pain, memory, appetite, mood, and peripheral nervous system.

The goal of the endocannabinoid system is to always promote homeostasis, which is a state of stability and balance. By interacting with that system and promoting homeostasis, CBD may help you feel your best.

Although much is still to be learned about the effects of CBD, studies suggest that it may provide a powerful, safe, natural treatment for many health issues.

Nature's Ultra website adds: When it comes to your health and wellness, it's natural to ask questions about safety. If you're nervous about the risk of overdosing on CBD, you can rest easy! According to the National Cancer Institute, cannabinoid receptors are not located in the areas of the brainstem that regulate breathing, so CBD does not cause fatal overdoses. That should assuage any concerns you may have about potential overdoses from CBD.

If you're wondering if you'll form a dependency on CBD, you can rest easy there, too! According to this 2018 World Health Organization critical review of cannabidiols, "In humans, CBD exhibits no effects indicative of any abuse or dependence potential." Unlike its cousin THC, CBD is not psychoactive and does not cause euphoria. Because there's no euphoric side effects to CBD, you can safely use it without forming a dependency on it. Of course, the quality of the products that you use makes a big difference in the overall safety profile. That's why we developed world-class quality assurance systems to ensure that all of our Nature's Ultra CBD oils are safe and effective. All of our ingredients are natural, organic, vegan-approved, and gluten-free, and we have a Seed to Seal® certified partner farm, so we can provide you with the highest-quality product.

Certified by a third-party lab: Vegan, Gluten-free, 99% Pure CBD, Non-GMO, No THC, Natural ingredients

MEDICAL PROPERTIES & USES:

Pain relieving, antianxiety, antidepressant, cancer symptom relieving, possible anticancer properties, anti-inflammatory, antiacne, neuroprotective, eases symptoms related to epilepsy and Parkinson's disease, possible reduction of the progression of Alzheimer's disease, may benefit heart health, antipsychotic, substance abuse treatment, antitumoral, antidiabetic, sleep enhancing, skin care

POSSIBLE SIDE EFFECTS:

Diarrhea, changes in appetite and weight, fatigue, possible interference with medications

DIRECTIONS:

Shake well before use. To preserve freshness, store away from heat, light, and humidity. For best results, keep refrigerated after opening.

CBD BLENDS (CINNAMON)
(500 mg and 1000 mg strengths)

MEDICAL PROPERTIES & USES:
Cinnamon CBD Oil is perfect when you need a boost.

INGREDIENTS:
MCT coconut oil, Cannabidiol (CBD), Cinnamon Bark, Organic stevia leaf extract

DIRECTIONS:
Apply 1 full dropper to desired area.

CAUTIONS:

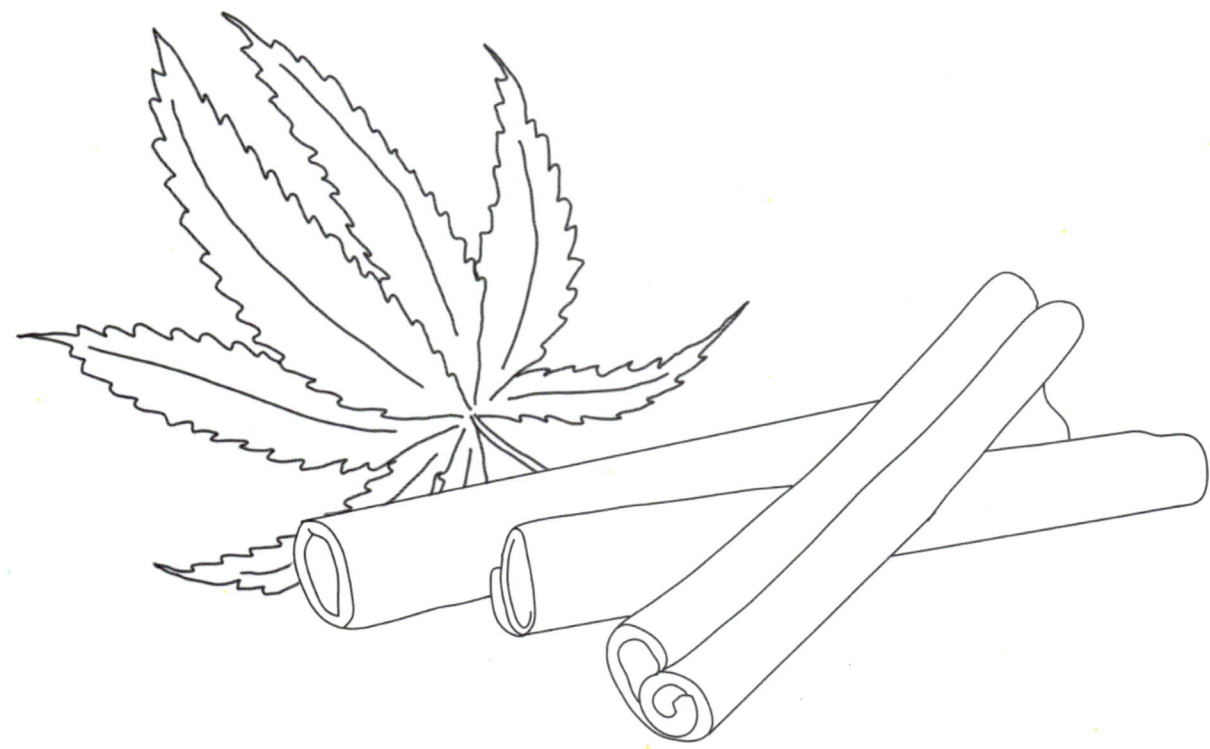

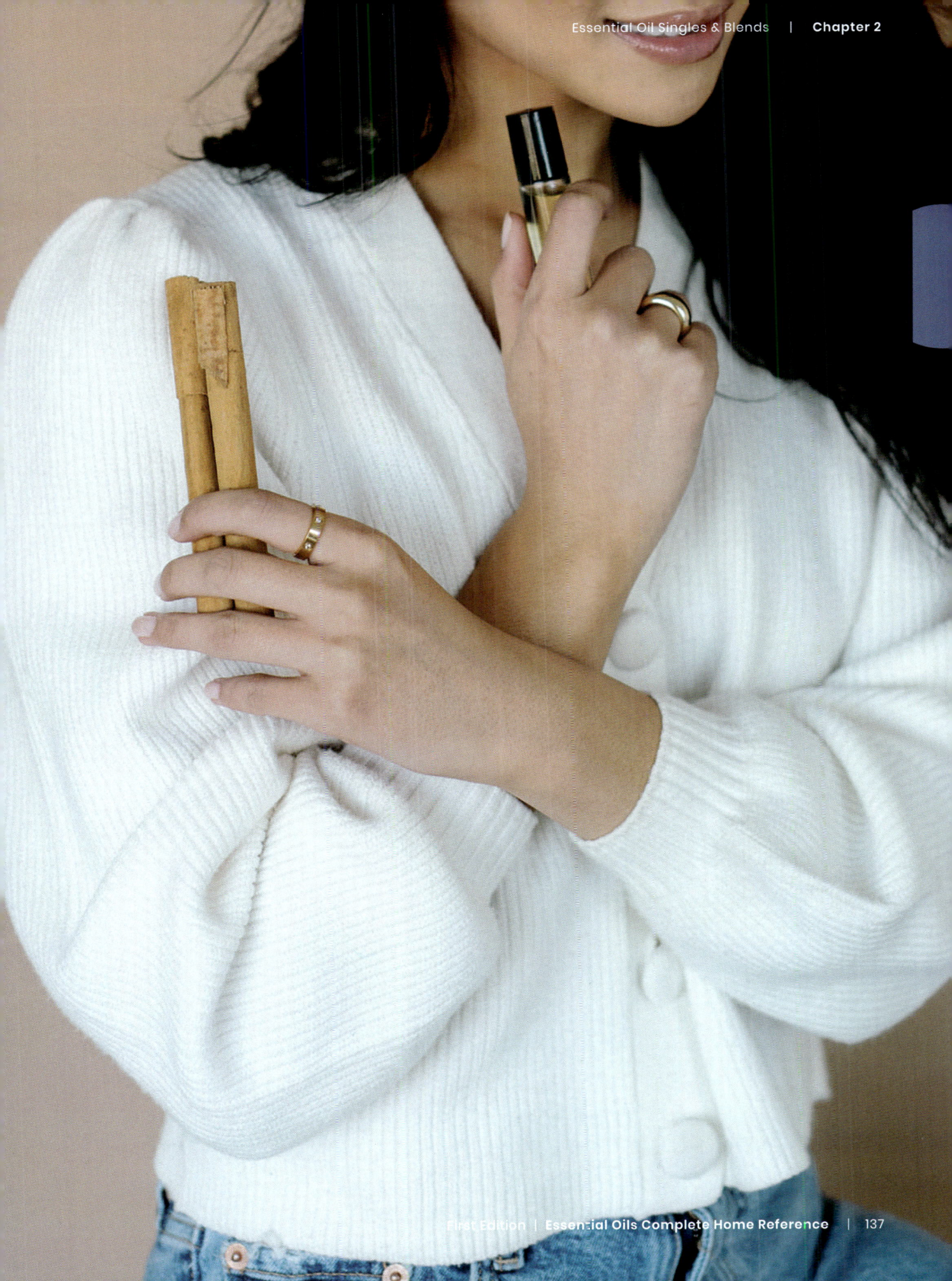

CBD BLENDS (CITRUS)
(500 mg and 1000 mg strengths)

MEDICAL PROPERTIES & USES:
Citrus CBD Oil is perfect when you need more energy.

INGREDIENTS:
MCT coconut oil, Cannabidiol (CBD), Cinnamon Bark, Organic stevia leaf extract

DIRECTIONS:
Apply 1 full dropper to desired area.

CAUTIONS:

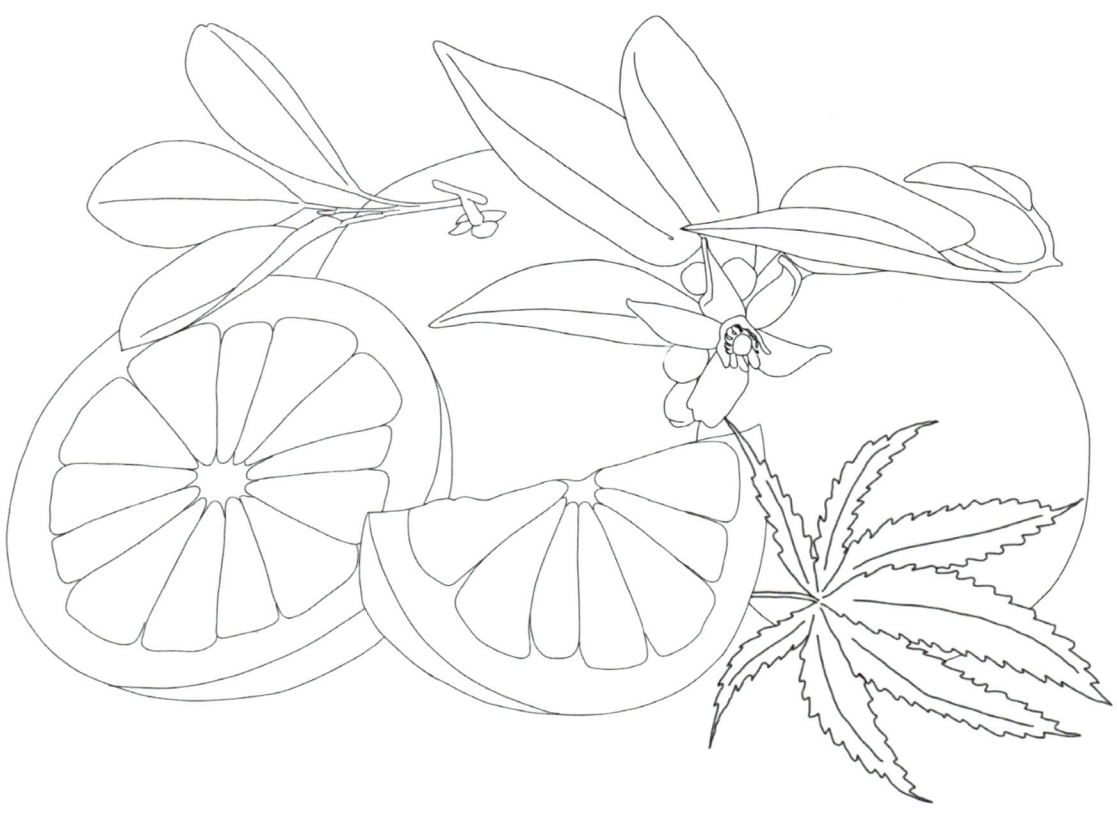

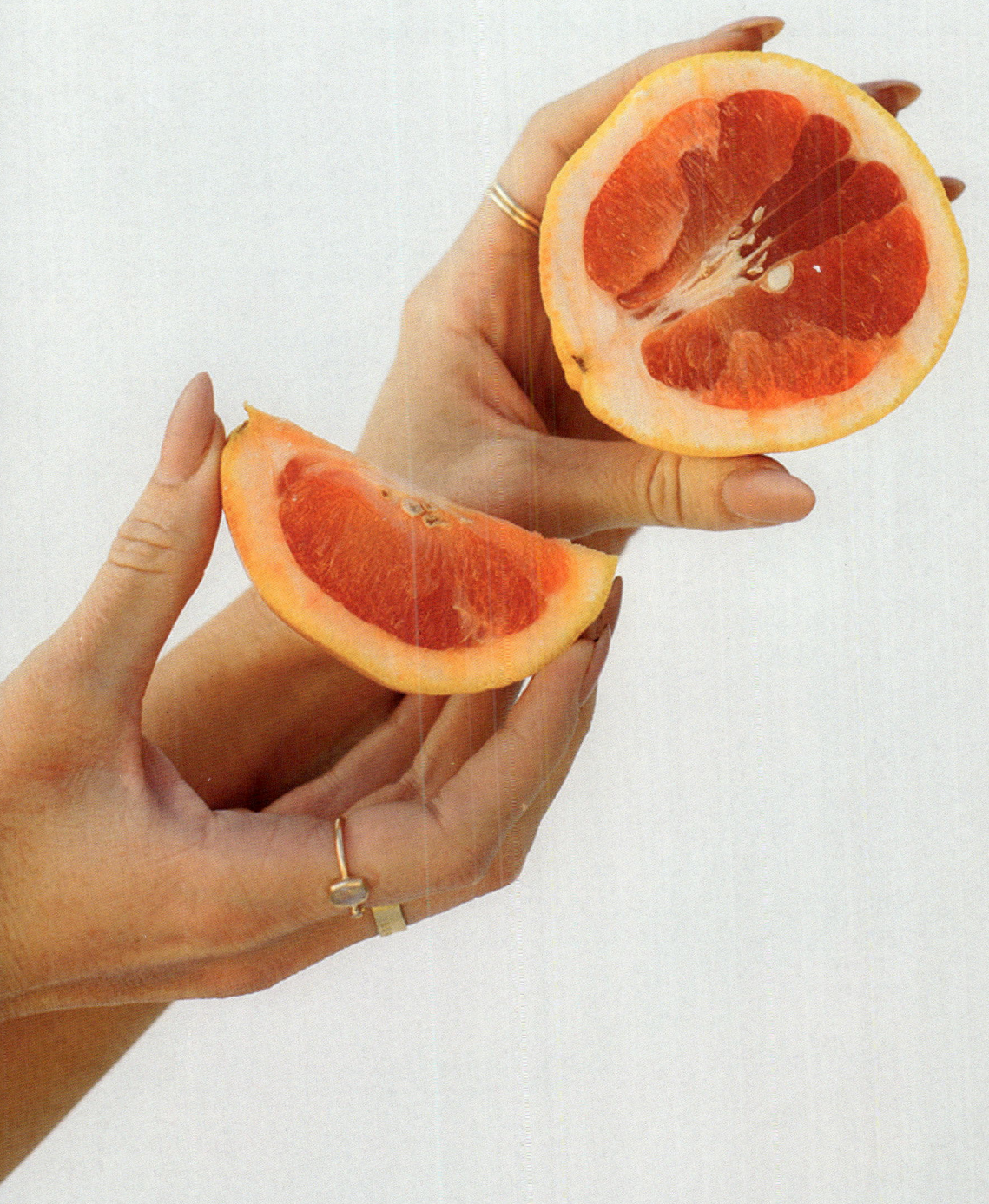

CBD BLENDS (COOL MINT)
(500 mg and 1000 mg strengths)

MEDICAL PROPERTIES & USES:
Cool Mint CBD Oil is great when you're looking for an uplifting scent.

INGREDIENTS:
MCT coconut oil, Cannabidiol (CBD), Peppermint, Spearmint, Organic stevia leaf extract

DIRECTIONS:
Apply 1 full dropper to desired area.

CAUTIONS:

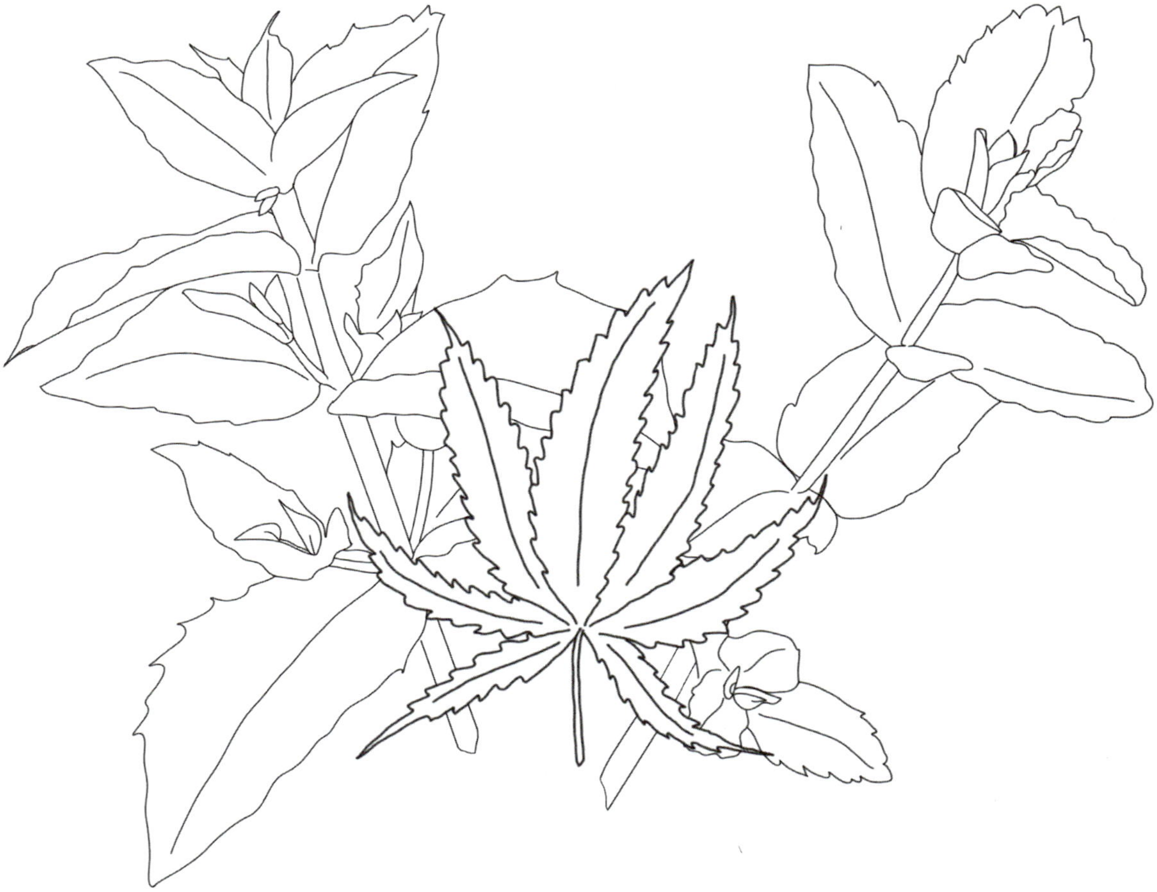

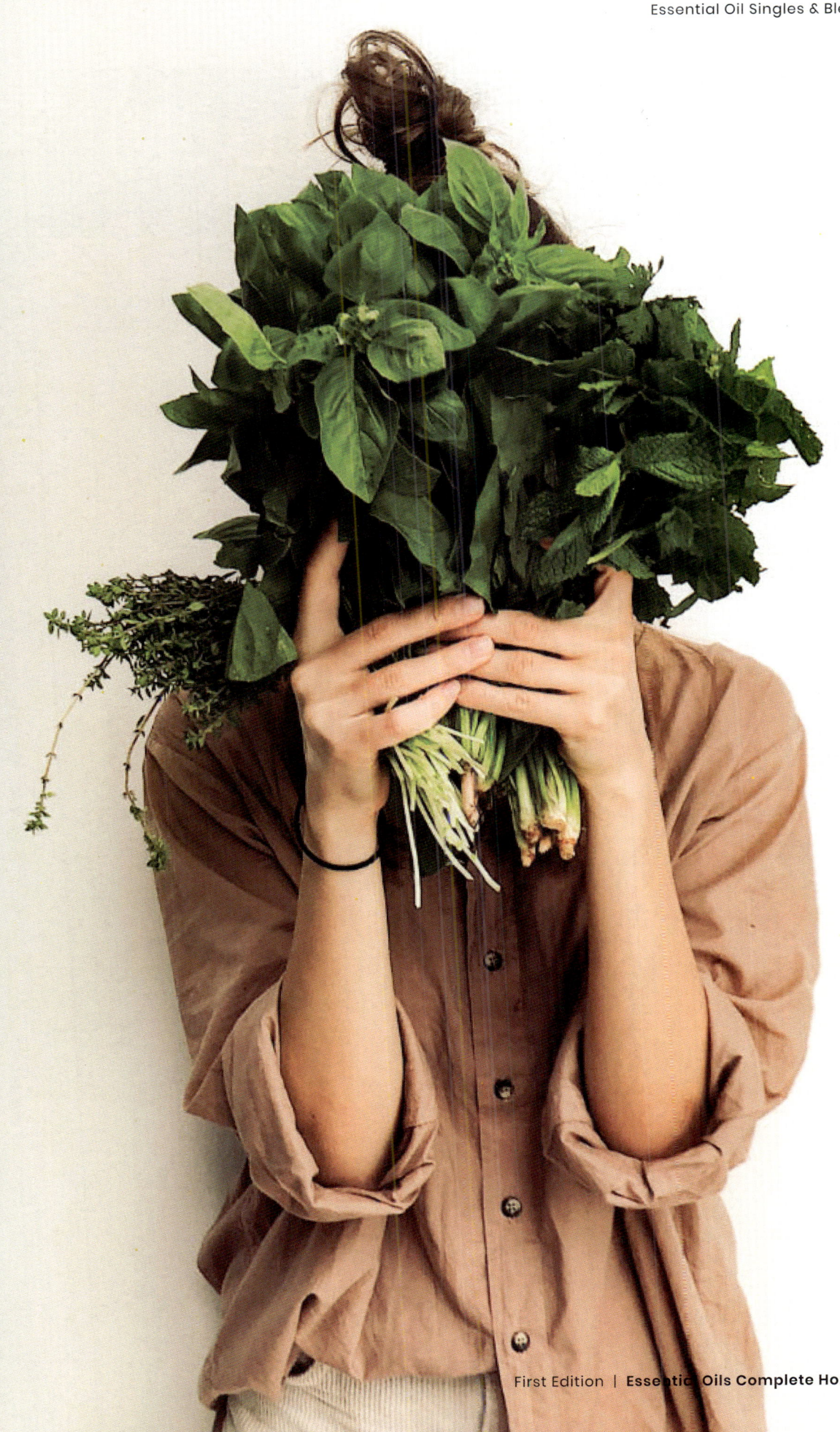

CBD BLENDS (CALM ROLL-ON)
(300 mg and 600 mg strengths)

MEDICAL PROPERTIES & USES:

Our Calm CBD Roll-On combines CBD oil and Young Living essential oils that work together to quiet and relax your mind and help you wind down for the night and enjoy a restful night's sleep.

INGREDIENTS:

Carrier oil blend: Apricot kernel oil,† Argan oil,† Avocado oil,† Camellia seed oil,† Evening primrose oil,† Hempseed oil,† Neem oil,† Rosehip seed oil,† Sweet almond oil,† Cannabidiol (CBD) oil,† Lavender, Vetiver, Eucalyptus Globulus, Frankincense, Orange, Ylang Ylang

DIRECTIONS:

Apply generously to chest and neck as desired.

CAUTIONS:

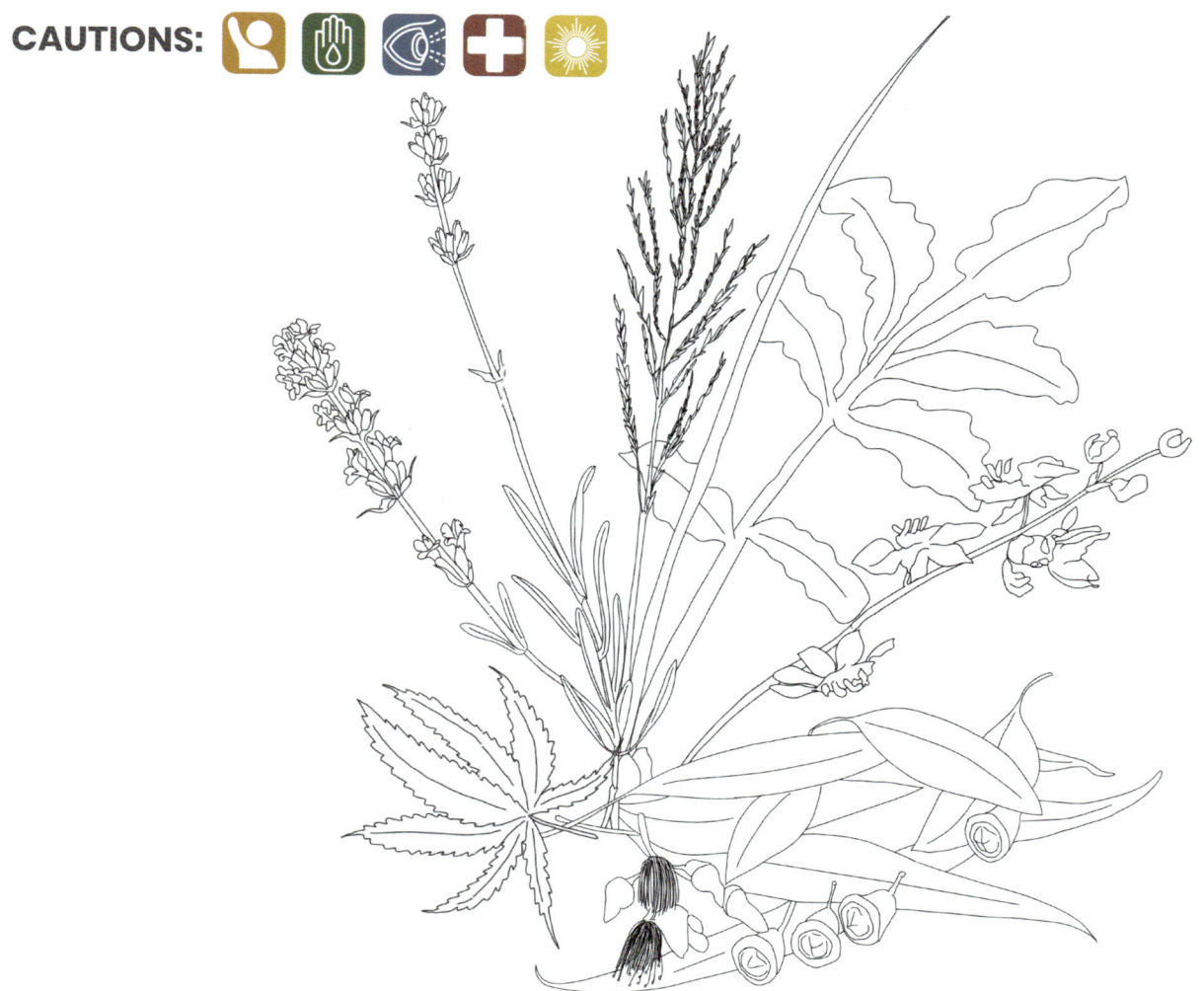

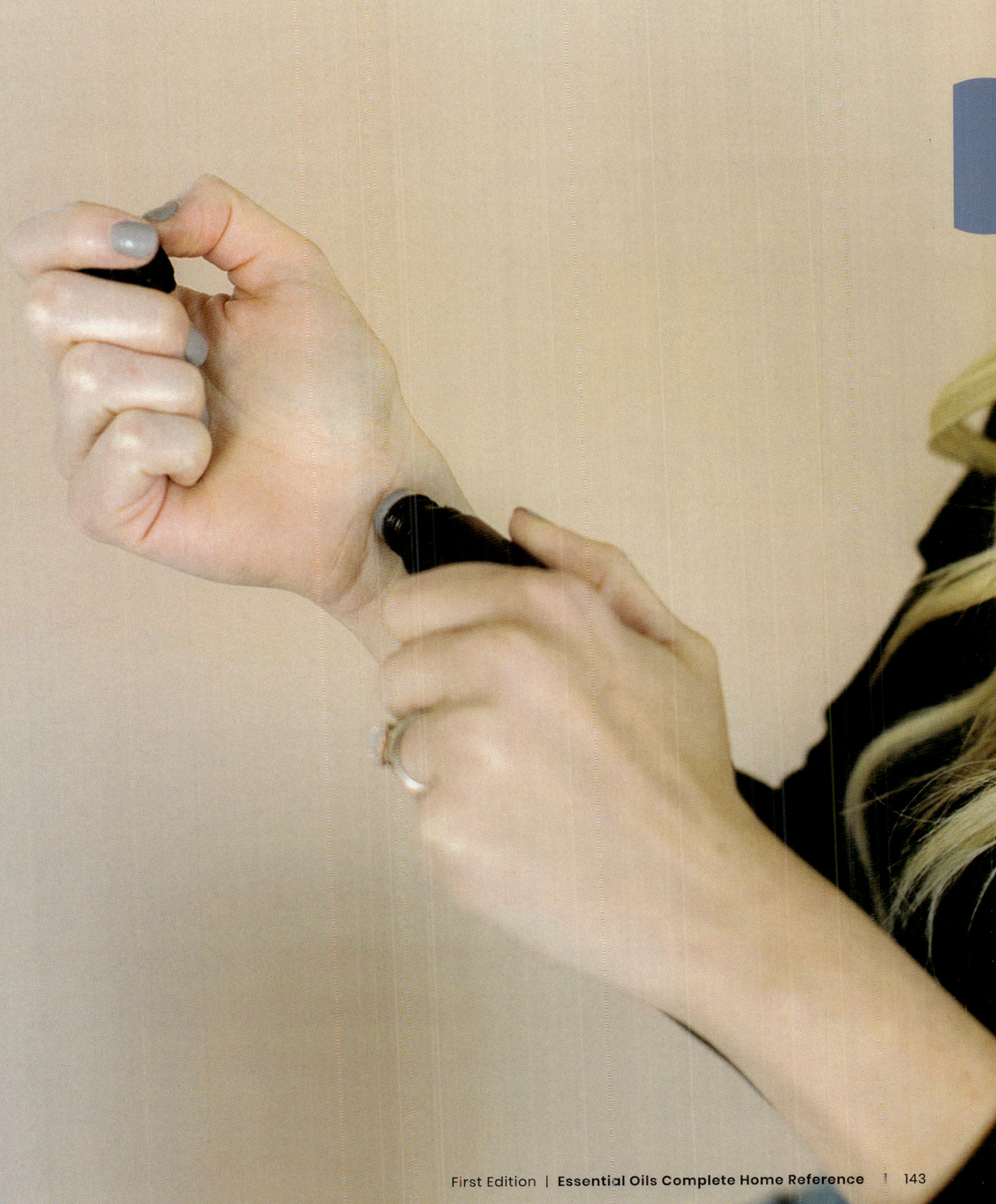

BOTANICAL FAMILY: Pinaceae

PLANT ORIGIN: Morocco; Cedrus atlantica is the species most closely related to the biblical Cedars of Lebanon

EXTRACTION METHOD: Steam distilled from the wood

KEY CONSTITUENTS: Beta-Himachalene (39-53%), Alpha-Himachalene (13-20%), Gamma-Himachalene (8-16%), Trans-Alpha-Atlantone (up to 4%), Delta-Cadinene (up to 4%)

CEDARWOOD
(Cedrus atlantica)

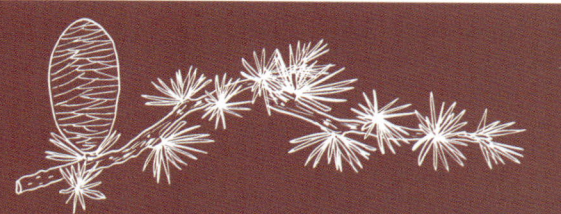

Throughout antiquity, cedarwood has been used in medicines. The Egyptians used it for embalming the dead. It was used as both a traditional medicine and incense in Tibet.

MEDICAL PROPERTIES:
Antibacterial, antifungal, lymphatic stimulant, inhibits proliferation of leukemia cells, antiparasitic, insecticide

USES:
Treats alopecia areata, sedative/relaxant, hair loss, arteriosclerosis, ADHD, skin problems (acne, eczema)

FRAGRANT INFLUENCE:
Centered, balanced aroma; stimulates the limbic region of the brain (the center of emotions), stimulates the pineal gland, which releases melatonin. Terry Friedmann, MD, found in clinical tests that this oil may treat ADD and ADHD (attention deficit disorders) in children. It is recognized for its calming, purifying properties.

DIRECTIONS:
Aromatic: 6o. Topical: Neat. Dietary: Take as a dietary supplement.

CAUTIONS:

SELECTED RESEARCH:

Powers CN, Satyal P, Mayo JA, McFeeters H, McFeeters RL. Bigger Data Approach to Analysis of Essential Oils and Their Antifungal Activity against Aspergillus niger, Candida albicans, and Cryptococcus neoformans. Molecules. 2019 Aug; 24(16): 2868. Published online 2019 Aug 7.

Martins DF, Emer AA, Batisti AP, Donatello N, Carlesso MG, Mazzardo-Martins L, Venzke D, Micke GA, Pizzolatti MG, Piovezan AP, dos Santos ARS. Inhalation of Cedrus atlantica essential oil alleviates pain behavior through activation of descending pain modulation pathways in a mouse model of postoperative pain. J Ethnopharmacol. 2015 Dec 4;175:30-38.

Saab Am, Lampronti I, Borgatti M, Finotti A, Harb F, Safi S, Gambari R. In vitro evaluation of the anti-proliferative activities of the wood essential oils of three Cedrus species against K562 human chronic myelogenous leukemia cells. Nat Prod Res. 2012;26(23):2227-31. Epub 2011 Dec 16.

Friedmann T. Attention deficit and hyperactivity disorder (ADHD). 2002. (Unpublished study). Available from: http://files.meetup.com/1481956/ADHD%20Research%20by%20Dr.%20Terry%20Friedmann.pdf.

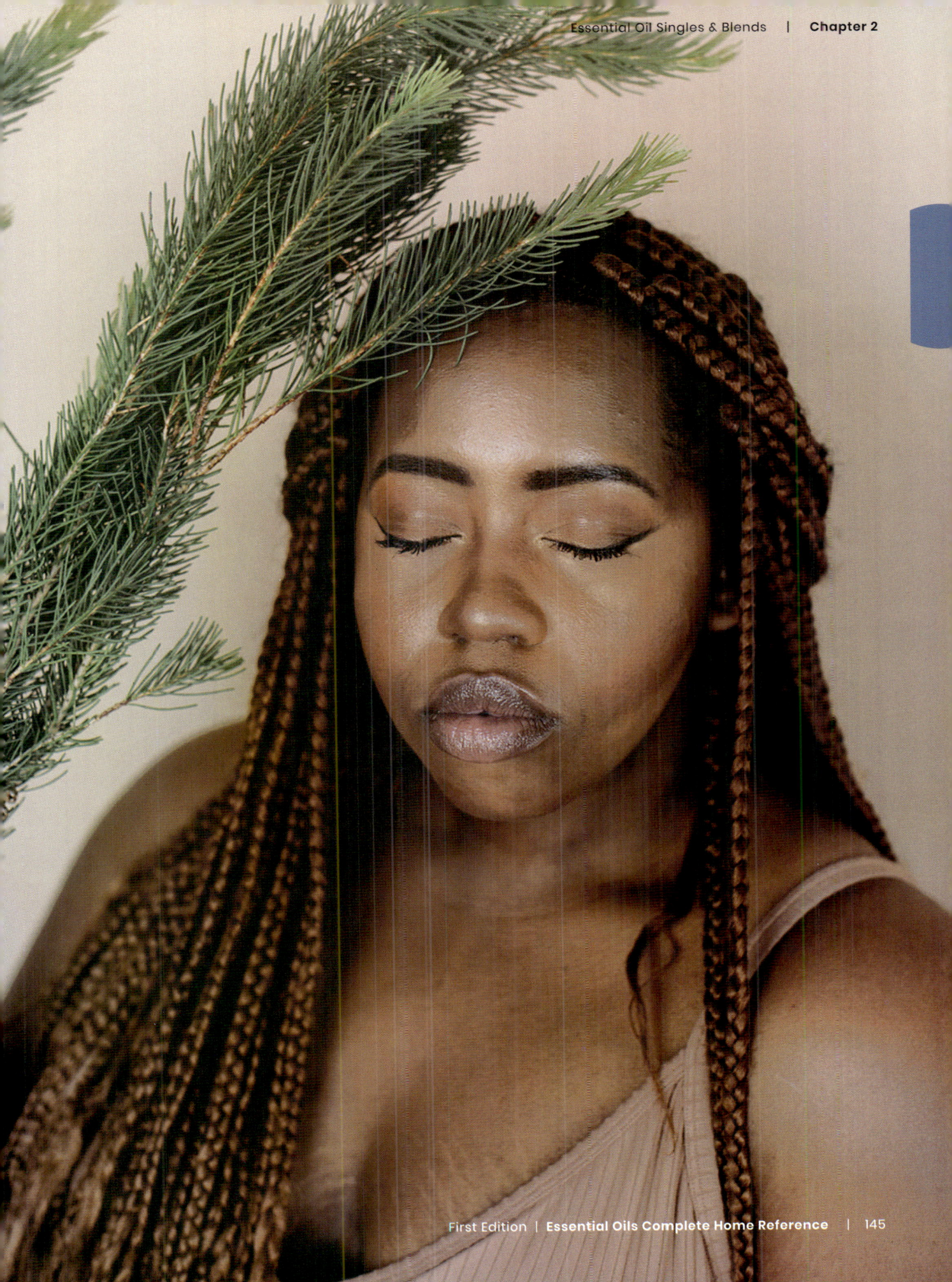

CELEBRATION™
(Essential Oil Blend)

This blend, full of essential oils known for their analgesic, calming, and antibacterial effects, will create harmonic balance for you, encourage positive emotions, alleviate mental fatigue and nervous strain, and reinvigorate you.

MEDICAL PROPERTIES & USES:

Anti-inflammatory, antimicrobial, antioxidative, calming, disease inhibitory, organ protective, pain or swelling reducing, performance enhancing/stimulating, respiratory system supportive, sleep improving, emotion supporting

INGREDIENTS:

Lavender, Angelica, German Chamomile, Cardamom, Rosemary, Peppermint, Dill, Sacred Sandalwood, Ylang Ylang, Frankincense, Orange, Geranium, Hyssop, Spanish Sage, Northern Lights Black Spruce, Coriander, Bergamot, Lemon, Jasmine, Roman Chamomile, Palmarosa, Rose

DIRECTIONS:

Aromatic: 30. Topical: Neat.

CAUTIONS:

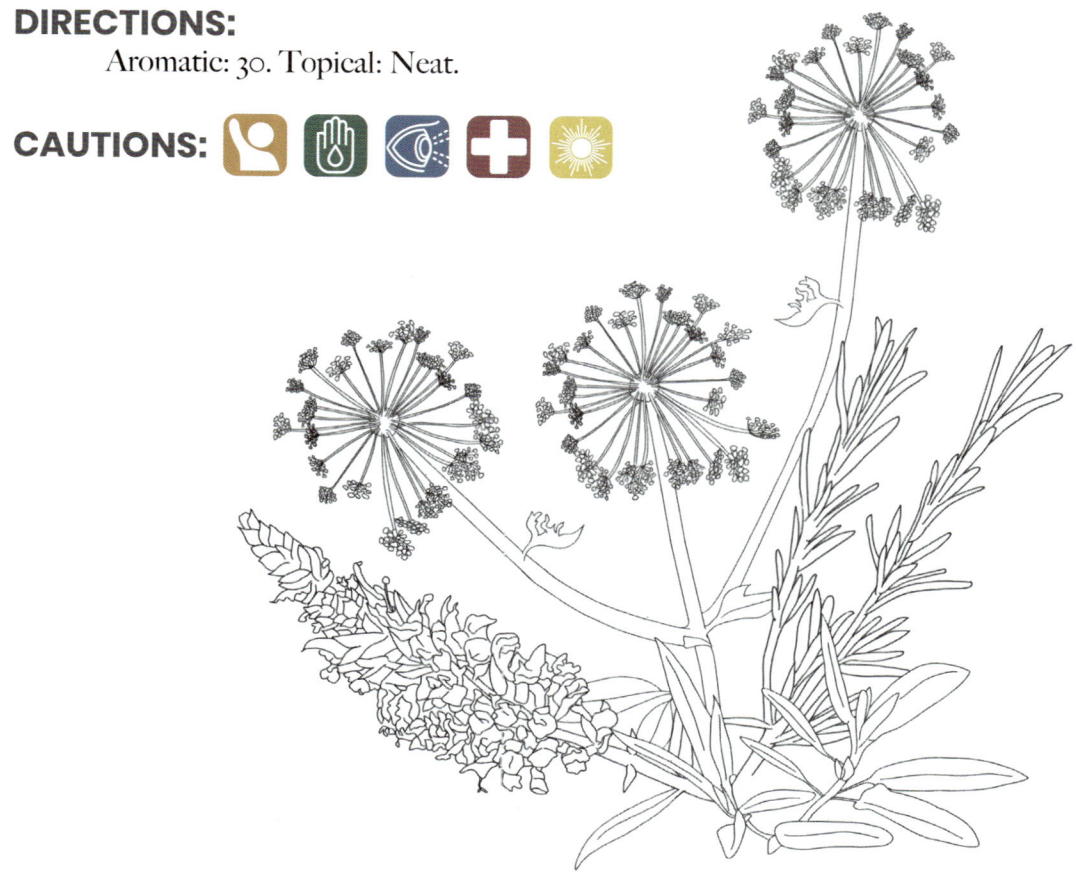

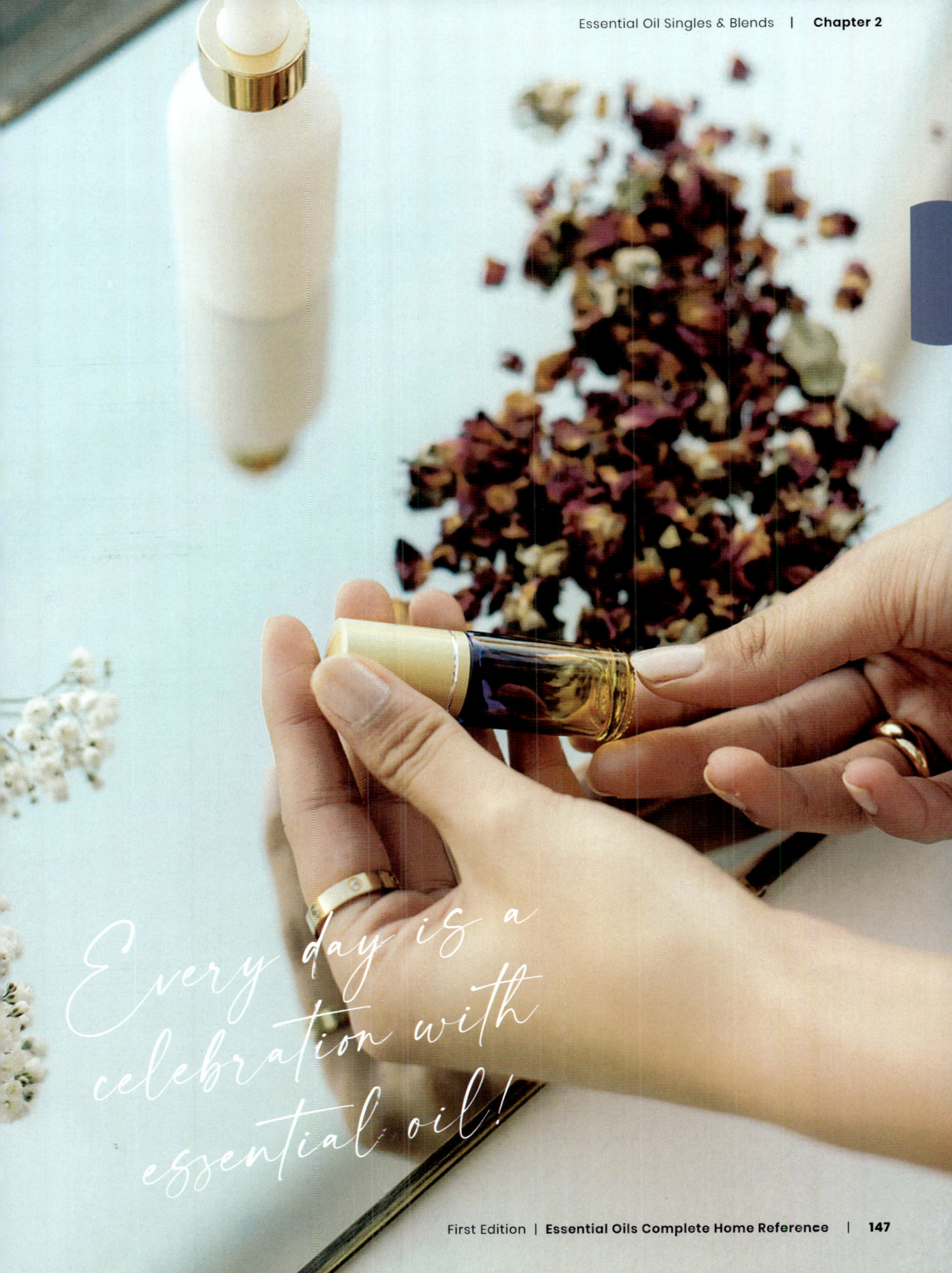

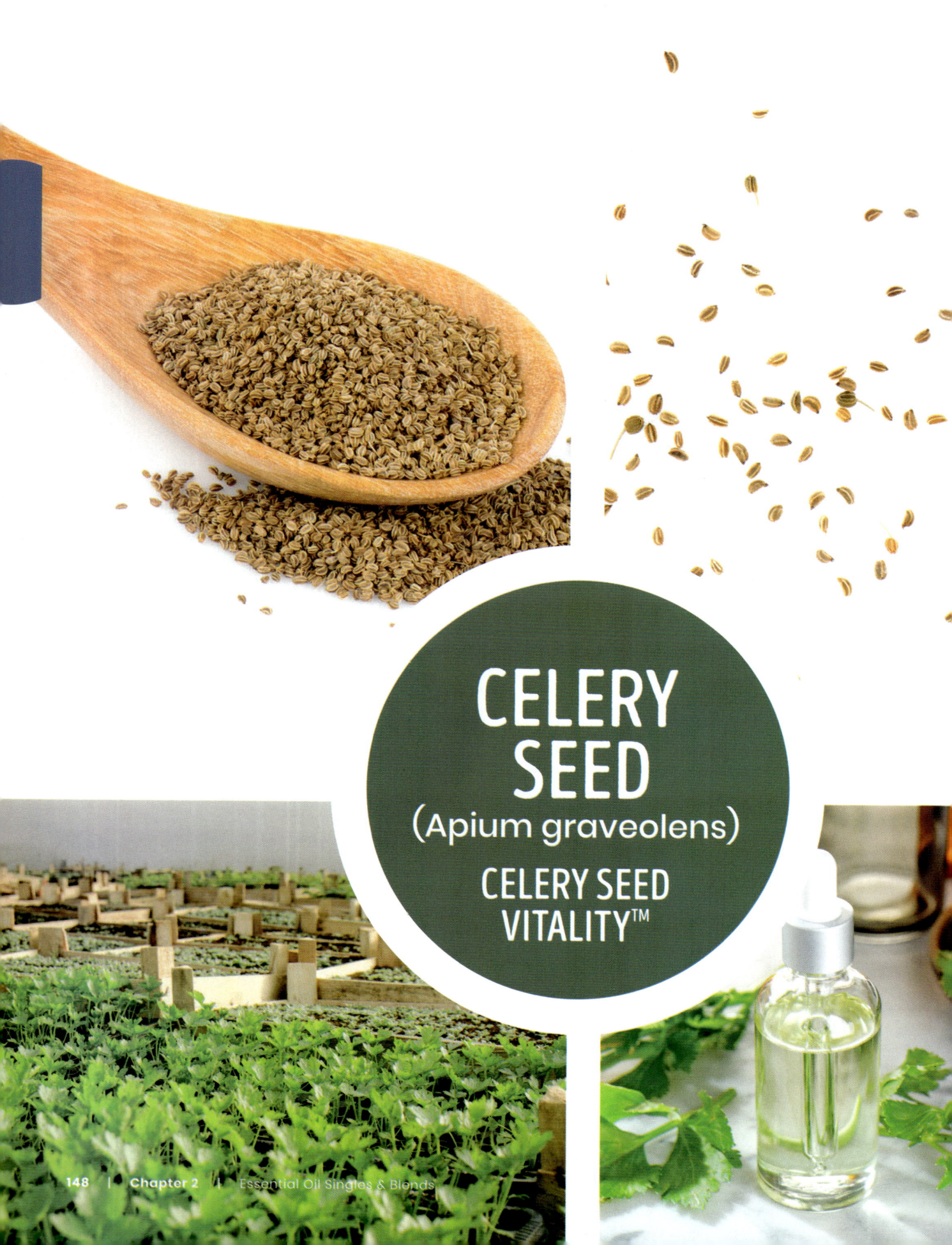

CELERY SEED
(Apium graveolens)

CELERY SEED VITALITY™

BOTANICAL FAMILY:
Apiaceae

PLANT ORIGIN:
India

EXTRACTION METHOD:
Steam distilled from fruit/seeds

KEY CONSTITUENTS:
Limonene (55-86%), Beta Selinene (4-21%), Sedanenolide (up to 10%)

HISTORICAL DATA:
Long recognized as helpful in digestion, liver cleansing, and urinary tract support. It is also said to increase milk flow in nursing mothers.

MEDICAL PROPERTIES:
Antibacterial, antioxidant, antirheumatic, digestive aid, diuretic, liver protectant

USES:
Arthritis/rheumatism, antioxidant, asthma, dizziness, digestive problems, liver problems/hepatitis, facilitates elimination of toxins, inflammation, pain relief

FRAGRANT INFLUENCE:
Insect repellent

DIRECTIONS:
Aromatic: 6o. Topical: 50-50. Dietary (Vitality): Dilute 2 drops with 2 drops of V-6 or other carrier oil. Put in a capsule and take up to 3 times daily or as needed.

CAUTIONS: Do not use if pregnant.

SELECTED RESEARCH:

Hirai M, Ito M. Sedative effects of the essential oil and headspace air of Ocimum basilicum by inhalation in mice. J Nat Med. 2019 Jan;73(1):283-288.

Kavoosi G, Amirghofran Z. Chemical composition, radical scavenging and anti-oxidant capacity of Ocimum basilicum essential oil. Journal of Essential Oil Research. 2017;29(2):189-199.

Basil (Ocimum basilicum L.) essential oil. Journal of Essential Oil Bearing Plants. 2017 Nov 02;20(6):1557-1569. Epub 2018 Jan 17.

Snoussi M, Dehmani A, Noumi E, Flamini G, Papetti A. Chemical composition and antibiofilm activity of Petroselinum crispum and Ocimum basilicum essential oils against Vibrio spp. strains. Microb Pathog. 2016 Jan;90:13-21. Epub 2015 Nov 16.

Ogaly HA, Eltablawy NA, El-Behairy AM, El-Hindi H, Abd-Elsalam RM. Hepatocyte growth factor mediates the antifibrogenic action of Ocimum basilicum essential oil against CCl4-induced liver fibrosis in rats. Molecules. 2015 Jul 23;20(8):13518-35.

Shirazi MT, Gholami H, Kavoosi G, Rowshan V, Tafsiry A. Chemical composition, antioxidant, antimicrobial and cytotoxic activities of Tagetes minuta and Ocimum basilicum essential oils. Food Sci & Nutr. 2014 Mar;2(2):146-55. Epub 2014 Jan 16.

Siddiqui BS, Bhatti HA, Begum S, Perwaiz S. Evaluation of the antimycobacterium activity of the constituents from Ocimum basilicum against Mycobacterium tuberculosis. J Ethnopharmacol. 2012 Oct 31;144(1):220-2. Epub 2012 Aug 17.

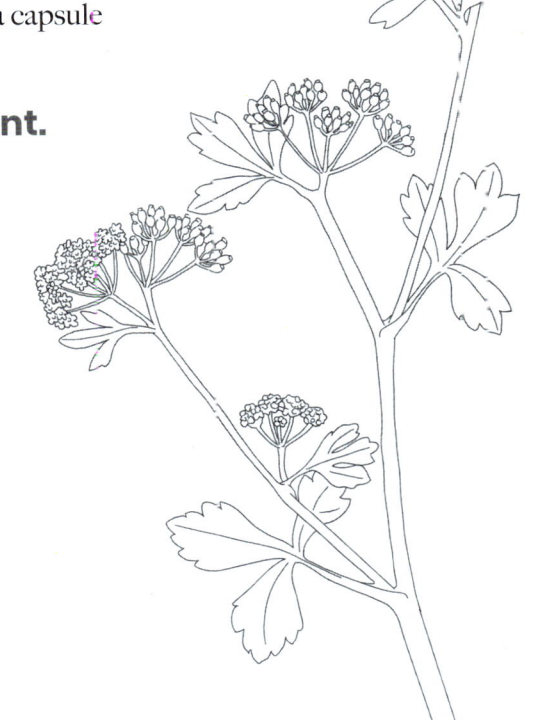

BOTANICAL FAMILY: Asteraceae

PLANT ORIGIN: Egypt

EXTRACTION METHOD: Steam distilled from flowers

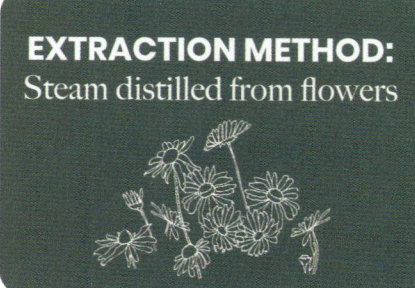

KEY CONSTITUENTS: Alpha-Bisabolol Oxide A (35-50%), Trans-Beta-Farnesene (15-35%), Alpha-Bisabolol (1-10%), Alpha-Bisabolol Oxide B (2-8%), Bisabolone Oxide A (2-7%), Chamazulene (2-5%)

CHAMOMILE, GERMAN & CHAMOMILE, GERMAN VITALITY™
(Chamomilla recutita) (Syn. Matricaria recutita; Matricaria chamomilla)

Listed in Dioscorides' De Materia Medica (AD 78), Europe's first authoritative guide to medicines, which became the standard reference work for herbal treatments for over 1,700 years.

MEDICAL PROPERTIES:
Antioxidant, chemoprotective, antibacterial, inhibits lipid peroxidation, antitumoral, anti-inflammatory, relaxant, anesthetic; promotes digestion, liver, and gallbladder health.

USES:
Migraines, atopic determatitis, reduces pain and edema, stimulating, hepatitis/fatty liver, arteriosclerosis, insomnia, nervous tension, arthritis, carpal tunnel syndrome, skin problems such as acne, eczema, scar tissue

FRAGRANT INFLUENCE:
Rich, earthy, floral aroma that helps create a more focused environment. Dispels anger, stabilizes emotions, and helps release emotions linked to the past. Soothes and clears the mind.

DIRECTIONS:
Aromatic: 6o. Topical: Neat. Dietary (Vitality): Put 2 drops in a capsule. Take 3 times daily or as needed.

CAUTIONS: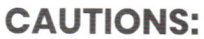

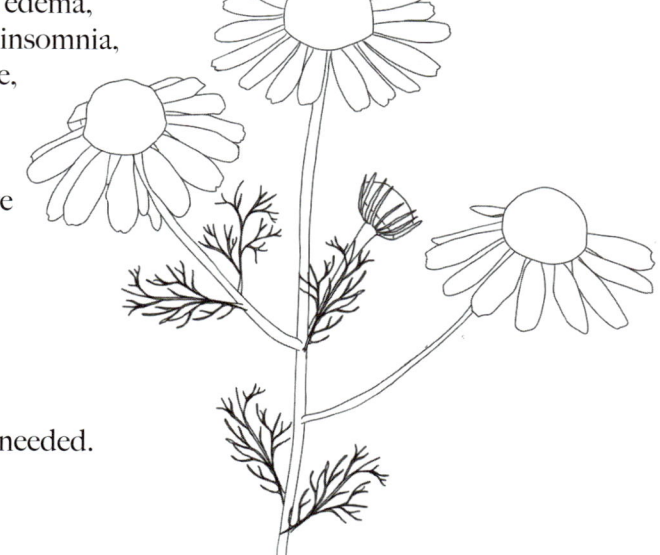

SELECTED RESEARCH:

de Franco EPD, Contesini FJ, da Silva BL, de Piloto Fernandes AMA, Leme CW, Cirino JPG, Campos PRB, de Oliveira Carvalho P. Enzyme-assisted modificantion of flavonoids from Matricaria chamomilla: antioxidant activity and inhibitory effect on digestive enzymes. J Enzyme Inhib Med Chem. 2020; 35(1): 42-49.

Al-Dabbagh B, Elhaty IA, Elhaw M, Murali C, Al Mansoori A, Awad B, Amin A. Antioxidant and anticancer activities of chamomile (Matricaria recutita L.). BMC Res Notes. 2019 Jan 3;12(1):3.

Dadashpour M, Firouzi-Amandi A, Pourhassan-Moghaddam M, Maleki MJ, Soozangar N, Jeddi F, Nouri M, Zarghami N, Pilehvar-Soltanahmadi Y. Biomimetic synthesis of silver nanoparticles using Matricaria chamomilla extract and their potential anticancer activity against human lung cancer cells. Mater Sci Eng C Mater Biol Appl. 2018 Nov 1;92:902-12. Epub 2018 Jul 21.

Kandelous HM, Salimi M, Khori V, Rastkari N, Amanzadeh A, Salimi M. Mitochondrial Apoptosis Induced by Chamaemelum Nobile Extract in Breast Cancer Cells. Iran J Pharm Res. 2016 Winter; 15(Suppl): 197-204.

Sebai H, Jabri MA, Souli A, Hosni K, Rtibi K, Tebourbi O, El-Benna J, Sakly M. Chemical composition, antioxidant properties and hepatoprotective effects of chamomile (Matricaria recutita L.) decoction extract against alcohol-induced oxidative stress in rat. Gen Physiol Biophys. 2015 Jul;34(3):263-75. Epub 2015 Mar 27.

Capuzzo A, Occhipinti A, Maffei ME. Antioxidant and radical scavenging activities of chamazulene. Nat Prod Res. 2014 Dec 17;28(24):2321-2323. Epub 2014 Jul 2.

Ranjbar A, Mohsenzadeh F, Chehregani A, Khajavi F, Zijoud SM, Ghasemi H. Ameliorative effect of Matricaria chamomilla L. on paraquat: induced oxidative damage in lung rats [sic: rat lungs]. Pharmacognosy Res. 2014 Jul;6(3):199-203.

Tomić M, Popović V, Petrović S, Stepanović-Petrović R, Micov A, Pavlović-Drobac M, Couladis M. Antihyperalgesic and antiedematous activities of bisabolol-oxides-rich matricaria oil in a rat model of inflammation. Phytother Res. 2014 May;28(5):759-66.

Zargaran A, Borhani-Haghighi A, Faridi P, Daneshamouz S, Kordafshari G, Mohagheghzadeh A. Potential effect and mechanism of action of topical chamomile (Matricaria chammomila L.) on migraine headache: a medical hypothesis. Med Hypotheses. 2014 Nov;83(5):566-569. [chammolia is an Iranian mistake]

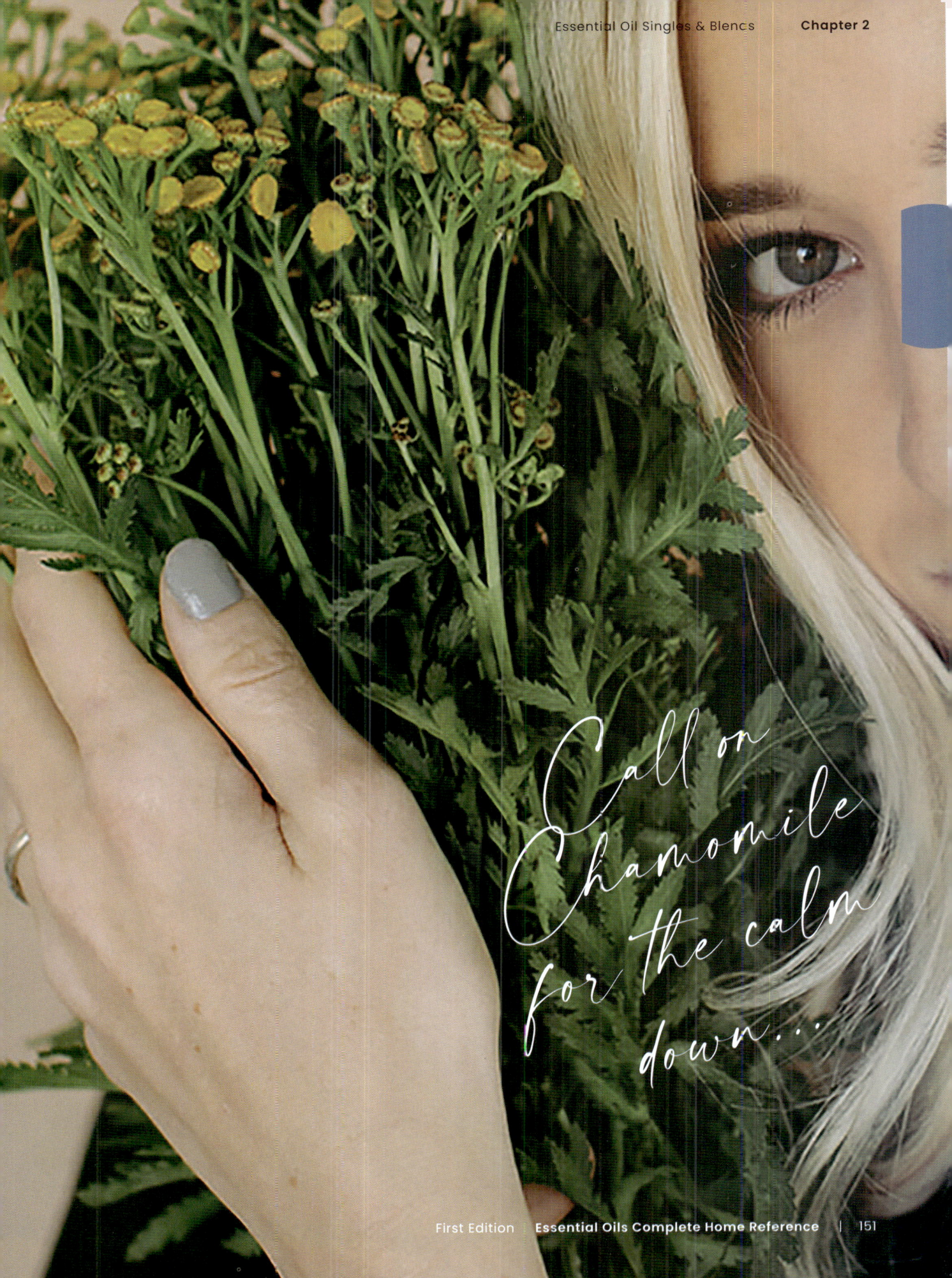

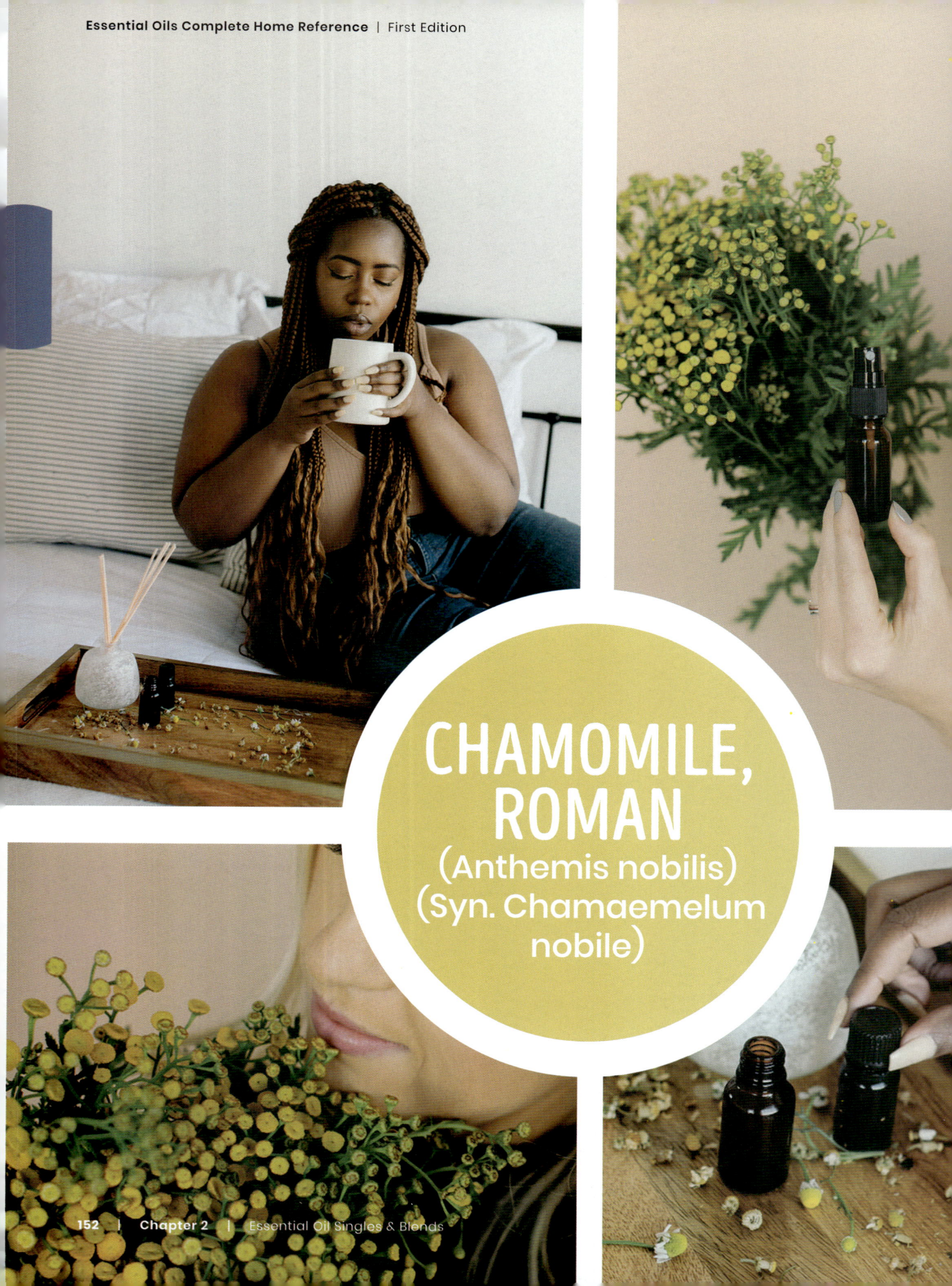

CHAMOMILE, ROMAN
(Anthemis nobilis)
(Syn. Chamaemelum nobile)

Essential Oil Singles & Blends | Chapter 2

BOTANICAL FAMILY: Asteraceae

PLANT ORIGIN: Bulgaria, France, Italy, Spain

EXTRACTION METHOD: Steam distilled from flowers

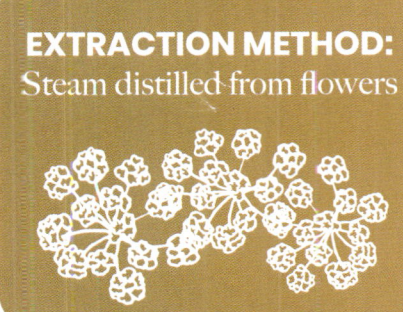

KEY CONSTITUENTS: Isobutyl Angelate + Isoamyl Methacrylate (29-40%), (E)-Isoamyl Angelate (10-22%), Methyl Allyl Angelate (6-10%), Trans-Pinocarveol (1-9%), Isobutyl Isobutyrate (3-9%), Pinocarvone (up to 7%), 2-Methyl Butyl Angelate (2-6%)

HISTORICAL DATA: Used in Europe for skin regeneration. For centuries, mothers have used chamomile to calm crying children, combat digestive and liver ailments, and relieve toothaches.

MEDICAL PROPERTIES:
Antioxidant, anti-inflammatory, antimicrobial, antiparasitic, antibacterial, anesthetic

USES:
Relieves restlessness, anxiety, ADHD, depression, insomnia, skin conditions (acne, dermatitis, eczema), cleansing, calming

FRAGRANT INFLUENCE:
Because it is calming and relaxing, it can combat depression, insomnia, and stress. It minimizes anxiety, irritability, and nervousness. It may also dispel anger, stabilize the emotions, and help to release emotions that are linked to the past. It also freshens the air.

DIRECTIONS:
Aromatic: 6o. Topical: Neat.

CAUTIONS:

SELECTED RESEARCH:

Kazemian H, Ghafourian S, Sadeghifard N, Houshmandfar R, Badakhsh B, Taji A, Shavalipour A, Mohebi R, Ebrahim-Saraie HS, Houri H, Heidari H. In vivo antibacterial and wound healing activities of Roman chamomile (Chamaemelum nobile). Infect Disord Drug Targets. 2018;18(1):41-45.

Kong Y, Wang T, Wang R, Ma Y, Song S, Liu J, Hu W, Li S. Inhalation of Roman chamomile essential oil attenuates depressive-like behaviors in Wistar Kyoto rats. Sci China Life Sci. 2017 Jun;60(6):647-655. Epub 2017 May 16.

Guimarães R, Calhelha RC, Froufe HJ, Areu RM, Carvalho AM, Queiroz MJ, Ferreira IC. Wild Roman chamomile extracts and phenolic compounds: enzymatic assays and molecular modelling studies with VEGFR-2 tyrosine kinase. Food Funct. 2016 Jan;7(1):79-83.

Kazemian H, Ghafourian S, Heidari H, Amiri P, Yamchi JK, Shavalipour A, Houri H, Maleki A Sadeghifard N. Antibacterial, anti-swarming and anti-biofilm formation activities of Chamaemelum nobile against Pseudomonas aeruginosa. Rev Soc Bras Med Trop. 2015 Jul-Aug;48(4):432-6.

Zhao J, Khan SI, Wang M, Vasquez Y, Yang MH, Avula B, Wang YH, Avonto C, Smillie TJ, Khan IA. Octulosonic acid derivatives from Roman chamomile (Chamaemelum nobile) with activities against inflammation and metabolic disorder. J Nat Prod. 2014 Mar 28;77(3):509-15. Epub 2014 Jan 28.

Zeggwagh NA, Michel JB, Eddouks M. Vascular effects of aqueous extract of Chamaemelum nobile: in vitro pharmacological studies in rats. Clin Exp Hypertens. 2013;35(3):200-6. Epub 2012 Aug 6.

Srivastava JK, Shankar E, Gupta S. Chamomile: a herbal medicine of the past with bright future. Mol Med Res. 2010 Nov 1;3(6):895-901.

Bail S, Buchbauer G, Jirovetz L. Denkova Z, Slavchev A, Stoyanova A. Schmidt E, Geissler M. Antimicrobial activities of Roman chamomile oil from France and its main compounds. Journal of Essential Oil Research. 2009 May 1;21(3):283-286.

Eddouks M, Lemhadri A, Zeggwagh NA, Michel JB. Potent hypoglycemic activity of the aqueous extract of Chamaemelum nobile in normal and streptozotocin-induced diabetic rats. Diabetes Res Clin Pract. 2005 Mar;67(3):189-95.

Garg SC. Essential oils as therapeutics. Natural Product Radiance. 2005 Jan-Feb;4(1):18-26.

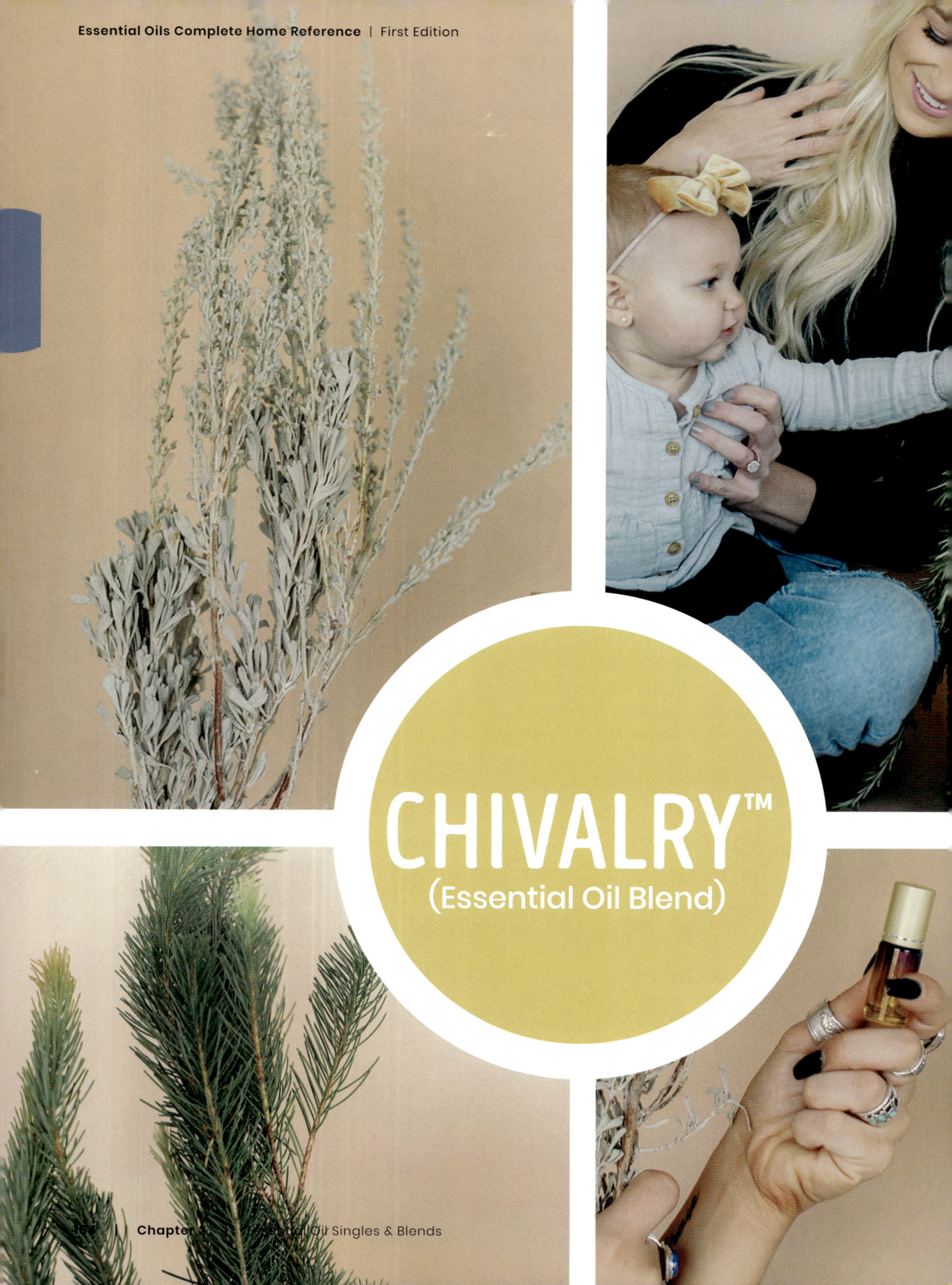

ABOUT CHIVALRY:

Harkening back to stories of gallant knights of old, Chivalry instills respect, honor, and integrity and empowers you to reach for higher ideals. It contains 23 essential oils known for their restorative properties and reminds the wearer to uphold values of benevolence and civility to others.

MEDICAL PROPERTIES & USES:

Anti-inflammatory, antimicrobial, antioxidative, emotion supporting, calming, cardiovascular supportive, disease inhibitory, organ-protective, pain or swelling reducing, respiratory system supportive, sleep improving

INGREDIENTS:

Fractionated coconut oil, Ylang Ylang, Black Spruce, Geranium, Rose, Camphor (Ho Wood), Bergamot (Furocoumarin-free), Frankincense, Idaho Grand Fir, Blue Tansy, Coriander, Lemon, Sacred Sandalwood, Lavender, Tangerine, Orange, Angelica, Myrrh, Hyssop, Spanish Sage, Jasmine, Roman Chamomile, Northern Lights Black Spruce, Palmarosa, Vetiver

DIRECTIONS:

Aromatic: (30). Topical: 50-50.

CAUTIONS:

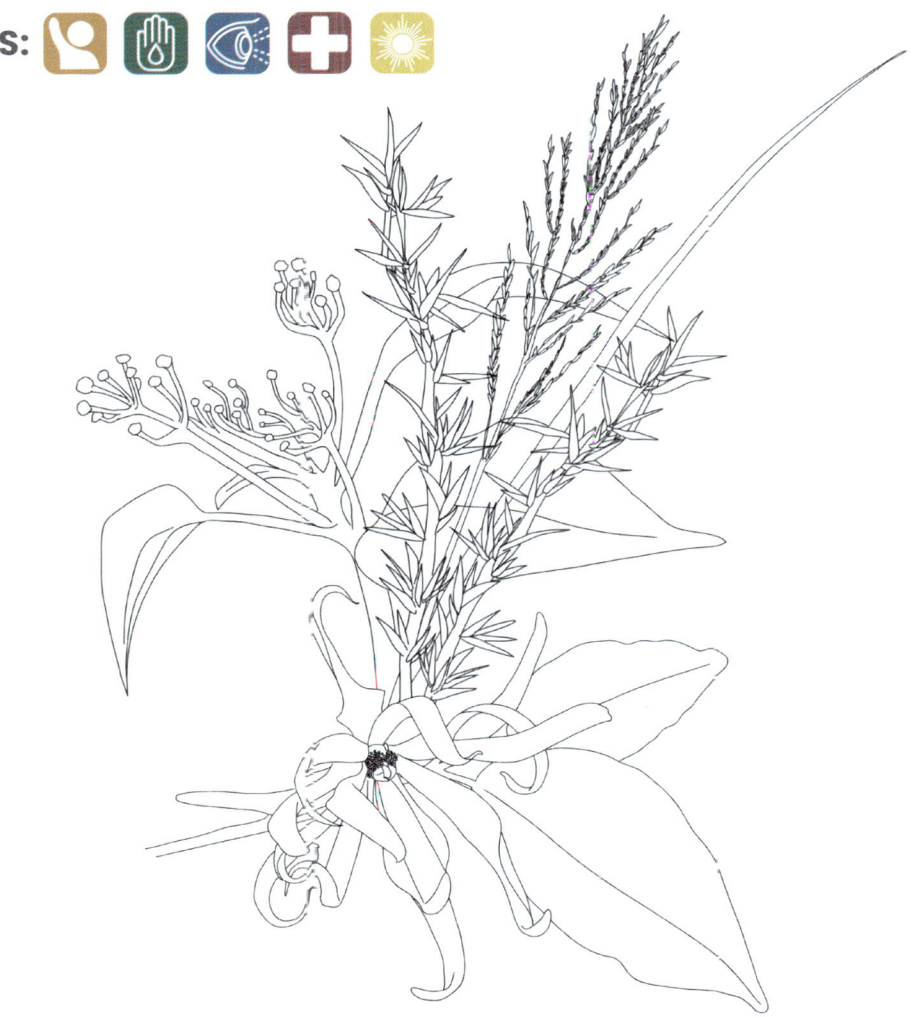

CHRISTMAS SPIRIT™
(Essential Oil Blend)

Christmas Spirit is a purifying blend of evergreen, citrus, and spice, reminiscent of winter holidays, and brings joy, peace, happiness, and security.

MEDICAL PROPERTIES & USES:
Anti-inflammatory, antimicrobial, antioxidative, emotionally uplifting, calming, disease inhibitory, insecticidal, pain or swelling reducing, skin and hair improving

INGREDIENTS:
Orange, Cinnamon Bark, Black Spruce

DIRECTIONS:
Aromatic: 30. Also, sprinkle on logs in the fireplace, on Christmas trees, on cedar chips for dresser drawers, or on potpourri. Use all year round. Topical: 20-80.

CAUTIONS:

Avoid using on infants and very small children.

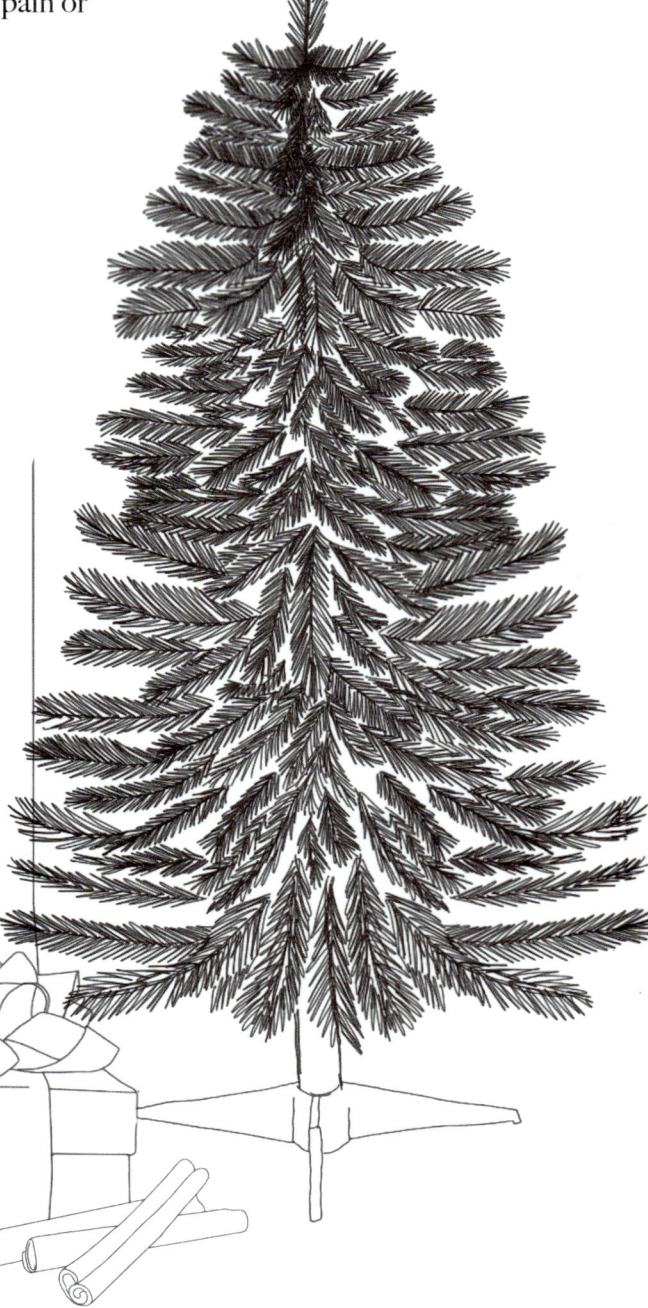

Essential Oil Singles & Blends | **Chapter 2**

Because every day needs a bit of Christmas!

BOTANICAL FAMILY: Apiaceae

PLANT ORIGIN: Egypt

EXTRACTION METHOD: Steam distilled from leaves/herbs/aerial parts of flowering plant

KEY CONSTITUENTS: Trans-2-Tetradecenal (33-39%), Decenal (12-22%), Linalool (10-21%), 2-dodecanal (2-10%), 2-undecenal (3-5%), Trans-2-Tetradecenal (2-4%)

CILANTRO & CILANTRO VITALITY™
(Coriandrum sativum)

Cilantro has cultivaton history that dates back to at least 1500 BC, as Sanskrit writings from that time indicate.
Cilantro Vitality offers a major immune-system boost and offers a bright, piquant flavor to Latin American and South Asian recipes.

MEDICAL PROPERTIES:
Antimicrobial, antioxidant, antibacterial, antianxiety, anti-inflammatory

USES:
Candida, skin irritations, cleansing, neurological inflammation, cardiovascular disease, digestion-aiding, endocrine gland function, hormones, immune system, anxiety, sleep problems, blood sugar problems, heart health, urinary tract infections, toxic metal cleansing

FRAGRANT INFLUENCE:
Herbal, sleep aid

DIRECTIONS:
Aromatic: 30. Topical: 50-50. Dietary (Vitality): Dilute 1 drop with 1 drop of carrier oil. Put in a capsule and take up to 3 times daily. Add 1 drop of Cilantro Vitality plus 1 drop of Lime Vitality to boost flavor in recipes.

CAUTIONS:

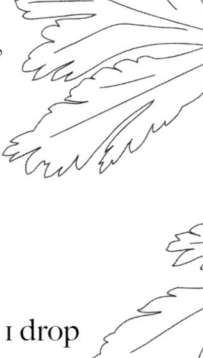

SELECTED RESEARCH:

Kačániová M, Galovičova L, Ivanišová E, Vukovic NL, Štefániková J, Valková V, Borotová P, Žiarovská J, Terentjeva M, Felšöciová S, Tvrdá E. Antioxidant, Antimicrobial and Antibiofilm Activity of Coriander (Coriander sativum L.) Essential Oil for its Application in Foods. Foods. 2020 Mar; 9(3): 282.

Kajal A, Singh R. Coriandrum sativum seeds extract mitigate progression of diabetic nephropathy in experimental rats via AGEs inhibition. PLoS One. 2019 Mar 7;14(3:e0213147. eCollection 2019.

Nishio R, Tamano H, Morioka H, Takeuchi A, Takeda A. Intake of heated leaf extract of Coriandrum sativum contributes to resistance to oxidative stress via decreases in heavy metal concentrations in the kidney. Plant Foods Hum Nutr. 2019 Feb 19. [Epub ahead of print].

Hussain F, Jahan N, Rahman KU, Sultana B, Jamil S. Identification of hypotensive biofunctional compounds of Coriandrum sativum and evaluation of their angiotensin-converting enzyme (ACE) inhibition potential. Oxid Med Cell Longev. 2018 Nov 15;2018:4643736. eCollection 2018.

Mansouri N, Aoun L, Dalichaouche N, Hadri D. Yields, chemical composition, and antimicrobial activity of two Algerian essential oils against 40 avian multidrug-resistant Escherichia coli strains. Vet World. 2018 Nov;11(11):1539-1550. Epub 2018 Nov 6.

Moghadam MH, Imenshahidi M, Mohajeri SA. Antihypertensive effect of celery seed on rat blood pressure in chronic administration. J Med Food. 2013 Jun;16(6):558-63. Epub 2013 Jun 4.

Find your missing superpower in a bottle of Cilantro!

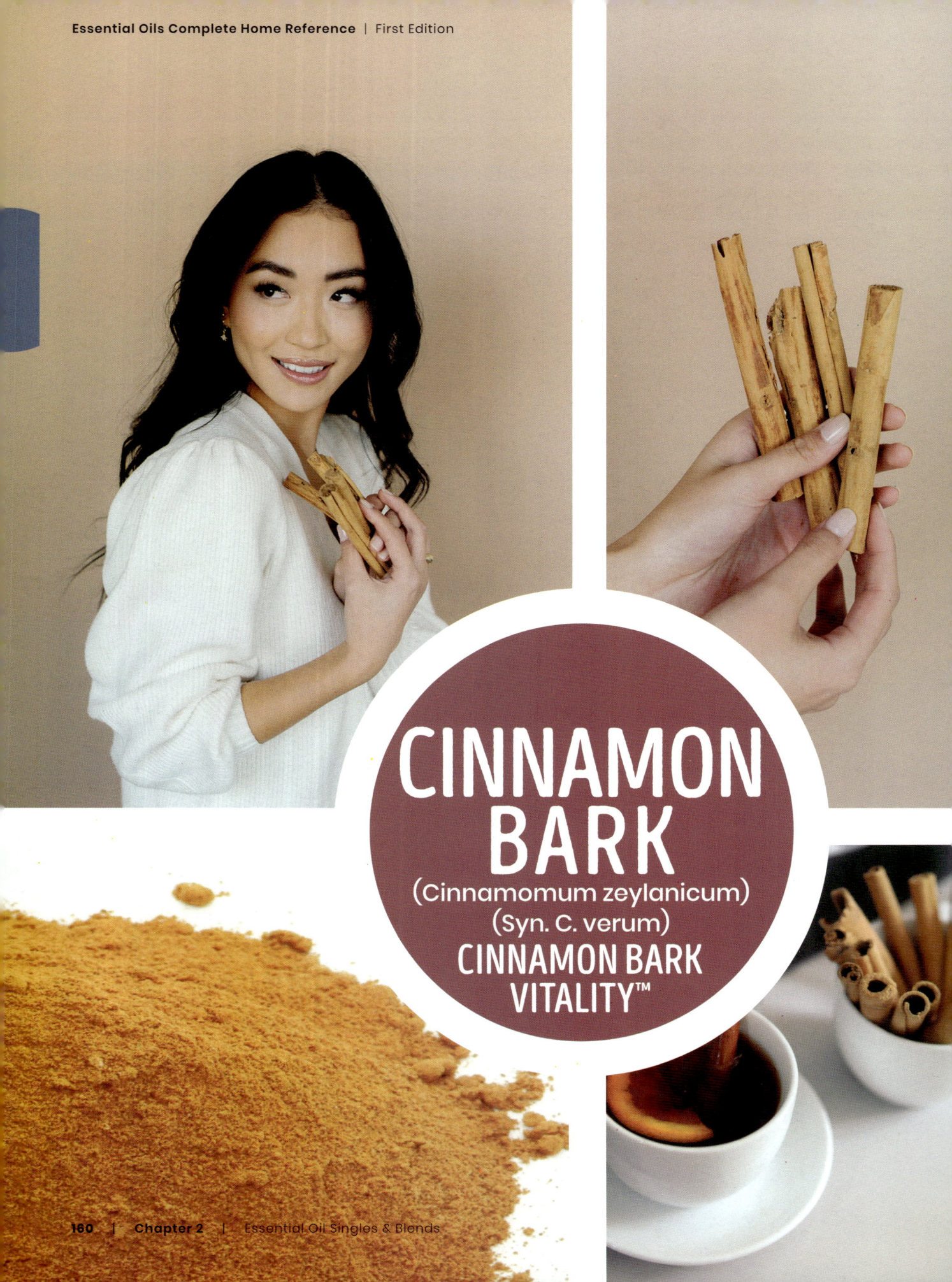

Essential Oil Singles & Blends | **Chapter 2**

BOTANICAL FAMILY:
Lauraceae

PLANT ORIGIN:
Sri Lanka, Madagascar

EXTRACTION METHOD:
Steam distilled from bark

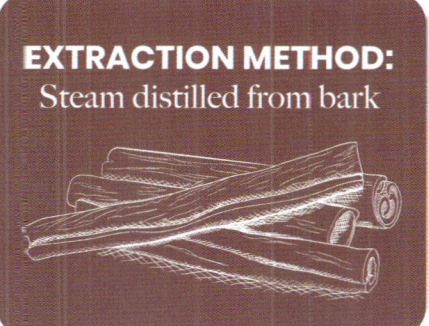

KEY CONSTITUENTS:
Trans-Cinnamaldehyde (61-82%),
Eugenol (1-11%),
Linalool (1-10%),
Cinnamyl Acetate (up to 10%),
Beta-Caryophyllene (up to 9%)

HISTORICAL DATA:
Listed in Dioscorides' De Materia Medica (AD 78), Europe's first authoritative guide to medicines, which became the standard reference work for herbal treatments for over 1,700 years.

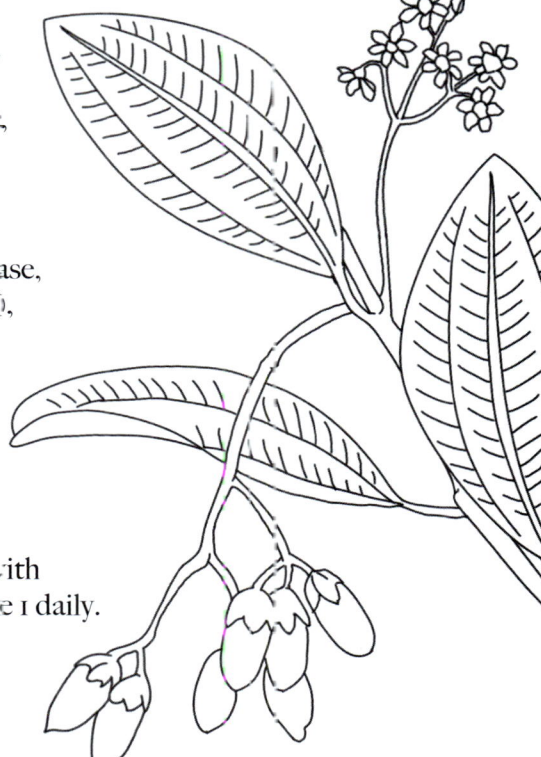

MEDICAL PROPERTIES:
Anti-inflammatory (COX-2 inhibitor), powerfully antibacterial, antiviral, antifungal, anticoagulant, antiparasitic (worms), antioxidant, antimicrobial, antitumoral, antiseptic, antidiabetic, circulatory stimulant, stomach protectant (ulcers)

USES:
Urinary tract infections, influenza, tumors, cardiovascular disease, infectious diseases, type-2 diabetes, viral infections (herpes, etc.), digestive complaints, ulcers, and warts

FRAGRANT INFLUENCE:
Spicy, enriching aroma; influenza, infections

DIRECTIONS:
Aromatic: 10. Topical: 20-80. Dietary (Vitality): Dilute 1 drop with 4 drops of V-6 or other pure carrier oil. Put in a capsule and take 1 daily.

CAUTIONS: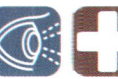

SELECTED RESEARCH:

Behbahani BA, Falah F, Arab FL, Vasiee M, Yazdi FT. Chemical Composition and Antioxidant, Antimicrobial, and Antiproliferative Activities of Cinnamomum zeylanicum Bark Essential Oil. Evid Based Complement Alternat Med. 2020; 2020: 5190603. Published online 2020 Apr 29.

Lira Neto JCG, Damasceno MMC, Ciol MA, de Freitas RWJF, de Araújo MFM, Teixeira CRdeS, Carvalho GCN, Coelho Lisboa KWdeS, de Souza DF, Nogueira JdeM, Marquex RLL, Garcia Alencar AMP. Analysis of the effectiveness of cinnamon (Cinnamomum verum) in the reduction of glycemic and lipidic levels of adults with type 2 diabetes: A study protocol. Medicine (Baltimore). 2020 Jan; 99(1): e18553. Published online 2020 Jan 3.

Yang S-J, Yusoff K, Ajat M, Thomas W, Abushelaibi A, Erin Kim S-H, Lai K-S. Disruption of KPC-producing Klebsiella pneumoniae membrane via induction of oxidative stress by cinnamon bark (Cinnamomum verum J. Presl) essential oil. PLoS one. 2019; 14(4): e0214326. Published online 2019 Apr 2.

Firmino DF, Cavalcante TTA, Gomes GA, Firmino NCS, Rosa LD, de Carvalho MG, Catunda FEA Jr. Antibacterial and antibiofilm activities of Cinnamomum sp. essential oil and cinnamaldehyde: antimicrobial activities. Scientific World Journal. 2018 Jun 6;2018:7405736. eCollection 2018.

Cui H, Li W, Li C, Vittayapadung S, Lin L. Liposome containing cinnamon oil with antibacterial activity against methicillin-resistant Staphylococcus aureus biofilm. Biofouling. 2016 Feb;32(2):215-25.

Davis PA, Yokoyama W. Cinnamon intake lowers fasting blood glucose: meta-analysis. J Med Food. 2011 Sep;14(9):884-9. Epub 2011 Apr 13.

Malik J, Munjal K, Deshmukh R. Attenuating effect of standardized lyophilized Cinnamomum zeylanicum bark extract against streptozotocin-induced experimental dementia of Alzheimer's type. J Basic Clin Physiol Pharmacol. 2015 May;26(3):275-85.

Yap PS, Krishnan T, Chan KG, Lim SH. Antibacterial mode of action of Cinnamomum verum bark essential oil, alone and in combination with piperacillin, against a multi-drug-resistant Escherichia coli strain. J Microbiol Biotechnol. 2015 Aug 28;25(8):1299-306. Epub Nov 11.

Sartorius T, Peter A, Schulz N, Drescher A, Bergheim I, Machann J, Schick F, Siegel-Axel D, Schürmann A, Weigert C, Häring HU, Hennige AM. Cinnamon extract improves insulin sensitivity in the brain and lowers liver fat in mouse models of obesity. PLoS One. 2014 Mar 18;9(3):e92358.

Yüce A, Türk G, Çeribaşi S, Güvenç M, Çiftçi M, Sönmez M, Özer Kaya Ş, Çay M, Aksakal M. Effectiveness of cinnamon (Cinnamomum zeylanicum) bark oil in the prevention of carbon tetrachloride-induced damages on the male reproductive system. Andrologia. 2014 Apr;46(3):263-72.

BOTANICAL FAMILY: Cistaceae

PLANT ORIGIN: Spain

EXTRACTION METHOD: Steam distilled from branches and branchlets

KEY CONSTITUENTS: Alpha-Pinene (21-55%), Camphene (up to 9%), Limonene (up to 9%), Para Cymene (up to 8%), Trans-Pinocarveol (1-7%), Viridiflorol (up to 6%)

CISTUS
(Cistus ladanifer/ladaniferus)

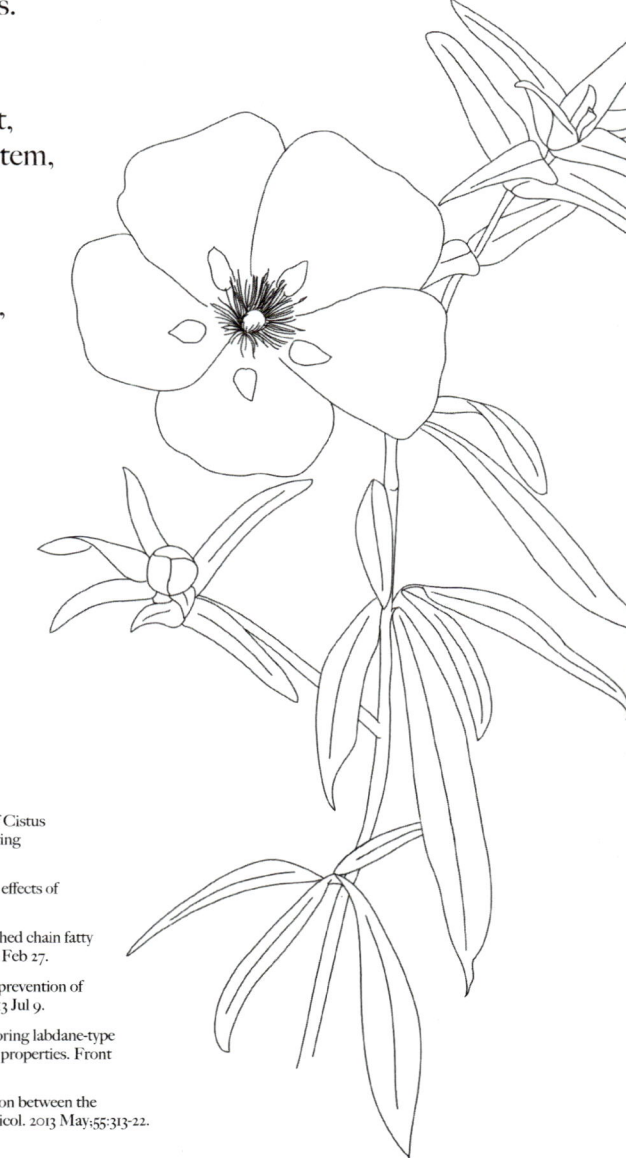

Cistus is also known as "rock rose" and "Rose of Sharon" and has been studied for its effects on the regeneration of cells.

MEDICAL PROPERTIES:
Antiviral, antibacterial, antihemorrhagic, antioxidant, anti-inflammatory, supports sympathetic nervous system, immune stimulant, skin protective

USES:
Hemorrhages, arthritis, viral and bacterial infections, immune system

FRAGRANT INFLUENCE:
Calming to the nerves, elevates the emotions

DIRECTIONS:
Aromatic: 6o. Topical: Neat. Dietary: Take 4 drops as dietary supplement.

CAUTIONS:

SELECTED RESEARCH:

Gawel-Bęben K, Kukula-Koch W, Hoian U, Czop M, Strzępek-Gomółka M, Antosiewicz B. Characterization of Cistus x incanus L. and Cistus ladanifer L. Extracts as Potential Multifunctional Antioxidant Ingredients for Skin Protecting Cosmetics. Antioxidants (Basel). 2020 Mar; 9(3): 202.

El Hamsas El Youbi A, El Mansouri L, Boukhira S, Daoudi A, Bousta D. In vivo anti-inflammatory and analgesic effects of aqueous extract of Cistus ladanifer L. from Morocco. Am J Ther. 2016 Nov/Dec;23(6):e1554-e1559.

Guerreiro O, Alves SP, Duarte MF, Bessa RJ, Jerónimo E. Cistus ladanifer L. shrub is rich in saturated and branched chain fatty acids and their concentration increases in the Mediterranean dry season. Lipids. 2015 May;50(5):493-501. Epub 2015 Feb 27.

Loizzo MR, Ben Jemia M, Senatore F, Bruno M, Menichini F, Tundis R. Chemistry and functional properties in prevention of neurodegenerative disorders of five Cistus species essential oils. Food Chem Toxicol. 2013 Sep;59:586-94. Epub 2013 Jul 9.

Papaefthimiou D, Papanikolaou A, Falara V, Givanoudi S, Kostas S, Kanellis AK. Genus Cistus: a model for exploring labdane-type diterpenes' biosynthesis and a natural source of high value products with biological, aromatic, and pharmacological properties. Front Chem. 2014 Jun 11;2:35. Epub 2014 Jun 27.

Tomás-Menor L, Morales-Soto A, Barrajón-Catalán E, Roldán-SeguraC, Segura-Carretero A, Micol V. Correlation between the antibacterial activity and the composition of extracts derived from various Spanish Cistus species. Food Chem Toxicol. 2013 May;55:313-22. Epub 2013 Jan 22.

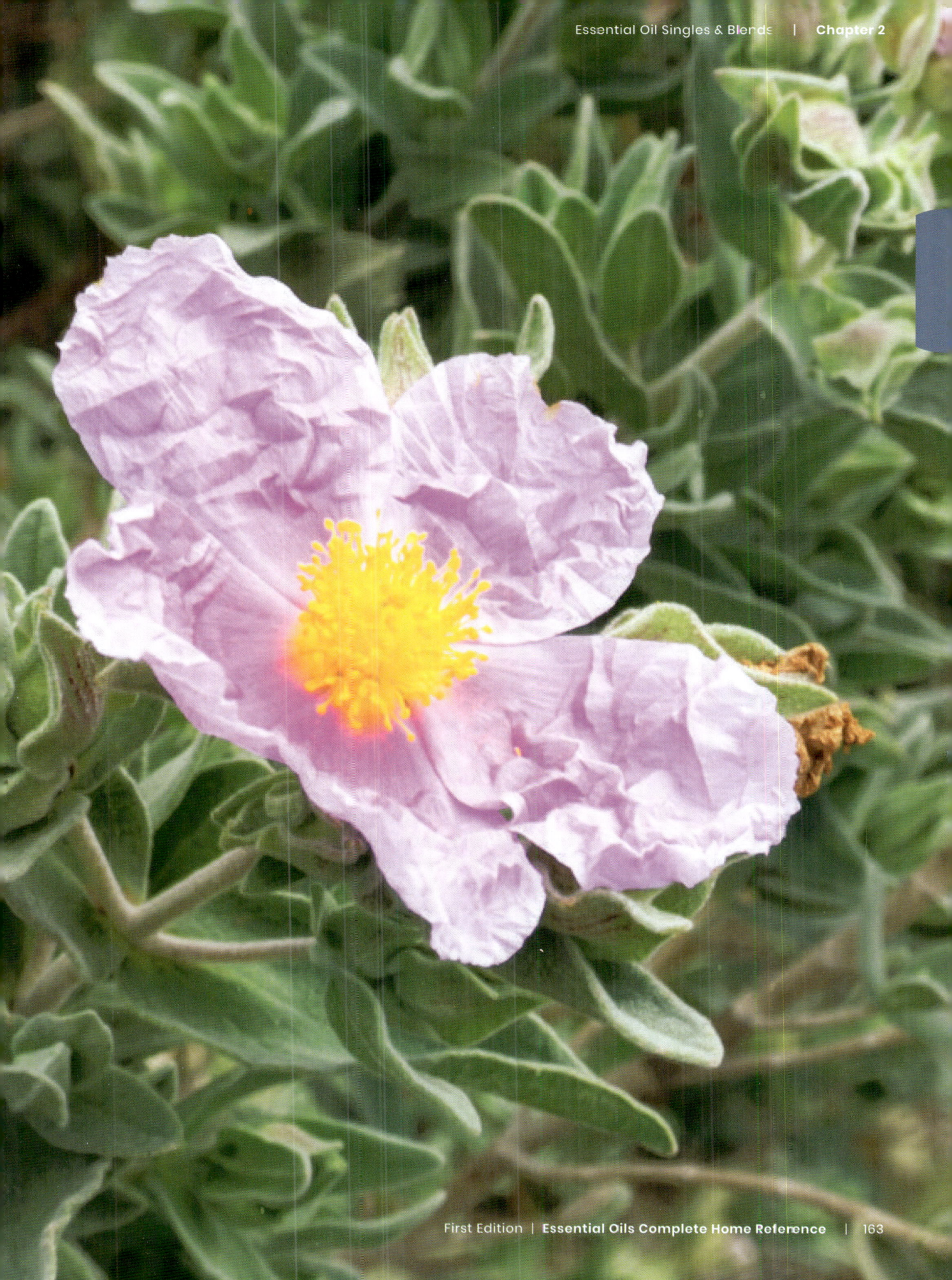

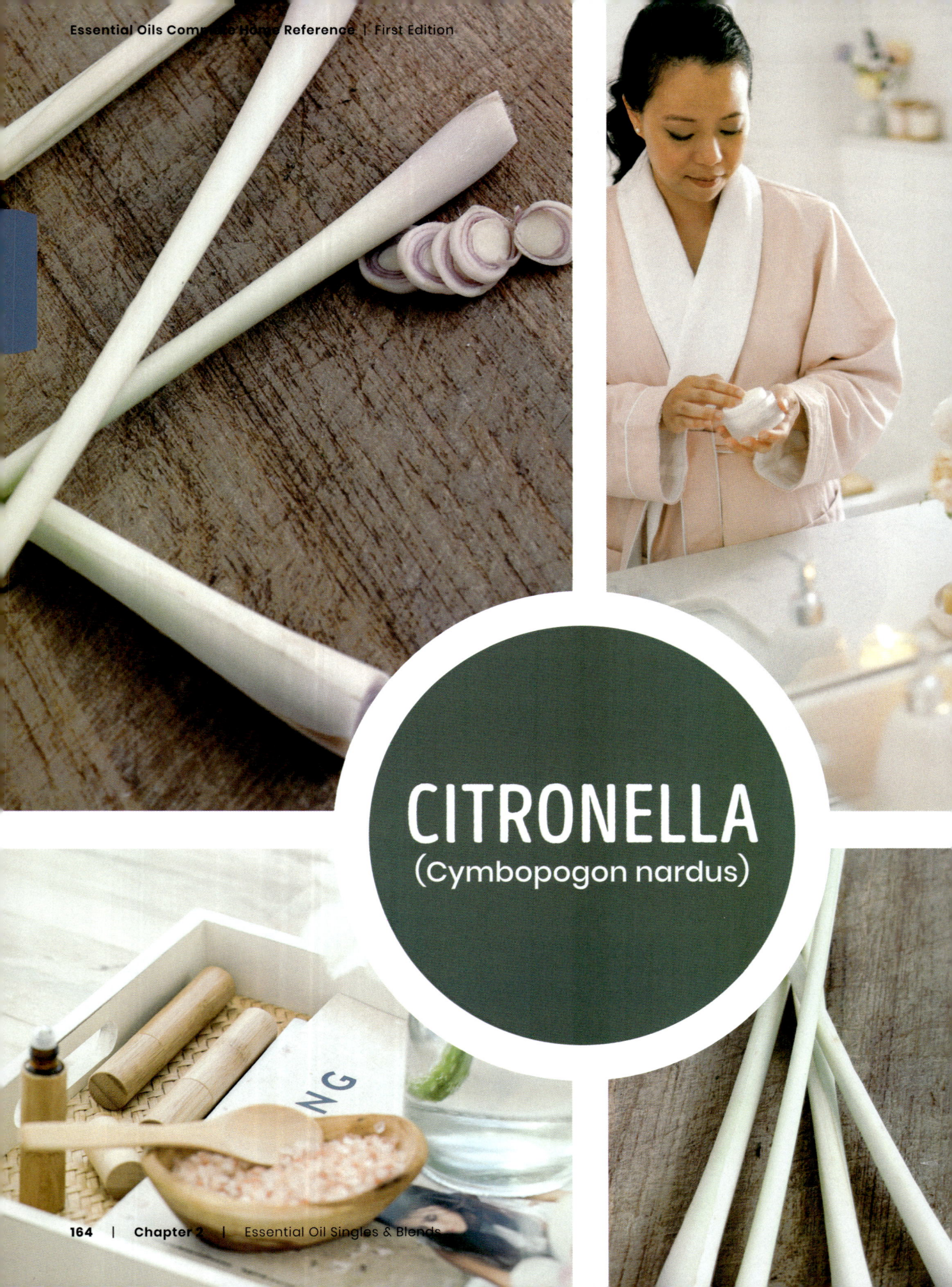

CITRONELLA
(Cymbopogon nardus)

BOTANICAL FAMILY:
Poaceae

PLANT ORIGIN:
Sri Lanka

EXTRACTION METHOD:
Steam distilled from aerial parts and leaves

KEY CONSTITUENTS:
Geraniol (15-23%),
Limonene (7-12%),
Methyl Isoeugenol (3-11%),
Camphene (7-10%),
Citronellol (3-9%),
Borneol (2-7%),
Citronellal (3-6%)

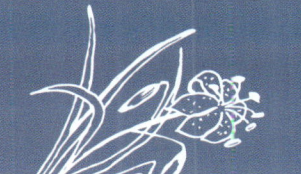

HISTORICAL DATA:
Used by various cultures to treat intestinal parasites, menstrual problems, and as a stimulant. Historically used to sanitize and deodorize surfaces. Enhanced insect repelling properties when combined with cedarwood.

MEDICAL PROPERTIES:
Powerful antioxidant, antibacterial, antifungal, anti-inflammatory, antispasmodic, antiparasitic (worms), relaxant, insecticidal

USES:
Insect repellent, head lice repellent, respiratory infections, muscle/nerve pain, digestive/intestinal problems, anxiety, skin problems (acne, eczema, oily skin), skin-penetration enhancer

FRAGRANT INFLUENCE:
Refreshing and uplifting, respiratory system, calming

DIRECTIONS:
Aromatic: 30. Topical: 50-50. Dietary: Dilute 1 drop essential oil with 1 drop V-6 or other pure carrier oil, put in a capsule, and take up to 3 times daily or as needed as a dietary supplement.

CAUTIONS:

SELECTED RESEARCH:
Pontes EKU, Melo HM, Nogueira JW, Firmino NCS, de Carvalho MG, Cantunda Júnior FEA, Cavalcante TTA. Antibiofilm activity of the essential oil of citronella (Cymbopogon nardus) and its major component, geraniol, on the bacterial biofilms of Staphylococcus aureus. Food Sci Biotechnol. 2019 Jun; 28(3): 633-5639. Published online 2018 Oct. 30.

De Toledo LG, Ramos MA, Spósito L, Castilho EM, Pavan FR, Lopes Éde O, Zocolo GJ, Silva FA, Soares TH, Dos Santos AG, Bauab TM, De Almeida MT. Essential oil of Cymbopogon nardus (L.) rendle: a strategy to combat fungal infections caused by candida species. Int J Mol Sci. 2016 Aug 9;17(8). Epub Aug 16.

Trindade LA, de Araújo Oliveira J, de Castro RD, de Oliveira Lima E. Inhibition of adherence of C. albicans to dental implants and cover screws by Cymbopogon nardus essential oil and citronellal. Clin Oral Investig. 2015 Dec;19(9):2223-31. Epub 2015 Mar 26.

Batubara I, Suparto IH, Sa'diah S, Matsuoka R, Mitsunaga T. Effects of inhaled citronella oil and related compounds on rat body weight and brown adipose tissue sympathetic nerve. Nutrients. 2015 Mar 12;7(3):1859-70.

Wei LS, Wee W. Chemical composition and antimicrobial activity of Cymbopogon nardus citronella essential oil against systematic bacteria of aquatic animals. Iran J Microbiol. 2013 Jun;5(2):147-52. Epub Jul 5.

Li WR, Shi QS, Ouyang YS, Chen YB, Duan SS. Antifungal effects of citronella oil against Aspergillus niger ATCC 16404. Appl Microbiol Biotechnol. 2013 Aug;97(16):7483-92. Epub 2012 Oct 19.

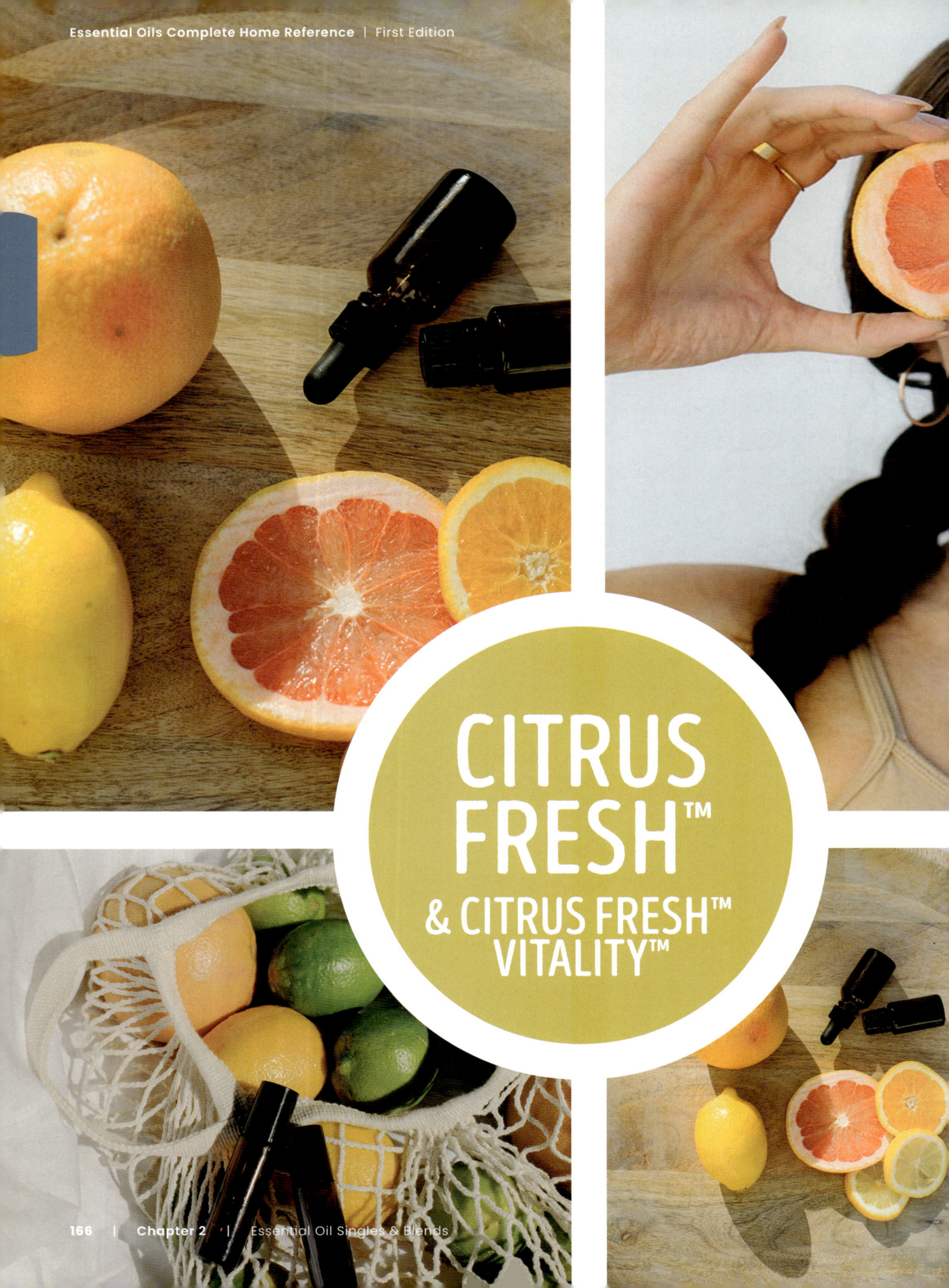

ABOUT CITRUS FRESH™ & CITRUS FRESH VITALITY™:

Citrus Fresh stimulates the right brain to amplify creativity and well-being, eradicates anxiety, and works well as an air purifier. When diffused, it adds a clean, fresh scent to any environment.

MEDICAL PROPERTIES & USES:

Antimicrobial, antioxidative, calming, cardiovascular supportive, dietary, digestion or elimination supportive/nausea reducing, disease inhibitory, insecticidal, organ protective, pain or swelling reducing, skin and hair improving, wellness supportive

INGREDIENTS:

Orange, Tangerine, Grapefruit, Lemon, Mandarin, Spearmint

DIRECTIONS:

Aromatic: 6o. Also, add a few drops onto cotton balls and place them in drawers, in air vents, under garbage cans, and in shoes for freshness. Topical: 50-50. Dietary (Vitality): Put 2 drops in a capsule and take 3 times daily. Great for culinary use.

CAUTIONS:

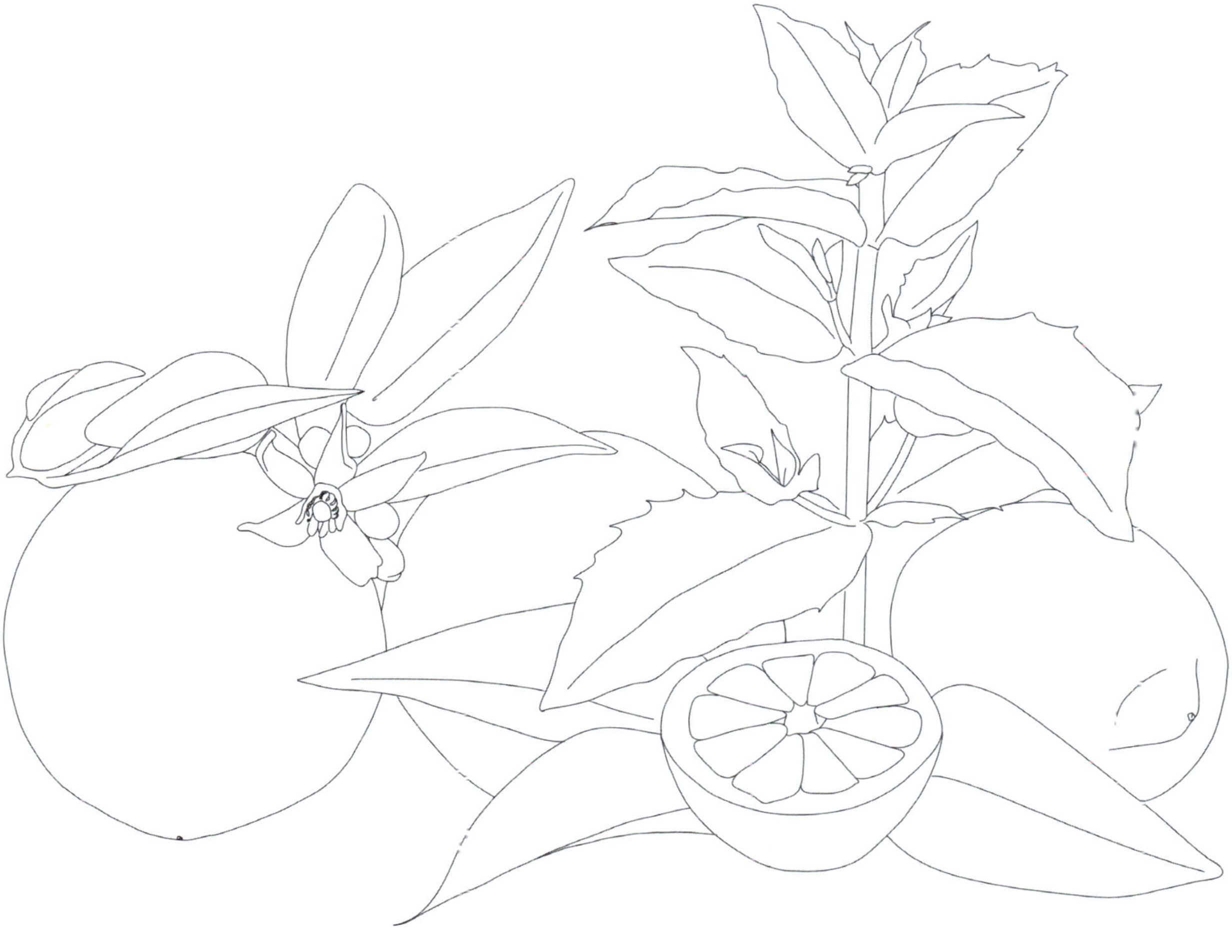

BOTANICAL FAMILY: Rutaceae

PLANT ORIGIN: Madagascar

EXTRACTION METHOD: Steam distilled from leaves/twigs

KEY CONSTITUENTS: Citronnellal (61-85%), Linalool (2-7%), Isopulegol (up to 6%), Citronellol (1-6%), Neoisopulegol (up to 5%)

CITRUS HYSTRIX/COMBAVA
(Citrus hystrix)

(also known as Thai lime, kaffir lime, or makrut lime)
Used as a flavorant and as a nausea, fainting, and headache treatment. Also used for stomachaches and dyspepsia.

MEDICAL PROPERTIES:
Anti-inflammatory, anti-infectious, antimicrobial, antidepressant, relaxant, antitumoral, antioxidant, rich in citronellal, possesses calmative properties, antibacterial, anticancer

USES:
Stress, anxiety, trauma, pain, cleanser for energy work, skin care, head lice

FRAGRANT INFLUENCE:
Freshens the air for rest and contemplation, uplifting, clarity, calming

DIRECTIONS:
Aromatic: 30. Topical: 50-50. Dietary: Take as a dietary supplement. Use as flavoring in foods.

CAUTIONS:

SELECTED RESEARCH:

Anuchapreeda S, Chueahongthong F, Viriyaadhammaa N, Panyajai P, Anzawa R, Tima S, Ampasavate C, Saiai A, Rungrojsakul M, Usuki T, Okonogi S. Antileukemic Cell Proliferation of Active Compounds from Kaffir Lime (Citrus hystrix) Leaves. Molecules. 2020 Mar; 25(6): 1300. Published online 2020 Mar 12.

Wongsariya K, Phanthong P, Bunyapraphatsara N, Srisukh V, Chomnawang MT. Synergistic interaction and mode of action of Citrus hystrix essential oil against bacteria causing periodontal diseases. Pharm Biol. 2014 Mar;52(3):273-80. Epub 2013 Oct 10.

Panthong K, Srisud Y, Rukachaisirikul V, Hutadilok-Towatana N, Voravuthikunchai SP, Tewtrakul S. Benzene, coumarin and quinolinone derivatives from roots of Citrus hystrix. Phytochemistry. 2013 Apr;88:79-84. Epub 2013 Jan 24.

Putri H, Nagadi S, Larasati YA, Wulandari N, Hermawan A, Nugroho AE. Cardioprotective and hepatoprotective effects of Citrus hystrix peels extract on rats model. Asian Pac J Trop Biomed. 2013 May;3(5):371-5.

Waikedre J, Dugay A, Barrachina I, Herrenknecht C, Cabalion P, Fournet A. Chemical composition and antimicrobial activity of the essential oils from New Caledonian Citrus macroptera and Citrus hystrix. Chem Biodivers. 2010 Apr;7(4):871-7.

Essential Oil Singles & Blends | **Chapter 2**

The rind and crushed leaves emit an intense citrus fragrance.

CLARITY™
(Essential Oil Blend)

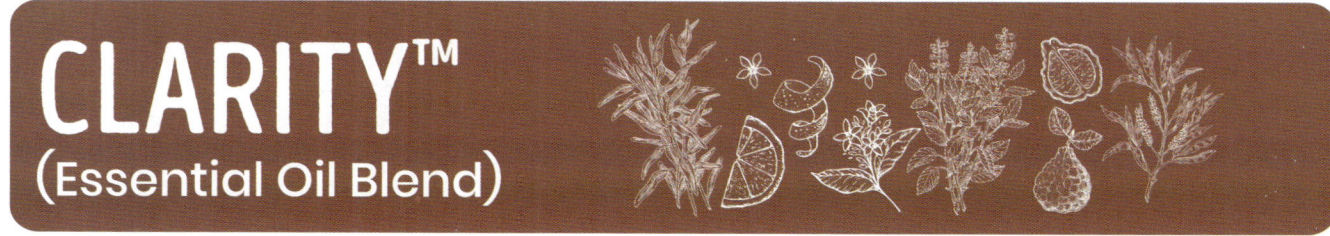

Clarity promotes a clear mind and amplifies mental alertness and vitality. It increases energy when overly tired and brings greater focus to the spirit and mind.

MEDICAL PROPERTIES & USES:
Anti-inflammatory, antimicrobial, antioxidative, clarity of mind, calming, cardiovascular supportive, digestion or elimination supportive/nausea reducing, disease inhibitory, muscle relaxant/bone-joint preservative, organ protective, pain or swelling reducing, performance enhancing/stimulating, wellness supportive

INGREDIENTS:
Basil, Cardamom, Rosemary, Peppermint, Coriander, Geranium, Bergamot (Furocoumarin-free), Lemon, Ylang Ylang, Jasmine, Roman Chamomile, Palmarosa

DIRECTIONS:
Aromatic: 3o. Topical: 50-50. Clarity works well with Brain Power, Palo Santo, Lemon, or Peppermint, as they enhance its effects.

CAUTIONS:

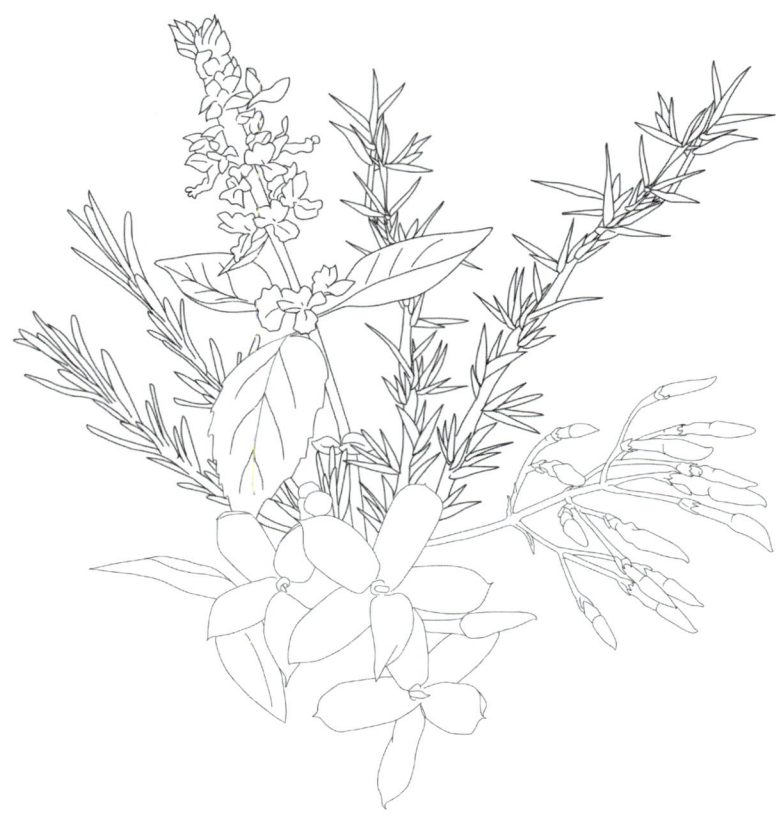

Essential Oil Singles & Blends | Chapter 2

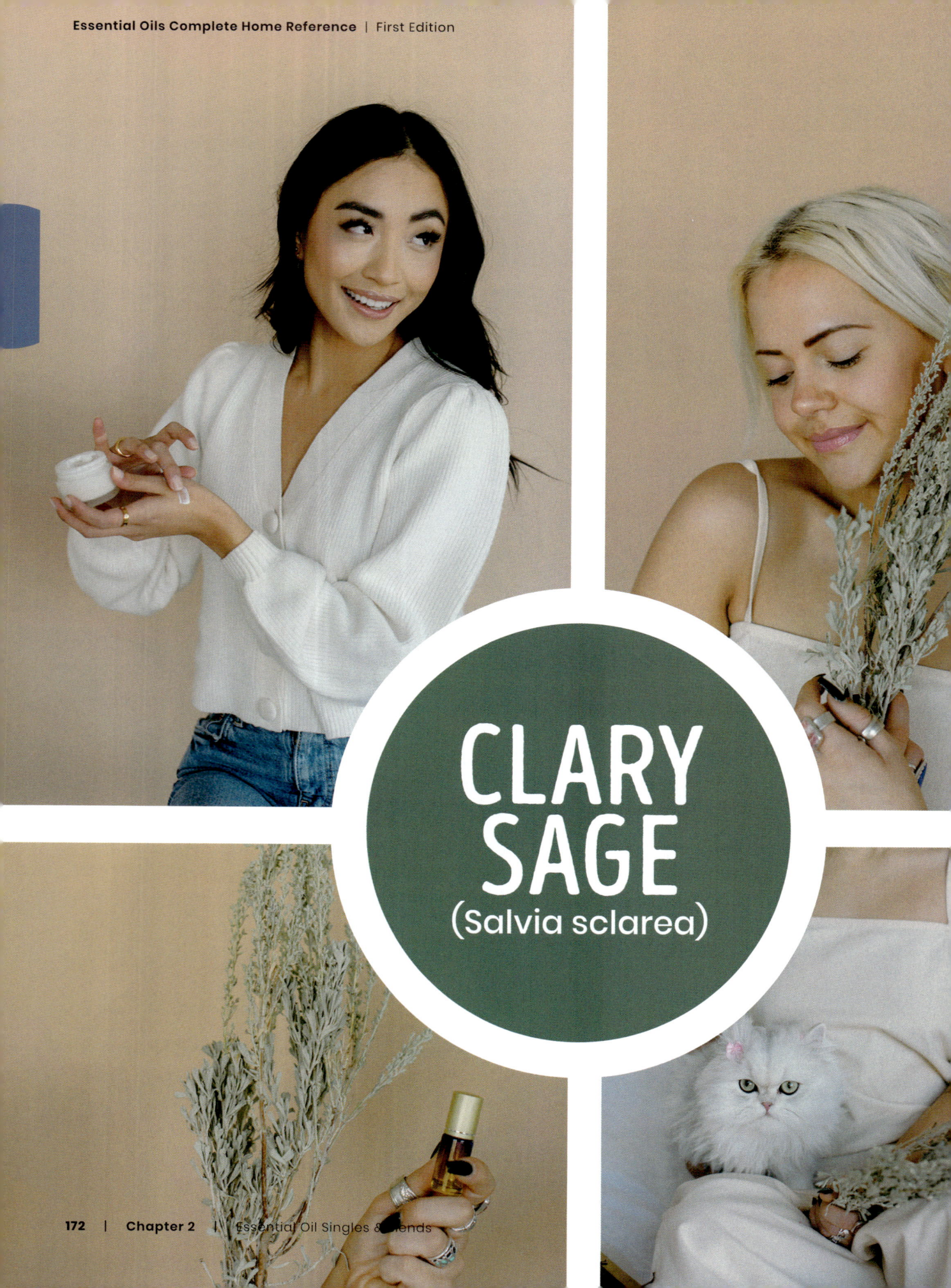

CLARY SAGE
(Salvia sclarea)

Essential Oil Singles & Blends | Chapter 2

BOTANICAL FAMILY:
Lamiaceae

PLANT ORIGIN:
Utah, France

EXTRACTION METHOD:
Steam distilled from flowering tops

KEY CONSTITUENTS:
Linalyl Acetate (44-79%),
Linalool (3-31%),
Germacrene D (up to 17%),
Alpha-Terpineol (up to 5%)

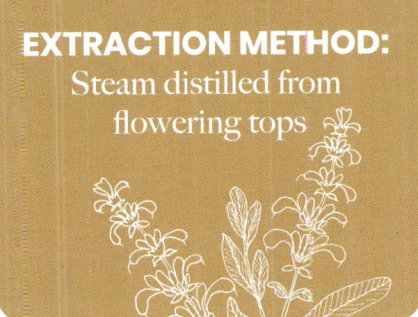

HISTORICAL DATA:
Clary sage seeds were historically soaked, and the mucilage was used as an eyewash and to draw thorns or splinters from the skin. It was also used to treat skin infections, acne, digestive disorders, women's ailments, and to soothe and calm the skin. Aromatically, clary sage was used to enhance the immune system, calm digestive disorders, reduce inflammation such as eczema, calm muscle spasms, and treat respiratory conditions.

MEDICAL PROPERTIES:
Anticoagulant, antioxidant, antimicrobial, antibacterial

USES:
Migraines, throat/lung infections, insect bites

FRAGRANT INFLUENCE:
Herbaceous, slightly floral aroma; enhances one's ability to dream; calming; stress relieving; anxiety; immune system; digestive disorders; inflammation; respiratory system

DIRECTIONS:
Aromatic: 3O. Topical: 50-50. Rub 6-8 drops on lower back during PMS. Dietary: Take as a dietary supplement: 1-10 drops in a capsule or 1-2 drops under the tongue or add to drinking water.

CAUTIONS:

SELECTED RESEARCH:
Llurba-Montesino N, Schmidt TJ. Salvia Species as Sources of Natural Products with Antiprotozoal Activity. In J Mol Sci. 2018 Jan; 19(1): 264.

Živković J, Ristić M, Kschonsek J, Westphal A, Mihailović M, Filipović V, Böhm V. Comparison of chemical profile and antioxidant capacity of seeds and oils from Salvia sclarea and Salvia officinalis. Chem Biodivers. 2017 Dec;14(12). Epub 2017 Dec 5.

Chovanová R, Mikulášová M, Vaverková Š. Modulation of mecA gene expression by essential oil from Salvia sclerea and synergism with oxacillin in methicillin resistant Staphylococcus epidermis carrying different types of Staphylococcal chromosomal cassette mec. Int J Microbiol. 2016:2016:6475837. Epub 2016 Feb 18.

Sienkiewicz M, Glowacka A, Poznańska-Kurowska K, Kaszuba A, Urbaniak A, Kowalczyk E. The effect of clary sage oil on staphylococci responsible for wound infections. Postepy Dermatol Alergol. 2015 Feb;32(1):21-6. Epub 2015 Mar 31.

Yuce E, Yildirim N, Yildirim NC, Paksoy MY, Bagci E. Essential oil composition, antioxidant and antifungal activities of Salvia sclarea L. from Munzur Valley in Tunceli, Turkey. Cell Mol Biol (Noisy-le-grand). 2014 Jun 15;60(2):1-5.

Lee KB, Cho E, Kang YS. Changes in 5-hydroxytryptamine and cortisol plasma levels in menopausal women after inhalation of clary sage oil. Phytother Res. 2014 Nov;28(11):1599-605. Epub 2014 May 8.

Seol GH, Shim HS, Kim PJ, Moon HK, Lee KH, Shim I, Suh SH, Min SS. Antidepressant-like effect of Salvia sclarea is explained by modulation of dopamine activities in rats. J Ethnopharmacol. 2010 Jul 6;130(1):187-90. Epub 2010 May 6.

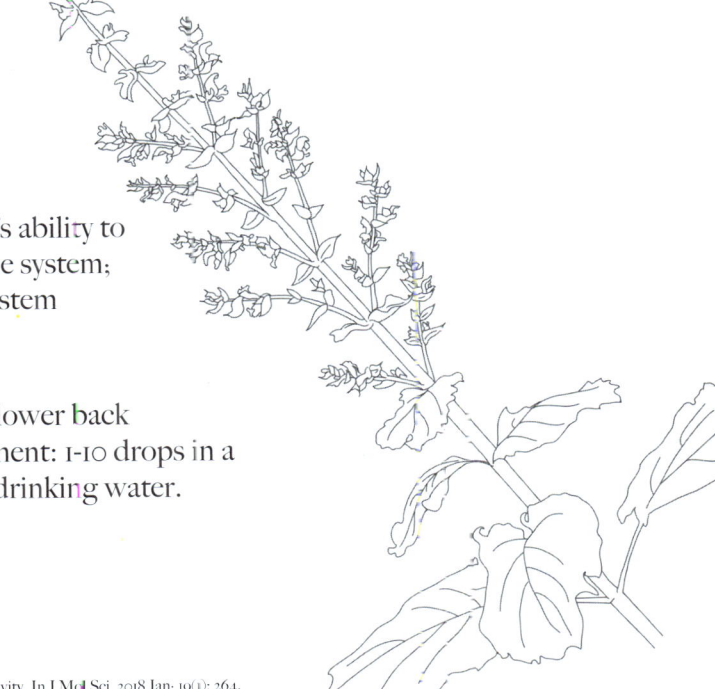

BOTANICAL FAMILY: Myrtaceae

PLANT ORIGIN: Madagascar

EXTRACTION METHOD: Steam distilled from dried flower buds

KEY CONSTITUENTS: Eugenol (75-89%), Eugenyl Acetate (2-15%), Beta-Caryophyllene (2-9%)

CLOVE & CLOVE VITALITY™
(Syzygium aromaticum) (Syn. Eugenia caryophyllus)

The people on the island of Ternate were free from epidemics until the 16th century, when Dutch conquerors destroyed the clove trees that flourished on the islands. Many of the islanders died from the epidemics that followed. Cloves were reputed to be part of the "Marseilles Vinegar" or "Four Thieves Vinegar" that bandits who robbed the dead and dying used to protect themselves during the 15th century plague.

Clove was listed in Hildegard's Medicine, a compilation of early German medicines by highly regarded Benedictine herbalist Hildegard of Bingen (1098-1179). Healers in China and India have used clove buds since ancient times as part of their treatments. Eugenol, clove's principal constituent, was used in the dental industry for years to numb gums.

MEDICAL PROPERTIES:
Antioxidant, antibacterial, antiviral, antifungal, antiseptic, analgesic, antiaging, antitumoral, antimicrobial, anticoagulant, anti-inflammatory, stomach protectant (ulcers), antiparasitic (worms), anticonvulsant, bone preserving

USES:
Immune system support, cardiovascular disease, blood clots, diabetes, arthritis/rheumatism, hepatitis, intestinal parasites, infections, for numbing all types of pain, throat/sinus/lung infections, cataracts, ulcers, lice, toothache

FRAGRANT INFLUENCE:
Clean, warm, mentally stimulating, encourages sleep, stimulates dreams, creates a sense of protection and courage

DIRECTIONS:
Aromatic: 30. Topical: 20-80. Dietary (Vitality): Dilute 1 drop with 1 drop of V-6 or other pure carrier oil. Put in a capsule and take up to 3 times daily.

CAUTIONS:  Anticoagulant properties may be enhanced when combined with aspirin, etc.

SELECTED RESEARCH:

El-Shouny WA, Ali SS, Hegazy HM, Elnabi MKA, Ali A, Sun J. Syzygium aromaticum L.: Traditional herbal medicine against cagA and vacA toxin genes-producing drug resistant Helicobacter pylori. J Tradi Complement Med. 2020 Jul; 10(4): 366-377.

Faujdar SS, Bishi D, Sharma A. Antibacterial activity of Syzygium aromaticum (cloveo against uropathogens producing ESBL, MBL, and AmpCbeta-lactamase: Are we getting closer to a new antibacterial agent? J Family Med Prim Care. 2020 Jan; 9(1): 180-186.

Radünz M, da Trindade MLM, Camargo TM, Radünz AL, Borges CD, Gandra EA, Helbig E. Antimicrobial and antioxidant activity of unencapsulated and encapsulated clove (Syzygium aromaticum, L.) essential oil. Food Chem. 2019 Mar 15;276:180-186. Epub 2018 Oct 4.

Issac A, Gopakumar G, Kuttan R, Maliakel B, Krishnakumar IM. Safety and anti-ulcerogenic activity of a novel polyphenol-rich extract of clove buds (Syzygium aromaticum L). Food Funct. 2015 Mar;6(3):842-52.

Sultana B, Anwar F, Mushtaq M, Aslam M, Ijaz S. In vitro antimutagenic, antioxidant activities and total phenolics of clove (Syzygium aromaticum L.) seed extracts. Pak J Pharm Sci. 2014 Jul;27(4):893-9

Kumar PS, Febriyanti RM, Sofyan FF, Luftimas DE, Abdulah R. Anticancer potential of Syzygium aromaticum L. in MCF-7 human breast cancer cell lines. Pharmacognosy Res. 2014 Oct;6(4):350-4.

Gupta A, Duhan J, Tewari S, Sangwan P, Yadav A, Singh G, Juneja R, Saini H. Comparative evaluation of antimicrobial efficacy of Syzygium aromaticum, Ocimum sanctum and Cinnamomum zeylanicum plant extracts against Enterococcus faecalis: a preliminary study. Int Endod J. 2013 Aug;46(8):775-83. Epub 2013 Mar 18.

Khathi A, Serumula MR, Myburg RB, Van Heerden FR, Musabayane CT. Effects of Syzygium aromaticum-derived triterpenes on postprandial blood glucose in streptozotocin-induced diabetic rats following carbohydrate challenge. PLoS One. 2013 Nov 22;8(11):e816323. Epub 2013 Nov 28.

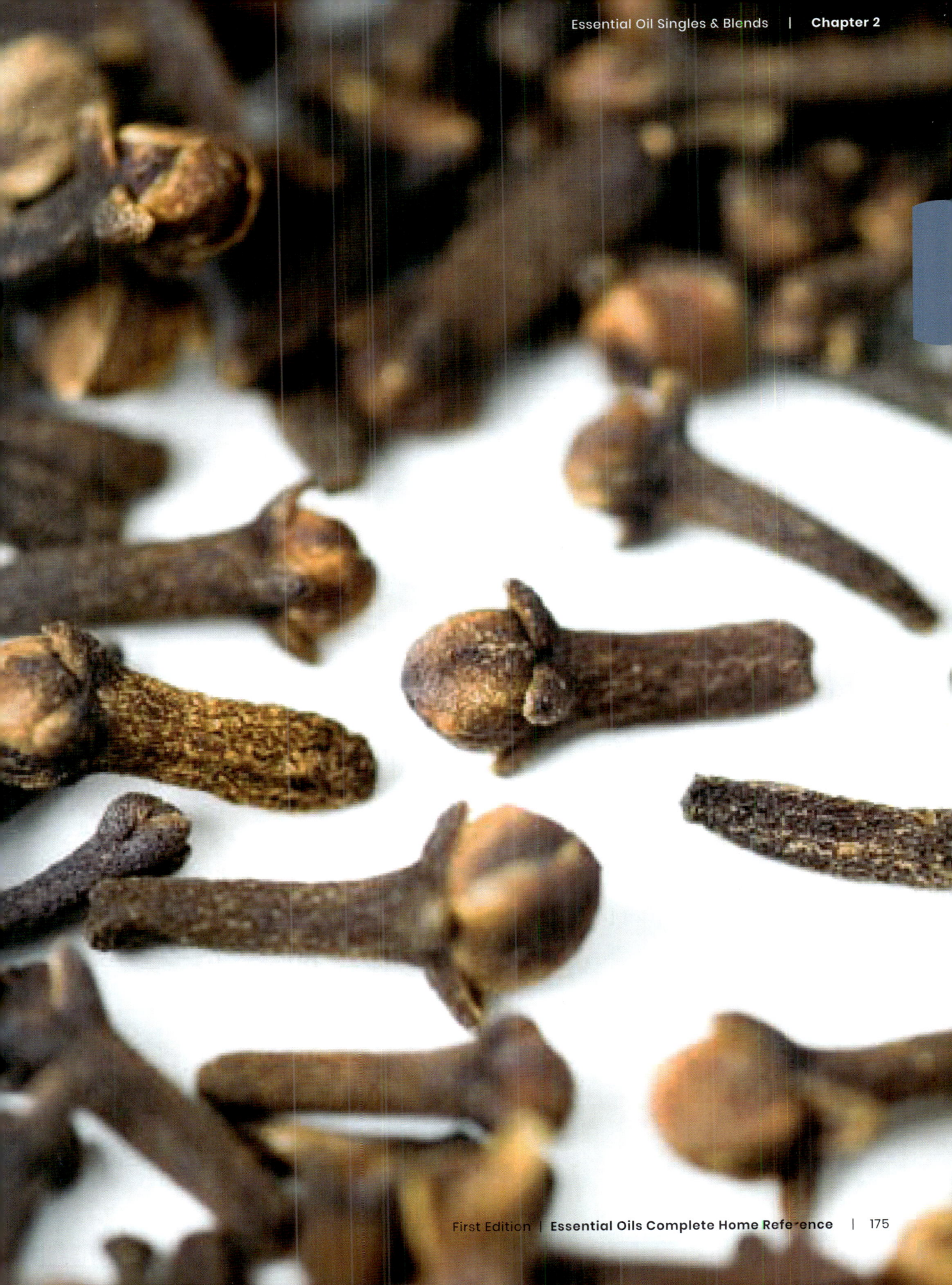

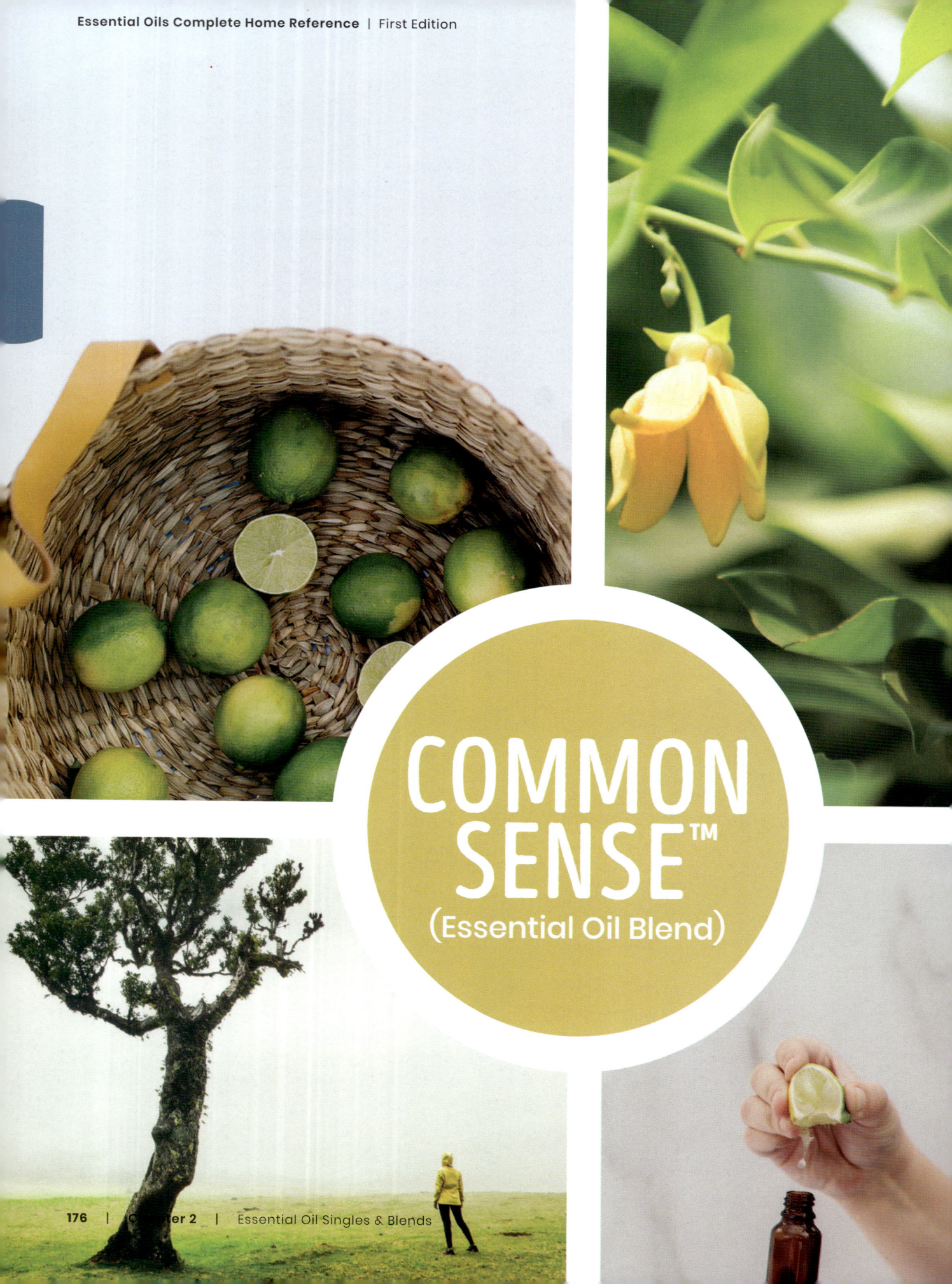

COMMON SENSE™
(Essential Oil Blend)

ABOUT COMMON SENSE™:

Common Sense is a proprietary blend of pure Young Living essential oils specially formulated by D. Gary Young to increase mental acuity, improve decision-making abilities, and strengthen everyday thinking skills.

MEDICAL PROPERTIES & USES:
Anti-inflammatory, antimicrobial, clarity of mind, calming, strengthening, organ protective, skin and hair improving

INGREDIENTS:
Frankincense, Ylang Ylang, Ocotea, Goldenrod, Rue, Dorado Azul, Lime

DIRECTIONS:
Aromatic: 30. Topical: 20-80.

CAUTIONS:
Do not use this product if you are pregnant, planning a pregnancy, or could possibly be pregnant.

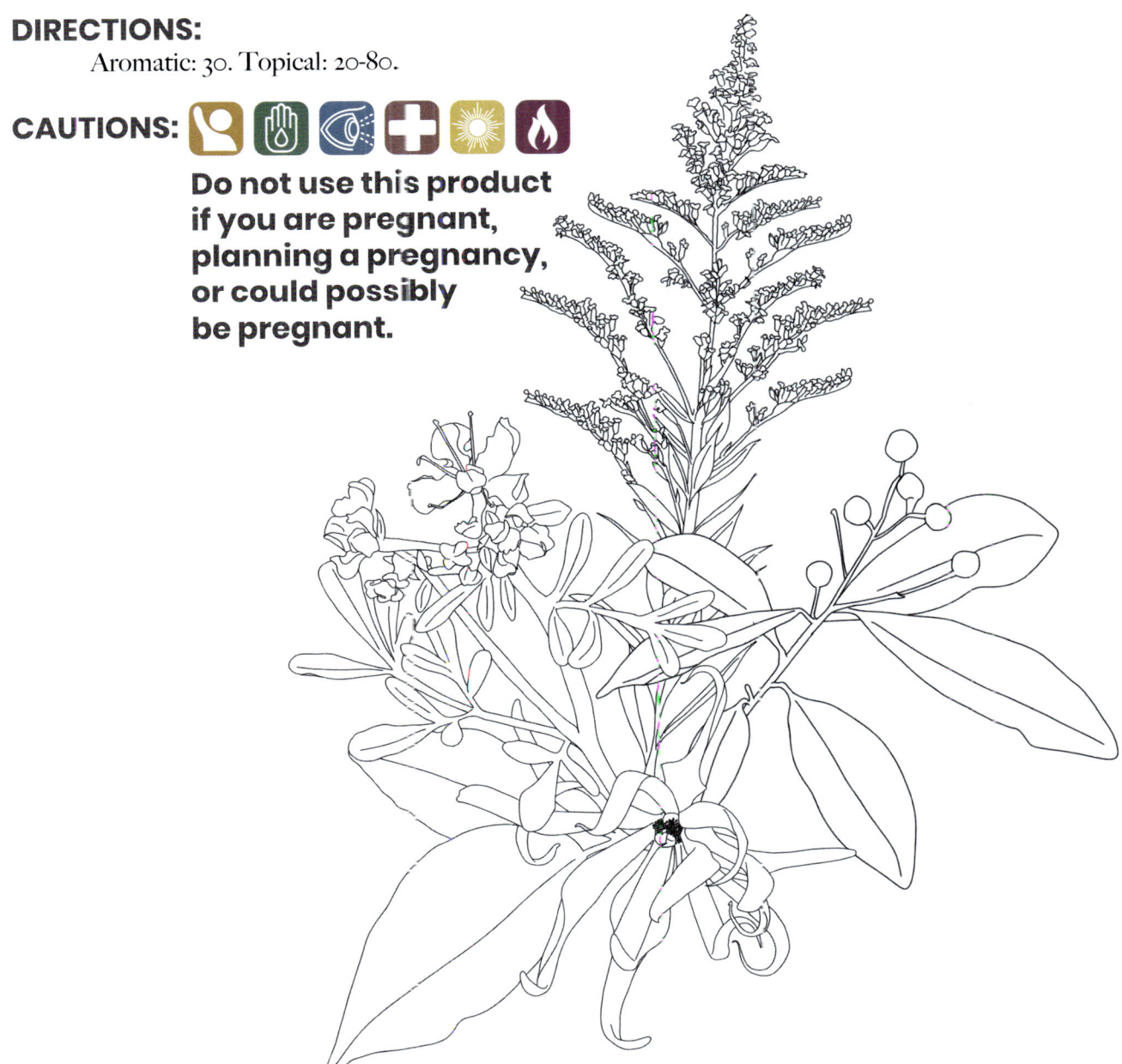

COOL AZUL™
(Essential Oil Blend)

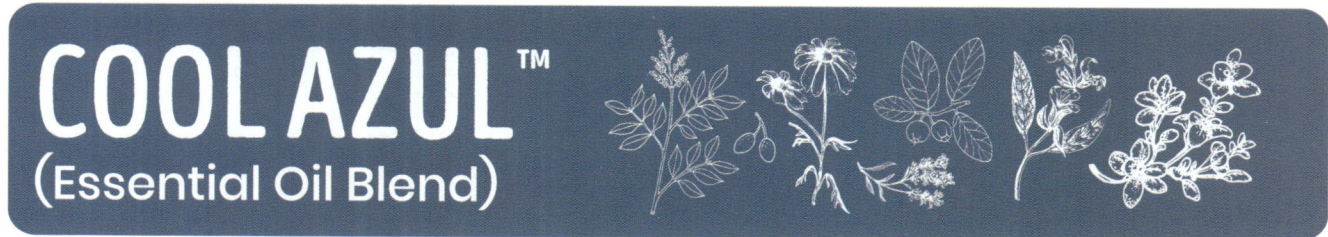

Cool Azul may be applied topically after physical activities to relieve sore or stressed muscles or for a cooling, aromatic sensation.

MEDICAL PROPERTIES & USES:
Anti-inflammatory, antimicrobial, antioxidative, calming, digestion or elimination supportive/nausea reducing, disease inhibitory, hormone supporting, oral protective, pain or swelling reducing, performance enhancing/stimulating, skin and hair improving

INGREDIENTS:
Wintergreen, Peppermint, Sage, Balsam Copaiba, Oregano, Melaleuca Quinquenervia (Niaouli), Ecuadorian (Plectranthus) Oregano, Lavender, Blue Cypress, Elemi, Vetiver, Caraway, Dorado Azul, Matricaria (German Chamomile).

DIRECTIONS:
Dilute as needed with V-6 or other pure carrier oil and apply topically.

CAUTIONS:    **Not intended for children under the age of six without the advice of a health care professional.**

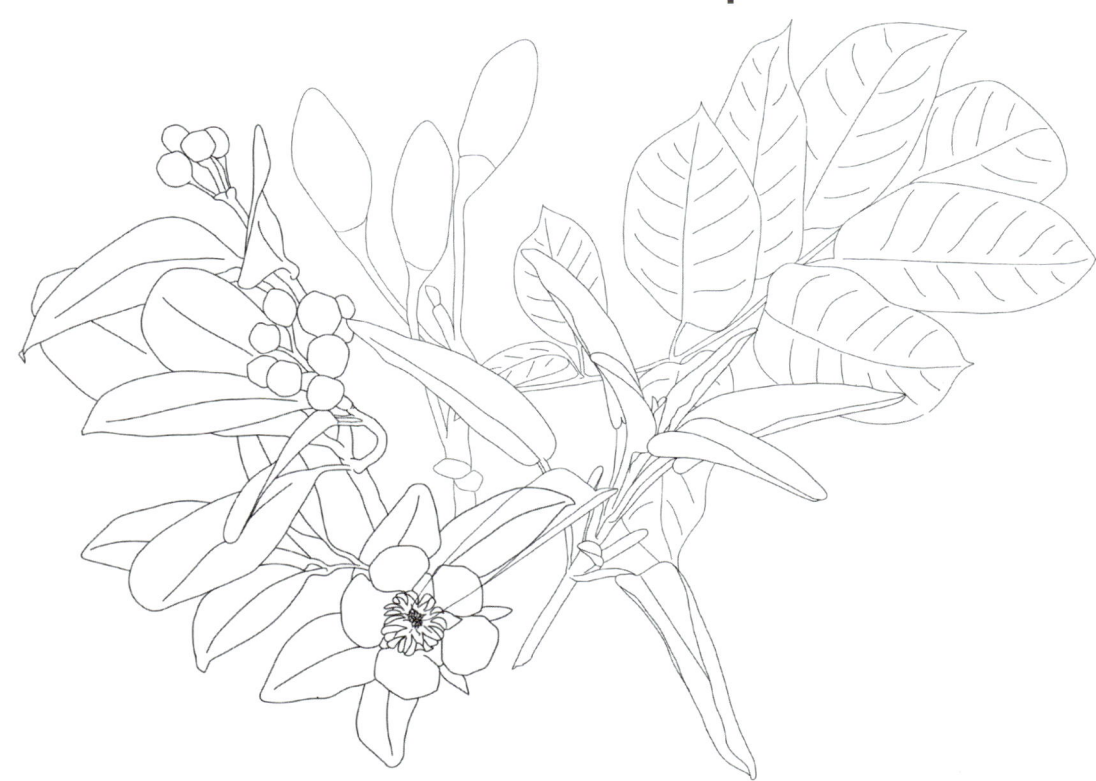

Essential Oil Singles & Blends | **Chapter 2**

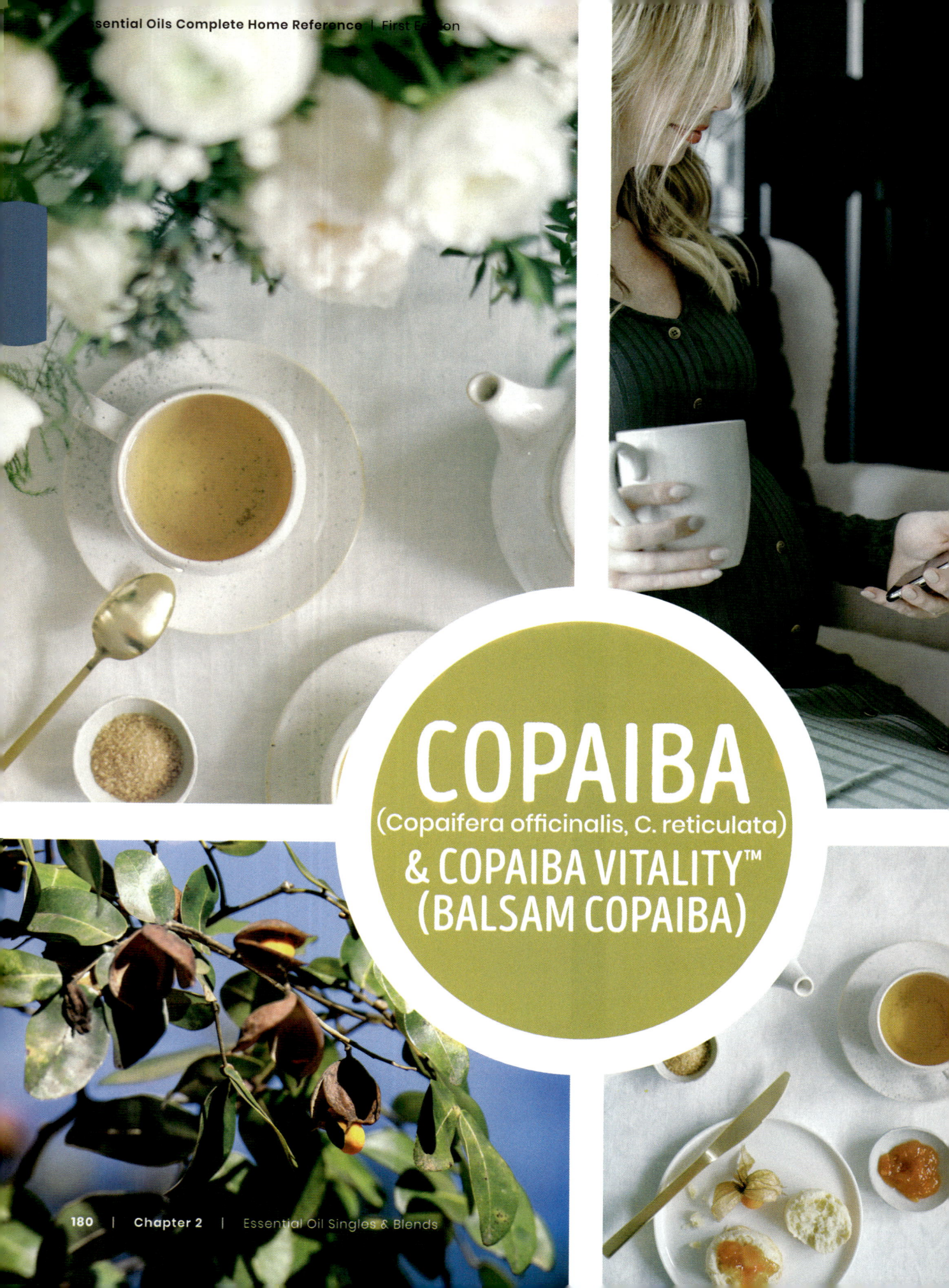

BOTANICAL FAMILY:
Fabaceae

PLANT ORIGIN:
Brazil

EXTRACTION METHOD:
Vacuum distilled from gum resin exudate

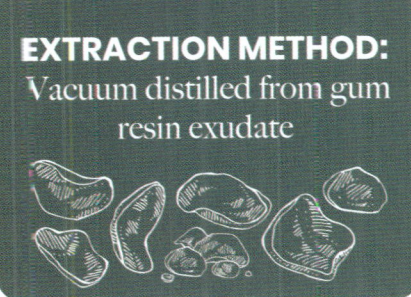

KEY CONSTITUENTS:
Beta-Caryophyllene (45-72%), Trans-Alpha-Bergamotene (up to 12%), Alpha-Humulene (6-10%), Gamma-Elemene (1-9%), Alpha-Copaene (2-6%)

HISTORICAL DATA:

Healers and curanderos in the Amazon use copaiba resin for all types of pain and inflammatory disorders, both internal (stomach ulcers and cancer) and external (skin disorders and insect bites).

In Peruvian traditional medicine, three or four drops of the resin are mixed with a spoonful of honey and taken as a natural sore throat remedy. It is also employed in Peruvian and Brazilian herbal medicine systems as an anti-inflammatory and antiseptic for the urinary tract (cystitis, bladder, and kidney disorders) and in the treatment of urinary problems, stomach ulcers, syphilis, tetanus, bronchitis, and tuberculosis.

In Brazilian herbal medicine, the resin is highly regarded as a strong antiseptic and expectorant for the respiratory tract (including bronchitis and sinusitis) and as an antiseptic gargle. It is a popular home remedy in Brazil for sore throats and tonsillitis (½ teaspoon of resin added to warm water).

Note: The word "copal" is derived from the Nahuatl (Aztec) word for incense (copelli) and can refer to any number of different resinous gums or exudates from trees in Malaysia and South America. Copals are known as black (Protium copal), white (blanco) (Bursera bipinnata), gold (oro) (H. courbaril), and Brazilian (Copaifera langsdorffii or reticulata). Only the Brazilian copal or copaiba has a GRAS distinction in the U.S. and has the most published research on anti-inflammatory effects.

MEDICAL PROPERTIES:
Anti-inflammatory (powerful), neuroprotective, antimicrobial, anesthetic, anxiolytic, mucolytic, antiulcer, anticancerous, antiseptic, kidney stone preventative

USES:
May treat Leishmaniosis, may reduce tumors, pain relief (strong anti-inflammatory), arthritis, rheumatism, cancer, aphrodisiac, contraception, cosmetic products, kidney stones, wound healing, skin disorders (psoriasis), insect bites, stomach distress, urinary disorders, sore throat, anxiety. Approved as a food additive in the U.S.

FRAGRANT INFLUENCE:
Calming, throat infections

DIRECTIONS:
Aromatic: 6o. Topical: Neat. Dietary (Vitality): Put 2 drops in a capsule. Take 3 times daily or as needed. As an alternative, add to food or rice milk, etc., as a dietary supplement.

CAUTIONS: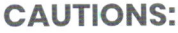

SELECTED RESEARCH:

Urasaki Y, Beaumont C, Workman M, Talbot JN, Hill DK, Le TT. Fast-Acting and Receptor-Mediated Regulation of Neuronal Signaling Pathways by Copaiba Essential Oil. Int J Mol Sci. 2020 Apr; 21(7): 2259. Published online 2020 Mar 25.

Morguette AEB, Bigotto BG, de Lima Varella R, Andriani GM, de Almeida Spoladori LF, Pereira PML, de Adrade FG, Lancheros CAC, Nakamura CV, Arakawa NS, Bruschi ML, Tomaz JC, Lonni AASG, Kerbauy G, Tavares ER, Yamauchi LM, Yamada-Ogatta SF. Hydrogel Containing Oleoresin from Copaifera officinalis Presents Antibacterial Activity Against Streptococcus agalactiae. Front Microbiol. 2019; 10: 2806. Published online 2019 Dec 4.

Diefenbach AL, Muniz FWMG, Oballe HJR, Rösing CK. Antimicrobial activity of copaiba oil (Copaifera ssp.) on oral pathogens: systematic review. Phytother Res. 2018 Apr;32(4):586-596. Epub 2017 Dec 2.

Santiago KB, Conti BJ, Murbach Teles Andrade BF, Mangabeira da Silva JJ, Rogez HLJ, Crevelin EJ, Beraldo de Moraes LA, Veneziani R, Ambrósio SR, Bastos JK, Sforcin JM. Immunomodulatory action of Copaifera spp oleoresins on cytokine production by human monocytes. Biomed & Pharmacother. 2015 Mar;70:12-8. Epub 2015 Jan 9.

Guimarães-Santos A, Santos DS, Santos IR, Lima RR, Pereira A, de Moura LS, Carvalho RN Jr, Lameira O, Gomes-Leal W. Copaiba oil-resin treatment is neuroprotective and reduces neutrophil recruitment and microglia activation after motor cortex excitotoxic injury. Evid Based Complement Alternat Med. 2012;2012:918174. doi: 10.1155/2012/918174. Epub 2012 Mar31.

Santos AO, Ueda-Nakamura T, Dias Filho BP, Veiga Junior VF, Pinto AC, Nakamura CV. Antimicrobial activity of Brazilian copaiba oils obtained from different species of the Copaifera genus. Mem Inst Oswaldo Cruz. 2008 May;103(3):277-81. Epub 2008 Jun 12.

BOTANICAL FAMILY: Apiaceae

PLANT ORIGIN: Russia

EXTRACTION METHOD: Steam distilled from seeds/fruit

KEY CONSTITUENTS: Linalool (65-78%), Alpha-Pinene (3-7%), Gamma-Terpinene (2-7%), Camphor (4-6%), Limonene (2-5%), Geranyl Acetate (1-4%), Geraniol (up to 3%), Myrcene (up to 2%), Alpha-Terpineol (up to 2%)

CORIANDER & CORIANDER VITALITY™
(Coriandrum sativum)

Coriander seeds were found in the ancient Egyptian tomb of Ramses II. This oil has been researched at Cairo University for its effects in lowering glucose and insulin levels and supporting pancreatic function. It has also been studied for its effects in strengthening the pancreas.

MEDICAL PROPERTIES:
Anti-inflammatory, antioxidant, sedative, analgesic, antimicrobial, antifungal, antibacterial, hepatoprotective, liver protectant, anti-migraine

USES:
Supports oral health, diabetes, arthritis, intestinal problems, skin conditions

FRAGRANT INFLUENCE:
Sweet, slightly spicy aroma; soothing and calming; cleansing

DIRECTIONS:
Aromatic: 30. Topical: 50-50. Dietary (Vitality): Dilute 1 drop with 1 drop of V-6 or other pure carrier oil. Put in a capsule and take up to 3 times daily or as needed.

CAUTIONS:

SELECTED RESEARCH:

Kačániová M, Galovičová L, Ivanišová E, Vukovic NL, Štefániková J, Valkova V, Borotova P, Žiarovská J, Terentijeva M, Felšöciová S, Tvrdá E. Antioxidant, Antimicrobial and Antibiofilm Activity of Coriander (Coriandrum sativum L.) Essential Oil for Its Application in Foods. Foods. 2020 Mar; 9(3): 282.

Elmas L, Secme M, Mammadov R, Fahrioglu U, Dodurga Y. The determination of the potential anticancer effects of Coriandrum sativum in PC-3 and LNCaP prostate cancer cell lines. J Cell Biochem. 2019 Mar;120(3)3506-3513. Epub 2018 Nov 11.

Kasmaei HD, Ghorbanifar Z, Zayeri F, Minaei B, Kamali SH, Rezaeizadeh H, Amin G, Ghobadi A, Mirzaei Z. Effects of Coriandrum sativum Syrup on Migraine: A Randomized, Triple-Blind, Placebo-Controlled Trial. Iran Red Crescent Med. J. 2016 Jan; 18(1): e20759. Published online 2016 Jan 2.

Alves S, Duarte A, Sousa S, Domingues FC. Study of the major essential oil compounds of Coriandrum sativum against Acinetobacter baumannii and the effect of linalool on adhesion, biofilms and quorum sensing. Biofouling. 2016 Feb;32(2):155-65.

Cioanca O, Hritcu L, Mihasan M, Hancianu M. Cognitive-enhancing and antioxidant activities of inhaled coriander volatile oil in amyloid β(1-42) rat model of Alzheimer's disease. Physiol Behav. 2013 Aug 15;120:193-202. Epub 2013 Aug 21.

Casetti F, Bartelke S, Biehler K, Augustin M, Schempp CM, Frank U. Antimicrobial activity against bacteria with dermatological relevance and skin tolerance of the essential oil from Coriandrum sativum L. fruits. Phytother Res. 2012 Mar;26(3):420-4. Epub 2011 Aug 5.

Aissaoui A, Zizi S, Israili ZH, Lyoussi B. Hypoglycemic and hypolipidemic effects of Coriandrum sativum L. in Meriones shawi rats. J Ethnopharmacol. 2011 Sep 1;137(1):652-61. Epub 2011 Jun 28.

Mahendra P, Bisht S. Anti-anxiety activity of Coriandrum sativum assessed using different experimental anxiety models. Indian J Pharmacol. 2011 Sep;43(5):574-7.

Pandey A, Bigoniya P, Raj V, Patel KK. Pharmacological screening of Coriandrum sativum Linn. for hepatoprotective activity. J Pharm Bioallied Sci. 2011 Jul;3(3):435-41.

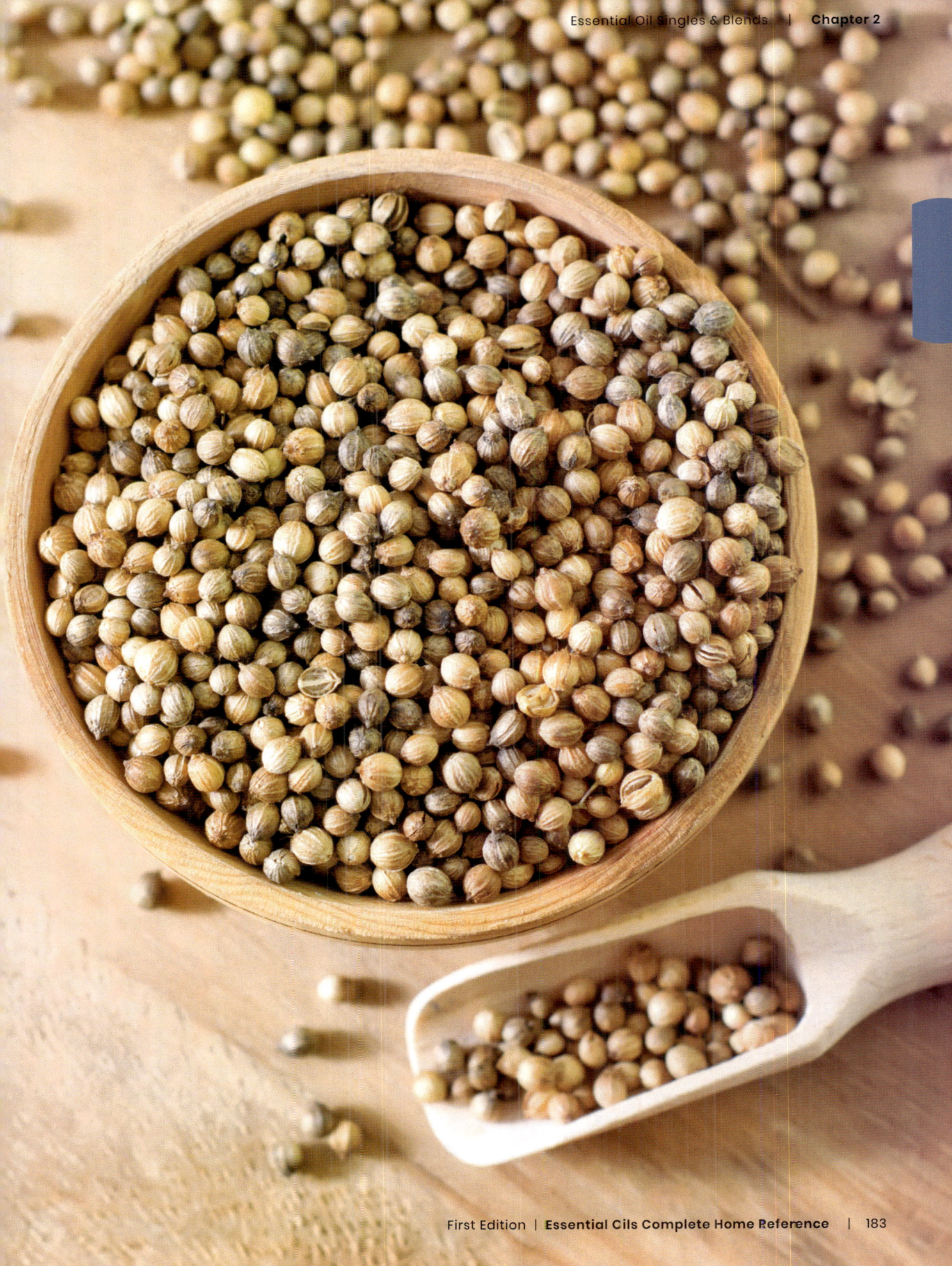

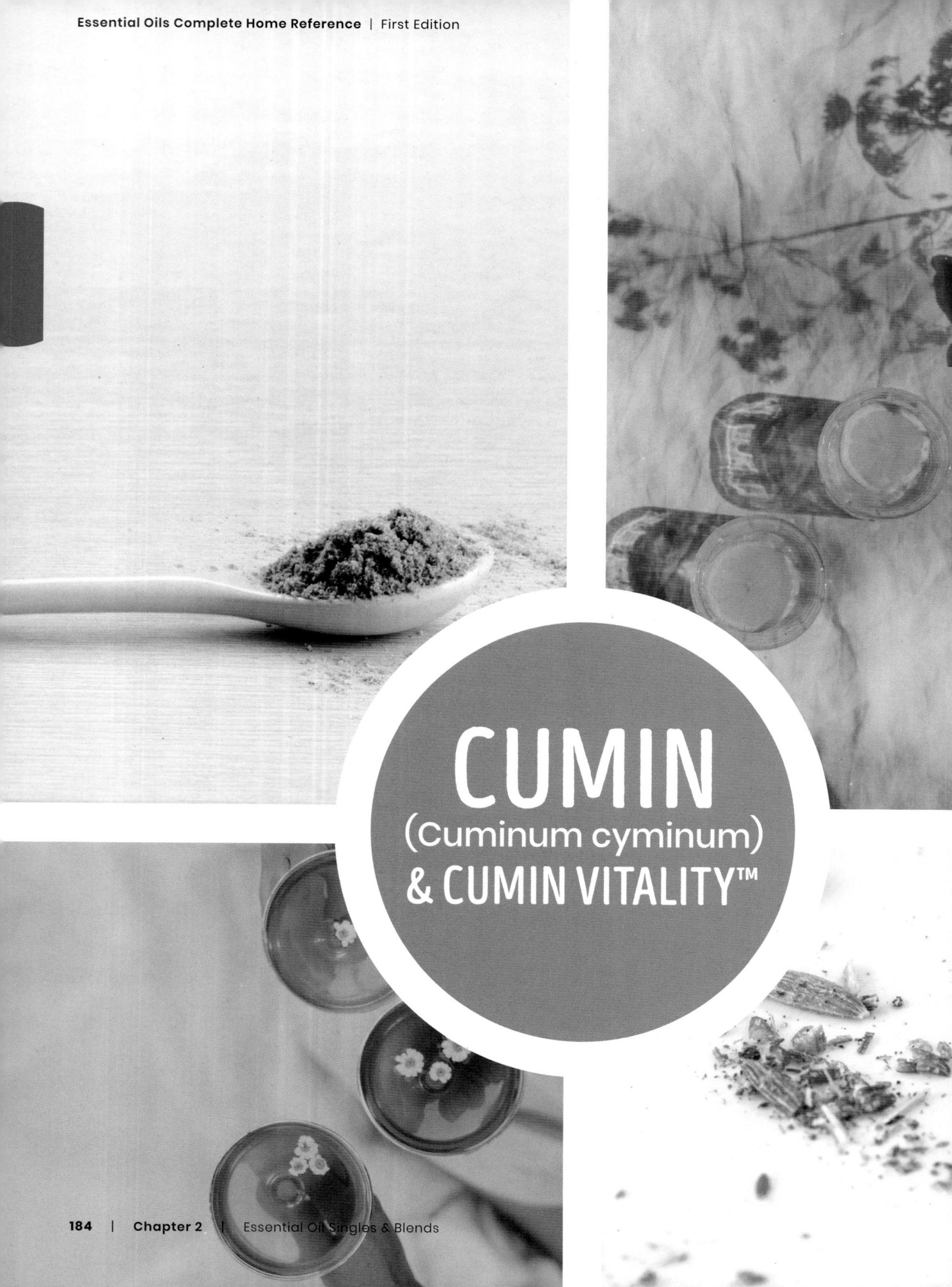

CUMIN (Cuminum cyminum) & CUMIN VITALITY™

Essential Oil Singles & Blends | Chapter 2

BOTANICAL FAMILY:
Apiaceae

PLANT ORIGIN:
Egypt

EXTRACTION METHOD:
Steam distilled from seeds

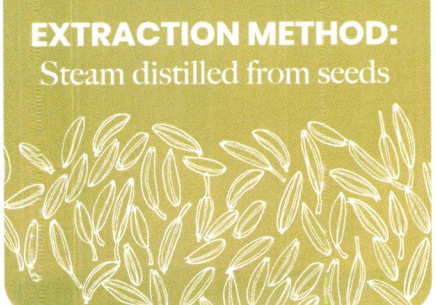

KEY CONSTITUENTS:
Cuminic Aldehyde (13-33%),
Gamma-Terpinene (16-23%),
Para-Mentha-1,4-dien-7-al (1-21%),
Para-Mentha-1,3-dien-7-al (9-21%),
Beta-Pinene (14-18%),
Para-Cymene (2-11%)

HISTORICAL DATA:
The Hebrews used cumin as an antiseptic for circumcision. In ancient Egypt, cumin was used for cooking and mummification.

MEDICAL PROPERTIES:
Antitumoral, anti-inflammatory, antioxidant, antiviral, antifungal, antimicrobial, digestive aid, liver protectant, immune stimulant

USES:
Cancer, infectious disease, diabetes, digestive problems, weight loss, inflammation, reduces bad cholesterol

FRAGRANT INFLUENCE:
Intense, spicy, herbaceous, supports respiratory health

DIRECTIONS:
Aromatic: 30. Topical: 20-80. Dietary (Vitality): Dilute as described under topical. Put in a capsule and take 1 daily or as directed by a health professional. Add 1-2 drops to water or hot tea to take advantage of its cleansing properties. Add to boost flavor in many recipes.

CAUTIONS:

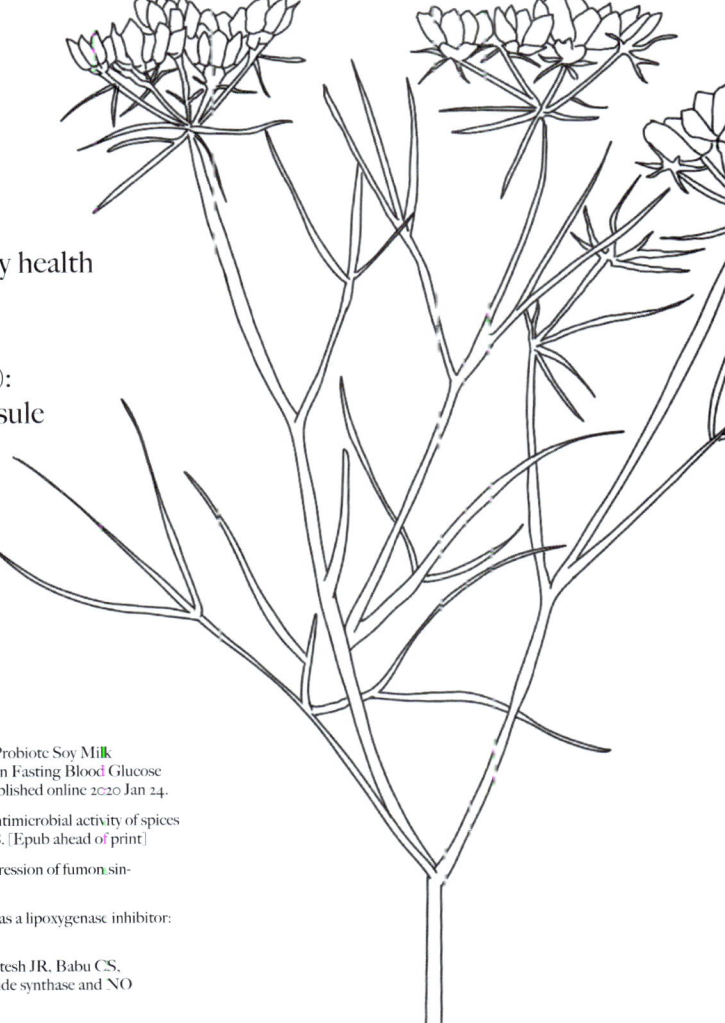

SELECTED RESEARCH:
Babashahi M, Mirlohi M, Ghiasvand R, Azadbakht L, Mosharaf L, Torki-Baghbadorani S. Effects of Probiotic Soy Milk Fermented by Lactobacillus plantarum A7 (KC 355240) added with Cuminum cyminum Essential Oil on Fasting Blood Glucose Levels, Serum Lipid Profile and Body Weight in Diabetic Wistar Ratrs. Int J Prev Med. 2020; 11: 8. Published online 2020 Jan 24.

Condò C, Anacarso I, Sabia C, Iseppi R, Anfelli I, Forti L, de Niederhäusern S, Bondi M, Messi P. Antimicrobial activity of spices essential oils and its effectiveness on mature biofilms of human pathogens. Nat Prod Res. 2018 Oct 13:1-8. [Epub ahead of print]

Khosravi AR, Shokri H, Mokhtari AR. Efficacy of Cuminum cyminum essential oil on FUM1 gene expression of fumonisin-producing Fusarium verticillioides strains. Avicenna J Phytomed. 2015 Jan Feb;5(1):34-42.

Tomy MJ, Dileep KV, Prasanth S, Preethidan DS, Sabu A, Sadasivan C, Haridas M. Cuminaldehyde as a lipoxygenase inhibitor: in vitro and in silico validation. Appl Biochem Biotechnol. 2014 Sep;174(1):388-97. Epub 2014 Jul 31.

Kalaivani P, Saranya RB, Ramakrishnan G, Ranju V, Sathiya S, Gayathri V, Thiyagarajan LK, Venkhatesh JR, Babu CS, Thanikachalam S. Cuminum cyminum, a dietary spice, attenuates hypertension via endothelial nitric oxide synthase and NO pathway in renovascular hypertensive rats. Clin Exp Hypertens. 2013;35(7):534-42. Epub 2013 Feb 12.

Patil SB, Takalikar SS, Joglekar MM, Haldavnekar VS, Arvindekar AU. Insulinotropic and β-cell protective action of cuminaldehyde, cuminol and an inhibitor isolated from Cuminum cyminum in streptozotocin-induced diabetic rats. Br J Nutr. 2013 Oct;110(8):1434-43. Epub 2013 Mar 14.

BOTANICAL FAMILY: Cupressaceae

PLANT ORIGIN: France, Spain

EXTRACTION METHOD: Steam distilled from branches

KEY CONSTITUENTS: Alpha-Pinene (40-65%), Delta-3-Carene (12-29%), Cedrol (up to 7%), Limonene (1-5%), Alpha-Terpenyl Acetate (1-4%)

CYPRESS
(Cupressus sempervirens)

The Phoenicians and Cretans used cypress for building ships and bows, while the Egyptians made sarcophagi from the wood. The Greeks used cypress to carve statues of their gods. The Greek word "sempervivens," from which the botanical name is derived, means "live forever." The tree shares its name with the island of Cypress, where it is used for worship. Cypress wood is noted for its durability, as it was used most famously for the original doors of St. Peter's Basilica at the Vatican that legends say lasted over 1,000 years.

MEDICAL PROPERTIES:
Antibacterial, antimicrobial, antiviral, anti-infectious, antispasmodic, antioxidant, circulatory

USES:
Kidney and liver function, diabetes, circulatory disorders, grounding, stabilizing, fluid retention, respiration, liver health

FRAGRANT INFLUENCE:
Fresh, clean, woodsy aroma. Eases the feeling of loss and creates a sense of security and grounding. Also helps heal emotional trauma, calms, soothes anger, and helps life flow better. Can help soothe irritating coughs and minor chest discomfort.

DIRECTIONS:
Aromatic: 6o. Topical: Neat. Use in Raindrop Technique. Massage toward center of body. Dietary: Take as a dietary supplement: 1-10 drops in a capsule, 1-2 drops under the tongue, or add to drinking water.

CAUTIONS:

SELECTED RESEARCH:

Ibrahim TA, El-Hela AA, El-Hefnawy HM, Al-Taweel AM, Perveen S. Chemical Composition and Antimicrobial Activities of Essential Oils of Some Coniferous Plants Cultivated in Egypt. Iran J Pharm Res. 2017 Winter; 16(1):328-337.

Senol FS, Orhan IE, Ustun O. In vitro cholinesterase inhibitory and antioxidant effect of selected coniferous tree species. Asian Pac J Trop Med. 2015 Apr;8(4):269-75.

Koriem KM, Gad IB, Nasiry ZK. Protective effect of Cupressus sempervirens extract against indomethacin-induced gastric ulcer in rats. Interdiscip Toxicol. 2015 Mar;8(1):25-34.

Selim SA, Adam ME, Hassan SM, Albalawi AR. Chemical composition, antimicrobial and antibiofilm activity of the essential oil and methanol extract of the Mediterranean cypress (Cupressus sempervirens L.). BMC Complement Altern Med. 2014 Jun 2;14:179.

Nejia H, Séverine C, Jalloul B, Mehrez R, Stéphane CJ. Extraction of essential oil from Cupressus sempervirens: comparison of global yields, chemical composition and antioxidant activity obtained by hydrodistillation and supercritical extraction. Nat Prod Res. 2013;27(19):1795-9. Epub 2013 Jan 14.

Tumen I, Süntar I, Keleş H, Akkol EK. A Therapeutic Approach for Wound Healing by Using Essential Oils of Cupressus and Juniperus species Growing in Turkey. Evid Based Complement Alternat Med. 2012; 2012: 728281. Published online 2011 Sep 18.

Essential Oil Singles & Blends | **Chapter 2**

When the storm is strong, hold on to the strength of Cypress!

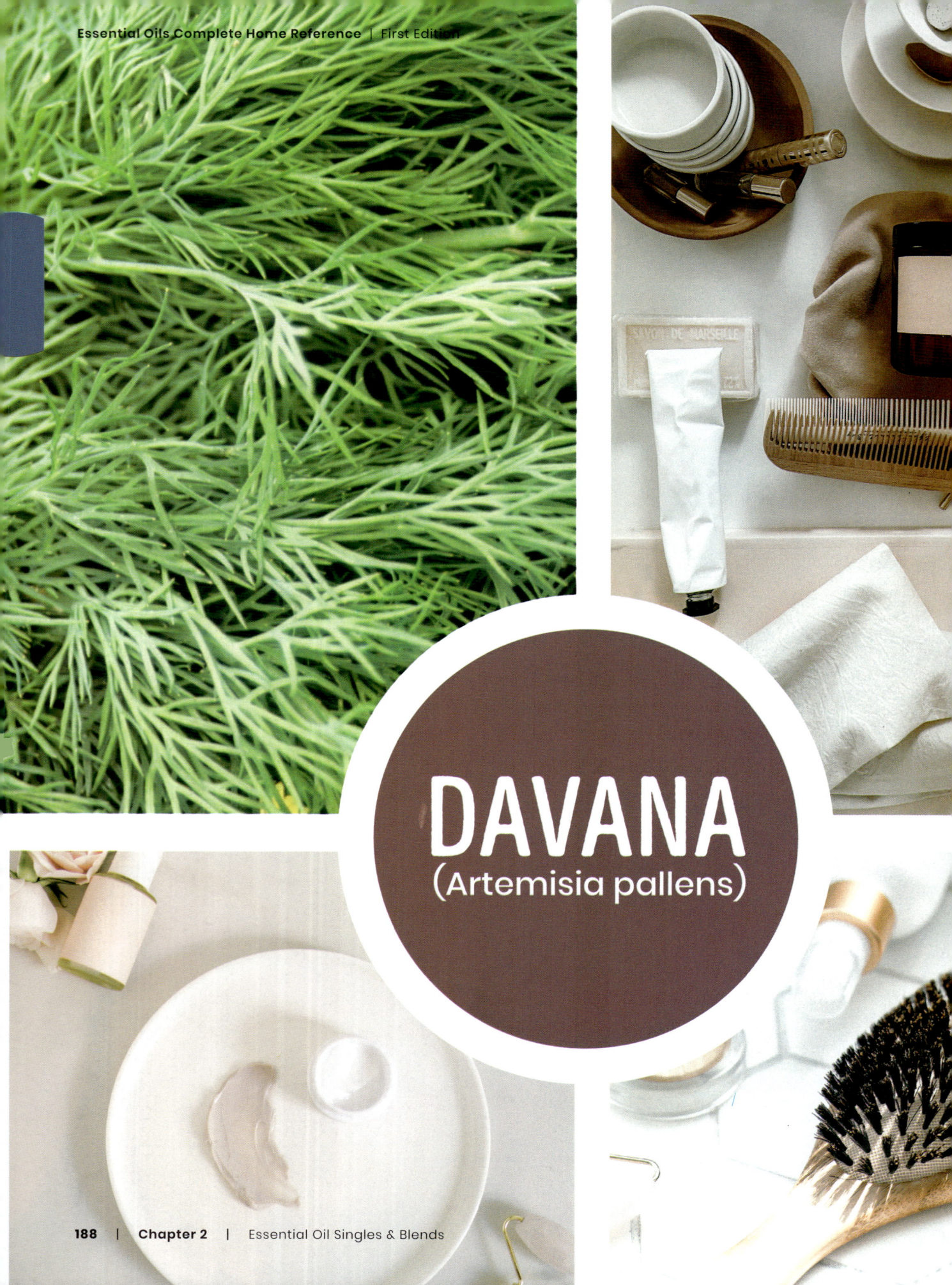

DAVANA
(Artemisia pallens)

BOTANICAL FAMILY:
Asteraceae

PLANT ORIGIN:
India

EXTRACTION METHOD:
Steam distilled from aerial parts

KEY CONSTITUENTS:
Davanone (40-61%),
Bicyclogermacrene (4-18%),
Davana Ether 2 (up to 8%),
I-Ethyl Cinnamate (2-7%),
Germacrene D (up to 3%)

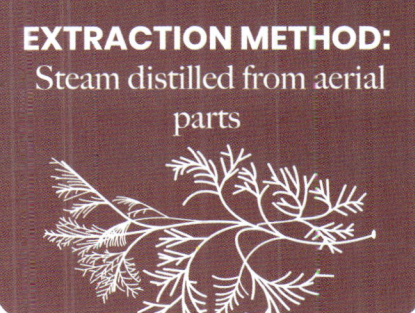

HISTORICAL DATA:
Davana grows in the same areas of India as sandalwood. It has been used in India for diabetes, digestive problems (expels parasites), fighting infections, and calming anger. It has been recommended as an aphrodisiac and is often used in perfumery. It has a very rich, concentrated aroma, is usually used in only very small quantities, and is usually used as a complement in very small amounts in essential oil blends. It has been known to heighten spiritual senses. Davana should always be diluted because it is high in ketones. The aroma tends to develop differently, depending on the individual chemistry of the person wearing the oil.

MEDICAL PROPERTIES:
Antioxidant, antimicrobial, anxiolytic, anti-infectious, antiviral, aphrodisiac, anthelmintic, calmative, analgesic, anti-inflammatory, anti-diabetes

USES:
Skin infections and blemishes, headaches, emotional stress, worm infestations, sugar metabolism, menopausal changes, muscle spasms, stress

FRAGRANT INFLUENCE:
Sweet, warm, rich, exotic, calming, heightens spiritual senses, boosts positive outlook on life

DIRECTIONS:
Aromatic: 30. Topical: Neat.

CAUTIONS:

SELECTED RESEARCH:

Salehi B, Ata A, Kumar NVA, Sharopov F, Ramirez-Alarcón K, Ruiz-Ortega A, Ayatollahi SA, Fokou PVT, Kobarfard F, Zakaria ZA, Iriti M, Taheri Y, Martorell M, Sureda A, Setzer WN, Durazzo A, Lucarini M, Santini A, Capasso R, Ostrander EA, Atta-Ur-Rahman, Choudhary MI, Cho WC, Sharifi-Rad J. Antidiabetic Potential of Medicinal Plants and Their Active Components. Biomolecules. 2019 Oct; 9(10): 551. Published online 2019 Sep 30.

Mukherjee AA, Kandhare AD, Rojatkar SR, Bodhankar SL. Ameliorative effects of Artemisia pallens in a murine model of ovalbumin-induced allergic asthma via modulation of biochemical perturbations. Biomed Pharmacother. 2017 Oct;94:880-889. Epub 2017 Aug 16.

Alok A, Shukla V, Pala Z, Kumar J, Kudale S, Desai N. In vitro regeneration and optimization of factors affecting Agrobacterium mediated transformation in Artemisia pallens, an important medicinal plant. Physiol Mol Biol Plants. 2016 Apr;22(2):261-9. Epub 2016 Apr 25.

Honmore V, Kandhare A, Zanwar AA, Rojatkar S, Bodhankar S, Natu A. Artemisia pallens alleviates acetaminophen induced toxicity via modulation of endogenous biomarkers. Pharm Biol. 2015 Apr;53(4):571-81. Epub 2014 Oct 24.

Ruikar AD, Khatiwora E, Ghayal NA, Misar AV, Mujumdar AM, Puranik VG, Deshpande NR. Studies on aerial parts of Artemisia pallens wall for phenol, flavonoid and evaluation of antioxidant activity. J Pharm Bioallied Sci. 2011 Apr;3(2):302-5.

Ruikar AD, Misar AV, Jadhav RB, Rojatkar SR, Mujumdar AM, Puranik VG, Deshpande NR. Sesquiterpene Lactone, a potent drug model from Artemisia pallens wall with anti-inflammatory activity. Arzneimittelforschung. 2011;61(9):510-4.

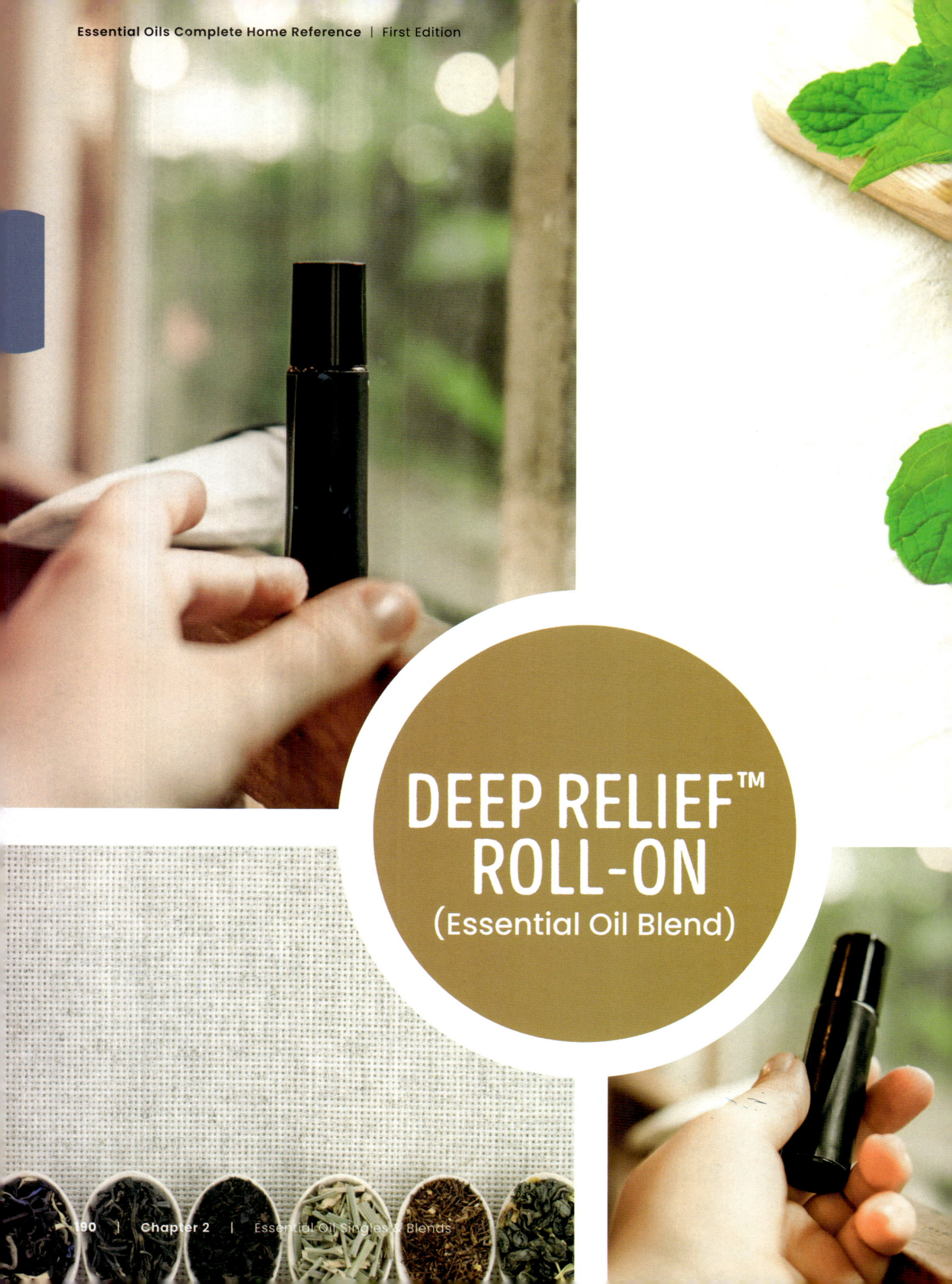

DEEP RELIEF™ ROLL-ON
(Essential Oil Blend)

ABOUT DEEP RELIEF™ ROLL ON™:

This convenient roll-on relieves muscle soreness and tension, soothes sore joints and ligaments, helps calm stressed nerves, and reduces inflammation. This powerful blend contains nine essential oils, most of which are known for their anti-inflammatory and pain-relieving characteristics.

This highly portable roll-on with its no-mess application is easy to carry in your pocket, purse, briefcase, etc. It also passes through airport security for "easy breathing" while flying high.

MEDICAL PROPERTIES & USES:

Anti-inflammatory, antimicrobial, antioxidative, cardiovascular supportive, digestion or elimination supportive/nausea reducing, disease inhibitory, organ protective, pain or swelling reducing, performance enhancing/stimulating, skin and hair improving

INGREDIENTS:

Peppermint, Caprylic/capric triglyceride,† Lemon, Idaho Grand Fir, Clove, Balsam Copaiba, Coconut oil,† Wintergreen, Helichrysum, Vetiver

DIRECTIONS:

Topical: Neat. For head tension, apply on temples, back of neck, and forehead.

CAUTIONS:

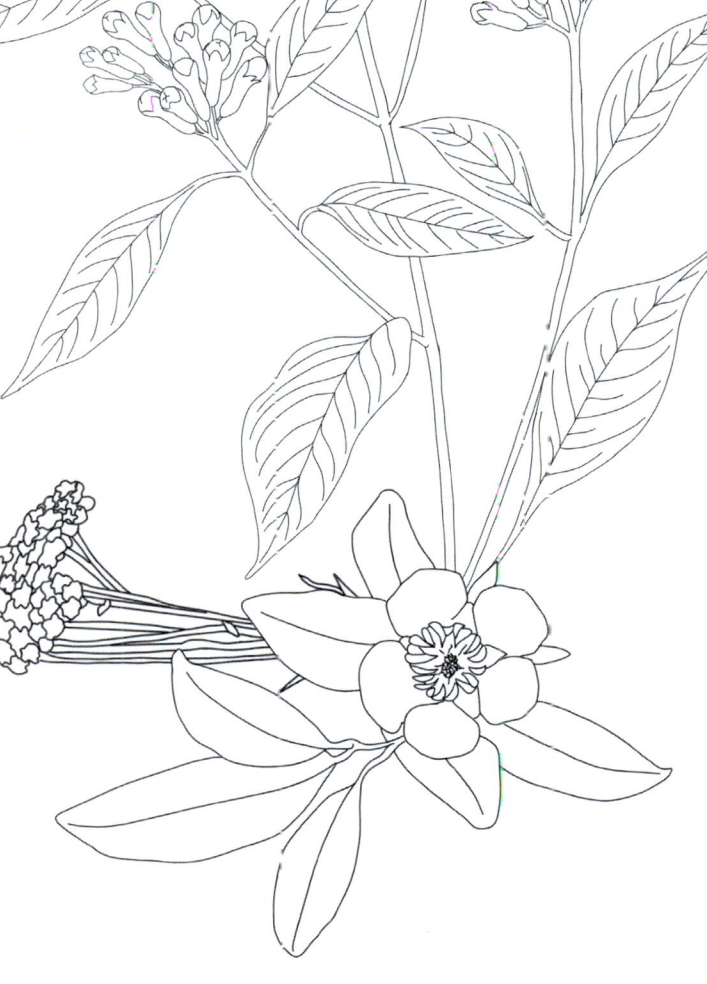

DIGIZE™ & DIGIZE™ VITALITY™
(Essential Oil Blend)

This blend relieves digestive problems, including indigestion, heartburn, gas, and bloating. It helps fight candida as it kills and digests parasite infestation.

MEDICAL PROPERTIES & USES:

Anti-allergy, antimicrobial, calming, cardiovascular supportive, dietary, digestion or elimination supportive/nausea reducing, disease inhibitory, muscle relaxant/bone-joint preservative, nervous system supportive, organ protective, pain or swelling reducing, performance enhancing/stimulating

INGREDIENTS:

Tarragon, Ginger, Peppermint, Juniper, Fennel, Lemongrass, Anise, Patchouli

DIRECTIONS:

Aromatic: 30. Topical: 50-50. Dietary (Vitality): Dilute 1 drop with 4 drops of V-6 or other pure carrier oil. Put in a capsule and take 1 daily or as directed by a health care professional. Apply to Vita Flex points on feet and ankles for stomach and intestinal relief or on desired location as needed. Massage or use as a compress on the stomach.

CAUTIONS:

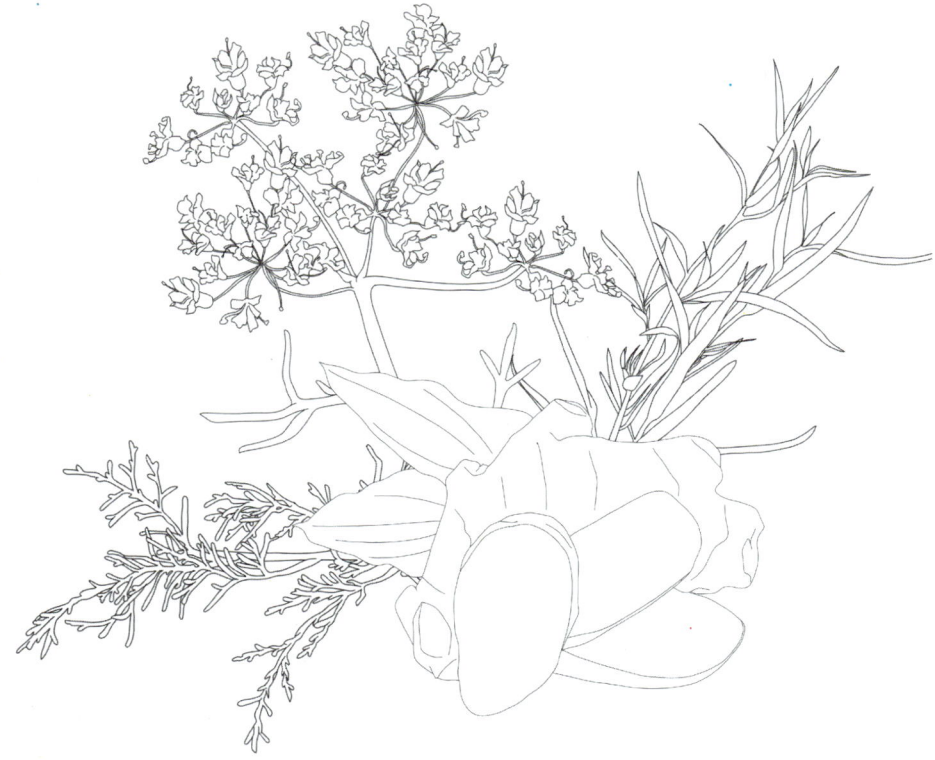

Essential Oil Singles & Blends | **Chapter 2**

DiGize your troubles away!

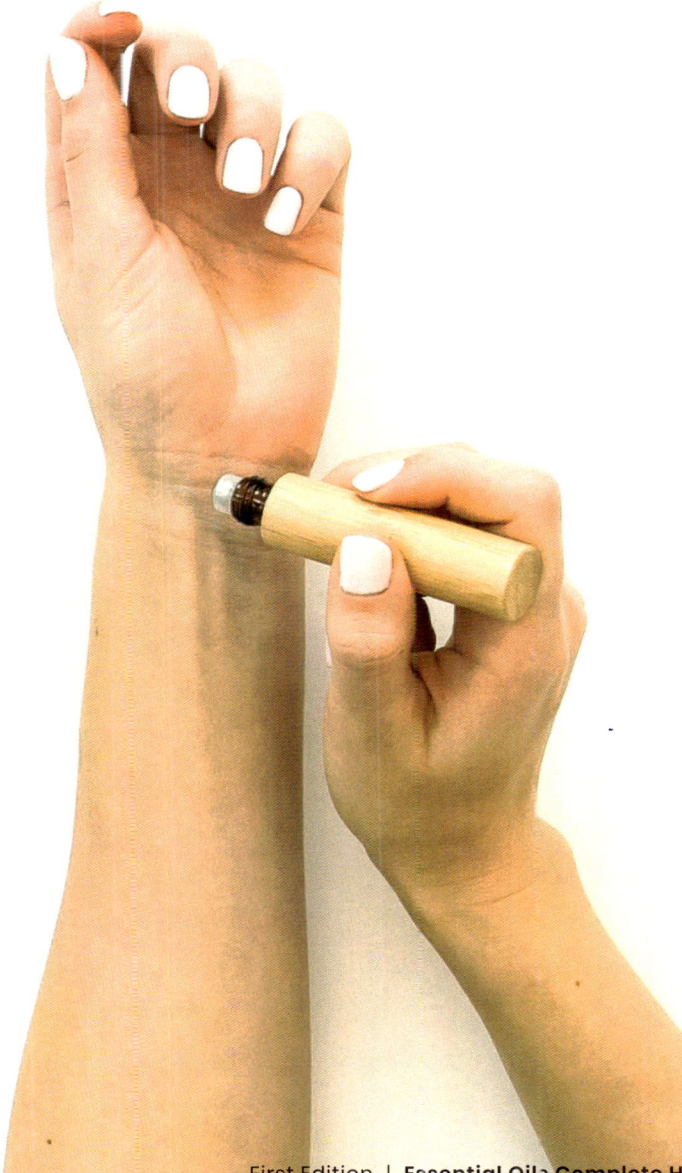

BOTANICAL FAMILY:
Apiaceae

PLANT ORIGIN:
Russia

EXTRACTION METHOD:
Steam distilled from dried fruit/seeds

KEY CONSTITUENTS:
Carvone (28-42%), Limonene (8-40%), Alpha-Phellandrene (15-34%), Dill Ether (4-9%), Beta-Phellandrene (up to 6%), Limonene, (up to 3%), Trans-Dihydrocarvone (up to 3%), Alpha-Pinene (up to 2%), Cis-Dihydrocarvone (up to 2%)

DILL & DILL VITALITY™
(Anethum graveolens)

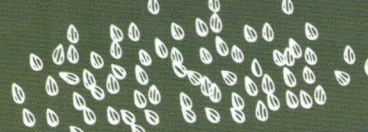

The dill plant is mentioned in the Papyrus of Ebers from Egypt (1550 BC). Roman gladiators rubbed their skin with dill before each match. It is listed in Dioscorides' De Materia Medica (AD 78), Europe's first authoritative guide to medicines, which became the standard reference work for herbal treatments for over 1,700 years. It was listed in Hildegard's Medicine, a compilation of early German medicines by highly regarded Benedictine herbalist Hildegard of Bingen (1098-1179).

MEDICAL PROPERTIES:
Antidiabetic, antispasmodic, antifungal, antibacterial, expectorant, pancreatic stimulant, insulin/blood sugar regulator, anti-inflammatory, antioxidant, hepatoprotective, hypolipidemic

USES:
Diabetes, digestive problems, liver deficiencies, infections, blood sugar, inflammation

FRAGRANT INFLUENCE:
Calms the autonomic nervous system and, when diffused with Roman Chamomile, combats ADHD

DIRECTIONS:
Aromatic: 3O. Topical: 50-50. Dietary (Vitality): Dilute 1 drop with 1 drop of carrier oil. Put in a capsule and take up to 3 times daily.

CAUTIONS:

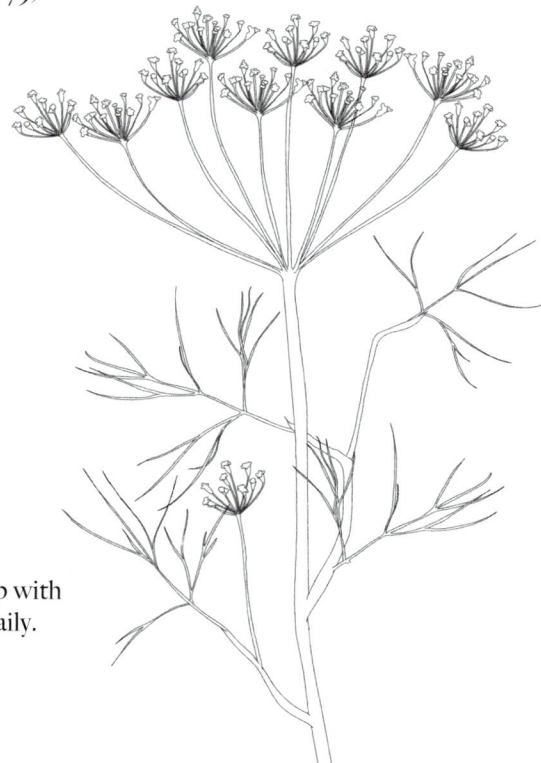

SELECTED RESEARCH:

Haidari F, Zakerkish M, Borazjani F, Angali KA, Foroushani GA. The effects of Anethum graveolens (dill) powder supplementation on clinical and metabolic status in patients with type 2 diabetes. Trials. 2020; 21:483. Published online 2020 Jun 5.

Mohammed FA, Elkady AI, Syed FQ, Mirza MB, Hakeem KR, Alkarim S. Anethum graveolens (dill) - A medicinal herb induces apoptosis and cell cycle arrest in HepG2 cell line. J Ethnopharmacol. 2018 Jun 12;219:15-22. Epub 2018 Mar 9.

Goodarzi MT, Khodadadi I, Tavilani H, Abbasi Oshaghi E. The role of Anethum graveolens L. (Dill) in the management of diabetes. J Trop Med. 2016;2016:1098916. Epub 2016 Oct 18.

Kazemi M. Phenolic profile, antioxidant capacity and anti-inflammatory activity of Anethum graveolens L. essential oil. Nat Prod Res. 2015 Mar 19;29(6):551-553.

Chen Y, Zeng H, Tian J, Ban X, Ma B, Wang Y. Dill (Anethum graveolens L.) seed essential oil induces Candida albicans apoptosis in a metacaspase-dependent manner. Fungal Biol. 2014 Apr 1;118(4):394-401.

Setorki M, Rafieian-Kopaei M, Merikhi A, Heidarian E, Shahinfard N, Ansari R, Nasri H, Esmael N, Baradaran A. Suppressive impact of Anethum graveolens consumption on biochemical risk factors of atherosclerosis in hypercholesterolemic rabbits. Int J Prev Med. 2013 Aug;4(8):889-95.

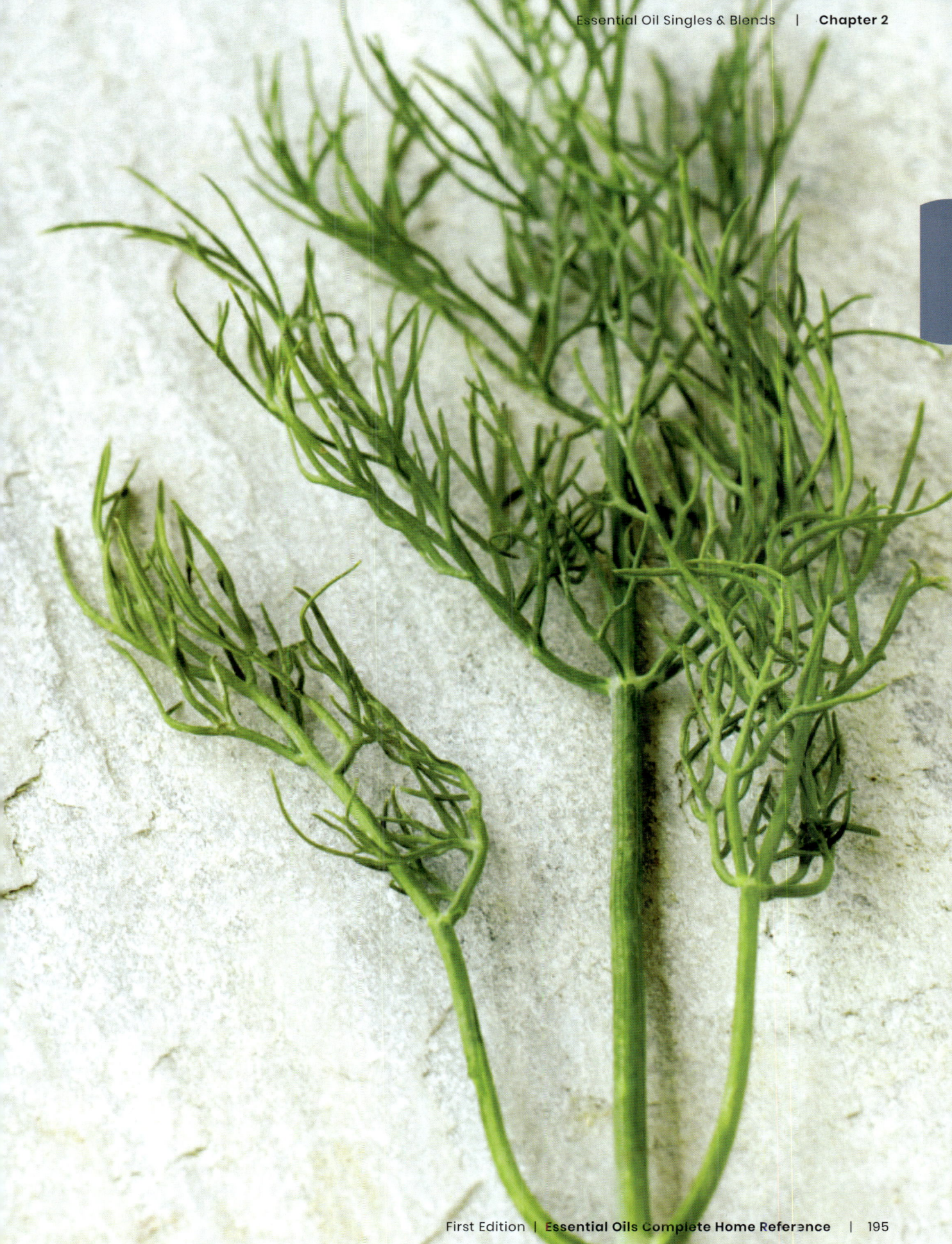

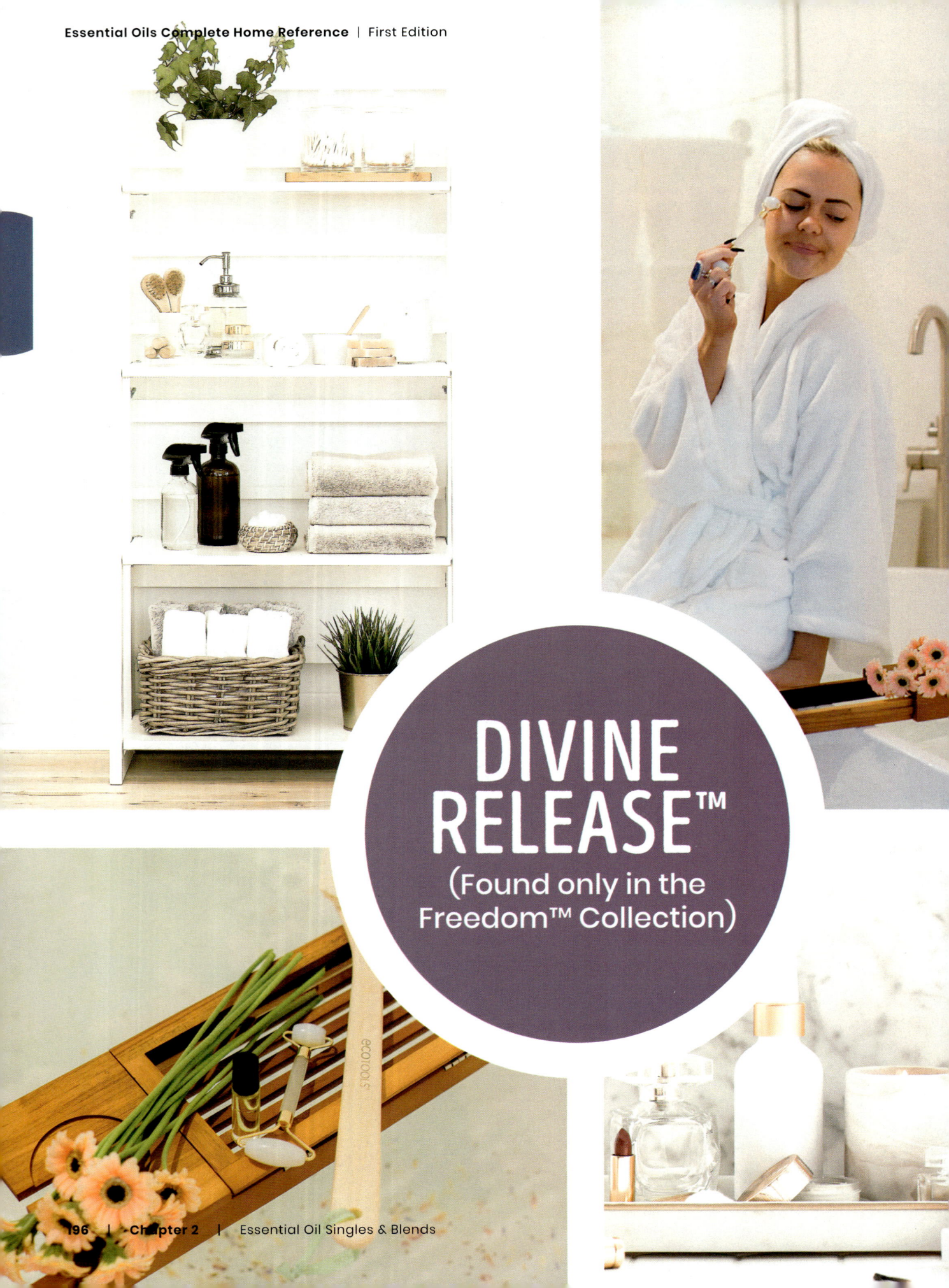

ABOUT DIVINE RELEASE™:
Divine Release is an elevating blend that helps release feelings of anger and promotes forgiveness to encourage the gentle characteristics within oneself for a positive outlook on life.

MEDICAL PROPERTIES & USES:
Antibacterial, antiviral, antifungal, immuno-stimulant, emotion supporting, uplifting, relaxing, antispasmodic, anti-inflammatory, antidepressant, muscle relaxing, antioxidant

INGREDIENTS:
Royal Hawaiian Sandalwood, Roman Chamomile, Frankincense, Melissa, Geranium, Grapefruit, Blue Cypress, Hinoki, Helichrysum, Bergamot, Rose, Ledum, Angelica

DIRECTIONS:
Aromatic: 6o. Topical: Neat.

CAUTIONS:

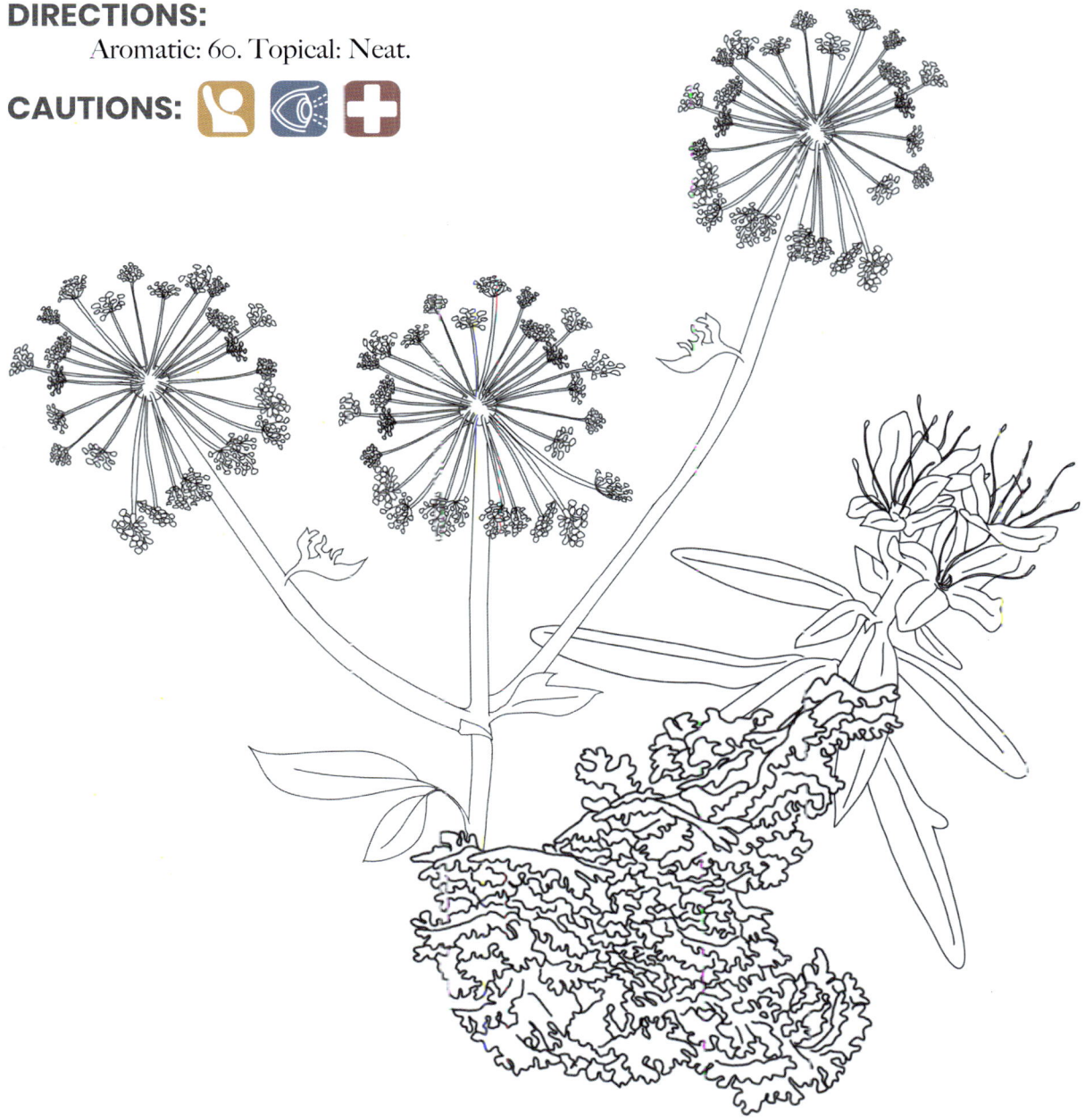

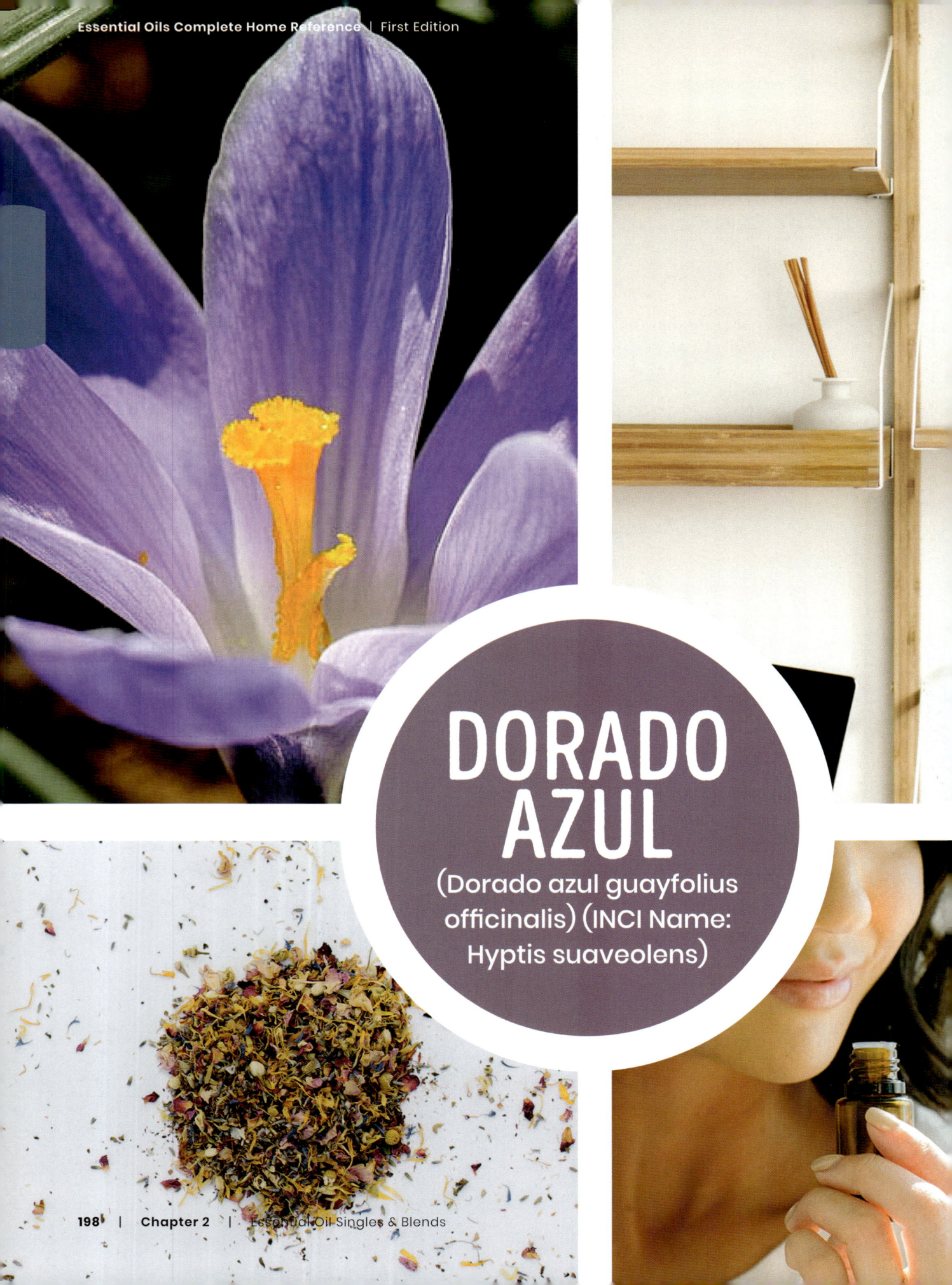

DORADO AZUL

(Dorado azul guayfolius officinalis) (INCI Name: Hyptis suaveolens)

Essential Oil Singles & Blends | Chapter 2

BOTANICAL FAMILY:
Lamiaceae

PLANT ORIGIN:
Ecuador

EXTRACTION METHOD:
Steam distilled from aerial parts

KEY CONSTITUENTS:
Eucalyptol (32-45),
Alpha-Fenchol (9-16%),
Sabinene (5-15%),
Bicyclogermacrene (3-10%),
Beta-Pinene (4-9%),
Limonene (up to 4%)

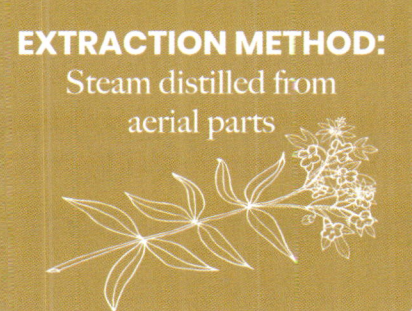

HISTORICAL DATA:
Until about 2006, Dorado Azul was recognized in Ecuador as only a weed. It did not even have a botanical name until D. Gary Young distilled and analyzed it for the first time and gave it its identity. It is a red liquid when distilled, and the natives use it to reverse cancer.

MEDICAL PROPERTIES:
Anti-inflammatory, anticancerous, antioxidant, antimicrobial, antiseptic, antihyperglycemic, gastroprotective, liver protectant, respiratory stimulant, mosquito repellent

USES:
Colds, coughs, flu, bronchitis, asthma, allergic reactions that cause constriction and compromised breathing, any compromise to the respiratory tract, hormone balance, diabetes, vascular dilator, circulatory stimulant, arthritic and rheumatoid-type pain, reducing candida and other intestinal tract problems, digestion, hygienic action for the mouth, enhances mood, spiritual and emotional balance

FRAGRANT INFLUENCE:
Freshens the air, uplifts, clears, builds confidence

DIRECTIONS:
Aromatic: 30. Topical: 50-50. Dietary: Take as a dietary supplement: 1-10 drops in a capsule or 1-2 drops under the tongue or add to drinking water. Dietary (Vitality): Dilute 1 drop with 4 drops of carrier oil. Put in a capsule and take 1 daily.

CAUTIONS: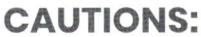

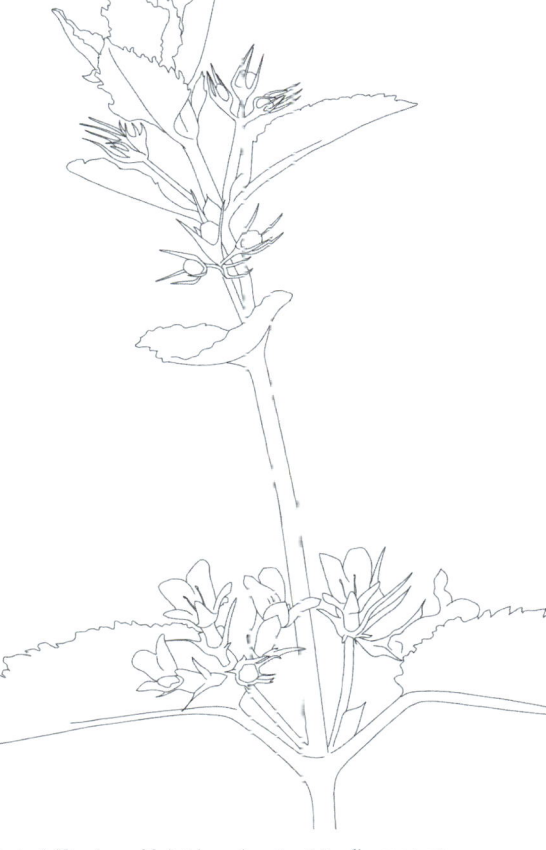

SELECTED RESEARCH:

Sharifi-Rad M, Fokou PVT, Sharopov F, Martorelli M, Ademuyi AO, Lajkovic J, Salehi B, Martins N, Iriti M, Sharifi-Rad J. Antiulcer Agents: From Plant Extracts to Phytochemicals in Healing Promotion. Molecules. 2018 Jul;23(7): 1751.

Ghaffari H, Ghassam BJ, Nayaka SC, Kini KR, Prakash HS. Antioxidant and neuroprotective activities of Hyptis suaveolens (L.) Poit. against oxidative stress-induced neurotoxicity. Asian Pac J Trop Med. 2014 Apr;34(3):323-31. Epub 2014 Jan 14.

Jesus NZ, Falcão HS, Lima GR, Caldas Filho MR, Sales IR, Gomes IF, Santos SG, Tavares JF, Barbosa-Filho JM, Batista LM. Hyptis suaveolens (L.) Poit. (Lamiaceae), a medicinal plant protects the stomach against several gastric ulcer models. J Ethnopharmacol. 2013 Dec. 12;150(3):982-8. Epub 2013 Nov 5.

Ghaffari H, Ghassam BJ, Prakash HS. Hepatoprotective and cytoprotective properties of Hyptis suaveolens against oxidative stress-induced damage by CCl(4) and H(2)O(2). Asian Pac J Trop Med. 2012 Nov;5(11):868-74.

Mishra SB, Verma A, Mukerjee A, Vijayakumar M. Anti-hyperglycemic activity of leaves extract of Hyptis suaveolens L. Poit in streptozotocin induced diabetic rats. Asian Pac J Trop Med. 2011 Sep;4(9):689-93.

Mueller M, Cavarkapa A, Unger FM, Viernstein H, Praznik W. Prebiotic potential of neutral oligo- and polysaccharides from seed mucilage of Hyptis suaveolens. Food Chem. 2017 Apr 15;221:508-514. Epub 2016 Oct 18.

Salini R, Sindhulakshmi M, Poongothai T, Pandian SK. Inhibition of quorum sensing mediated biofilm development and virulence in uropathogens by Hyptis suaveolens. Antonie Van Leeuwenhoek. 2015 Apr;107(4): 07(4):1095-106. Epub 2015 Feb 7.

BOTANICAL FAMILY:
Pinaceae

PLANT ORIGIN:
Idaho, USA

EXTRACTION METHOD:
Steam distilled from wood/bark/twigs/needles

KEY CONSTITUENTS:
Alpha-Pinene (25-40%),
Beta-Pinene (7-15%),
Limonene (6-11%),
Bornyl Acetate (8-15%)

DOUGLAS FIR
(Pseudotsuga menziesii)

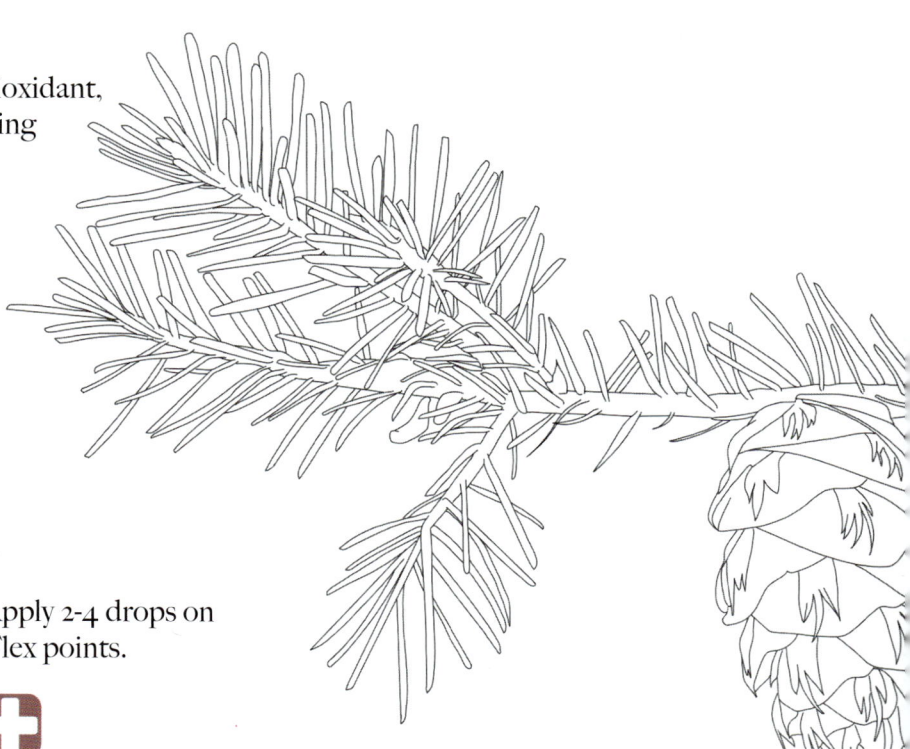

American Indians not only used Douglas fir for building and basketry but also medicinally for ailments like headaches, stomachaches, the common cold, and rheumatism.

MEDICAL PROPERTIES:
antimicrobial, antitumoral, antioxidant, antifungal, antiviral, pain relieving

USES:
Respiratory/sinus infections, cough, asthma, rheumatism, headache, arthritis, skin care, strengthens immune system

FRAGRANT INFLUENCE:
Focus, clarity, purifying air, uplifting, grounding

DIRECTIONS:
Aromatic: 60. Topical: 50-50. Apply 2-4 drops on location, chakras, and/or Vita Flex points.

CAUTIONS:

SELECTED RESEARCH:

Krauze-Baranowska M, Sowiński P, Kawiak A, Sparzak B. Flavonoids from Pseudotsuga menziesii. Z Naturforsch C. 2013 Mar-Apr;68(3-4):87-96.

Johnston WH, Karchesy JJ, Constantine GH, Craig AM. Antimicrobial activity of some Pacific Northwest woods against anaerobic bacteria and yeast. Phytother Res. 2001 Nov;15(7):586-8.

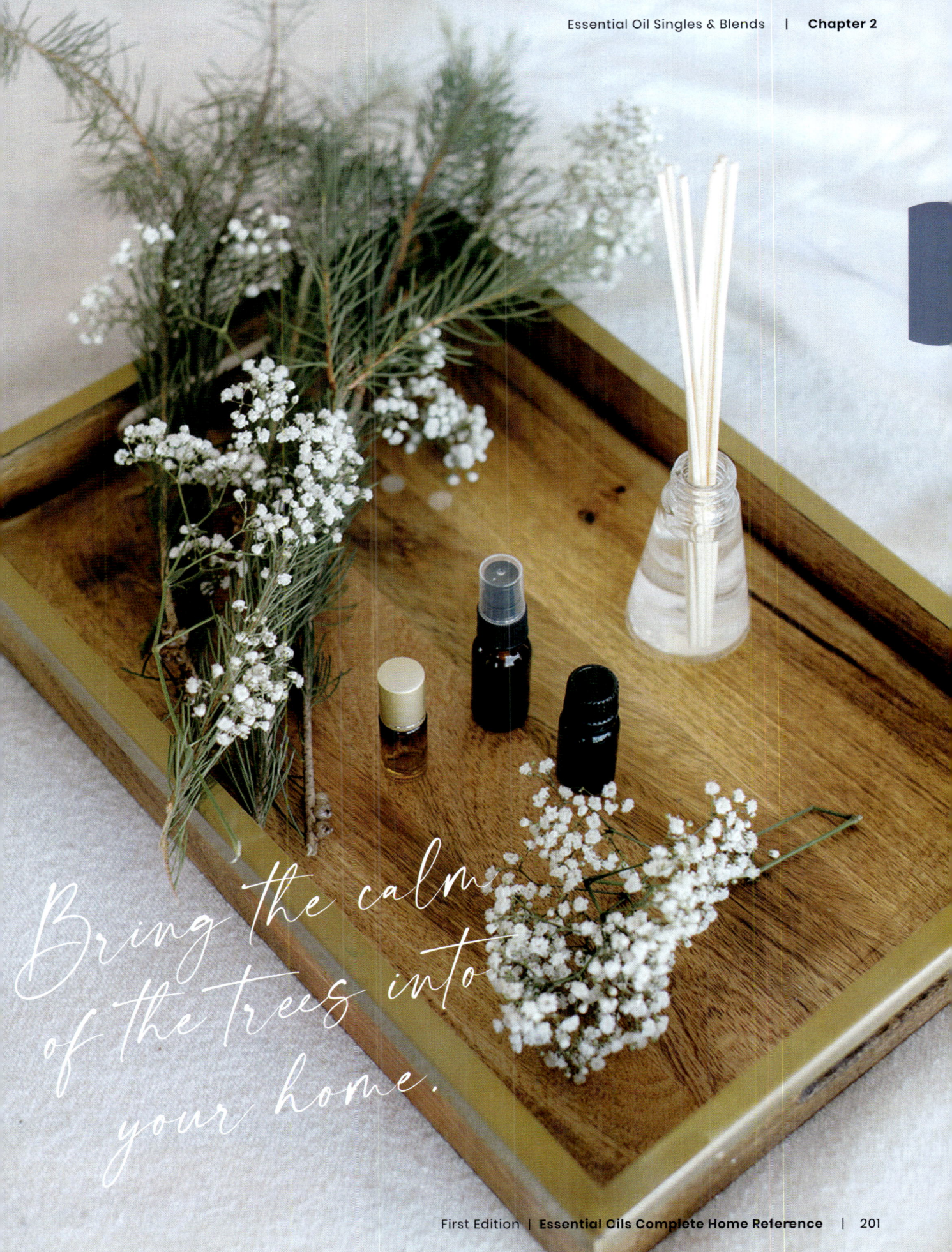

Essential Oil Singles & Blends | **Chapter 2**

Bring the calm of the trees into your home.

First Edition | **Essential Oils Complete Home Reference**

DRAGON TIME™
(Essential Oil Blend)

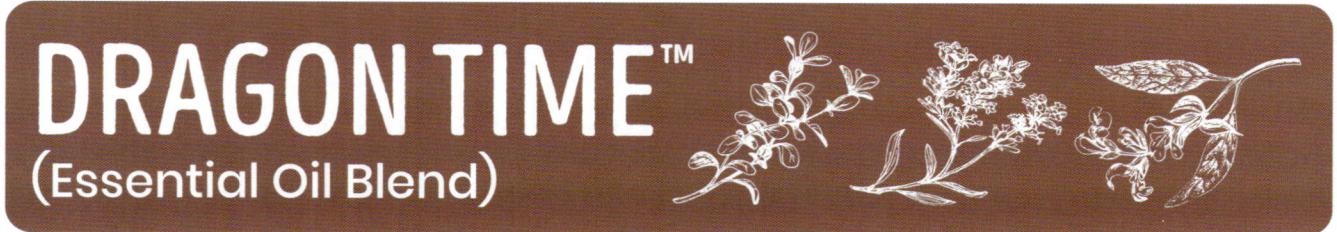

This blend relieves PMS symptoms and menstrual discomforts, including cramping and irregular periods. It helps balance emotions, alleviating mood swings and headaches caused by hormonal imbalance.

MEDICAL PROPERTIES & USES:
Anti-inflammatory, antimicrobial, antioxidative, hormone balancing, calming, cardiovascular supportive, digestion or elimination supportive/nausea reducing, organ protective, emotion supportive

INGREDIENTS:
Fennel, Clary Sage, Marjoram, Lavender, Yarrow, Jasmine

DIRECTIONS:
Aromatic: 30. Topical: 50-50. Apply with a hot compress or directly over lower abdomen, across lower back, or on location of pain. Use on both sides of ankles and feet.

CAUTIONS:

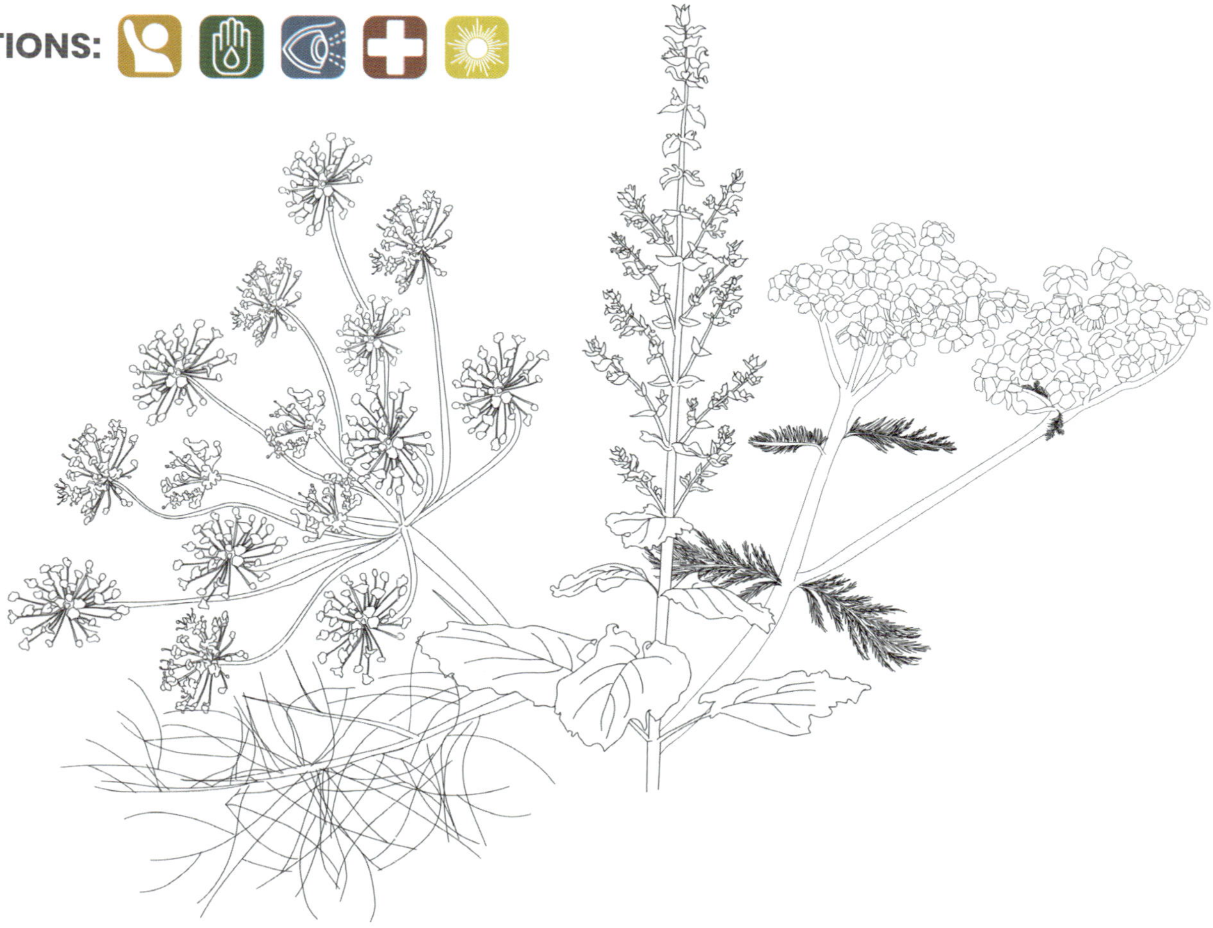

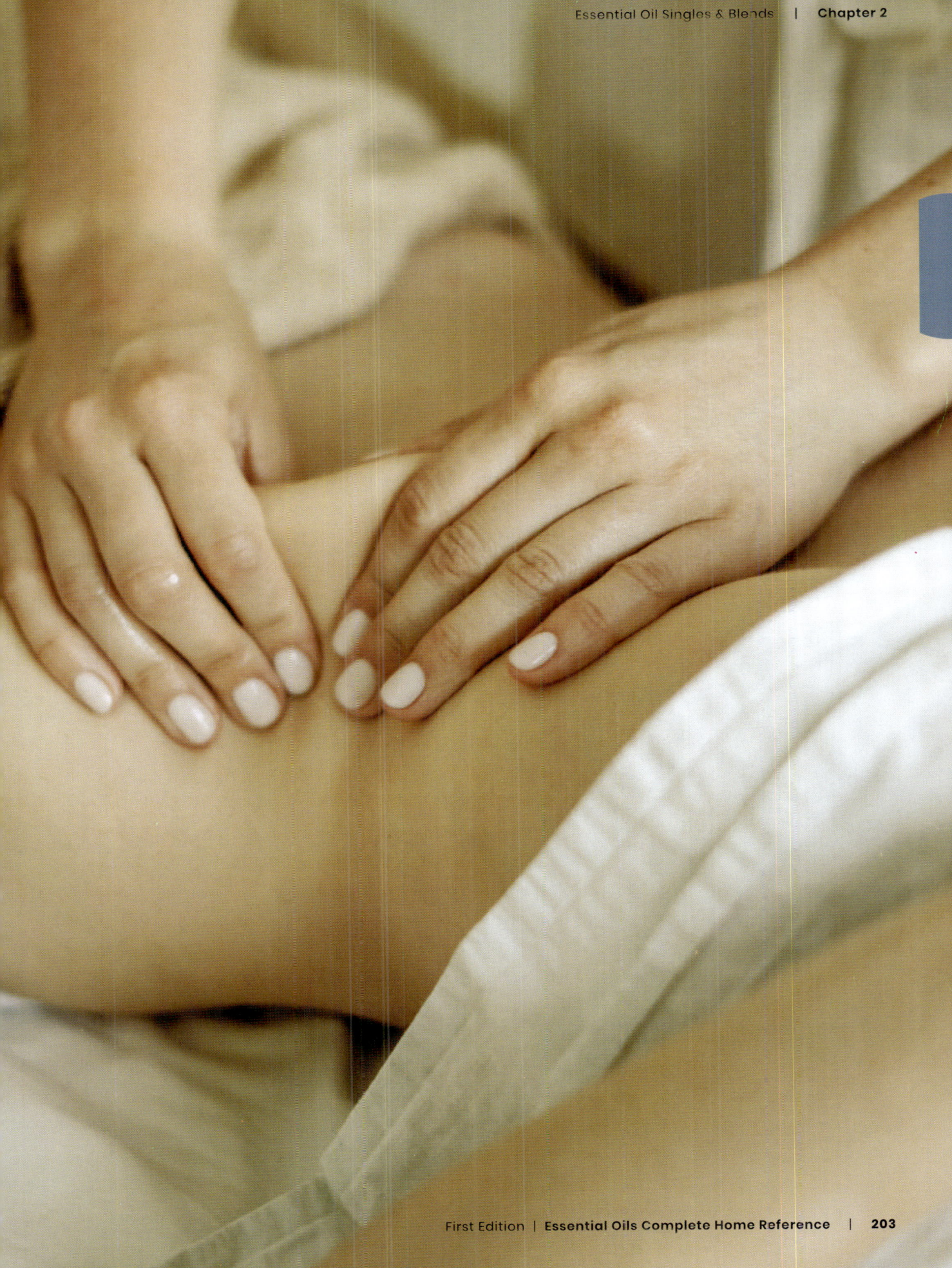

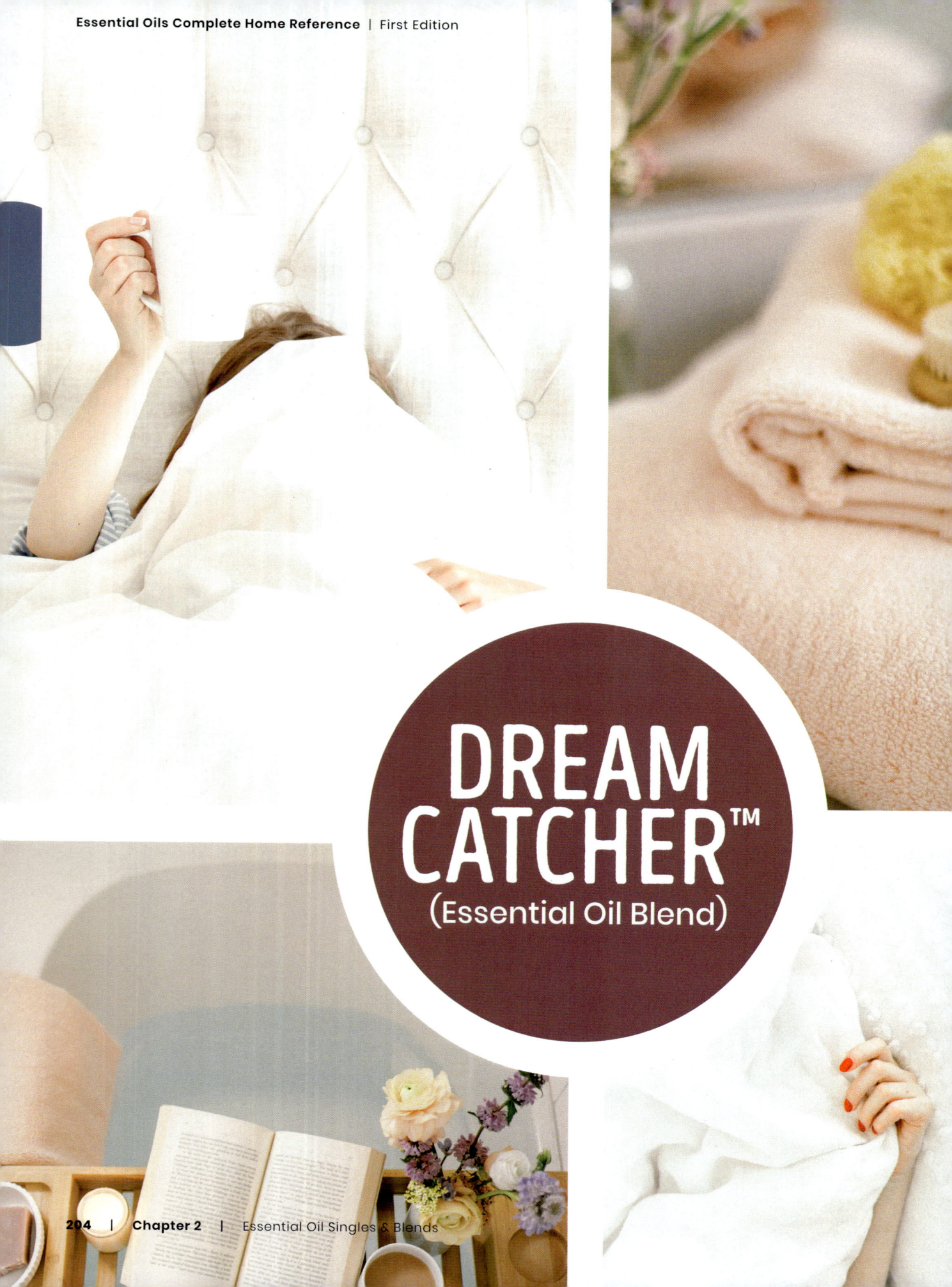

ABOUT DREAM CATCHER™:

This blend stimulates the emotional centers of the brain, awakening creative thoughts and enhancing dreams and visualizations, promoting greater potential for realizing your dreams and staying on your path. It also protects from negative thoughts and dreams that might cloud your vision.

MEDICAL PROPERTIES & USES:
Anti-inflammatory, antimicrobial, antioxidative, emotion supporting, uplifting, calming, digestion or elimination supportive/nausea reducing, muscle relaxant/bone-joint preserving, organ protective, mental clarity

INGREDIENTS:
Sacred Sandalwood, Tangerine, Ylang Ylang, Black Pepper, Bergamot, Anise, Juniper, Geranium, Blue Cypress, Davana, Citrus Hystrix, Jasmine, Matricaria (German Chamomile), Blue Tansy, Rose, Grapefruit, Spearmint, Lemon, Ocotea

DIRECTIONS:
Aromatic: 6o. Most effective before and during sleep. Topical: 50-50. Also, use during meditation, in saunas, or just before sleeping.

CAUTIONS: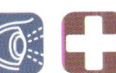

NOTE:
If unpleasant dreams occur, continue to use, since subconscious memories and thoughts will still need to be resolved. Hold on to your dreams and visualize the problems being solved. It may be helpful to write down the dreams upon rising.

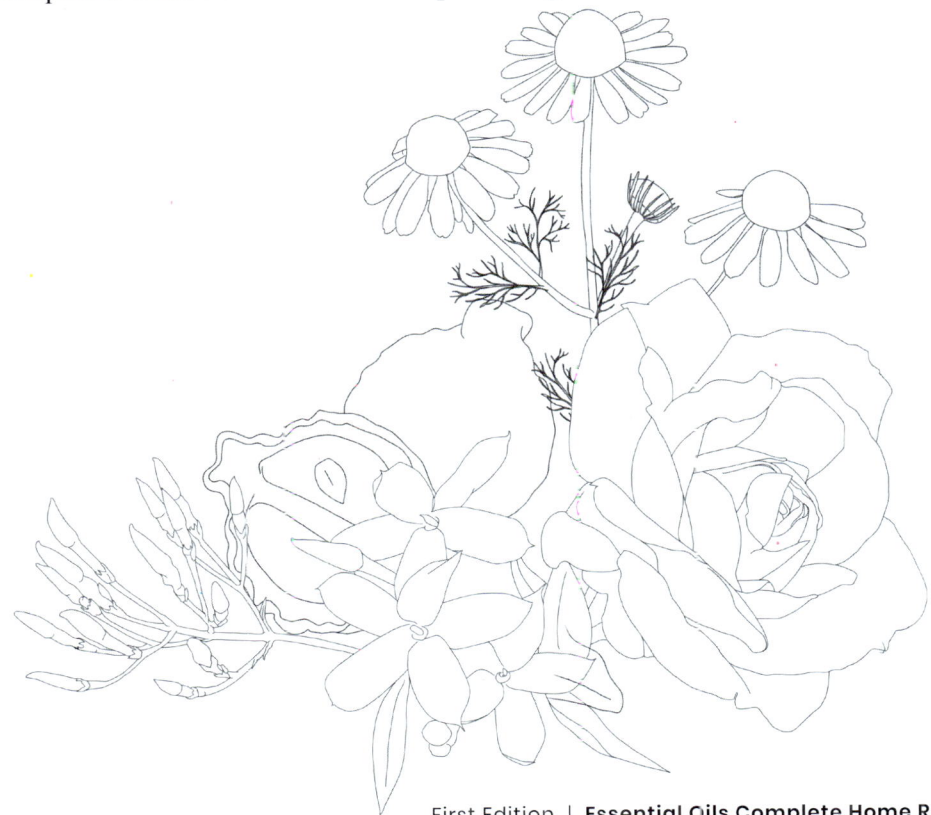

EGYPTIAN GOLD™
(Essential Oil Blend)

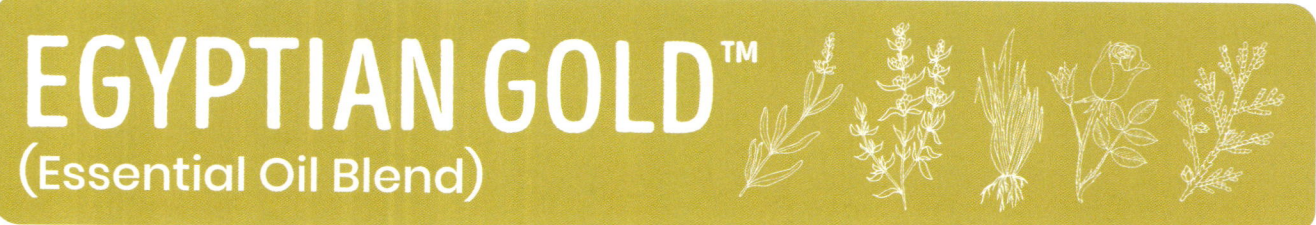

This is a very unique blend that combines the most valuable essences of the Middle East and Central Europe. It offers a truly enchanting aromatic effect that stimulates the central nervous system and the immune and respiratory systems.

MEDICAL PROPERTIES & USES:
Anti-inflammatory, antimicrobial, calming, immune system supportive, respiratory system supportive, nervous system supportive, organ protective

INGREDIENTS:
Frankincense, Idaho Grand Fir, Lavender, Myrrh, Hyssop, Northern Lights Black Spruce, Cedarwood, Vetiver, Rose, Cinnamon Bark

DIRECTIONS:
Aromatic: 10. Topical: 20-80.

CAUTIONS:

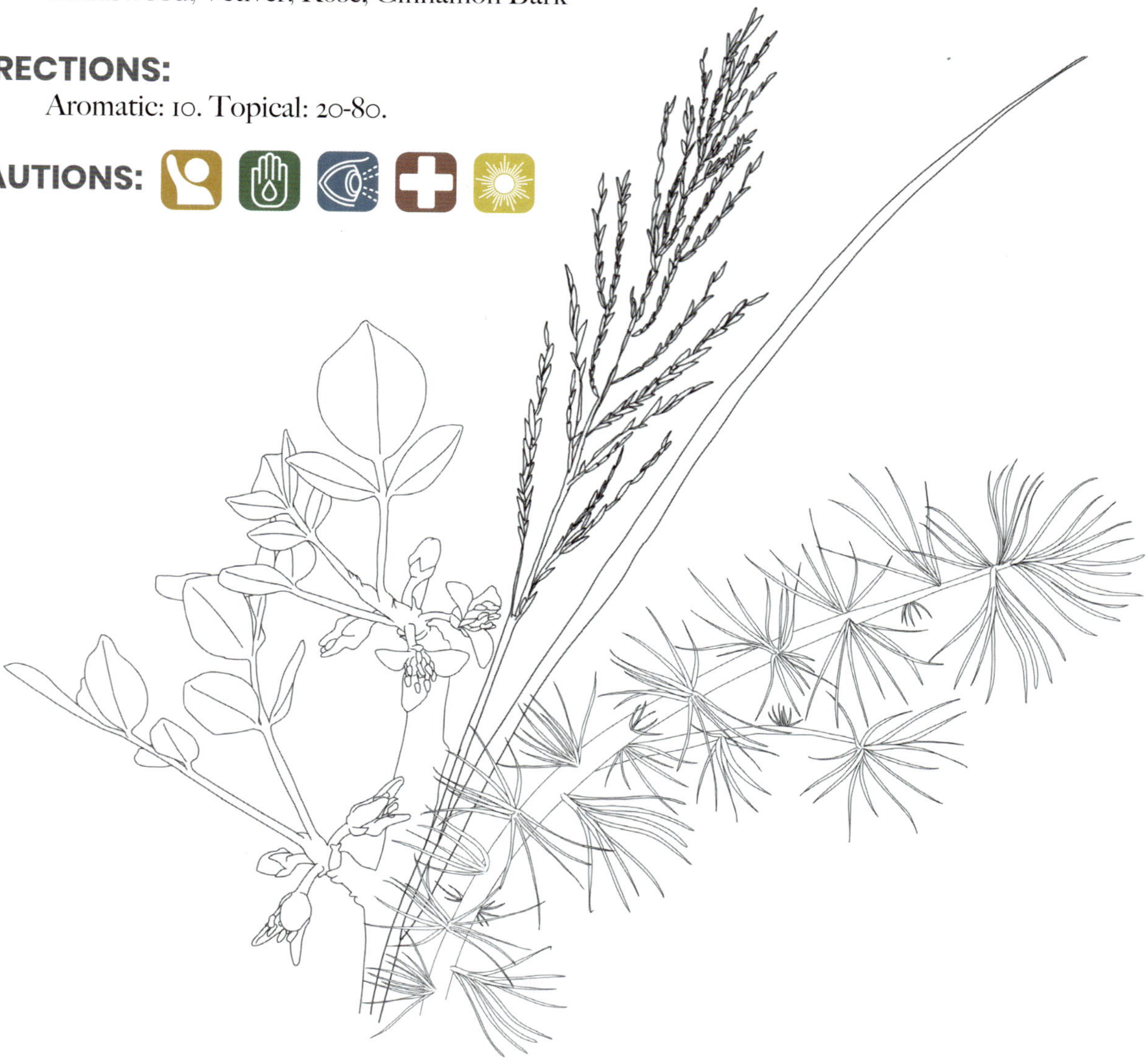

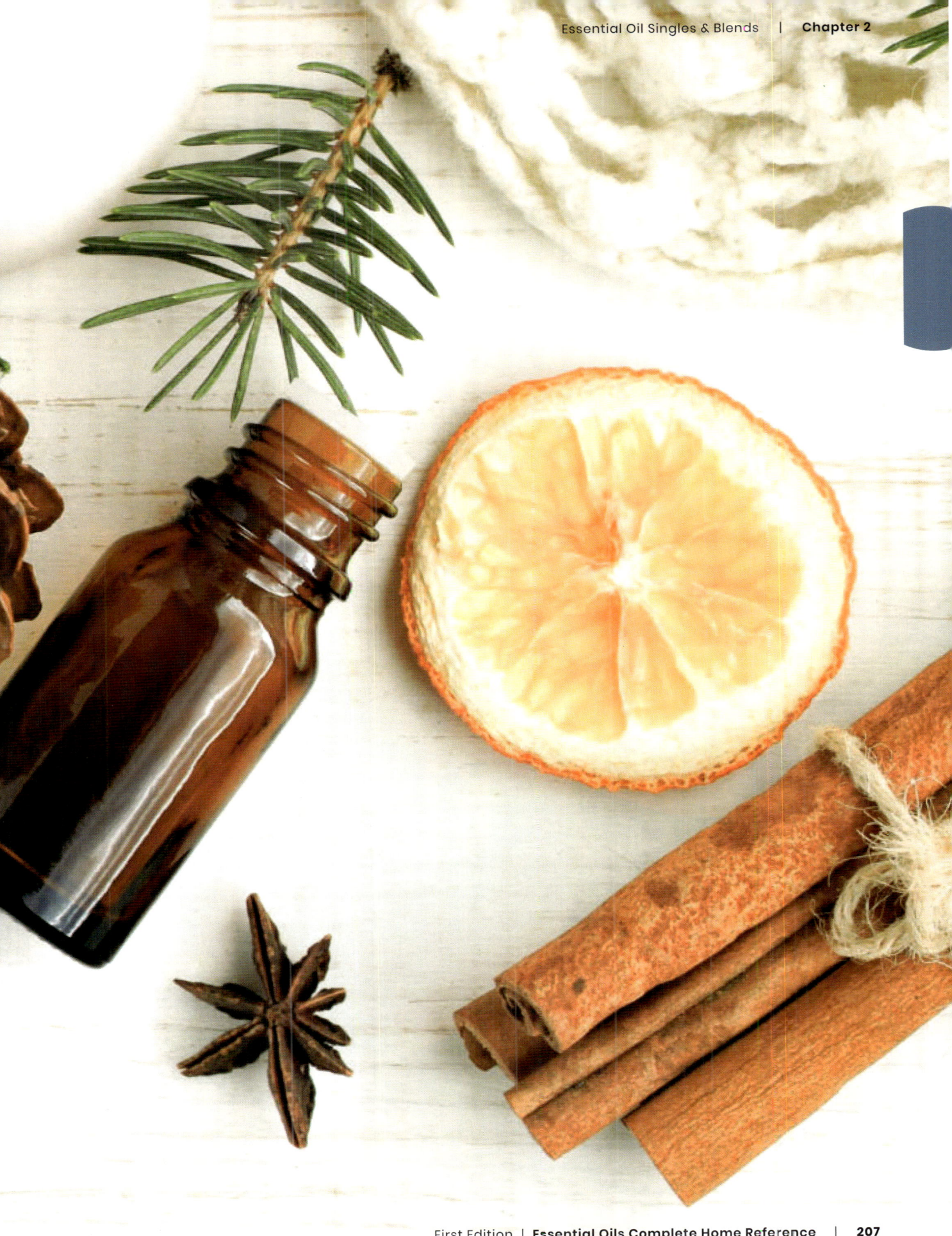

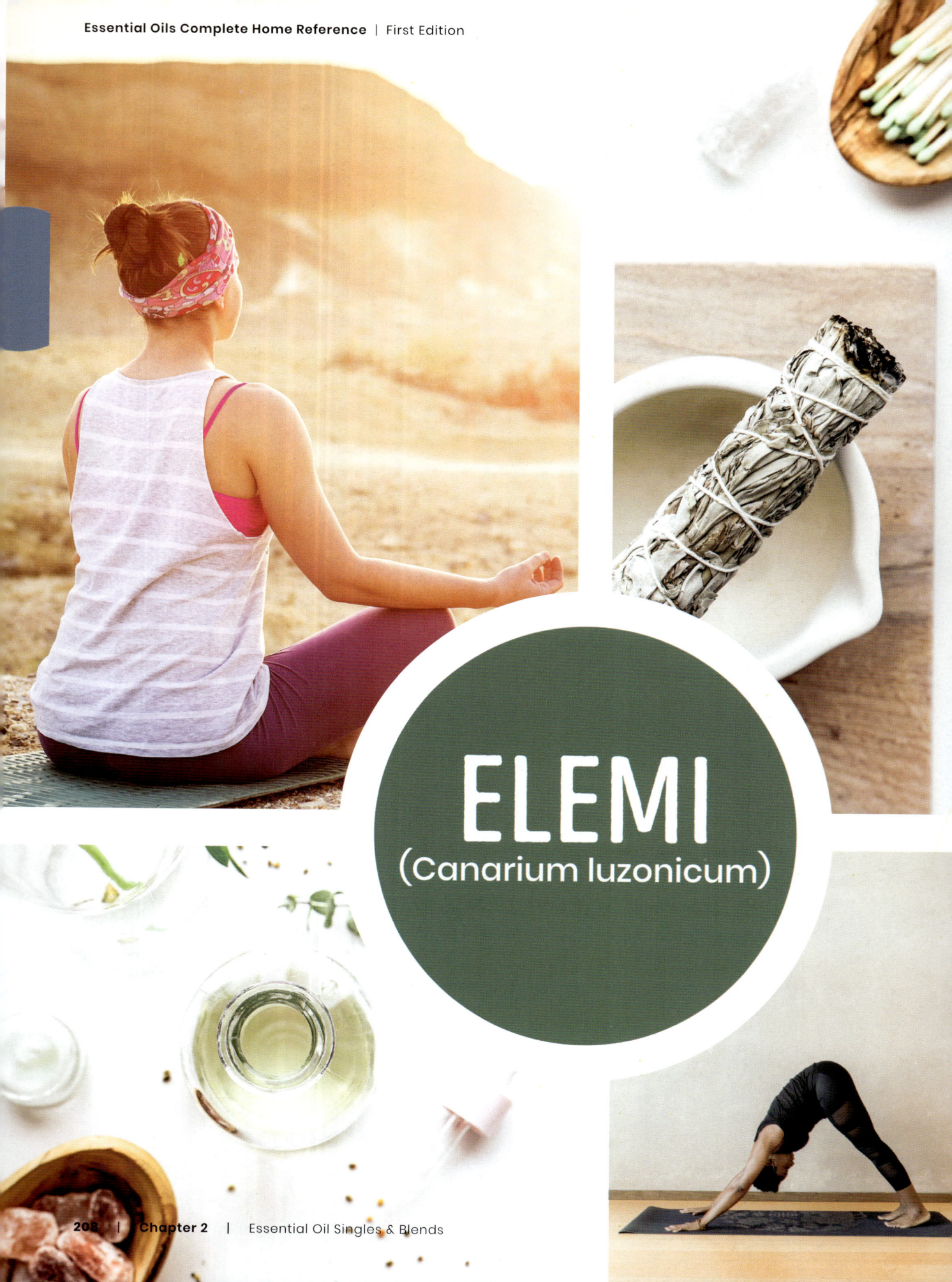

ELEMI
(Canarium luzonicum)

BOTANICAL FAMILY:
Burseraceae

PLANT ORIGIN:
Philippines

EXTRACTION METHOD:
Steam distilled from the gum/resin of the tree

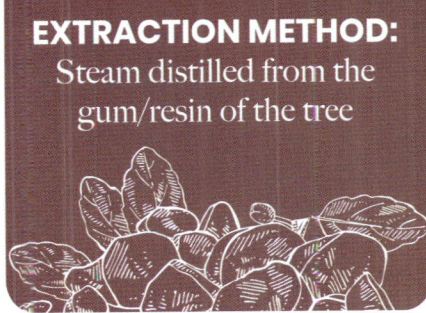

KEY CONSTITUENTS:
Limonene (40-74%),
Alpha-Phellandrene (4-24%),
Elemol (2-13%),
Sabinene (2-8%),
Elemicine (up to 9%)

HISTORICAL DATA:

Elemi has been used in Europe for hundreds of years in salves for skin and is included in celebrated healing ointments such as baum paralytique. Used by 17th century physician J. J. Wecker on the battle wounds of soldiers, Elemi belongs to the same botanical family as Frankincense (Boswellia carterii) and Myrrh (Commiphora myrrha). The Egyptians used Elemi for embalming, and subsequent cultures (particularly in Europe) used it for skin care and for reducing fine lines and wrinkles and improving skin tone.

MEDICAL PROPERTIES:
Antispasmodic, anti-inflammatory, antimicrobial, antiseptic, anticancerous

USES:
Muscle/nerve pain, skin problems (scars, wrinkles), meditation, prayer, calming, rejuvenating

FRAGRANT INFLUENCE:
Woodsy, fresh, incense-like aroma great for meditation, can be grounding and used to clear the mind.

DIRECTIONS:
Aromatic: 6o. Topical: Neat. Dietary: Use as a dietary supplement: put 1 drop in a capsule and take or put 1 drop in 4 ounces of liquid (rice milk, etc.).

CAUTIONS: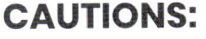

SELECTED RESEARCH:

Nikolic M, Smiljkovic M, Markovic T, Cirica A, Glamoclija J, Markovic D, Sokovic M. Sensitivity of clinical isolates of Candida to essential oils from Burseraceae family. EXCLI J. 2016 Apr 19;15:280-9. eCollection 2016.

Mogana R, Wiart C. Canarium L.: a phytochemical and pharmacological review. J Pharm Res. 2011;4(8):2482-89.

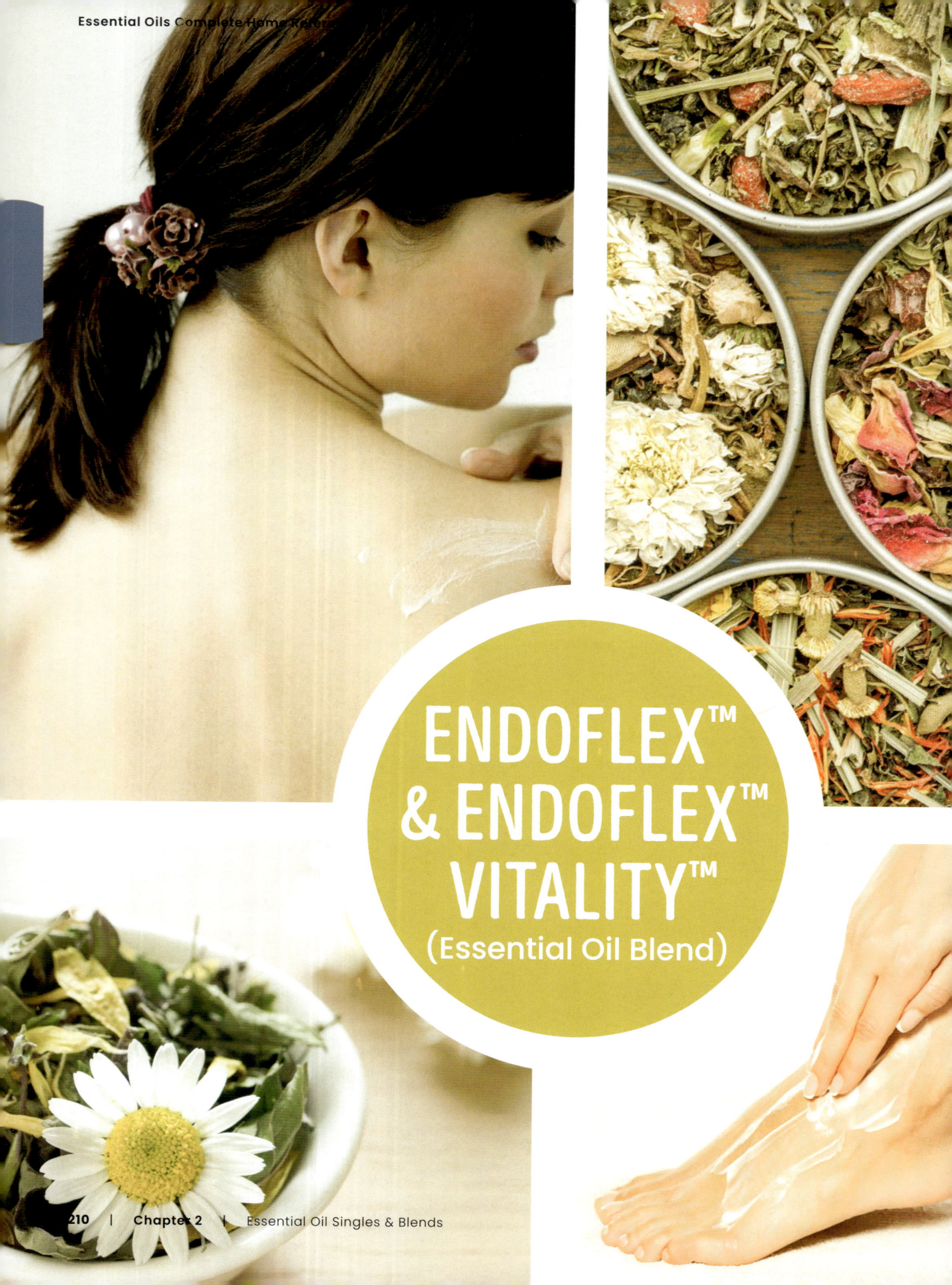

ENDOFLEX™ & ENDOFLEX™ VITALITY™
(Essential Oil Blend)

ABOUT ENDOFLEX™ & ENDOFLEX™ VITALITY™:
This blend amplifies metabolism and vitality and creates hormonal balance.

MEDICAL PROPERTIES & USES:
Anti-inflammatory, antimicrobial, antioxidative, calming, digestion-or-elimination supportive/nausea reducing, hormone balancing, uplifting

INGREDIENTS:
Spearmint, Sesame seed oil, Sage, Geranium, Myrtle, Matricaria (German Chamomile), Nutmeg

DIRECTIONS:
Aromatic: 30. Topical: 50-50. Apply over lower back, thyroid, kidneys, liver, feet, glandular locations, foot Vita Flex points, or desired location as needed. Dietary (Vitality): Dilute 1 drop with 1 drop of V-6 or other pure carrier oil. Put in a capsule and take up to 3 times daily.

CAUTIONS:

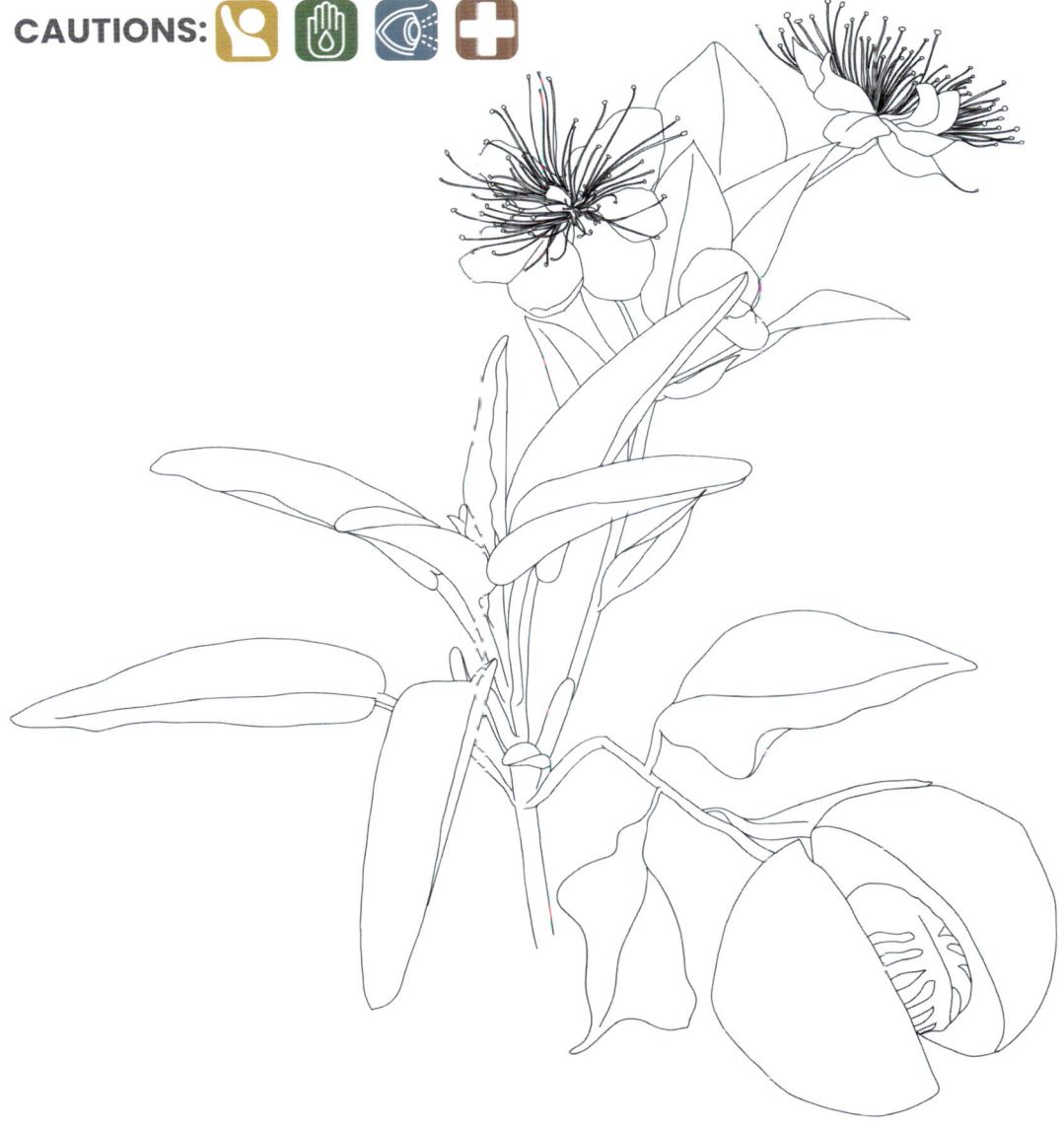

EN-R-GEE™
(Essential Oil Blend)

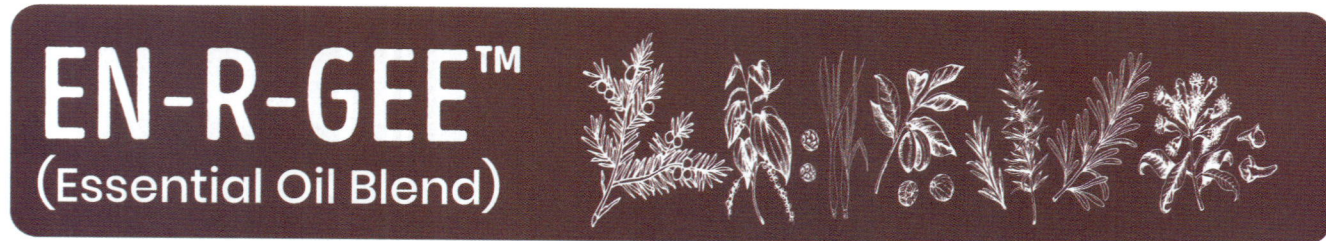

This blend increases vitality, circulation, and alertness.

MEDICAL PROPERTIES & USES:
Antimicrobial, antioxidative, calming, cardiovascular supportive, dietary supportive, digestion or elimination supportive/nausea reducing, disease inhibitory, muscle relaxant/bone-joint preservative, organ protective, pain or swelling reducing, performance enhancing/stimulating, wellness supportive

INGREDIENTS:
Rosemary, Juniper, Lemongrass, Nutmeg, Idaho Grand Fir, Clove, Black Pepper

DIRECTIONS:
Aromatic: 30. Topical: 20-80. It may also be used with Raindrop Technique. Rub En-R-Gee on feet and Awaken on temples for intensified effect.

CAUTIONS:

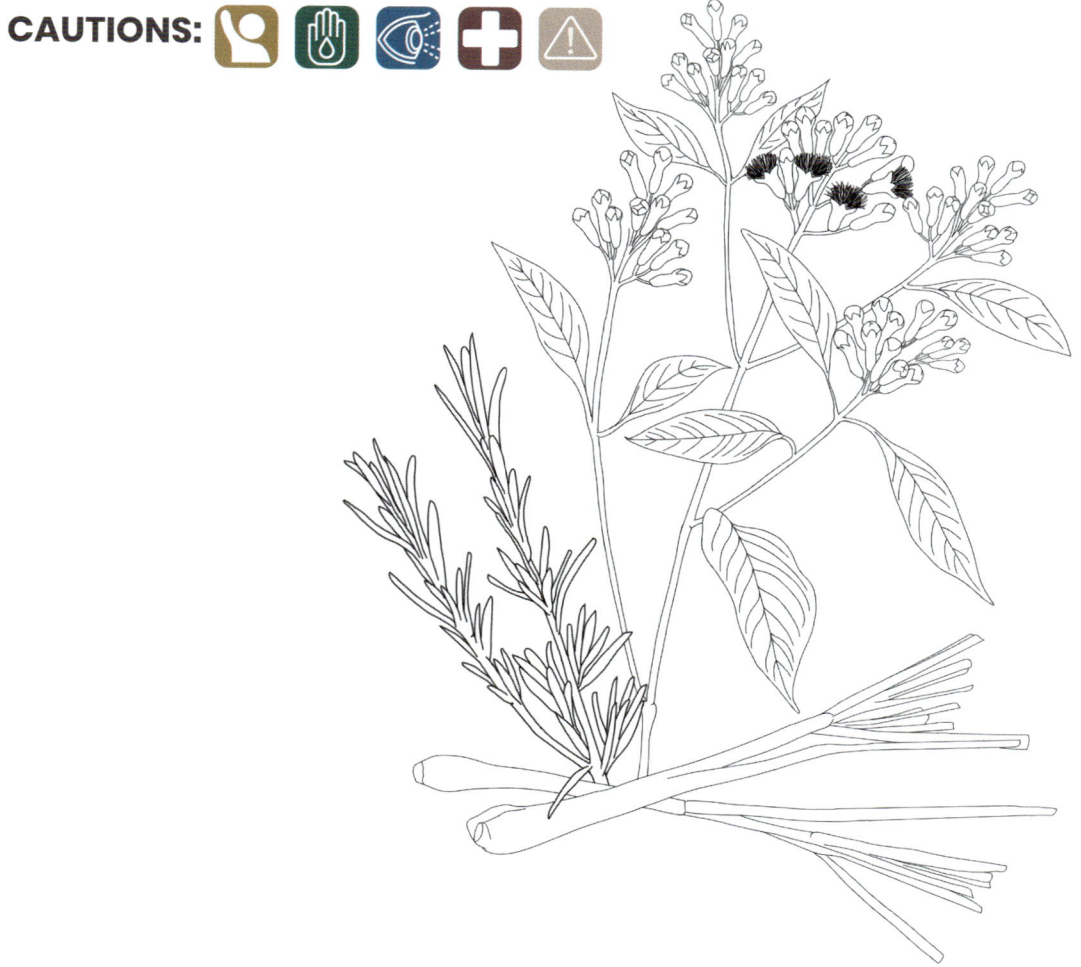

Essential Oil Singles & Blends | **Chapter 2**

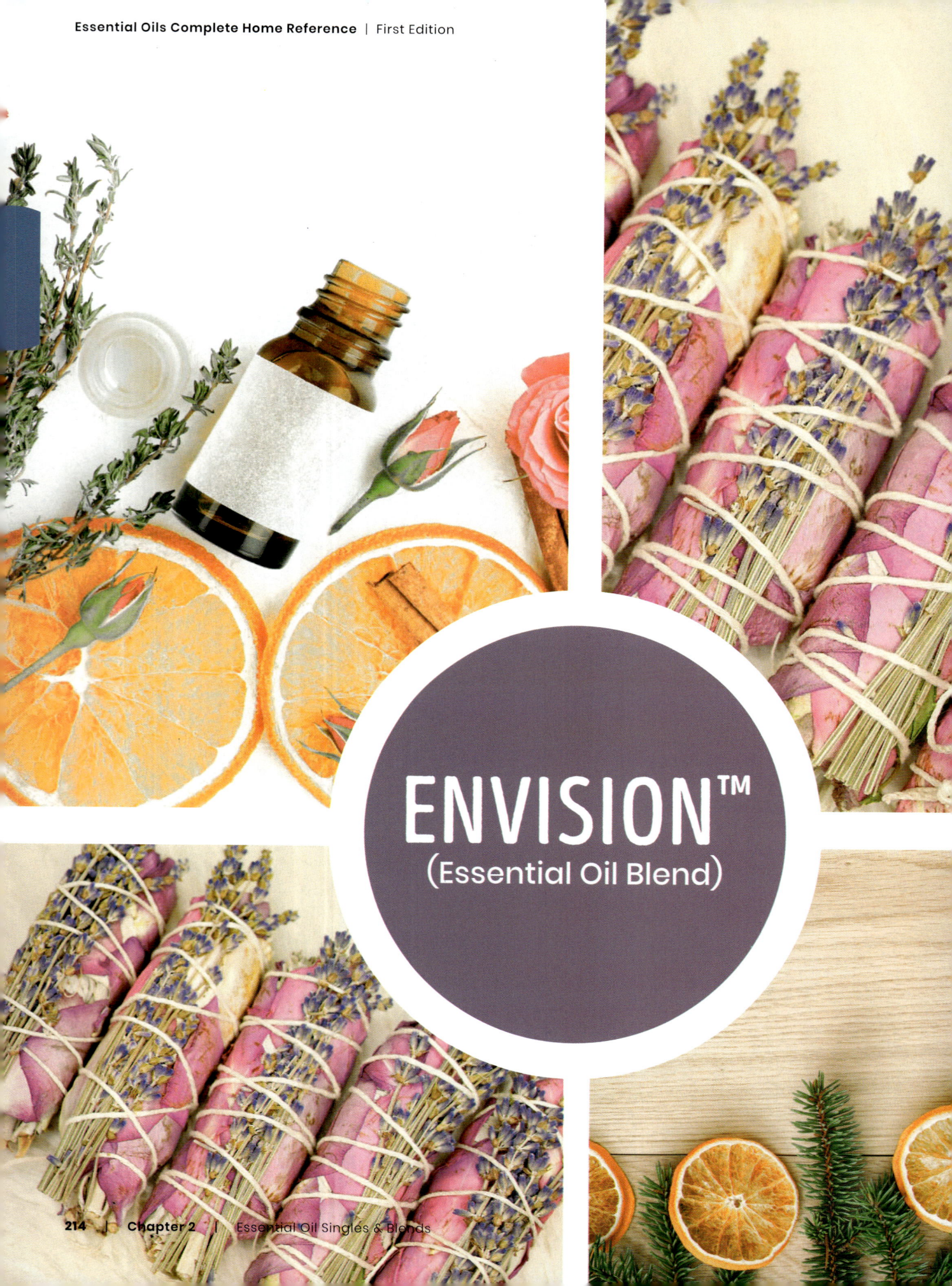

ENVISION™
(Essential Oil Blend)

ABOUT ENVISION™:

This blend renews focus and stimulates creative and intuitive abilities needed to achieve goals and dreams. It helps to reawaken internal drive and independence and to overcome fears and emotional blocks.

MEDICAL PROPERTIES & USES:

Anti-inflammatory, antimicrobial, antioxidative, uplifting, emotion supporting, calming, disease inhibitory, glandular/hormonal supportive, insecticidal/antiparasitic, pain or swelling reducing

INGREDIENTS:

Black Spruce, Geranium, Orange, Lavender, Sage, Rose

DIRECTIONS:

Aromatic: 30. Topical: 50-50.

CAUTIONS:

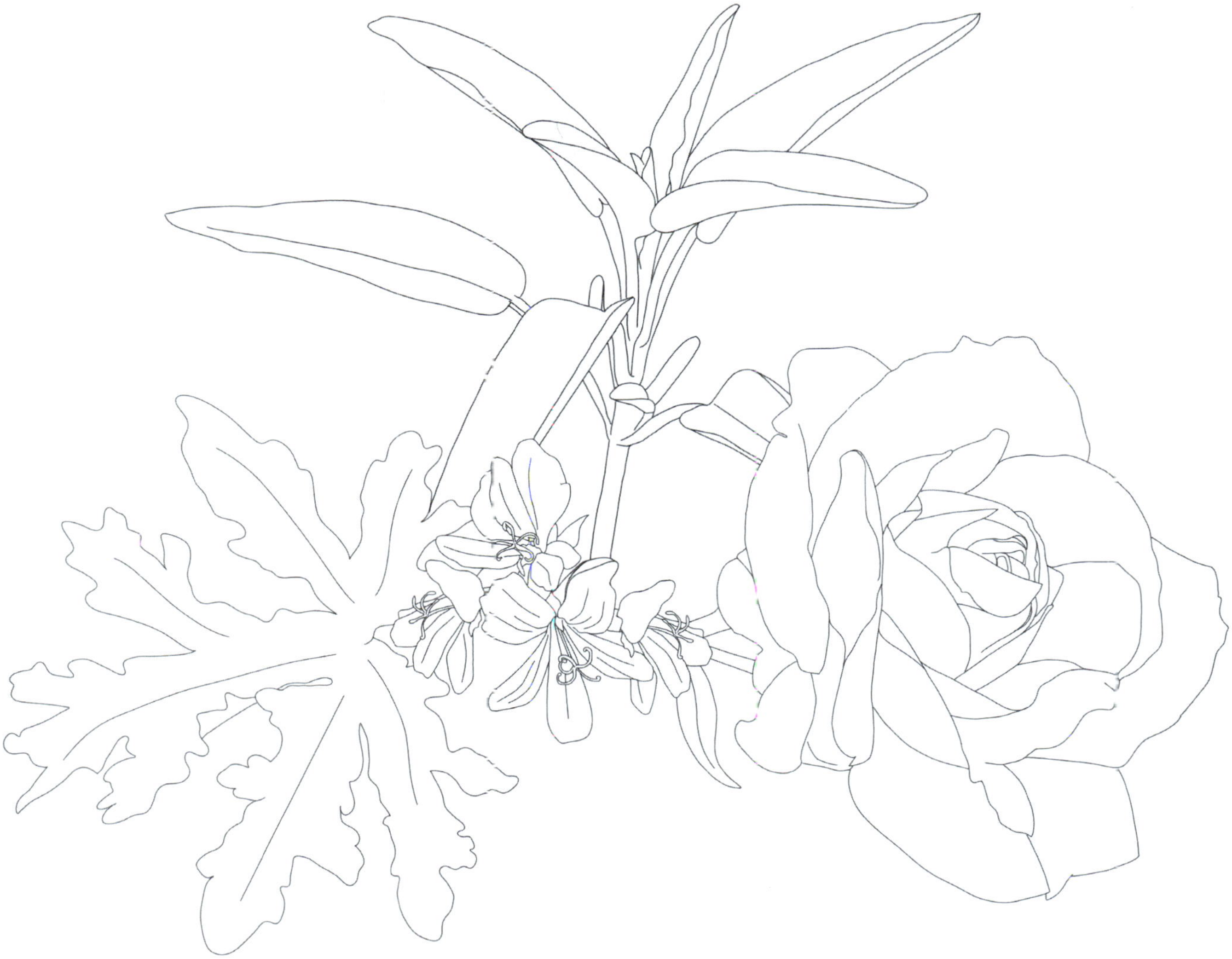

BOTANICAL FAMILY: Myrtaceae

PLANT ORIGIN: Ecuador

EXTRACTION METHOD: Steam distilled from the leaves and branches

KEY CONSTITUENTS: Eucalyptol (40-84%), Alpha-Pinene (7-34%), Limonene (3-8%), Aromadendrene (up to 7%)

EUCALYPTUS BLUE
(Eucalyptus bicostata)

Eucalyptus blue is grown and distilled on Young Living's farm in Ecuador. It is called "blue gum" and is a tree from the wilds of the Andean Mountains. It has been a crossbreed of Eucalyptus citriodora and Eucalyptus globulus for 250 years. The native people of Ecuador have used the disinfecting leaves to cover wounds and repel insects.

Although it contains a high percentage of eucalyptol, because of its balanced chemical constituents within the eucalyptus, it is the only eucalyptus that has been found in the world today that does not cause an allergic reaction in people who have allergies to eucalyptol. Eucalyptus Blue is preferred over many of the eucalyptus species, simply because of its well-balanced chemistry and its non-allergic effect for all types of respiratory conditions. In a recent study of eight eucalyptus species, Eucalyptus bicostata had the best antiviral activity. It is a great companion to Dorado Azul.

MEDICAL PROPERTIES:
Expectorant, diaphoretic, insecticidal, oestrogenic, antifungal, antiviral, antibacterial

USES:
Supports respiratory function to promote normal breathing, relieves sore muscles, calming, detoxing, invigorating

FRAGRANT INFLUENCE:
Fresh, balanced, invigorating before trauma or anger was experienced

DIRECTIONS:
Aromatic: 30. Topical: 50-50.

CAUTIONS: 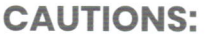   Do not use as a dietary supplement. Large amounts of any eucalyptus oil may be toxic.

SELECTED RESEARCH:
Ma L, Yao L. Antiviral Effects of Plant-Derived Essential Oils and Their Component Parts: An Updated Review. Molecules. 2020 Jun; 25(11): 2627.

Sebei K, Sakouhi F, Herchi W, Khouja ML, Boukhchina S. Chemical composition and antibacterial activities of seven Eucalyptus species essential oils leaves. Biol Res. 2015 Jan 19;48(1):7.

Elaissi A, Rouis Z, Salem NA, Mabrouk S, ben Salem Y, Salah KB, Aouni M, Farhat F, Chemli R, Harzallah-Skhiri F, Khouja ML. Chemical composition of 8 eucalyptus species' essential oils and the evaluation of their antibacterial, antifungal and antiviral activities. BMC Complement Alternat Med. 2012 Jun 28;12:81.

Elaissi A, Salah KH, Mabrouk S, Larbi KM, Chemli R, Harzallah-Skhiri F. Antibacterial activity and chemical composition of 20 Eucalyptus species' essential oils. Food Chem. 2011 Dec 15;129(4):1427-1434.

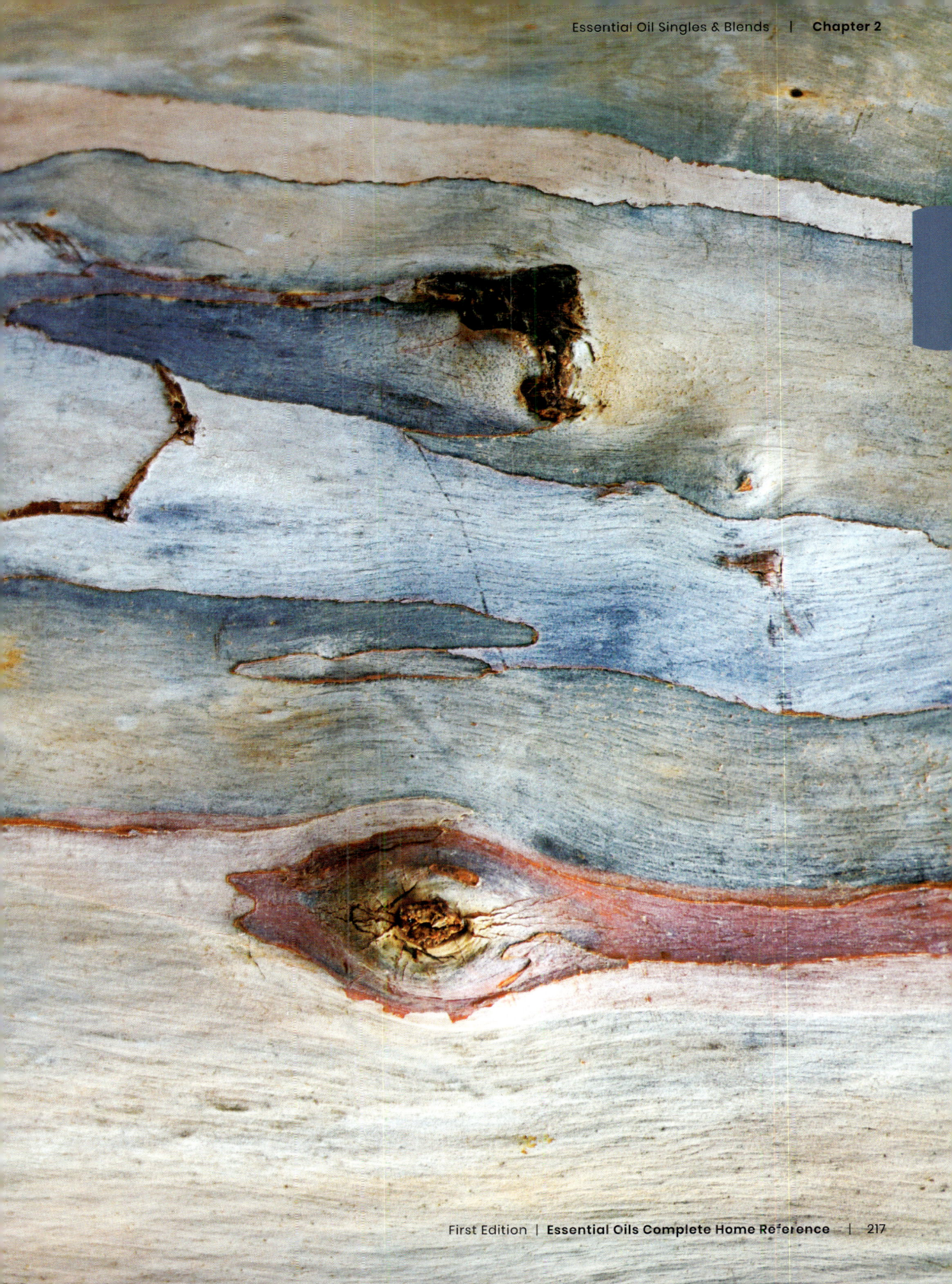

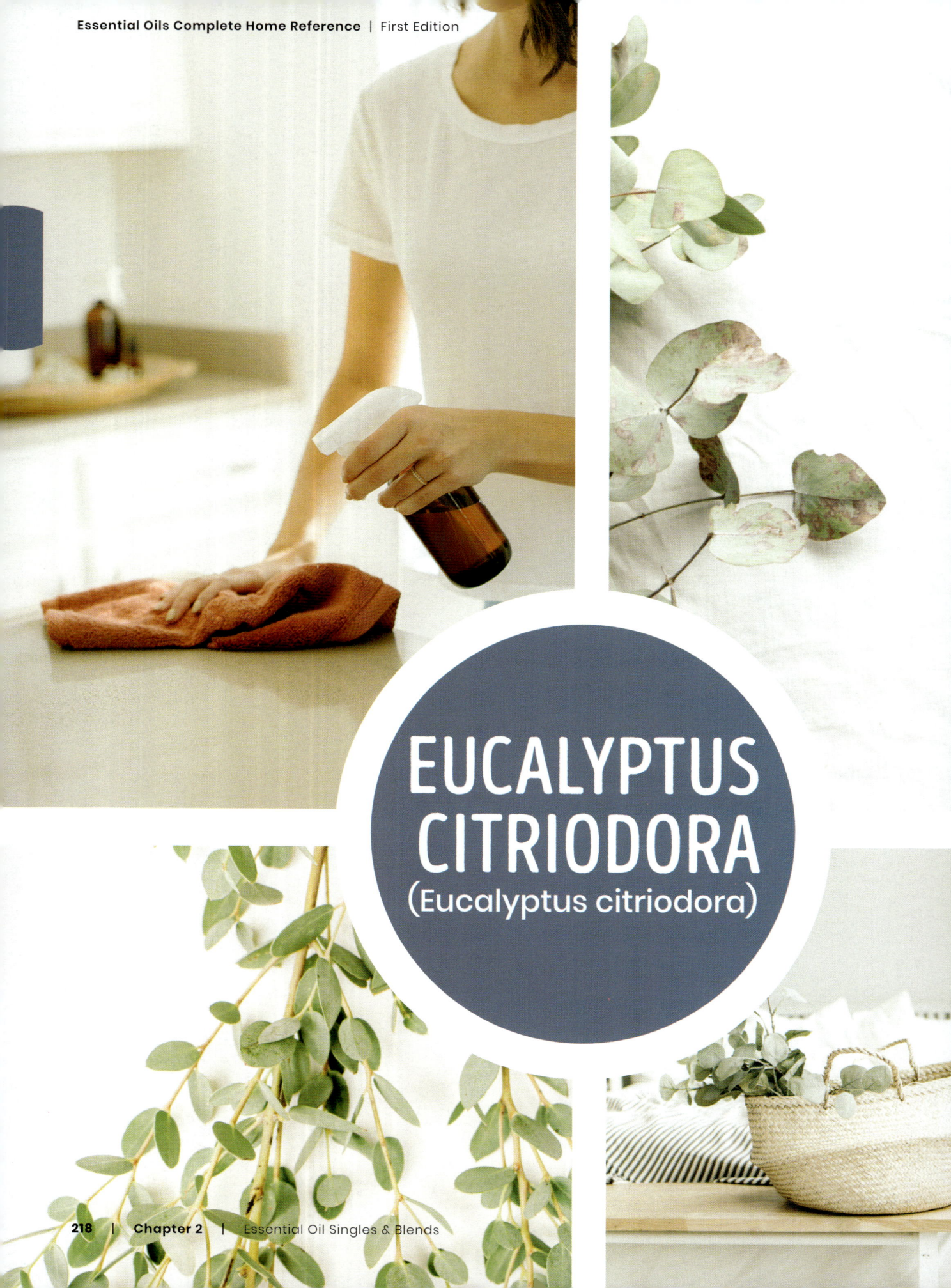

BOTANICAL FAMILY:
Myrtaceae

PLANT ORIGIN:
Madagascar

EXTRACTION METHOD:
Steam distilled from leaves

KEY CONSTITUENTS:
Citronellal (71-86%),
Isopulegol (1-9%),
Neo-isopulegol (up to 5%)

HISTORICAL DATA:
Traditionally used to perfume linen closets and as an insect repellent.

MEDICAL PROPERTIES:
Analgesic, antiviral, antibacterial, antifungal, anticancerous, liver protectant, expectorant, insecticidal, highly anti-inflammatory

USES:
Fungal infections (ringworm, candida), respiratory infections, viral infections (herpes, shingles), bug repellent (especially mosquitoes), supports immunity, joints and muscles, cuts, wounds, dandruff, removing negative energies, releasing grief

FRAGRANT INFLUENCE:
Clear mind, respiratory system, cleanse air and surfaces, calming

DIRECTIONS:
Aromatic: 30. Topical: 50-50.

CAUTIONS: Do not ingest.

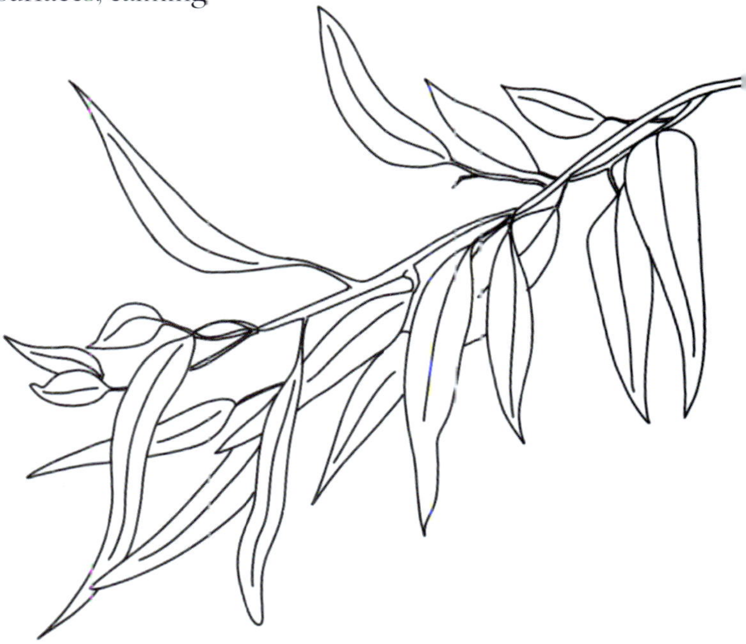

SELECTED RESEARCH:

Ho C-L, Li L-H, Weng Y-C, Hua K-F, Ju T-C. Eucalyptus essential oils inhibit the lipopolysaccharide-induced inflammatory response to RAW264.7 microphages through reducing MAPK and NF-κB pathways. BMC Complement Med Ther. 2020; 20: 200. Published online 2020 Jun 29.

Al-Sayed E, El-Naga RN. Protective role of ellagitannins from Eucalyptus citriodora against ethanol-induced gastric ulcer in rats: impact on oxidative stress, inflammation and calcitonin-gene related peptide. Phytomedicine. 2015 Jan 15;22(1):5-15. Epub 2014 Oct 24.

Lin L, Cui H, Zhou H, Zhang X, Bortolini C, Chen M, Liu L, Dong M. Nanoliposomes containing Eucalyptus citriodora as antibiotic with specific antimicrobial activity. Chem Commun (Camb). 2015 Feb 14;51(13):2653-5.

Ramos Alvarenga RF, Wan B, Inui T, Franzblau SG, Pauli GF, Jaki BU. Airborne antituberculosis activity of Eucalyptus citriodora essential oil. J Nat Prod. 2014 Mar 28;77(3):603-10. Epub 2014 Mar 20.

Siddique YH, Mujtaba SF, Jyoti S, Naz F. GC-MS analysis of Eucalyptus citriodora leaf extract and its role on the dietary supplementation in transgenic Drosophila model of Parkinson's disease. Food Chem Toxicol. 2013 May;55:29-35. Epub 2013 Jan 11.

Bhagat M, Sharma V, Saxena AK. Anti-proliferative effect of leaf extracts of Eucalyptus citriodora against human cancer cells in vitro and in vivo. Indian J Biochem Biophys. 2012 Dec;49(6):451-7. Epub 2013 Jan 29.

BOTANICAL FAMILY: Myrtaceae

PLANT ORIGIN: China

EXTRACTION METHOD: Steam distilled from rectified leaves

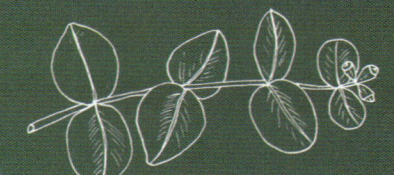

KEY CONSTITUENTS: Eucalyptol (up to 70%), Limonene (2-15%), Alpha-Pinene (1-10%), Alpha-Pinene (1-10%), Para-Cymene (1-6%), Trans-Pinocarveol (up to 5%), Aromadendrene (up to 2%), Alpha-Phellandrene (up to 2%)

EUCALYPTUS GLOBULUS
(Eucalyptus globulus)

For centuries, Australian Aborigines used the disinfecting leaves of this plant to cover wounds. Shown by laboratory tests to be a powerful antimicrobial agent, E. globulus contains a high percentage of eucalyptol (a key ingredient in many antiseptic mouth rinses). It is often used for the respiratory system. Eucalyptus has also been investigated for its powerful insect repellent effects (Trigg, 1996). Eucalyptus trees have been planted throughout parts of North Africa to successsfully block the spread of malaria. According to Jean Valnet, MD, a solution of 2 percent eucalyptus oil sprayed on the skin will kill 70 percent of ambient staph bacteria. Some doctors still use solutions of eucalyptus oil in surgical dressings.

MEDICAL PROPERTIES:
Expectorant, mucolytic, antimicrobial, antibacterial, antifungal, antiviral, antiaging, antiulcer, antidiabetic, antioxidant, anti-inflammatory, disinfectant, hypotensive, renal protective

USES:
Respiratory/sinus infections, decongestant, rheumatism/arthritis, soothe sore muscles

FRAGRANT INFLUENCE:
Sharp, clean, refreshing aroma; promotes health, well-being, purification, and healing

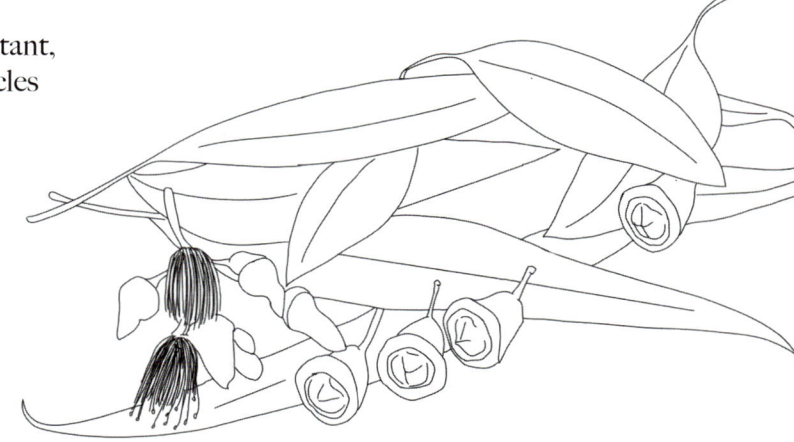

DIRECTIONS:
Aromatic: 30. Topical: 50-50.

CAUTIONS:

SELECTED RESEARCH:

Ghareeb MA, Sobeh M, El-Maadawy WH, Mohammed WH, Khalil H, Botros S, Wink M. Chemical profiling of Polyphenolics in Eucalyptus globulus and Evaluation of Its Hepato-Renal Protective Potential Against Cyclophosphamide Induced Toxicity in Mice. Antioxidants (Basel). 2019 Sep; 8(9): 415.

Chaleshtori FS, Saholi M, Chaleshtori RS. Chemical Composition, Antioxidant and Antibacterial Activity of Bunium persicum, Eucalyptus globulous, and Rose Water on Multidrug-Resistant Listeria Species. J Evid Based Integ Med. 2018; 23: 2515690X1775131.

Brezáni V, Leláková V, Hassan STS, Berchová-Bimová K, Nový P, Klouček P, Maršik P, Dall'Acqua S, Hošek J, Šmejkal K. Anti-Infectivity against Herpes Simplex Virus and Selected Microbes and Anti-Inflammatory Activities of Compounds Isolated from Eucalyptus globulus Labill. Viruses. 2018 Jul; 10(7): 360.

Dhibi S, Mbarki S, Elfeki A, Hfaiedh N. Eucalyptus globulus extract protects upon acetaminophen-induced kidney damages in male rat. Bosn J Basic Med Sci. 2014 May;14(2):99-104.

Juergens UR. Anti-inflammatory properties of the monoterpene 1,8-cineole: current evidence for co-medication in inflammatory airway diseases. Drug Res (Stuttg). 2014 May 15;64(12):638-46. Epub 2014 May 17.

Bachir RG, Benali M. Antibacterial activity of the essential oils from the leaves of Eucalyptus globulus against Escherichia coli and Staphylococcus aureus. Asian Pac J Trop Biomed. 2012 Sep;2(9):739-42. Epub Apr 10.

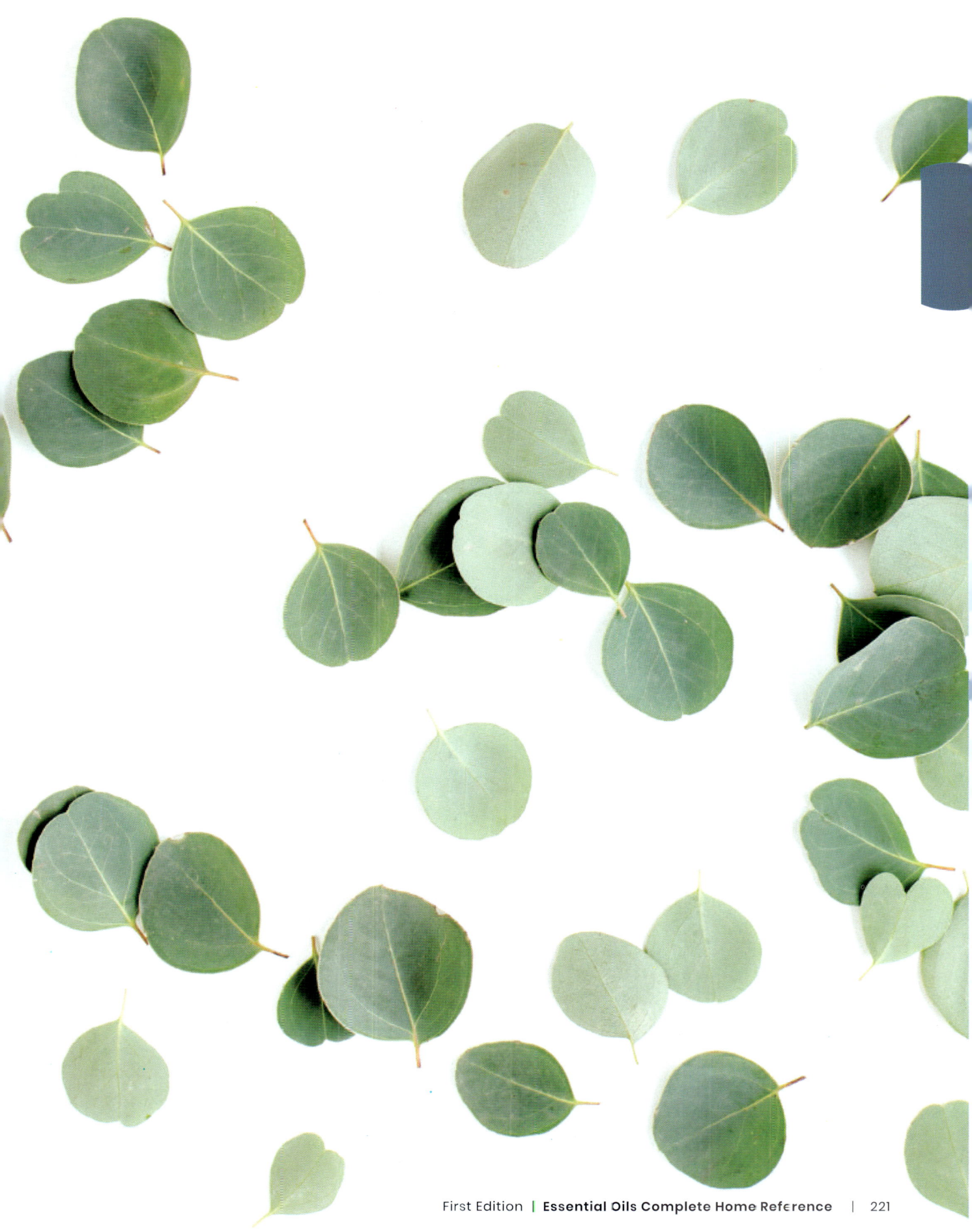

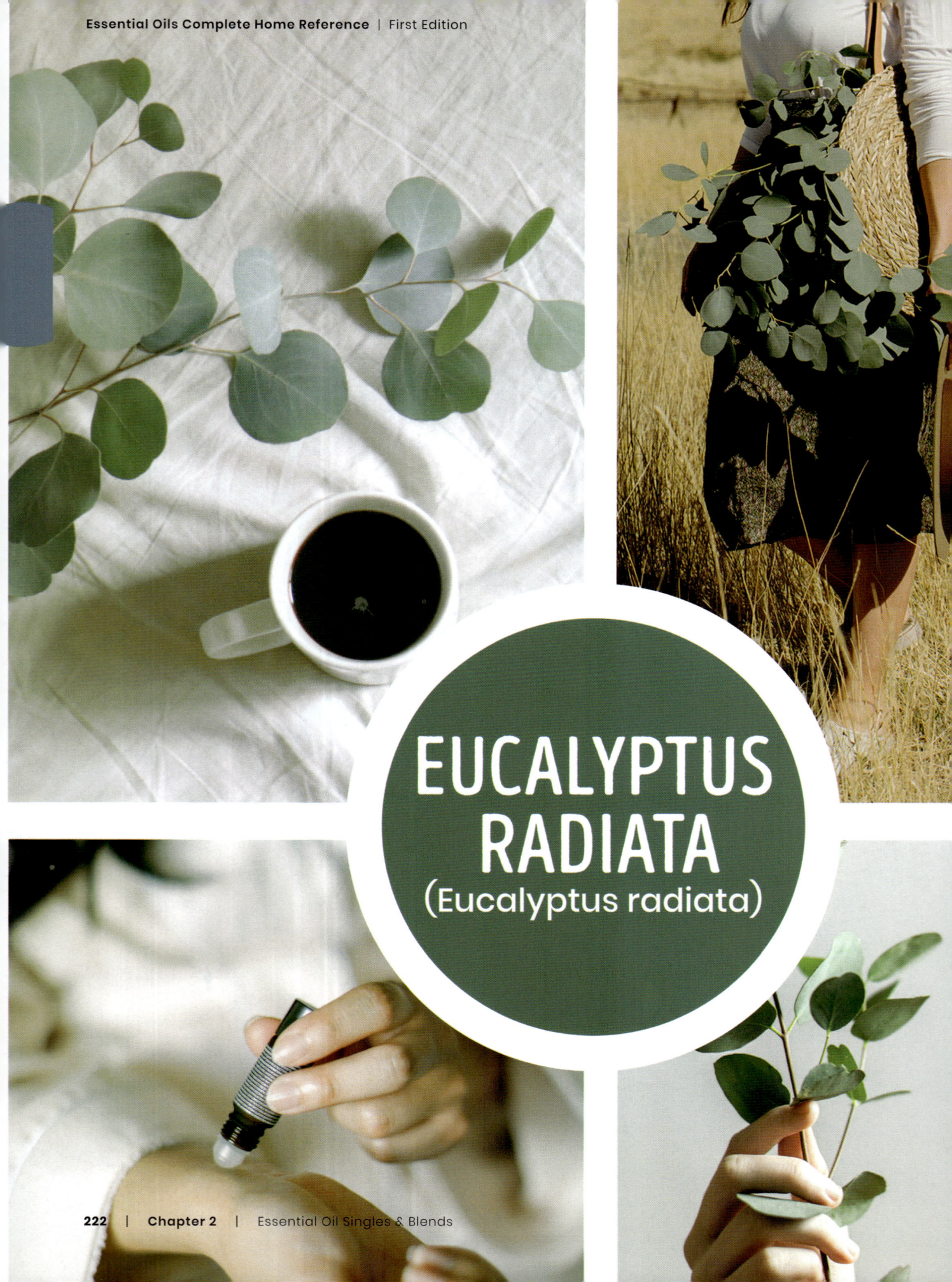

EUCALYPTUS RADIATA
(Eucalyptus radiata)

Essential Oil Singles & Blends | Chapter 2

BOTANICAL FAMILY:
Myrtaceae

PLANT ORIGIN:
Australia, South Africa

EXTRACTION METHOD:
Steam distilled from leaves

KEY CONSTITUENTS:
Eucalyptol (60-83%),
Alpha-Terpineol (2-14%),
Limonene (4-9%),
Alpha-Pinene (up to 5%),
Alpha-Terpinyl Acetate (up to 4%),
Myrcene (up to 2%)

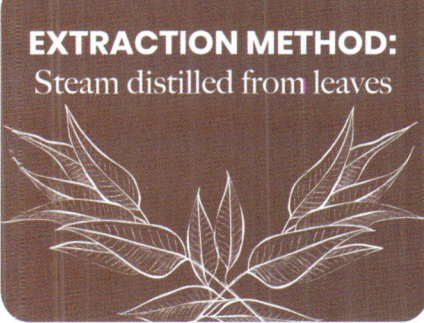

HISTORICAL DATA:
This eucalyptus species has been treasured in folk medicine. A 2011 study conducted at Heidelberg University found that Eucalyptus radiata has the second highest abundance of 1,8 cineole (Eucalyptol) after E. globulus.

MEDICAL PROPERTIES:
Antibacterial, anesthetic, antiseptic, antimicrobial, antiviral, expectorant, anti-inflammatory

USES:
Respiratory/sinus infections, sore muscles, viral infections, fights herpes simplex when combined with bergamot

FRAGRANT INFLUENCE:
Sharp, clean, fresh aroma; energizing; soothing

DIRECTIONS:
Aromatic: 30. Topical: 50-50.

CAUTIONS:

SELECTED RESEARCH:

Ângelo L., Duarte AP, Pereira L., Domingues F. Chemical Profiling and Evaluation of Antioxidant and Anti-Microbial Properties of Selected Commercial Essential Oils: A Comparative Study. Medicines (Basel). 2017 Jun; 4(2): 36.

Luis A, Duarte A., Gominho J., Domingues F., Duarte A.P. Chemical composition, antioxidant, antibacterial and anti-quorum sensing activities of Eucalyptus globulus and Eucalyptus radiata essential oils. Ind. Crops Prod. 2016;79:274–282.

Sugumar S, Ghosh V, Nirmala MJ, Mukherjee A, Chandrasekaran N. Ultrasonic emulsification of eucalyptus oil nanoemulsion: antibacterial activity against Staphylococcus aureus and wound healing activity in Wistar rats. Ultrason Sonochem. 2014 May;21(3):1044-9. Epub 2013 Nov 6.

Murata S, Shiragami R, Kosugi C, Tezuka T, Yamazaki M, Hirano A, Yoshimura Y, Suzuki M, Shuto K, Ohkohchi N, Koda K. Antitumor effect of 1, 8 cineole against colon cancer. Oncol Rep. 2013 Dec;30(6):2647-52. Epub 2013 Oct 1.

Bendaoud H, Bouajila J, Rhouma A, Savagnac A, Romdhane M. GC/MS analysis and antimicrobial and antioxidant activities of essential oil of Eucalyptus radiata. J Sci Food Agric. 2009 Jun;89(8):1292-127.

Chao S, Young DG, Oberg C, Nakaoka K. Inhibition of methicillin-resistant Staphylococcus aureus (MRSA) by essential oils. FLAVOUR Fragr. J. 2008; 23: 444-449.

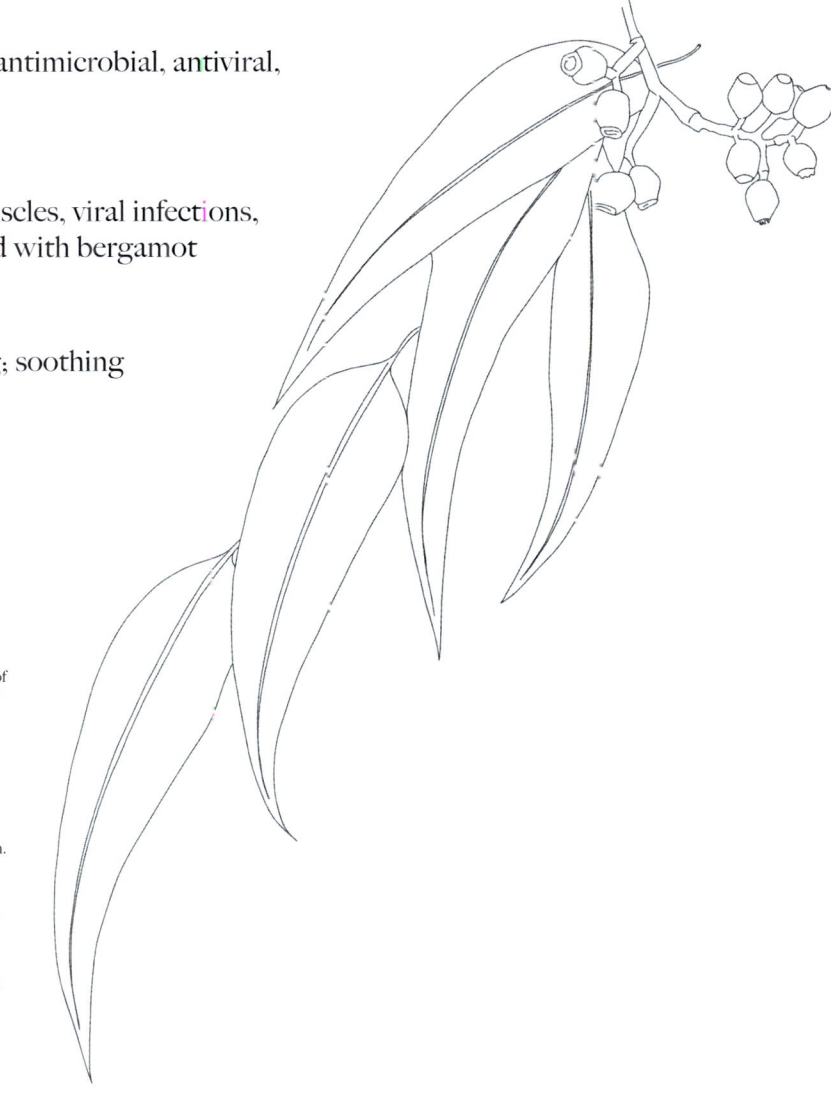

BOTANICAL FAMILY:
Apiaceae

PLANT ORIGIN:
Belgium, Bulgaria, Netherlands

EXTRACTION METHOD:
Steam distilled from root

KEY CONSTITUENTS:
Beta-Phellandrene (≤30%), Alpha-Phellandrene (7-28%), Alpha-Pinene (10-27%), Delta-3-Carene (8-15%), Limonene (3-13%), Sabinene (≤12%), Trans-Beta Ocimene (≤7%), Cis-Beta-Ocimene (≤4%)

EUCALYPTUS STAIGERIANA
(Eucalyptus staigeriana)

This gentle eucalyptus species was valued by Australian Aborigines as a general cure-all. By 1788 it was introduced in Europe, where it was valued for treating respiratory conditions and for colic. Recent research documents E. staigeriana as a powerful antiparasitic as well as being highly antimicrobial.

MEDICAL PROPERTIES:
Antibacterial, diuretic, decongestant, expectorant, antiparasitic, analgesic, antispasmodic, anti-inflammatory, insecticidal

USES:
Helps wounds, burns, and insect bites heal; insect repellent; suppresses coughs; relieves muscle aches, suitable for use with children, cleaning

FRAGRANT INFLUENCE:
Eucalyptus staigeriana, also known as lemon iron bark, has a lemon-scented aroma, without the medicine-like scent of other eucalyptus oils. Lifts spirits. It can be used on people with sensitive skin.

DIRECTIONS:
Aromatic: 30. Topical: 50-50.

CAUTIONS: Avoid use when pregnant.

SELECTED RESEARCH:

Barbosa LC, Filomeno CA, Teixeira RR. Chemical variability and Biological Activities of Eucalyptus spp. Essential Oils. Molecules. 2016 Dec; 21(12): 1671.

Ribeiro WL, Camurça-Vasconcelos AL, Macedo IT, dos Santos JM, de Araújo-Filho JV, Ribeiro Jde C, Pereira Vde A, Viana Dde A, de Paula HC, Bevilaqua CM. In vitro effects of Eucalyptus staigeriana nanoemulsion on Haemonchus contortus and toxicity in rodents. Vet Parasitol. 2015 Sep 15;212(3-4):444-7. Epub 2015 Jul 26.

Gilles M., Zhao J., An M., Agboola S. Chemical composition and antimicrobial properties of EOs of three Australian Eucalyptus species. Food Chem. 2010;119:731–737.

Gilles M, Zhao J, An M, Agboola S. Chemical composition and antimicrobial properties of essential oils of three Australian Eucalyptus species. Food Chem. 2010 15 Mar;119(2):731-7.

Zhao Q, Bowles EJ, Zhang HY. Antioxidant activities of eleven Australian essential oils. Nat Prod Comm. 2008;3(5):837-842.

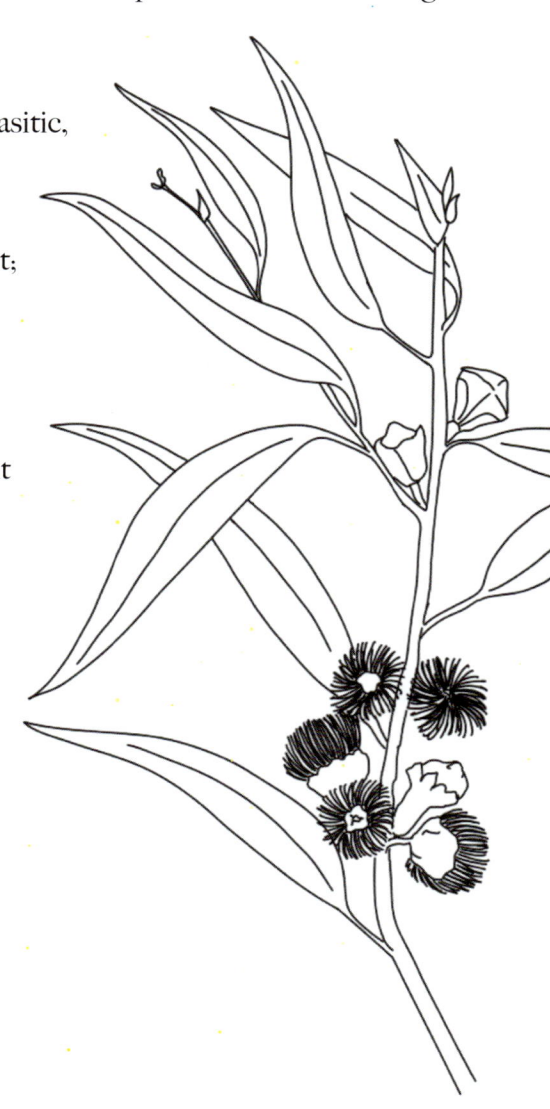

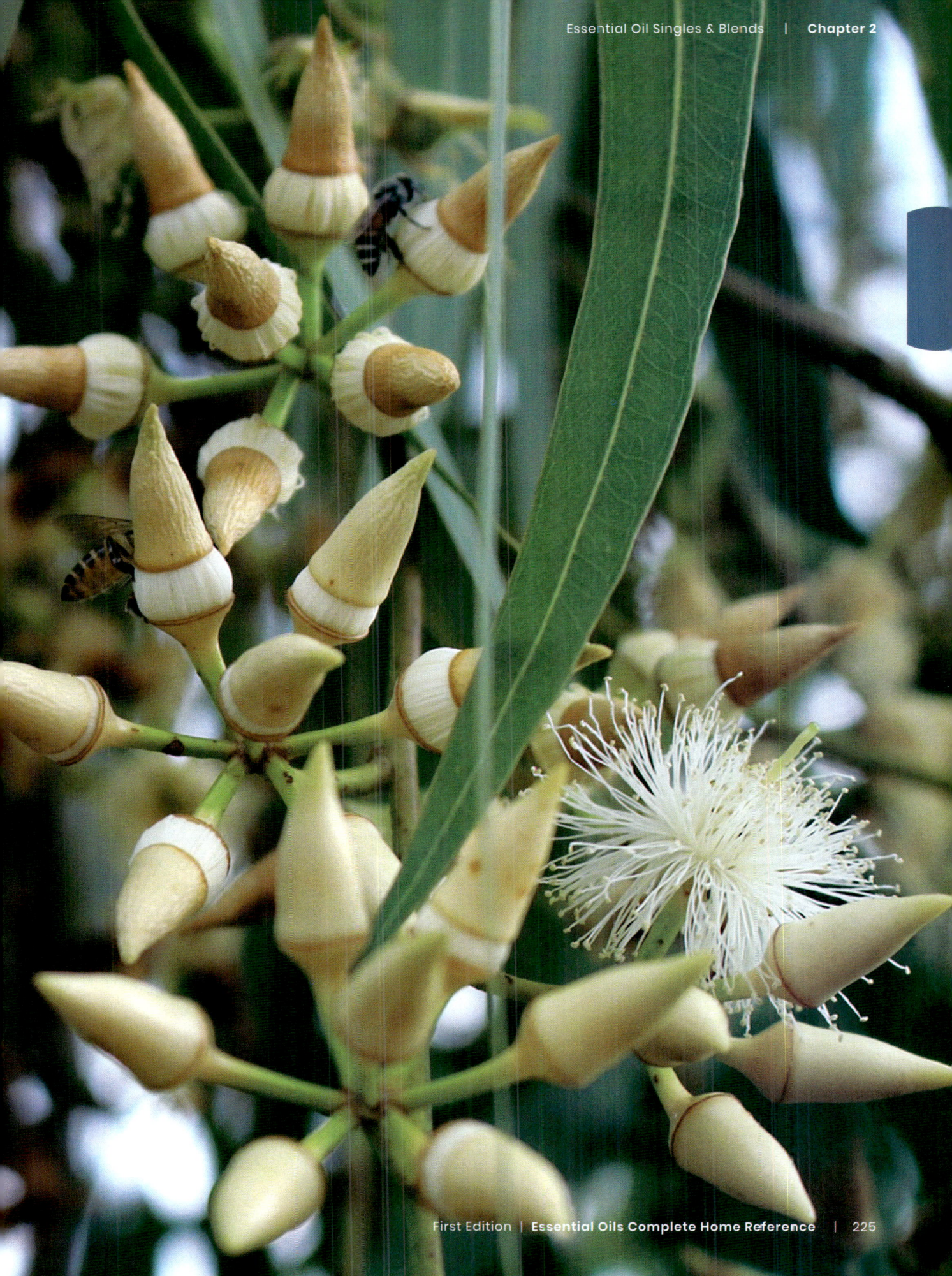

EVERGREEN ESSENCE™
(Essential Oil Blend)

Evergreen Essence essential oil blend has a refreshing, crisp scent that is invigorating and emotionally strengthening. With an arrangement of popular evergreen trees, the scents of pine, fir, and spruce complement one another and may assist in the release of occasional emotional blocks. Refreshing to the senses, Evergreen Essence brings a feeling of balance, peace, and security. The relaxing scent may also help clear the mind for a calming sense of meditation and reflection.

MEDICAL PROPERTIES & USES:
Antinociceptive (analgesic; reduces sensitivity to pain), antioxidative, antibacterial, antimicrobial, anti-inflammatory, balancing, uplifting, calming, meditation

INGREDIENTS:
Idaho Blue Spruce, Ponderosa Pine, Scotch Pine, Red Fir, Western Red Cedar, White Fir, Black Pine, Pinyon Pine, Lodgepole Pine

DIRECTIONS:
Aromatic: 6o. Topical: 50-50.

CAUTIONS:

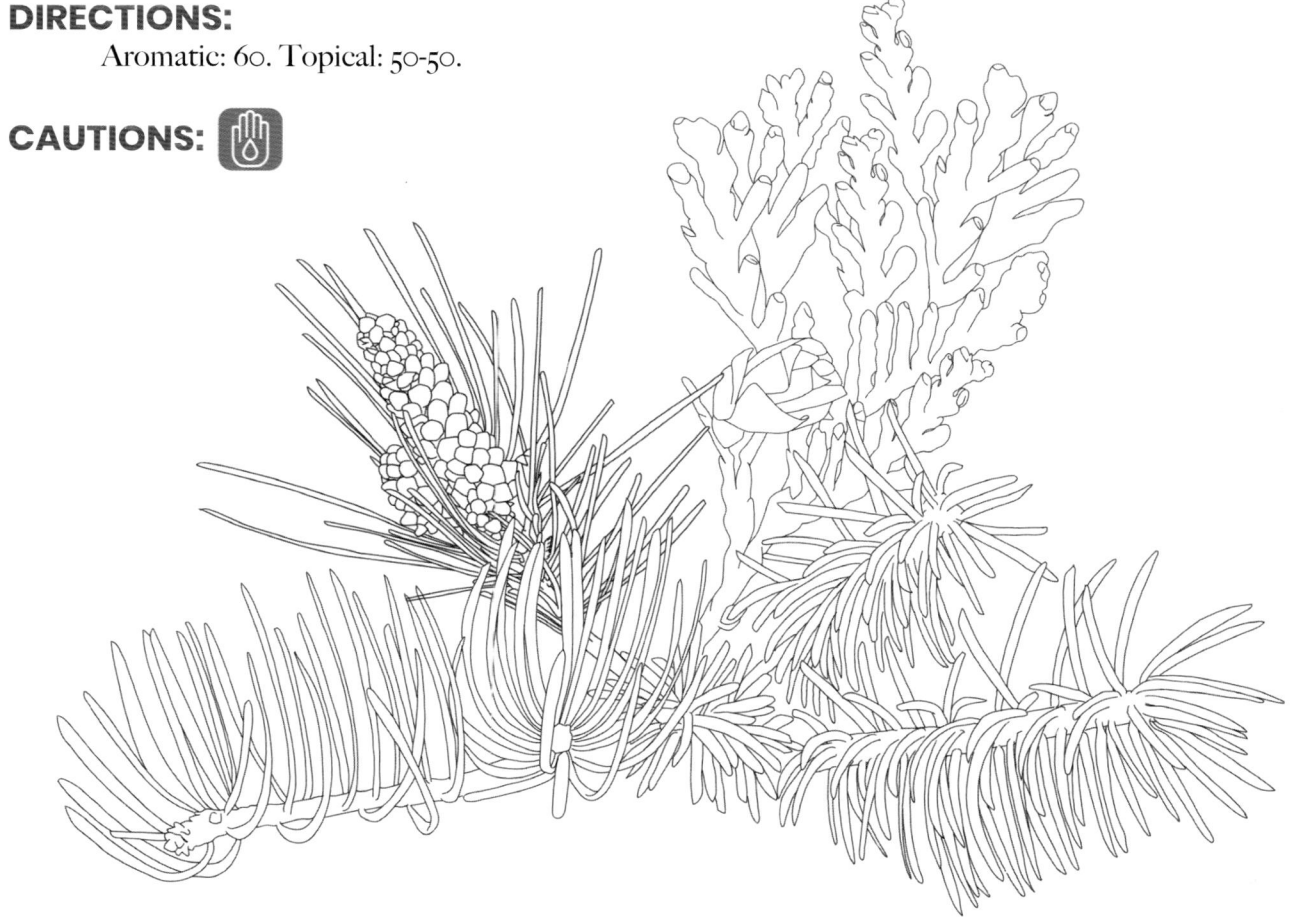

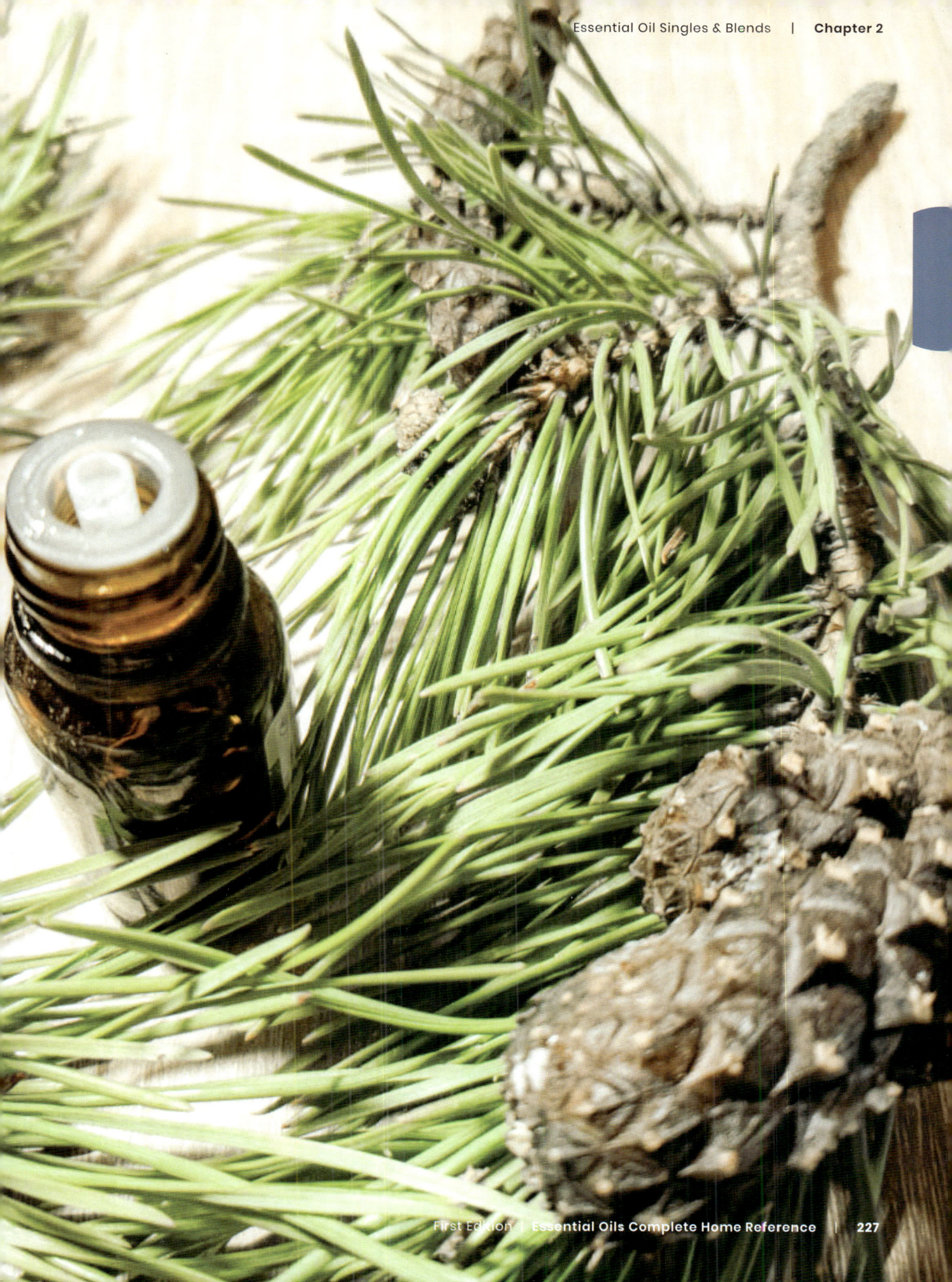

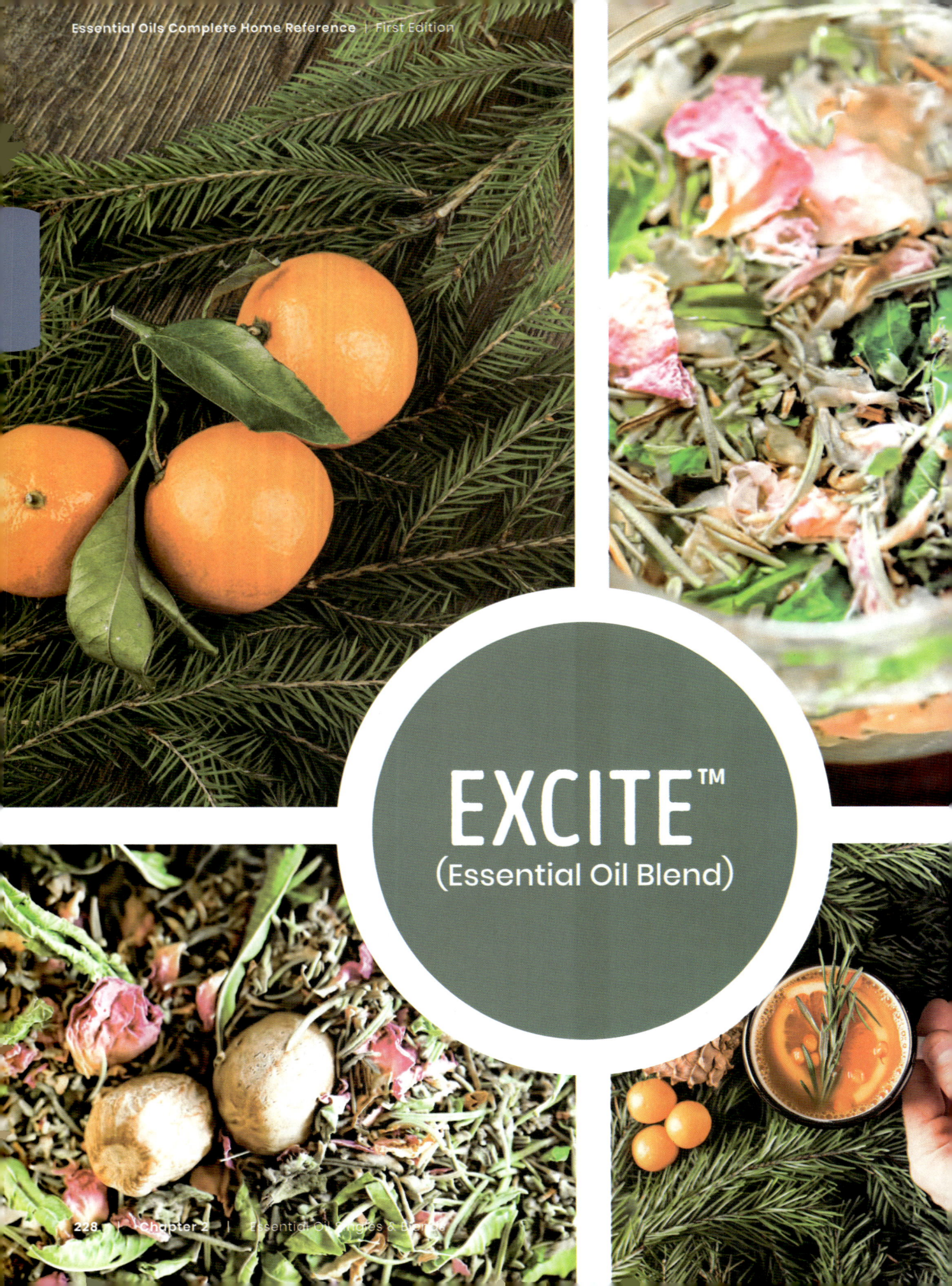

ABOUT EXCITE™:

This blend was specially crafted by D. Gary Young and combines the uplifting aromas of Jade Lemon and Tangerine with the sharp scents of Black Pepper and Northern Lights Black Spruce. Essential oils like Spearmint, Hinoki, and Nutmeg add brightness and warmth.

MEDICAL PROPERTIES & USES:

Antimicrobial, antioxidative, calming, uplifting, disease inhibitory, pain or swelling reducing, performance enhancing/stimulating

INGREDIENTS:

Spearmint, Cassia, Mastrante, Nutmeg, Ocotea, Canadian Fleabane, Jade Lemon, Tangerine, Black Pepper, Northern Lights Black Spruce

DIRECTIONS:

Aromatic: 10. Topical: 20-80.

CAUTIONS:

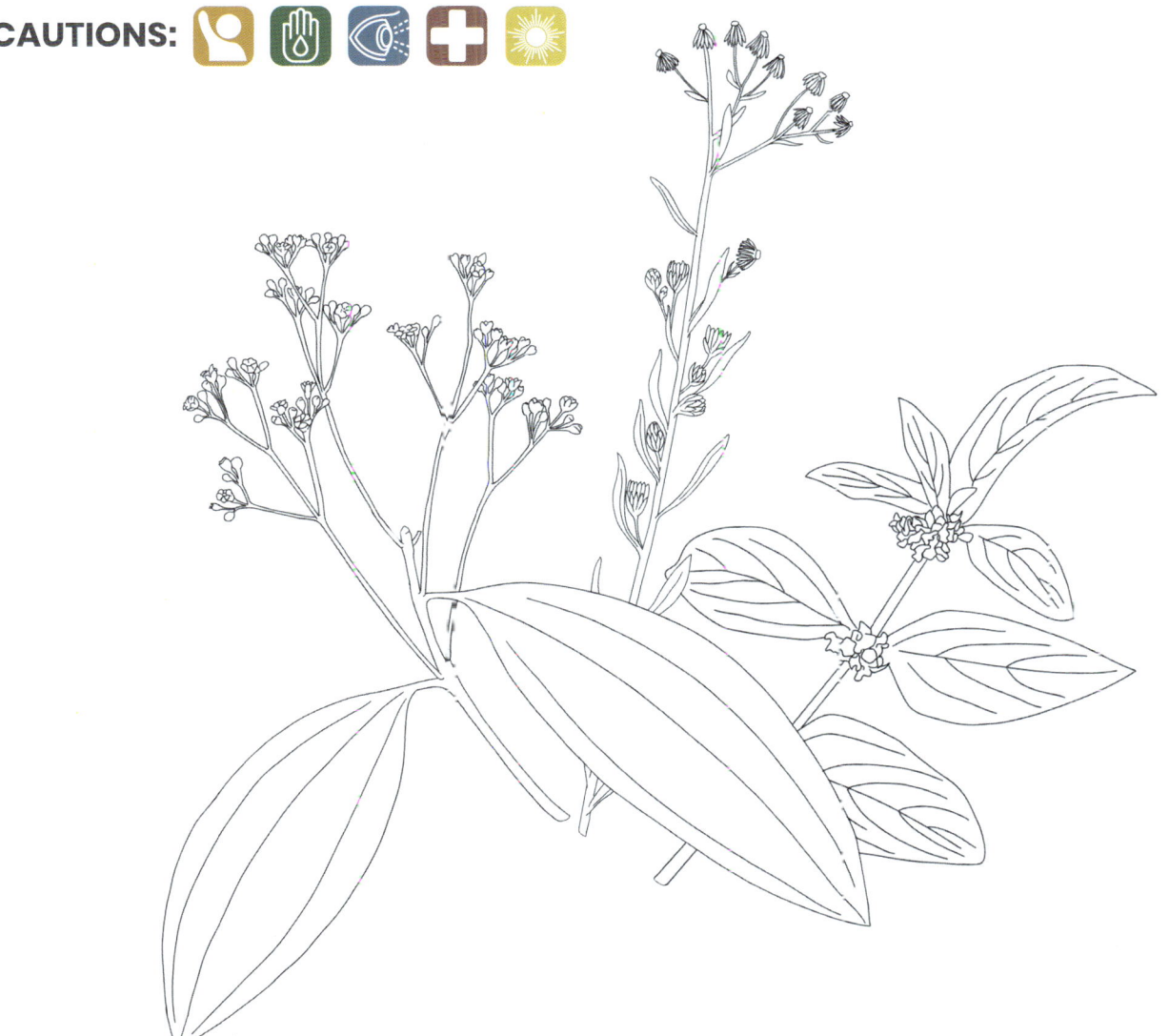

EXODUS II™
(Essential Oil Blend)

Some researchers believe that some of these aromatics were used by Aaron, the brother of Moses, to protect the Israelites from a plague. Modern science shows that these oils contain immune-stimulating and antimicrobial compounds. Because of the complex chemistry of essential oils, it is very difficult for viruses and bacteria to mutate and acquire resistance to them.

MEDICAL PROPERTIES & USES:
Anti-inflammatory, antimicrobial, antioxidative, calming, cardiovascular supportive, disease inhibitory, insecticidal/antiparasitic, organ protective, performance enhancing/stimulating

INGREDIENTS:
Olive oil, Myrrh, Cassia, Cinnamon Bark, Calamus, Northern Lights Black Spruce, Hyssop, Vetiver, Frankincense

DIRECTIONS:
Aromatic: 10. Topical: 20-80.

CAUTIONS:

Not intended for children under 12 years of age, unless directed by a health care professional.

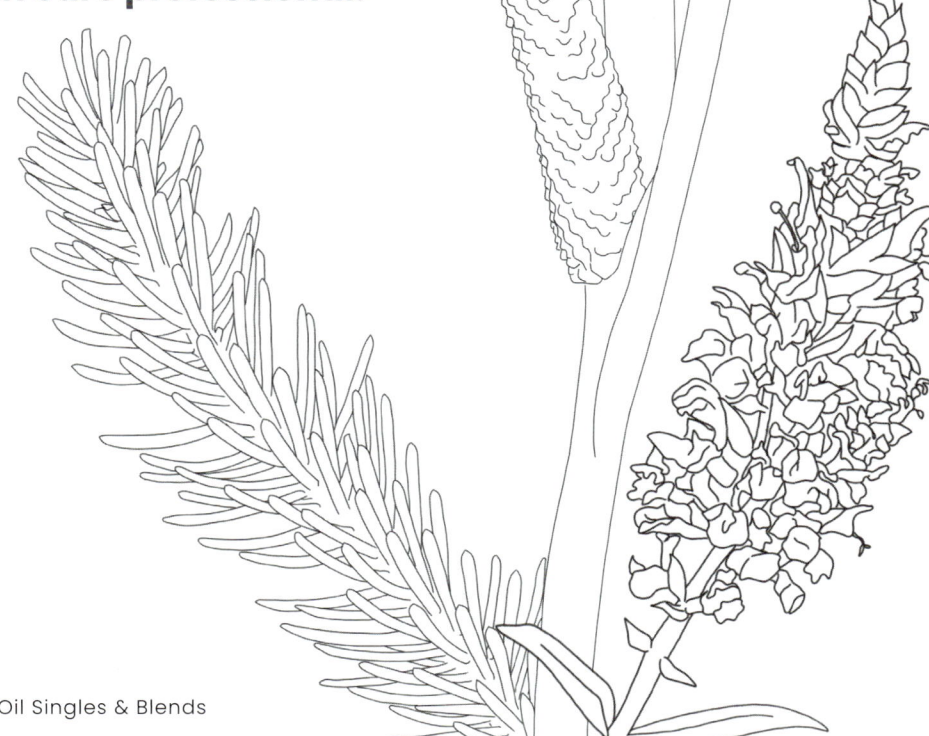

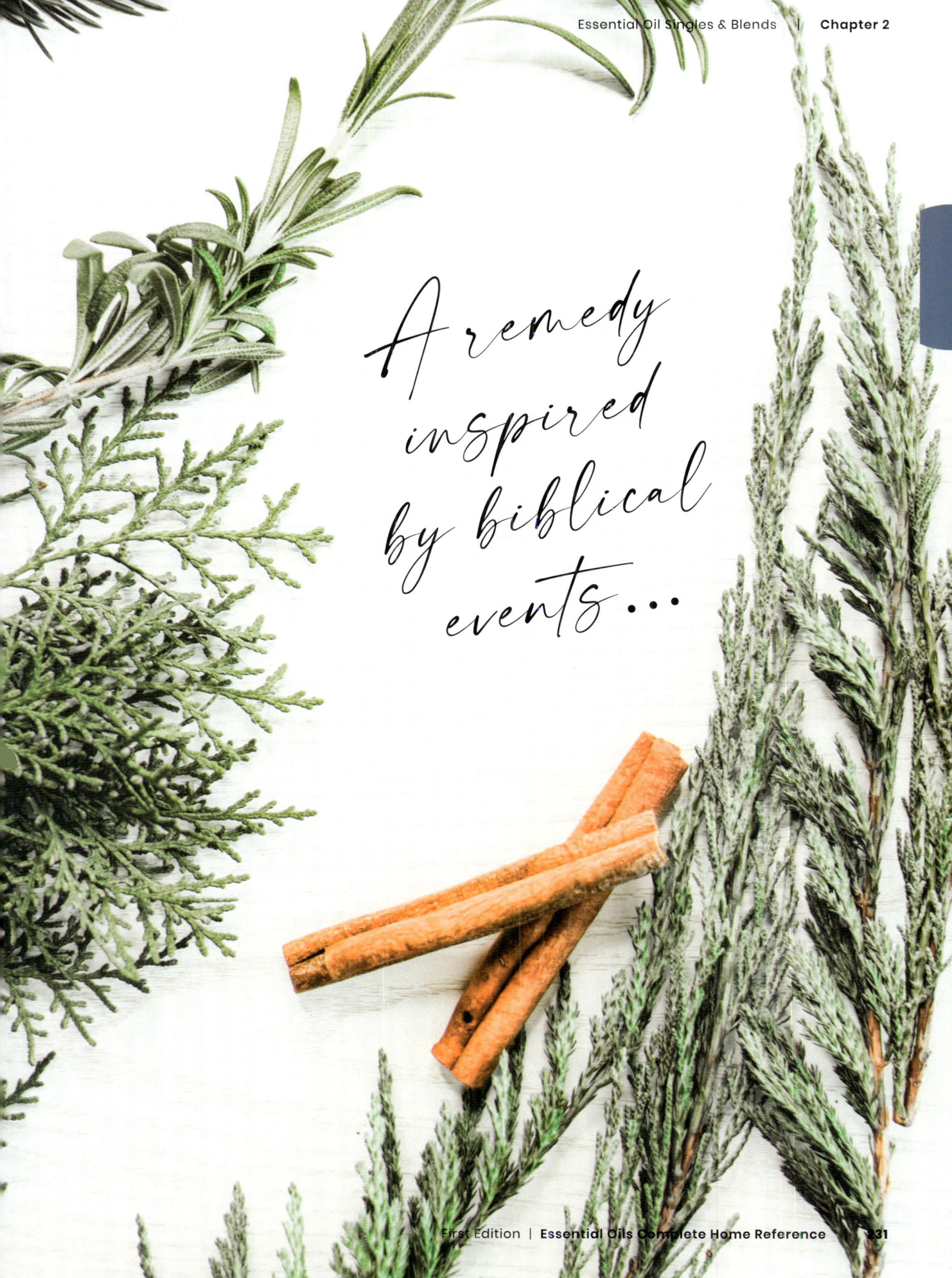

A remedy inspired by biblical events...

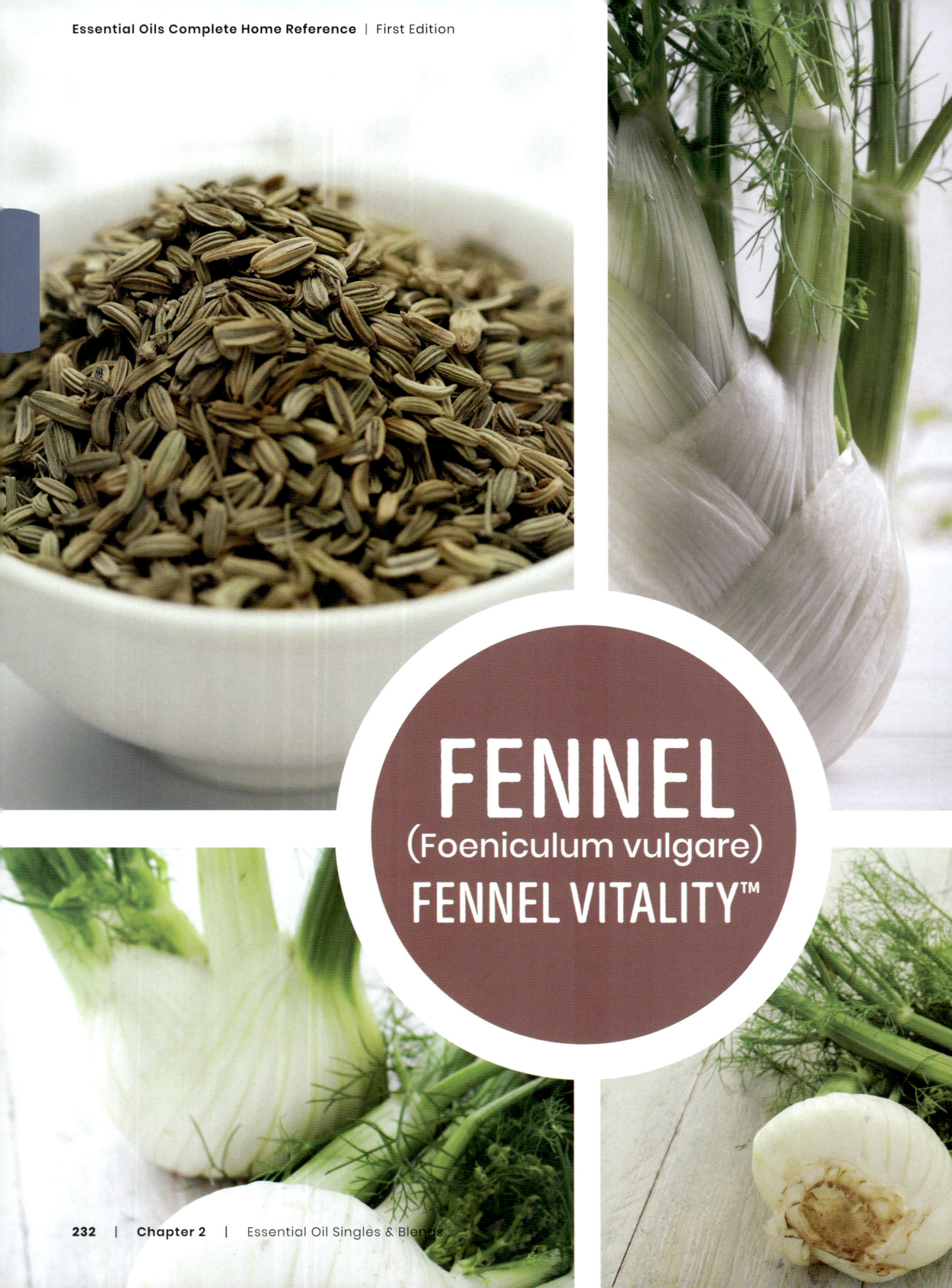

FENNEL
(Foeniculum vulgare)
FENNEL VITALITY™

Essential Oil Singles & Blends | Chapter 2

BOTANICAL FAMILY:
Apiaceae

PLANT ORIGIN:
Australia, Hungary

EXTRACTION METHOD:
Steam distilled from the seeds (fruit)

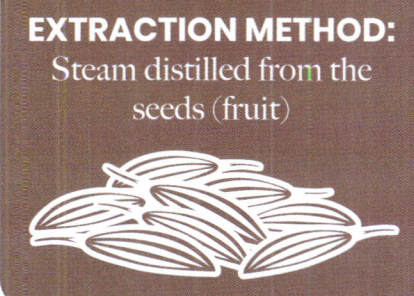

KEY CONSTITUENTS:
Trans-Anethole (50-79%),
Fenchone (7-25%),
Alpha-Pinene (1-11%),
Alpha-Phellandrene (up to 9%),
Methyl Chavicol (1-6%),
Limonene (1-6%),
Myrcene (up to 2%)

HISTORICAL DATA:
Fennel was believed to ward off evil spirits and to protect against spells cast by witches during medieval times. Sprigs were hung over doors to fend off evil phantasms. For hundreds of years, fennel seeds have been used as a digestive aid and to balance menstrual cycles. It is mentioned in one of the oldest known medical records, the Ebers Papyrus (dating from 16th century BC), an ancient Egyptian list of 877 prescriptions and recipes. It was listed in Hildegard's Medicine, a compilation of early German medicines by highly regarded Benedictine herbalist Hildegard of Bingen (1098-1179).

MEDICAL PROPERTIES:
Bronchodilator, antimicrobial, antifungal, hepatoprotective, inhibits genotoxicity and oxidative stress, antidiabetic, anti-inflammatory, antitumoral, estrogen-like, antiparasitic (worms), antiseptic, antispasmodic, analgesic

USES:
Anxiety, infantile colic, irritable bowel syndrome, anxiety, dysmenorrhea, reduces formation of blood clots, diabetes, cancer, obesity, arthritis/rheumatism, urinary tract infection, fluid retention, intestinal parasites, skin cleansing, metabolism, menstrual problems/PMS, digestive aid

FRAGRANT INFLUENCE:
Smells like black licorice, grounding

DIRECTIONS:
Aromatic: 3O. Topical: Neat. Dietary (Vitality): Dilute 1 drop with 1 drop of V-6 or other pure carrier oil. Put in a capsule and take up to 3 times daily or as needed.

CAUTIONS: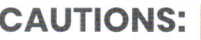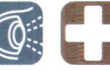
Avoid using if epileptic.
Not intended for use during pregnancy.

SELECTED RESEARCH:
Mahboubi M. Foeniculum vulgare as Valuable Plant in Management of Women's Health. J Menopausal Med. 2019 Apr; 25(1): 1-14.

Di Ciaula A, Portincasa P, Maes N, Albert A. Efficacy of bio-optimized extracts of turmeric and essential fennel oil on the quality of life in patients with irritable bowel syndrome. Ann Gastroenterol. 2018 Nov-Dec;31(6):685-691. Epub 2018 Aug 6.

Keskin I, Gunal Y, Ayla S, Kolbasi B, Sakul A, Kilic U, Gok O, Koroglu K, Ozbek H. Effects of Foeniculum vulgare essential oil compounds, fenchone and limonene, on experimental wound healing. Biotech Histochem. 2017;92(4):274-82. Epub 2017 Apr 20.

Portincasa P, Bonfrate L, Scribano ML, Kohn A, Caporaso N, Festi D, Campanale MC, Di Rienzo T, Guarino M, Taddia M, Fogli MV, Grimaldi M, Gasbarrini A. Curcumin and fennel essential oil improve symptoms and quality of life in patients with irritable bowel syndrome. J Gastrointestin Liver Dis. 2016 Jun;25(2):151-7.

Mota AS, Martins MR, Arantes S, Lopes VR, Bettencourt E, Pombal S, Gomes AC, Silva LA. Antimicrobial activity and chemical composition of the essential oils of Portuguese Foeniculum vulgare fruits. Nat Prod Commun. 2015 Apr;10(4):673-6.

Goswami N, Chatterjee S. Assessment of free radical scavenging potential and oxidative DNA damage preventive activity of Trachyspermum ammi L. (carom) and Foeniculum vulgare Mill. (fennel) seed extracts. Biomed Res Int. 2014;2014:582767. Epub 2014 Jul 23.

Mesfin M, Asres K, Shibeshi W. Evaluation of anxiolytic activity of the essential oil of the aerial part of Foeniculum vulgare Miller in mice. BMC Complement Altern Med. 2014 Aug 23;14(1):310. doi: 10.1186/1472-6882-14-310. Epub 2014 Aug 26.

Senatore F, Oliveira F, Scandolera E, Taglialatela-Seafati O, Roscigno C, Zaccardelli M, De Falco E. Chemical composition, antimicrobial and antioxidant activites of anethole-rich oil from leaves of selected varieties of fennel [Foeniculum vulgare Mill. Ssp. Vulgare var. azoricum (Mill.) Thell]. Fitoterapia. 2013 Oct;90:214-9. Epub 2013 Aug 13.

Omidvar S, Esmailzadeh S, Baradaran M, Basirat Z. Effect of fennel on pain intensity in dysmenorrhea: a placebo-controlled trial. Ayu. 2012 Apr;33(2):311-3. Epub 2013 Apr 6.

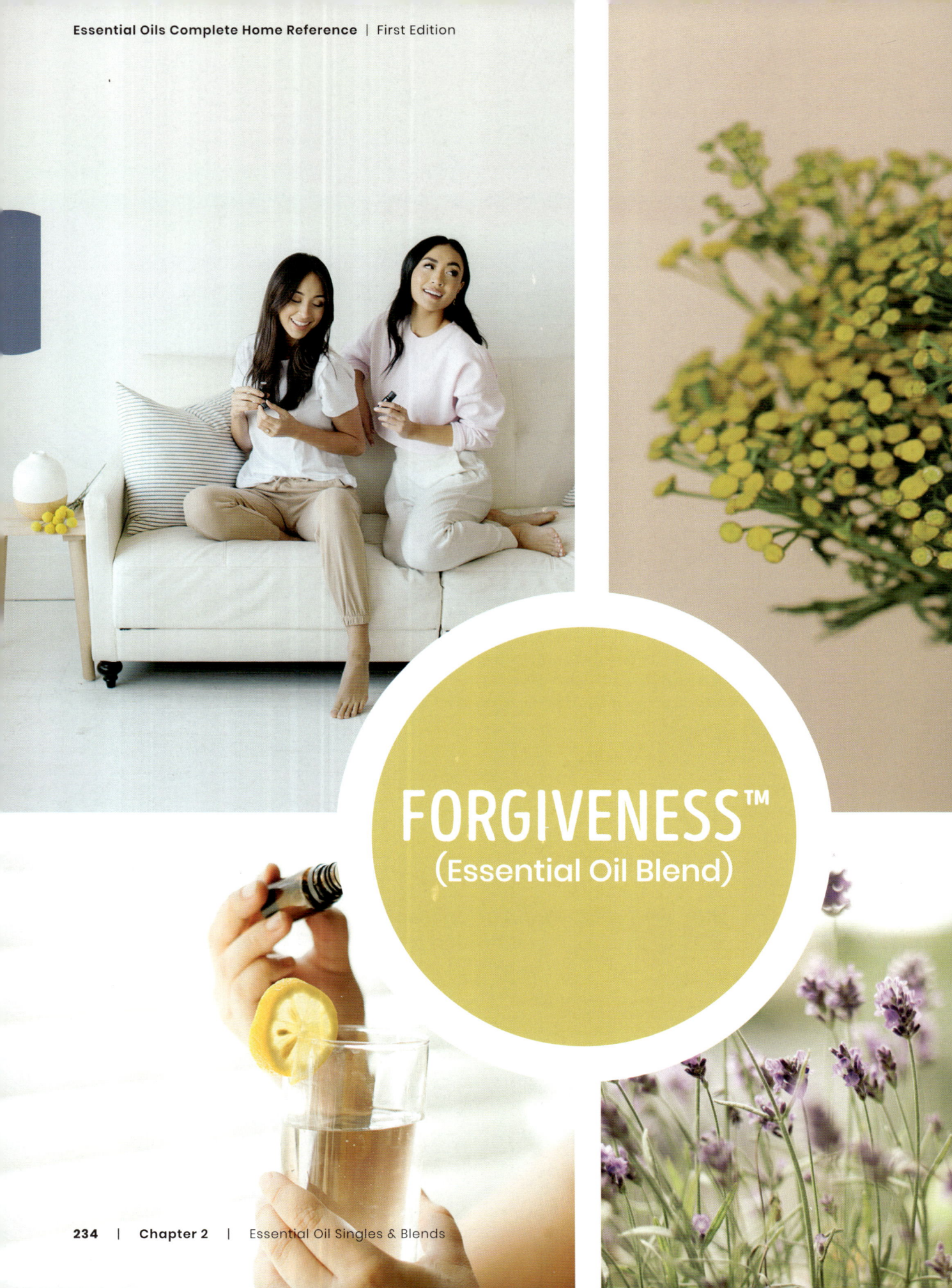

| Essential Oil Singles & Blends | **Chapter 2**

ABOUT FORGIVENESS™:
This blend helps to release hurt feelings and negative emotions. It also helps release negative memories, allowing one to move past emotional barriers and attain higher awareness, assisting the person to forgive and let go.

MEDICAL PROPERTIES & USES:
Anti-inflammatory, antimicrobial, antioxidative, emotion supporting, uplifting, calming, cardiovascular supportive, digestion or elimination supportive/nausea reducing, disease inhibitory

INGREDIENTS:
Sesame seed oil, Melissa, Geranium, Frankincense, Royal Hawaiian Sandalwood, Coriander, Angelica, Lavender, Bergamot (Furocoumarin-free), Lemon, Ylang Ylang, Jasmine, Helichrysum, Roman Chamomile, Palmarosa, Rose

DIRECTIONS:
Aromatic: 6o. Topical: Neat.

CAUTIONS:

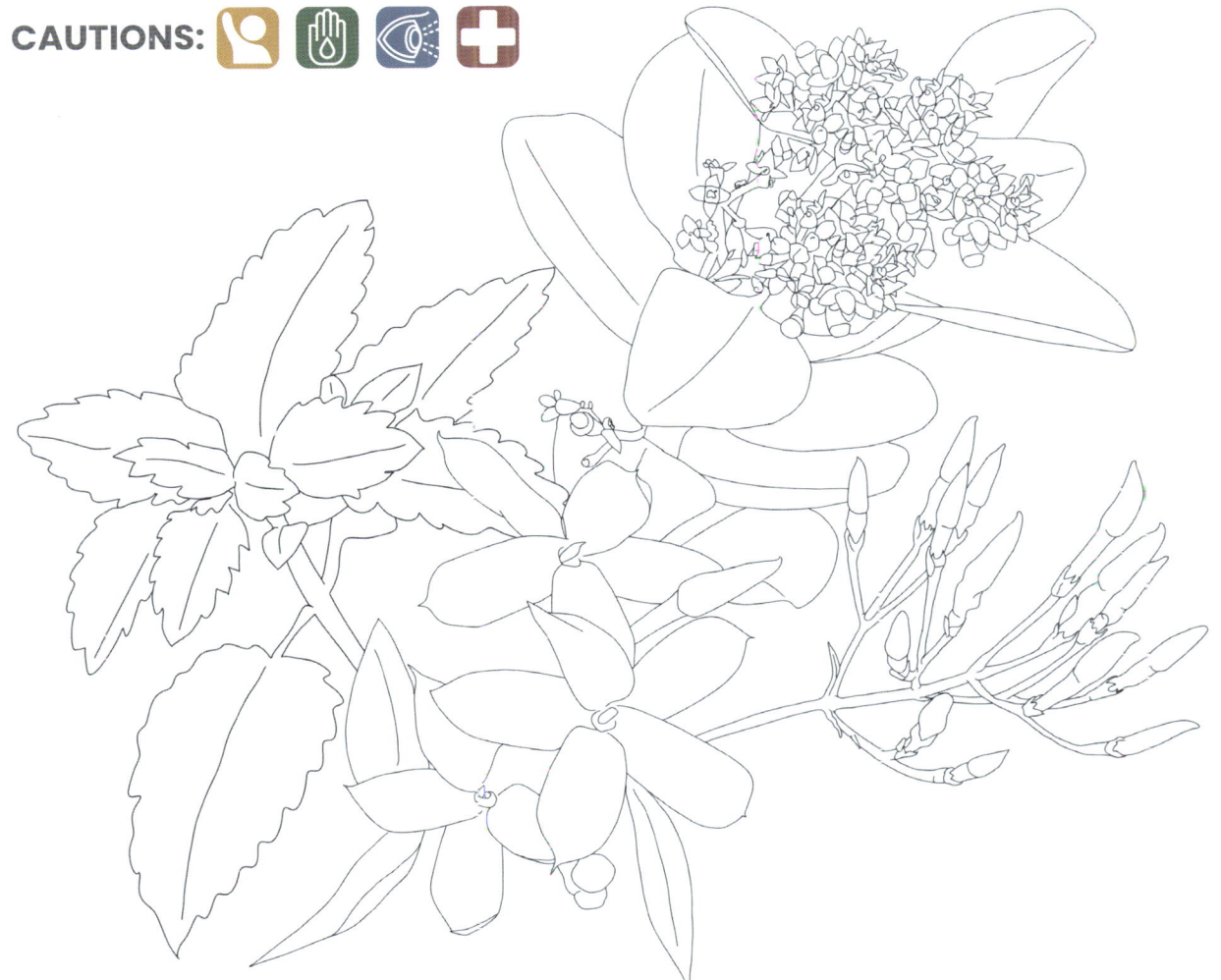

First Edition | **Essential Oils Complete Home Reference** | 235

BOTANICAL FAMILY: Myrtaceae

PLANT ORIGIN: Western Australia

EXTRACTION METHOD: Steam distilled from leaves and stems

KEY CONSTITUENTS: Oxides [29.52% 1,8-cineole (eucalyptol)], Monoterpene alcohols (9.21% linalool, 3.21% tepinene-ol, 7.02 a-terpineol, 3.58% myrtenol), Monoterpene hydrocrbons (25.06% a-pinene)

FRAGONIA
(Agonis fragrans; Taxandria fragrans)

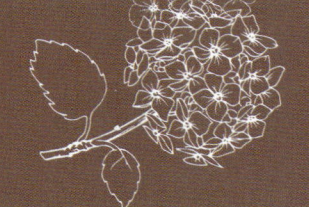

Fragonia essential oil has a soft scent reminiscent of floral Tea Tree oil. This sweet, herbaceous scent will be a favorite during seasonal changes and will be a favorite for cleansing and soothing. It balances the emotions, decreases grief and anxiety, promotes inner peace, and is calming to the mind.

MEDICAL PROPERTIES:
Antioxidant, antibacterial, antimicrobial, anti-inflammatory, antifungal, analgesic, immune stimulant, expectorant

USES:
Emotional balancing, removes scars from negative emotions, skin care, hair care, sleep disturbances, hydrating, respiratory conditions, bronchitis, catarrh, sinus congestion, sore joints, pain, acne, bacterial and fungal infections, sore muscles, immune system, unbalanced chakras, significant relief to the discomfort of menstrual periods, improve connection to the Divine during meditation and prayer, enhance dignity and strength

FRAGRANT INFLUENCE:
Calming, unblocks negative emotions, improves sleep, clears the air, supports the respiratory system, generates sense of well-being, balancing

DIRECTIONS:
Aromatic: 6o. Topical: Neat.

CAUTIONS:

SELECTED RESEARCH:

Ramsey JT, Shropshire BC, Nagy TR, Chambers KD, Li Y, Korach KS. Essential oils and health. Yale J Biol Med. 2020 Jun; 93(2): 291-305. Published online 2020 Jun 29.

Powers CN, Satyal P, Mayo JA, McFeeters H, McFeeters RL.. Bigger Data Approach to Analysis of Essential Oils and Their Antifungal Activity against Aspergillus niger, Candida albicans, and Cryptococcus neoformans. Molecules. 2019 Aug; 24(16): 2868. Published online 2019 Aug 7.

Hammer KA, Carson CF, Dunstan JA, Hale J, Lehmann H, Robinson CJ, Prescott SL, Riley TV. Antimicrobial and anti-inflammatory activity of five Taxandria fragrans oils in vitro. Microbiol Immunol. 2008 Nov;52(11):522-30.

J.R. Wheeler et N.G. Marchant. Lowe RF, Russell MF, Southwell IA, Robinson CJ, Day J. Composition of an Essential Oil from Agonis fragrans. Journal of Essential Oil Research. June 2007,19(4):342-344.

Essential Oil Singles & Blends | **Chapter 2**

Your restful nights will thank Fragonia.

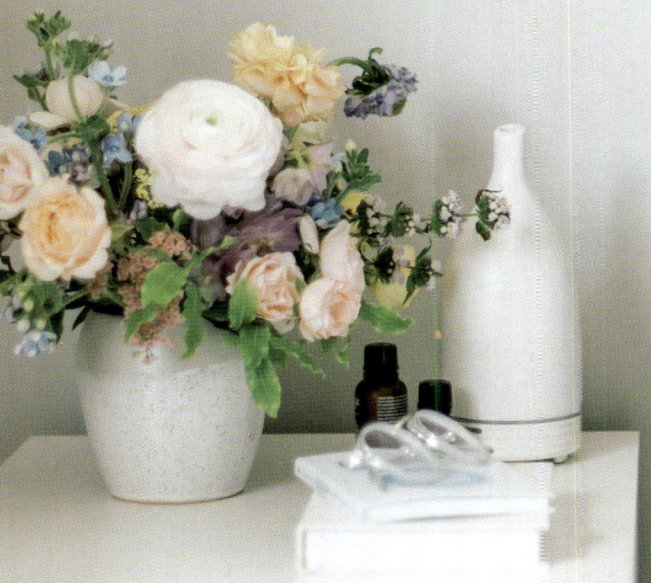

First Edition | **Essential Oils Complete Home Reference** | 237

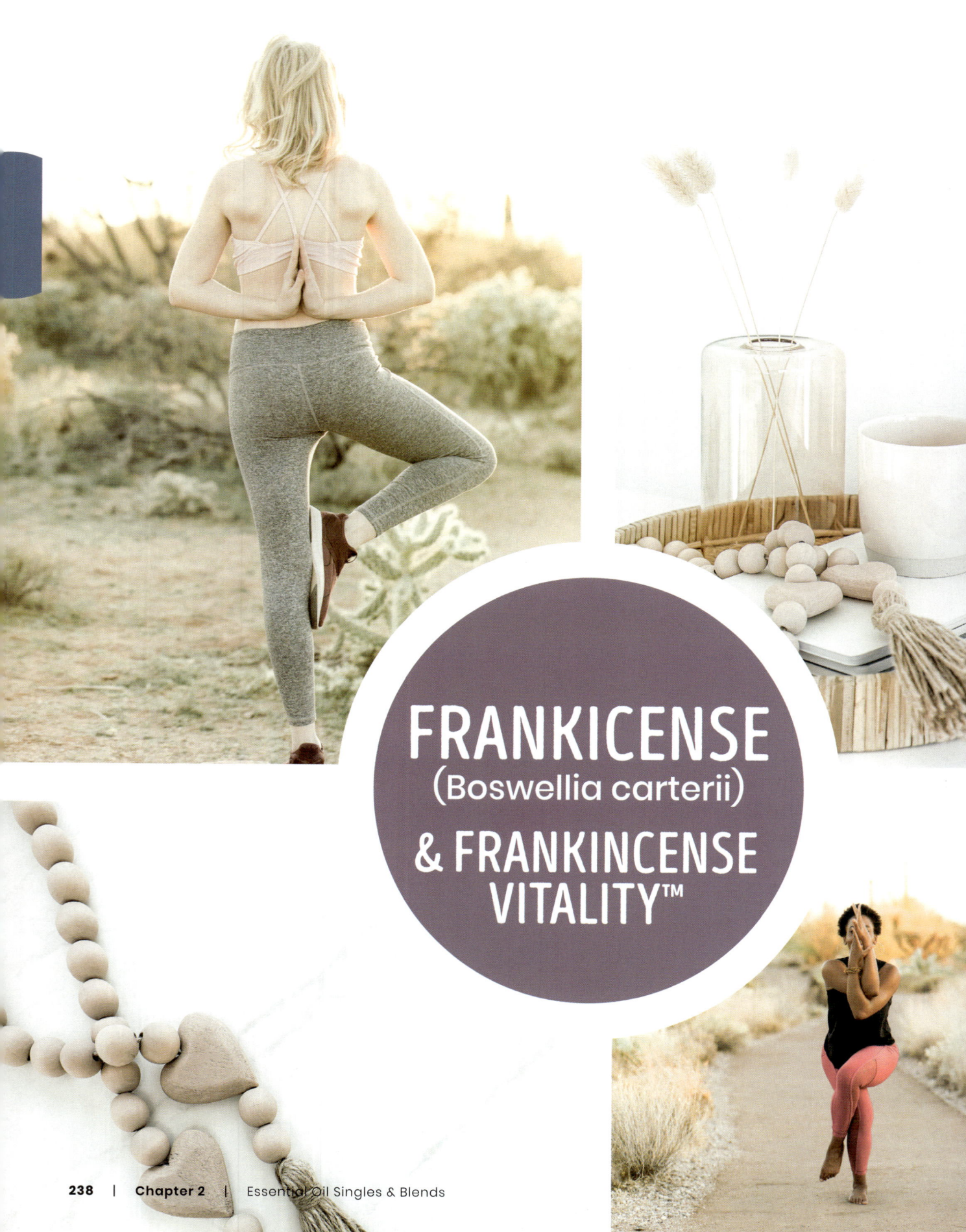

BOTANICAL FAMILY:
Burseraceae

PLANT ORIGIN:
Somalia

EXTRACTION METHOD:
Steam distilled from gum/resin

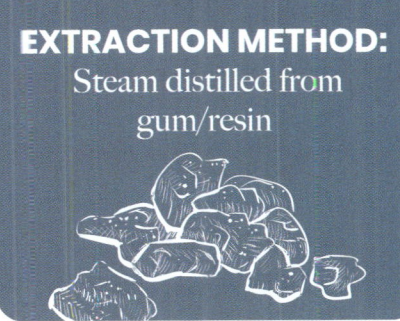

KEY CONSTITUENTS:
Alpha-Pinene (35-75%),
Alpha-Thujene (up to 20%),
Limonene (up to 18%),
Myrcene (up to 13%),
Sabinene (1-6%),
Decyl Methyl Ether (up to 2%),
Octyl Acetate (up to 2%)

HISTORICAL DATA:

Also known as "olibanum," the name frankincense is derived from the medieval French word for "real incense." Frankincense is considered the "holy anointing oil" in the Middle East and has been used in religious ceremonies for thousands of years. It was well known during the time of Christ for anointing and healing powers and was one of the gifts given to Christ at His birth. Used to treat every conceivable ill known to man, frankincense was valued more than gold during ancient times, and only those with great wealth and abundance possessed it. It is mentioned in one of the oldest known medical records, Ebers Papyrus (dating from 16th century BC), an ancient Egyptian list of 877 prescriptions and recipes.

MEDICAL PROPERTIES:
Antitumoral, immuno-stimulant, antidepressant, muscle relaxing, antifungal, anti-inflammatory, anticancerous

USES:
Arthritis, depression, cancer, respiratory infections, inflammation, helps maintain normal brain function, immune stimulating

FRAGRANT INFLUENCE:
Stimulating aroma, increases spiritual awareness, promotes meditation, improves attitude, and uplifts spirits

DIRECTIONS:
Aromatic: 6o. Topical: Neat. Dietary (Vitality): Put 2 drops in a capsule and take 3 times daily.

CAUTIONS: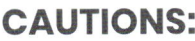

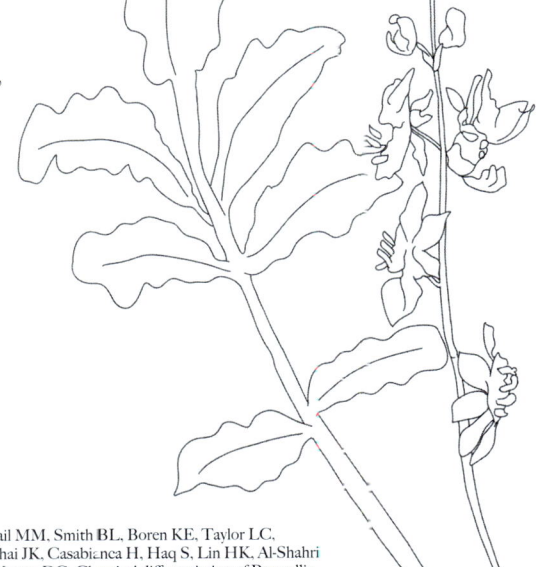

SELECTED RESEARCH:

Sharifi-Rad J, Ozleyen A, Tumer TB, Adetunji CO, El Omari N, Balahbib A, Taheri Y, Bouyahya A, Martorell M, Martins N, Cho WC. Natural Products and Synthetic Analogs as a Source of Antitumor Drugs. Biomolecules. 2019 Nov; 9(11) 679.

Reis D, Jones TT. Frankincense essential oil as a supportive therapy for cancer-related fatigue: a case study. Holist Nurs Pract. 2018 May/Jun;32(3):140-142.

Wang YG, Ma QG, Tian J, Ren J, Wang AG, Ji TF, Yang JB, Su YL. Hepatoprotective triterpenes from the gum resin of Boswellia carterii. Fitoterapia. 2016 Mar;109:266-73. Epub 2015 Dec 29.

Al-Yasiry AR, Kiczorowska B. Frankincense—therapeutic properties. Postepy Hig Med Dosw (Online). 2016 Jan 4;70:380-91. Kazemian A, Toghiani A, Shafiei K, Afshar H, Rafiei R, Memari M, Adibi P. Evaluating the efficacy of mixture of Boswellia carterii, Zingiber officinale, and Achillea millefolium on severity of symptoms, anxiety, and depression in irritable bowel syndrome patients. J Res Med Sci. 2017 Nov 28;22:120. eCollection 2017.

Mostafa DM, Ammar NM, Basha M, Hussein RA, El Awdan S, Awad G. Transdermal microemulsions of Boswellia carterii Bird: formulation, characterization and in vivo evaluation of anti-inflammatory activity. Drug Deliv. 2015 Aug 18;22(6):748-56.

Zaki AA, Hashish NE, Amer MA, Lahloub MF. Cardioprotective and antioxidant effects of oleogum resin "Olibanum" from Boswellia carteri Birdw. (Burseraceae). Chin J Nat Med. 2014 May;12(5):345-50.

Woolley CL, Suhail MM, Smith BL, Boren KE, Taylor LC, Schreuder MF, Chai JK, Casabianca H, Haq S, Lin HK, Al-Shahri AA, Al-Hatmi S, Young DG. Chemical differentiation of Boswellia sacra and Boswellia carterii essential oils by gas chromatography and chiral gas chromatography-mass spectrometry. J Chromatogr A. 2012 Oct 26;1261:158-63. Epub 2012 Jun 26.

Moussaieff A, Rimmerman N, Bregman T, Straiker A, Felder CC, Shoham S, Kashman Y, Huang SM, Lee H, Shohami E, Mackie K, Caterina MJ, Walker JM, Fride E, Mechoulam R. Incensole acetate, an incense component, elicits psychoactivity by activating TRPV3 channels in the brain. FASEB J. 2008 Aug 1;22(8):3024-34. Epub 2008 May 22.

Moussaieff A, Shein NA, Tsenter J, Grigoriadis S, Simeonidou C, Alexandrovich AG, Trembovler V, Ben-Neriah Y, Schmitz ML, Fiebich BL, Munoz E, Mechoulam R, Shohami E. Incensole acetate: a novel neuroprotective agent isolated from Boswellia carterii. J Cereb Blood Flow Metab. 2008 Jul;28(7):1341-52. Epub 2008 Apr 16.

BOTANICAL FAMILY: Burseraceae

PLANT ORIGIN: Somalia

EXTRACTION METHOD: Steam distilled from gum/resin

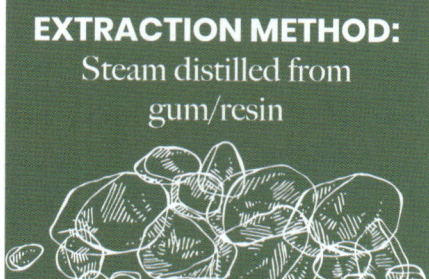

KEY CONSTITUENTS: Alpha-Thujene (23-45%), Alpha-Pinene (5-9%), Sabinene (1-8%), Para-Cymene (10-20%), Terpinen-4-ol (2-9%)

FRANKINCENSE, FREREANA
(Boswellia frereana)

This species of frankincense is native to northern Somalia, where the locals call it "Maydi" and the "King of Frankincense." Frereana incense has been a part of Eastern Orthodox and Catholic worship for hundreds of years. Since Boswellia carterii also grows in Somalia, it is hard to explain why B. frereana has such a unique chemical composition, so different from B. carterii and other frankincense species. As shown by Frank and Unger, as well as E. J. Blain, frereana contains no boswellic acids. S. Hamm reports that frereana "is devoid of diterpenes of the incensole family." Now that a pure source can be guaranteed, it is hoped researchers will delve into the benefits of frereana.

There are unique constituents of frereana—found in no other frankincense—that have mostly been overlooked by researchers. Two frereana studies in 2010 and 2006 reported strong anti-inflammatory activity. Sadly, some trusting purchasers have received an amalgamation of cheaper frankincense resins rather than pure Boswellia frereana. Political conditions in Somalia make it essential for a "feet on the ground" presence in order to secure contracts to obtain pure, high quality frereana resin. For this reason, D. Gary Young personally visited Somalia in November 2013 to contract with local clans of harvesters.

MEDICAL PROPERTIES:
Anti-inflammatory, antibacterial, antispasmodic, analgesic

USES:
Arthritis/rheumatism, skin supporting, resin used for chewing gum

FRAGRANT INFLUENCE:
The aroma of Frereana Frankincense has a more lemony scent than carterii and is uplifting, grounding, and cheering; spiritually elevating before trauma or anger was experienced

DIRECTIONS:
Aromatic: 6o. Topical: Neat. Dietary: 2o-8o. Put in a capsule and take 1 capsule before each meal or as desired

CAUTIONS:

SELECTED RESEARCH:

Schmiech M, Lang SJ, Werner K, Rashan LJ, Syrovets T, Simmet T. Comparative Analysis of Pentacyclic Triterpenic Acid Compositions in Oleogum Resins of Different Boswellia Species and Their In Vitro Cytotoxicity against Treatment-Resistant Human Breast Cancer Cells. Molecules. 2019 Jun; 24(11): 2153.

Parr C, Ali AY. Boswellia frereana suppresses HGF-mediated breast cancer cell invasion and migration through inhibition of c-Met signaling. J Transl Med. 2018 Oct 12;16(1):281.

Niebler J, Buettner A. Frankincense revisited, part I: comparative analysis of volatiles in commercially relevant Boswellia species. Chem Biodivers. 2016 May;13(5):613-29.

Blain EJ, Ali AY, Duance VC. Boswellia frereana (frankincense) suppresses cytokine-induced matrix metalloproteinase expression and production of pro-inflammatory molecules in articular cartilage. Phytother Res. 2010 Jun;24(6):905-12.

Frank A, Unger M. Analysis of frankincense from various Boswellia species with inhibitory activity on human drug metabolising cytochrome P450 enzymes using liquid chromatography mass spectrometry after automated on-line extraction. J Chromatogr A. 2006 Apr 21;1112(1-2):255-62. Epub 2005 Dec 20.

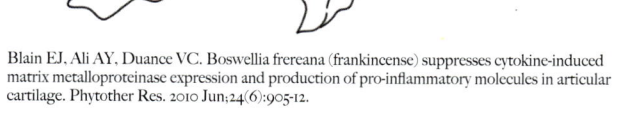

Frereana – the "lemony" Frankincense

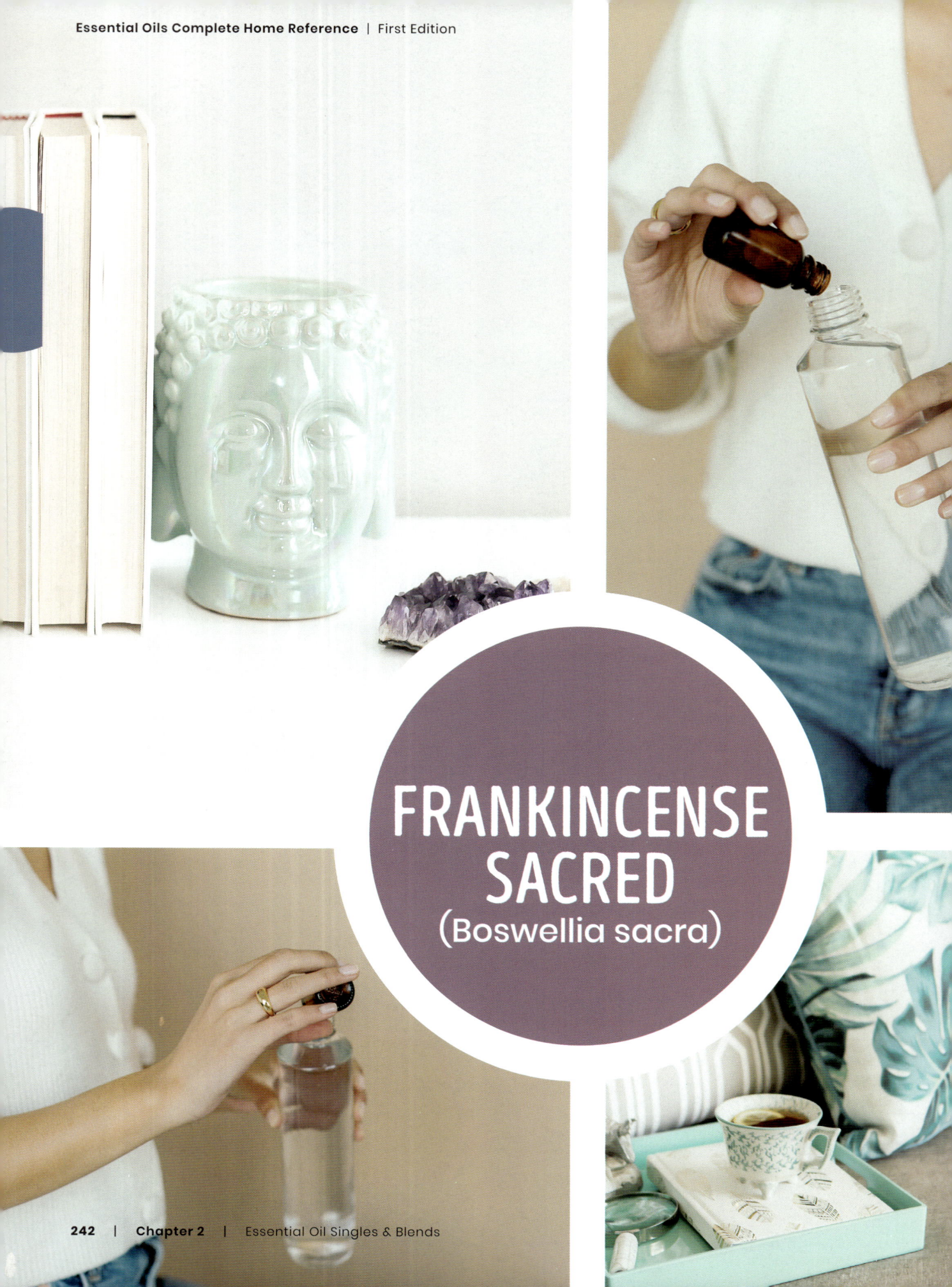

FRANKINCENSE SACRED
(Boswellia sacra)

BOTANICAL FAMILY:
Burseraceae

PLANT ORIGIN:
Oman

EXTRACTION METHOD:
Hydro distilled from resin

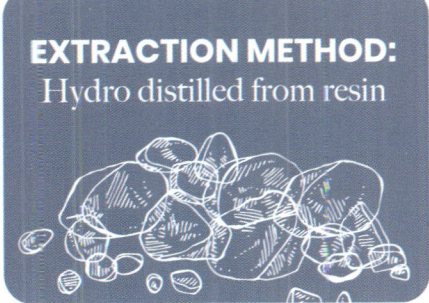

KEY CONSTITUENTS:
Alpha-pinene (63-92%),
Myrcene (up to 15%),
Limonene (up to 15%),
Sabinene (up to 5%),
Para-Cymene (up to 5%),
Camphene (1-3%)

HISTORICAL DATA:

Young Living's Sacred Frankincense essential oil is the first Omani Frankincense oil to be available to those outside of Saudi royals or the privileged of Oman. It is regarded the world over as the rarest, most sought-after aromatic in existence.

After 15 years of research, 15 trips to Oman, and numerous meetings and negotiations with Omani officials, D. Gary Young was granted the first export permit in the modern history of Oman for the release and export of the oil and permission to build a Young Living distillery in the country and to export the resulting essential oil out of Oman. Gary Young was on-site to supervise the building of Young Living's Omani distillery, and Young Living has contracted with local harvesters to secure our supply of Omani resin. This marks the first time any Westerners have been able to experience the unique spiritual properties of Sacred Frankincense essential oil. Omani Frankincense is highly regarded as the Frankincense of the ancients and the traditional spiritual oil of biblical times. Historically, it is believed that this beautiful, white hojari resin produced the Frankincense that was taken to the Christ Child. Science continues to document the oil's immense healing properties which users of this oil already know.

Complement to: Frankincense, Boswellia carterii

MEDICAL PROPERTIES:
Antimicrobial, anti-inflammatory, analgesic. Frankincense has been tested as an anticancer agent (Ni, et al., 2012; Suhail, et al., 2011). Therapeutic-grade Frankincense oil contains boswellic acids, which are potent anti-inflammatory agents against rheumatoid arthritis and osteoporosis.

USES:
Tumor-suppressive, skin health, stomach disorders, ulcers, cancer, dental and gum diseases, bad blood, infections, mental disorders, insect bites

FRAGRANT INFLUENCE:
Calming, meditative, relaxing, promotes higher states of spiritual awareness and higher levels of consciousness and sensitivity.

DIRECTIONS:
Aromatic: 6o. Topical: Neat. Dietary: Put 2 drops in a capsule and take 3 times daily or as needed or put 1-2 drops in water and drink.

CAUTIONS: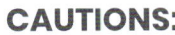

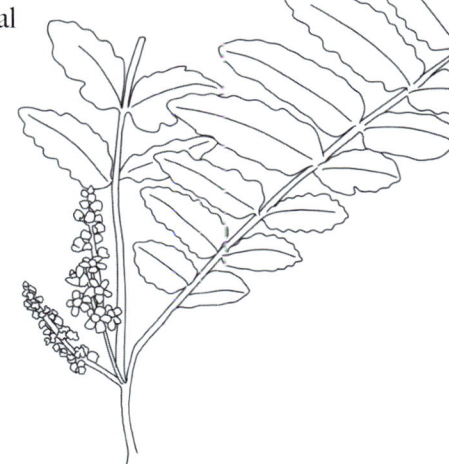

SELECTED RESEARCH:

Kieliszek M, Edris A, Kot AM, Piwowarek K. Biological Activity of Some Aromatic Plants and Their Metabolites, with an Emphasis on Health-Promoting Properties. Molecules. 2020 Jun; 25(11): 2478. Published online 2020 May 27.

Xia D, Lou W, Fung KM, Woolley CL, Suhail MM, Lin HK. Cancer chemopreventive effects of Boswellia sacra gum resin hydrodistillates on invasive urothelial cell carcinoma: report of a case. Integr Cancer Ther. 2017 Dec;16(4):605-611. Epub 2016 Aug 16.

Niebler J, Buettner A. Identification of odorants in frankincense (Boswellia sacra Flueck.) by aroma extract dilution analysis and two-dimensional gas chromatography-mass spectrometry/olfactometry. Phytochemistry. 2015 Jan;109:66-75. Epub 2014 Nov 18.

Al-Harrasi A, Ali L, Hussain J, Rehman NU, Mehjabeen, Ahmed M, Al-Rawahi A. Analgesic effects of crude extracts and fractions of Omani frankincense obtained from traditional medicinal plant Boswellia sacra on animal models. Asian Pac J Trop Med. 2014 Sep 7S1:S485-90.

Woolley CL, Suhail MM, Smith BL, Boren KE, Taylor LC, Schreuder MF, Chai JK, Casabianca H, Haq S, Lin HK, Al-Shahri AA, Al-Hatmi S, Young DG. Chemical differentiation of Boswellia sacra and Boswellia carterii essential oils by gas chromatography and chiral gas chromatography-mass spectrometry. J Chromatogr A. 2012 Oct 26;1261:158-63. Epub 2012 Jun 28.

Ni X, Suhail MM, Yang Q, Cao A, Fung KM, Postier RG, Woolley C, Young DG, Zhang J, Lin HK. Frankincense essential oil prepared from hydrodistillation of Boswellia sacra gum resins induces human pancreatic cancer cell death in cultures and in a xenograft murine model. BMC Complement Alternat Med. 2012 Dec 13;12:253.

Suhail MM, Wu W, Cao A, Mondalek FG, Fung KM, Shih PT, Fang YT, Woolley C, Young DG, Lin HK. Boswellia sacra essential oil induces tumor cell-specific apoptosis and suppresses tumor aggressiveness in cultured human breast cancer cells. BMC Complement Alternat Med. 2011 Dec 15;11:129.

FREEDOM™
(Essential Oil Blend)

This liberating blend was created to help re-establish a positive energy flow through the body to promote a sense of balance. It is part of the Freedom Collection Bundle.

MEDICAL PROPERTIES & USES:
Anti-inflammatory, neuroprotective, antimicrobial, antioxidative, relaxant, emotion supportive, balancing

INGREDIENTS:
Caprylic/capric triglyceride, Balsam Copaiba, Lavender, Sacred Frankincense, Vetiver, Idaho Blue Spruce, Peppermint, Palo Santo, Valerian, Rue

DIRECTIONS:
Aromatic: 6o. Topical: Neat.

CAUTIONS:

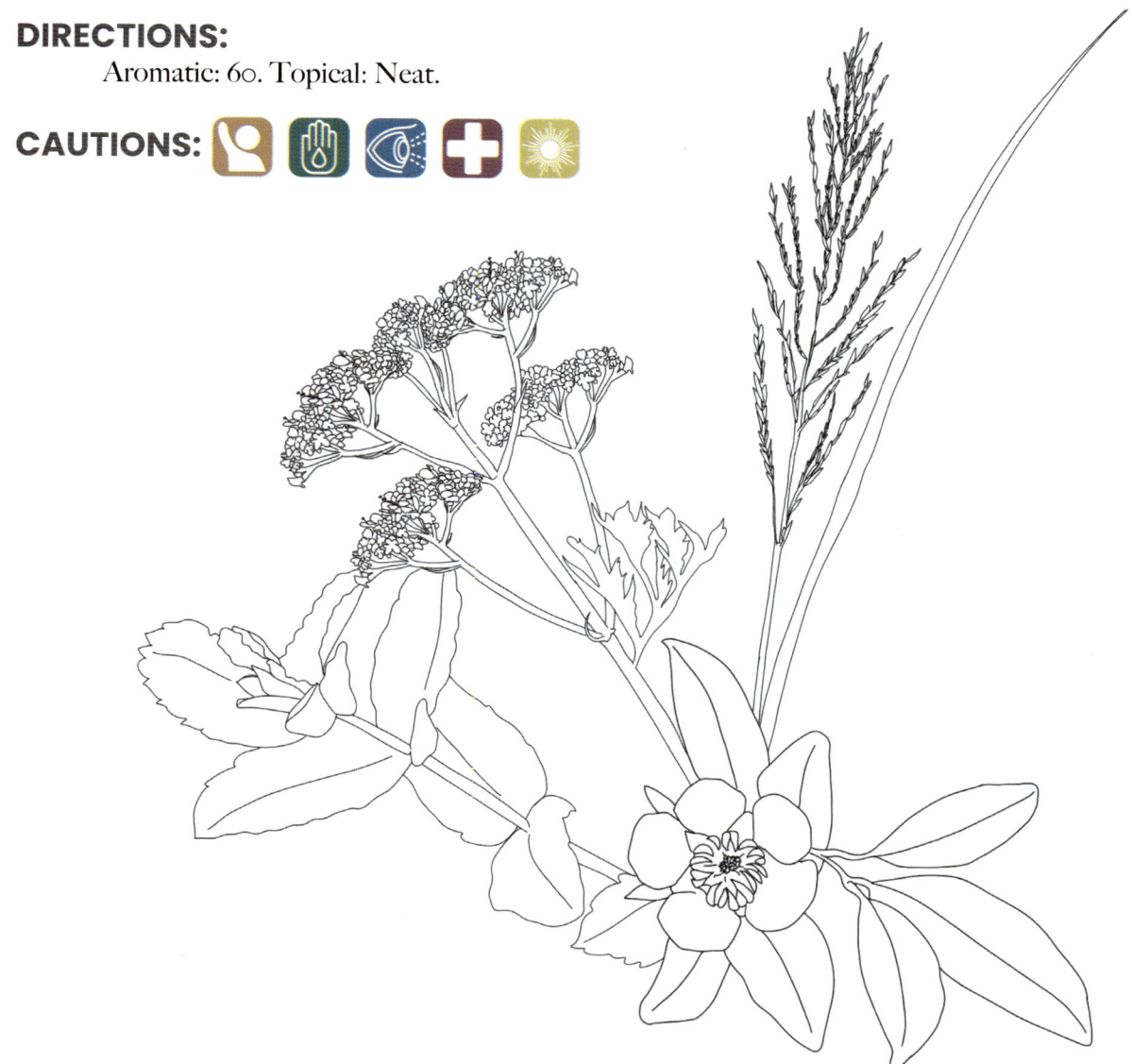

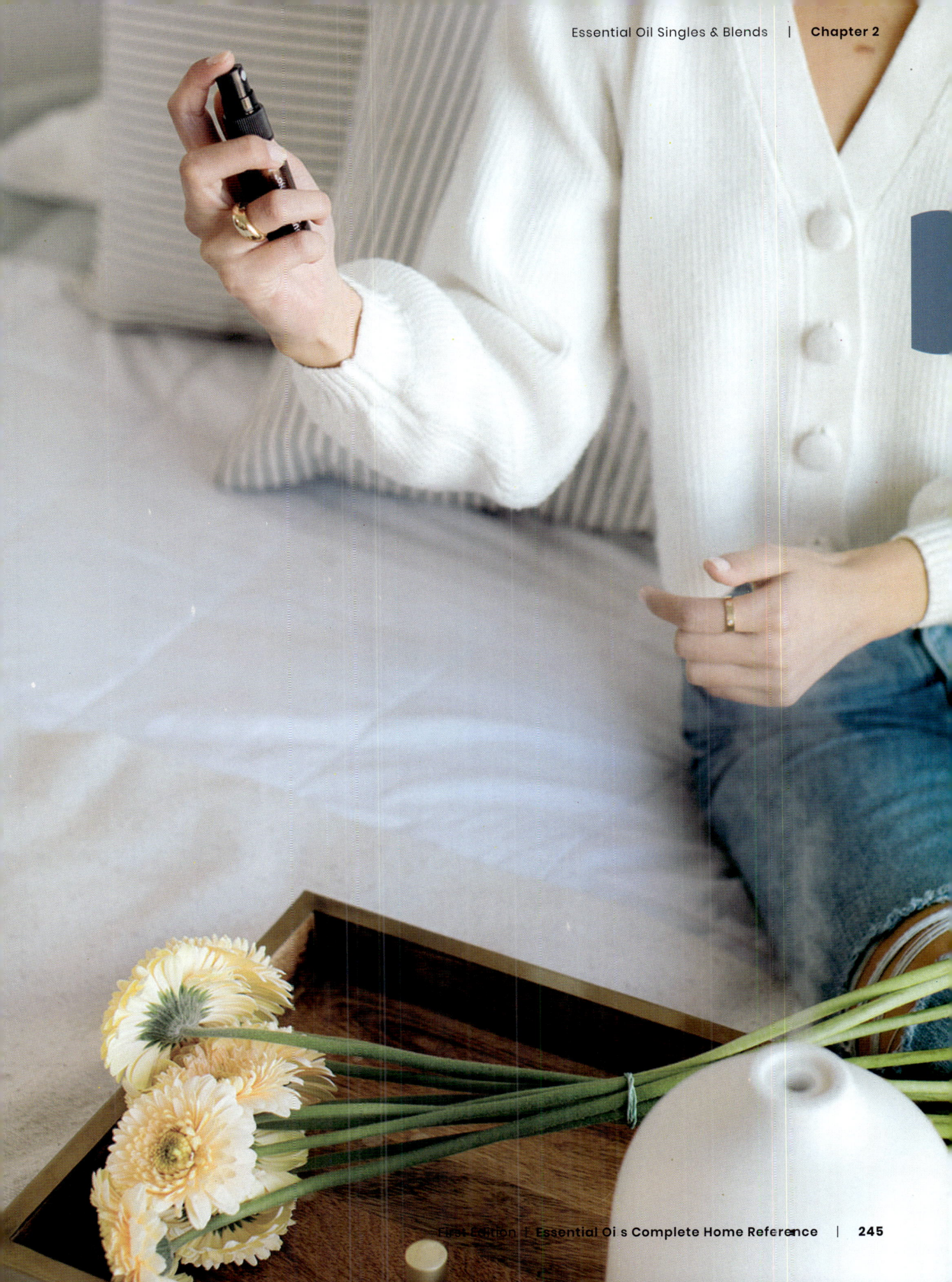

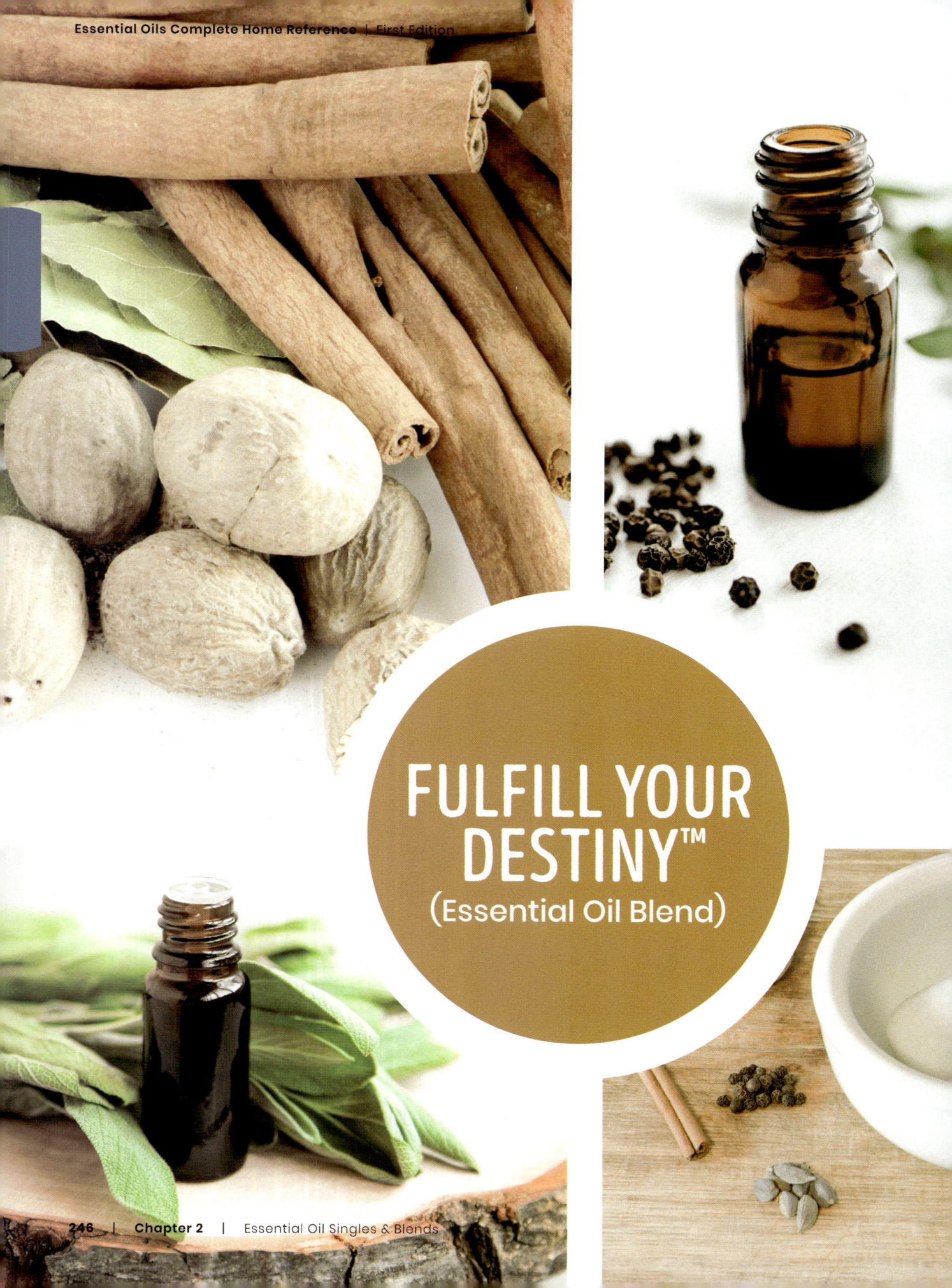

ABOUT FULFILL YOUR DESTINY™:

Do your dreams seem impossible? Is your destiny predetermined? Gary Young's life-story says otherwise! His 2017 Convention blend, Fulfill Your Destiny, supports your power and agency to claim the destiny of your choice. Use this blend created by Gary to choose the course of events that will lead to your true destiny.

MEDICAL PROPERTIES & USES:

Anti-inflammatory, antimicrobial, antioxidative, uplifting, calming, digestion or elimination supportive/nausea reducing, disease inhibitory, performance enhancing/stimulating, wellness supportive

INGREDIENTS:

Tangerine, Frankincense, Nutmeg, Cassia, Cardamom, Clary Sage, Black Pepper, Idaho Blue Spruce, Bitter Orange (Neroli)

DIRECTIONS:

Aromatic: 10. Topical: 20-80.

CAUTIONS:

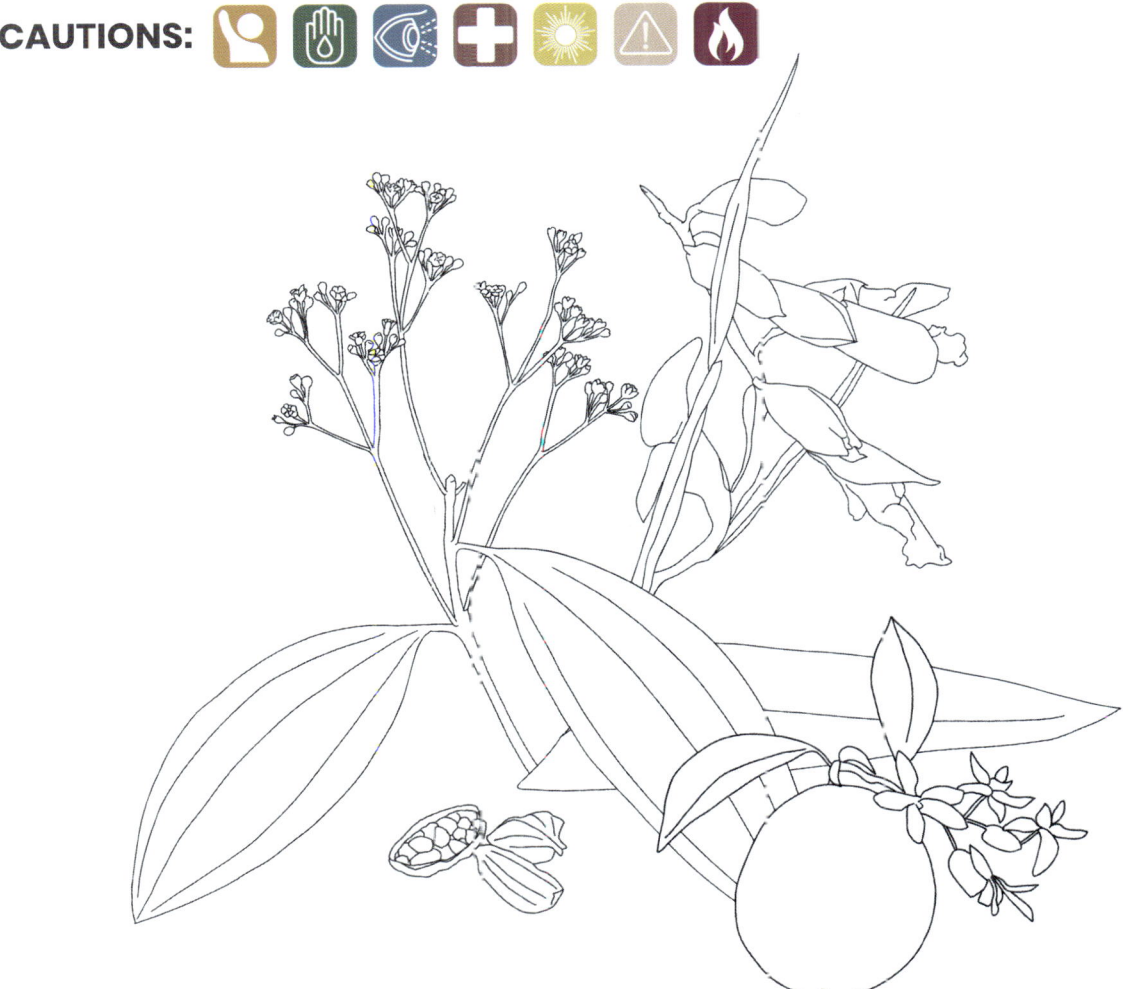

GARY'S LIGHT™
(Essential Oil Blend)

Gary's Light was formulated to enlighten our minds to a greater awareness of truth and discernment—certainly something we need today.

Mary often thinks about new blends based on formulas Gary made at home and because of their close relationship; she often brings new things to light through her understanding of Gary and impressions she has.

Some of the oils in this formula have a rich history of ancient usage, and others are relatively new in their discovery; but the combination of these oils has a fascinating array of different constituents that support different physical and emotional needs.

The aroma is so smooth and elegant and so perfectly balanced that there is no mistake that it's Gary's formula. This blend is very special and gives a calming feeling of strength that makes you feel grounded and protected; and at the same time, your heart will be filled with joy and peace.

MEDICAL PROPERTIES & USES:
Emotional clearing, calming, harmonizing, cleansing, invigorating, restorative, inspires a healthy lifestyle

INGREDIENTS:
Sacred Frankincense, Cistus, Lemongrass, Cinnamon Bark, Myrrh, Dorado Azul, Eucalypts Radiata, Hyssop, Bitter Orange

DIRECTIONS:
Aromatic: 6o. Topical: Neat.

CAUTIONS:

Flammable: Do not use near fire, flame, heat, or sparks. Do not store above room temperature.

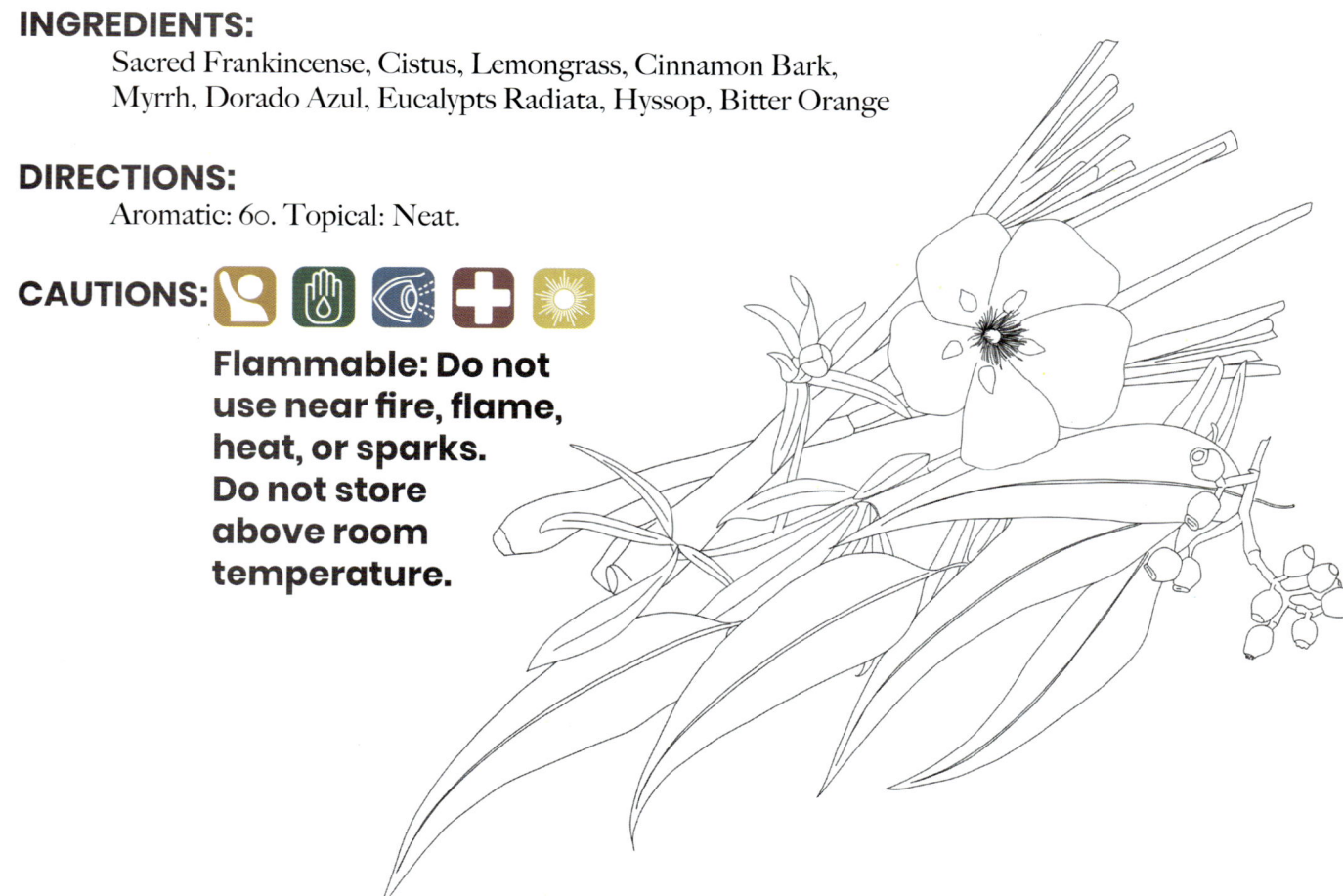

Essential Oil Singles & Blends | **Chapter 2**

Fill your heart with joy and peace

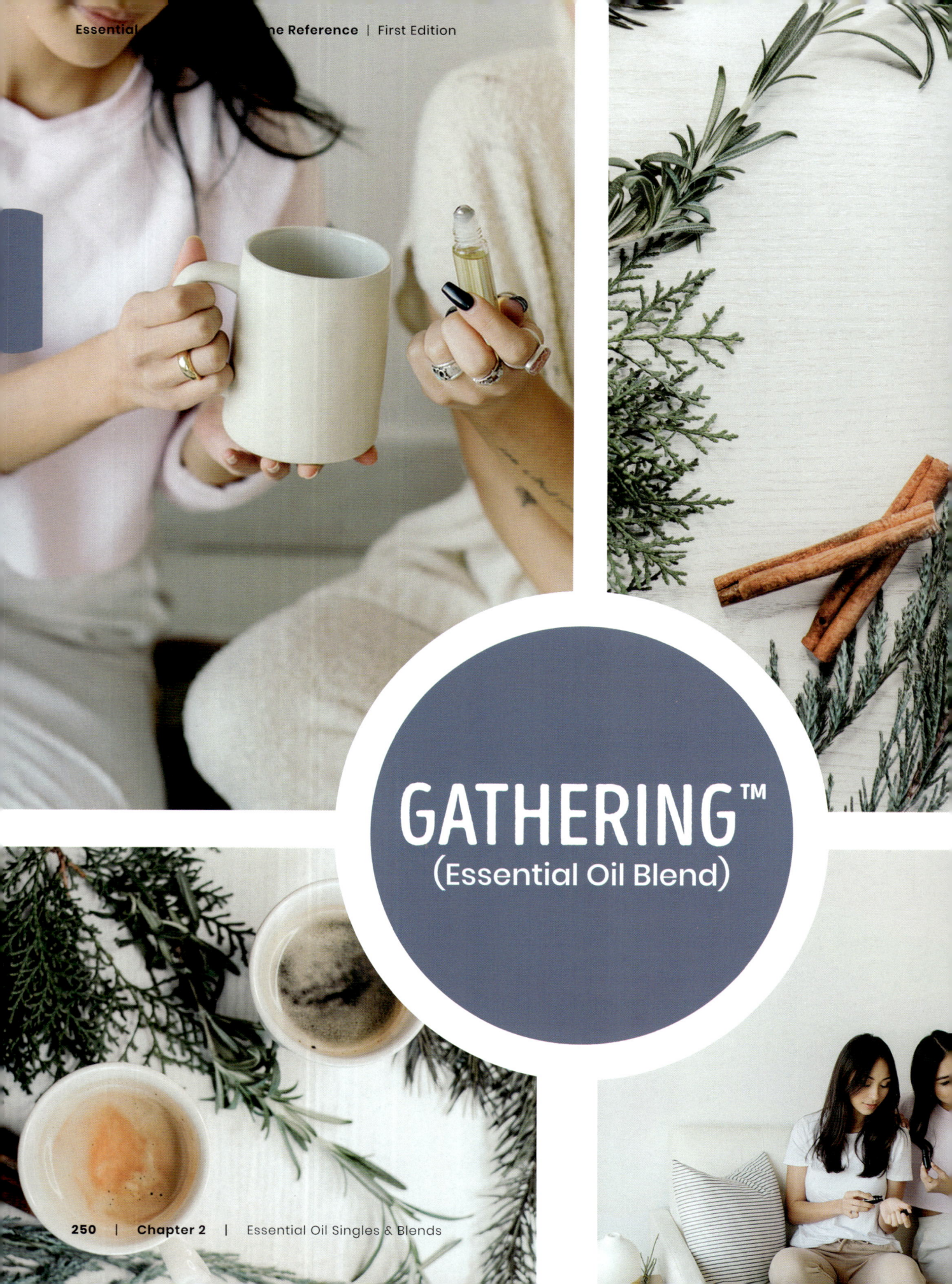

GATHERING™
(Essential Oil Blend)

ABOUT GATHERING™:

This blend is created to help us overcome the bombardment of chaotic energy that alters our focus and puts us on our path toward higher achievements. Northern Lights Black Spruce and Vetiver have a strong effect when blended with Frankincense and Sandalwood in gathering our emotional and spiritual thoughts, helping us to achieve our potential. These oils help increase the oxygen around the pineal and pituitary glands, bringing greater harmonic frequency to receive the communication we desire.

This blend helps bring people together on a physical, emotional, and spiritual level for greater focus and clarity. It helps one stay focused, grounded, and clear in gathering motivation for self-improvement.

MEDICAL PROPERTIES & USES:

Anti-inflammatory, antioxidative, calming, uplifting, emotion supportive, clarity of mind, disease inhibitory, organ protective, pain or swelling reducing, performance enhancing/stimulating

INGREDIENTS:

Lavender, Northern Lights Black Spruce, Geranium, Frankincense, Royal Hawaiian Sandalwood, Ylang Ylang, Vetiver, Cinnamon Bark, Rose

DIRECTIONS:

Aromatic: 6o. Topical: Neat. Apply 1-2 drops on edge of ears, wrists, neck, temples, or along the spine as in Raindrop Technique. Also use Forgiveness on the navel; The Gift and Sacred Mountain on the crown (to clear negative attitudes); Valor on the crown or feet; 3 Wise Men on the crown; Clarity on the temples; and Dream Catcher on the forehead, ears, throat, eyebrows, base of neck, and under the nose.

CAUTIONS:

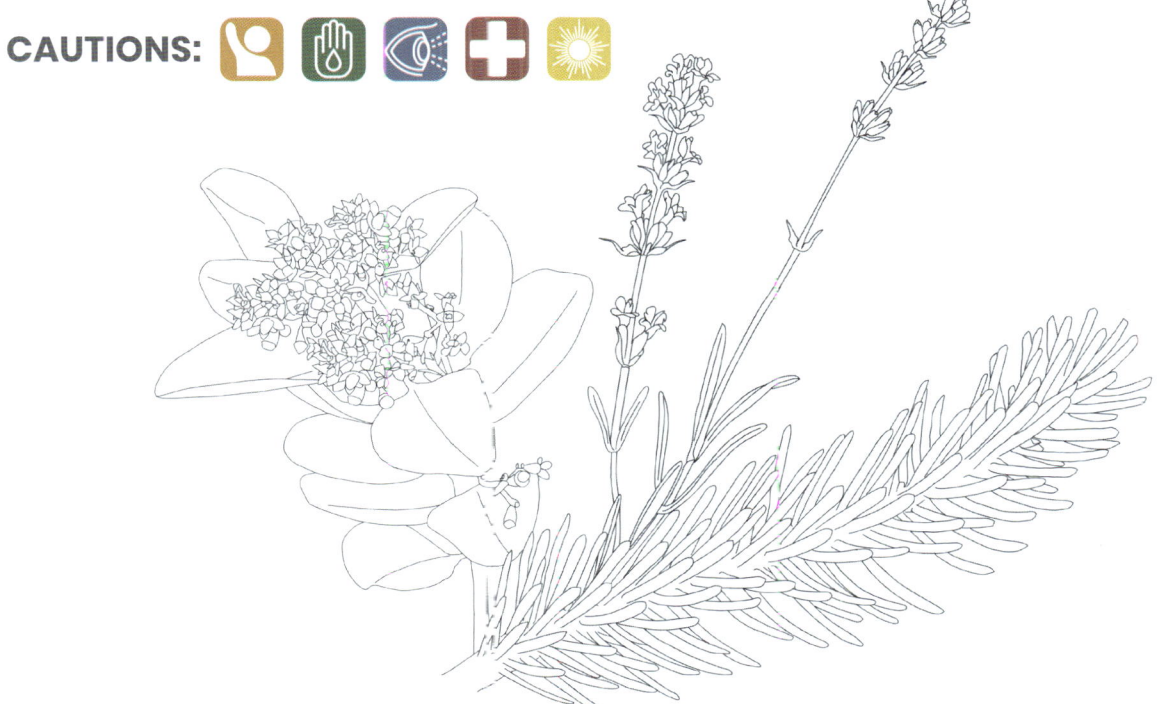

GENTLE BABY™
(Essential Oil Blend)

This blend is comforting, soothing, relaxing, and beneficial for reducing stress during pregnancy. It helps reduce stretch marks and scar tissue, rejuvenates the skin, improves elasticity, and helps to reduce wrinkles.

It is particularly soothing to babies with dry, chapped skin and diaper rash. Skin issues improve when using Gentle Baby with Rose Ointment on top of it. Gentle Baby is calming and brings a feeling of peace for tiny babies, children, and adults.

MEDICAL PROPERTIES & USES:

Anti-inflammatory, antimicrobial, antioxidative, calming, digestion or elimination supportive/nausea reducing, disease inhibitory, pain or swelling reducing, skin improving

INGREDIENTS:

Coriander, Geranium, Palmarosa, Lavender, Ylang Ylang, Roman Chamomile, Bergamot (Furocoumarin-free), Lemon, Jasmine, Rose

DIRECTIONS:

Aromatic: 30. Topical: 50-50. Dilute 1 part essential oil to 1 part V-6 or other pure carrier oil for body massage and for applying on baby's skin. Apply over mother's abdomen, on feet, lower back, face, and neck locations; apply on location for dry, chapped skin or diaper rash. Use as needed. For Pregnancy and Delivery: Use for massage throughout entire pregnancy for relieving stress and anxiety, creating serenity, and preventing scarring. Massage on the perineum to help it stretch for easier birthing.

CAUTIONS:

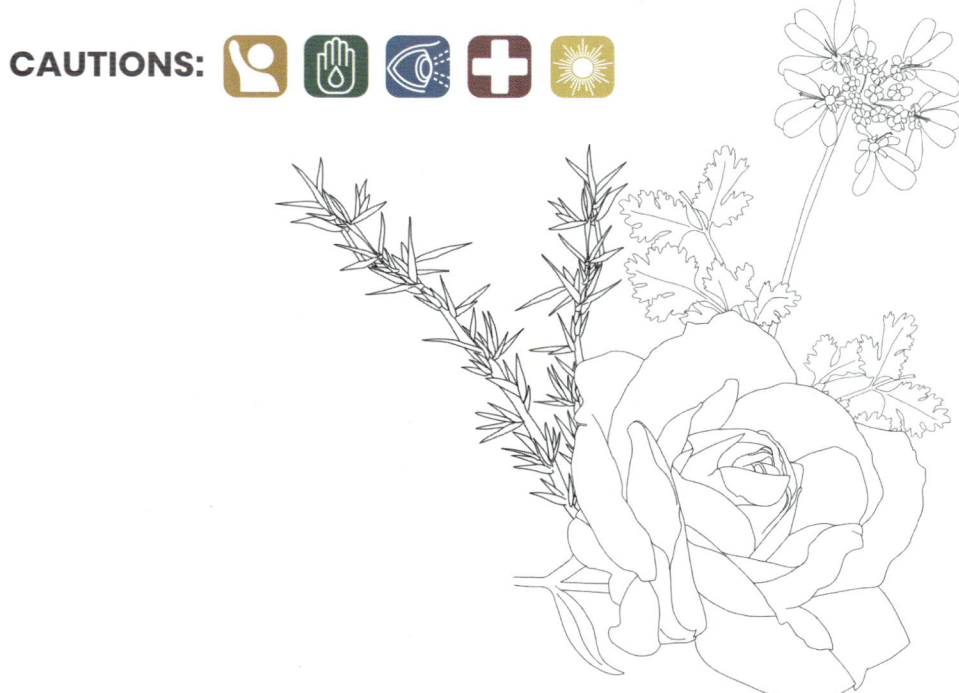

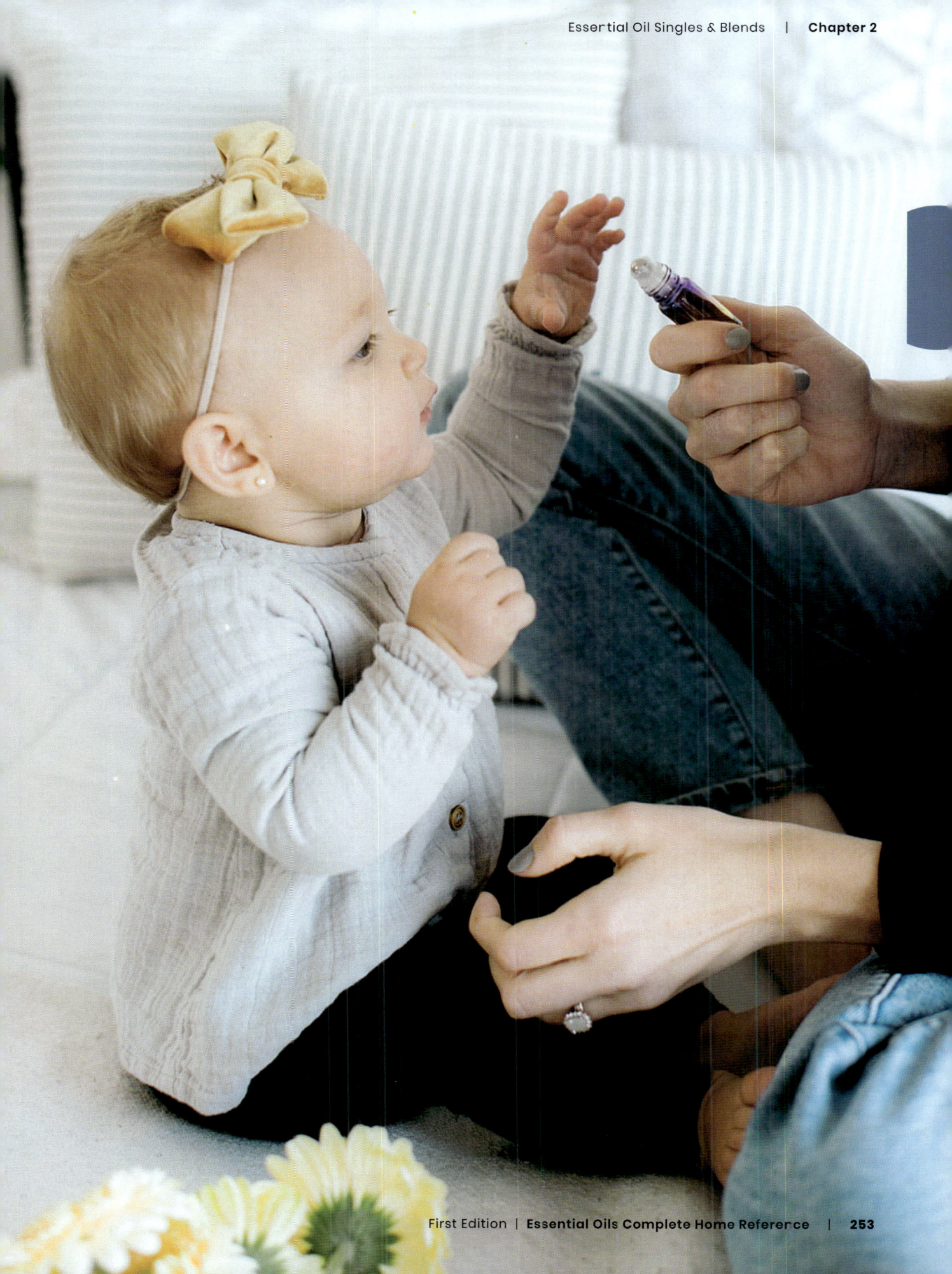

BOTANICAL FAMILY:
Geraniaceae

PLANT ORIGIN:
Egypt

EXTRACTION METHOD:
Steam distilled from the leaves

KEY CONSTITUENTS:
Citronellol (25-36%),
Geraniol (10-18%),
Linalool (4-9%),
Isomenthone (4-8%),
Citronellyl Formate (4-8%),
Geranyl Formate (2-7%),
10-Epi-Gamma-Eudesmol (3-7%)

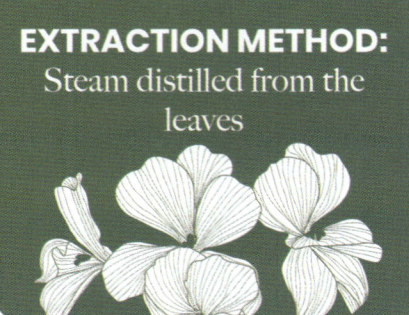

GERANIUM
(Pelargonium graveolens)

Geranium has been used for centuries for regenerating and healing skin conditions.

MEDICAL PROPERTIES:
Anti-inflammatory, antihyperglycemic, antiviral, antimicrobial, antispasmodic, antioxidant, antitumoral, anticancerous, hemostatic (stops bleeding), antibacterial, antifungal, improves blood flow, liver and pancreas stimulant, dilates bile ducts for liver detoxification, helps cleanse oily skin; revitalizes skin cells

USES:
Denture stomatitis, postherpetic neuralgia pain, hepatitis/fatty liver (Jean Valnet, MD), skin conditions (dermatitis, eczema, psoriasis, acne, vitiligo), fungal infections (ringworm), viral infections (herpes, shingles), hormone imbalances, circulatory problems (improves blood flow), menstrual problems/PMS

FRAGRANT INFLUENCE:
Uplifting floral fragrance, helps release negative memories and eases nervous tension; balances the emotions, lifts the spirit, and fosters peace, well-being, and hope

DIRECTIONS:
Aromatic: 6o. Topical: Neat. Dietary: Dilute 1 drop of Geranium in 4 drops V-6 or other pure carrier oil. Put in a capsule and take 1 capsule before each meal or as desired.

CAUTIONS:

SELECTED RESEARCH:

Lohani A, Mishra AK, Verma A. Cosmeceutical potential of geranium and calendula essential oil: determination of antioxidant activity and in vitro sun protection factor. J Cosmet Dermatol. 2018 Sept 24. [Epub ahead of print]

Lotfipur-Rafsanjani SM, Ravari A, Ghorashi Z, Haji-Maghsoudi S, Akbarinasab J, Bekhradi R. Effects of geranium aromatherapy massage on premenstrual syndrome: a clinical trial. Int J Prev Med. 2018 Nov 5;9:98. eCollection 2018.

Ren P, Ren X, Cheng L, Xu L. Frankincense, pine needle and geranium essential oils suppress tumor progression through the regulation of the AMPK/mTOR pathway in breast cancer. Oncol Rep. 2018 Jan;39(1):129-137. Epub 2017 Nov 1.

Łysakowska ME, Sienkiewicz M, Banaszek K, Sokołowski J. The Sensitivity of Endodontic Enterococcus spp. Strains to Geranium Essential Oil. Molecules. 2015 Dec; 20(12): 22881-22889. Published online 2015 Dec 21.

Rashidi Fakari F, Tabatabaeichehr M, Kamali H, Rashidi Fakari F, Naseri M. Effect of inhalation of aroma of geranium essence on anxiety and physiological parameters during first stage of labor in nulliparous women: a randomized clinical trial. J Caring Sci. 2015 Jun 1;4(2):135-41. eCollection 2015 Jun.

Budzyńska A, Sadowska B, Więckowska-Szakiel M, Różalska B. Enzymatic profile, adhesive and invasive properties of Candida albicans under the influence of selected plant essential oils. Acta Biochim Pol. 2014;61(1):115-21. Epub 2014 Mar 20.

Bigos M, Wasiela M, Kalemba D, Sienkiewicz M. Antimicrobial activity of geranium oil against clinical strains of Staphylococcus aureus. Molecules. 2012 Aug 28;17(9):10276-91. Epub Aug 30.

Malik T, Singh P, Pant S, Chauhan N, Lohani H. Potentiation of antimicrobial activity of ciprofloxacin by Pelargonium graveolens essential oil against selected uropathogens. Phytother Res. 2011 Aug;25(8):1225-8. Epub 2011 May 28.

Geranium is the ultimate pregnancy sleep hack

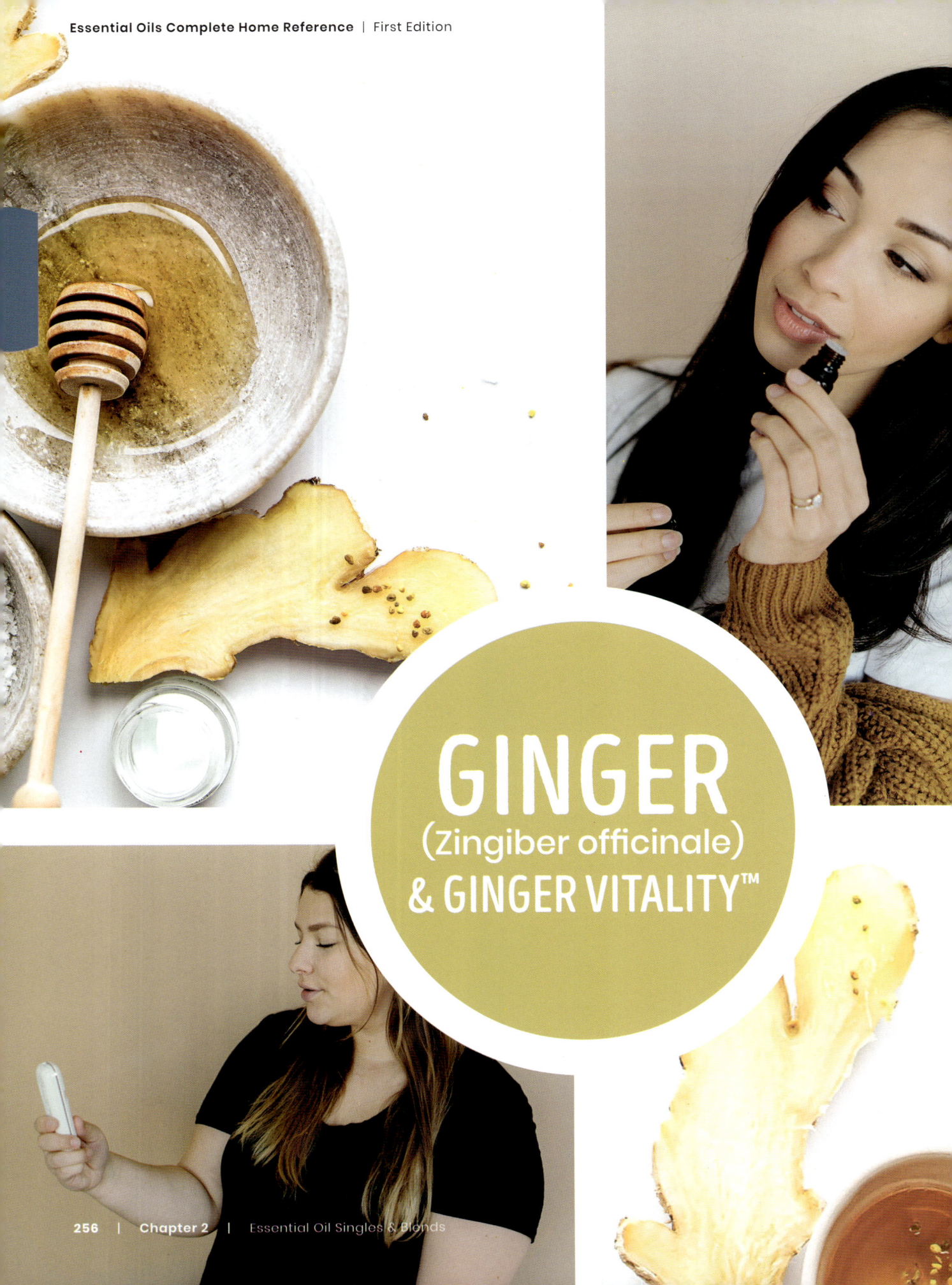

GINGER
(Zingiber officinale)
& GINGER VITALITY™

BOTANICAL FAMILY:
Zingiberaceae

PLANT ORIGIN:
China

EXTRACTION METHOD:
Steam distilled from rhizomes/root

KEY CONSTITUENTS:
Zingiberene (28-39%), Beta-Sesquiphellandrene (8-17%), Curcumene (5-11%), Eucalyptol + Beta Phellandrene (4-11%), T,T-Alpha-Farnesene + Bicyclosesquiphellandrene (2-10%), Camphene (4-9%), Beta Bisabolene (4-9%) (4-9%)

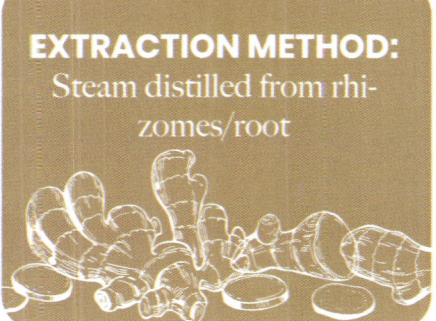

HISTORICAL DATA:
Traditionally used to combat nausea. Women in the West African country of Senegal weave belts of ginger root to restore their mates' sexual potency.

MEDICAL PROPERTIES:
Anti-inflammatory, antitumoral, anticoagulant, anti-aging, digestive aid, anesthetic, expectorant, antifungal

USES:
Rheumatism/arthritis, digestive disorders, decongests the lymphatic system, respiratory infections/congestion, muscular/menstrual aches/pains, nausea

FRAGRANT INFLUENCE:
Gentle, stimulating, endowing physical energy, courage

DIRECTIONS:
Aromatic: 30. Topical: 50-50. Dietary (Vitality): Dilute 1 drop with 1 drop of V-6 or other pure carrier oil. Put in a capsule and take up to 3 times daily.

CAUTIONS: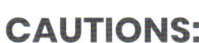
Anticoagulant properties can be enhanced when combined with aspirin, etc.

SELECTED RESEARCH:

Mohd Sahardi NFN, Jaafar F, Nordin MFM, Makpol S. Zingiber Officinale Roscoe Prevents Cellular Senescence of Myoblasts in Culture and Promotes Muscle Regeneration. Evid Based Complement Alternat Med. 2020; 2020: 1787342. Published online 2020 Apr 29.

Mohd Sahardi NFN, Makpol S. Ginger (Zingiber officinale Roscoe) in the Prevention of Ageing and Degenerative Diseases: Review of Current Evidence. Evid Based Complement Alternat Med. 2019; 2019: 5054395. Published online 2019 Aug 20.

Tóth B, Lantos T, Hegyi P, Viola R, Vasas A, Benkő R, Gyöngyi Z, Vincze Á, Csécsei P, Mikó A, Hegyi D, Szentesi A, Matuz M, Csupor D. Ginger (Zingiber officinale): an alternative for the prevention of postoperative nausea and vomiting. A meta-analysis. Phytomedicine. 2018 Nov 15;50:8-18. Epub 2018 Sep 5.

Lai YS, Lee WC, Lin YE, Ho CT, Lu KH, Lin SH, Panyod S, Chu YL, Sheen LY. Ginger essential oil ameliorates hepatic injury and lipid accumulation in high fat diet-induced nonalcoholic fatty liver disease. J Agric Food Chem. 2016 Mar 16;64(10):2062-71. Epub 2016 Mar 3.

Lee YR, Shin HS. Effectiveness of ginger essential oil on postoperative nausea and vomiting in abdominal surgery patients. J Altern Complement Med. 2017 Mar;23(3):196-200. Epub 2016 Nov 14.

Santos PA, Avanço GB, Nerilo SB, Marcelino RI, Janeiro V, Valadares MC, Machinski M. Assessment of cytotoxic activity of rosemary (Rosmarinus officinalis L.), turmeric (Curcuma longa L.), and ginger (Zingiber oficinale R.) essential oils in cervical cancer Cells (HeLa). ScientificWorldJournal. 2016;2016:9273078. Epub 2016 Nov 30.

Bartels EM, Folmer VN, Bliddal H, Altman RD, Juhl C, Tarp S, Zhang W, Christensen R. Efficacy and safety of ginger in osteoarthritis patients: a meta-analysis of randomized placebo-controlled trials. Osteoarthritis Cartilage. 2015 Jan;23(1):13-21. Epub 2014 Oct 11.

Lua PL, Salihah N, Mazlan N. Effects of inhaled ginger aromatherapy on chemotherapy-induced nausea and vomiting and health-related quality of life in women with breast cancer. Complement Ther Med. 2015 Jun;23(3):396-404. Epub 2015 Jun 9.

Khayat S, Kheirkhah M, Behboodi Moghadam Z, Fanaei H, Kasaeian A, Javadimehr M. Effect of treatment with ginger on the severity of premenstrual syndrome symptoms. ISRN Obstet Gynecol. 2014 May 4;2014:792708. Epub Jun 20.

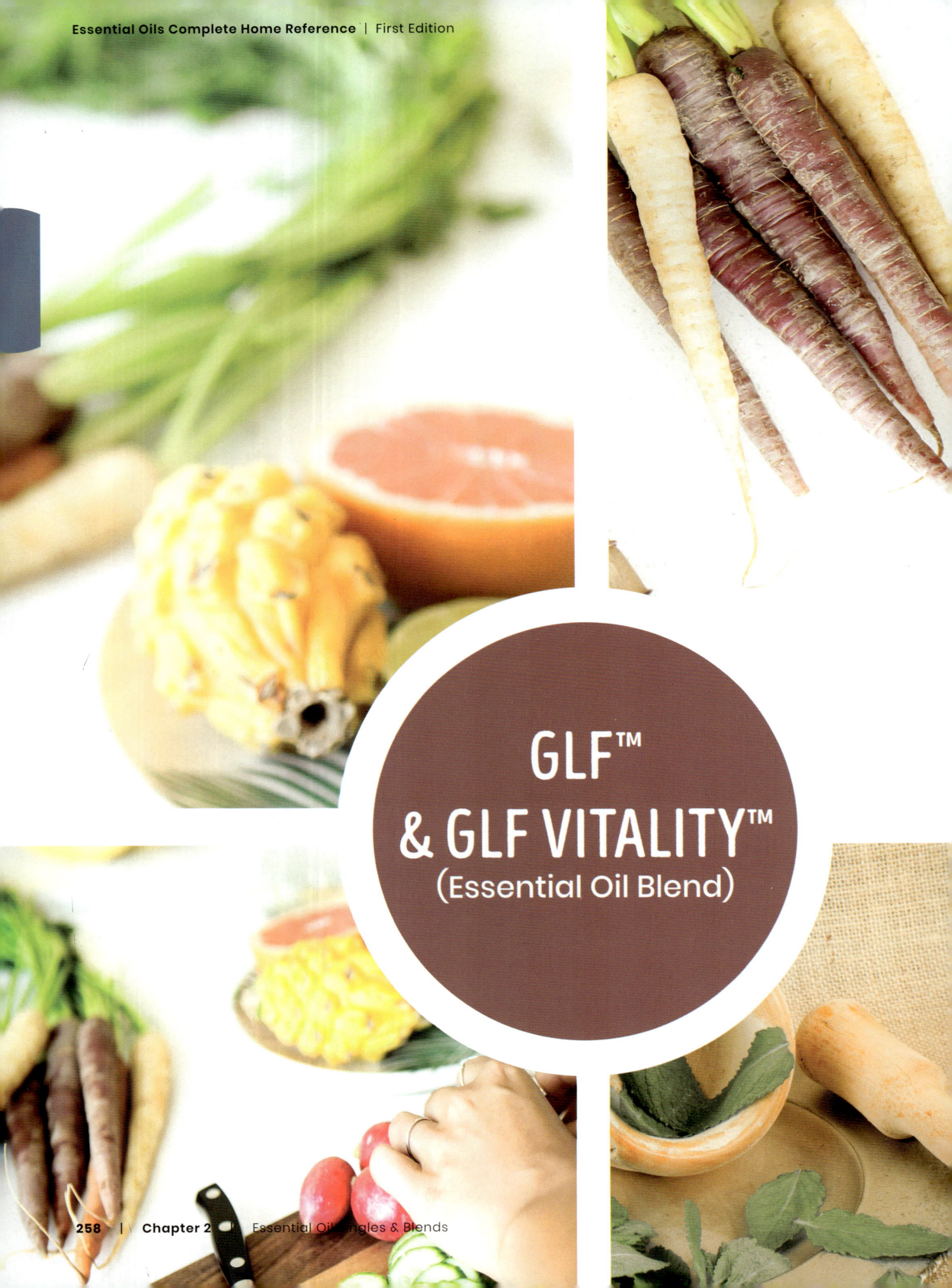

ABOUT GLF™ & GLF VITALITY™:

The initials of this essential oil blend stand for Gallbladder and Liver Flush. It is formulated with oils that help to cleanse and restore liver and gallbladder function when taken in capsules as a dietary supplement.

MEDICAL PROPERTIES & USES:
Anti-inflammatory, antimicrobial, antioxidative, dietary, wellness supportive

INGREDIENTS:
Grapefruit, Ledum, Helichrysum, Celery Seed, Hyssop, Spearmint

DIRECTIONS:
Topical: 50-50. Dietary (Vitality): Dilute 1 drop with 4 drops of V-6 or other pure carrier oil. Put in a capsule and take 1 before each meal or as desired.

CAUTIONS:

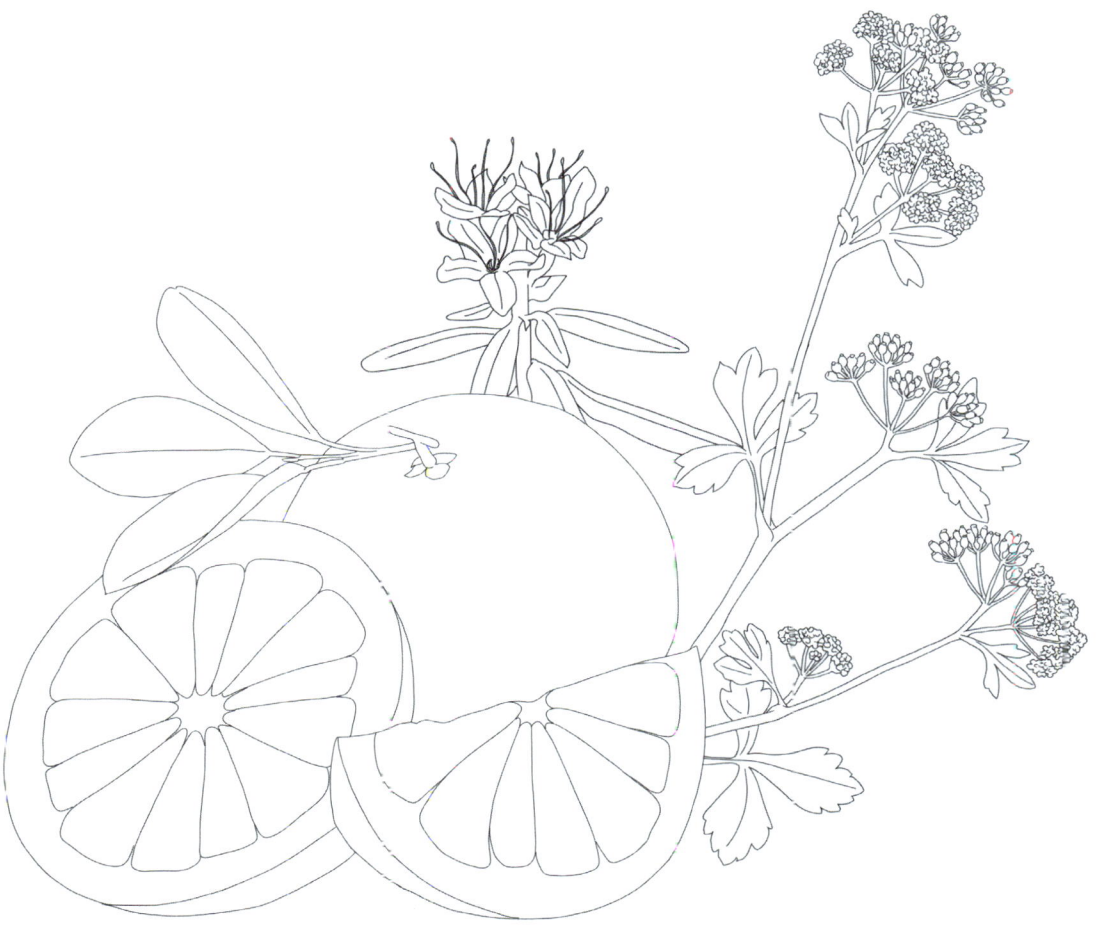

BOTANICAL FAMILY:
Asteraceae

PLANT ORIGIN:
Canada, USA

EXTRACTION METHOD:
Steam distilled from flowering tops

KEY CONSTITUENTS:
Germacrene D (11-38%),
Limonene (9-21%),
Alpha-Pinene (9-21%),
Sabinene (2-21%),
Myrcene (2-13%)

GOLDENROD
(Solidago canadensis)

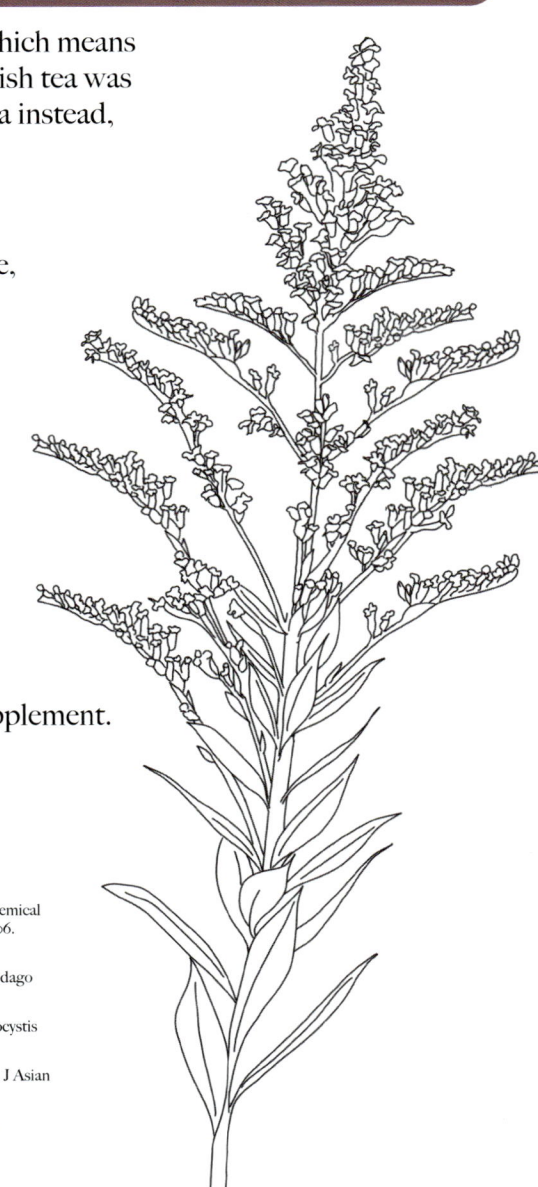

The genus name, Solidago, comes from the Latin solide, which means "to make whole." During the Boston Tea Party, when English tea was dumped into Boston Harbor, colonists drank goldenrod tea instead, which gave it the nickname "Liberty Tea."

MEDICAL PROPERTIES:
Diuretic, anti-inflammatory, antimicrobial, antihypertensive, liver stimulant, antihistamine, antioxidant

USES:
Hypertension, liver congestion, hepatitis/fatty liver, circulatory conditions, urinary tract/bladder conditions, enhances appearance of healthy-looking skin, congestion

FRAGRANT INFLUENCE:
Calming

DIRECTIONS:
Aromatic: 30. Topical: 50-50. Dietary: Take as a dietary supplement.

CAUTIONS:

SELECTED RESEARCH:

Elshafie HS, Grulova D, Baranová B, Caputo L, De Martino L, Sedlák V, Camele I, De Feo V. Antimicrobial Activity and Chemical Composition of Essential Oil Extracted from Solidago canadensis L. Growing Wild in Slovakia. Molecules. 2019 Apr; 24(7): 1206. Published online 2019 Mar 27.

Marksa M, Radušienė J, Jakštas V, Ivanauskas L, Marksienė. Development of an HPLC post-column antioxidant assay for Solidago canadensis radical scavengers. Nat Prod Res. 2016;30(5):536-43. Epub 2015 Apr 2.

Huang Y, Bai Y, Wang Y, Kong H. Allelopathic effects of the extracts from an invasive species Solidago canadensis L. on Microcystis aeruginosa. Lett Appl Microbiol. 2013 Nov;57(5):451-8. Epub 2013 Aug 1.

Huang Y, Hao YL, Mai XY. Chemical constituents from Solidago canadensis with hypolipidemic effects in HFD-fed hamsters. J Asian Nat Prod Res. 2013;15(4):319-24. Epub 2013 Apr 22.

Mishra D, Joshi S, Bisht G, Pilkhwal S. Chemical Composition and Antimicrobial Activity of Solidago canadensis Linn. Root Essential Oil. J Basic Clin Pharm. June 2010-August 2010;1(3): 187-190.

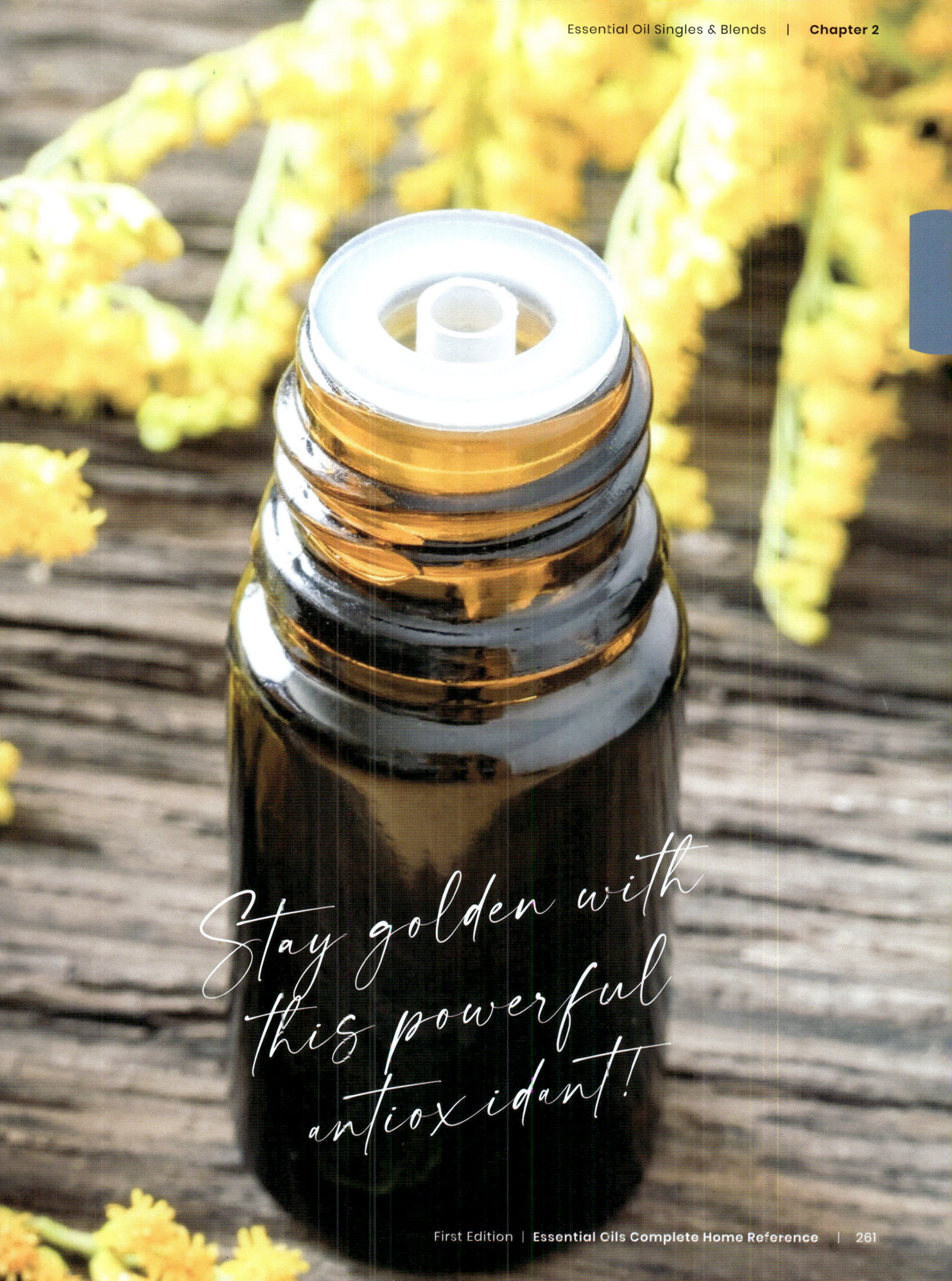

Stay golden with this powerful antioxidant!

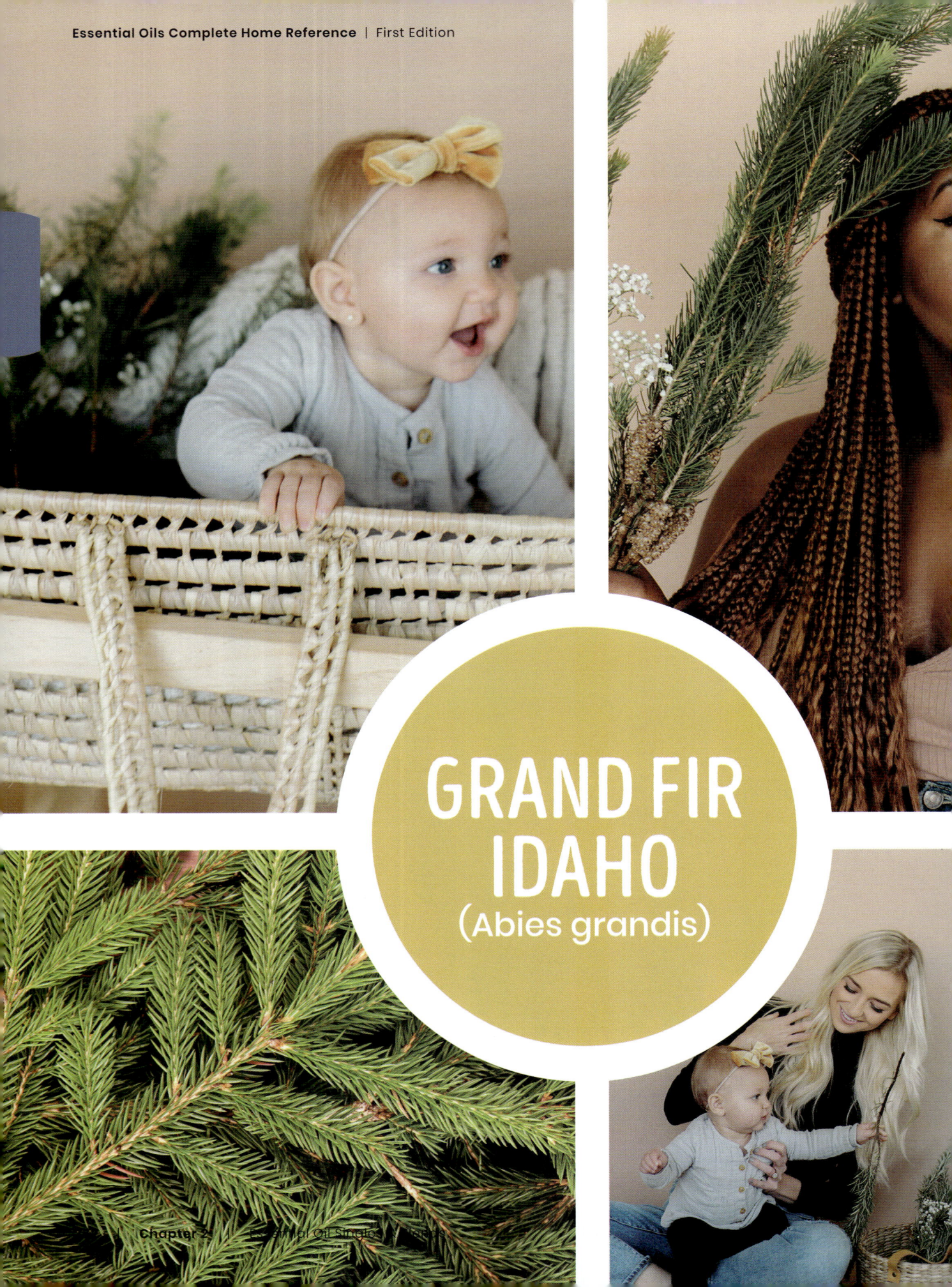

Essential Oil Singles & Blends | Chapter 2

BOTANICAL FAMILY:
Pinaceae

PLANT ORIGIN:
USA, Highland Flats in Naples, Idaho

EXTRACTION METHOD:
Steam distilled from whole tree

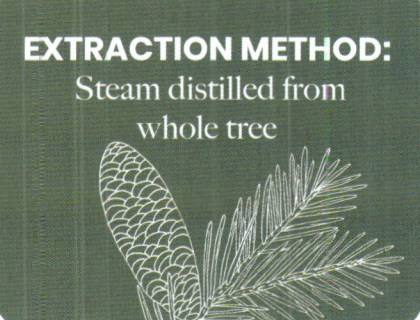

KEY CONSTITUENTS:
Beta-Pinene (18-30%), Bornyl Acetate (10-18%), Beta Phellandrene (8-15%), Camphene (9-15%), Alpha-Pinene (6-11%), Delta-Cadinene (1-8%), Limonene (2-5%), Delta-3-Carene (up to 2%)

HISTORICAL DATA:
Idaho Grand Fir, formerly known as Idaho Balsam Fir, is a favorite essential oil. The oil, aroma, and benefits are unchanged, offering a woodsy, refreshing aroma reminiscent of a freshly cut Christmas tree. It has been prized through the ages for its medicinal effects and ability to heal respiratory conditions and muscular and rheumatic pain. Its Christmas-tree scent also soothes tired muscles, opens airways, and improves meditation. Young Living calls it Idaho Grand Fir because it comes from the Young Living Highland Flats Tree Farm in Naples, Idaho, where every year Young Living members participate in the annual Winter Harvest, allowing them to experience the Young Living Seed to Seal quality commitment firsthand.

MEDICAL PROPERTIES:
Antimicrobial, pulmonary antiseptic and antitussive, anxiolytic, insect repellent, anticoagulant, antibacterial, anti-inflammatory, antitumoral

USES:
Asthma, bronchitis, muscle tension, arthritis/rheumatism, urinary tract infections, throat/lung/sinus infections, fatigue, skin conditions, spirituality, relaxing and stress-relieving

FRAGRANT INFLUENCE:
Woodsy and refreshing aroma; grounding, stimulating to the mind, relaxing to the body

DIRECTIONS:
Aromatic: 6o. Topical: Neat. May use neat in Raindrop Technique. Dietary: Take as a dietary supplement.

CAUTIONS:

SELECTED RESEARCH:
Formighieri C, Melis A. Cyanobacterial production of plant essential oils. Planta. 2018 Oct;248(4):933-946. Epub 2018 Jul 4.

Turner NJ, Hebda RJ. Contemporary use of bark for medicine by two Salishan native elders of southeast Vancouver Island Canada. J Ethnopharmacol. 1990 Apr;29(1):59-72.

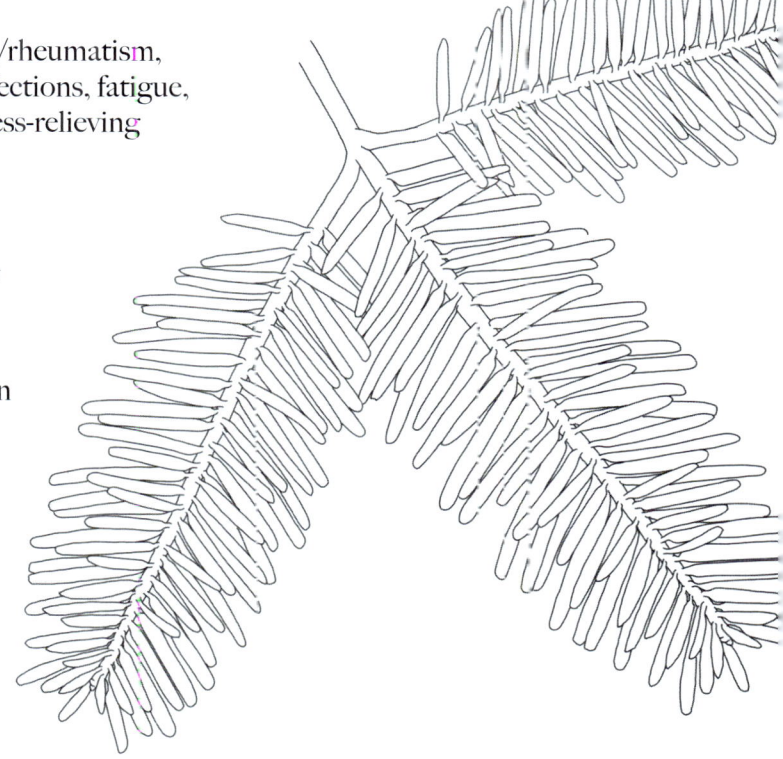

BOTANICAL FAMILY: Rutaceae

PLANT ORIGIN: Belgium, Bulgaria, Netherlands

EXTRACTION METHOD: Mexico, South Africa, USA. (Grapefruit is a hybrid between Citrus maxima and Citrus sinensis.)

KEY CONSTITUENTS: Cold pressed from rind; Key Constituents: Limonene (92-96%), Myrcene (1-3%)

GRAPEFRUIT & GRAPEFRUIT VITALITY™
(Citrus paradisi)

Grapefruit is believed to have originated in Barbados by an accidental crossing of sweet orange (Citrus sinensis) and pomelo (Citrus maxima). When it was discovered, it was called the "forbidden fruit."

MEDICAL PROPERTIES:
Antimicrobial, antioxidant, antitumoral, metabolic stimulant, antiseptic, detoxifying, diuretic, fat-dissolving, cleansing for kidneys, lymphatic and vascular system; antidepressant, rich in limonene, which has been extensively studied in over 50 clinical studies for ability to combat tumor growth.

USES:
Stimulates sympathic nervous system, suppresses weight gain; regulates blood sugar; Alzheimer's, fluid retention, depression, obesity, liver disorders, anxiety, cellulite

FRAGRANT INFLUENCE:
Refreshing and uplifting. A Mie University study found that citrus fragrances boosted immunity, induced relaxation, and reduced depression (Komori, et al., 1995).

DIRECTIONS:
Aromatic: 6o. Topical: 50-50. Dietary (Vitality): Put 2 drops in a capsule and take 3 times daily.

CAUTIONS: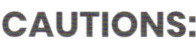

SELECTED RESEARCH:

Deng W, Liu K, Cao S, Sun J, Zhong B, Chun J. Chemical Compositionm, Antimicrobial, Antioxidant, and Antiproliferative Properties of Grapefruit Essential Oil Prepared by Molecular Distillation. Molecules. 2020 Jan; 25(1): 217.

Gupta V, Sharma R, Bansai P, Kaur G. Bioactivity-guided isolation of potent anxiolytic componds from leaves of Citrus paradisi. 2018 Jan-Mar; 39(1): 21-28.

Han C, Tian S, Liu Y, Xiao H, Wu X, Zhang Weiyue, Zhang Wei, Mao M. Beneficial effect of essential oil inhalation on central fatigue. BMC Complement Altern Med. 2018; 18: 309.

Cirmi S, Maugeri A, Ferlazzo N, Gangemi S, Calapai G, Schumacher U, Navarra M. Anticancer potential of Citrus juices and their extracts: a systematic review of both preclinical and clinical studies. Front Pharmacol. 2017 Jun 30;8:420. eCollection 2017.

Onakpoya I, O'Sullivan J, Heneghan C, Thompson M. The effect of grapefruits (Citrus paradisi) on body weight and cardiovascular risk factors: a systematic review and meta-analysis of randomized clinical trials. Crit Rev Food Sci Nutr. 2017 Feb 11;57(3):602-12.

Gamboa-Gómez C, Salgado LM, González-Gallardo A, Ramos-Gómez M, Loarca-Piña G, Reynoso-Camacho R. Consumption of Ocimum sanctum L. and Citrus paradisi infusions modulates lipid metabolism and insulin resistance in obese rats. Food Funct. 2014 May;5(5):927-35.

Adukwu EC, Allen SCH, Phillips CA. The anti-biofilm activity of lemongrass (Cymbopogon flexuosus) and grapefruit (Citrus paradisi) essential oils against five strains of Staphylococcus aureus. J Appl Microbiol. 2012 Nov;113(5):1217-27.

Murase T, Misawa K, Haramizu S, Minegishi Y, Hase T. Nootkatone, a characteristic constituent of grapefruit, stimulates energy metabolism and prevents diet-induced obesity by activating AMPK. Am J Physiol Endocrinol Metab. 2010 Aug;299(2):E266-75. Epub 2010 May 27.

Komori T, Fujiwara R, Tanida M, Nomura J, Yokoyama MM. Effects of citrus fragrance on immune function and depressive states. Neuroimmunomodulation. 1995 May-Jun;2(3):174-80. Epub May 1.

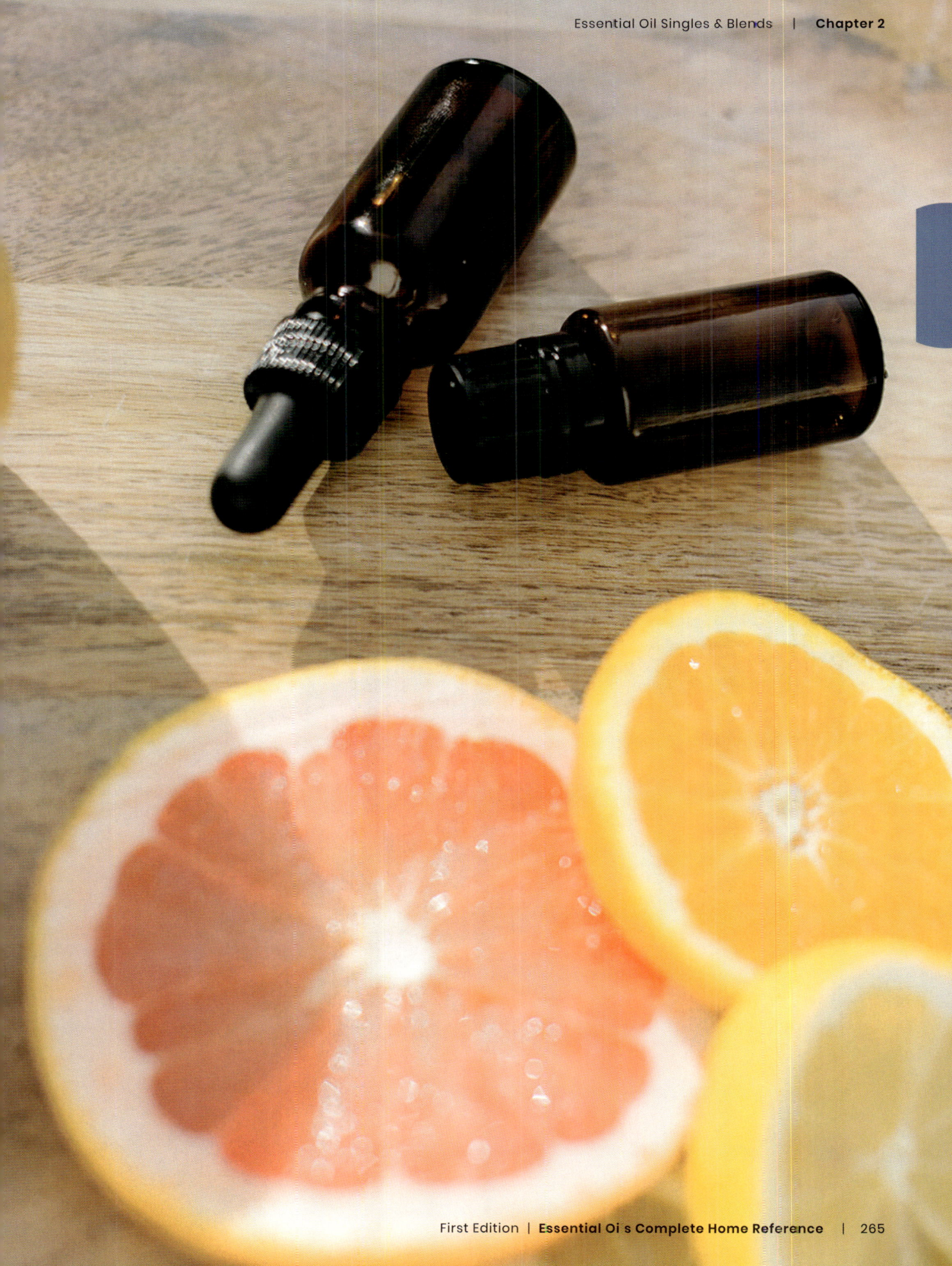

GRATITUDE™ (Essential Oil Blend)

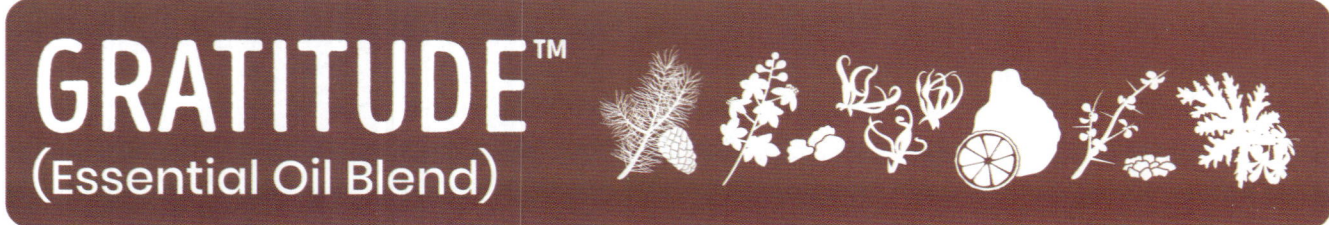

This delightful blend is designed to elevate, soothe, and bring relief to the body while helping to foster a grateful attitude. It is also nourishing and supportive to the skin. The New Testament tells us that on one occasion, Christ healed 10 lepers (Luke 17:12-19), but only one returned to express his thanks. This blend embodies the spirit of that grateful leper.

MEDICAL PROPERTIES & USES:

Anti-inflammatory, antimicrobial, antioxidative, calming, emotion supportive, uplifting, disease inhibitory, organ protective, pain or swelling reducing, performance enhancing/stimulating, skin improving

INGREDIENTS:

Idaho Grand Fir, Frankincense, Coriander, Myrrh, Ylang Ylang, Bergamot (Furocoumarin-free), Northern Lights Black Spruce, Vetiver, Geranium

DIRECTIONS:

Aromatic: 6o. Topical: Neat.

CAUTIONS:

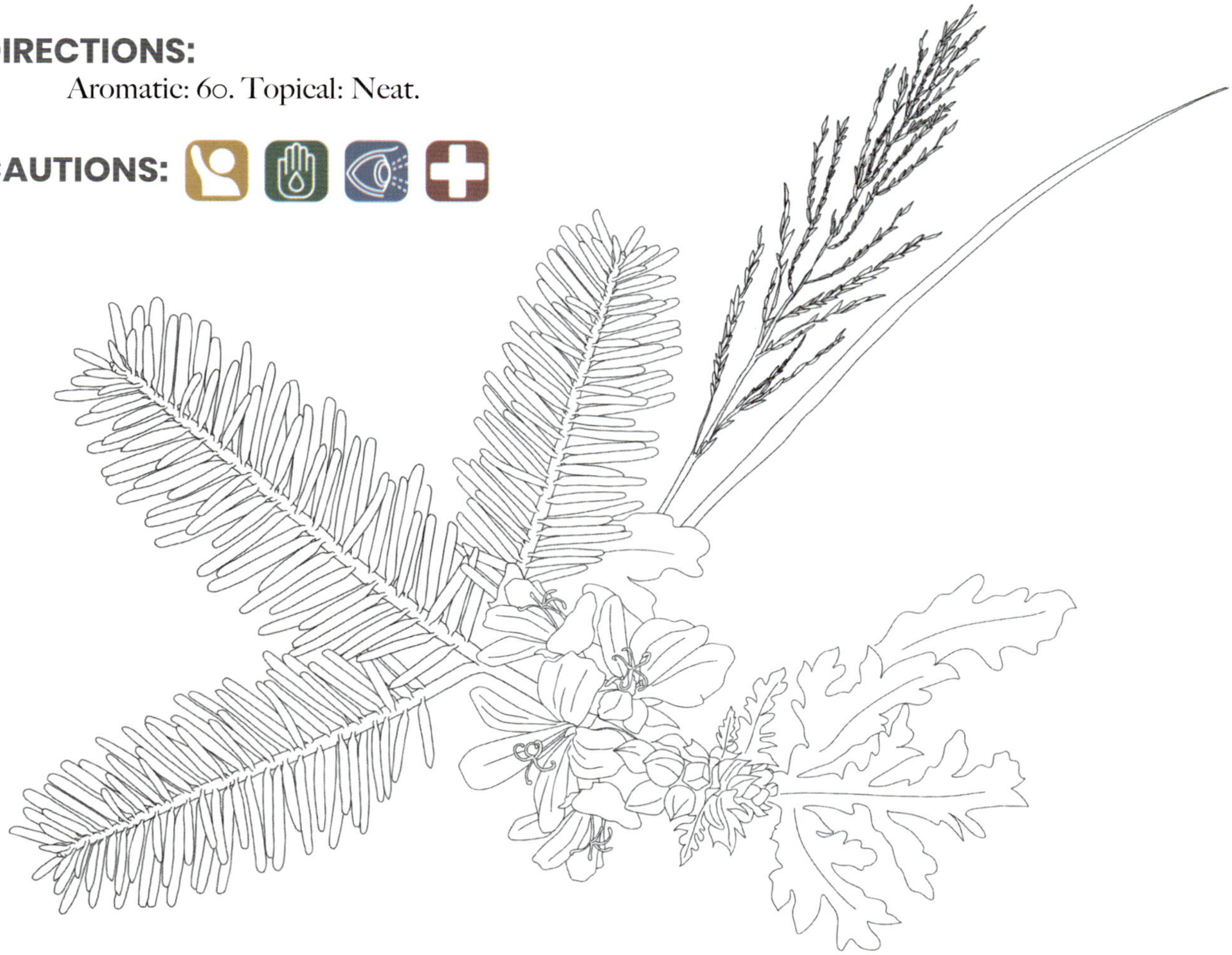

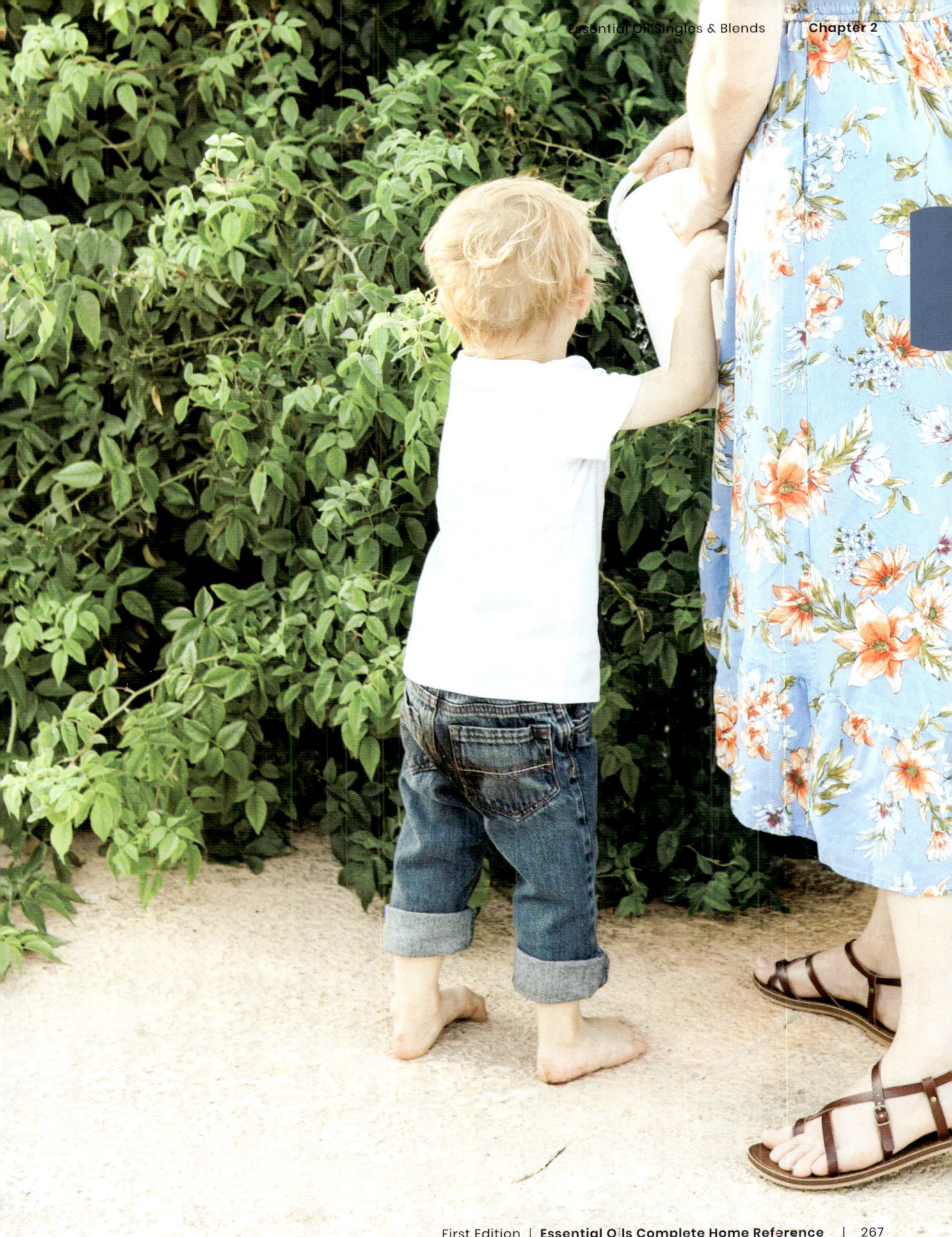

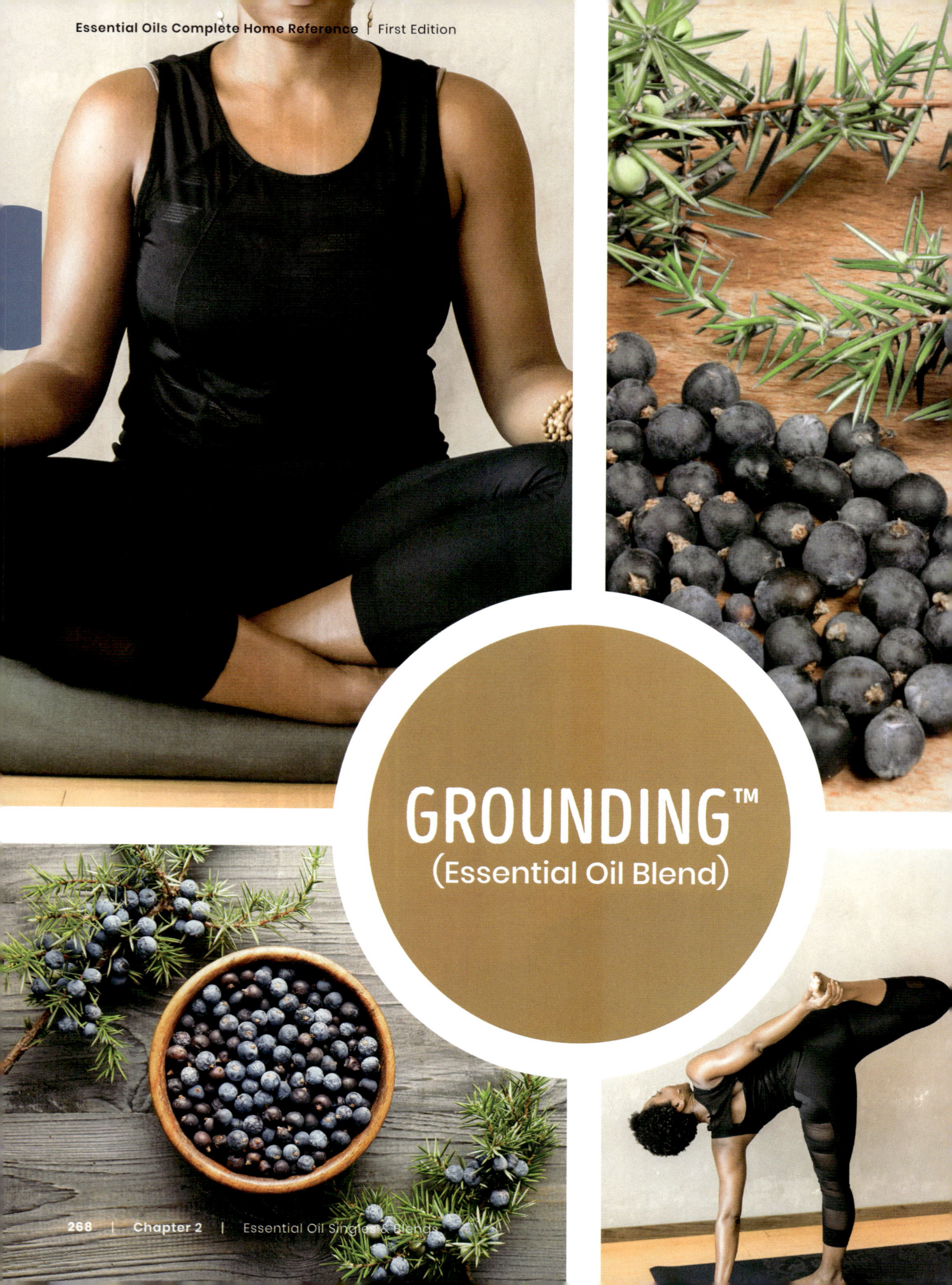

ABOUT GROUNDING™

This blend creates a feeling of solidarity and balance. It stabilizes and grounds us so we can cope constructively with reality. When we're hurting emotionally, we resort to avoidance. When this happens, it is easy to make poor choices that lead to unhealthy relationships and unwise business decisions. We seek to escape because we do not have anchoring or awareness to know how to deal with our emotions.

MEDICAL PROPERTIES & USES:

Anti-inflammatory, antioxidative, grounding, balancing, emotion supporting, calming, disease inhibitory

INGREDIENTS:

White Fir, Black Spruce, Ylang Ylang, Pine, Cedarwood, Angelica, Juniper

DIRECTIONS:

Aromatic: 30. Topical: 50-50.

CAUTIONS:

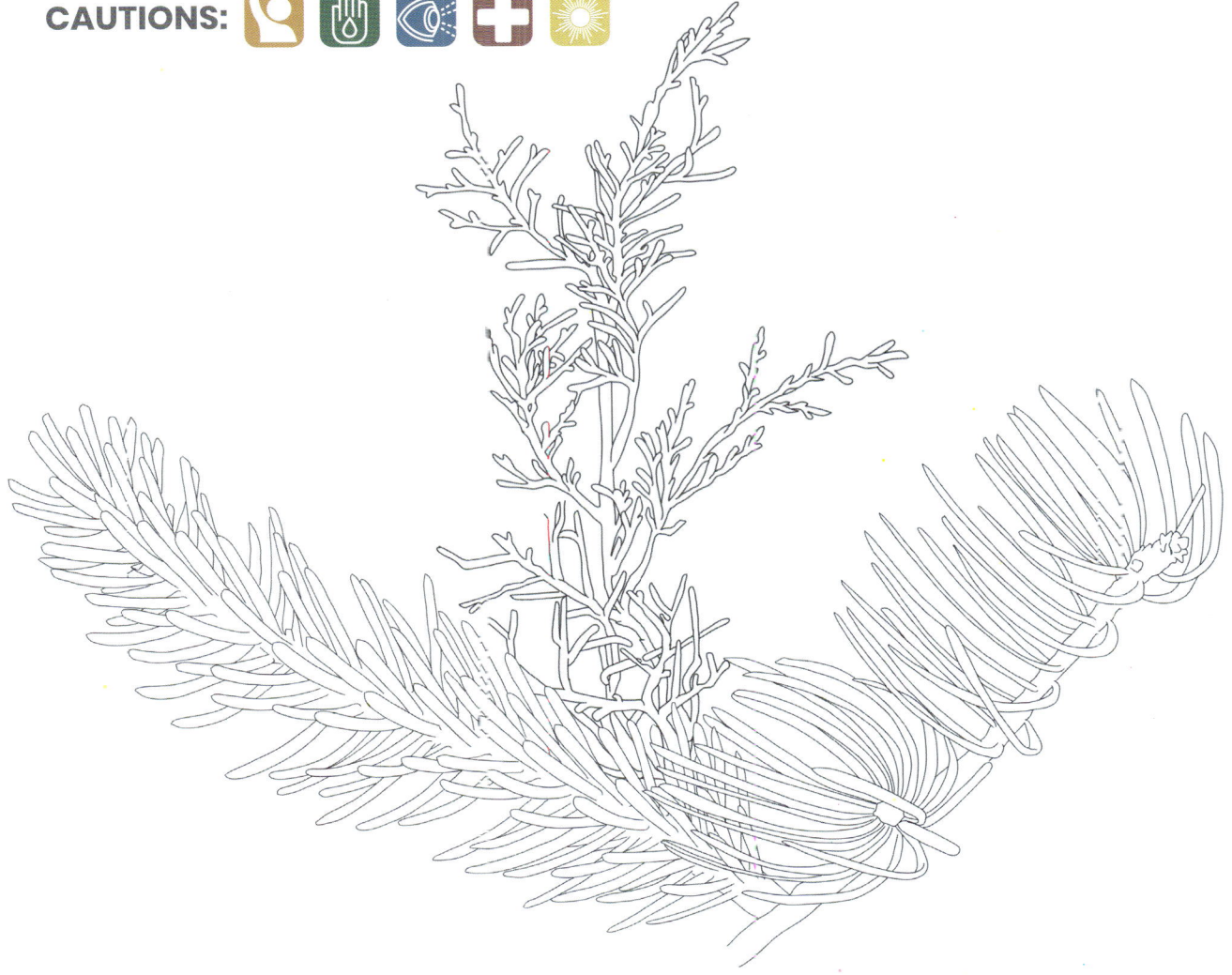

HARMONY™
(Essential Oil Blend)

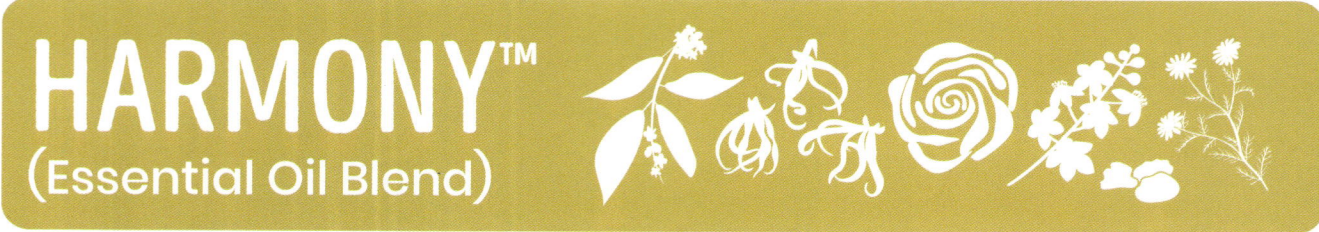

This blend promotes physical and emotional healing by creating a harmonic balance for the energy centers of the body. It brings us into harmony with all things, people, and cycles of life. It is beneficial in reducing stress, amplifying well-being, and dissipating feelings of discord. It is also uplifting and elevating to the mind, creating a positive attitude.

MEDICAL PROPERTIES & USES:
Anti-inflammatory, antimicrobial, antioxidative, uplifting, emotion supporting, calming, cardiovascular supportive, pain or swelling reducing

INGREDIENTS:
Sacred Sandalwood, Lavender, Ylang Ylang, Frankincense, Orange, Angelica, Geranium, Hyssop, Spanish Sage, Black Spruce, Coriander, Bergamot (Furocoumarin-free), Lemon, Jasmine, Roman Chamomile, Palmarosa, Rose

DIRECTIONS:
Aromatic: 6o. Topical: Neat.

CAUTIONS:

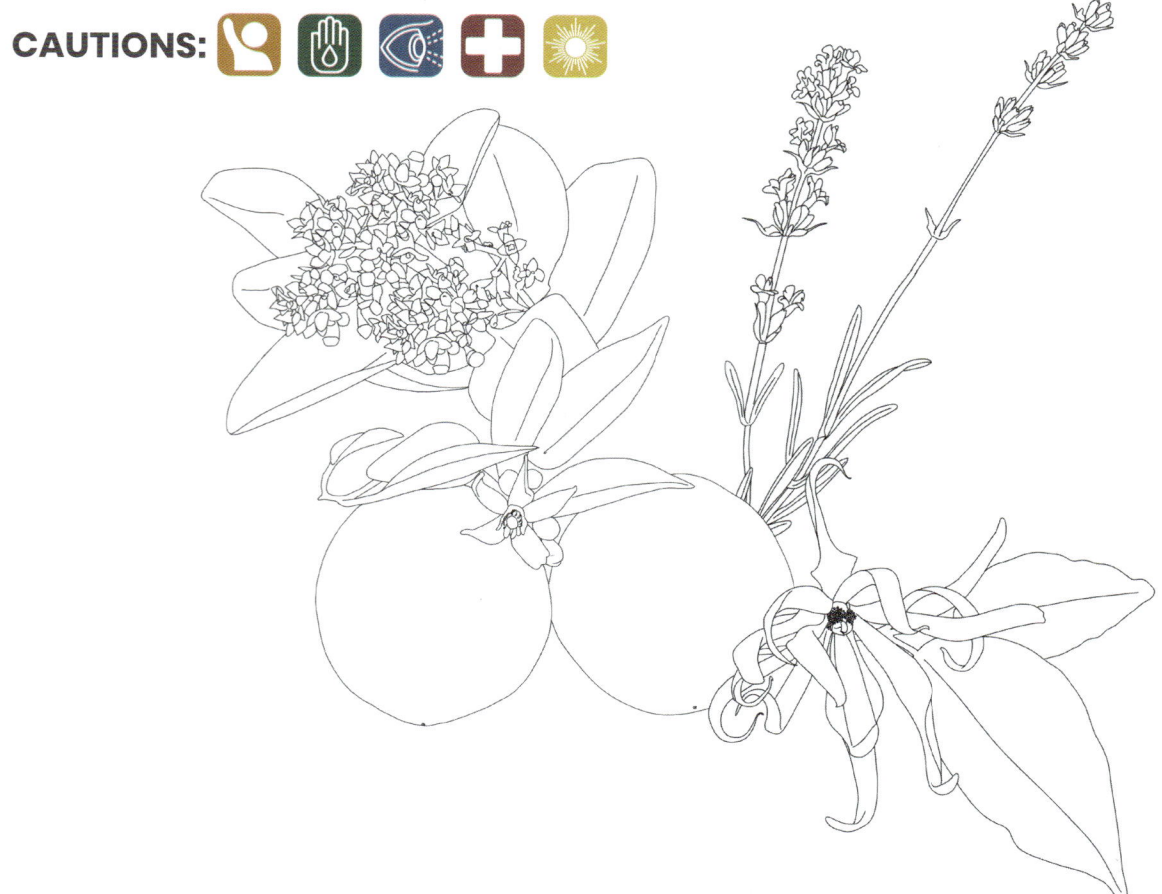

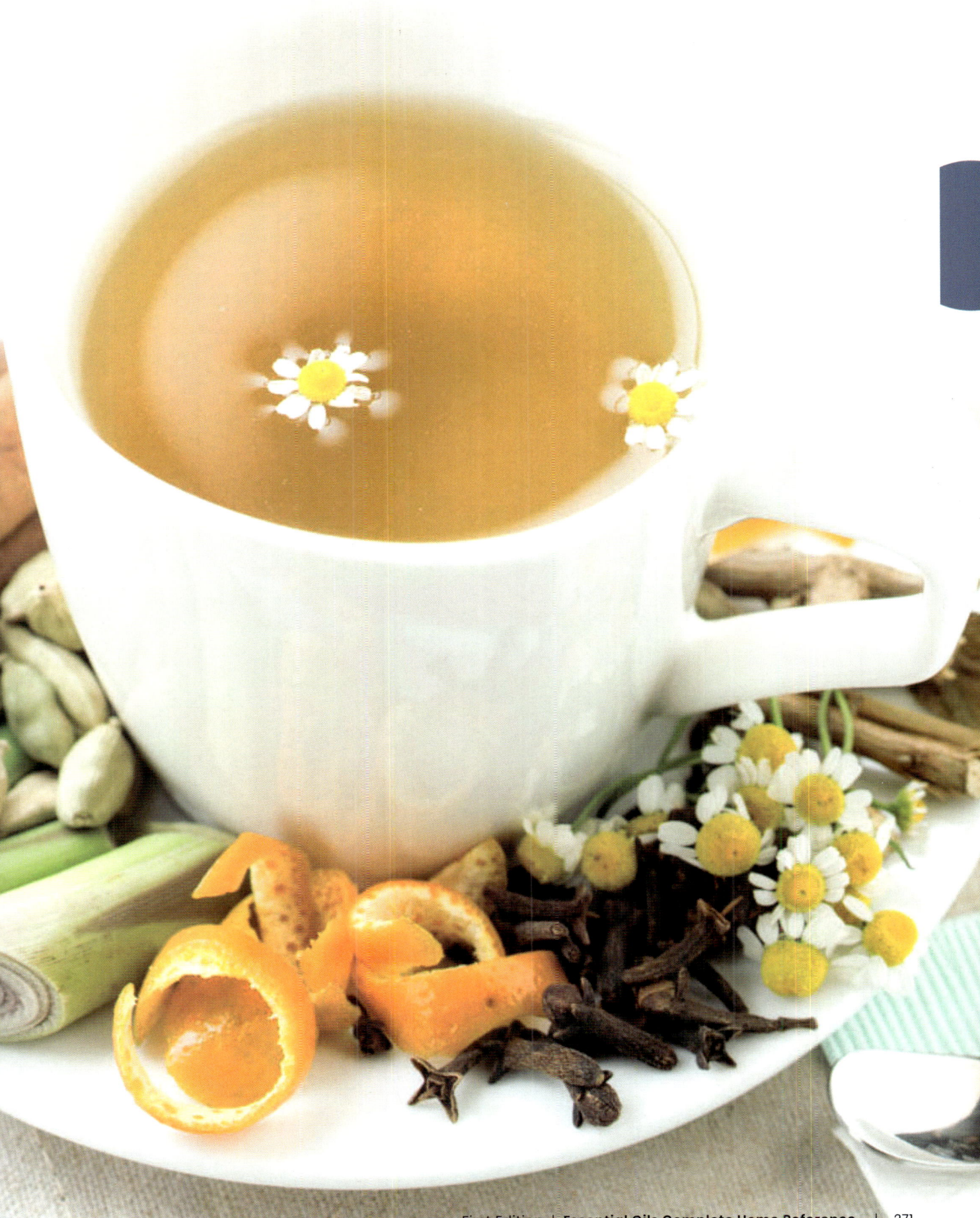

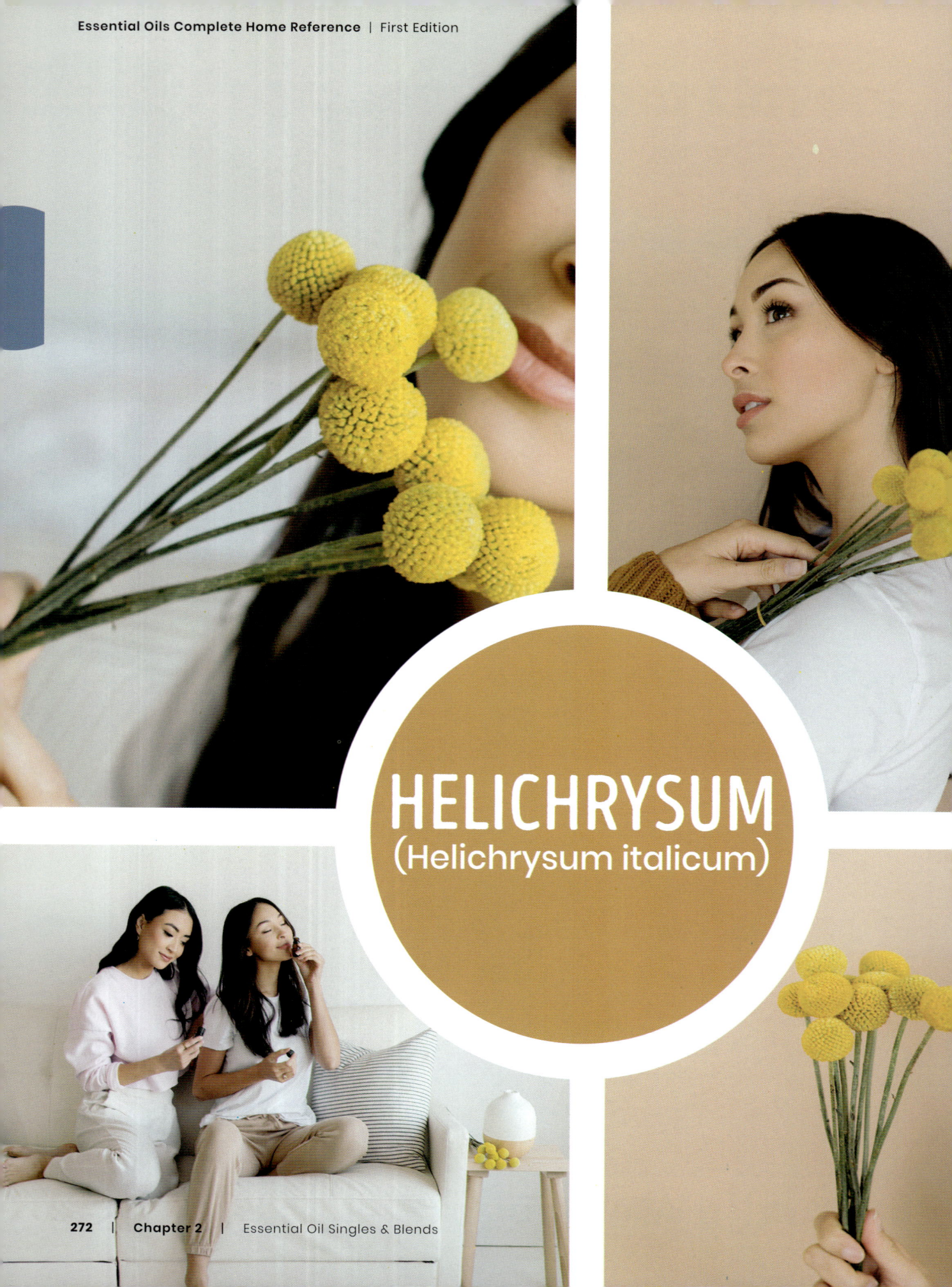

Essential Oil Singles & Blends | Chapter 2

BOTANICAL FAMILY:
Asteraceae

PLANT ORIGIN:
Croatia, France, Spain

EXTRACTION METHOD:
Steam distilled from flowers and flowering tops

KEY CONSTITUENTS:
Neryl Acetate (up to 35%),
Alpha-Pinene (13-30%),
Gamma-Curcumene (7-30%),
Beta-Caryophyllene (up to 11%),
Beta-Selinene (3-10%),
Italicene (2-8%),
Alpha-Curcumene (up to 6%),
Alpha-Selinene (2-6%),
Limonene (up to 5%)

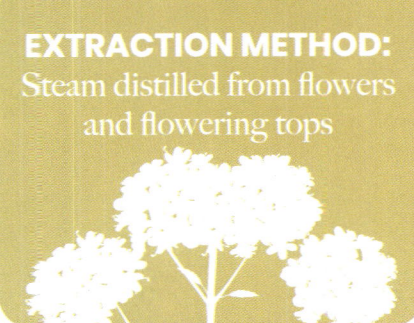

HISTORICAL DATA:
Helichrysum is also known by the names Immortelle and Everlasting. Helichrysum essential oil is renowned for its anti-inflammatory effects.

MEDICAL PROPERTIES:
Antimicrobial, antifungal, antioxidant, anti-inflammatory

USES:
Weight loss, regulates blood sugar, digestive support, herpes virus, arteriosclerosis, atherosclerosis, hypertension, blood clots, liver disorders, circulatory disorders, skin conditions (eczema, psoriasis, scar tissue, varicose veins)

FRAGRANT INFLUENCE:
Herbaceous and sweet aroma; uplifting to the subconscious

DIRECTIONS:
Aromatic: 6o. Topical: Neat. Dietary: Take as a dietary supplement.

CAUTIONS:

SELECTED RESEARCH:
Djihane B, Wafa N, Elkhamssa S, Pedro HJ, Maria AE, Mohamed Mihoub Z. Chemical constituents of Helichrysum italicum (Roth) G. Don essential oil and their antimicrobial activity against gram-positive and gram-negative bacteria, filamentous fungi and Candida albicans. Saudi Pharm J. 2017 Jul;25(5):780-787. Epub 2017 Jul 21.

Antunes Viegas D, Palmeira-de-Oliveira A, Salgueiro L, Martinez-de-Oliveira J, Palmeira-de-Oliveira R. Helichrysum italicum: from traditional use to scientific data. J Ethnopharmacol. 2014 Jan 10;151(1):54-65. Epub 2013 Nov 19.

Rigano D, Formisano C, Senatore F, Piacente S, Pagano E, Capasso R, Borrelli F, Izzo AA. Intestinal antispasmodic effects of Helichrysum italicum (Roth) Don ssp. italicum and chemical identification of the active ingredients. J Ethnopharmacol. 2013 Dec 12;150(3):901-6. Epub 2013 Oct 22.

Taglialatela-Scafati O, Pollastro F, Chianese G, Minassi A, Gibbons S, Arunotayanum W, Mabebie B, Ballero M, Appendino G. Antimicrobial phenolics and unusual glycerides from Helichrysum italicum subsp. microphyllum. J Nat Prod. 2013 Mar 22;76(3):346-53. Epub 2012 Dec 24.

Appendino G, Ottino M, Marquez N, Bianchi F, Giana A, Ballero M, Sterner O, Fiebich BL, Munoz E. Arzanol, an anti-inflammatory and anti-HIV-1 phloroglucinol alpha-Pyrone from Helichrysum italicum ssp. microphyllum. J Nat Prod. 2007 Apr;70(4):608-12. Epub 2007 Feb 24.

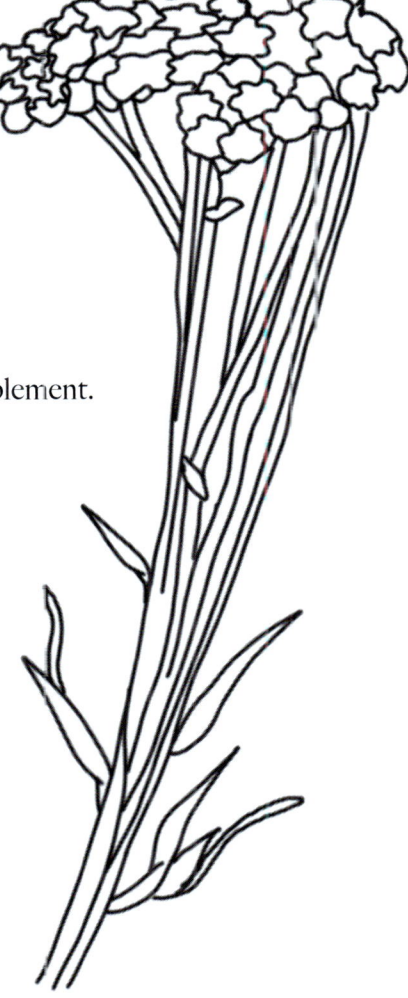

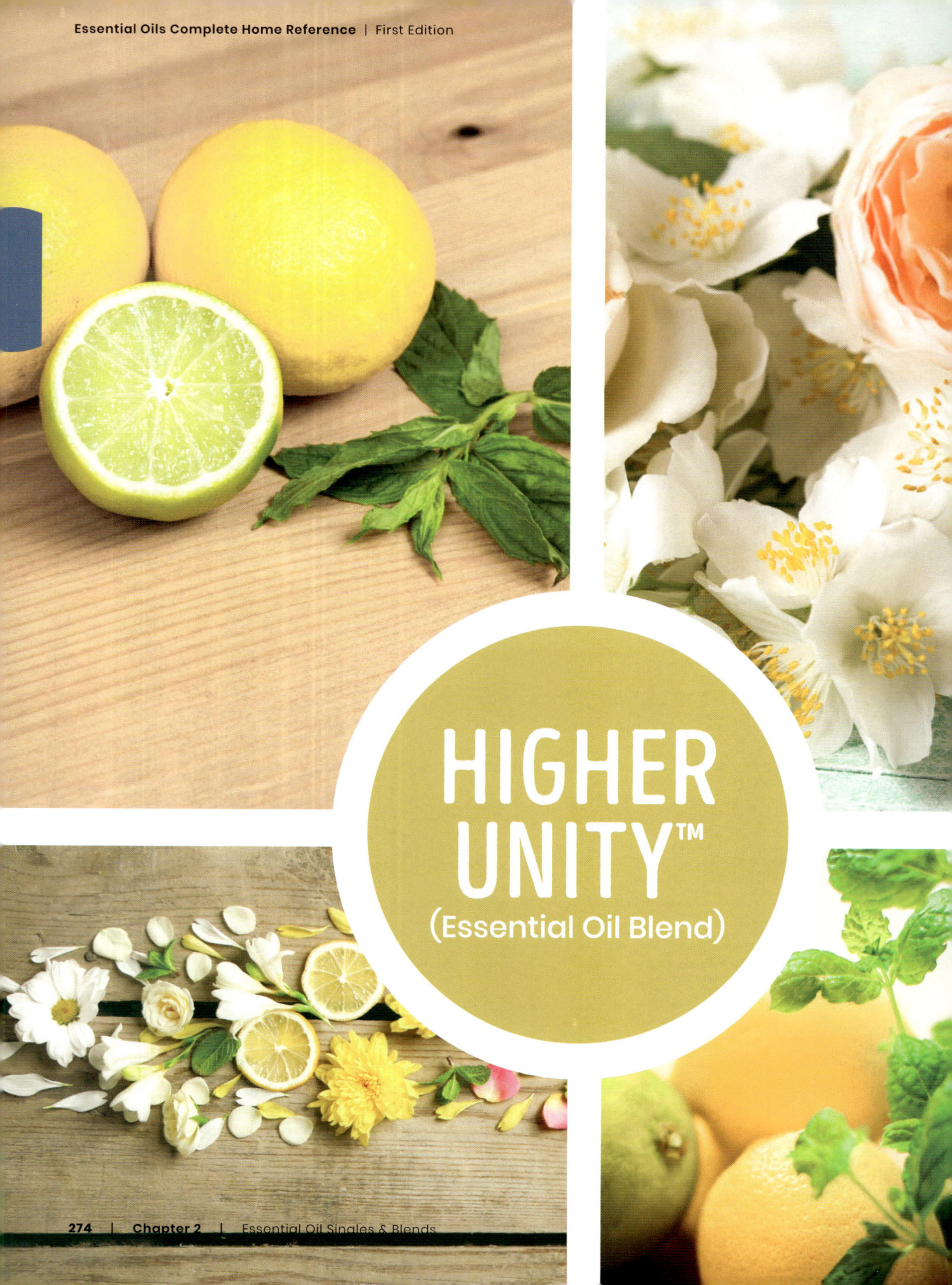

ABOUT HIGHER UNITY™:

This luxurious and rich blend has an aroma that strikes a delicate balance between sweet florals, uplifting citruses, and soothing woods. This makes it an ideal partner for your spiritual practice or meditation or to add a little peace to your daily life.

MEDICAL PROPERTIES & USES:

Anti-inflammatory, antimicrobial, antioxidant, calming, relaxing, cardiovascular supportive, digestion or elimination supportive/nausea reducing, disease inhibitory, pain or swelling reducing

INGREDIENTS:

Sacred Sandalwood, Lime, Sacred Frankincense, Spearmint, Northern Lights Black Spruce, Lemon, Jasmine, Rose

DIRECTIONS:

Aromatic: 30. Topical: 50-50.

CAUTIONS: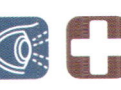

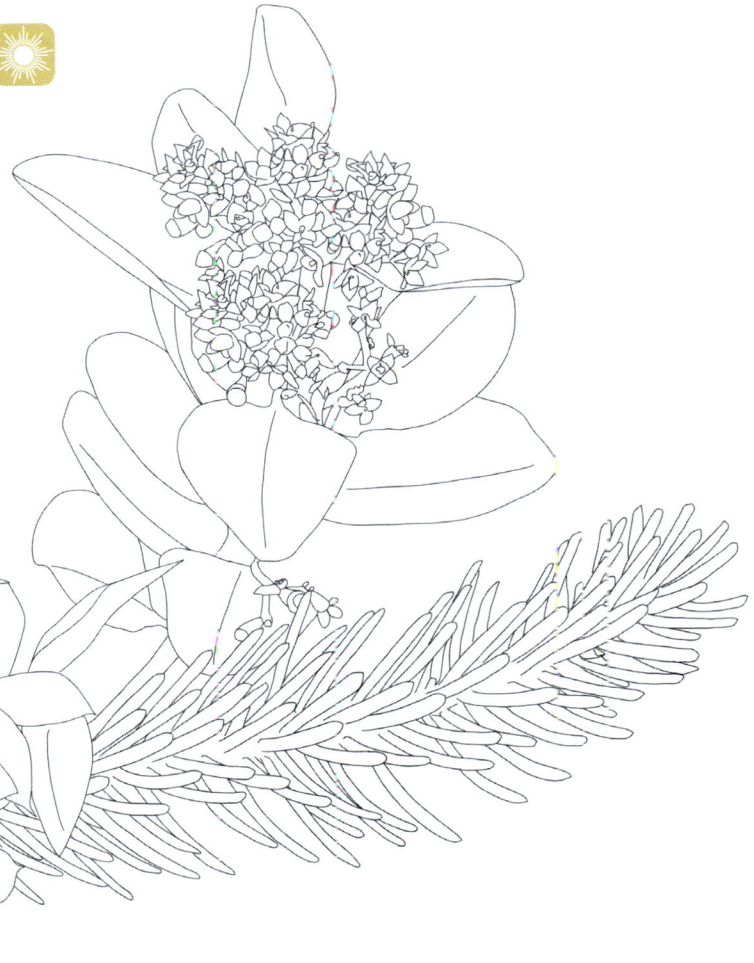

HIGHEST POTENTIAL™
(Essential Oil Blend)

This blend elevates the mind as you gather your thoughts and mental energy to achieve your highest potential. It harmonizes several grounding, calming, inspiring, and empowering essential oils into one intoxicating blend.

Biochemist R. W. Moncrieff wrote that Ylang Ylang "soothes and inhibits anger born of frustration," which removes roadblocks and opens new vistas. The uplifting fragrance of Jasmine spurs creativity, while Lavender clears the thought processes for focused intentions.

MEDICAL PROPERTIES & USES:
Anti-inflammatory, antimicrobial, antioxidative, emotion supporting, calming, cardiovascular supportive, digestion or elimination supportive/nausea reducing, disease inhibitory, performance enhancing, wellness supportive

INGREDIENTS:
Blue Cypress, Ylang Ylang, Jasmine, Cedarwood, Geranium, Lavender, Northern Lights Black Spruce, Frankincense, Royal Hawaiian Sandalwood, White Fir, Vetiver, Cinnamon Bark, Davana, Citrus Hystrix, Rose, German Chamomile, Blue Tansy, Grapefruit, Tangerine, Spearmint, Lemon, Ocotea

DIRECTIONS:
Aromatic: 30. Topical: Neat. In case of sensitivity, dilute 15 drops in 10 ml of V-6.

CAUTIONS:

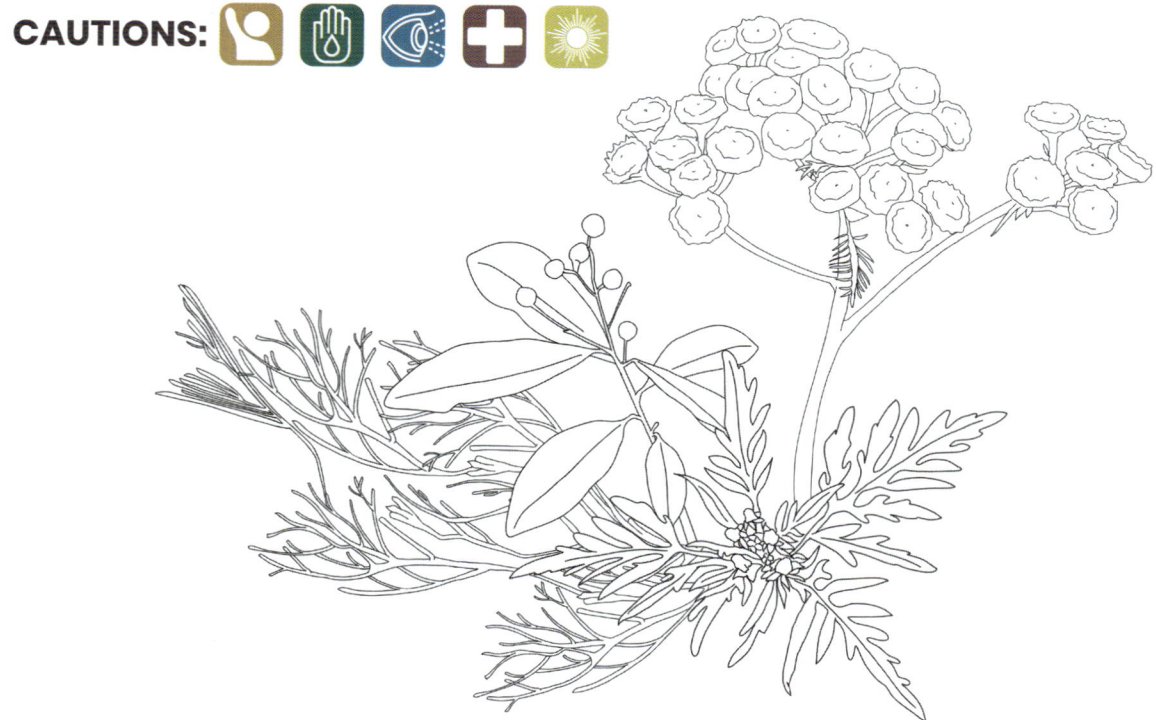

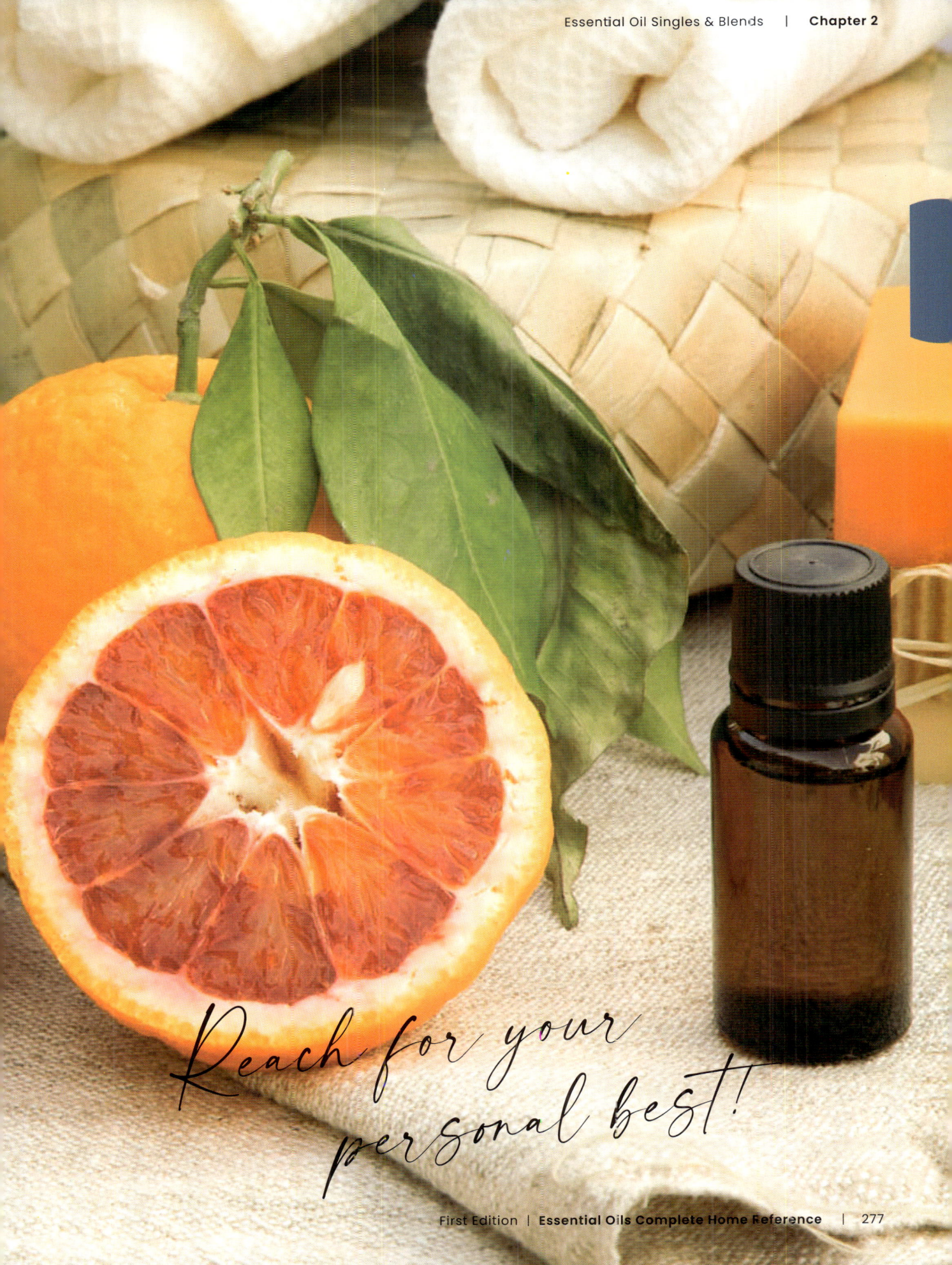

BOTANICAL FAMILY: Cupressaceae

PLANT ORIGIN: Japan

EXTRACTION METHOD: Steam distilled from wood/branches/leaves

KEY CONSTITUENTS: Alpha-Pinene (37-55%), T-Cadinol + Alpha-eadinol (6-13%), T-Muurolol (5-11%), Delta Cadinene (7-11%), Gamma Cadinene (3-6%), Alpha Muurolene (2-4%), Gamma Muurolene (1-3%), Sabinene (1-3%), Alpha Terpinyl Acetate (1-3%)

HINOKI
(Chamaecyparis obtusa)

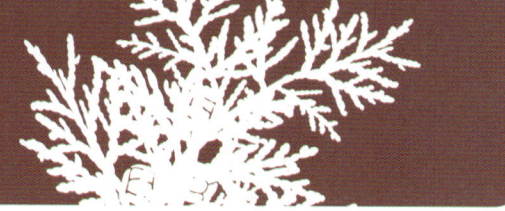

Hinoki wood has been used to construct many holy temples in Japan, including Horyuji Temple and Osaka Castle, and is said to be the "tree where God stayed." Hinoki wood is resistant to decay and carries a symbolic reputation of being immortal.

MEDICAL PROPERTIES:
Antibacterial, antiviral, antidepressant, anti-inflammatory, anti-diabetic, astringent, odor eliminator, promotes hair growth, stimulates digestion, relieves pain, anti-stress, relaxing

USES:
Contains tau-muurolene, a powerful antifungal compound; reduces agitation and hyperactivity

FRAGRANT INFLUENCE:
Calming, centering

DIRECTIONS:
Aromatic: 30. Topical: 50-50.

CAUTIONS:

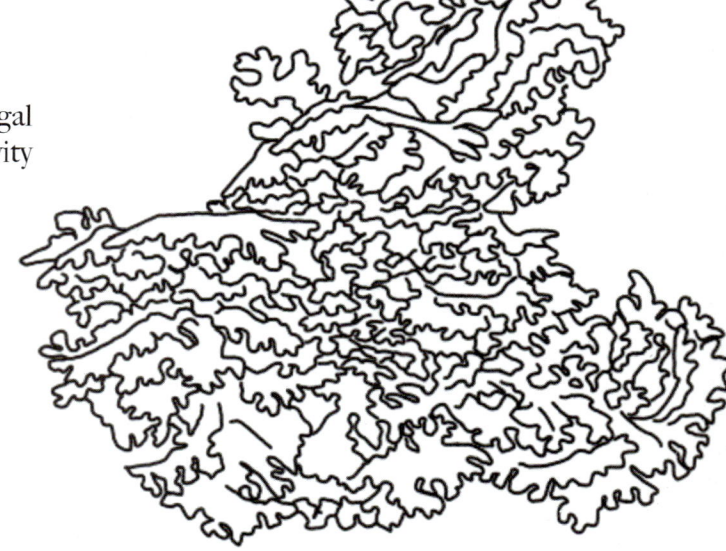

SELECTED RESEARCH:

Hsu C-Y, Lin G-M, Chang S-T. Hypoglycemic activity of extracts of Chamaecyparis obtusa var. Formosa leaf in rats with hyperglycemia induced by high-fat diets and streptozotocin. J Tradit Complement Med. 2020 Jul; 19(4): 389-395.

Kwak BM, Kim E-H, Kim Y-M, Kim H-T. Component analysis of four four-part exraxcts from Chamaecyparis obtusa Endl. by supercritical fluid extraction and anti-inflammatory effect on RAW 264.7 cells. J Exerc Rehabil. 2019 Oct; 15(5): 723-730.

Ahn C, Lee JH, Kim JW, Park MJ, Lee SS, Jeung EB. Alleviation effects of natural volatile organic compounds from Pinus densiflora and Chamaecyparis obtusa on systemic and pulmonary inflammation. Biomed Rep. 2018 Nov;9(5):405-414. Epub 2018 Sep 12.

Ikei H, Song C, Miyazaki Y. Physiological effect of olfactory stimulation by Hinoki cypress (Chamaecyparis obtusa) leaf oil. J. Physiol Anthropol. 2015; 34: 44. Published online 2015 Dec 22.

Kim ES, Kang SY, Kim YH, Lee YE, Choi NY, You YO, Kim KJ. Chamaecyparis obtusa essential oil inhibits methicillin-resistant Staphylococcus aureus biofilm formation and expression of virulence factors. J Med Food. 2015 Jul;18(7):810-7. Epub 2015 Apr 30.

Chien TC, Lo SF, Ho CL. Chemical composition and anti-inflammatory activity of Chamaecyparis obtusa formosana wood essential oil from Taiwan. Nat Prod Commun. 2014 May;9(5):723-6.

Kasuya H, Hata E, Satou T, Yoshikawa M, Hayashi S, Masuo Y, Koike K. Effect on emotional behavior and stress by inhalation of the essential oil from Chamaecyparis obtusa. Nat Prod Commun. 2013 Apr;8(4):515-8.

Bae D, Seol H, Yoon HG, Na JR, Oh K, Choi CY, Lee DW, Jun W, Youl Lee K, Lee J, Hwang K, Lee YH, Kim S. Inhaled essential oil from Chamaecyparis obtusa ameliorates the impairments of cognitive function induced by injection of β-amyloid in rats. Pharm Bull. 2012 Jul;50(7):900-10.

Lee GS, Hong EJ, Gwak KS, Park MJ, Choi KC, Choi IG, Jang JW, Jeung EB. The essential oil of Chamaecyparis obtusa promote[s] hair growth through the induction of vascular endothelial growth factor gene. Fitoterpia. 2010 Jan;81(1):17-24. Epub 2009 Jul 7.

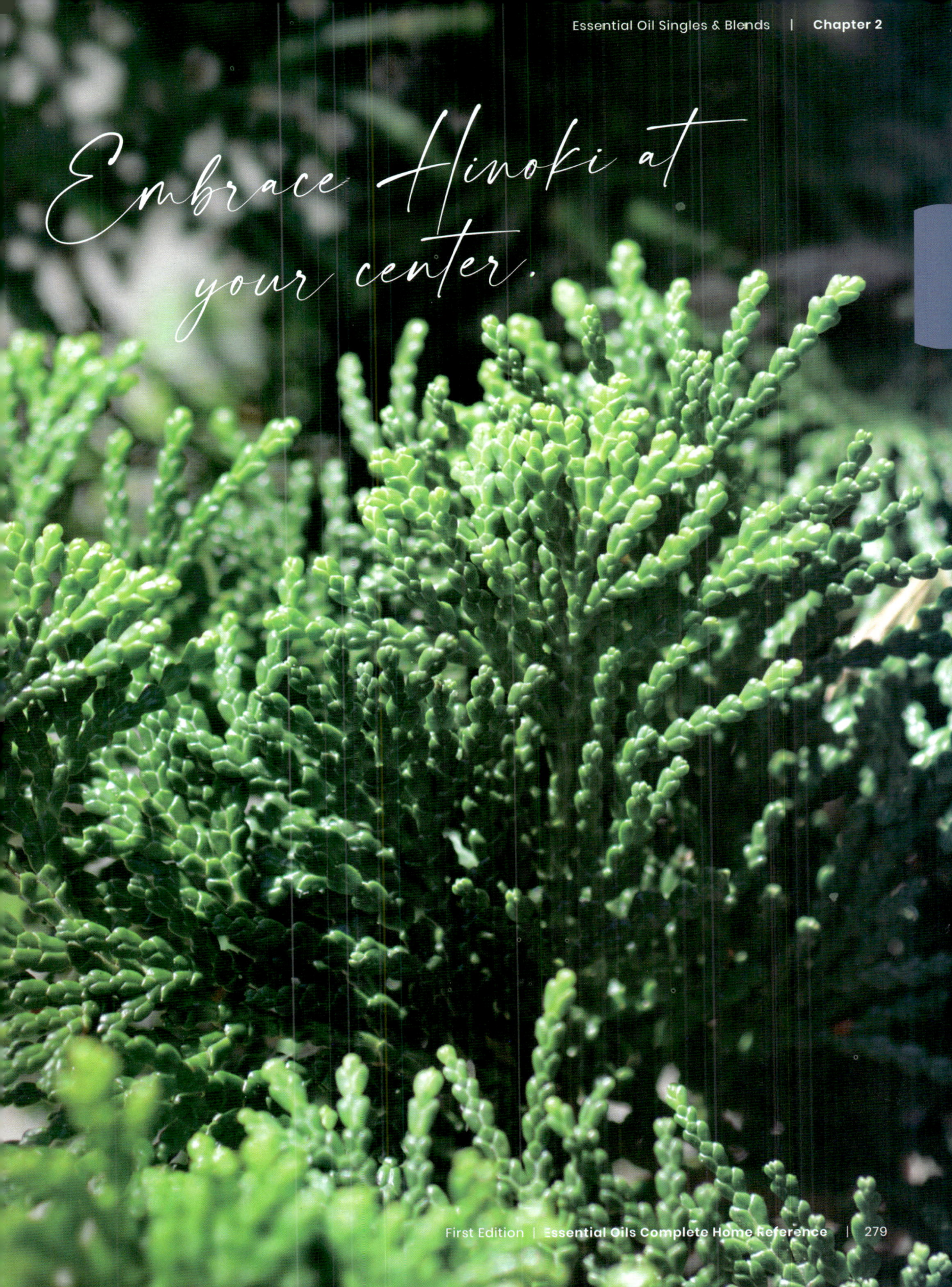

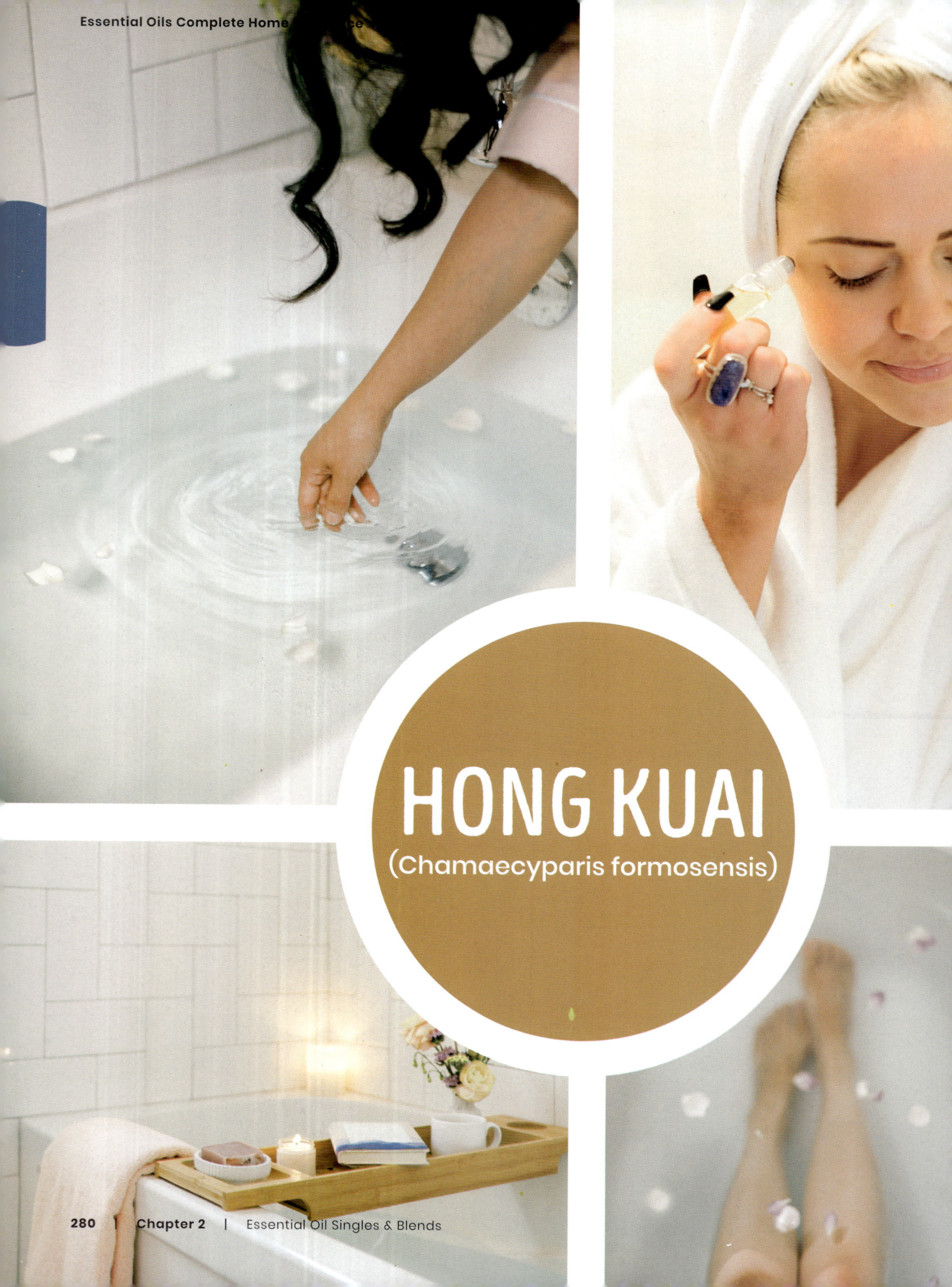

HONG KUAI
(Chamaecyparis formosensis)

BOTANICAL FAMILY:
Cupressaceae

PLANT ORIGIN:
Taiwan

EXTRACTION METHOD:
Steam distilled from wood

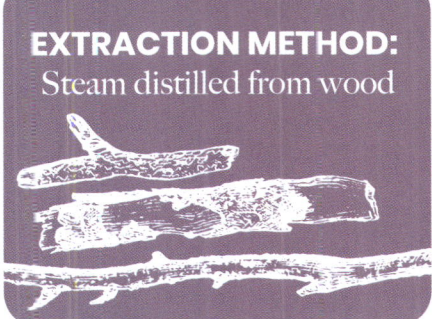

KEY CONSTITUENTS:
Myrtanol (12-20%), Myrtenol (10-19%), Delta-Cadinene (7-10%), Myrtenal (2-7%), Alpha-Pinene (3-6%), Tau-Muurolol (2-5%), Alpha-Elemol (2-4%), Beta-Elemene (1-3%)

HISTORICAL DATA:
Hong Kuai trees grow up to 55-60 meters tall in high altitude areas of Taiwan and can live over 1,000 years. The wood of these trees is highly resistant to decay and valued for building temples. The highly scented oil was known for supporting respiratory health.

MEDICAL PROPERTIES:
Antifungal, anticancerous, immune support, anti-diabetic

USES:
Fungal infections (ringworm), cancer, respiratory problems

FRAGRANT INFLUENCE:
Calming and centering, inspiration, confidence, respiratory health

DIRECTIONS:
Aromatic: 30. Topical: 20-80.

CAUTIONS:

SELECTED RESEARCH:

Hsu C-Y, Lin G-M, Chang S-T. Hypoglycemic activity of extracts of Chamaecyparis obtusa var. formosana leaf in rats with hyperglygemia induced by high-fat diets and streptozotocin. J Tradit Complement Med. 2020 Jul; 10(4): 389-395.

Kwak BM, Kim E-H, Kim Y-M, Kim H-T. Component analysis of four-part extracts from Chamaecyparis obtusa Endl. by supercritical fluid extraction and anti-inflammatory effect on RAW 264.7 cells. J Exerc Rhabil. 2019 Oct; 15(5): 723-730.

Ikei H, Song C, Miyazaki Y. Physiological effect of olfactory stimulation by Hinoki cypress (Chamaecyparis obtusa) leaf oil. J Physiol Anthropol. 2015; 34: 44.

Chen YJ, Lin CY, Cheng SS, Chang ST. Rapid discrimination and feature extraction of three Chamaecyparis species by static-HS/GC-MS. J Agric Food Chem. 2015 Jan 28;63(3):810-20.

Ho CL, Hua KF, Hsu KP, Wang EI, Su YC. Composition and antipathogenic activities of the twig essential oil of Chamaecyparis formosensis from Taiwan. Nat Prod Commun. 2012 Jul;7(7):933-6. Epub 2012 Aug 23.

Chen TH, Liau BC, Wang SY, Jong TT. Isolation and cytotoxicity of the lignanoids from Chamaecyparis formosensis. Planta Med. 2008 Dec;74(15):1806-11. Epub 2008 Nov 13.

Ieh YH, Kuo PM, Chien SC, Shyur LF, Wang SY. Effects of Chamaecyparis formosensis Matasumura extractives on lipopolysaccharide-induced release of nitrous oxide. Phytomedicine. 2007 Oct;14(10):675-80. Epub 2007 Feb 13.

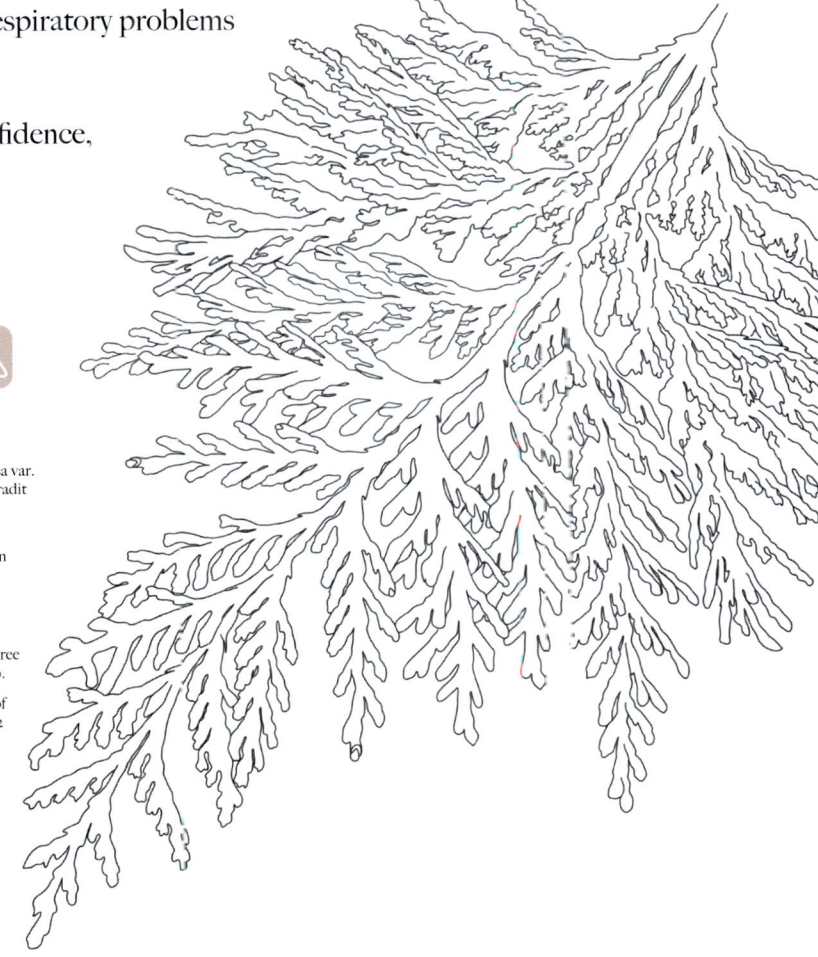

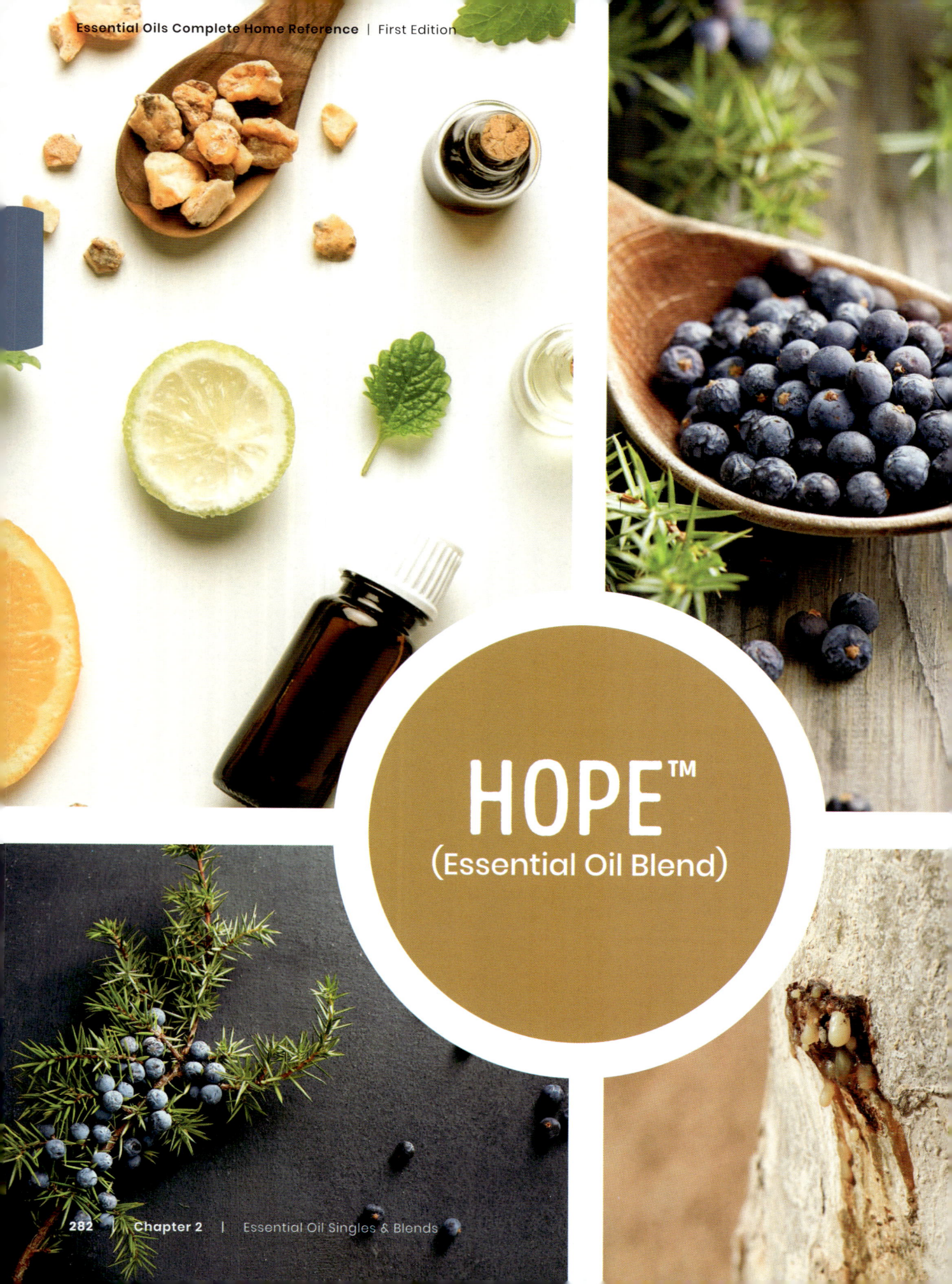

HOPE™
(Essential Oil Blend)

ABOUT HOPE™:

Hope is essential for moving forward in life. Hopelessness can cause a loss of vision, goals, and dreams. This blend helps you reconnect with a feeling of strength and grounding, restoring hope for tomorrow. It has helped many overcome suicidal depression.

MEDICAL PROPERTIES & USES:

Anti-inflammatory, uplifting, emotion supporting, antimicrobial, organ protective

INGREDIENTS:

Sweet almond oil, Melissa, Juniper, Myrrh, Black Spruce

DIRECTIONS:

Aromatic: 6o. Topical: Neat.

CAUTIONS: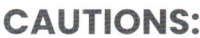

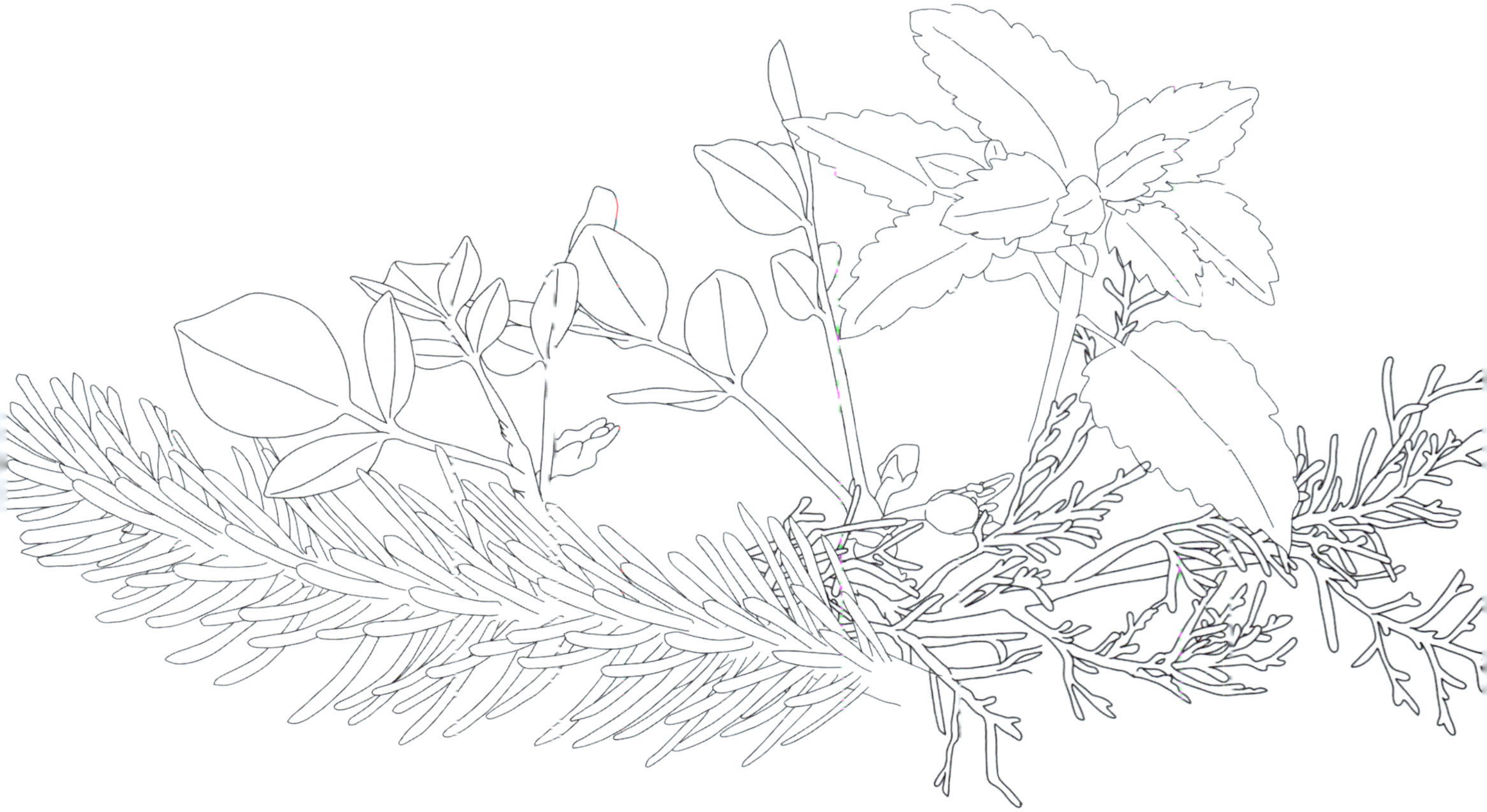

HUMILITY™
(Essential Oil Blend)

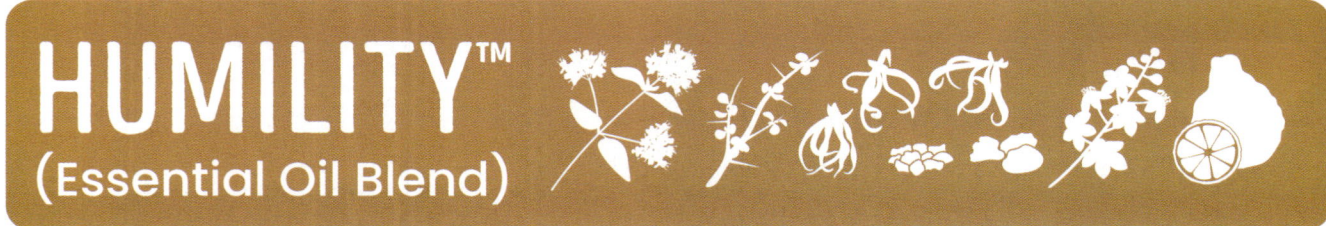

Having humility and forgiveness helps us heal ourselves and our earth (2 Chronicles 7:14). Humility is an integral component in obtaining forgiveness and is needed for a closer relationship with God. Through the frequency and fragrance of this blend, you may arrive at a place where healing can begin.

MEDICAL PROPERTIES & USES:
Anti-inflammatory, antimicrobial, antioxidative, emotion supporting, uplifting, calming, disease inhibitory, organ protective, pain or swelling reducing, performance enhancing/stimulating

INGREDIENTS:
Caprylic/capric triglyceride, Coriander, Ylang Ylang, Bergamot (Furocoumarin-free), Geranium, Melissa, Frankincense, Myrrh, Northern Lights Black Spruce, Vetiver, Bitter Orange (Neroli), Rose

DIRECTIONS:
Aromatic: 60. Topical: Neat.

CAUTIONS:

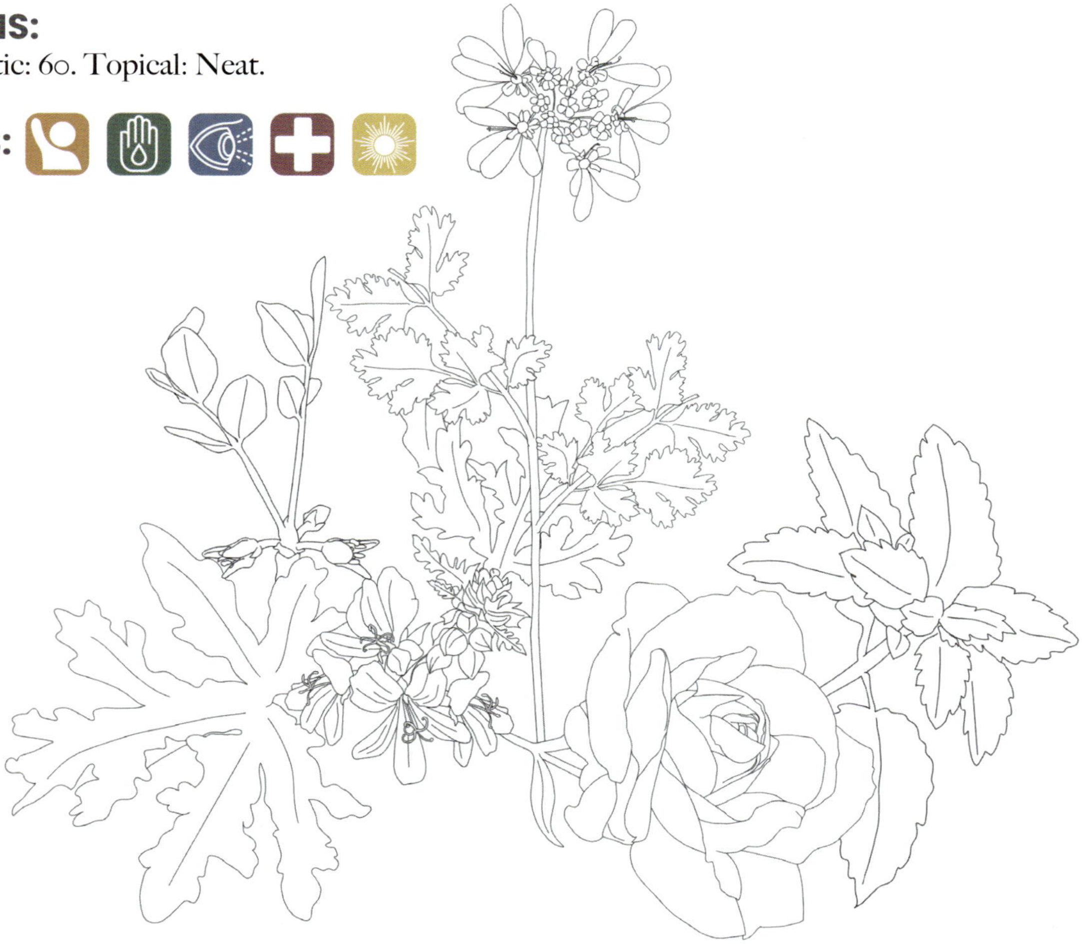

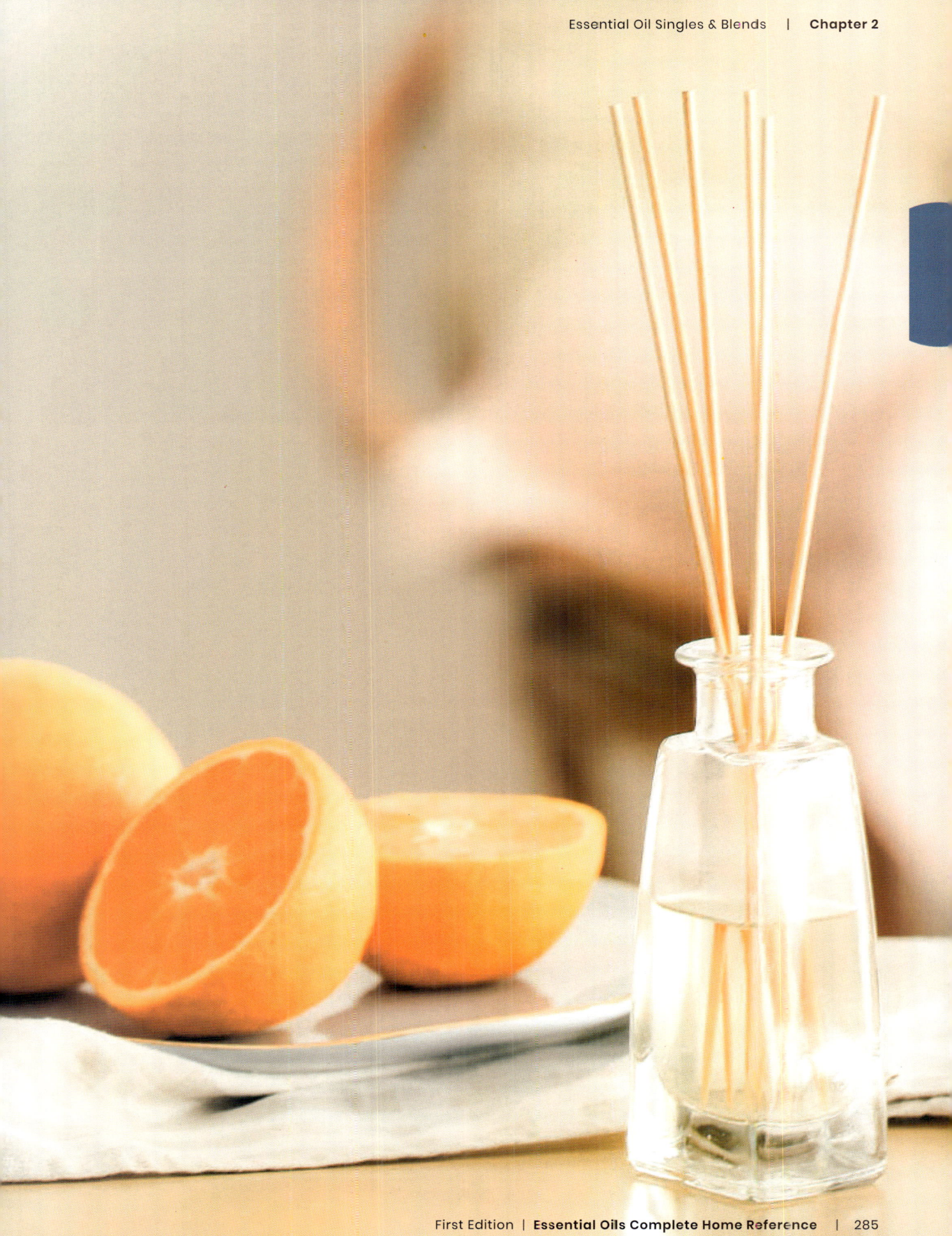

BOTANICAL FAMILY: Lamiaceae

PLANT ORIGIN: France, Moldova

EXTRACTION METHOD: Steam distilled from leaves and aerial parts

KEY CONSTITUENTS: Iso-Pinochamphone (33-53%), Pinocamphone (5-30%), Beta-Pinene (5-17%), Germacrene D (up to 4%), Beta-Caryophyllene (up to 2%)

HYSSOP
(Hyssopus officinalis)

While there is some uncertainty that Hyssopus officinalis is the same species of plant as the hyssop referred to in the Bible, there is no question that H. officinalis has been used medicinally for almost a millennium for antiseptic properties. It has also been used for opening the respiratory system.

MEDICAL PROPERTIES:
Mucolytic, decongestant, anti-inflammatory, regulates lipid metabolism, antiviral, antibacterial, antiparasitic, antispasmodic, antiseptic, astringent, antirheumatic, cicatrisant, digestive, diuretic, expectorant, carminative, hypertensive. antioxidant

USES:
Respiratory infections/congestion, parasites (expelling worms), viral infections, and circulatory disorders, digestive and intestinal problems, wounds, cuts, bruises, helps fade scars, regulates menstrual cycle, helps prevent muscles and skin from sagging, strengthens nervous system, stimulates body systems

FRAGRANT INFLUENCE:
Stimulates creativity, meditation, bronchitis, asthma

DIRECTIONS:
Aromatic: 10. Topical: 50-50.

CAUTIONS: 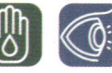 Avoid use if epileptic.

SELECTED RESEARCH:

Nile SH, Nile AS, Keum YS. Total phenolics, antioxidant, antitumor, and enzyme inhibitory activity of Indian medicinal and aromatic plants extracted with different extraction methods. 3 Biotech. 2017 May;7(1):76. Epub 2017 Apr 27.

Stappen I, Wanner J, Tabanca N, Wedge DE, Ali A, Kaul VK, Lal B, Jaitak V, Gochev VK, Schmidt E, Jirovetz L. Chemical composition and biological activity of essential oils of Dracocephalum heterophyllum and Hyssopus officinalis from Western Himalaya. Nat Prod Commun. 2015 Jan;10(1):133-8.

Ma X, Ma X, Ma Z, Wang J, Sun Z, Yu W, Li F, Ding J. Effect of Hyssopus officinalis L. on inhibiting airway inflammation and immune regulation in a chronic asthmatic mouse model. Exp Ther Med. 2014 Nov;8(5):1371-1374. Epub 2014 Oct 8.

Vlase L, Benedec D, Hanganu D, Damian G, Csillag I, Sevastre B, Mot AC, Silaghi-Dumitrescu R, Tilea I. Evaluation of antioxidant and antimicrobial activities and phenolic profile for Hyssopus officinalis, Ocimum basilicum and Teucrium chamedrys. Molecules. 2014 Apr 28;19(5):5490-507.

Fathiazad F, Mazandarani M, Hamedeyazdan S. Phytochemical analysis and antioxidant activity of Hyssopus officinalis L. from Iran. Adv Pharm Bull. 2011 Dec; 1(2): 63-67. Published online 2011 Dec. 15.

Miyazaki H, Matsuura H, Yanagiya C, Mizutani J, Tsuji M, Ishihara C. Inhibitory effects of hyssop (Hyssopus officinalis) extracts on intestinal alpha-glucosidase activity and postprandial hyperglycemia. J Nutr Sci Vitaminol (Tokyo). 2003 Oct;49(5):346-9.

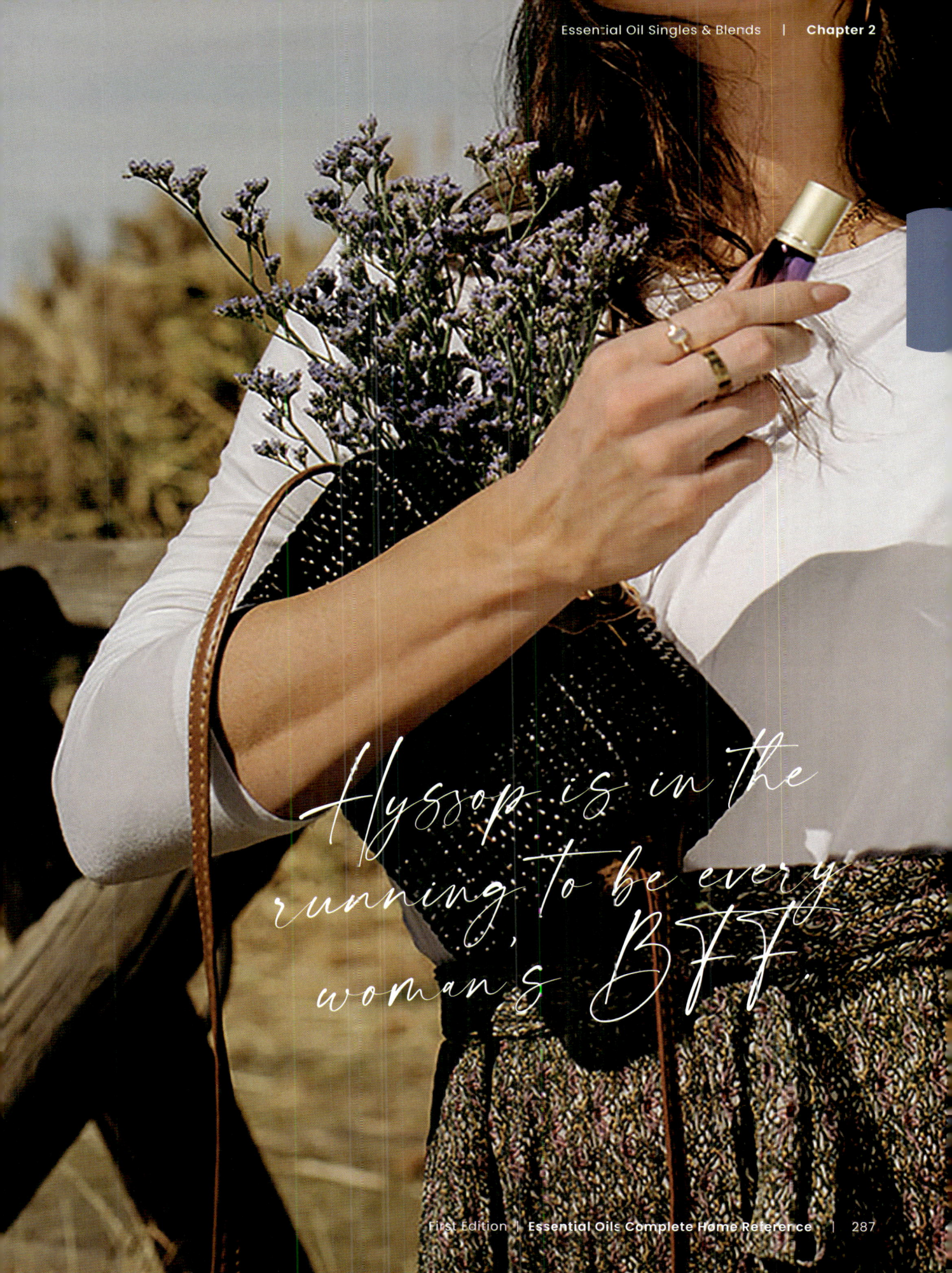

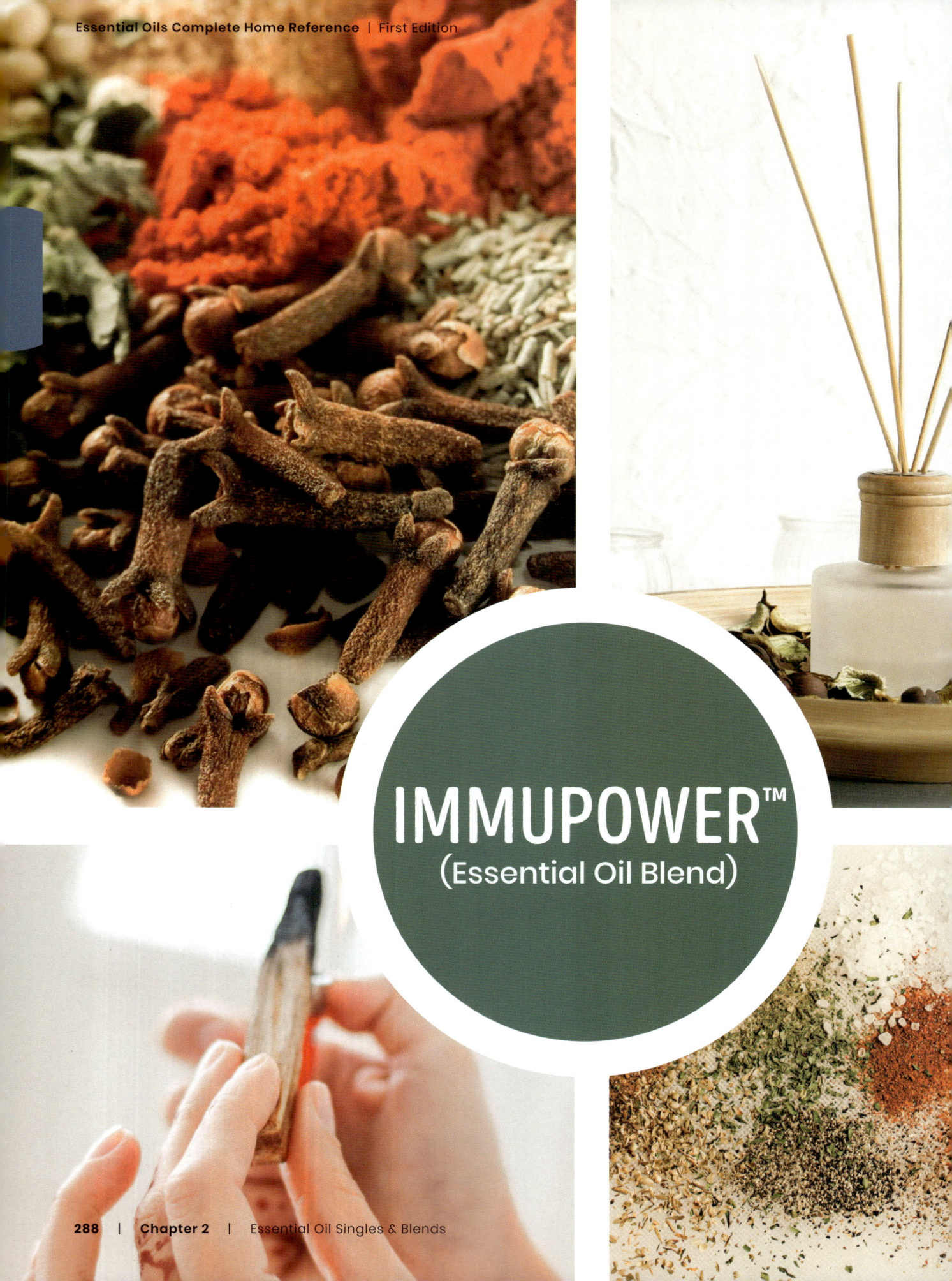

IMMUPOWER™
(Essential Oil Blend)

ABOUT IMMUPOWER:

This blend strengthens immunity and DNA repair in the cells. It is strongly antiseptic and anti-infectious.

MEDICAL PROPERTIES & USES:

Anti-inflammatory, antiseptic, anti-infectious, antimicrobial, antioxidative, calming, cardiovascular supportive, organ protective, pain or swelling reducing, wellness supportive

INGREDIENTS:

Hyssop, Mountain Savory, Cistus, Camphor (Ravintsara), Frankincense, Oregano, Clove, Cumin, Dorado Azul

DIRECTIONS:

Aromatic: 30. Alternate the diffused oils with Thieves and Exodus II. To enhance effects, add Melissa, Palo Santo, or more Clove, Cistus, or Dorado Azul. Topical: 20-80.

CAUTIONS: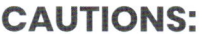

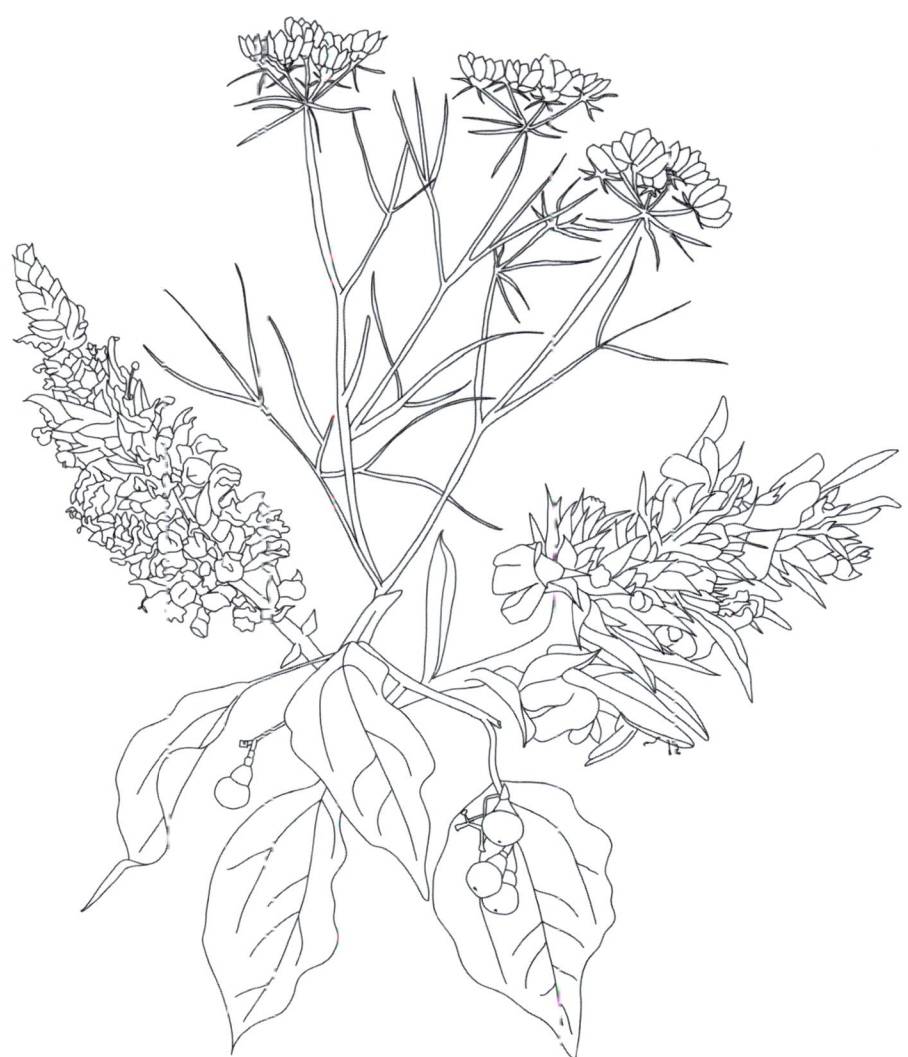

INNER CHILD™
(Essential Oil Blend)

When children have been abused, they become disconnected from their inner child, or identity, which causes confusion. This fractures the personality and creates problems that tend to surface in the early- to mid-adult years, often mislabeled as a midlife crisis. This fragrance stimulates memory response and helps one reconnect with the inner self or identity. This is one of the first steps to finding emotional balance.

MEDICAL PROPERTIES & USES:
Antimicrobial, emotion supporting, calming, disease inhibitory, muscle relaxant/bone-joint preservative, pain or swelling reducing

INGREDIENTS:
Orange, Tangerine, Ylang Ylang, Royal Hawaiian Sandalwood, Jasmine, Lemongrass, Black Spruce, Bitter Orange (Neroli)

DIRECTIONS:
Aromatic: 6o. Topical: 50-50.

CAUTIONS:

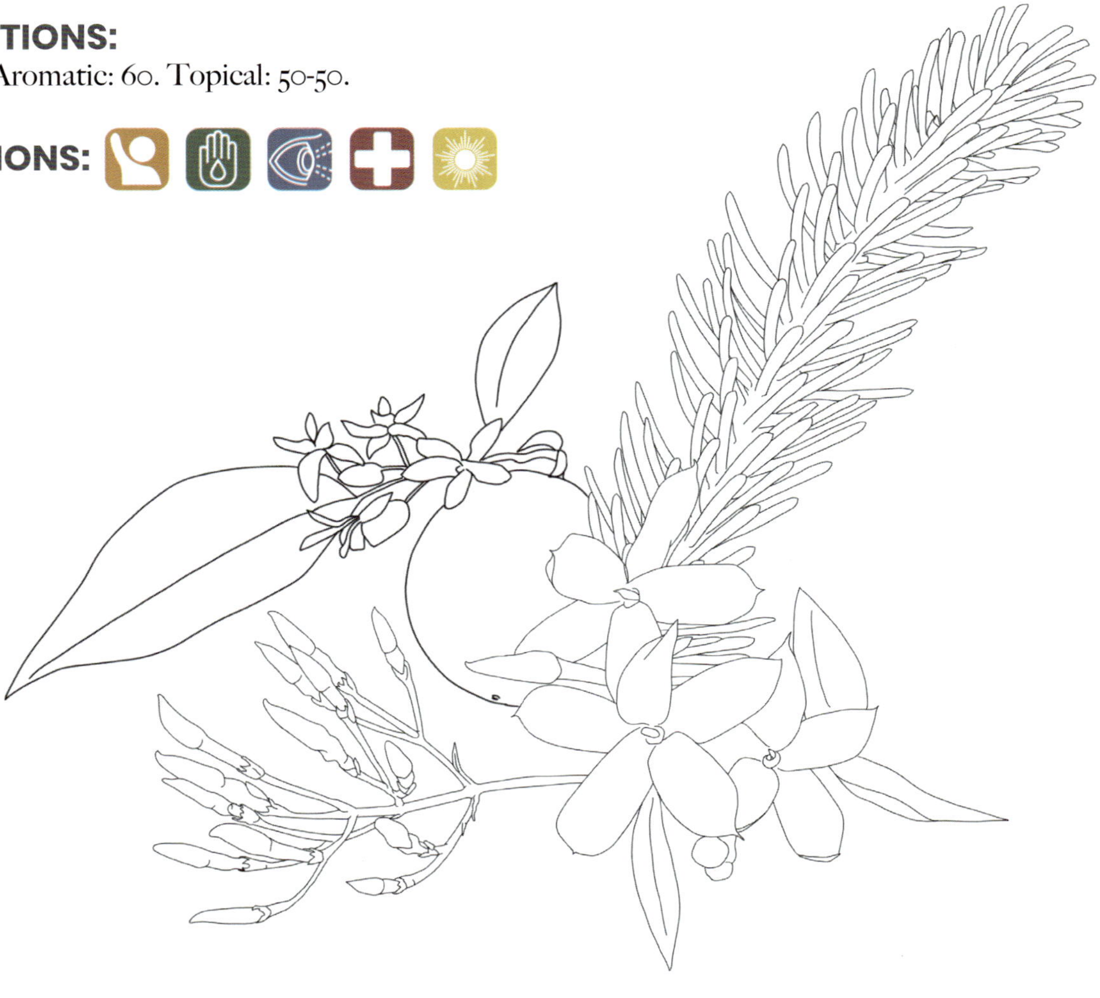

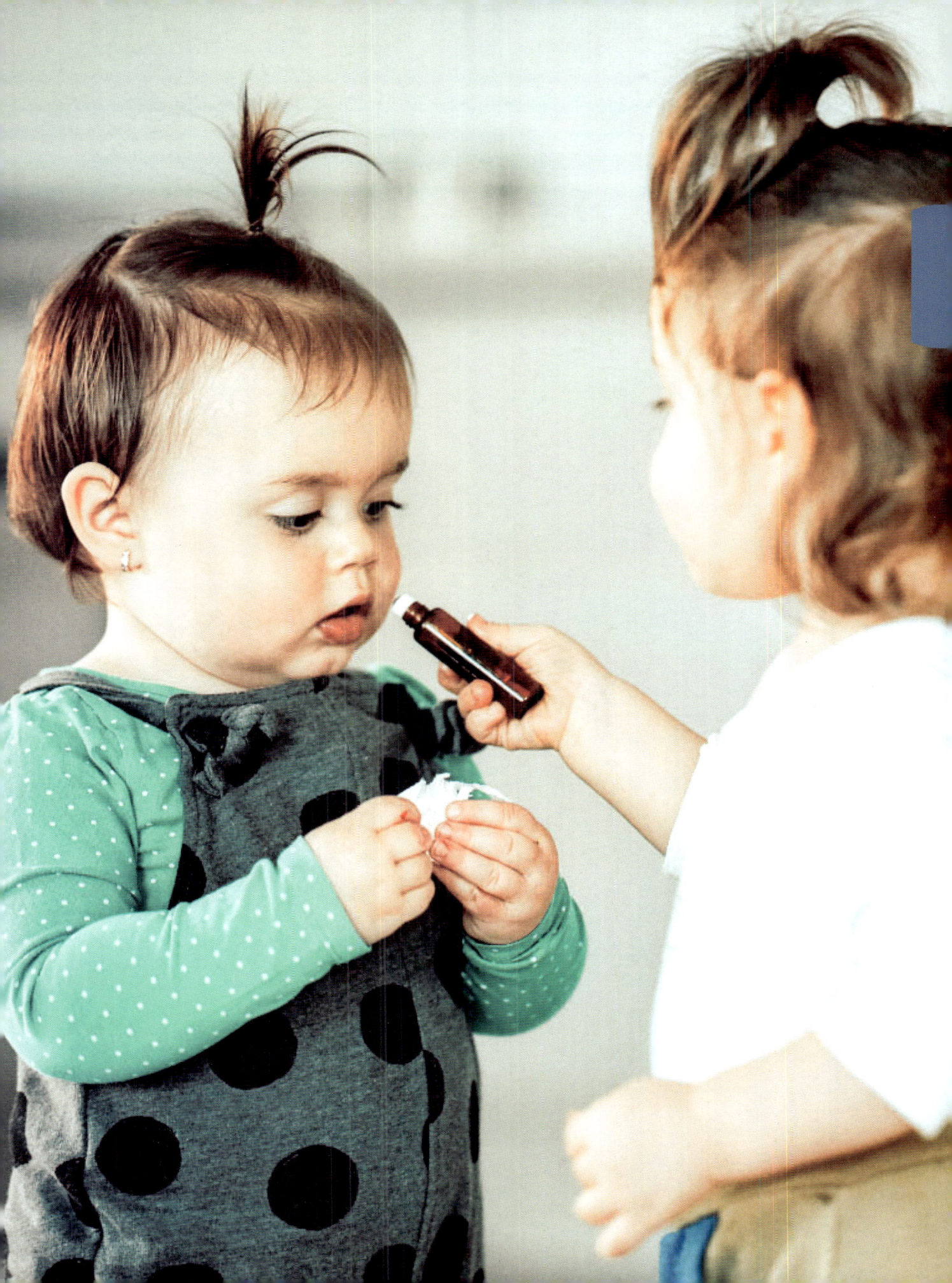

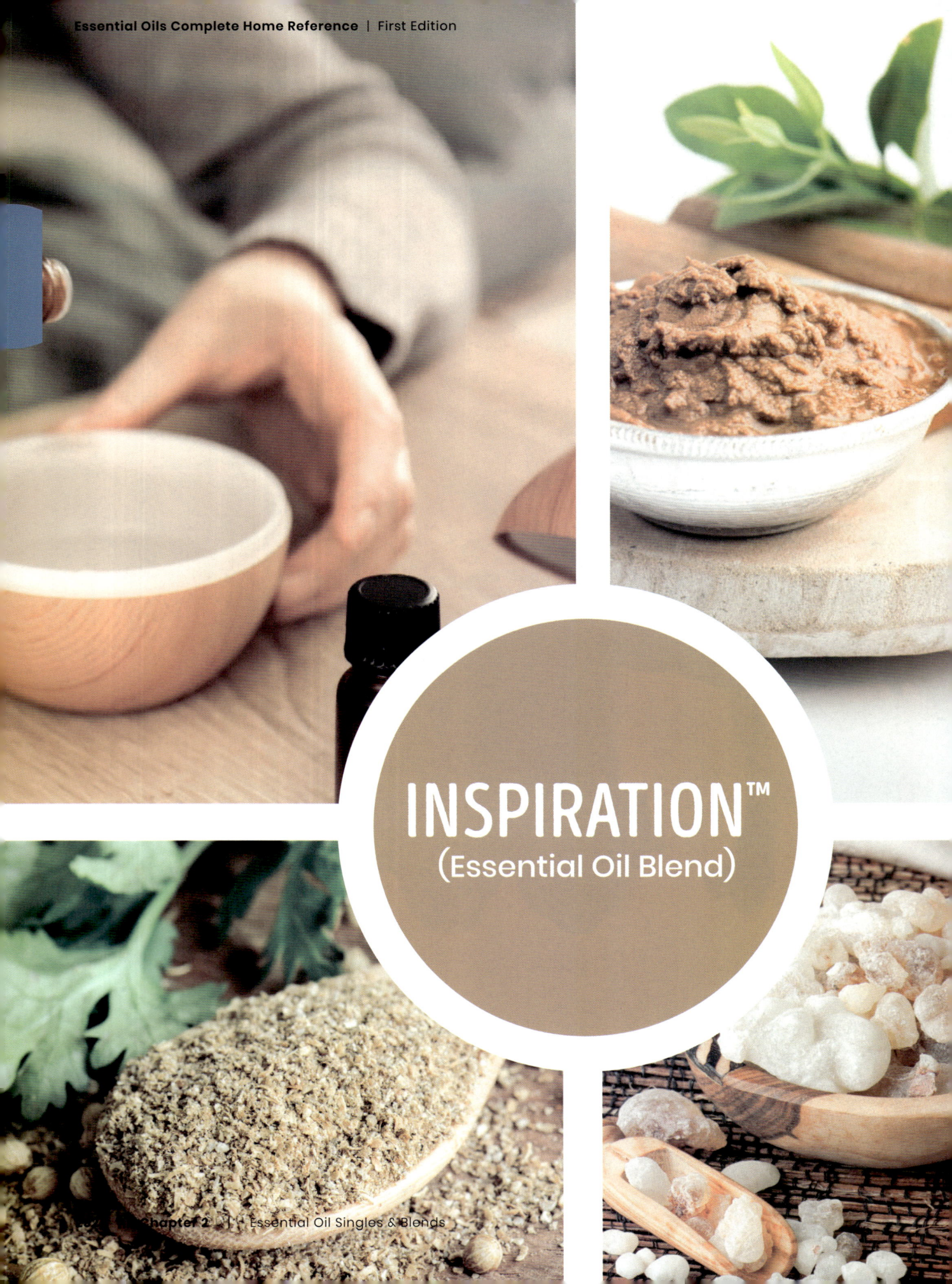

ABOUT INSPIRATION™:

This blend is formulated to help find a calm space in our minds and bring us closer to that creative center where our higher intuition operates. These oils were traditionally used by the Native Americans to enhance spirituality, prayer, and inner awareness.

MEDICAL PROPERTIES & USES:

Anti-inflammatory, antioxidative, emotion supporting, uplifting, calming, disease inhibitory, organ protective, pain or swelling reducing, performance enhancing/stimulating

INGREDIENTS:

Cedarwood, Black Spruce, Myrtle, Coriander, Royal Hawaiian Sandalwood, Frankincense, Bergamot (Furocoumarin-free), Vetiver, Ylang Ylang, Geranium

DIRECTIONS:

Aromatic: 6o. Topical: Neat.

CAUTIONS:

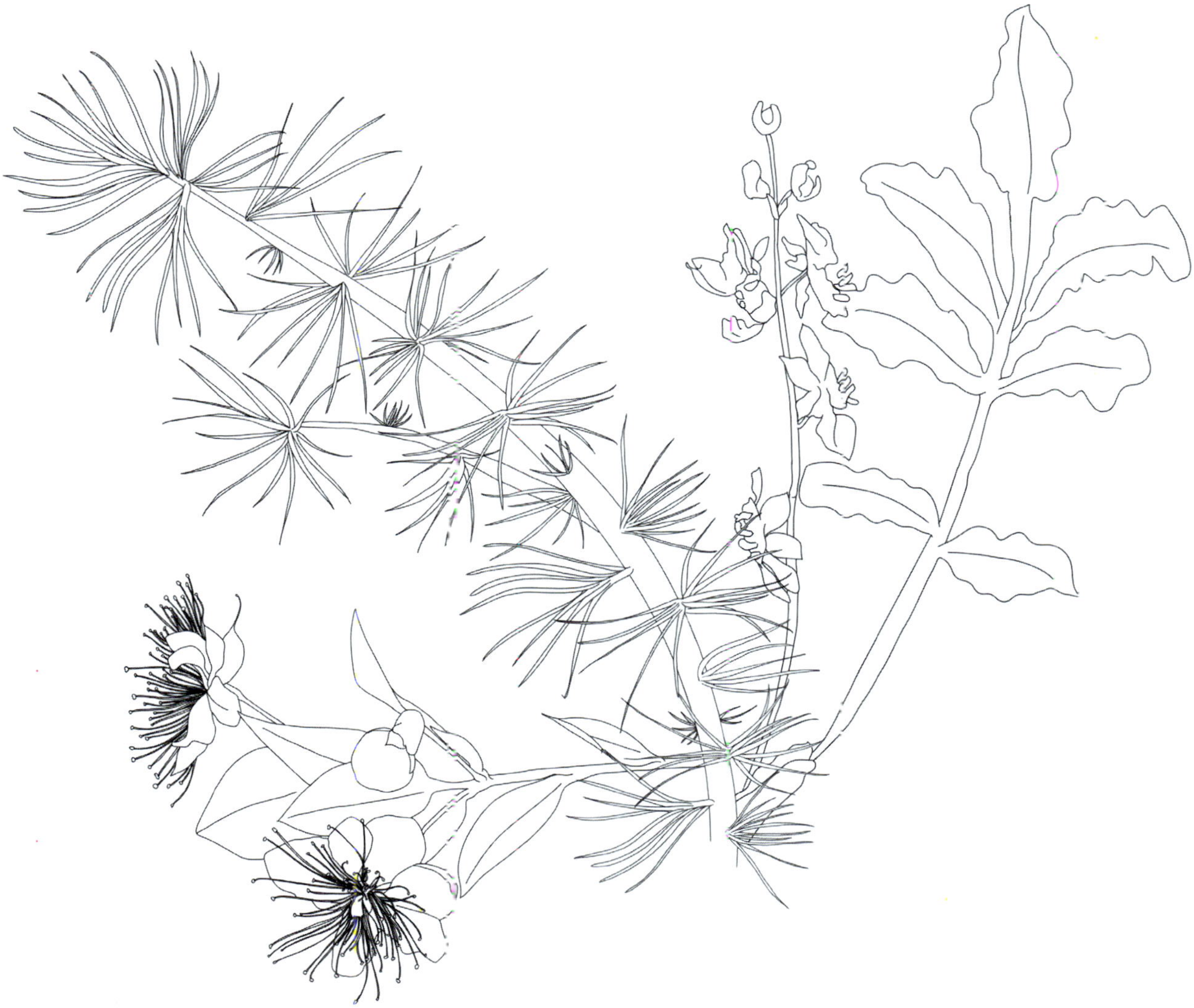

INTO THE FUTURE™
(Essential Oil Blend)

This blend helps one leave the past behind in order to progress with vision and excitement. So many times we find ourselves settling for mediocrity and sacrificing our own potential and success because of fear of the unknown and the future. This blend inspires determination and a pioneering spirit and creates a strong emotional feeling of being able to reach one's potential.

MEDICAL PROPERTIES & USES:
Anti-inflammatory, antimicrobial, antioxidative, emotion supporting, uplifting, calming, disease inhibitory, wellness supportive

INGREDIENTS:
Sweet almond oil, Clary Sage, Ylang Ylang, White Fir, Idaho Blue Spruce, Jasmine, Juniper, Frankincense, Orange, Cedarwood, White Lotus

DIRECTIONS:
Aromatic: 6o. Topical: 20-80.

CAUTIONS:

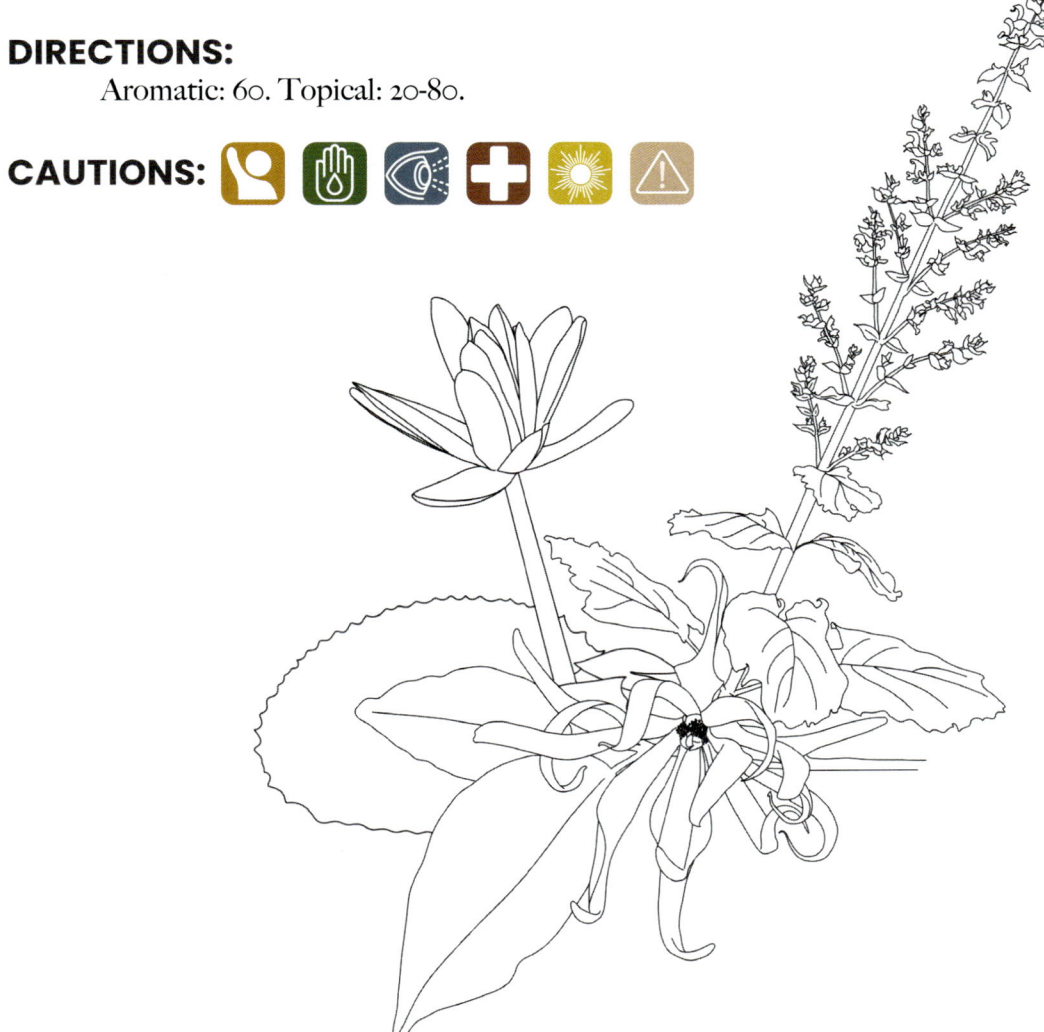

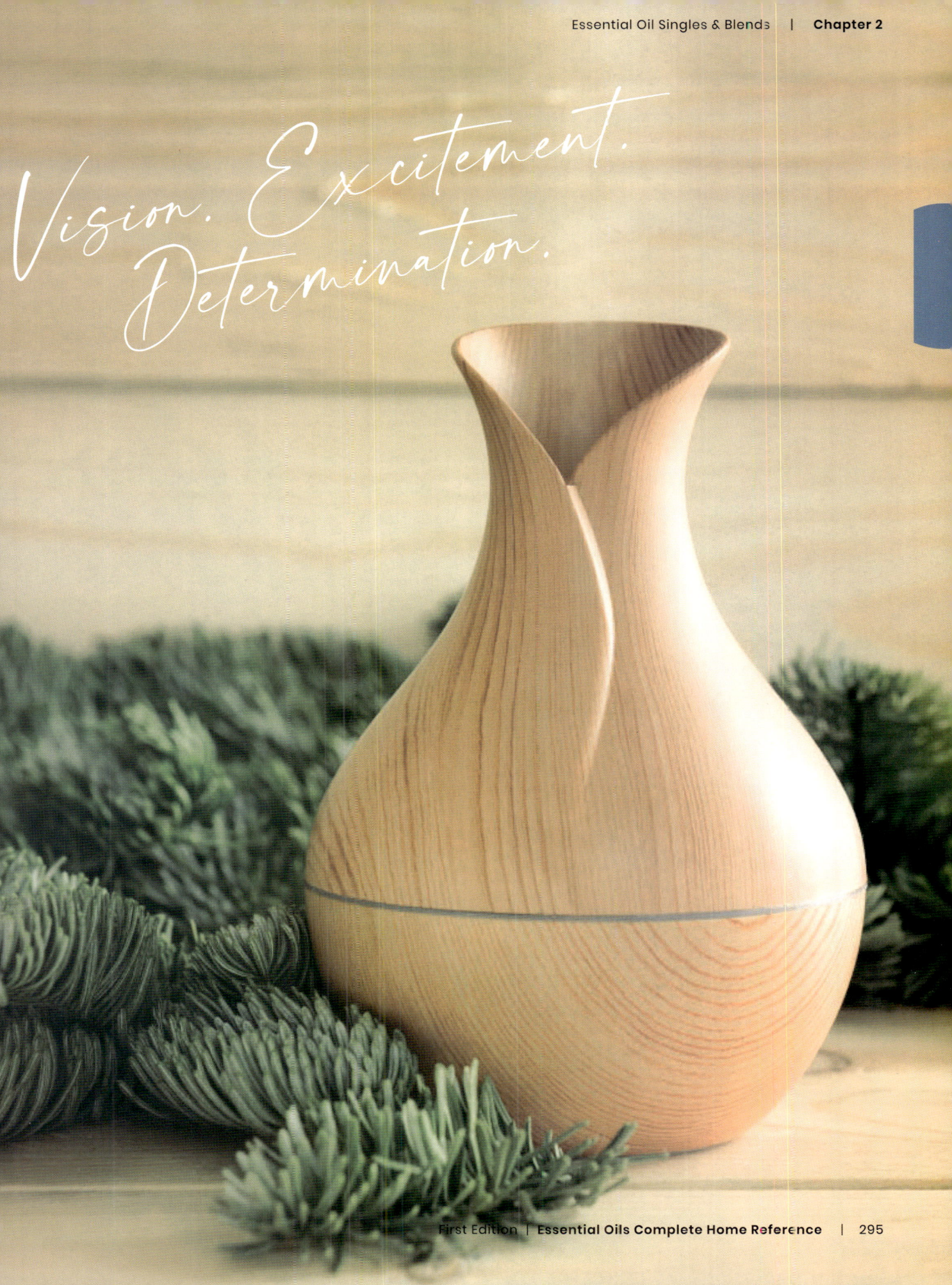

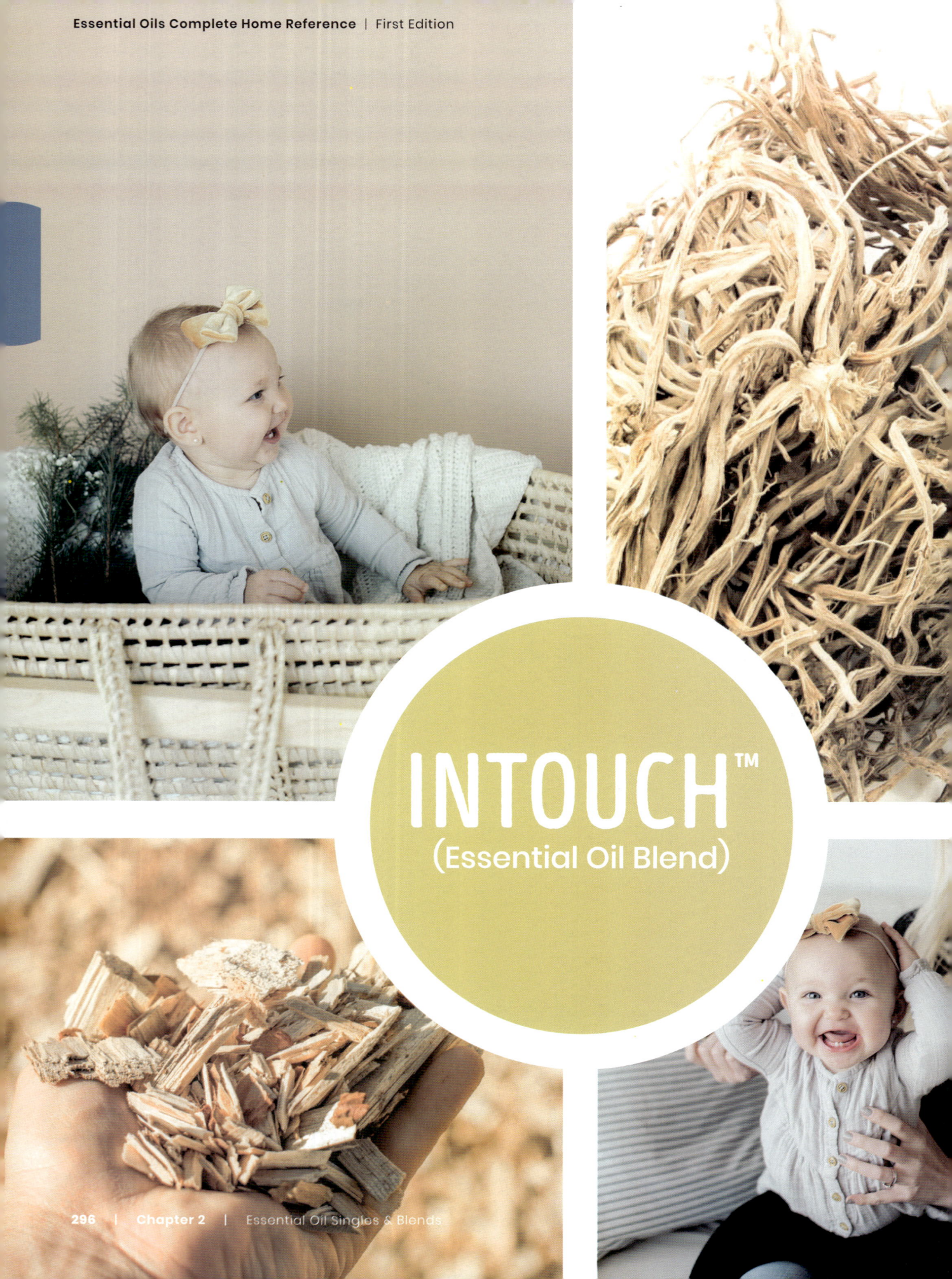

INTOUCH™
(Essential Oil Blend)

ABOUT INTOUCH™:
(found only in the Reconnect Collection)
This uplifting blend can help support mood by encouraging positive energy in times of restlessness and unease and to help ground and unite the body, mind, and spirit.

MEDICAL PROPERTIES & USES:
Antibacterial, antidepressant, anti-inflammatory, antioxidative, antiviral, relaxant, emotion supporting, cardiovascular supporting, nervous system supportive, insomnia, immune stimulant, ADD and ADHD (attention deficit disorders) in children, pain relieving

INGREDIENTS:
Caprylic/capric triglyceride, Vetiver, Melissa, Royal Hawaiian Sandalwood, Cedarwood, Idaho Blue Spruce

DIRECTIONS:
Aromatic: 6o. Topical: Neat.

CAUTIONS:

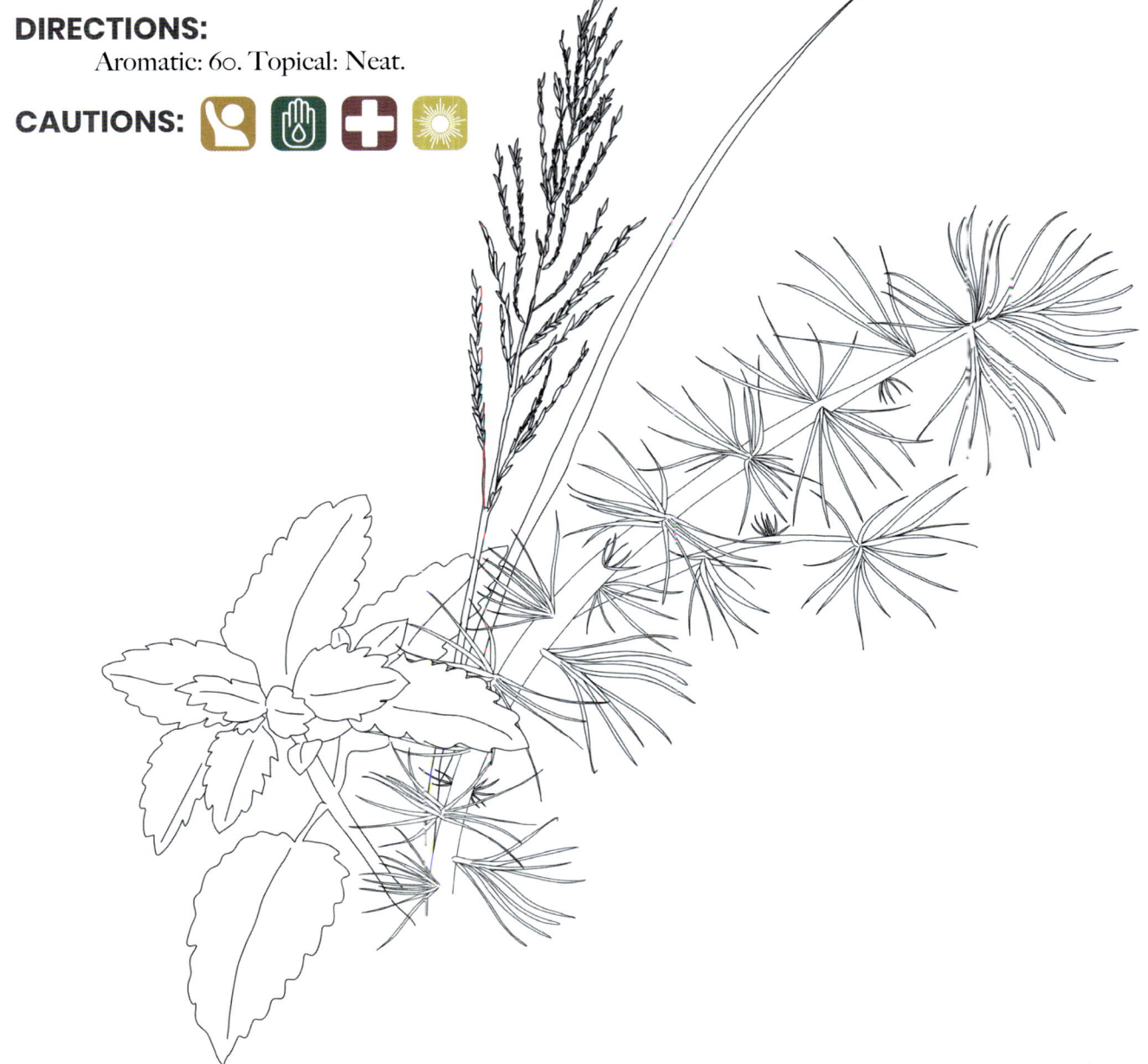

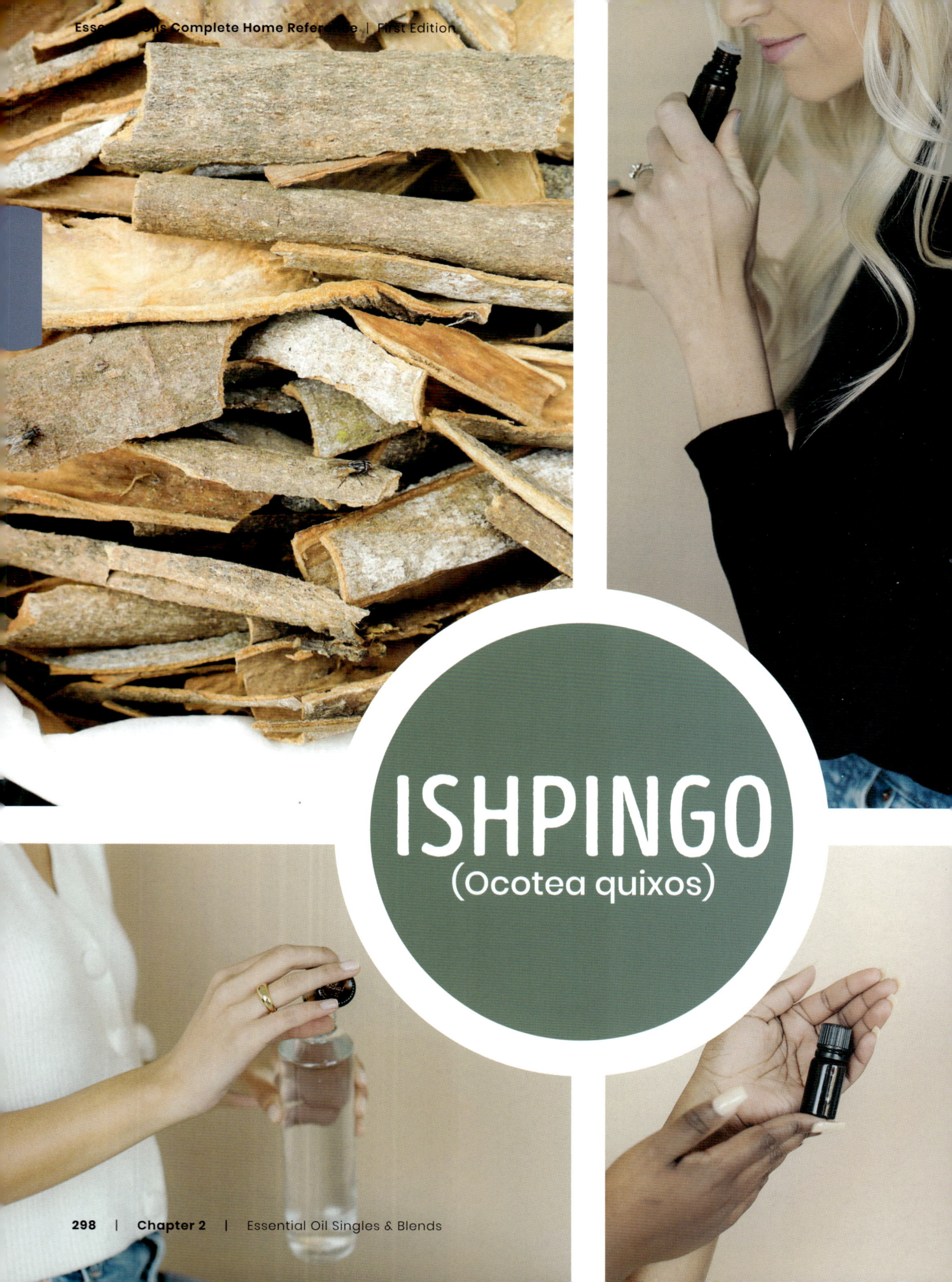

Essential Oil Singles & Blends | Chapter 2

BOTANICAL FAMILY:
Lauraceae

PLANT ORIGIN:
Ecuador

EXTRACTION METHOD:
Steam distilled from fruit

KEY CONSTITUENTS:
Cinnamyl Acetate (up to 55%),
Trans-Cinnamaldehyde (up to 42%),
Methyl Cinnamate (up to 33%),
Para-Cymene (up to 14%),
Alpha-Pinene (up to 13%),
Eucalyptol (up to 10%)

HISTORICAL DATA:

Ishpingo is a Hispanic name for Ocotea and is distilled from the flower and fruit of a tree found in the Amazon wilderness on the ranges of the west side of the Andes Mountains. It is commonly referred to by the native people throughout Ecuador as "false canilla" or "false cinnamon." The tree grows to a very large size, reaching up to 48 inches in diameter and over 60 feet tall, making a large canopy top. Historical usage of ocotea dates back more than 500 years, when it was used to aromatize sweets and cakes. Of 114 ocotea species' studies on PubMed, only two refer to the properties of ocotea essential oil distilled from flowers or fruit, as Young Living's Ishpingo essential oil is, rather than the leaves and bark of the tree.

MEDICAL PROPERTIES:
Antimicrobial, antioxidant, antifungal, antibacterial

USES:
Soap, food flavoring, cleansing, supporting, easing stress, cleansing, and purifying the spirit

FRAGRANT INFLUENCE:
Warm, mentally relaxing

DIRECTIONS:
Aromatic: 60. Topical: 20-80. Dietary: Dilute 1 drop essential oil with 4 drops V-6 or other pure carrier oil. Put in a capsule and take 1 daily or as directed by a health care professional.

CAUTIONS:

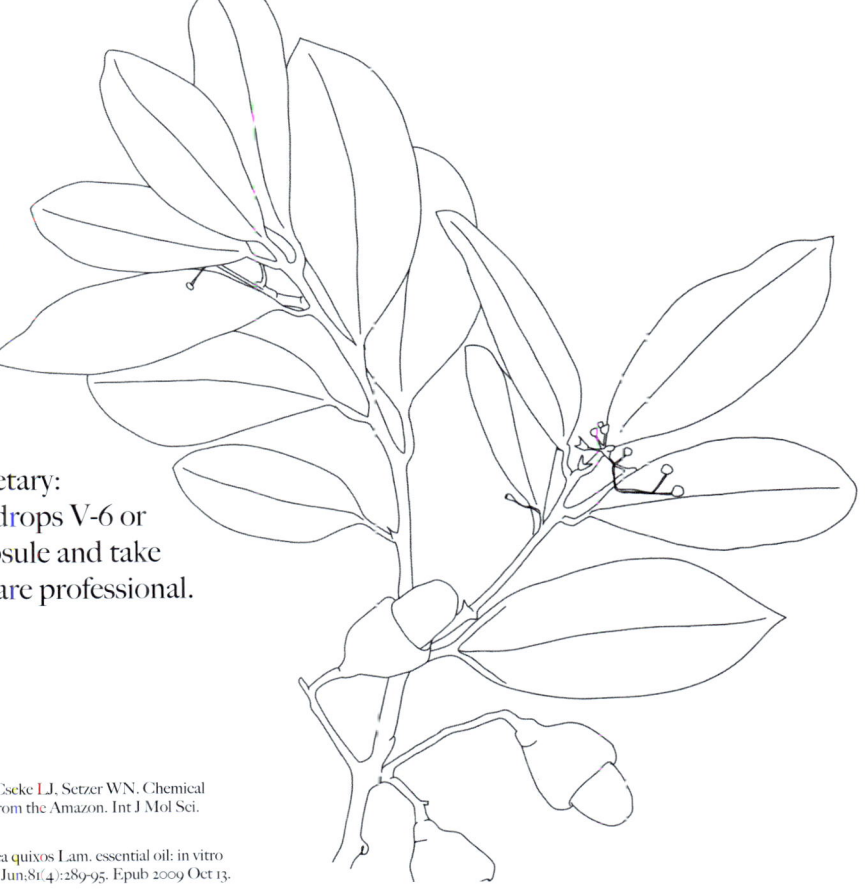

SELECTED RESEARCH:

a Silva JK, da Trindade R, Moreira EC, Maia JGS, Dosoky NS, Miller RS, Cseke LJ, Setzer WN. Chemical Diversity, Biological Activity, and Genetic Aspects of Three Ocotea Species from the Amazon. Int J Mol Sci. 2017 May; 18(5): 1081.

Ballabeni V, Tognolini M, Giorgio C, Bertoni S, Bruni R, Barocelli E. Ocotea quixos Lam. essential oil: in vitro and in vivo investigation on its anti-inflammatory properties. Fitoterapia. 2010 Jun;81(4):289-95. Epub 2009 Oct 13.

Guerrini A, Sacchetti G, Muzzoli M, Moreno Rueda G, Medici A, Besco E, Bruni R. Composition of the volatile fraction of Ocotea bofo Kunth (Lauraceae) calyces by GC MS and NMR fingerprinting and antimicrobial and antioxidant activity. J Agric Food Chem. 2006 Oct 4;54(20):7778-88.

Bruni R, Medici A, Andreotti E, Fantin C, Muzzoli M, Dehesa M, Romagnoli C, Sacchetti G. Chemical composition and biological activities of Ishpingo essential oil, a traditional Ecuadorian spice from Ocotea quixos (Lam.) Kosterm. (Lauraceae) flower calices. Food Chem. 2004 May;85(3):415-421.

BOTANICAL FAMILY: Rutaceae

PLANT ORIGIN: Taiwan

EXTRACTION METHOD: Cold pressed from peel; it takes 3,000 lemons to produce 1 kilo of oil

KEY CONSTITUENTS: Limonene (50-72%), Beta-Pinene (8-22%), Gamma-Terpinene (7-15%), Alpha-Pinene (1-3%), Geranial (up to 3%), Sabinene (up to 3%), Neral (up to 2%)

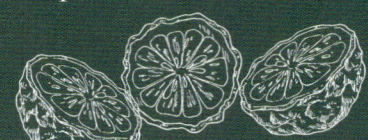

JADE LEMON & JADE LEMON VITALITY™
(Citrus limon Eureka var. formosensis)

Taiwan and China are home to this exquisitely scented lemon variety. Unique among lemons, when fully mature, it is a lovely green color; hence, the name Jade Lemon. Not only is the color of this lemon unique, this essential oil has a tantalizing lemon-lime scent. Introduced at the 2014 YL convention, it has become a most beloved essential oil. Jade Lemon contains the same major constituents as Lemon essential oil but in slightly different percentages.

MEDICAL PROPERTIES:
Antitumoral, antiseptic, improves microcirculation, immune stimulant (may increase white blood cells), improves memory, relaxation; rich in limonene, which has been extensively studied in over 50 clinical studies for ability to combat tumor growth.

USES:
Uplift and stimulate the mind and body. Can be used in household cleaning or mixed with Citronella essential oil for a pleasant, citrus-scented insect repellent.

FRAGRANT INFLUENCE:
Uplifting and stimulating, energizes the spirit

DIRECTIONS:
Aromatic: 60. Topical: 50-50. Combine 10-15 drops with lotions and shampoos to energize the spirit. Dietary (Vitality): Put 2 drops in a capsule. Take 3 times daily. Use as a flavoring in foods and beverages.

CAUTIONS:

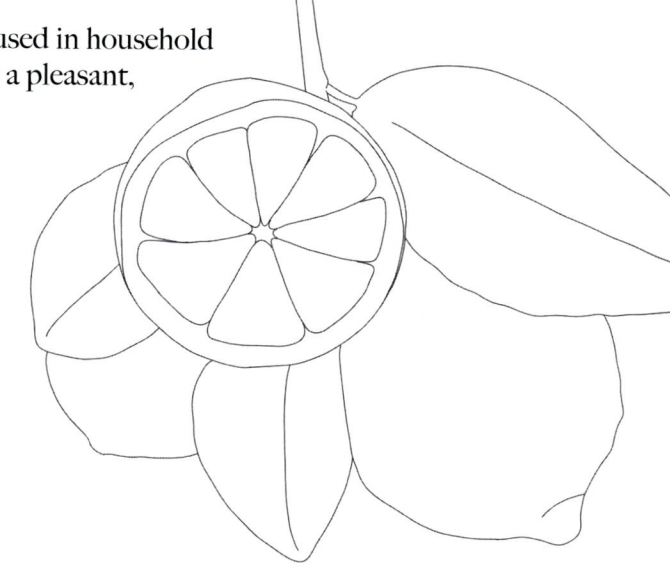

SELECTED RESEARCH:
Bouzenna H, Dhibi S, Samout N, Rjeibi I, Talarmin H, Elfeki A, Hfaiedh N. The protective effect of Citrus limon essential oil on hepatotoxicity on nephrotoxicity induced by aspirin in rats. Biomed Pharmacother. 2016 Oct;83:1327-1334. Epub 2016 Oct 25.

Khan RA, Riaz A. Behavioral effects of Citrus limon in rats. Metab Brain Dis. 2015 Apr;30(2):589-96. Epub 2014 Sep 17.

Oliveira SA, Zambrana JR, Iorio FB, Pereira CA, Jorge AO. The antimicrobial effects of Citrus limon and Citrus aurantium essential oils on multi-species biofilms. Braz Oral Res. 2014;28(1):22-7.

Yavari Kia P, Safajou F, Shahnazi M, Nazemiyeh H. The effect of lemon inhalation aromatherapy on nausea and vomiting of pregnancy: a double-blinded, randomized, controlled clinical trial. Iran Red Crescent Med J. 2014 Mar;16(3):e14360. Epub 2014 May 16.

Guerra FQ, Mendes JM, Sousa JP, Morais-Braga MF, Santos BH, Melo Coutinho HD, Lima Ede O. Increasing antibiotic activity against a multidrug-resistant Acinetobacter spp by essential oils of Citrus limon and Cinnamomum zeylanicum. Nat Prod Res. 2012;26(23):2235-8. Epub 2011 Dec 23.

Valgimigli L, Gabbanini S, Berlini E, Lucchi E, Beltramini C, Bertarelli YL. Lemon (Citrus limon Burm.f.) essential oil enhances the trans-epidermal release of lipid-(A, E) and water-(B6, C) soluble vitamins from topical emulsions in reconstructed human epidermis. Int J Cosmet Sci. 2012 Aug;34(4):347-56. Epub 2012 Apr 21.

Jade's got it. She's serving up cleansing, protection & prosperity.

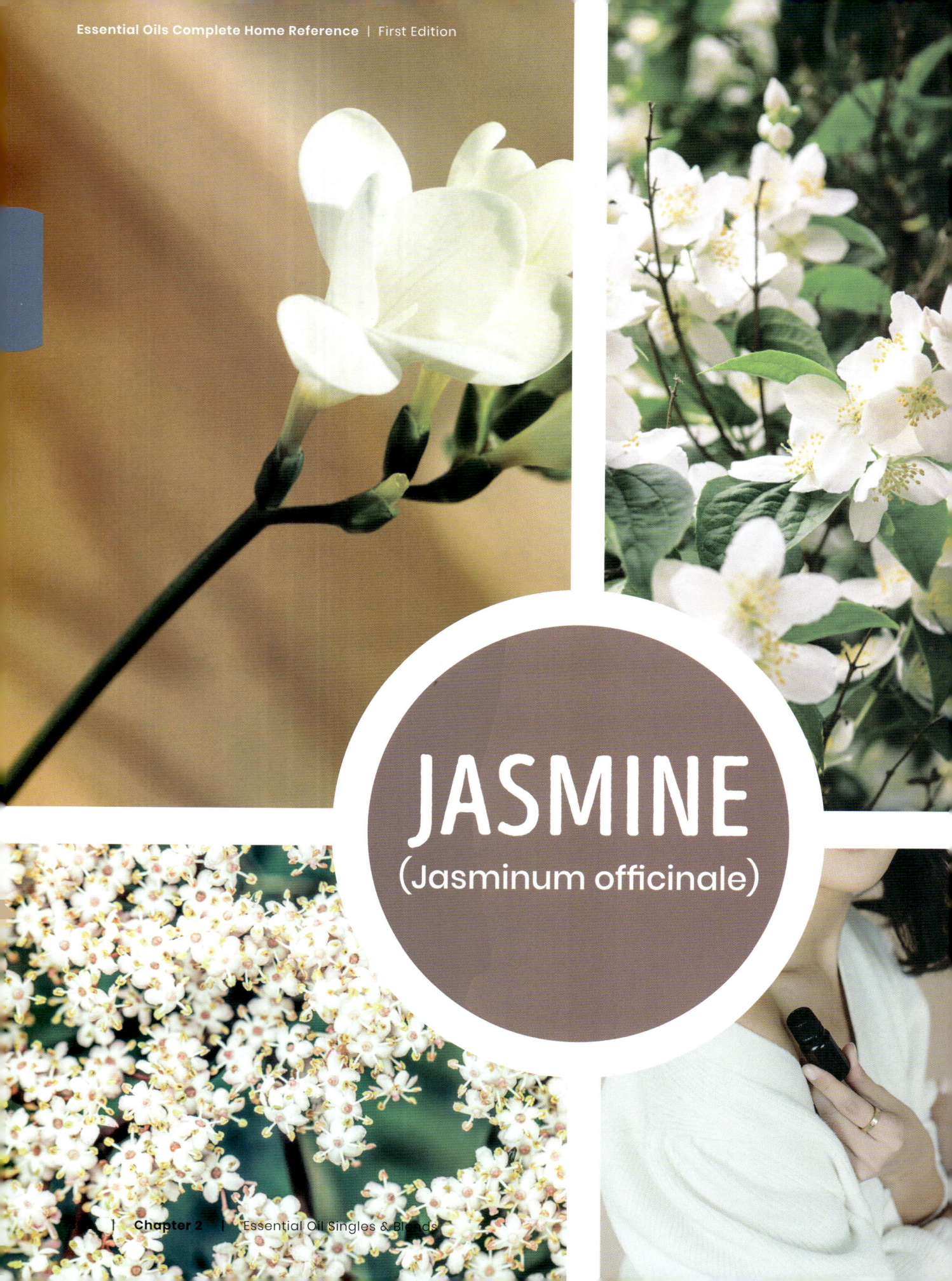

Essential Oils Complete Home Reference | First Edition

JASMINE
(Jasminum officinale)

Chapter 2 | Essential Oil Singles & Blends

BOTANICAL FAMILY:
Oleaceae

PLANT ORIGIN:
Egypt

EXTRACTION METHOD:
Absolute extraction from flower

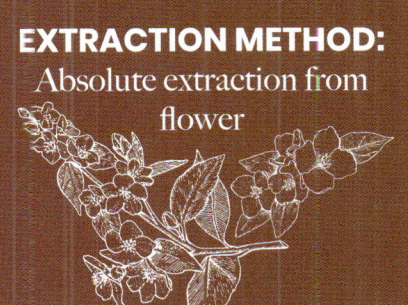

KEY CONSTITUENTS:
Benzyl Benzoate (4-32%), Benzyl Acetate (14-31%), Phytol (3-18%), Isophytol (3-11%), Linalool (2-11%), Phytyl Acetate (3-9%), Cis-Jasmone (up to 7%), Geranyl Linalol (up to 7%), Indole (up to 5%)

HISTORICAL DATA:

Jasmine is nicknamed the "queen of the night" and "moonlight of the grove." For centuries, women have treasured jasmine for its beautiful, seductive fragrance. It is an absolute, or essence, rather than an essential oil.
Note: One pound of Jasmine oil requires about 1,000 pounds of jasmine or 3.6 million fresh, unpacked blossoms. The blossoms must be collected before sunrise, or much of the fragrance will have evaporated. The quality of the blossoms may also be compromised if they are crushed. A single pound of pure Jasmine oil may cost between $1,200 and $4,500. In contrast, synthetic jasmine oils can be obtained for $3.50 per pound, but they do not possess the therapeutic qualities of the pure oil.

MEDICAL PROPERTIES:
Antidepressant, stimulating, antibacterial, antiviral, antiseptic, aphrodisiac, antispasmodic, cicatrizant, sedative

USES:
Anxiety, depression, menstrual problems/PMS, may improve lactation, menopause symptoms, skin problems (eczema, wrinkles, greasy), frigidity, uplifting, food ingredient, perfume, sedating

FRAGRANT INFLUENCE:
Uplifting, counteracts hopelessness, nervous exhaustion, anxiety, depression, indifference, and listlessness

DIRECTIONS:
Aromatic: 60. Topical: Neat. In case of sensitivity, dilute 2 drops in 15 ml of V-6.

CAUTIONS: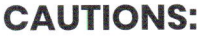

SELECTED RESEARCH:

Gunasekara T, Radhika N, Ragunathan KK, Gunathilaka D, Weerasekera MM, Hewageegana H, Arawwawala LADM, Fernando S. Determination of antimicrobial potential of five herbs used in Ayurveda practices against Candida albicans, Candida parapsilosis and Methicillin resistant Staphylococcus aureus. Anc Sci Life. 2017 Apr-Jun;36(4):187-90.

Kaviani M, Maghbool S, Azima S. Tabaei MH. Comparison of the effect of aromatherapy with Jasminum officinale and Salvia officinale on pain severity and labor outcome in nulliparous women. Iran J Nurs Midwifery Res. 2014 Nov;19(6):666-72.

Uniyal V, Saxena S, Bhatt RP. Screening of some essential oils against Trichosporon species. J Environ Biol. 2013 Jan;34(1):17-22.

Zhao G, Yin Z, Dong J. Antiviral efficacy against hepatitis B virus replication of oleuropein isolated from Jasminium officinale L. var. grandiflorum. J Ethnopharmacol. 2009 Sep 7;125(2):265-8. Epub 2009 Jul 4.

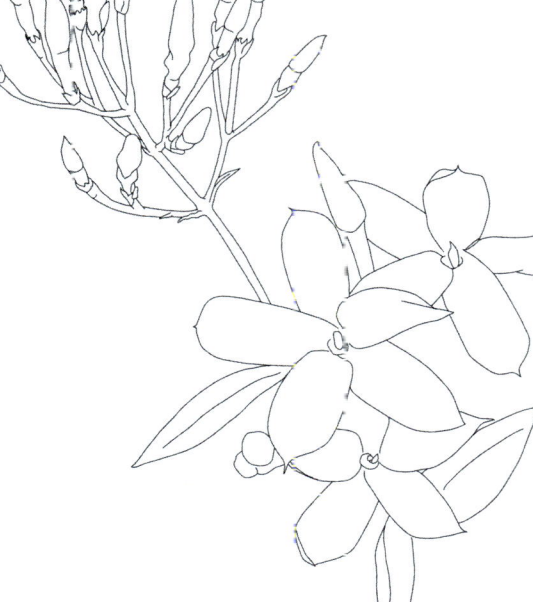

JOURNEY ON™
(Essential Oil Blend)

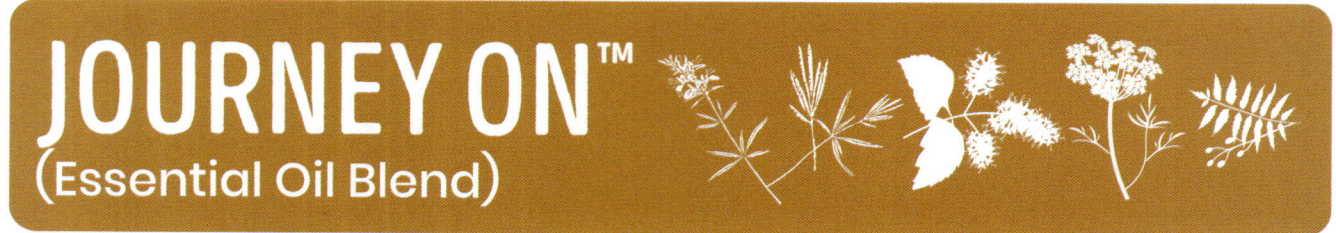

This special blend formulated by Gary encourages us to pick up his standard and Journey On. His mission of taking Young Living's pure essential oils to the world is our journey as well.

MEDICAL PROPERTIES & USES:
Anti-inflammatory, antimicrobial, antioxidative, emotion supporting, calming, cardiovascular supportive, digestion or elimination supportive/nausea reducing, disease inhibitory, muscle relaxant/bone-joint preservative, organ protective, pain or swelling reducing, performance enhancing/stimulating, respiratory system supportive, wellness supportive

INGREDIENTS:
Peppermint, Balsam Copaiba, Hyssop, Mountain Savory, Cistus, Camphor (Ravintsara), Frankincense, Oregano, Sacred Sandalwood, Tangerine, Ylang Ylang, Cinnamon Bark, Clove, Cumin, Black Pepper, Roman Chamomile, Bergamot, Anise, Juniper, Black Spruce, Geranium, Lavender, Dorado Azul, Blue Cypress, Davana, Citrus Hystrix, Jasmine, Matricaria (German Chamomile), Blue Tansy, Rose, Grapefruit, Spearmint, Lemon, Ocotea

DIRECTIONS:
Aromatic: 30. Topical: 20-80.

CAUTIONS:

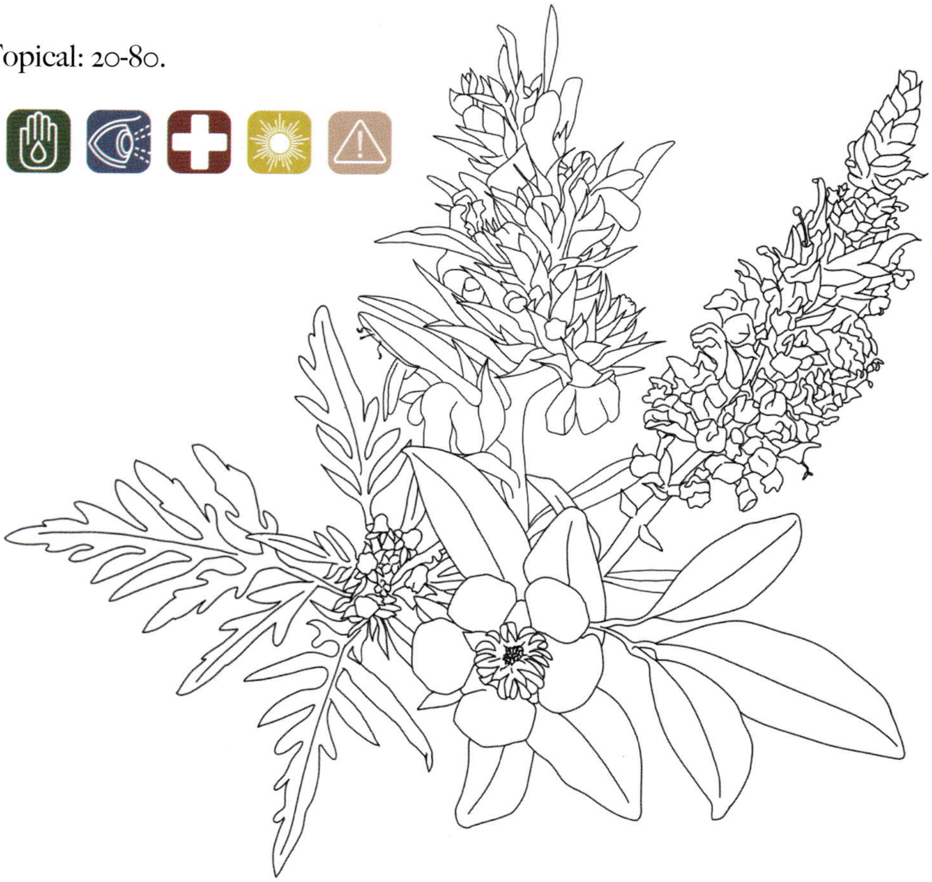

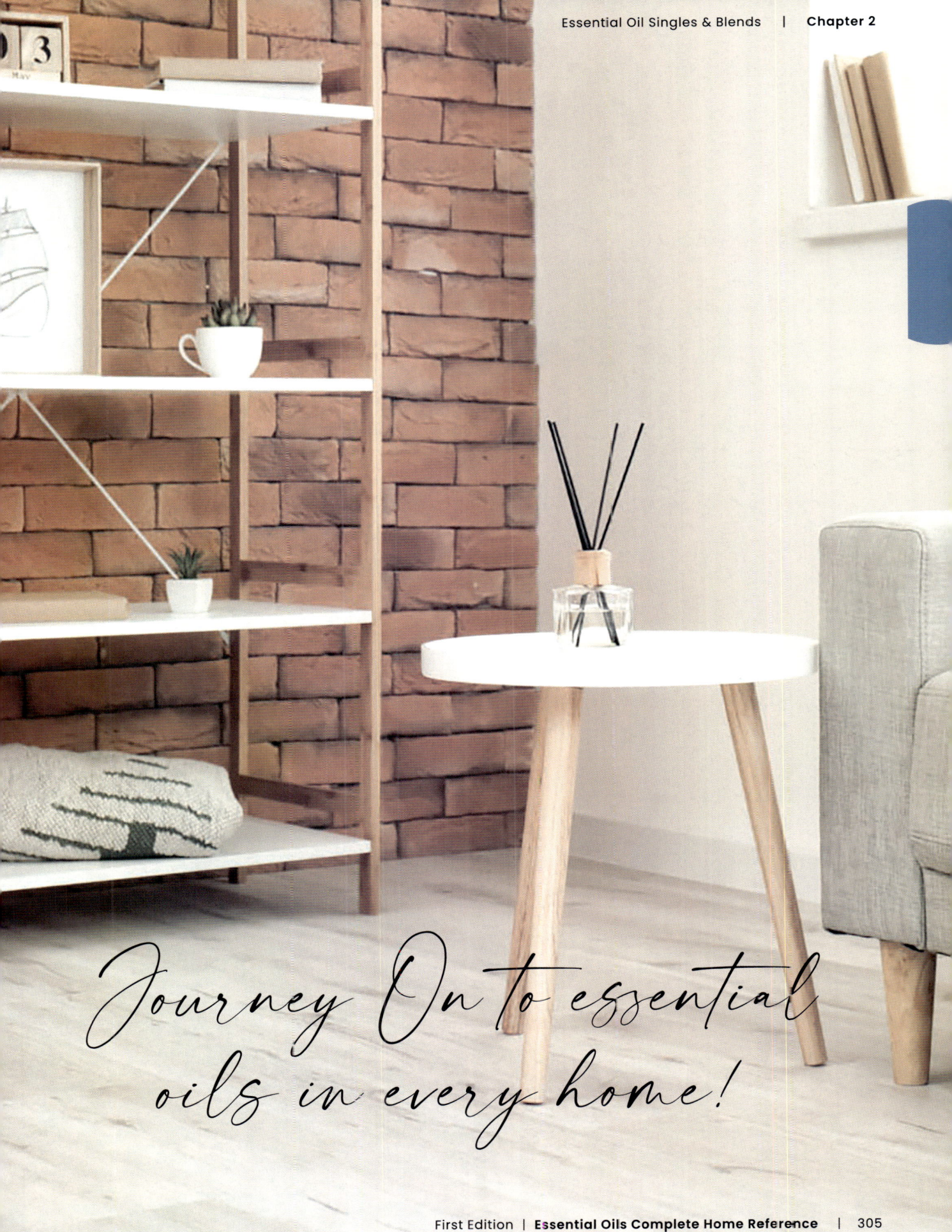

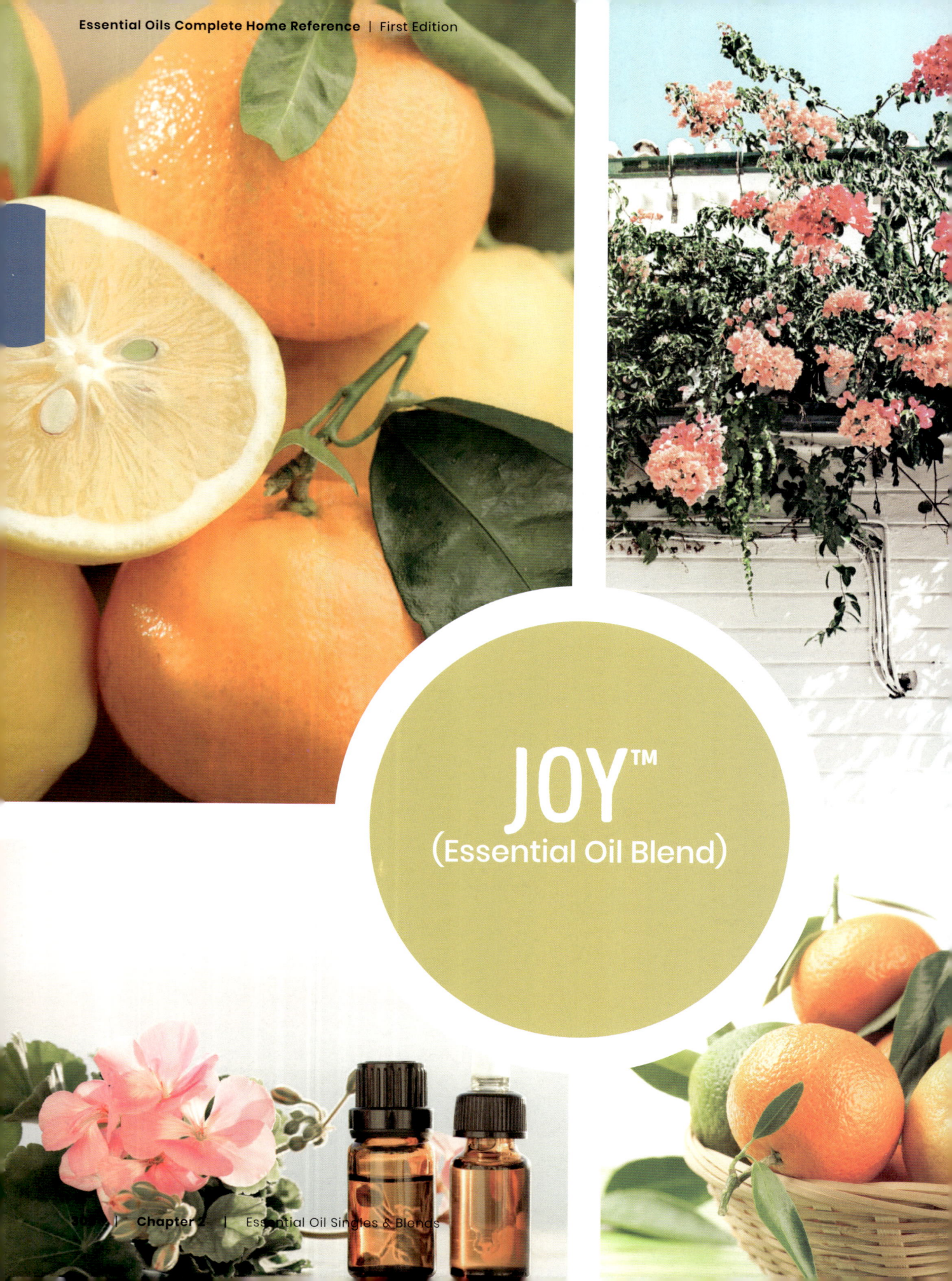

ABOUT JOY™:

This beautiful blend produces a magnetic energy that brings joy to the heart, mind, and soul. It inspires romance and helps overcome deep-seated grief and depression.

MEDICAL PROPERTIES & USES:

Anti-inflammatory, antimicrobial, antioxidative, emotion supporting, uplifting, calming, cardiovascular supportive, organ protective, pain or swelling reducing, skin and hair improving

INGREDIENTS:

Bergamot, Ylang Ylang, Geranium, Lemon, Coriander, Tangerine, Jasmine, Roman Chamomile, Palmarosa, Rose

DIRECTIONS:

Aromatic: 6o. Topical: Neat.

CAUTIONS: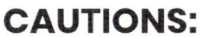

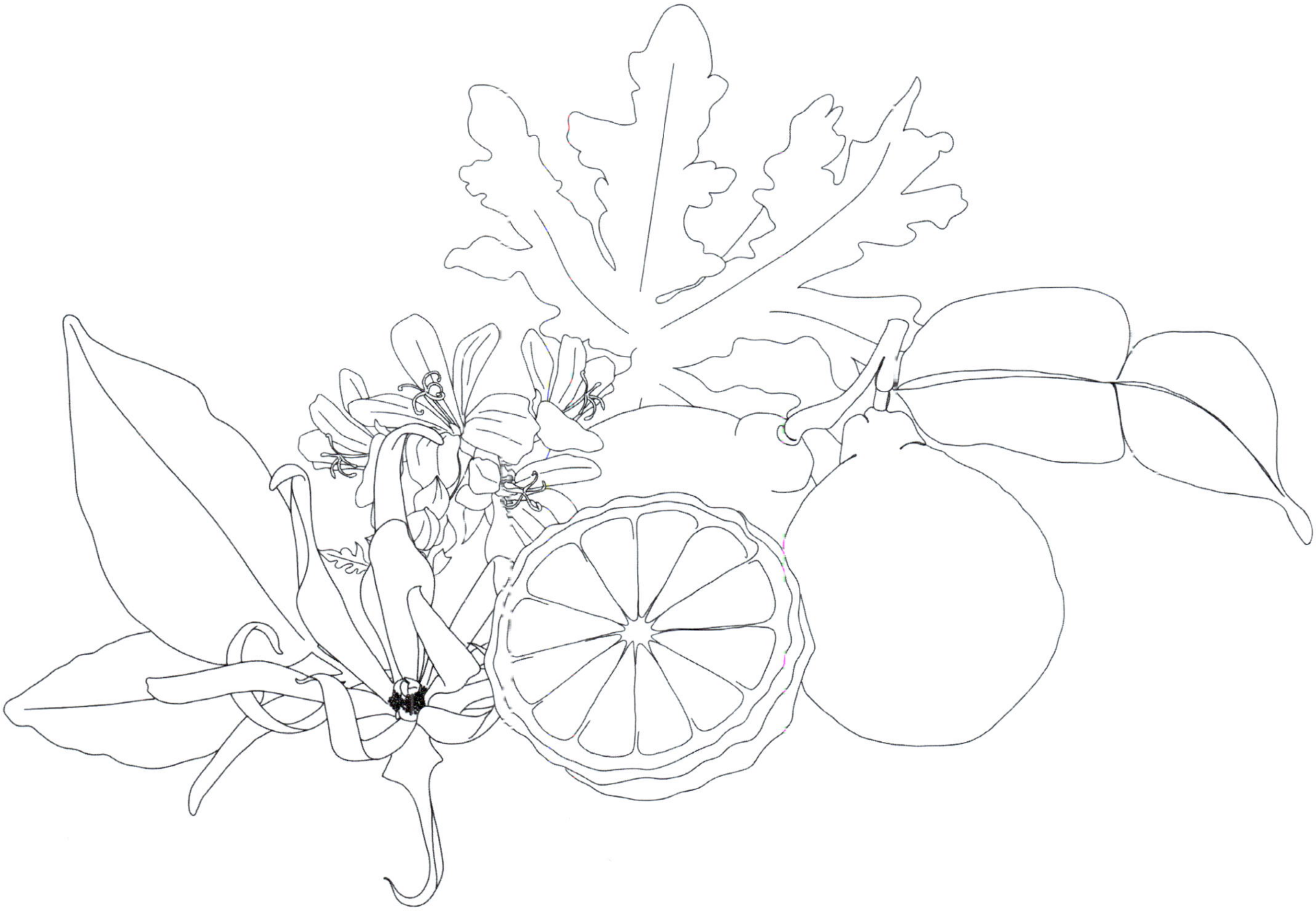

BOTANICAL FAMILY:
Cupressaceae

PLANT ORIGIN:
Croatia, USA, Utah

EXTRACTION METHOD:
Steam distilled from trunks/branches/leaves

KEY CONSTITUENTS:
Alpha-Pinene (15-35%), Widdrol + Cedrol (3-13%), Cis Thujopsene (5-12%), Bornyl Acetate (5-11%), Camphor (3-9%), Sabinene (1-7%), Limonene (2-6%)

JUNIPER
(Juniperus osteosperma)

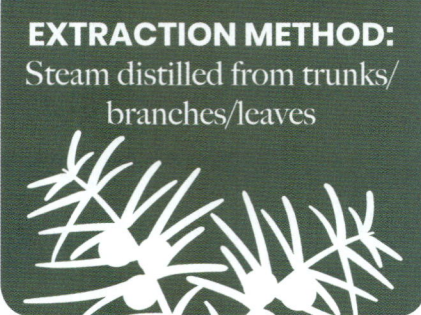

Bundles of juniper berries were hung over doorways to ward off witches during medieval times. Juniper has been used for centuries as a diuretic. Until recently, French hospital wards burned sprigs of juniper and rosemary to protect from infection.

MEDICAL PROPERTIES:
Antiseptic, digestive cleanser/stimulant, purifying, detoxifying, increases circulation through the kidneys and promotes excretion of toxins, promotes nerve regeneration

USES:
Skin conditions (eczema), liver problems, urinary/bladder infections, fluid retention

FRAGRANT INFLUENCE:
Evokes feelings of health, love, and peace and may help to elevate one's spiritual awareness

DIRECTIONS:
Aromatic: 30. Topical: 50-50.

CAUTIONS:

SELECTED RESEARCH:
Acuña UM, Atha DE, Ma J, Nee MH, Kennelly EJ. Antioxidant capacities of ten edible North American plants. Phytother Res. 2002 Feb;16(1):63-5.

Takácsová M, Pribela A, Faktorová M. Study of the antioxidative effects of thyme, sage, juniper and oregano. Nahrung. 1995;39(3):241-3.

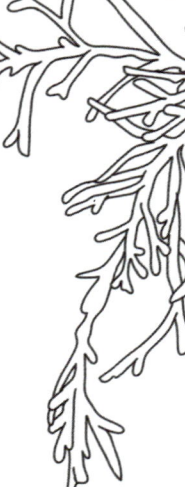

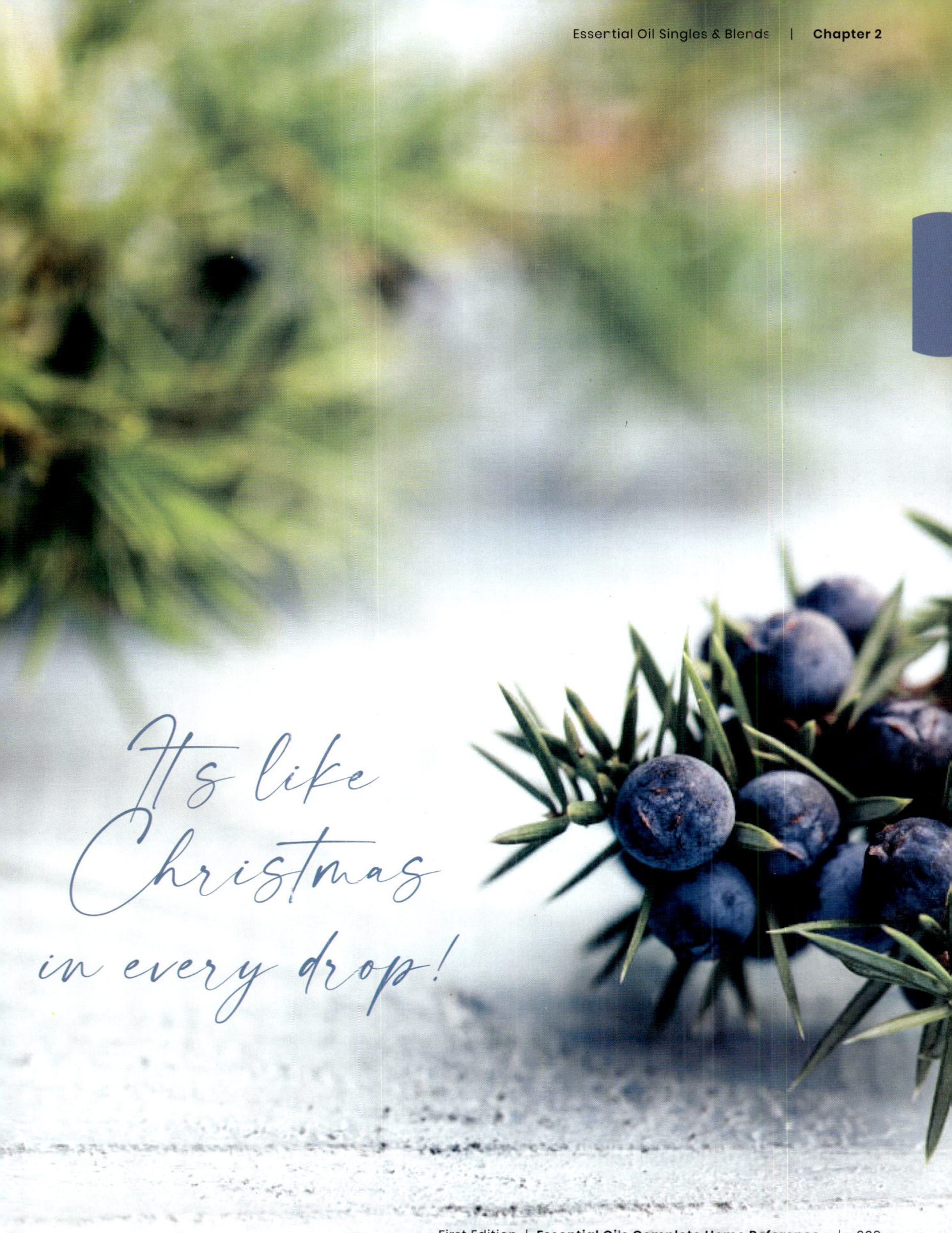

It's like Christmas in every drop!

JUVACLEANSE® & JUVACLEANSE® VITALITY®
(Essential Oil Blend)

The liver is the body's largest internal organ and major detoxifier. Even the toxins in the air we breathe are filtered by the liver, including chemicals from aerosol cleaners, paint, insect sprays, etc.; but eventually those filters need to be cleaned. The essential oils of Ledum, Celery Seed, and Helichrysum have long been known for their liver-cleansing properties. JuvaCleanse was clinically tested in 2003 for removing mercury from body tissues.

In 2003 a study conducted by Roger Lewis, MD, at the Young Life Research Clinic in Springville, Utah, evaluated the efficacy of Helichrysum, Ledum, and Celery Seed in treating cases of advanced Hepatitis C.

In one case, a 20-year-old male diagnosed with Hepatitis C had a viral count of 13,200. After taking two capsules (approx. 750 mg each) of JuvaCleanse per day for one month with no other intervention, the patient's viral count dropped more than 80 percent to 2,580.

MEDICAL PROPERTIES & USES:
Anti-inflammatory, antimicrobial, antioxidative, dietary, digestion or elimination supportive/nausea reducing, cleansing, disease inhibitory

INGREDIENTS:
Helichrysum, Ledum, Celery Seed

DIRECTIONS:
Aromatic: 3O. Topical: 50-50. Use with Raindrop Technique. Dietary (Vitality): Dilute 1 drop with 4 drops of V-6 or other pure carrier oil. Put in a capsule and take 1 daily or as needed.

CAUTIONS:

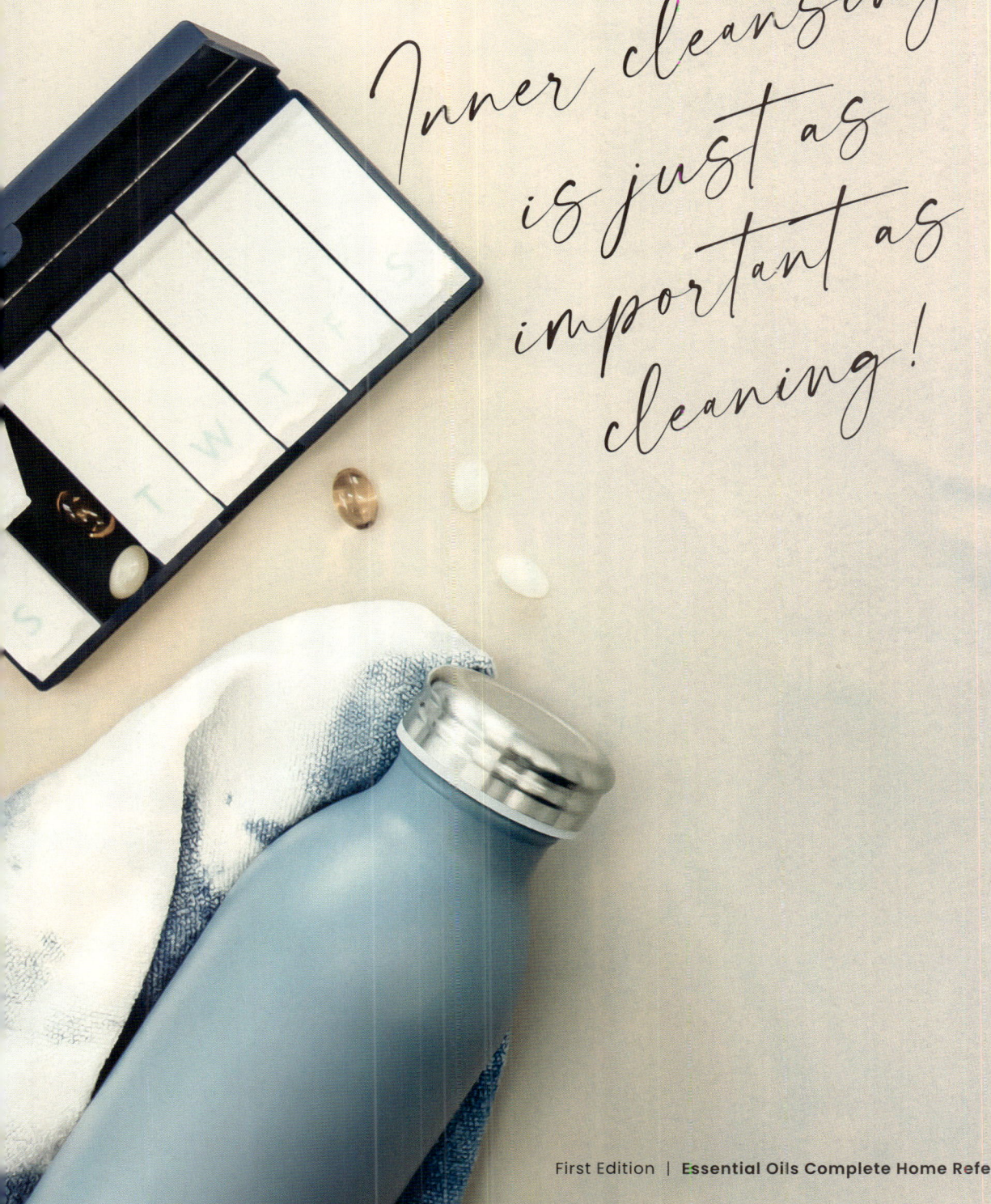

Inner cleansing is just as important as cleaning!

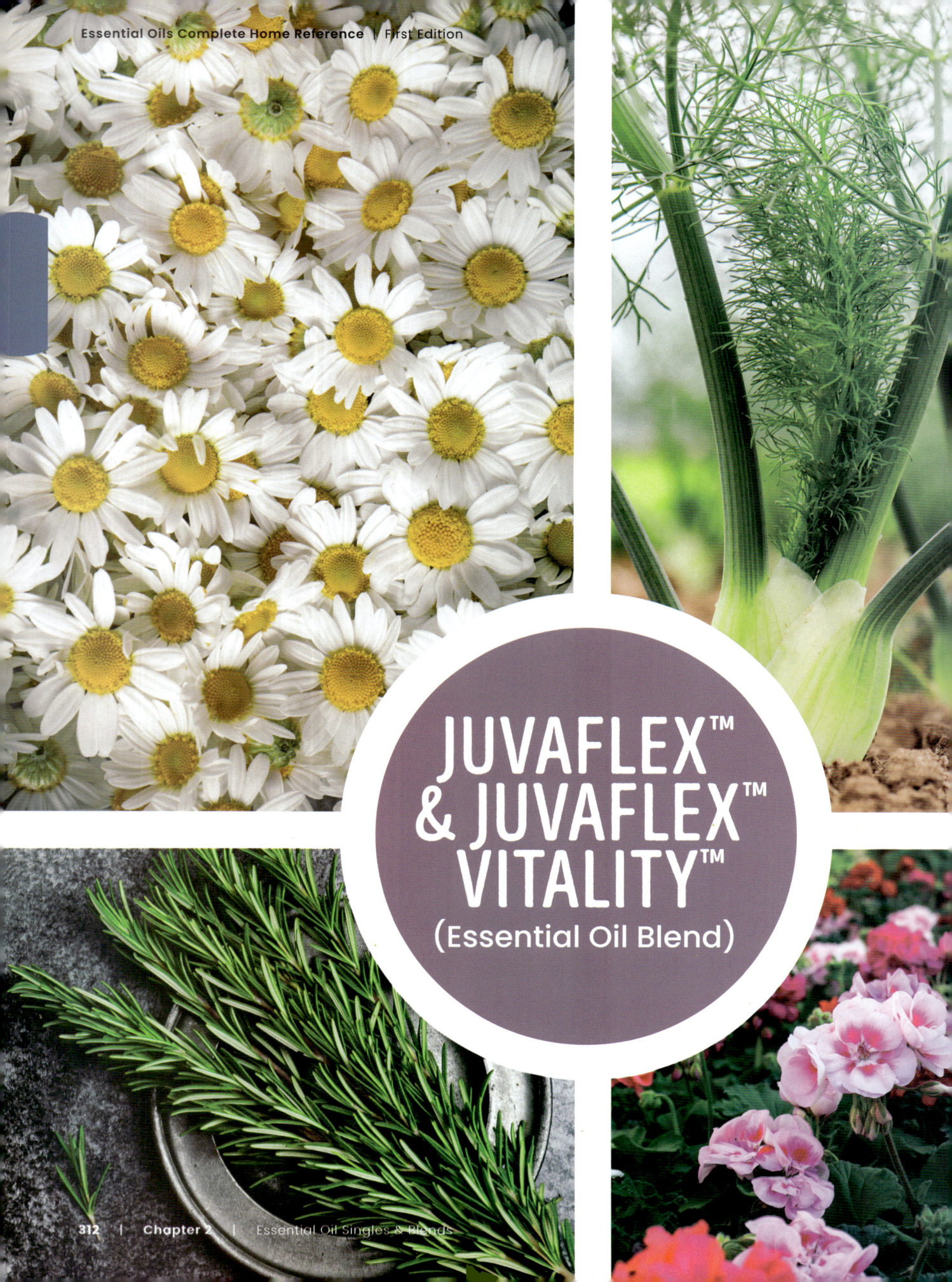

JUVAFLEX™ & JUVAFLEX VITALITY™
(Essential Oil Blend)

ABOUT JUVAFLEX™ & JUVAFLEX™ VITALITY™:

This blend helps with liver and lymphatic detoxification. The emotions of anger and hate create toxins that are stored in the liver, which can lead to sickness and disease. JuvaFlex helps break addictions to coffee, alcohol, drugs, and tobacco.

MEDICAL PROPERTIES & USES:

Anti-inflammatory, antimicrobial, antioxidative, addiction relieving, emotion supporting, calming, cardiovascular supportive, dietary, digestion or elimination supportive/nausea reducing, disease inhibitory, organ protective, pain or swelling reducing, performance enhancing/stimulating, respiratory system supportive, wellness supportive

INGREDIENTS:

Sesame seed oil, Fennel, Geranium, Rosemary, Roman Chamomile, Blue Tansy, Helichrysum

DIRECTIONS:

Aromatic: 30. Topical: Neat. Use a warm compress with 3-4 drops of oils with Ortho Sport or Ortho Ease massage oils. Dietary (Vitality): Put 2 drops in a capsule. Take 3 times daily or as needed.

CAUTIONS:

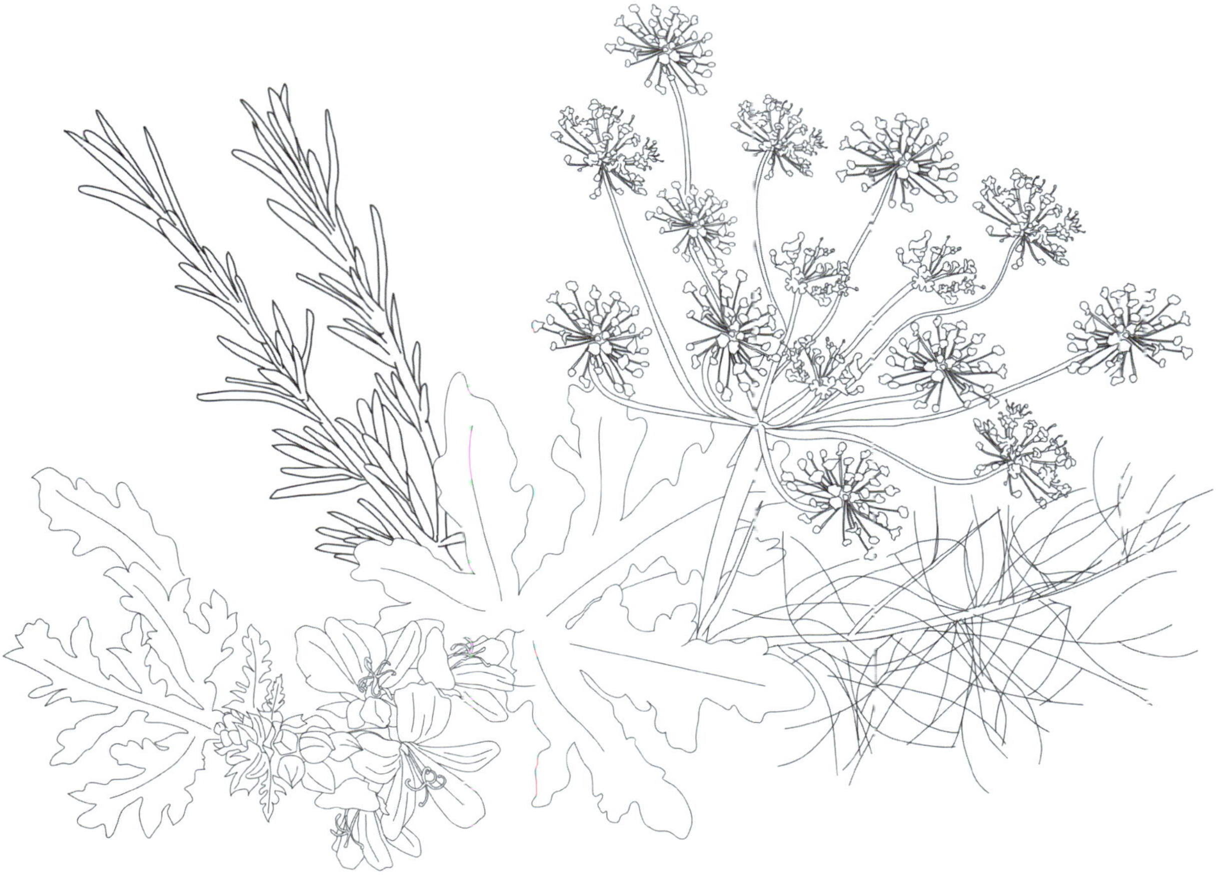

KIDSCENTS® GENEYUS™ & KIDSCENTS® GENEYUS™ ROLL-ON
(Essential Oil Blend)

Diffuse KidScents GeneYus or use the roll-on to help minds focus and concentrate on projects.

MEDICAL PROPERTIES & USES:
Anti-inflammatory, antimicrobial, antioxidative, uplifting, calming, clarity of mind supportive, cardiovascular supportive, disease inhibitory, organ protective, performance enhancing/stimulating

INGREDIENTS:
Caprylic/capric triglyceride,† Sacred Frankincense, Blue Cypress, Cedarwood, Idaho Blue Spruce, Melissa, Palo Santo, Northern Lights Black Spruce, Sweet almond oil,† Vetiver, Bergamot, Myrrh, Geranium, Sacred Sandalwood, Ylang Ylang, Coriander, Black Spruce, Hyssop, Rose

DIRECTIONS:
Aromatic: 6o. Topical: Neat. Recommended application is for children ages 2-12. To be applied only by a trusted adult or under adult supervision.

CAUTIONS: 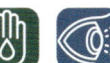 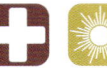   **Allergen Warnings: Contains coconut product.**

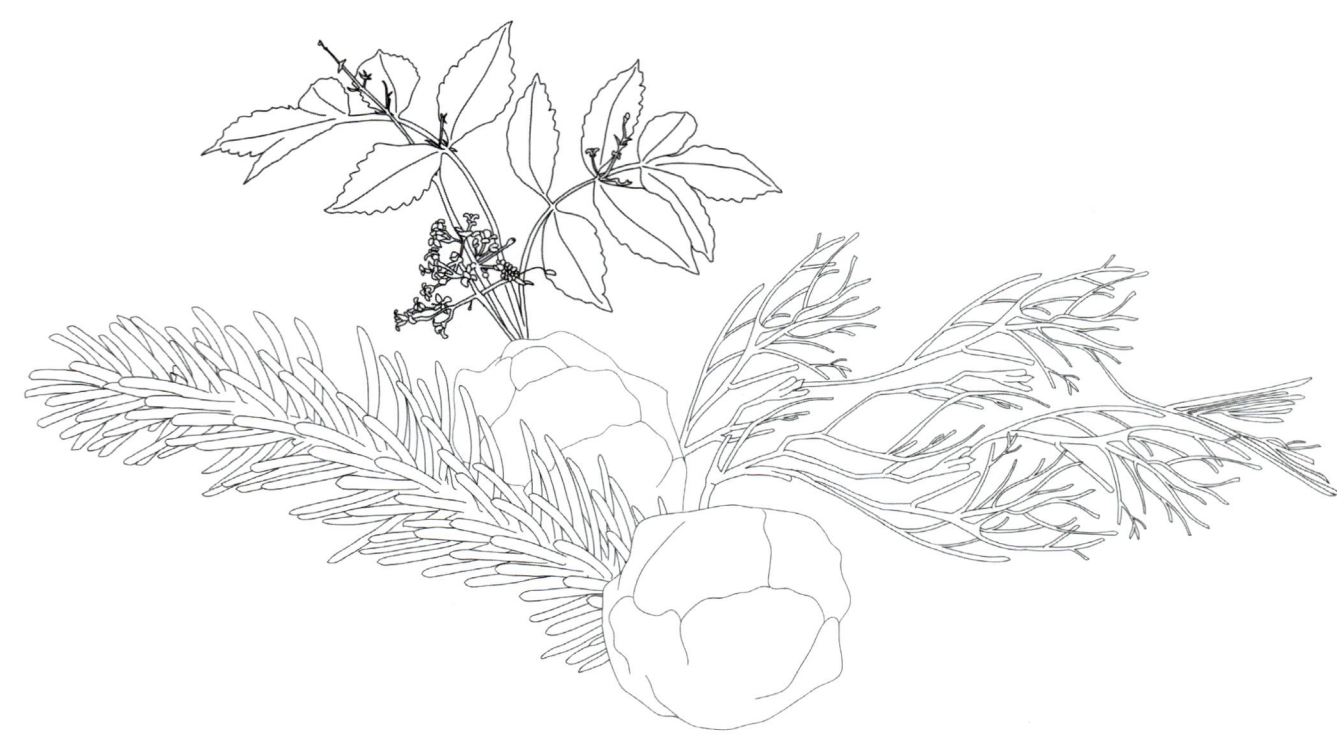

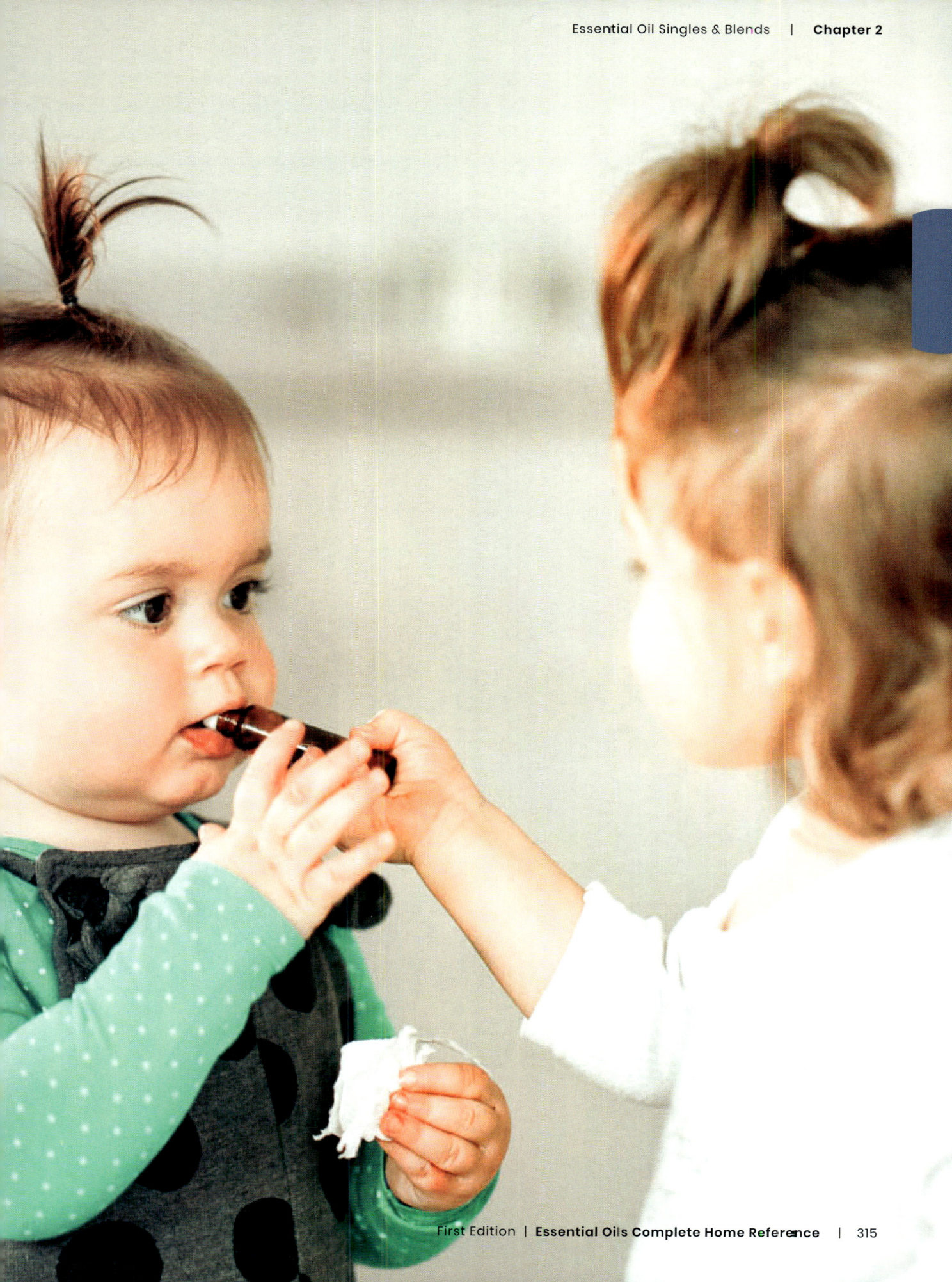

KIDSCENTS® KIDPOWER™ & KIDSCENTS® KIDPOWER™ ROLL-ON
(Essential Oil Blend)

KidPower is a unique, everyday blend formulated to help inspire feelings of confidence, courage, and positivity at home, at school, or at play. Apply KidPower on your children's wrists or back of their necks to inspire, motivate, and empower them for their best day every day or diffuse daily to promote feelings of courage and inspire positivity to help them find their power within.

MEDICAL PROPERTIES & USES:
Promotes peaceful feelings, prompts spiritual feelings, balances the senses, energizes, relaxes, promotes a comforting environment, uplifting

INGREDIENTS:
Fractionated coconut oil,† Orange, Vanilla, Black Spruce, Ho Wood, Blue Tansy, Frankincense, Geranium

DIRECTIONS:
Aromatic: 6o. Topical: Neat. Recommended application is for children ages 2-12. To be applied only by a trusted adult or under adult supervision.

CAUTIONS: Allergen Warnings: Contains coconut product.

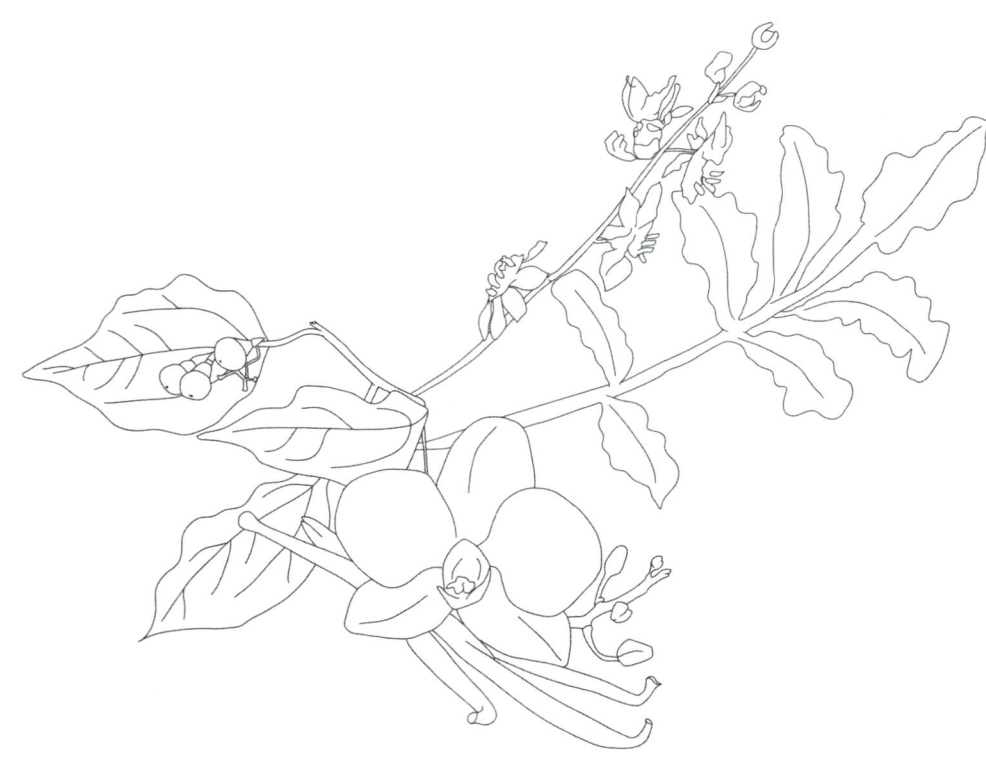

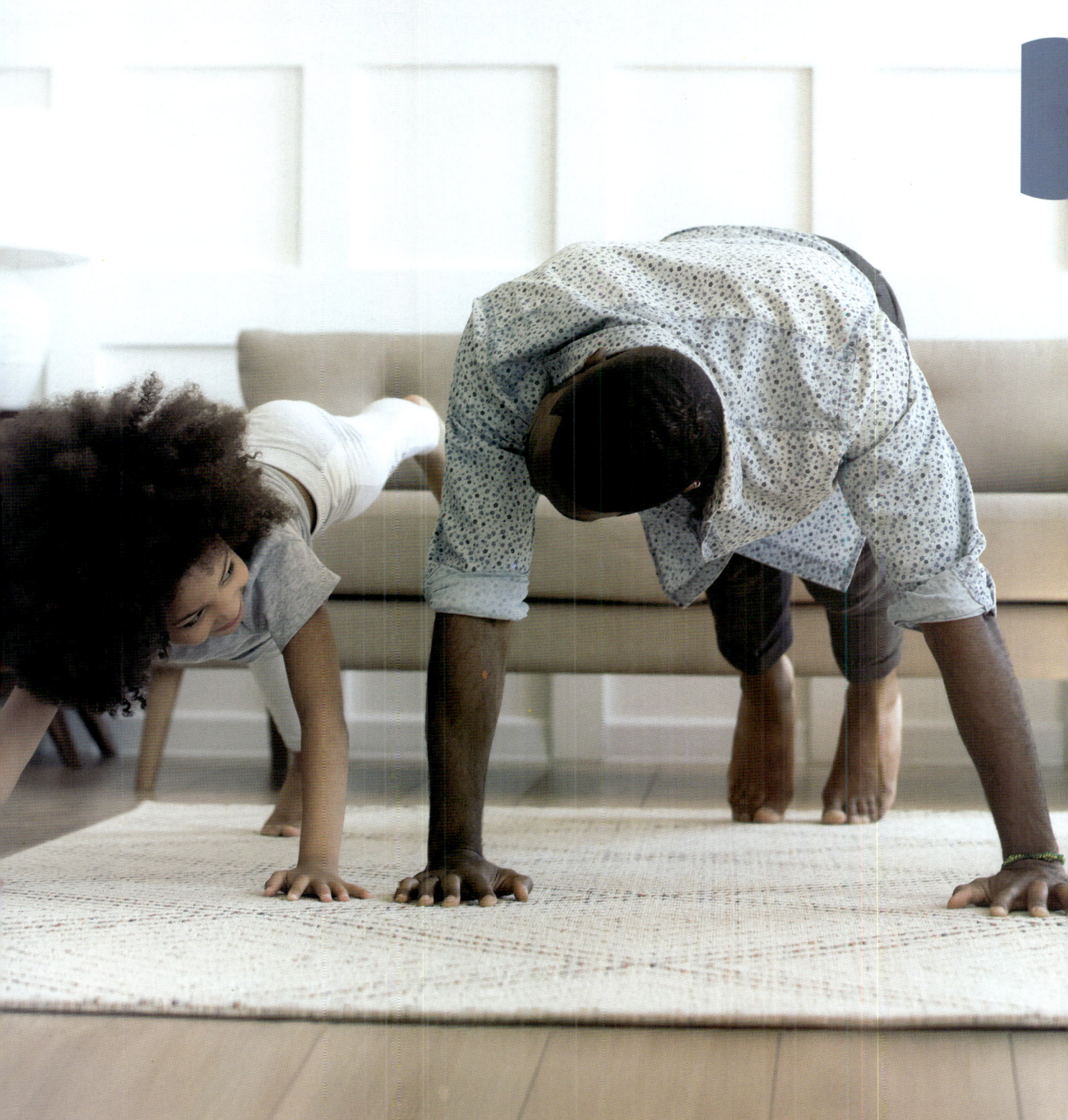

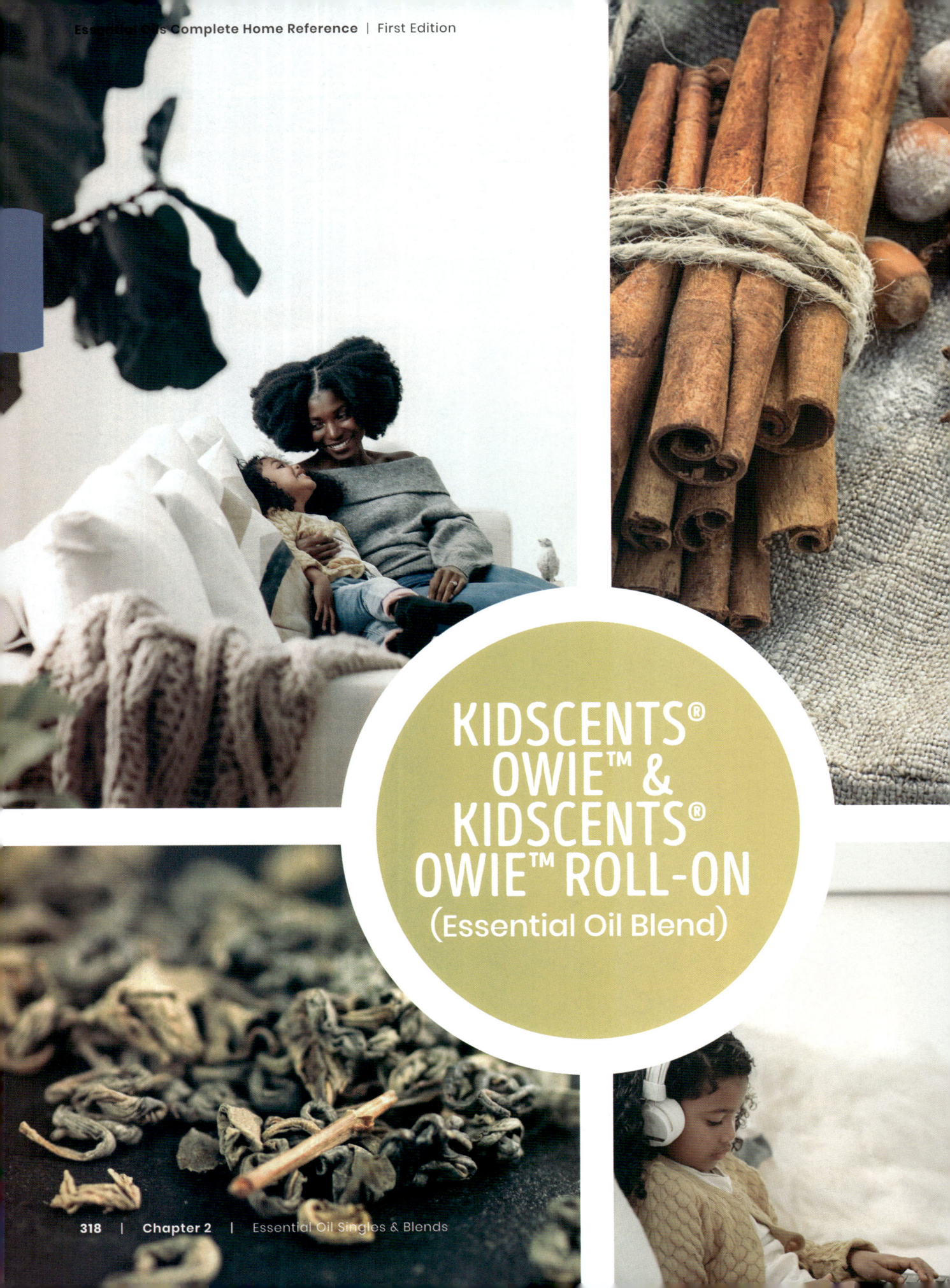

Chapter 2 | Essential Oil Singles & Blends

ABOUT KIDSCENTS® OWIE™ & KIDSCENTS® OWIE™ ROLL-ON

Apply Owie topically to improve the appearance of your child's skin and to help heal a wound.

MEDICAL PROPERTIES & USES:
Anti-inflammatory, antimicrobial, antioxidative, cardiovascular supportive, pain or swelling reducing, skin improving, wellness supportive

INGREDIENTS:
Caprylic/capric triglycerides, Idaho Grand Fir, Tea Tree, Helichrysum, Elemi, Cistus, Clove

DIRECTIONS:
Aromatic: 6o. Topical: Neat. Recommended application is for children ages 2-12. To be applied only by a trusted adult or under adult supervision.

CAUTIONS: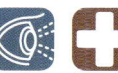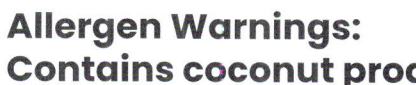

Allergen Warnings: Contains coconut product.

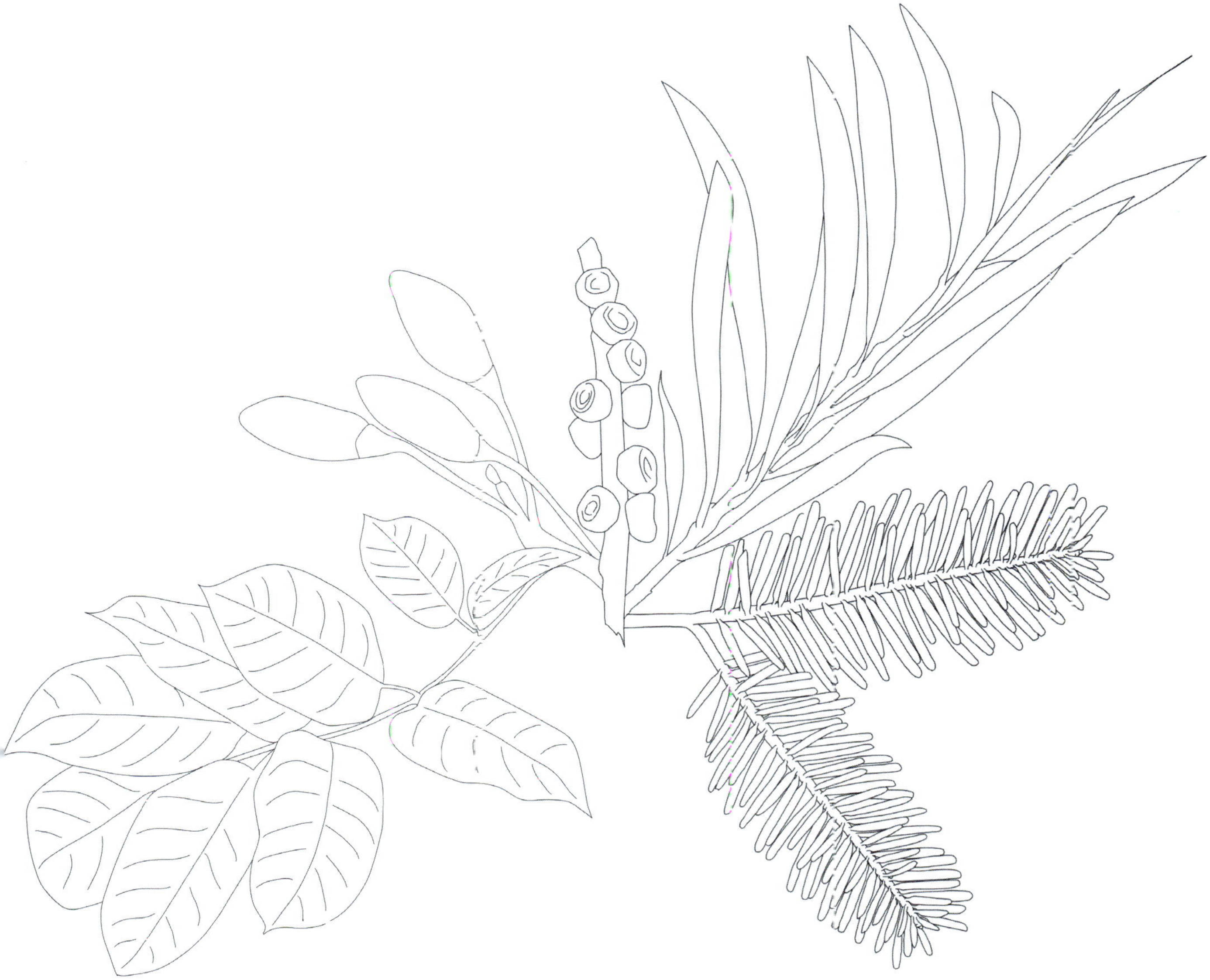

KIDSCENTS® SLEEPYIZE™ & KIDSCENTS® SLEEPYIZE™ ROLL-ON
(Essential Oil Blend)

SleepyIze calms and relaxes the mind and body prior to children's bedtime.

MEDICAL PROPERTIES & USES:

Anti-inflammatory, antimicrobial, antioxidative, calming, disease inhibitory, glandular/hormonal support, performance enhancing/stimulating, sleep improving

INGREDIENTS:

Caprylic/capric glycerides,‡ Lavender, Geranium, Roman Chamomile, Bergamot, Tangerine, Sacred Frankincense, Valerian, Rue

DIRECTIONS:

Aromatic: 6o Topical: Neat. Recommended application is for children ages 2-12. To be applied only by a trusted adult or under adult supervision.

CAUTIONS:

Do not use this product if you are pregnant, planning a pregnancy, or could possibly be pregnant.
Allergen Warnings:
Contains coconut product.

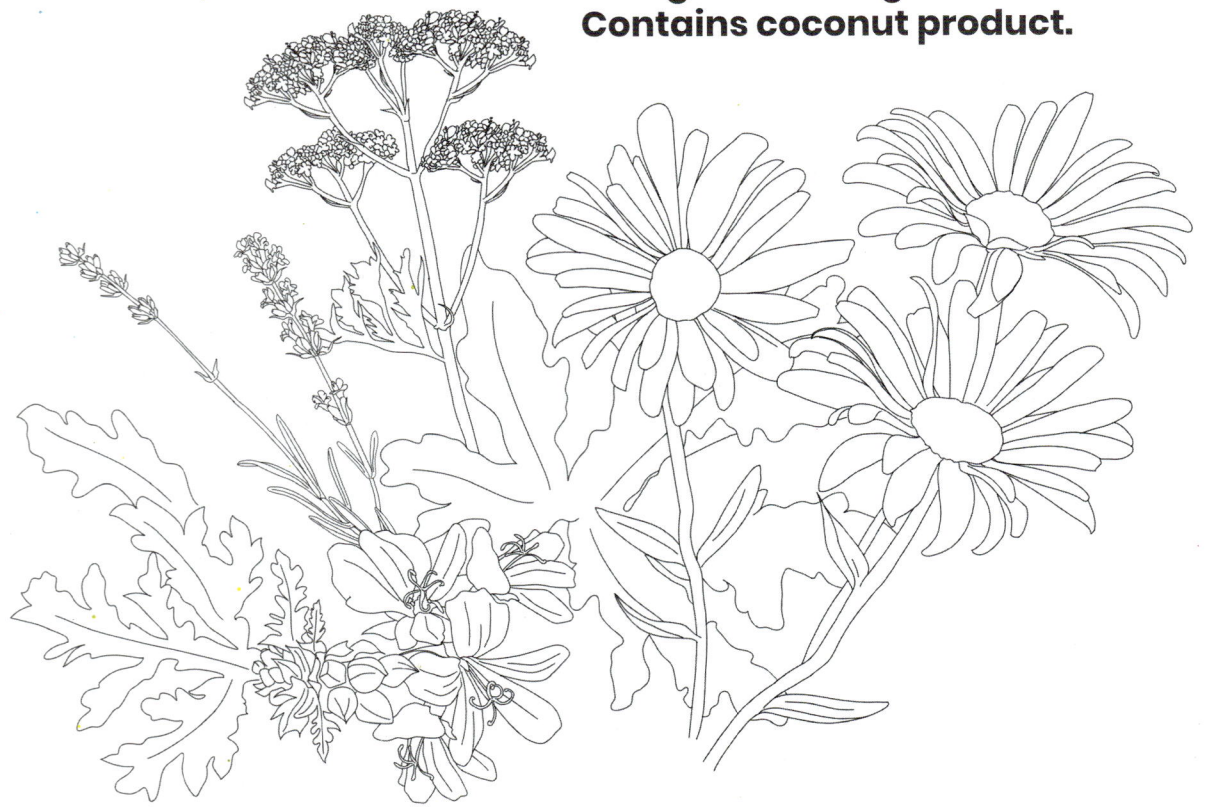

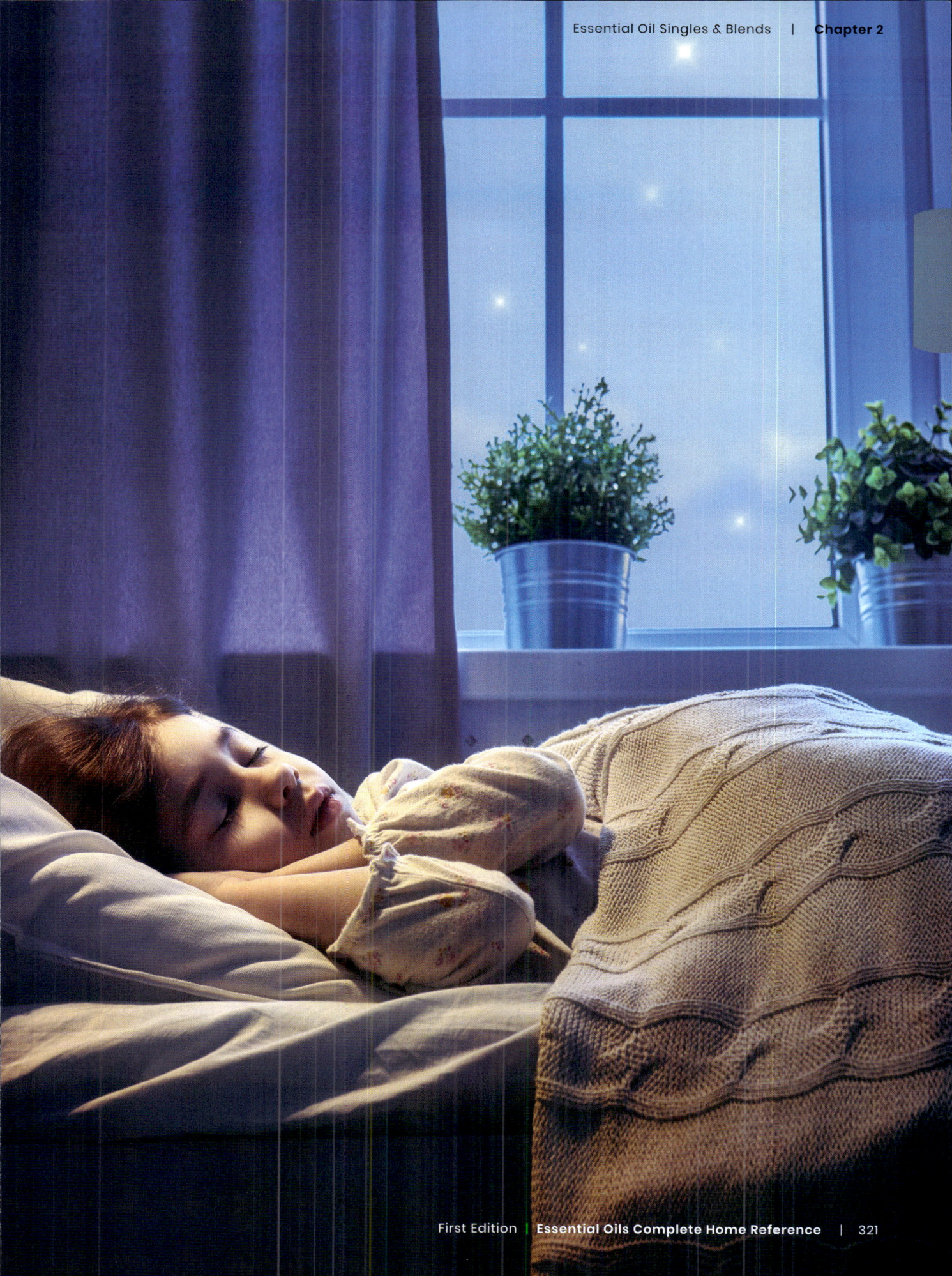

KIDSCENTS® SNIFFLEEASE™ & KIDSCENTS® SNIFFLEEASE™ ROLL-ON
(Essential Oil Blend)

SniffleEase is a refreshing, rejuvenating blend formulated just for kids for when they have congestion.

MEDICAL PROPERTIES & USES:

Supports respiratory function, expectorant, anti-inflammatory, antifungal, antiviral, antibacterial, calming, lymphatic stimulant, throat/lung/sinus infections, fluid retention, headaches

INGREDIENTS:

Caprylic/capric triglyceride,‡ Eucalyptus Blue, Palo Santo, Lavender, Dorado Azul, Camphor (Ravintsara), Eucalyptus Globulus, Myrtle, Pine, Marjoram, Eucalyptus Radiata, Eucalyptus Citriodora, Cypress, Black Spruce, Peppermint

DIRECTIONS:

Aromatic: 60. Topical: Neat. Recommended application is for children ages 2-12. To be applied only by a trusted adult or under adult supervision.

CAUTIONS: **Allergen Warnings: Contains coconut product.**

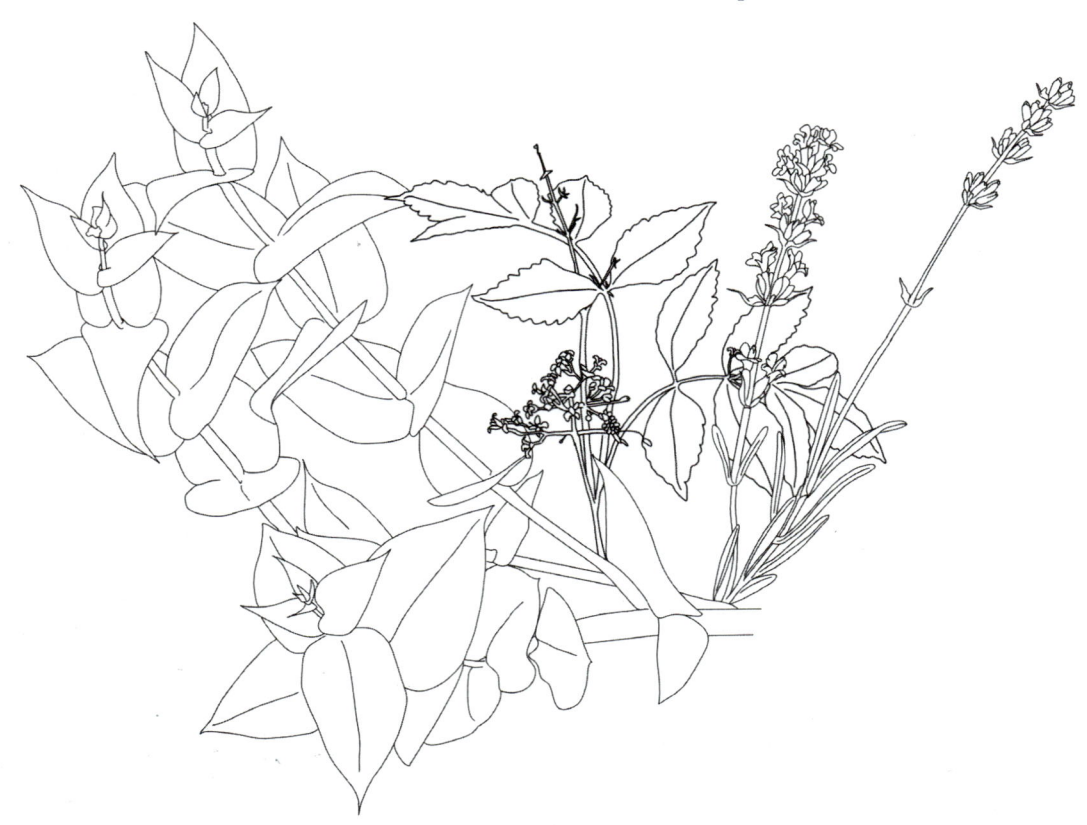

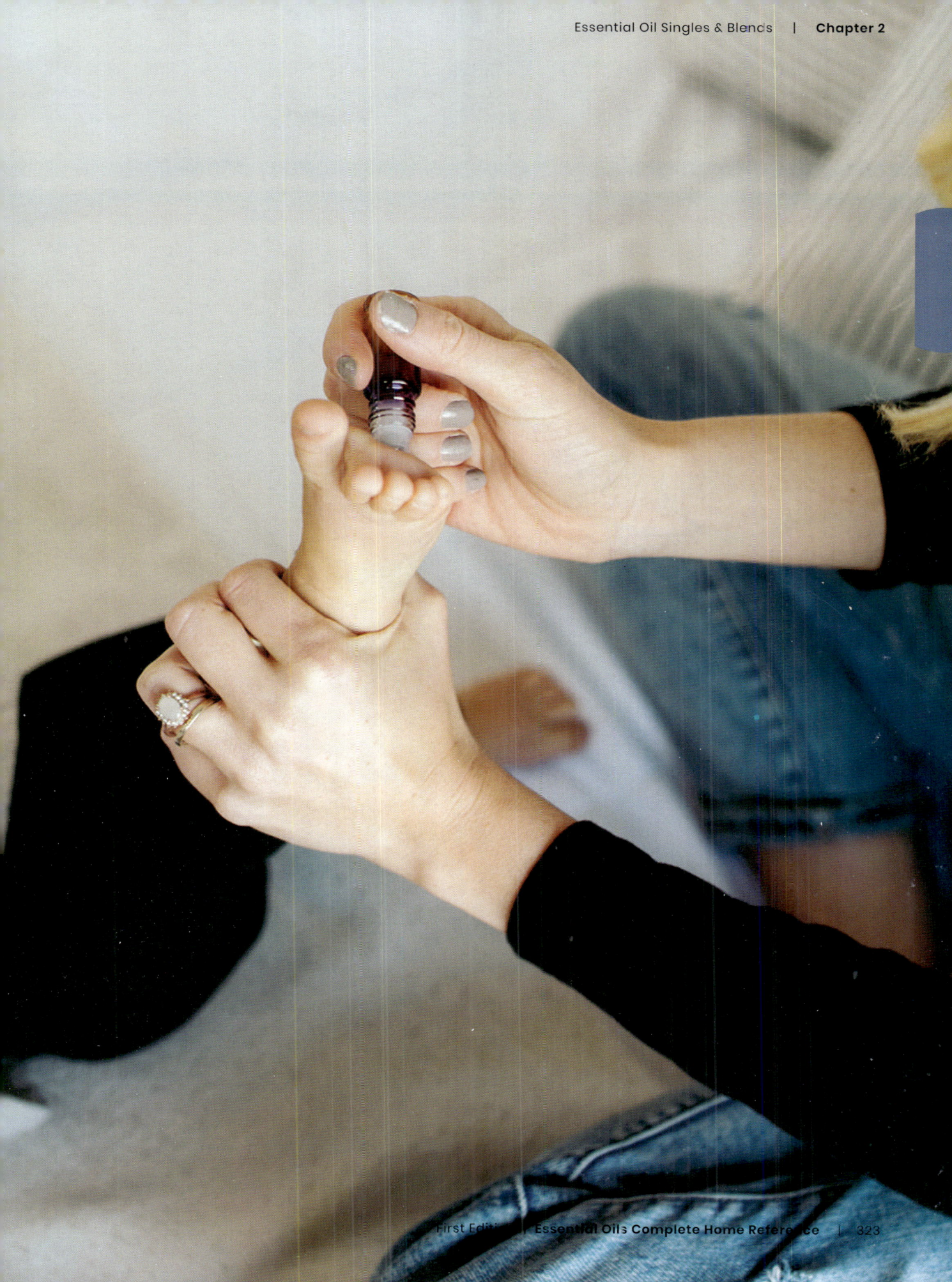

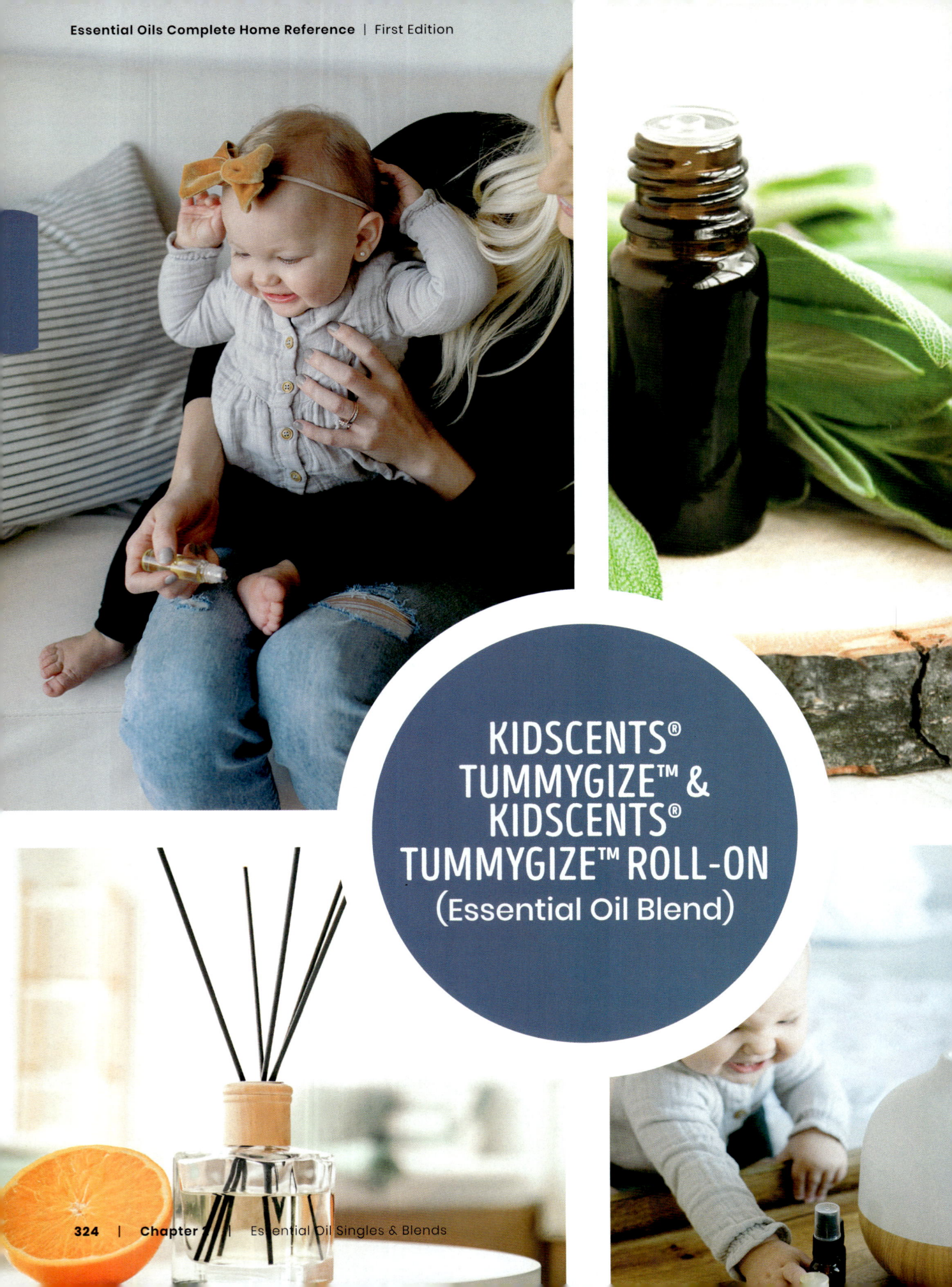

ABOUT KIDSCENTS TUMMYGIZE™ & KIDSCENTS TUMMYGIZE™™ ROLL-ON

TummyGize is a quieting, relaxing blend that can be applied to little tummies that are upset. It also supports proper digestion.

MEDICAL PROPERTIES & USES:
Calming, digestive or elimination supportive/nausea reducing, anti-inflammatory, mucolytic, antitumor, antispasmodic, antibacterial, increases metabolism, relaxant, circulatory enhancer, encourages energy

INGREDIENTS:
Caprylic/capric triglyceride,‡ Spearmint, Peppermint, Tangerine, Anise, Fennel, Cardamom, Ginger

DIRECTIONS:
Aromatic: 6o. Topical: Neat. Recommended application is for children ages 2-12. To be applied only by a trusted adult or under adult supervision.

CAUTIONS: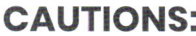

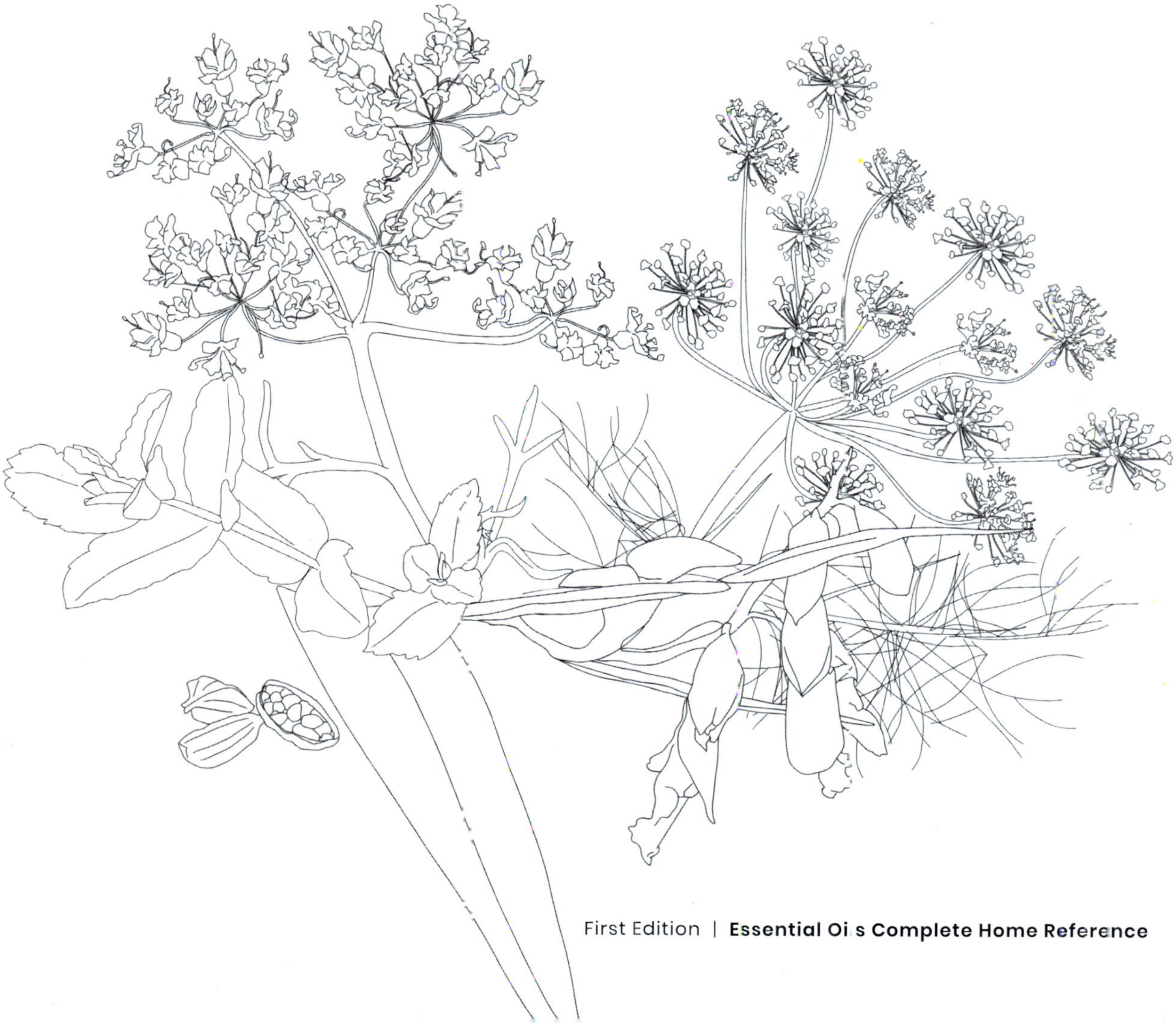

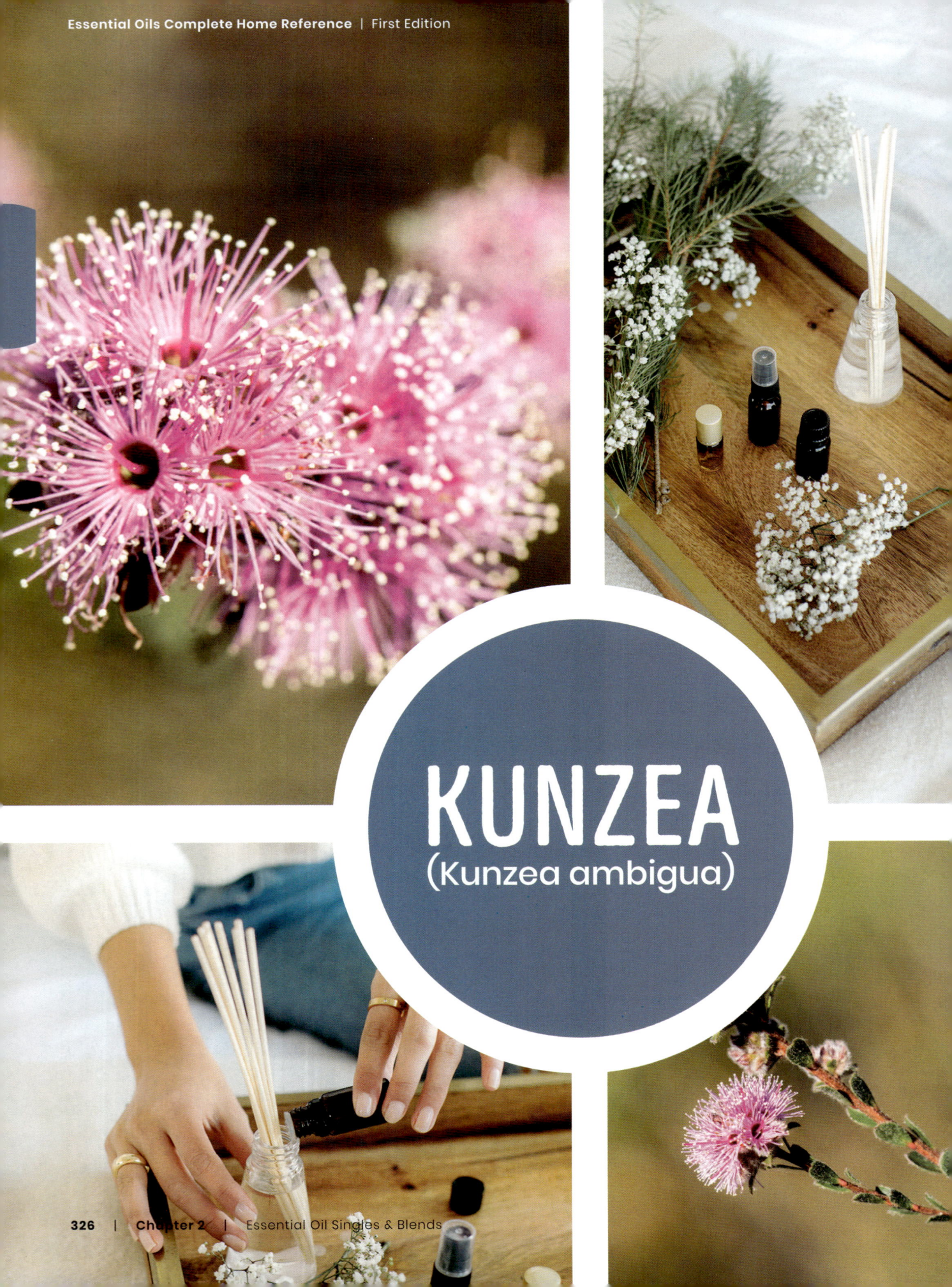

KUNZEA
(Kunzea ambigua)

Essential Oil Singles & Blends | Chapter 2

BOTANICAL FAMILY:
Myrtaceae

PLANT ORIGIN:
Australia

EXTRACTION METHOD:
steam distilled from leaves and branches

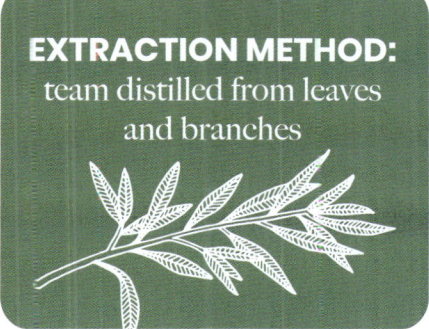

KEY CONSTITUENTS:
Alpha-Pinene (23-51%), Viridiflorol (10-22%), Eucalyptol (10-17%), Bicyclogermacrene (2-9%), Viridifloral (1-4%), Globulol (1-4%), Alpha-Terpineol (up to 3%), Citronellol (up to 2%), Allo-aromadedrene (up to 2%)

HISTORICAL DATA:
This shrub grows along the coasts of Australia and Tasmania. With narrow, green leaves and white, starburst flowers when it blooms, kunzea is sometimes called "white cloud." Australian Aboriginal communities traditionally used kunzea for relief from irritated skin, muscle tightness, and pain. Kunzea is registered with the Australian Therapeutic Administration (TGA) for providing temporary relief from arthritic pain. With several constituents similar to Tea Tree oil, Kunzea's aroma and effect on skin is milder.

MEDICAL PROPERTIES:
Antiviral, skin-supportive, insecticidal, antifungal, antiseptic, anti-inflammatory, antimicrobial

USES:
Appearance of blemishes, joint and muscle pain, dry skin

FRAGRANT INFLUENCE:
Uplifting, spicy, and woodsy aroma; purifies the air

DIRECTIONS:
Aromatic: 30. Topical: 50-50.

CAUTIONS:

SELECTED RESEARCH:

Powers CN, Satyal P, Mayo JA, McFeeters H, McFeeters RL. Bigger Data Approach to Analysis of Essential Oils and Their Antifungal Activity against Aspergillus niger, Candida albicans, and Cryptococcus neoformans. Molecules. 2019 Aug; 24(16): 2868. Published online 2019 Aug 7.

Park CG, Jang M, Shin E, Kim J. Myrtaceae plant essential oils and their β-triketone components as insecticides against Drosophila suzukii. Molecules. 2017 Jun 24;22(7).

Thomas J, Webb CE, Narkowicz C, Jacobson GA, Peterson GM, Davies NW, Russell RC. Evaluation of repellent properties of volatile extracts from the Australian native plant Kunzea ambigua against Aedes aegypti (Diptera: Culicidae). J Med Entomol. 2009 Nov;46(6):1387-91. Epub Dec 8.

Kasajima N, Ito H, Hatano T, Yoshida T. Phloroglucinol diglycosides accompanying hydrolyzable tannins from Kunzea ambigua. Phytochemistry. 2008 Dec;69(18):3080-3086.

Ito H, Kasajima N, Tokuda H, Nishino H, Yoshida T. Dimeric flavonol glycoside and galloylated C-glucosylchromones from Kunzea ambigua. J Nat Prod. 2004 Mar;67(3):411-5. Epub 2004 Mar 27.

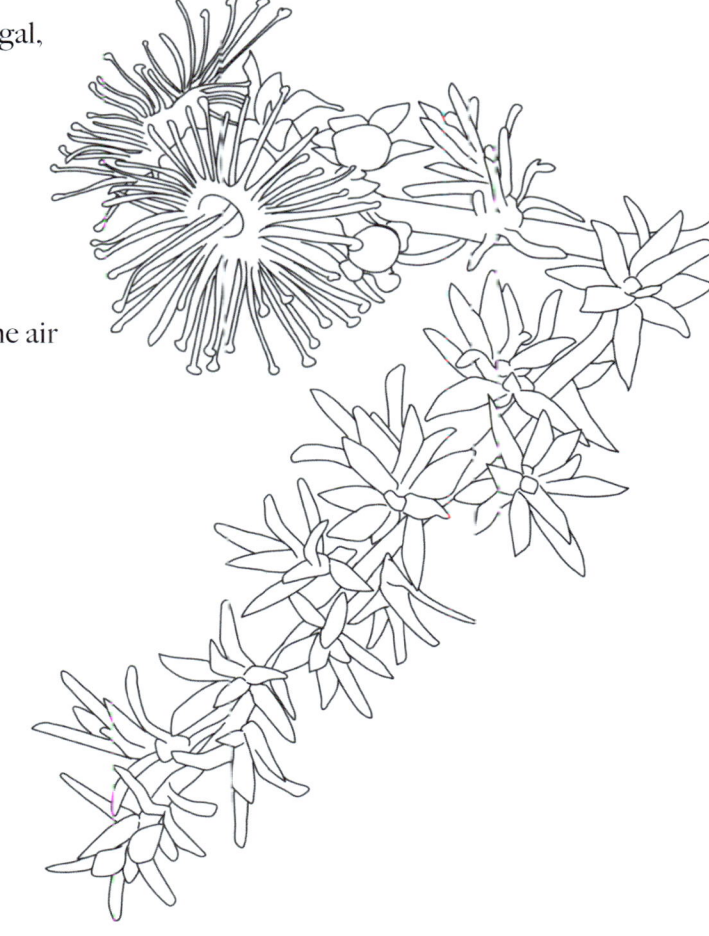

LADY SCLAREOL™
(Essential Oil Blend)

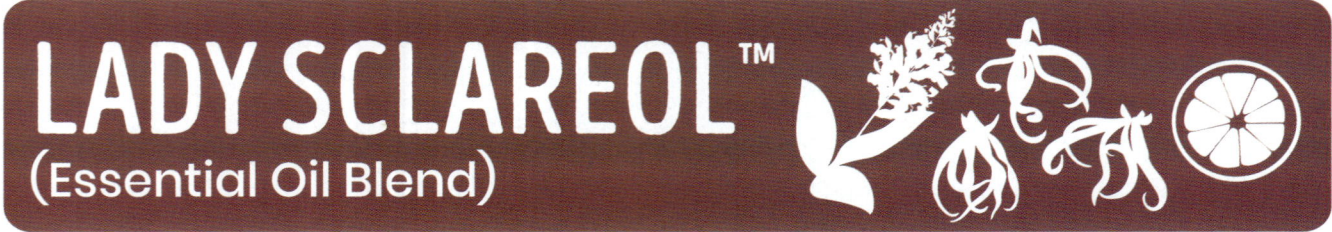

This oil, rich in phytoestrogens, is designed to be worn as an exquisite fragrance. It enhances the feminine nature by improving mood and raising estrogen levels. It may also provide relief for PMS symptoms.

MEDICAL PROPERTIES & USES:

Anti-inflammatory, antimicrobial, antioxidative, calming, disease inhibitory, insecticidal/antiparasitic, organ protective, pain or swelling reducing, performance enhancing, skin and hair improving

INGREDIENTS:

Geranium, Coriander, Vetiver, Orange, Clary Sage, Bergamot, Ylang Ylang, Royal Hawaiian Sandalwood, Spanish Sage, Jasmine, Idaho Blue Spruce, Spearmint

DIRECTIONS:

Aromatic: 6o. Topical: Neat. Apply 2-4 drops to Vita Flex points on the ankles, at the clavicle notch, to the abdomen for relief of premenstrual discomfort, or on desired location as needed.
Use as a fragrance.

CAUTIONS:

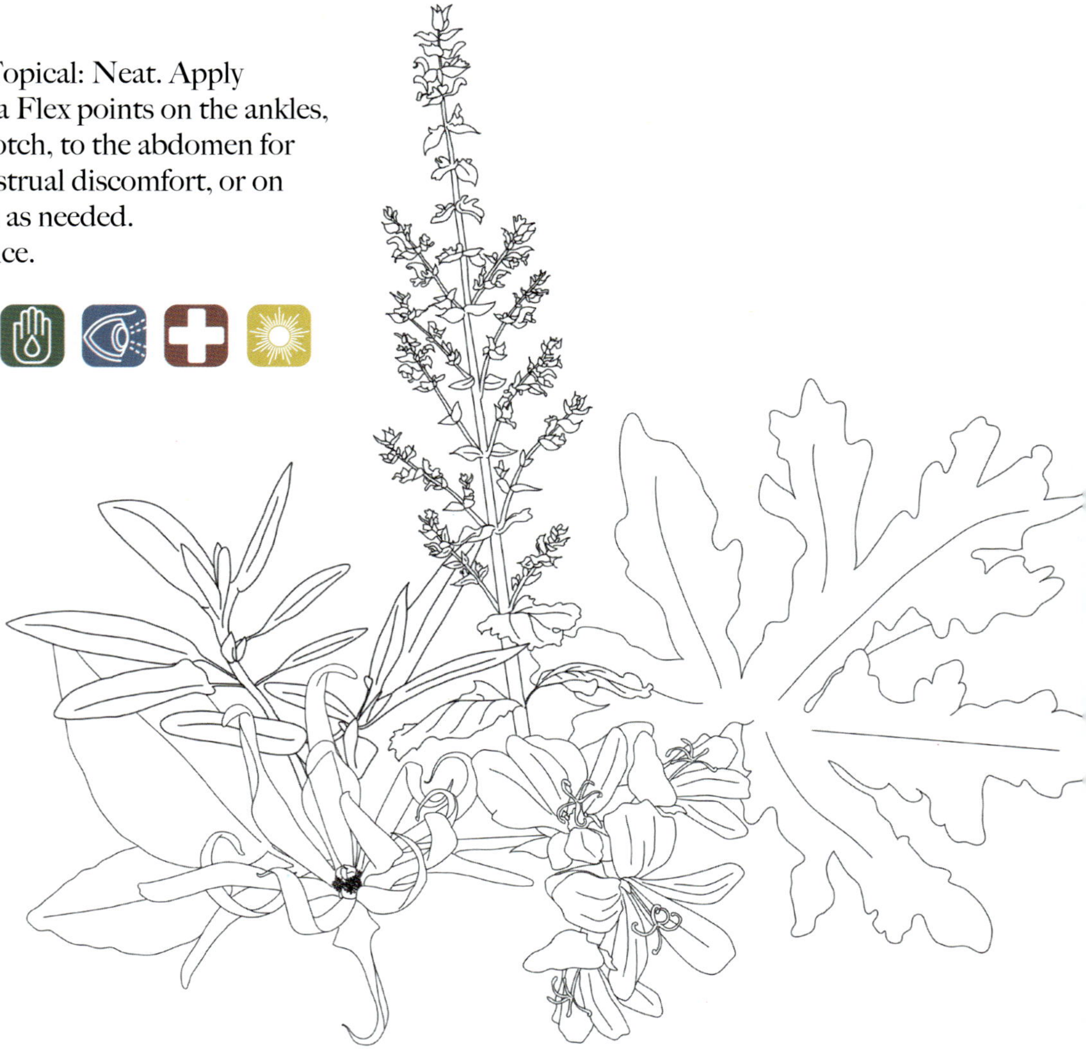

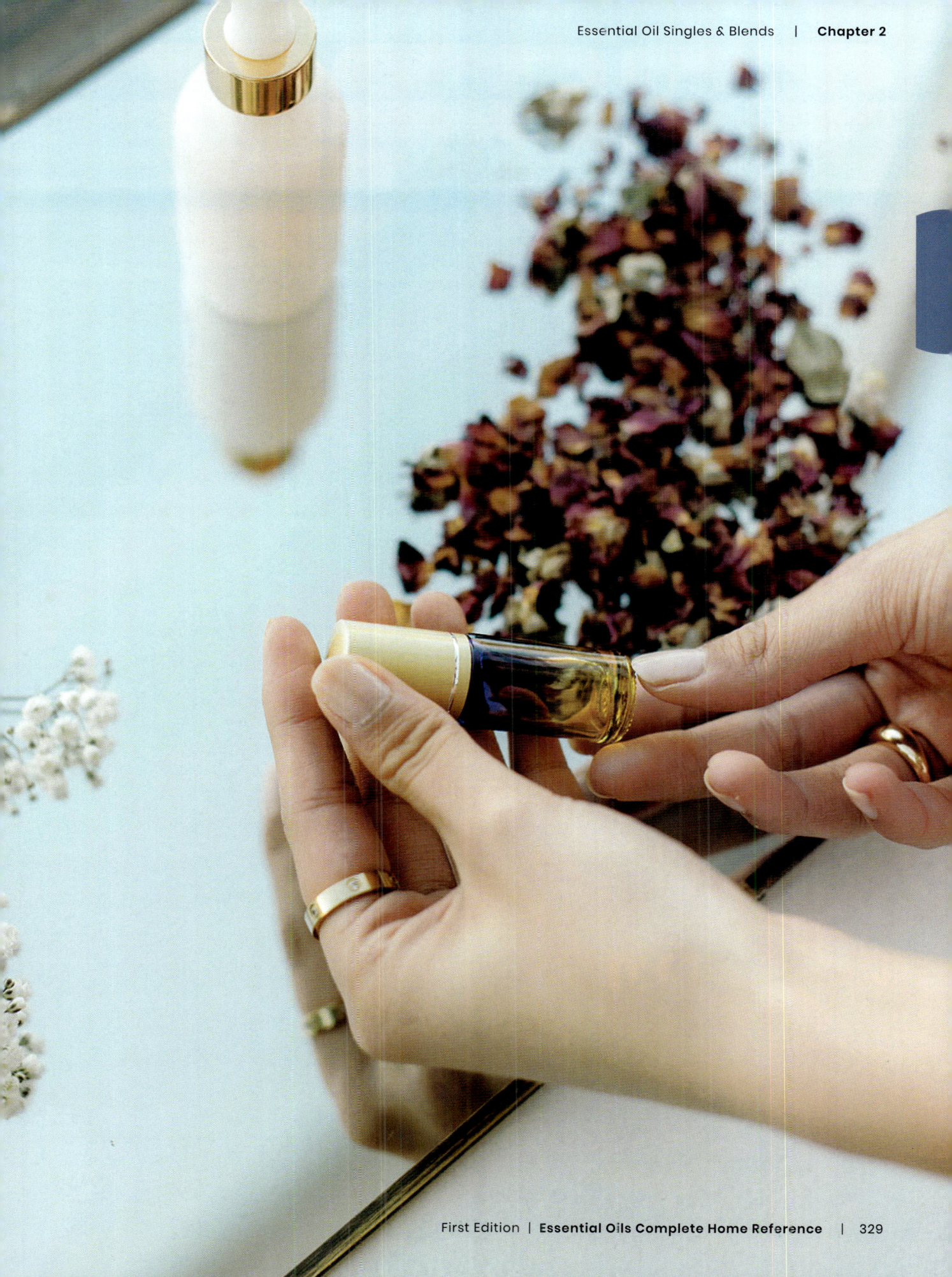

BOTANICAL FAMILY:
Lauraceae

PLANT ORIGIN:
Croatia, Montenegro

EXTRACTION METHOD:
Steam distilled from leaves

KEY CONSTITUENTS:
Eucalyptol (40-51%),
Alpha-Terpinyl Acetate (5-17%),
Sabinene (7-11%),
Alpha-Pinene (4-7%),
Linalool (2-7%),
Limonene (1-6%),
Beta-Pinene (3-6%),
Methyl Eugenol (1-5%)

LAURUS NOBILIS & LAURUS NOBILIS VITALITY™
(Laurus nobilis) (also Bay Laurel)

Both the leaves and the black berries were used to alleviate indigestion and loss of appetite. During the Middle Ages, Laurus nobilis was used for angina, migraine, heart palpitations, and liver and spleen complaints.

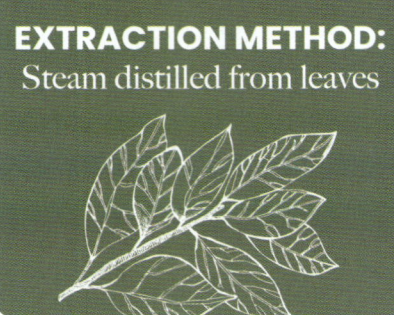

MEDICAL PROPERTIES:
Antimicrobial, antioxidant, anti-inflammatory, antiviral, anticonvulsant, antidiabetic, anti-acne

USES:
Nerve regeneration, arthritis (rheumatoid), oral infections (gingivitis), respiratory infections, viral infections, food flavoring, soap, protecting, cleansing

FRAGRANT INFLUENCE:
Protection, promoting success, relaxing, balancing, may increase intuition, enhances creativity

DIRECTIONS:
Aromatic: 3o. Topical: 50-50. Dietary (Vitality): Dilute 1 drop with 1 drop of V-6 or other pure carrier oil. Put in a capsule and take up to 3 times daily or as needed.

CAUTIONS:

SELECTED RESEARCH:

Nafis A, Kasrati A, Jamali CA, Custódio L, Vitalini S, Iriti M, Hassani L. A Comparative Study of the in Vitro Antimicrobial and Synergistic Effect of Essential Oils from Laurus nobilis L. and Prunus armeniaca L. from Morocco with Antimicrobial Drugs: New Approach for Health Promoting Products. Antibiotics (Basel): 2020 Apr; 9(4): 140. Published online 2020 Mar 25.

Heghes SC, Filip L, Vostinaru O, Mogosan C, Miere D, Iuga CA, Moldovan M. Essential Oil-Bearing Plants rom Balkan Peninsula: Promising Sources for New Drug Candidates for the Prevention and Treatment of Diabetes Mellitus and Dyslipidemia. Front Pharmacol. 2020; 11: 989.

Lee EH, Shin JH, Kim SS, Joo J-H, Choi E, Seo SR. Suppression of Propionibacterium acnes-Induced Skin Inflammation by Laurus nobilis Extract and Its Major Constituent Eucalyptol. Int J Mol Sci. 2019 Jul; 20(14): 3501. Published online 2019 Jul 17.

Merghni A, Marzouki H, Hentati H, Aouni M, Mastouri M. Antibacterial and antibiofilm activities of Laurus nobilis L. essential oil against Staphylococcus aureus strains associated with oral infections. Pathol Biol (Paris). 2015 Dec 4. [Epub ahead of print]

Lee T, Lee S, Ho Kim K, Oh KB, Shin J, Mar W. Effects of magnolialide isolated from the leaves of Laurus nobilis L. (Lauraceae) on immunoglobulin E-mediated type I hypersensitivity in vitro. J Ethnopharmacol. 2013 Sep 16;149(2):550-6. Epub 2013 Jul 24.

Basak SS, Candan F. Effect of Laurus nobilis L. essential oil and its main components on α-glucosidase and reactive oxygen species scavenging activity. Iran J Pharm Res. 2013 Spring;12(2):367-79.

Khan A, Zaman G, Anderson RA. Bay Leaves Improve Glucose and Lipid Profile of People with Type 2 Diabetes. J Clin Biochem Nutr. 2009 Jan; 44(1): 52-56. Published online 2008 Dec. 27.

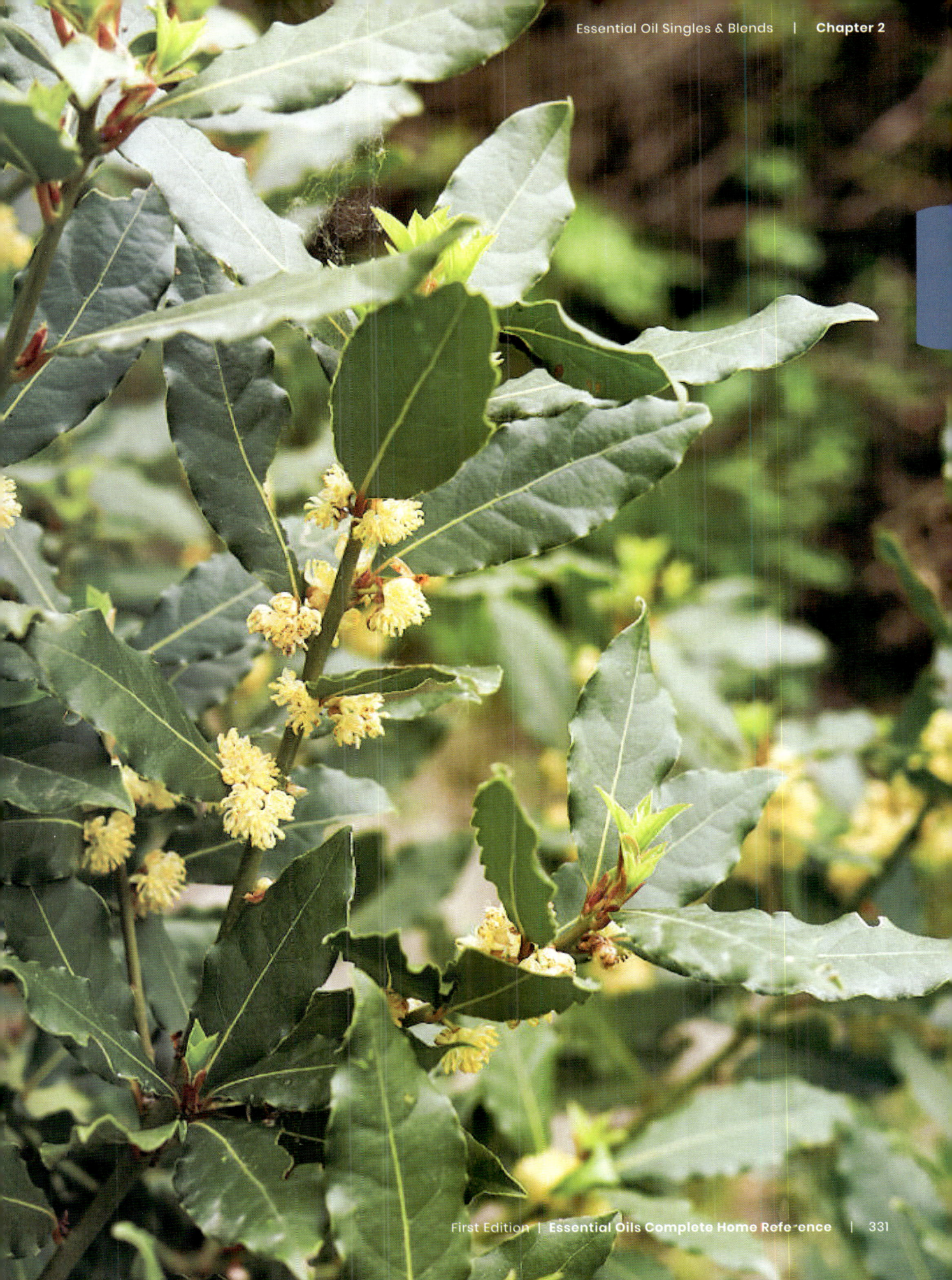

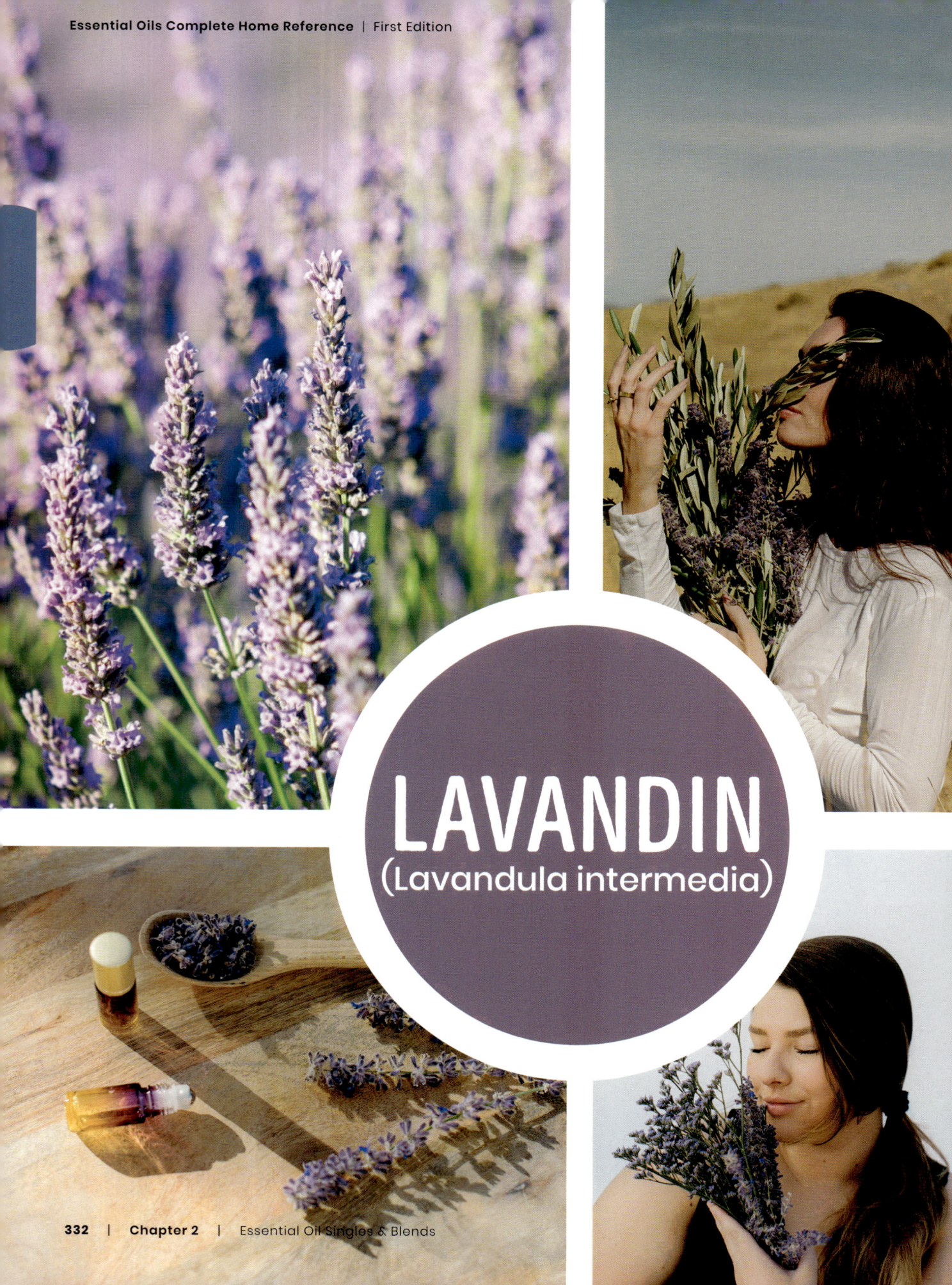

BOTANICAL FAMILY:
Lamiaceae

PLANT ORIGIN:
France

EXTRACTION METHOD:
Steam distilled from flowering tops

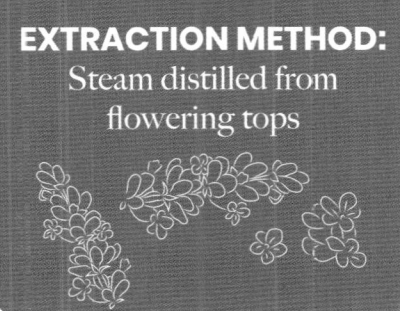

KEY CONSTITUENTS:
Cineole-1,8 (1-10%),
Linalool (24-44%),
Camphor (5-10%),
Linalyl Acetate (21-42%),
Lavandulyl Acetate (1-4%)

HISTORICAL DATA:
Also known as Lavandula x intermedia and Lavandula hybrida, lavandin is a hybrid plant developed by crossing true lavender (Lavandula angustifolia, also known as Lavandula officinalis) with spike lavender or aspic (Lavandula latifolia). It has been used to sterilize the animal cages in veterinary clinics and hospitals throughout Europe.

MEDICAL PROPERTIES:
Antibacterial, antifungal, anti-infectious, antioxidant, analgesic, anti-anxiety

USES:
Lavandin is a stronger antiseptic than lavender (Lavandula angustifolia). Reduces pain and inflammation. Its greater penetrating qualities make it well suited to help with respiratory, circulatory, and muscular conditions. Strengthens nervous system. Promotes cell regeneration. However, its camphor content invalidates its use to soothe burns.

FRAGRANT INFLUENCE:
Calming, strengthens respiratory system

DIRECTIONS:
Aromatic: 6o. Topical: Neat..

CAUTIONS: (Do not use for burns; instead, use pure Lavender (Lavandula angustifolia).

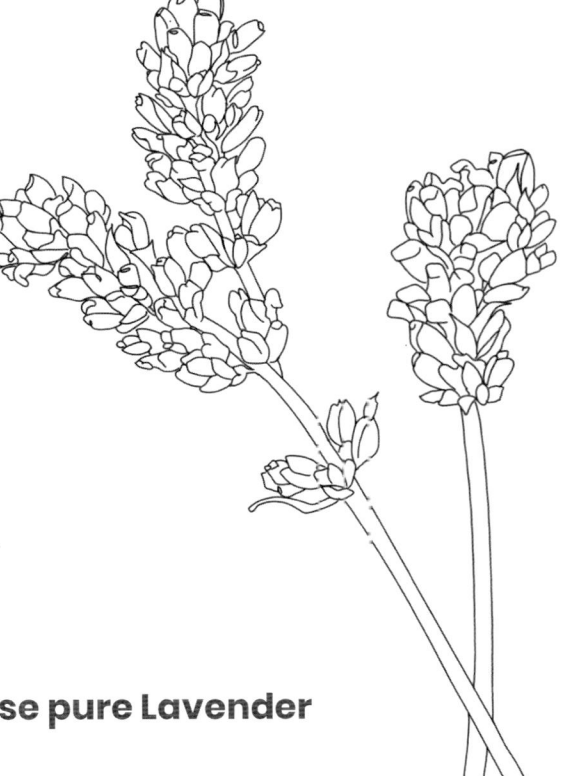

SELECTED RESEARCH:

Garzoli S, Turchetti G, Giacomello P, Tiezzi A, Masci VL, Ovidi E. Liquid and Vapour Phase of Lavandin (Lavandula x intermedia) Essential Oil: Chemical Composition and Antimicrobial Activity. Molecules. 2019 Aug; 24(15):2701.

Tardugno R, Serio A, Pellati F, D'Amato S, Chaves López C, Bellardi MG, Di Vito M, Savini V, Paparella A, Benvenuti S. Lavandula x Intermedia and Lavandula angustifolia essential oils: phytochemical composition and antimicrobial activity against foodborne pathogens. Nat Prod Res. 2018 May 21:1-6.

Carrasco A, Martinez-Gutierrez R, Tomas V, Tudela J. Lavandin (Lavandula x intermedia Emeric ex Loiseleur) essential oil from Spain: determination of aromatic profile by gas chromatography-mass spectrometry, antioxidant and lipoxygenase inhibitory bioactivities. Nat Prod Res. 2016;30(10):1123-30.

Végh A, Bencsik T, Molnár P, Böszörményi A, Lemberkovics E, Kovács K, Kocsis B, Horváth G. Composition and antipseudomonal effect of essential oils isolated from different lavender species. Nat Prod Commun. 2012 Oct;7(10):1393-6.

Blazeković B, Stanic G, Pepeljnjak S, Vladimir-Knezevic S. In vitro Antibacterial and Antifungal Activity of Lavandula x intermedia Emeric ex Loisel. 'Bucrovka.' Molecules. 2011 May; 16(5):4241-4253.

Blazeković B, Vladimir-Knezević S, Brantner A, Stefan MB. Evaluation of antioxidant potential of Lavandula x intermedia Emeric ex Loisel. 'Budrovka': a comparative study with L. angustifolia Mill. Molecules. 2010 Aug 30;15(9):5971-87.

Braden R, Reichow S, Halm MA. The use of the essential oil lavandin to reduce preoperative anxiety in surgical patients. J Perianesth Nurs. 2009 Dec;24(6):348-355.

BOTANICAL FAMILY: Lamiaceae

PLANT ORIGIN: USA, France

EXTRACTION METHOD: Steam distilled from flowering parts

KEY CONSTITUENTS: Linalyl Acetate (25-47%), Linalool (20-43%), Cis-Beta-Ocimene (1-10%), Terpinene-4-ol (up to 8%), Lavandulyl Acetate (up to 8%), Trans-Beta-Ocimene (1-6%), Camphor (up to 2%)

LAVENDER & LAVENDER VITALITY™
(Lavandula angustifolia)

The French scientist René Gattefossé was the first to discover lavender's ability to promote tissue regeneration and speed wound healing when he severely burned his arm in a laboratory explosion. Today, lavender is one of the few essential oils to still be listed in the British Pharmacopoeia.

MEDICAL PROPERTIES:
Sedative, antiseptic, antifungal, analgesic, antitumoral, anticonvulsant, vasodilating, relaxant, anti-inflammatory, reduces blood fat/cholesterol, combats excess sebum on skin

USES:
Cleanse and soothe minor burns, cuts, and other skin irritations; respiratory infections, high blood pressure, arteriosclerosis, menstrual problems/PMS, skin conditions (perineal repair, acne, eczema, psoriasis, scarring, stretch marks), burns, hair loss, insomnia, nervous tension

FRAGRANT INFLUENCE:
Fresh, floral, clean; calming, relaxing, and balancing, both physically and emotionally. Lavender has been documented to improve concentration and mental acuity.
University of Miami researchers found that inhalation of lavender oil increased beta waves in the brain, suggesting heightened relaxation. It also reduced depression and improved cognitive performance. A 2001 Osaka Kyoiku University study found that lavender reduced mental stress and increased alertness.

DIRECTIONS:
Aromatic 60. Topical: Neat. Dietary (Vitality): Put 2 drops in a capsule and take 3 times daily.

CAUTIONS: True lavender is often adulterated with hybrid lavender (lavandin), synthetic linalool and linalyl acetate, or synthetic fragrance chemicals like ethyl vanillin to increase volume.

SELECTED RESEARCH:

Kwiatkowski P, Łopusiewicz Ł, Kostek M, Drozłowska E, Pruss A, Wojciuk B, Sienkiewicz M, Zielińska-Bliźniewska H, Dołęgowska B. The Antibacterial Activity of Lavender Essential Oil Alone and in Combination with Octenidine Dihydrochloride against MRSA Strains. Molecules. 2020 Jan; 25(1): 95.

Araj-Khodaei M, Noorbala AA, Yarani R, Emadi F, Emaratkar E, Faghihzadeh S, Parsian Z, Alijaniha F, Kamalinejad M, Nasen M. A double-blind, randomized pilot study for comparison of Melissa officinalis L. and Lavandula angustifolia Mill. with Fluoxetine for the treatment of depression. BMC Complement Med Ther. 2020; 20: 207. Published online 2020 Jul 3. BMC Complement Altern Med.

Dyer J, Cleary L, McNeill S, Ragsdale-Lowe M, Osland C. The use of aromasticks to help with sleep problems: a patient experience survey. Complement Ther Clin Pract. 2016 Feb;22:51-8. Epub 2015 Dec 12. Prusinowska R, Smigielski K, Stobiecka A, Kunicka-Styczyńska A. Hydrolates from lavender (Lavandula angustifolia)—their chemical composition as well as aromatic, antimicrobial and antioxidant properties. Nat Prod Res. 2016;30(4):386-93. Epub 2015 Mar 4.

Hashemi SH, Hajbagheri A, Aghajani M. The effect of massage with lavender oil on restless leg syndrome in hemodialysis patients: a randomized controlled trial. Nurs Midwifery Stud. 2015 Dec;4(4):e29617. Epub 2015 Dec 1.

Raisi Dehkordi Z, Hosseini Baharanchi FS, Bekhradi R. Effect of lavender inhalation on the symptoms of primary dysmenorrhea and the amount of menstrual bleeding: a randomized clinical trial. Complement Ther Med. 2014 Apr;22(2):212-9. Epub 2014 Jan 6.

Tayarani-Najaran Z, Amiri A, Karimi G, Emami SA, Asili J, Mousavi SH. Comparative studies of cytotoxic and apoptotic properties of different extracts and essential oil of Lavandula angustifolia on malignant and normal cells. Nutr Cancer. 2014;66(3):424-34. Epub 2014 Feb 26.

Yap PS, Krishnan T, Yiap BC, Hu CP, Chan KG, Lim SH. Membrane disruption and anti-quorum sensing effects of synergistic interaction between Lavandula angustifolia (lavender oil) in combination with antibiotic against plasmid-conferred multi-drug-resistant Escherichia coli. J Appl Microbiol. 2014 May;116(5):1119-28. Epub 2014 Feb 14.

Vakili A, Sharifat S, Akhavan MM, Bandegi AR. Effect of lavender oil (Lavandula angustifolia) on cerebral edema and its possible mechanisms in an experimental model of stroke. Brain Res. 2014 Feb 22;1548:56-62. Epub 2013 Dec 30.

O'Connor DW, Eppingstall B, Taffe J, van der Ploeg ES. A randomized controlled cross-over trial of dermally applied lavender (Lavandula angustifolia) as a treatment of agitated behaviour in dementia. BMC Complement Altern Med. 2013 Nov 13;13:315.

Motomura N, Sakurai A, Yotsuya Y. Reduction of mental stress with lavender odorant. Percept Mot Skills. 2001 Dec;93(3):713-8.

Diego MA, Jones NA, Field T, Hernandez Reif M, Schanberg S, Kuhn C, McAdam V, Galamaga R, Galamaga M. Aromatherapy positively affects mood, EEG patterns of alertness and math computations. Int J Neurosci. 1998 Dec;96(3-4):217-24.

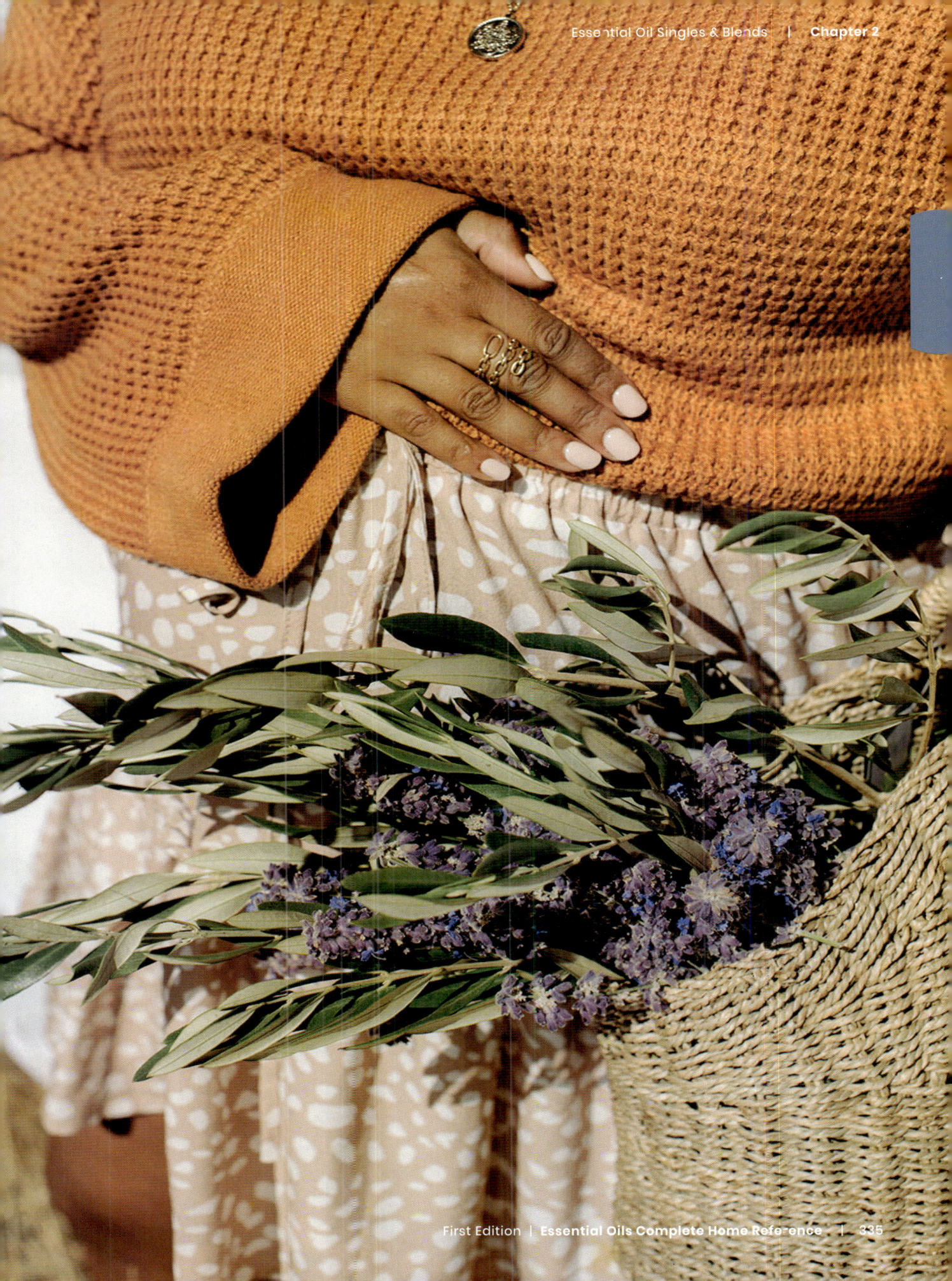

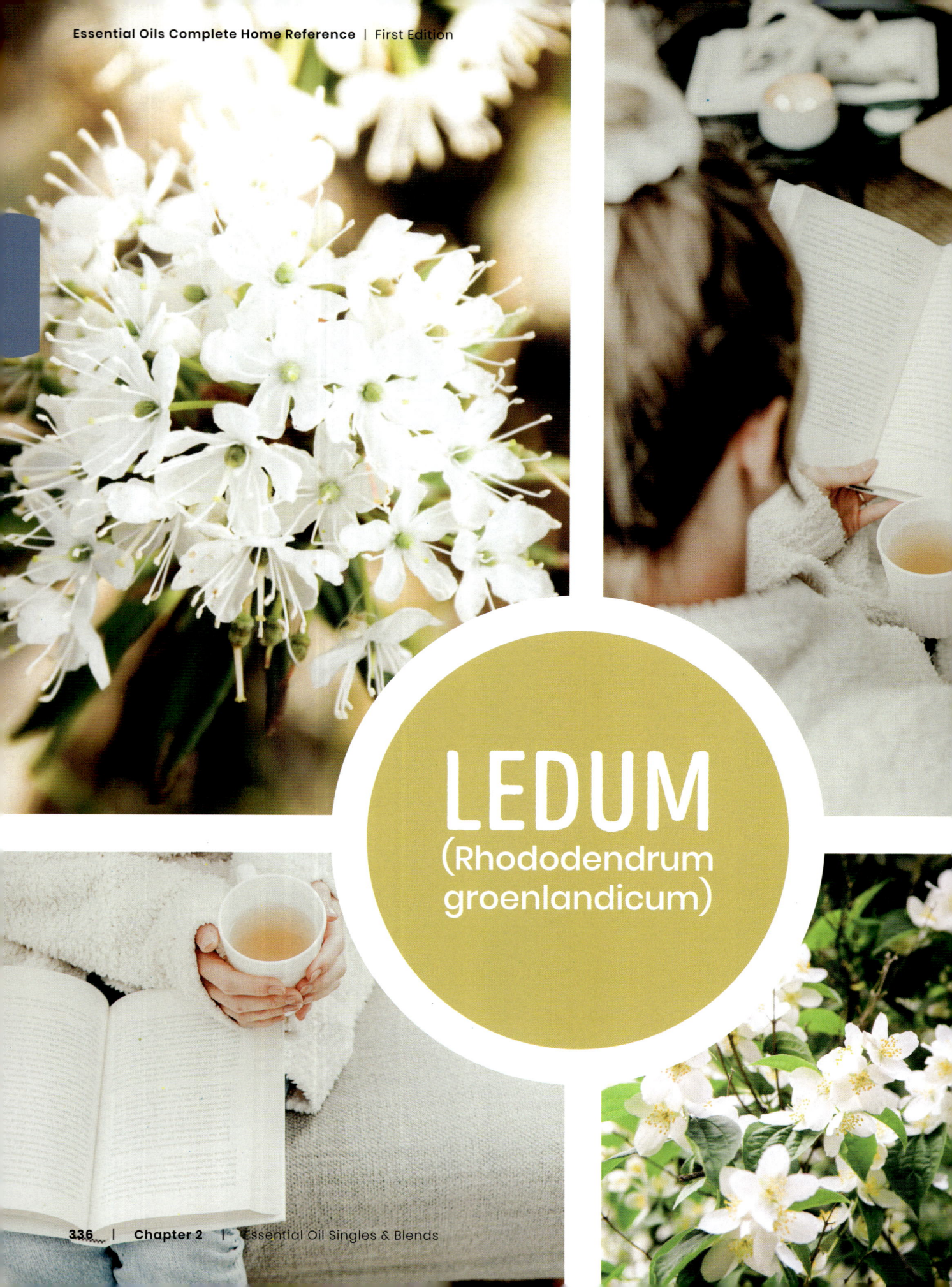
LEDUM
(Rhododendrum groenlandicum)

Essential Oil Singles & Blends | Chapter 2

BOTANICAL FAMILY:
Ericaceae

PLANT ORIGIN:
Canada

EXTRACTION METHOD:
Steam distilled from flowering tops

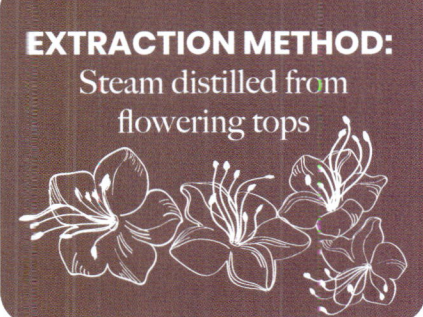

KEY CONSTITUENTS:
Sabinene (up to 40%), Limonene (up to 32%), Alpha-Selinene (up to 21%), Beta-Selinene (2-19%), Alpha-Pinene (1-12%), Cis-Para-Mentha-1(7),8-dien-8-ol (up to 11%), Terpinene-4-ol (up to 9%), Trans-Para-Mentha-1(7),8-dien-8-ol (up to 9%), Trans-Para-Mentha-1,3,8-triene (up to 8%)

HISTORICAL DATA:
Known colloquially as "Labrador tea," ledum has been reclassified from the genus Ledum and is now classified as Rhododendrum groenlandicum. It is a strongly aromatic herb that has been used for centuries in folk medicine. The native people of Eastern Canada used this herb for tea, as a general tonic, and to treat a variety of kidney-related problems. Ledum has helped protect the native people of North America against scurvy for more than 5,000 years. The Cree used it for fevers and colds.

MEDICAL PROPERTIES:
Anti-inflammatory, antitumoral, anticancerous, antibacterial, diuretic, liver-protectant

USES:
Liver problems/hepatitis/fatty liver, obesity, water retention, supports immune system, fights cancer, supports body systems, supports urinary tract, treats addiction-based disorders, fights ADD, treats skin conditions, bronchitis, flu

FRAGRANT INFLUENCE:
Harmonize and balance the body, relieves congestion and cough, calming

DIRECTIONS:
Aromatic: 30. Topical: 50-50. Dietary: Take as a dietary supplement or tea.

CAUTIONS:

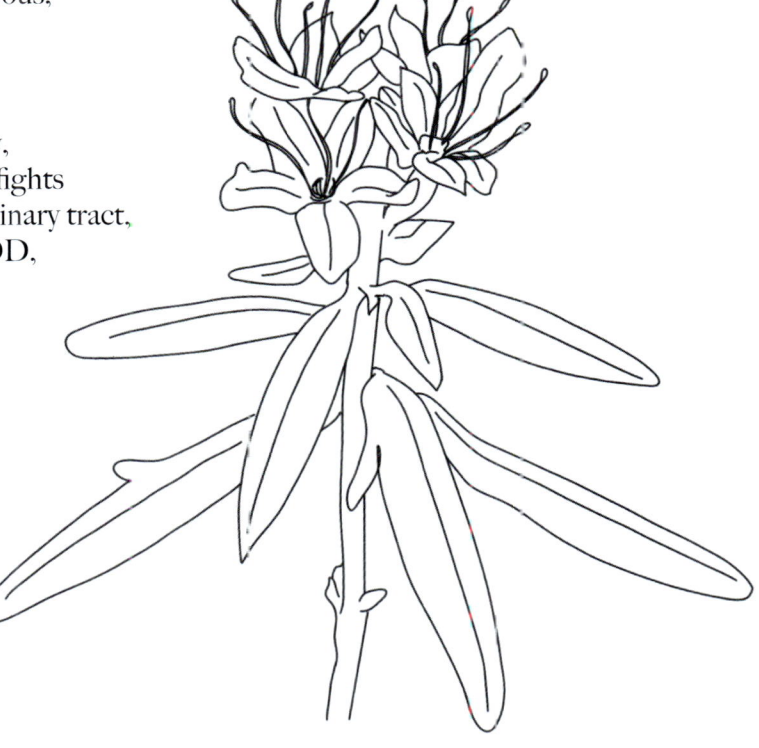

SELECTED RESEARCH:
Li S, Brault A, Sanchez Villavicencio M, Haddad PS. Rhododendron groenlandicum (Labrador tea), an antidiabetic plant from the traditional pharmacopoeia of the Canadian Eastern James Bay Cree, improves renal integrity in the diet-induced obese mouse model. Pharm Biol. 2016 Oct;54(10):1998-2006.

Ouchfoun M, Eid HM, Musallam L, Brault A, Li S, Vallerand D, Arnason JT, Haddad PS. Labrador tea (Rhododendron groenlandicum) attenuates insulin resistance in a diet-induced obesity mouse model. Eur J Nutr. 2016 Apr;55(3):941-54.

Rapinski M, Musallam L, Arnason JT, Haddad P, Cuerrier A. Adipogenic Activity of Wild Populations of Rhododendron groenlandicum, a Medicinal Shrub from the James Bay Cree Traditional Pharmacopeia. Evid Based Complement Alternat Med. 2015; 2015: 492458. Published online 2015 Oct 5.

Dampc A, Luczkiewicz M. Labrador tea—the aromatic beverage and spice: a review of origin, processing and safety. J Sci Food Agric. 2015 Jun;95(8):1577-83. Epub 2014 Sep 29.

Dufour D, Pichette A, Mshvildadze V, Bradette-Hébert ME, Lavoie S, Longtin A, Laprise C, Legault J. Antioxidant, anti-inflammatory and anticancer activities of methanolic extracts from Ledum groenlandicum Retzius. J Ethnopharmacol. 2007 Apr 20;111(1):22-8. Epub 2006 Oct 26.

BOTANICAL FAMILY: Rutaceae

PLANT ORIGIN: Argentina, South Africa, Spain

EXTRACTION METHOD: Cold pressed from peel. It takes 3,000 lemons to produce 1 kilo of oil.

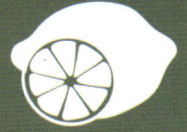

KEY CONSTITUENTS: Limonene (59-80%), Beta-Pinene (7-17%), Gamma-Terpinene (6-12%), Alpha-Pinene (1-3%), Sabinene (1-3%), Geranial (up to 2%), Neral (up to 2%)

LEMON & LEMON VITALITY™
(Citrus limon)

Lemon oil has been widely used in skin care to cleanse skin, reduce wrinkles, and combat acne. Lemon peel was used as an antiseptic, carminative, diuretic, eupeptic, a vascular stimulant and protector, and as a vitaminic (Arias, et al., 2005). It is also used as a flavorant for cleaning, cooking, and treating scurvy and a variety of other ailments.

MEDICAL PROPERTIES:
Antioxidant, analgesic, lipolytic, anticarcinogenic, antiviral, antitumoral, antimicrobial, antifungal, gastroprotective, antidementia, potential antihyperglycemic activity, antiseptic, antinociceptive

USES:
Helps manage LDLs; reduces stress, anxiety, and depression; inhibits apoptosis; enhances penetration of vitamins A, E, C, and B6 through the skin; reduces nausea and vomiting in pregnant women, circulatory problems, arteriosclerosis, obesity, parasites, urinary tract infections, varicose veins, immune stimulant (may increase white blood cells), improves memory, relaxation; rich in limonene, it has been extensively studied in over 50 clinical studies for ability to combat tumor growth, anxiety, hypertension, digestive problems, etc. Also helps remove adhesives. Also, Lemon's flavonoid eriocitrin blocks the detection of pain (antinociceptive).

FRAGRANT INFLUENCE:
Promotes clarity of thought and purpose with a fragrance that is invigorating, enhancing, and warming. A Mie University study found that citrus fragrances boosted immunity, induced relaxation, and reduced depression (Komori, et al., 1995).

DIRECTIONS:
Aromatic: 6o. Topical: 50-50. Dietary (Vitality): Put 2 drops in a capsule. Take 3 times daily or as needed.

CAUTIONS:

SELECTED RESEARCH:

Alghamdi S. Antinociceptive Effect of Citrus Flavonoid Eriocitrin on Postoperative Pain Conditions. J Pain Res. 2020; 13: 805-815.

Nikolić MM, Jovanović KK, Marković TL, Marković TL, Gligorijević NN, Radulović SS, Kostić M, Glamočlija JM, Soković MD. Antimicrobial synergism and cytotoxic properties of Citrus limon L., Piper nigrum L. and Melaleuca alternifolia (Maiden and Betche) Cheel essential oils. J Pharm Pharmacol. 2017 Nov;69(11):1606-14. Epub 2017 Aug 17.

Oliveira SA, Zambrana JR, Iorio FB, Pereira CA, Jorge AO. The antimicrobial effects of Citrus limon and Citrus aurantium essential oils on multi-species biofilms. Braz Oral Res. 2014;28:22-7.

Vandresen F, Falzirolli H, Almeida Batista SA, da Silva-Giardini AP, de Oliveira DN, Catharino RR, Ruiz AL, de Carvalho JE, Foglio MA, da Silva CC. Novel R-(+)-limonene-based thiosemicarbazones and their antitumor activity against human tumor cell lines. Eur J Med Chem. 2014 May 22;79:110-6. Epub 2014 Apr 1.

Yavari Kia P, Safajou F, Shahnazi M, Nazemiyeh H. The effect of lemon inhalation aromatherapy on nausea and vomiting of pregnancy: a double-blinded, randomized, controlled trial. Iran Red Crescent Med J. 2014 Mar;16(3):e14360. Epub 2014 Mar 5.

Guerra FQ, Mendes JM, Sousa JP, Morais-Braga MF, Santos BH, Melo Coutinho HD, Lima Ede O. Increasing antibiotic activity against a multidrug-resistant Acinetobacter spp by essential oils of Citrus limon and Cinnamomum zeylandicum. Nat Prod Res. 2012;26(23):2235-8.

Komori T, Fujiwara R, Tanida M, Nomura J, Yokoyama MM. Effects of citrus fragrance on immune function and depressive states. Neuroimmunomodulation. 1995 May-Jun;2(3):174-180.

Essential Oil Singles & Blends | **Chapter 2**

When life gives you lemons make an essential oil!

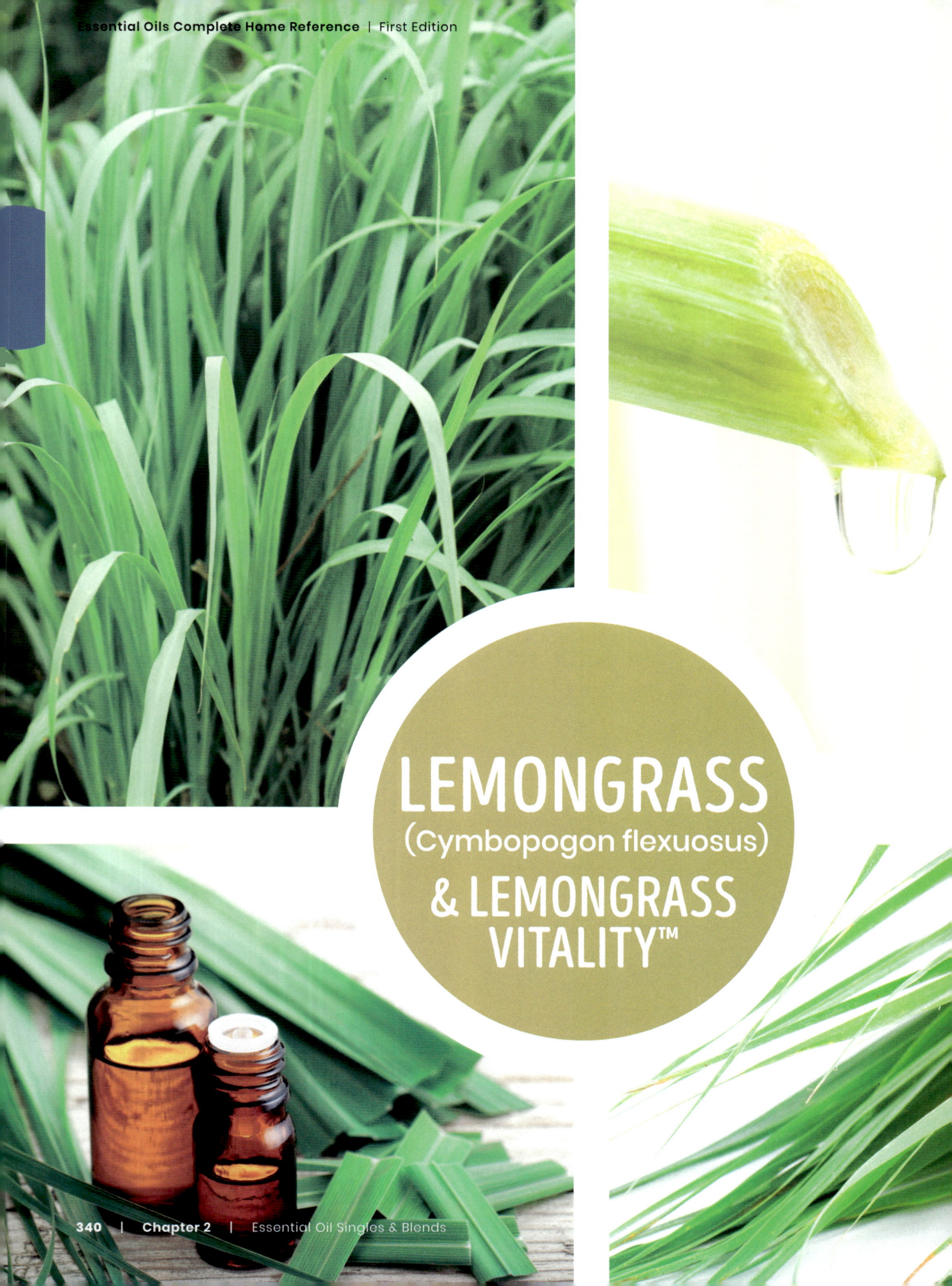

BOTANICAL FAMILY:
Poaceae

PLANT ORIGIN:
India

EXTRACTION METHOD:
Steam distilled from leaves

KEY CONSTITUENTS:
Geranial (30-47%),
Neral (25-35%),
Geraniol (1-8%),
Geranyl Acetate (up to 6%),
Limonene (up to 4%),
Beta-Caryophyllene (up to 4%),
6-Methyl-5-Heptene-2one (up to 2%)

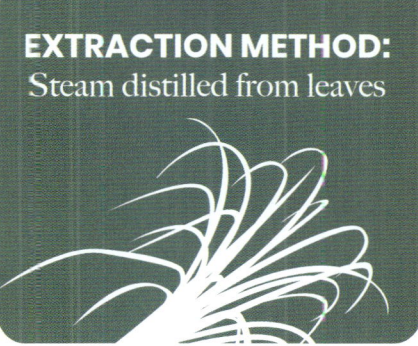

HISTORICAL DATA:
Lemongrass is used for purification and digestion. Historically, it was used for hypertension, inflammation, as a sedative, and for treatment of fevers and digestion. In a 2008 study, 91 single essential oils were tested against MRSA (Methicillin-resistant Staphylococcus aureus). The study found that "remarkably, lemongrass essential oil completely inhibited all MRSA growth on the plate" (Chao S, et al., 2008).

MEDICAL PROPERTIES:
Antimicrobial antifungal, antiviral, anticancerous, antispasmodic, antibacterial, antioxidant, antiparasitic, anti-inflammatory, promotes lymph flow. Several research articles document strong antifungal and antibacterial properties of lemongrass.

USES:
Supports weight loss and normal glucose levels in animals, bladder infections, respiratory/sinus infections, digestive problems, parasites, torn ligaments/muscles, fluid retention, varicose veins, circulation, salmonella, candida, relieves nausea, eases diarrhea

FRAGRANT INFLUENCE:
Citrus, promotes psychic awareness and purification, neutralizes air

DIRECTIONS:
Aromatic: 30. Topical: 20-80. In case of sensitivity, dilute 15 drops in up to 10 ml of V-6 or other pure carrier oil. Dietary (Vitality): Dilute 1 drop with 1 drop of carrier oil. Put in a capsule and take up to 3 times daily.

CAUTIONS: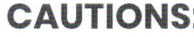

SELECTED RESEARCH:

Ortega-Ramirez LA, Gutiérrez-Pacheco MM, Vargas-Arispuro I, González-Aguilar GA, Martinez-Téllez MA, Ayala-Zavala JF. Inhibition of Glucosyltransferase Activity and Glucan Production as an Antibiofilm Mechanism of Lemongrass Essential Oil against Escherichia coli O157:H7. Antibiotics (Basel). 2020 Mar; 9(3): 102.

Basera P, Lavania M, Agnihotri A, Lal B. Analytical Investigation of Cymbopogon citratus and Exploiting the Potential of Developed Silver Nanoparticle Against the Dominating Species of Pathogenic Bacteria. Front Microbiol. 2019; 10: 282. Published online 2019 Feb 27.

Bustos C RO, Alberti R FV, Matiacevich SB. Edible antimicrobial films based on microencapsulated lemongrass oil. J Food Sci Technol. 2016 Jan;53(1):832-9. Epub 2015 Sep 16.

Goes TC, Ursulino FR, Almeida-Souza TH, Alves PB, Teixeira-Silva F. Effect of lemongrass aroma on experimental anxiety in humans. J Altern Complement Med. 2015 Dec;21(12):766-73. Epub 2015 Sep 14.

Boukhatem MN, Ferhat MA, Kameli A, Saidi F, Kebir HT. Lemon grass (Cymbopogon citratus) essential oil as potent anti-inflammatory and antifungal drugs. Libyan J Med. 2014; 9: 10.3402/ljm.

Katsukawa M, Nakata R, Takizawa Y, Hori K, Takahashi S, Inoue H. Citral, a component of lemongrass oil, activates PPARα and γ and suppresses COX-2 expression. Biochim Biophys Acta. 2010 Nov;1801(11):1214-20. Epub 2010 Jul 23.

Sharma PR, Mondhe DM, Muthiah S. Pal HC, Shahi AK, Saxena AK. Qazi GN. Anticancer activity of an essential oil from Cymbopogon flexuosus. Chem Biol Interact. 2009 May 15;179(2-3):160-8. Epub 2008 Dec 11.

Chao SC, Young DG, Oberg C, Nakaoka K. Inhibition of methicillin-resistant Staphylococcus aureus (MRSA) by essential oils. Flavour Fragr J. 2008 Nov/Dec;23(6):444-9.

BOTANICAL FAMILY:
Myrtaceae

PLANT ORIGIN:
Australia, France

EXTRACTION METHOD:
Steam distilled from leaves

KEY CONSTITUENTS:
Geranial (45-54%),
Neral (35-42%),
Cyclocitral B (2-4%),
Cyclocitral A (up to 4%)

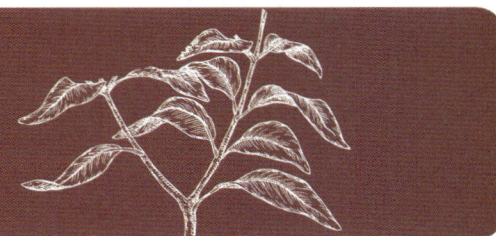

LEMON MYRTLE
(Backhousia citriodora)

The aboriginal people of Australia valued Lemon Myrtle's flavor in cooking, calling it "bush food." It is also known as the "queen of lemon herbs." Lemon Myrtle can replace lemon in milk-based foods, as it does not have Lemon's curdling problems. Lemon Myrtle was also widely used as a healing plant. It is the highest natural source of the constituent citral. Since citral, consisting of isomers geranial and neral, has a strong and sweet lemon scent, Lemon Myrtle continues to be valued in perfumery. It is used in health care and cleaning products such as soaps, shampoos, and lotions. Lemon Myrtle is cultivated in Queensland and the north coast of New South Wales, Australia.

MEDICAL PROPERTIES:
Antiseptic, antimicrobial, antifungal, anti-inflammatory, central nervous system stimulant

USES:
Weight loss, respiratory/sinus infection, treatment of MCV (molluscum contagiosum virus) in children

FRAGRANT INFLUENCE:
Uplifting and invigorating, Lemon Myrtle's fresh and sweet lemon scent encourages follow-through with goals.

DIRECTIONS:
Aromatic: 30. Topical: 50-50.

CAUTIONS:

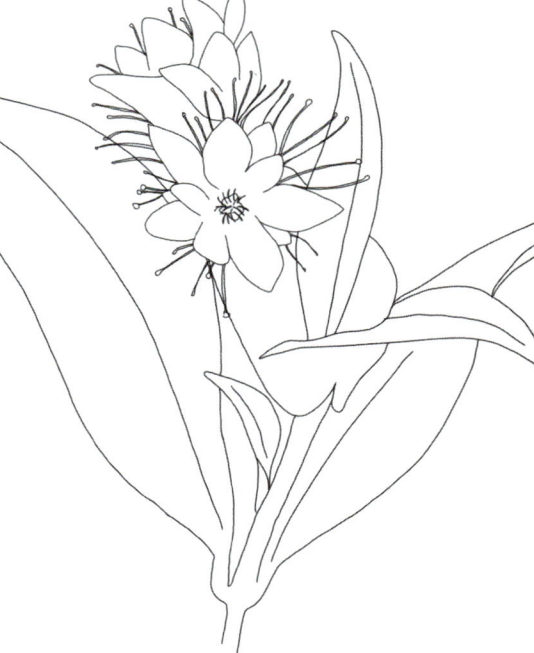

SELECTED RESEARCH:

Shim S-Y, Kim J-H, Kho K-H, Lee M. Anti-inflammatory and anti-oxidative activities of lemon myrtle (Backhousia citriodora) leaf extract. Toxicol Rep. 2020; 7: 277-281.

Yabuta Y, Mukoyama H, Kaneda Y, Kimura N, Bito T, Ichiyanagi T, Ishihara A, Watanabe F. A lemon myrtle extract inhibits glucosyltransferases activity of Streptococcus mutans. Biosci Biotechnol Biochem. 2018 Sept;82(9):1584-90. Epub 2018 May 26.

Sakulnarmrat K, Fenech M, Thomas P, Konczak I. Cytoprotective and pro-apoptotic activities of native Australian herbs polyphenolic-rich extracts. Food Chem. 2013 Jan 1;136(1):9-17. Epub 2012 Jul 27.

Modak T, Mukhopadhaya A. Effects of citral, a naturally occurring antiadipogenic molecule, on an energy-intense diet model of obesity. Indian J Pharmacol. 2011 May; 43(3):300-5.

Burke BE, Baillie JE, Olson RD. Essential oil of Australian lemon myrtle (Backhousia citriodora) in the treatment of molluscum contagiosum in children. Biomed Pharmacother. 2004 May;58(4):245-7.

Wilkinson JM, Hipwell M, Ryan T, Cavanagh HM. Bioactivity of Backhousia citriodora: antibacterial and antifungal activity. J. Agric Food Chem. 2003 Jan 1;51(1):76-81.

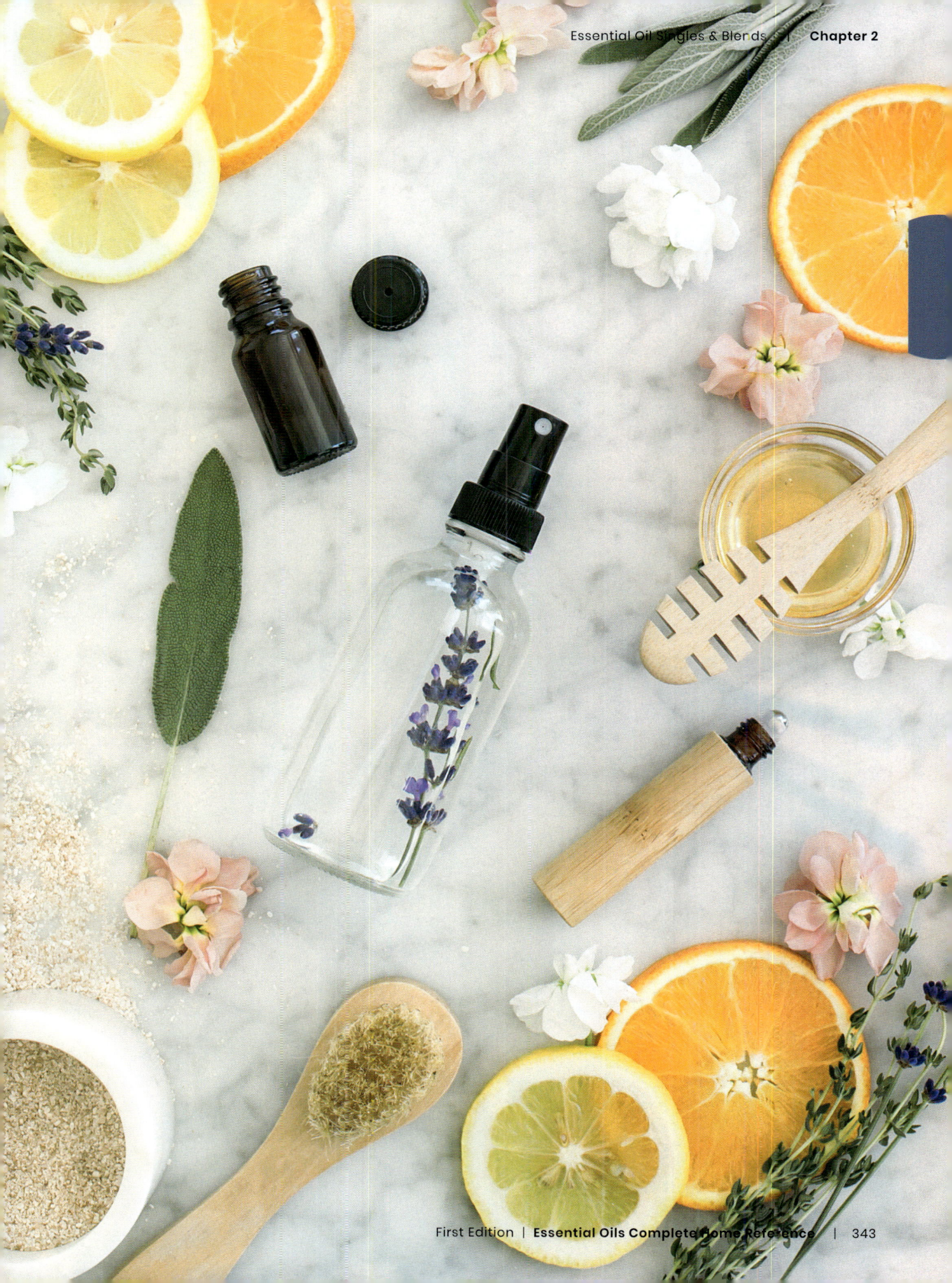

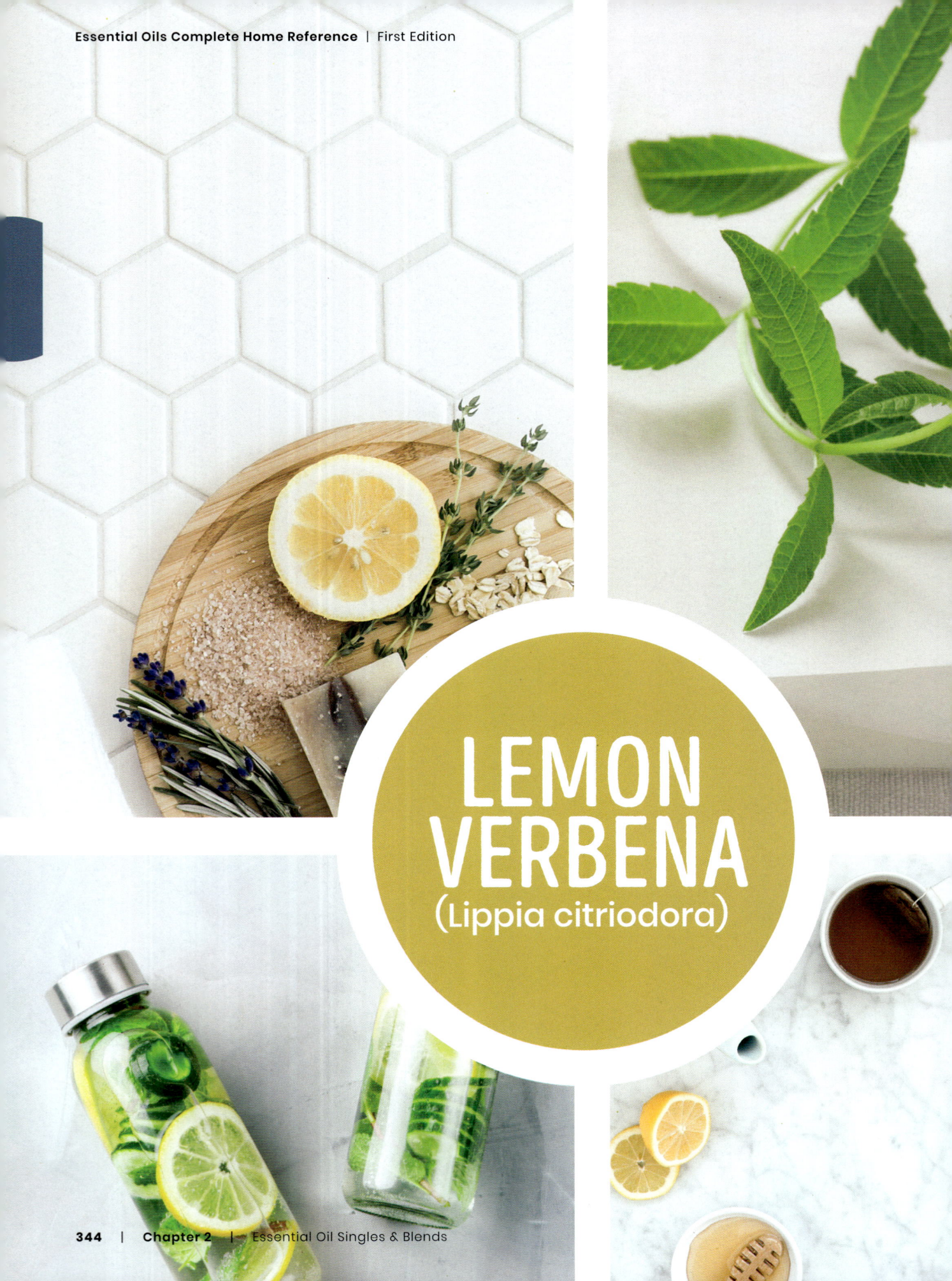

LEMON VERBENA
(Lippia citriodora)

BOTANICAL FAMILY:
Verbenaceae

PLANT ORIGIN:
South America

EXTRACTION METHOD:
Steam distillation

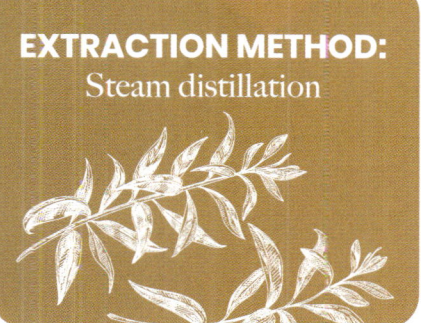

KEY CONSTITUENTS:
Eucalyptol + Limonene (12-34%), Geranial (4-18%), Neral (3-14%), Trans-beta-caryophyllene (3-9%), AR-curcumene (2-8%), Caryopllene Oxide (1-6%)

HISTORICAL DATA:
Lemon verbena has been used for centuries to stop muscle spasms, as a fever reducer and sedative, for indigestion, and to increase appetite, among other things. Its fragrance is used in perfumery, and its extract has demonstrated antioxidant activity. Lemon verbena essential oil also has some antimicrobial properties and has been studied for weight loss.

MEDICAL PROPERTIES:
Antimicrobial, anxiolytic, antiviral, gastroprotective, antioxidant, antiparasitic, sedating

USES:
Fatigued muscles, skin conditions, sleep problems, intestinal/digestive disorders/weight loss

FRAGRANT INFLUENCE:
Fresh, citrus, herbal aroma; relaxing; sedating; sleep aid

DIRECTIONS:
Aromatic: 30. Topical: 50-50.

CAUTIONS:

SELECTED RESEARCH:
Marhuenda J, Perez S, Victoria-Montesinos D, Abellán MS, Caturia N, Jones J, López-Román J. A Randomized, Double-Blind, Placebo Controlled Trial to Determine the Effectiveness [of] a Polyphenolic Extract (Hibiscus sabdariffa and lippia citriodora) in the Reduction of Body Fat Mass in Healthy Subjects. Foods. 2020 Jan; 9(1): 55.

Herranz-López M, Olivares-Vicente M, Boix-Castejón M, Caturia N, Roche E, Micol V. Differential effects of a combination of Hibiscus sabdariffa and Lippia citriodora polyphenols in overweight/obese subjects: A randomized controlled trial. Sci Rep. 2019; 9: 2999. Published online 2019 Feb. 28.

Fitsiou E, Mitropoulou G, Spyridopoulou K, Vamvakias M, Bardouki H, Galanis A, Pappa A. Chemical composition and evaluation of the biological properties of the essential oil of the dietary phytochemical Lippia citriodora. Molecules. 2018;23(1):123.

Tajik J, Kheirandish R, Azizi S, Amanollahi R, Mahmoudi T. The effects of aqueous extracts of Lippia citriodora, Trachyspermum copticum, Dracocepalum polychaetum on repair of ethanol induced gastric ulcer in rats. Comparative Clinical Pathology. 2016;25(1):117-123.

Paun G, Zrira S, Boutakiout A, Ungureanu O, Simion D, Chelaru C, Radu GL. Chemical composition, antioxidant and antibacterial activity of essential oils from Moroccan aromatic herbs. Revue Roumaine de Chimie. 2013;58(11-12):891-897.

Ohno T, Kita M, Yamaoka Y, Imamura S, Yamamoto T, Mitsufuji S, Imanishi J. Antimicrobial activity of essential oils against Helicobacter pylori. Helicobacter. 2003;8(3):207-215.

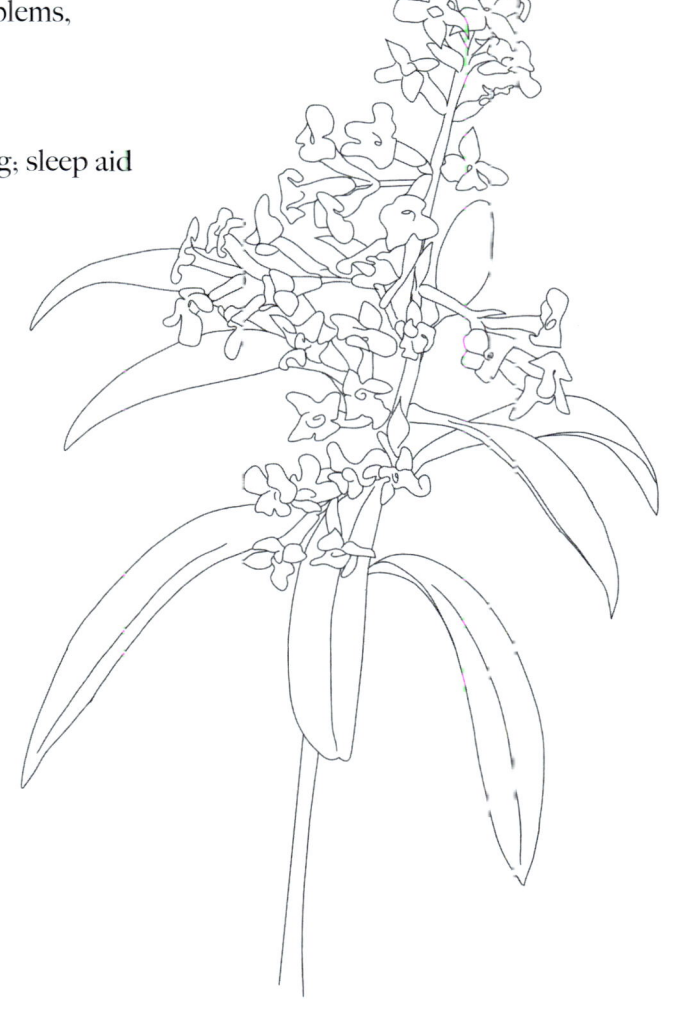

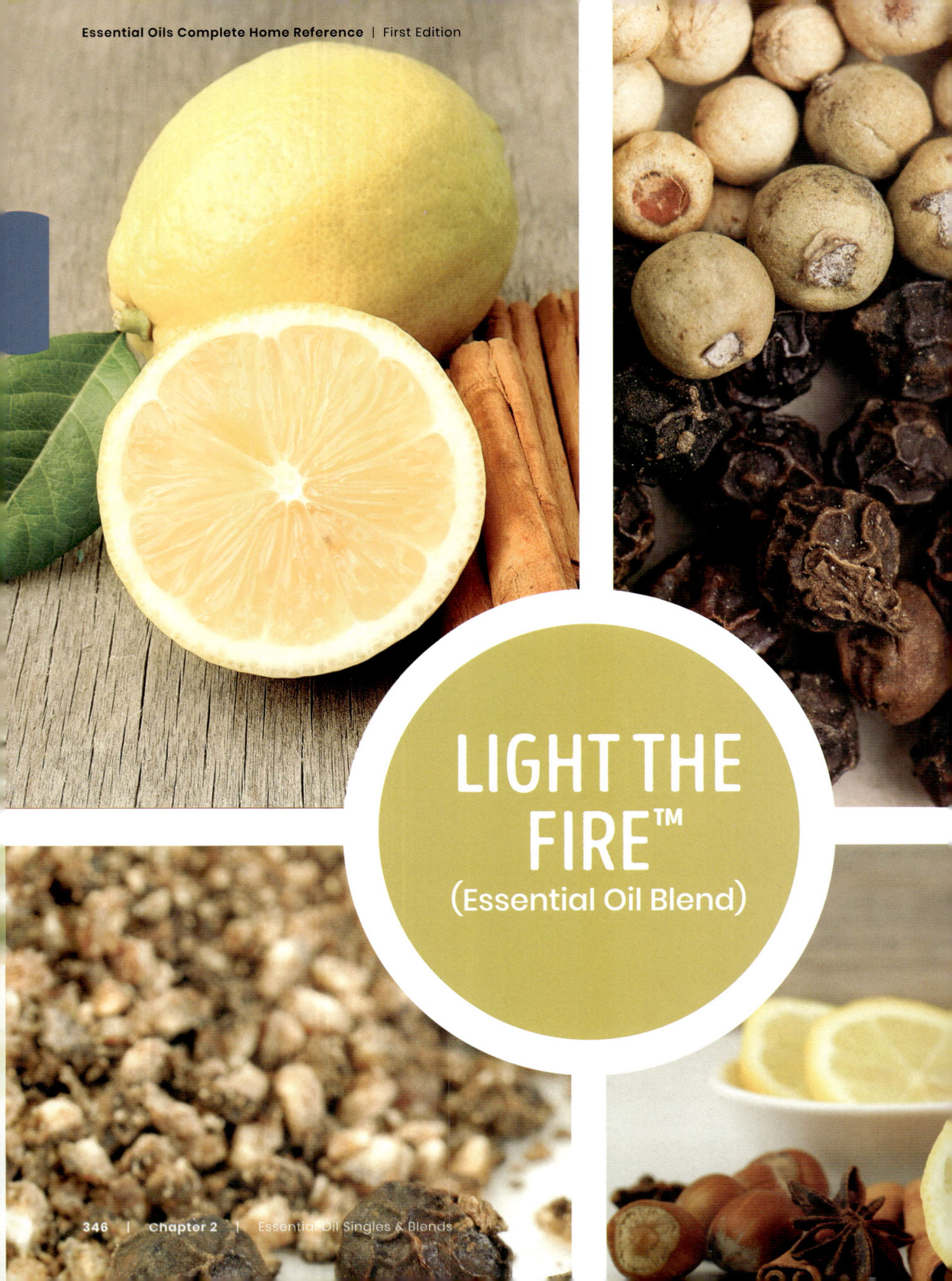

LIGHT THE FIRE™
(Essential Oil Blend)

ABOUT LIGHT THE FIRE™:

Light the Fire is an inspiring blend with a warm, spicy aroma that can encourage feelings of power and ambition.

MEDICAL PROPERTIES & USES:

Antimicrobial, antioxidative, calming, cardiovascular supportive, digestion or elimination supportive/nausea reducing, disease inhibitory, organ protective, pain or swelling reducing, performance enhancing/stimulating

INGREDIENTS:

Nutmeg, Cassia, Mastrante, Ocotea, Canadian Fleabane, Lemon, Black Pepper, Northern Lights Black Spruce

DIRECTIONS:

Aromatic: 10. Topical: 20-80.

CAUTIONS:

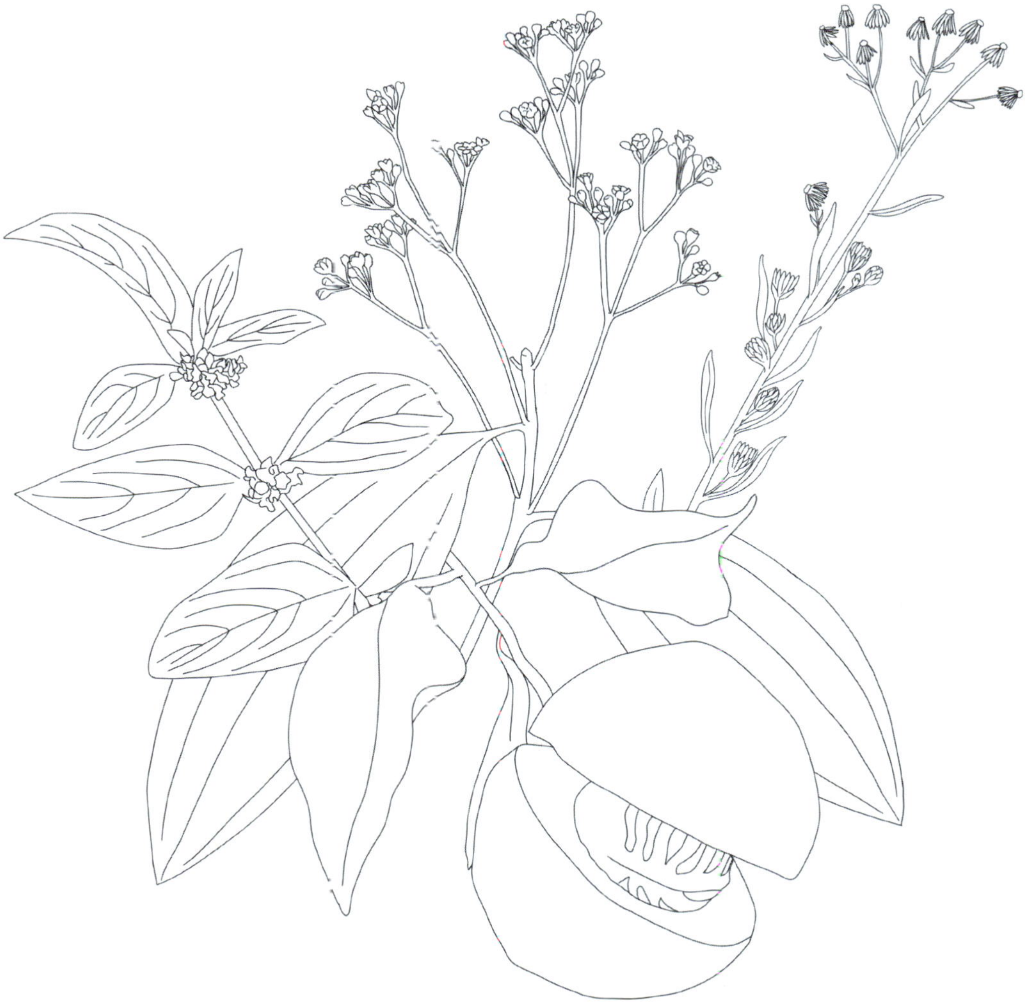

BOTANICAL FAMILY: Rutaceae

PLANT ORIGIN: Mexico

EXTRACTION METHOD: Cold pressed from rind

KEY CONSTITUENTS: Limonene (47-60%), Beta-Pinene (10-15%), Gamma-Terpinene (11-14%), Alpha-Pinene (2-3%), Geranial (2-3%), Myrcene (1-2%), Neral (1-2%), Beta-Bisabolene (1-2%), Neryl Acetate (up to 2%), Alpha-Bergamotene (up to 2%)

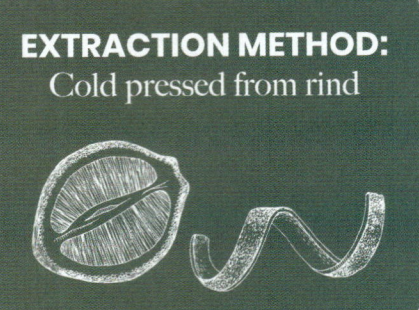

LIME & LIME VITALITY™
(Citrus aurantifolia or C. latifolia)

Primarily used in skin care and in supporting and strengthening the respiratory and immune systems.

MEDICAL PROPERTIES:
Antirheumatic, antiviral, antibacterial, antioxidant, antidiabetic, anticancer

USES:
Skin conditions (herpes), supports radiant skin, insect bites, respiratory problems, decongests the lymphatic system, weight loss, household cleaner, absorbs refrigerator odor

FRAGRANT INFLUENCE:
Inspiring, uplifting, refreshing

DIRECTIONS:
Aromatic: 30. Topical: 50-50. Dietary (Vitality): Dilute 1 drop with 1 drop of V-6 or other pure carrier oil. Put in a capsule and take up to 3 times daily.

CAUTIONS:

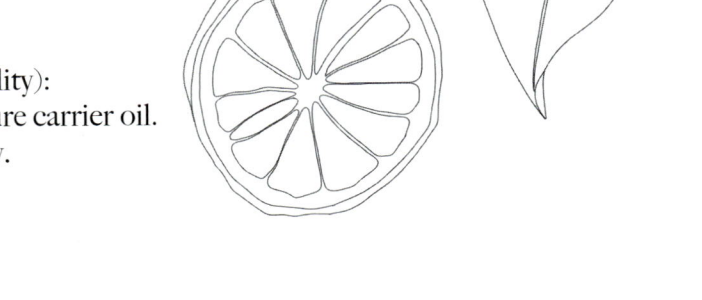

SELECTED RESEARCH:

Lin L-Y, Chuang C-H, Chen H-C, Chen HC, Yang K-M. Lime (Citrus aurantifolia (Christm.) Swingle) Essential Oils: Volatile Compounds, Antioxidant Capacity, and Hypolipideemic Effect. Foods. 2019 Sep 7. Published online 2019 Sep 7.

Ibrahim FA, Usman LA, Akolade JO, Idowu OA, Abdulazeez AT, Amuzat AO. Antidiabetic potentials of citrus aurantifolia leaf essential oil. Drug Res (stuttg). 2019 Apr;69(4):201-206. Epub 2018 Oct 1.

Lee S-M, Park S-Y, Kim M-J, Cho E-A, Jun E-A, Park C-H, Kim H-S, Choi S-K, Rew J-S. Key lime (Citrus aurantifolia) inhibits the growth of triple drug resistant Helicobacter pylori. Gut Pathog. 2018; 10: 16. Published online 2018 May 21.

Narang N, Jiraungkoorskul W. Anticancer Activity of Key Lime, Citrus aurantifolia. Pharmacogn Rev. 2016 Jul-Dec; 10(20): 118-122.

Ruiz-Pérez NJ, González-Ávila M, Sánchez-Navarrete J, Toscano-Garibay JD, Moreno-Eutimio MA, Sandoval-Hernández T. Arriaga-Alba M. Antimycotic activity and genotoxic evaluation of Citrus sinensis and Citrus latifolia essential oils. Sci Rep. 2016 May 3;6:25371.

Kummer R, Fachini-Queiroz FC, Estevão-Silva CF, Grespan R, Silva EL, Bersani-Amado CA, Cuman RK. Evaluation of anti-inflammatory activity of Citrus latifolia Tanaka essential oil and Limonene in experimental mouse models. Evid Based Complement Alternat Med. 2013;2013:859083. Epub 2013 May 15.

Meiyanto E, Hermawan A, Anindyajati. Natural products for cancer-targeted therapy: citrus flavonoids as potent chemopreventive agents. Asian Pac J Cancer Prev. 2012;13(2):427-436.

Essential Oil Singles & Blends | **Chapter 2**

While you're putting that Lime in the coconut, put some in the diffuser too.

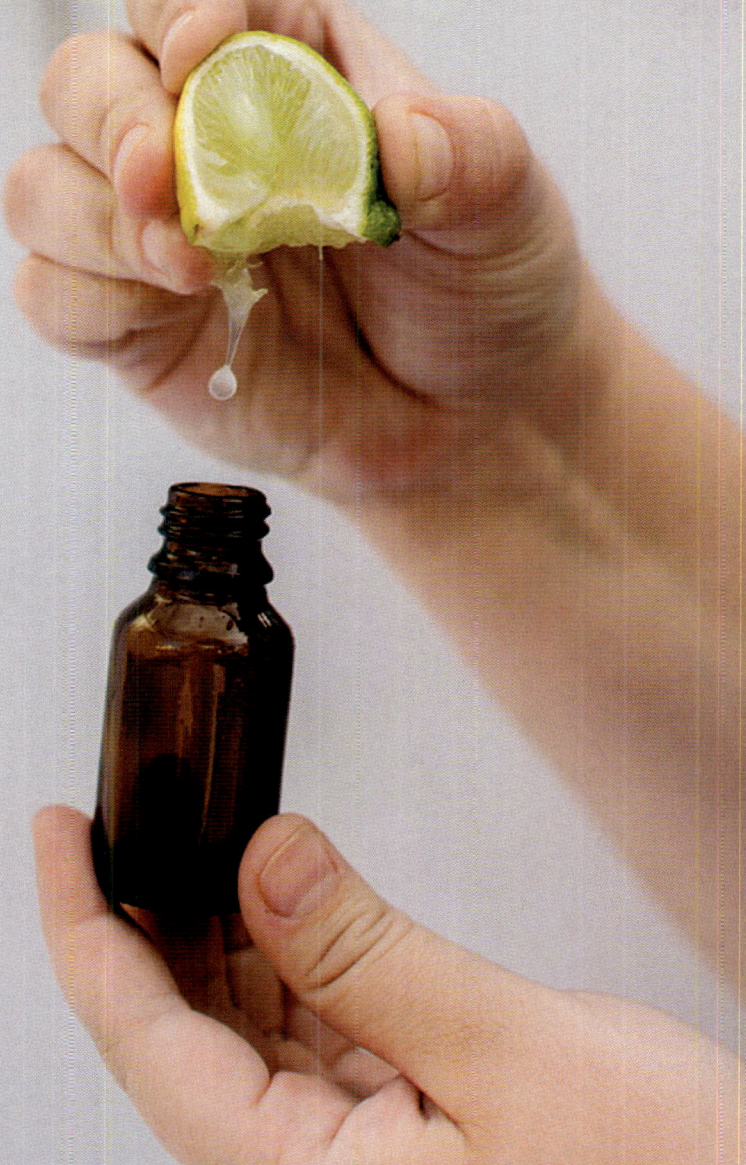

LIVE WITH PASSION™
(Essential Oil Blend)

This blend revives the zest for life and improves internal energy with a combination of essential oils formulated specifically to help people attain an optimistic attitude.

MEDICAL PROPERTIES & USES:
Antiallergy, anti-inflammatory, antimicrobial, antioxidative, calming, dietary, digestion or elimination supportive/nausea reducing, disease inhibitory, insecticidal/antiparasitic, nervous system supportive

INGREDIENTS:
Royal Hawaiian Sandalwood, Clary Sage, Ginger, Jasmine, Angelica, Patchouli, Cedarwood, Helichrysum, Melissa, Bitter Orange (Neroli)

DIRECTIONS:
Aromatic: 30. Topical: 50-50. Mix 2-4 drops of oil with 2 tablespoons of a bath and shower gel or mix with ½ cup bath salts water and pour into the tub. Soak for 20-30 minutes or until water cools.

CAUTIONS:

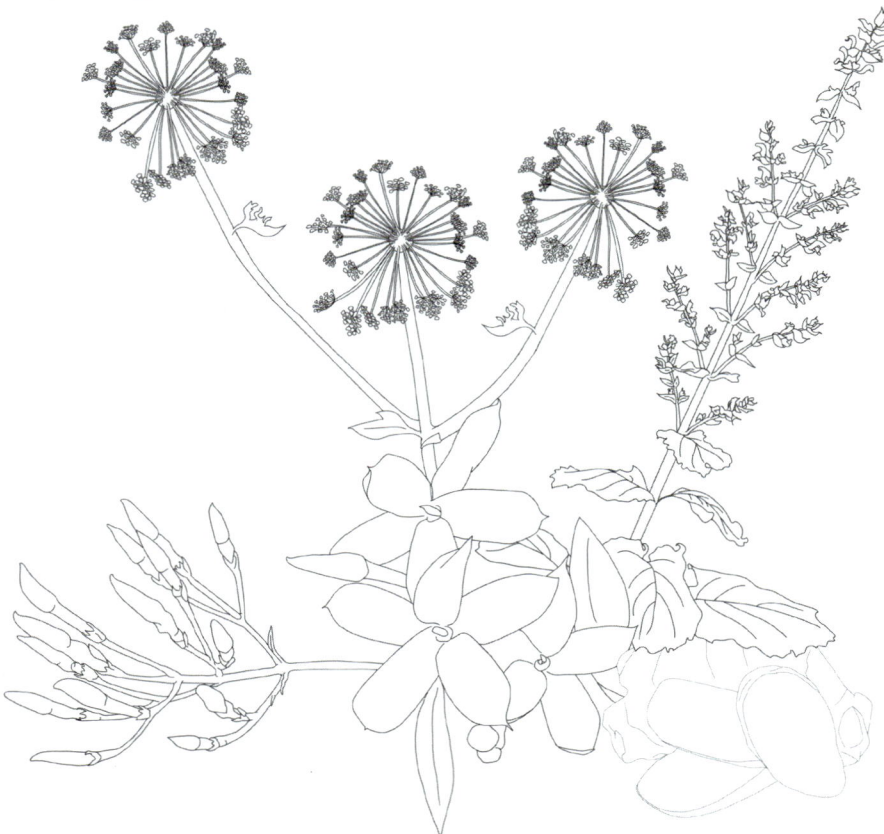

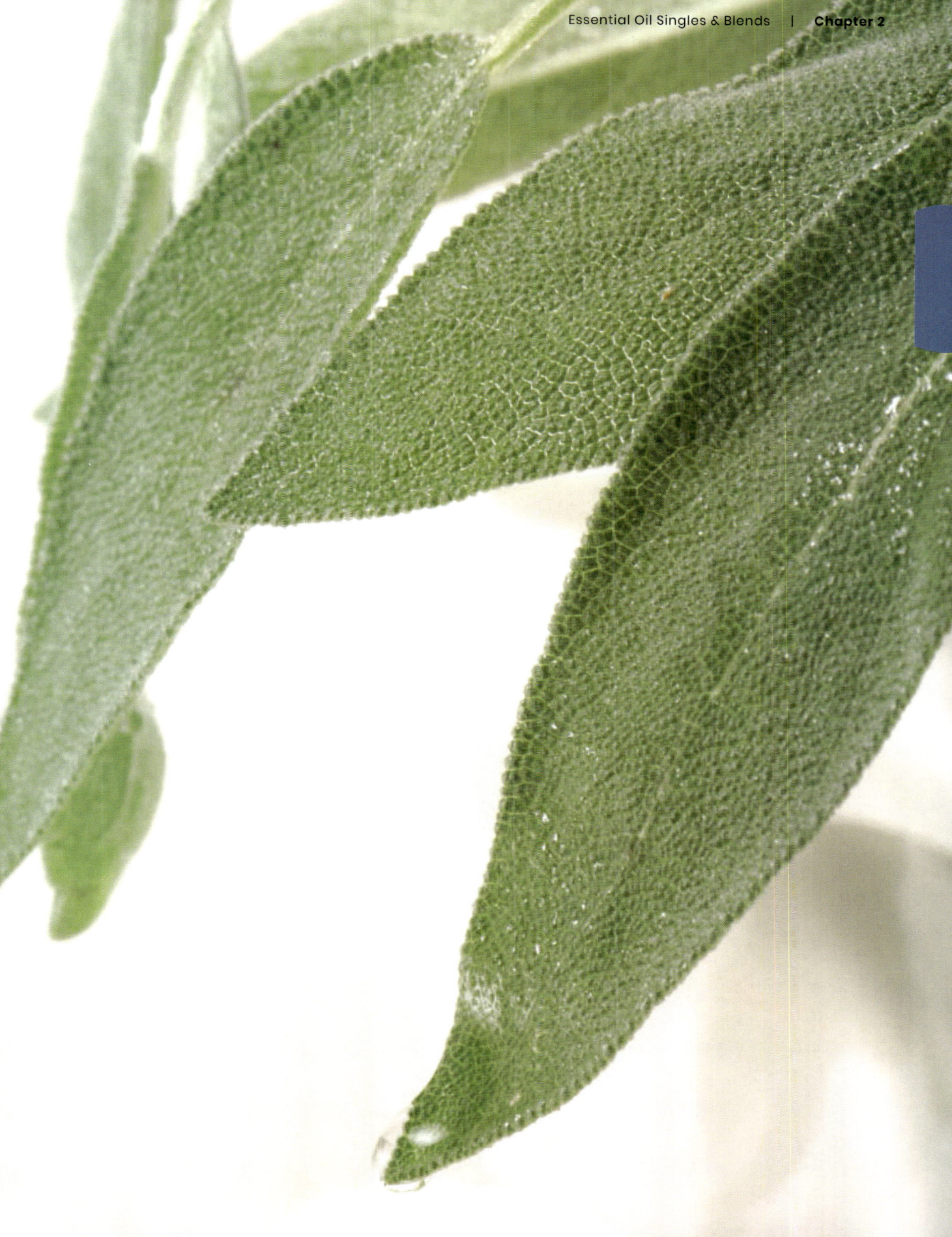

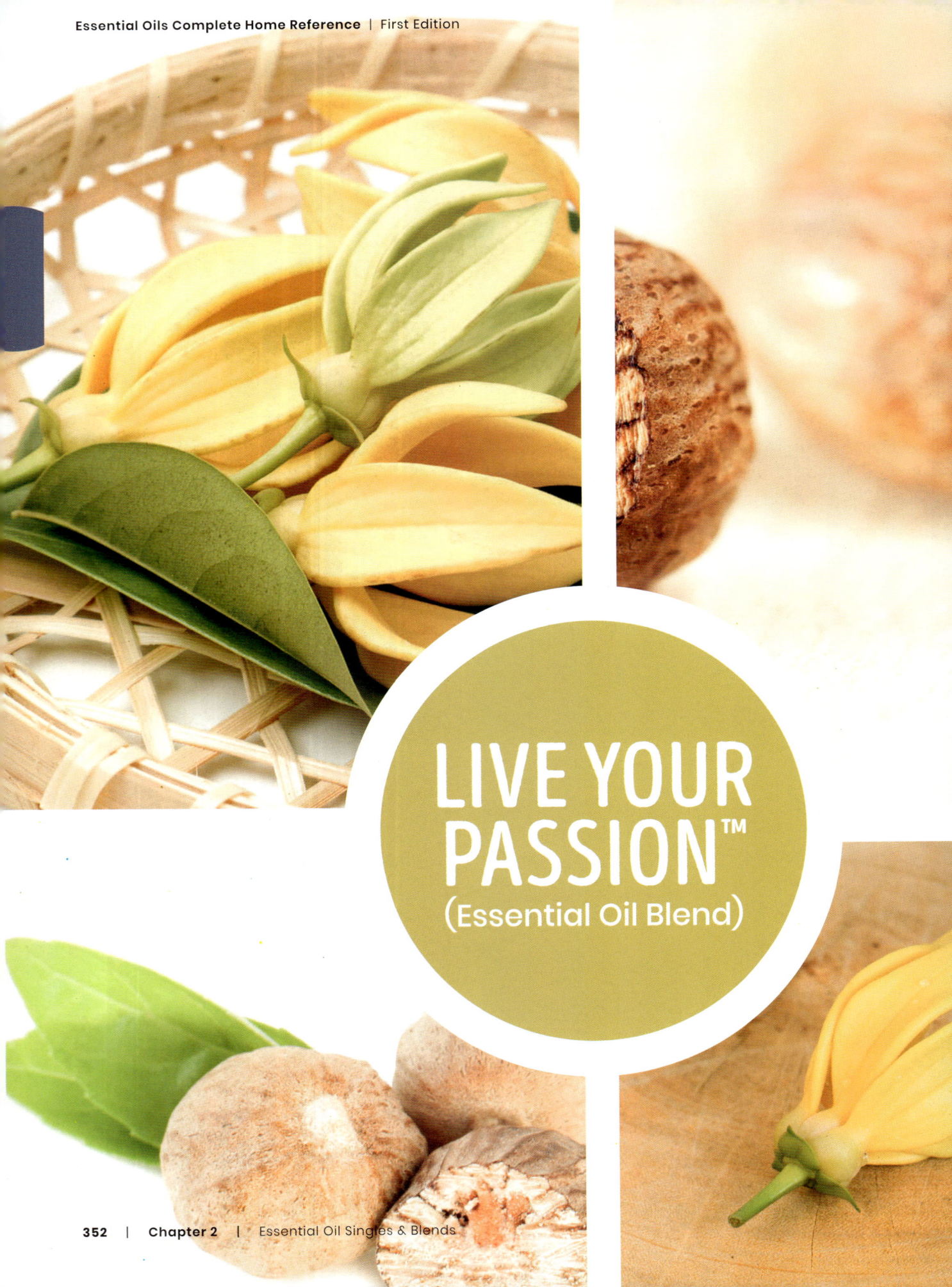

ABOUT LIVE YOUR PASSION™:

Live Your Passion enhances the zest for life and improves internal energy to specifically help people go forward with motivation and excitement.

MEDICAL PROPERTIES & USES:

Anti-inflammatory, antimicrobial, antioxidative, calming, digestion or elimination supportive/nausea reducing, disease inhibitory, insecticidal/antiparasitic, performance enhancing/stimulating, skin and hair improving

INGREDIENTS:

Orange, Royal Hawaiian Sandalwood, Nutmeg, Lime, Idaho Blue Spruce, Northern Lights Black Spruce, Ylang Ylang, Frankincense, Peppermint

DIRECTIONS:

Aromatic: 3o. Topical: 50-50.

CAUTIONS:

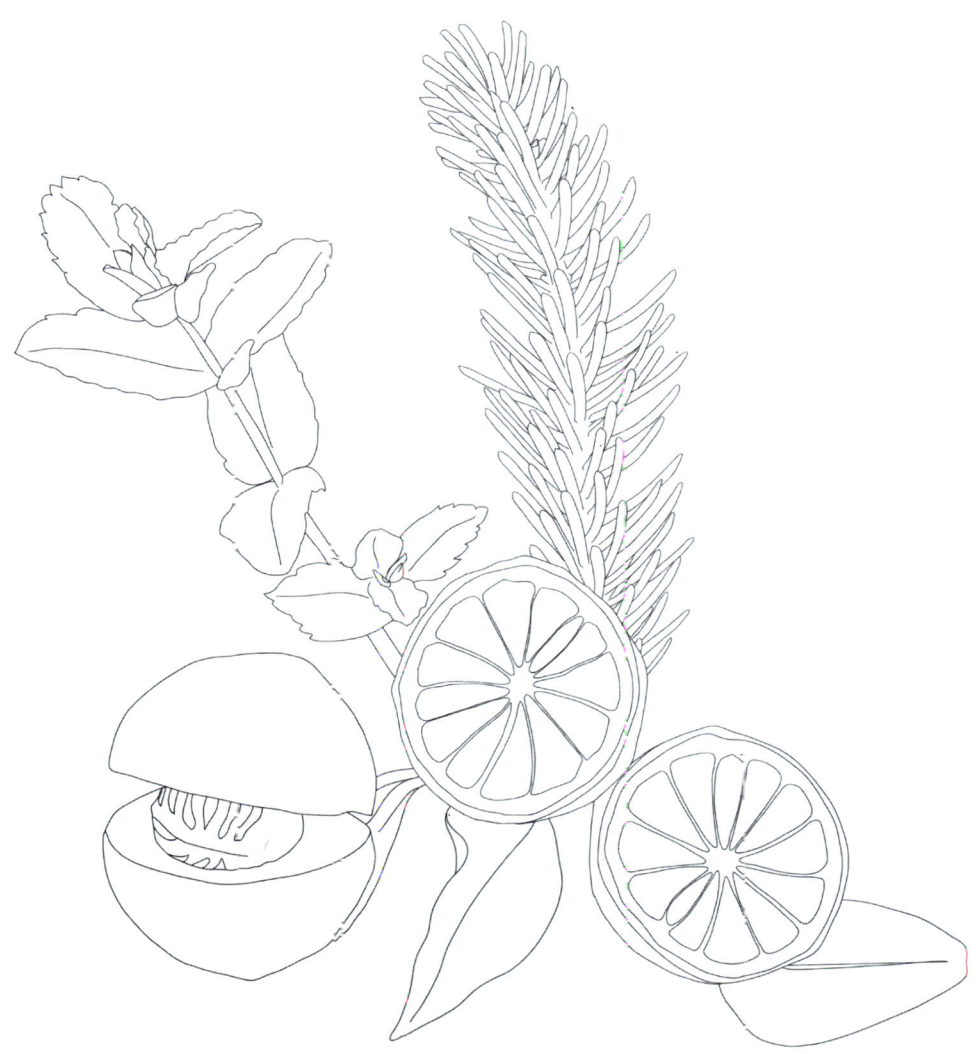

LONGEVITY™ & LONGEVITY™ VITALITY™
(Essential Oil Blend)

This oil contains the highest antioxidant and DNA-protecting essential oils. When taken as a dietary supplement, this blend promotes longevity and prevents premature aging (see Longevity™ Softgels in Chapter 8, Nutritional Support).

MEDICAL PROPERTIES & USES:
Anti-inflammatory, antimicrobial, antioxidative, calming, cardiovascular supportive, insecticidal/antiparasitic, organ protective, pain or swelling reducing, skin and hair improving, wellness supporting

INGREDIENTS:
Thyme, Orange, Clove, Frankincense

DIRECTIONS:
Aromatic: 10. Topical: 20-80. Dietary (Vitality): Dilute 1 drop with 4 drops of V-6 or other pure carrier oil. Put in a capsule and take 1 daily or as needed, or put 2-3 drops in Yacon Syrup, honey, or maple syrup in a spoon; mix and swallow; or mix in about 4 fl. oz. of NingXia Red, goat milk, or rice milk, etc.

CAUTIONS:

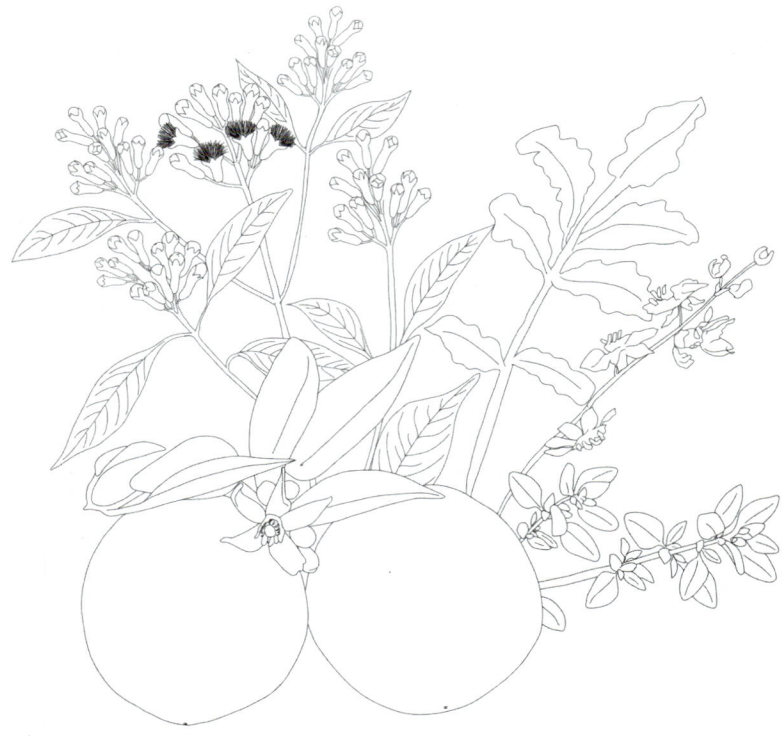

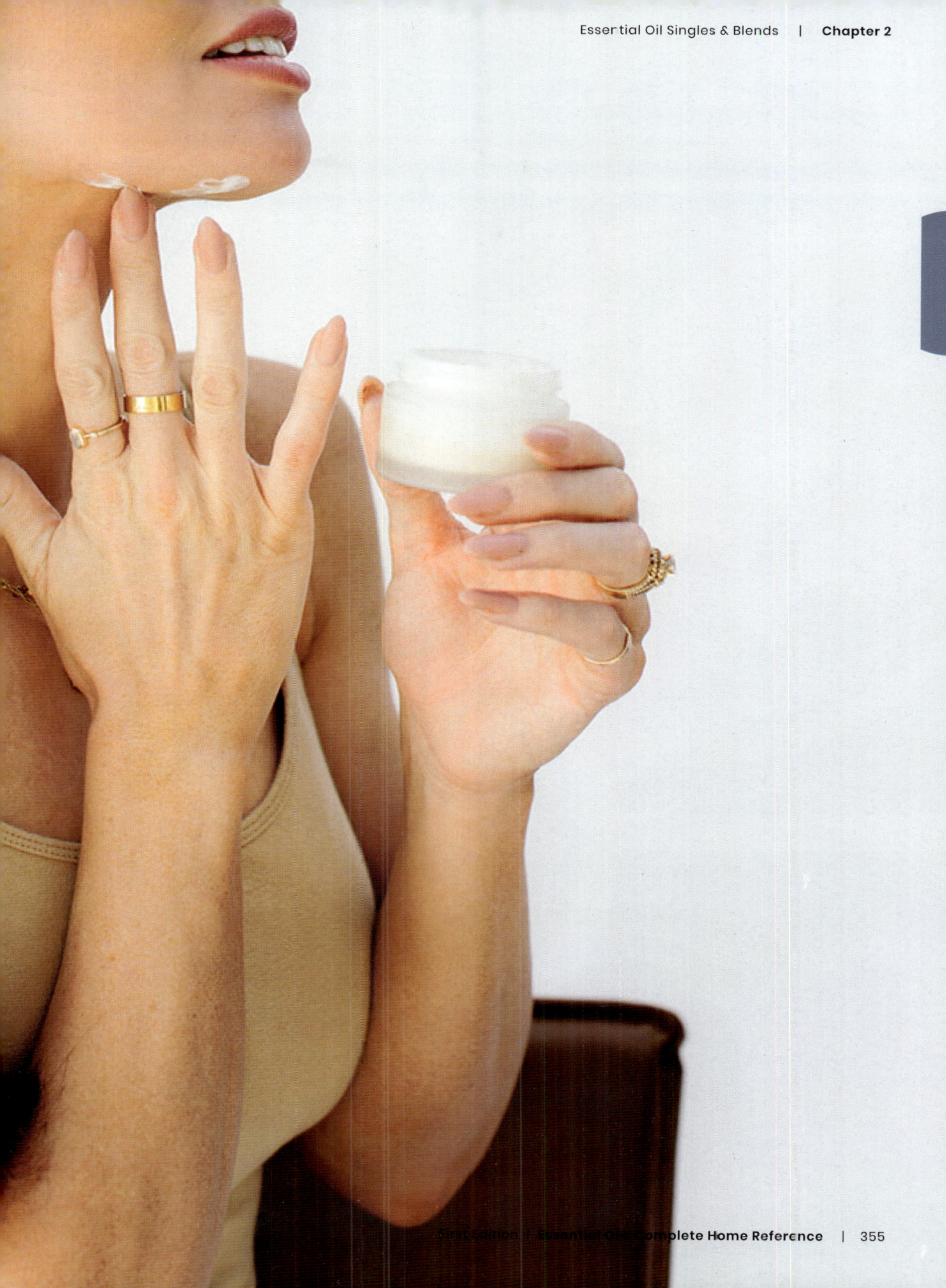

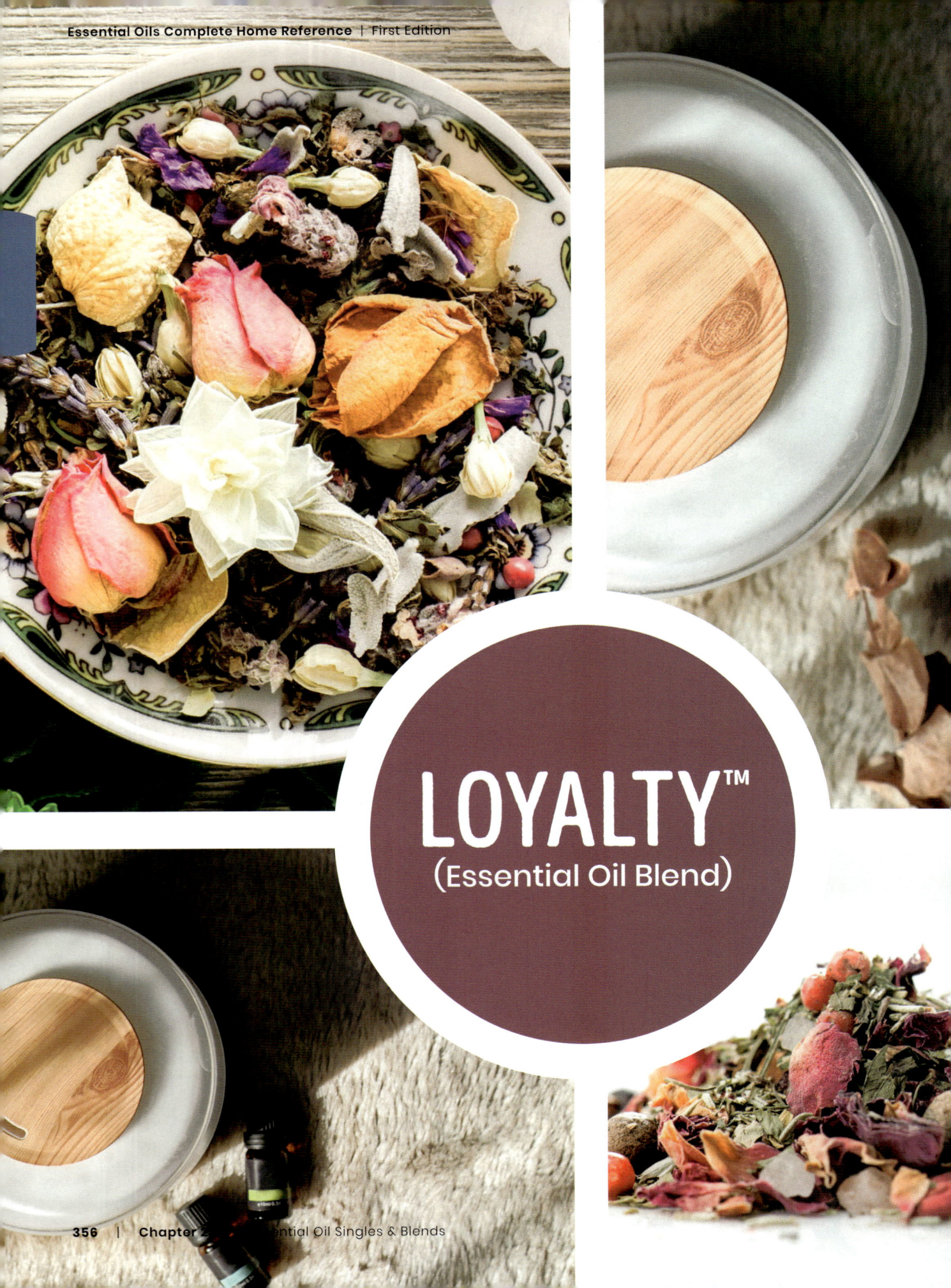

LOYALTY™
(Essential Oil Blend)

ABOUT LOYALTY™:

Loyalty essential oil blend will empower you to remain steadfast and faithful to all that you value. Uplifting and empowering oils cherished around the world such as Rose, Sacred Frankincense, and Sacred Sandalwood will strengthen your devotion.

MEDICAL PROPERTIES & USES:

Antiallergy, anti-inflammatory, antimicrobial, antioxidative, calming, digestion or elimination supportive/nausea reducing, disease inhibitory, insecticidal/antiparasitic, nervous system supporting, pain or swelling reducing, performance enhancing

INGREDIENTS:

Caprylic/capric triglyceride, Angelica, Ylang Ylang, Lavender, Idaho Blue Spruce, Cassia, Vetiver, Sacred Sandalwood, Geranium, Sacred Frankincense, Patchouli, Cardamom, Mastrante, Peppermint, Melissa, Rose

DIRECTIONS:

Aromatic: 6o. Topical: Neat.

CAUTIONS: Not intended for use on infants.

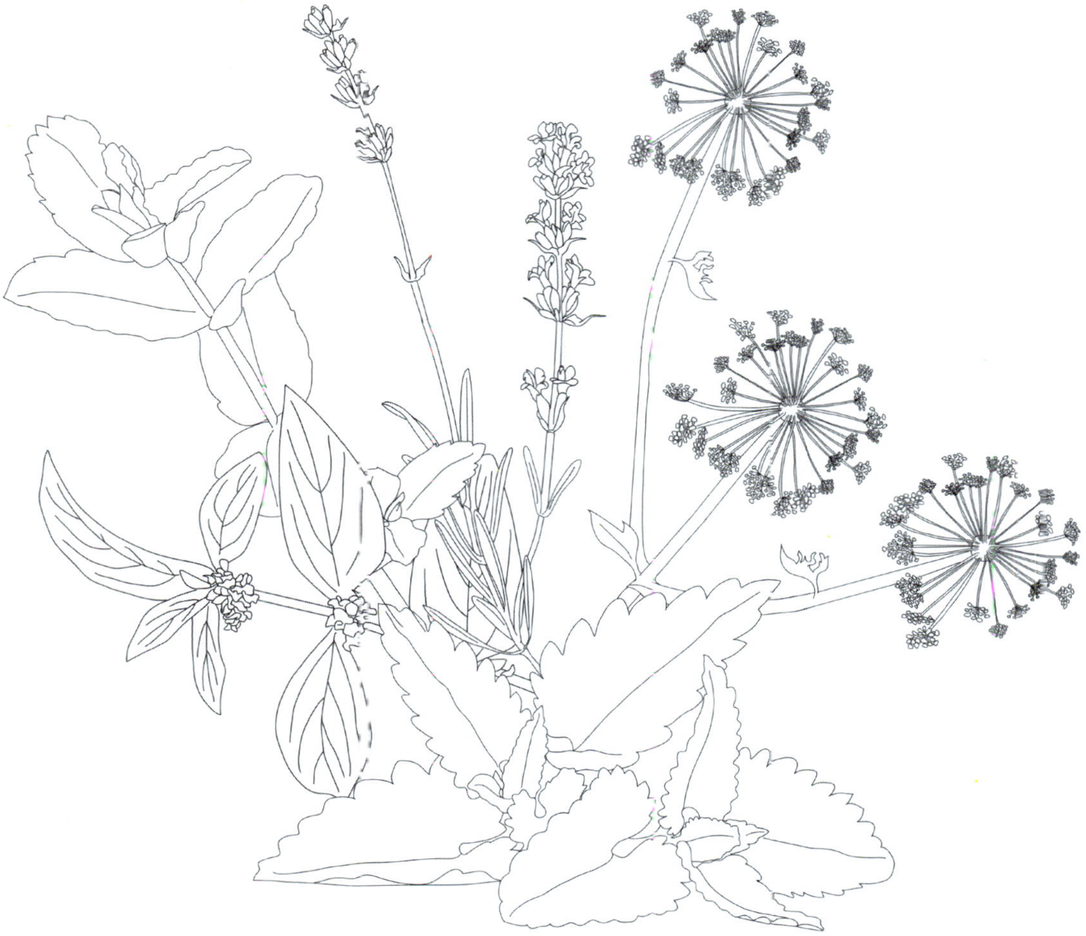

MAGNIFY YOUR PURPOSE™
(Essential Oil Blend)

This blend stimulates the endocrine system for greater energy flow to the right hemisphere of the brain, activating creativity, motivation, and focus. This helps strengthen commitment to purpose, desire, and intentions until you realize your goals.

MEDICAL PROPERTIES & USES:
Antiallergy, anti-inflammatory, antimicrobial, antioxidative, calming, digestion or elimination supportive/nausea reducing, disease inhibitory, glandular/hormonal supportive, insecticidal/antiparasitic, nervous system supportive, performance enhancing/stimulating, wellness supportive

INGREDIENTS:
Sacred Sandalwood, Sage, Coriander, Patchouli, Nutmeg, Bergamot, Cinnamon Bark, Ginger, Ylang Ylang, Geranium

DIRECTIONS:
Aromatic: 30. Topical: 50-50.

CAUTIONS:

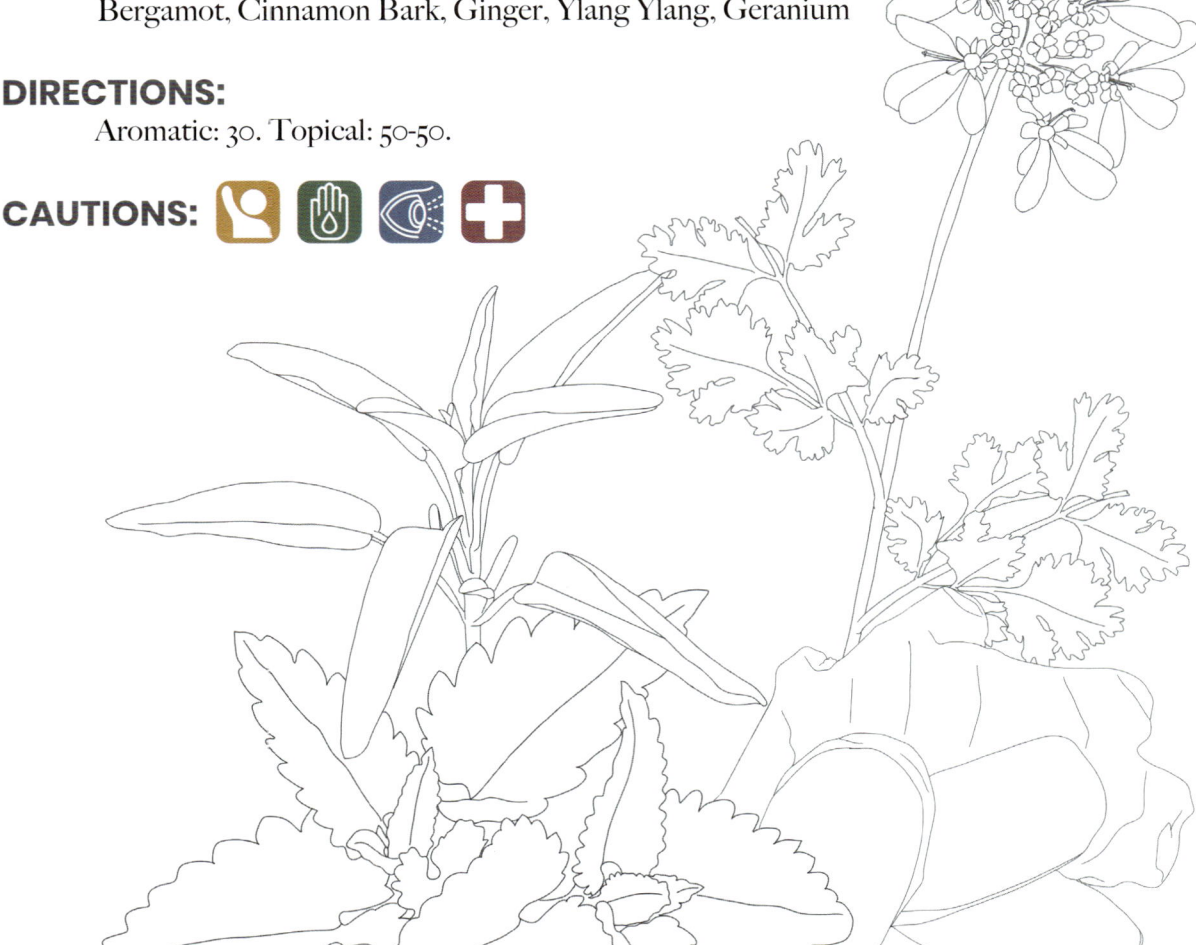

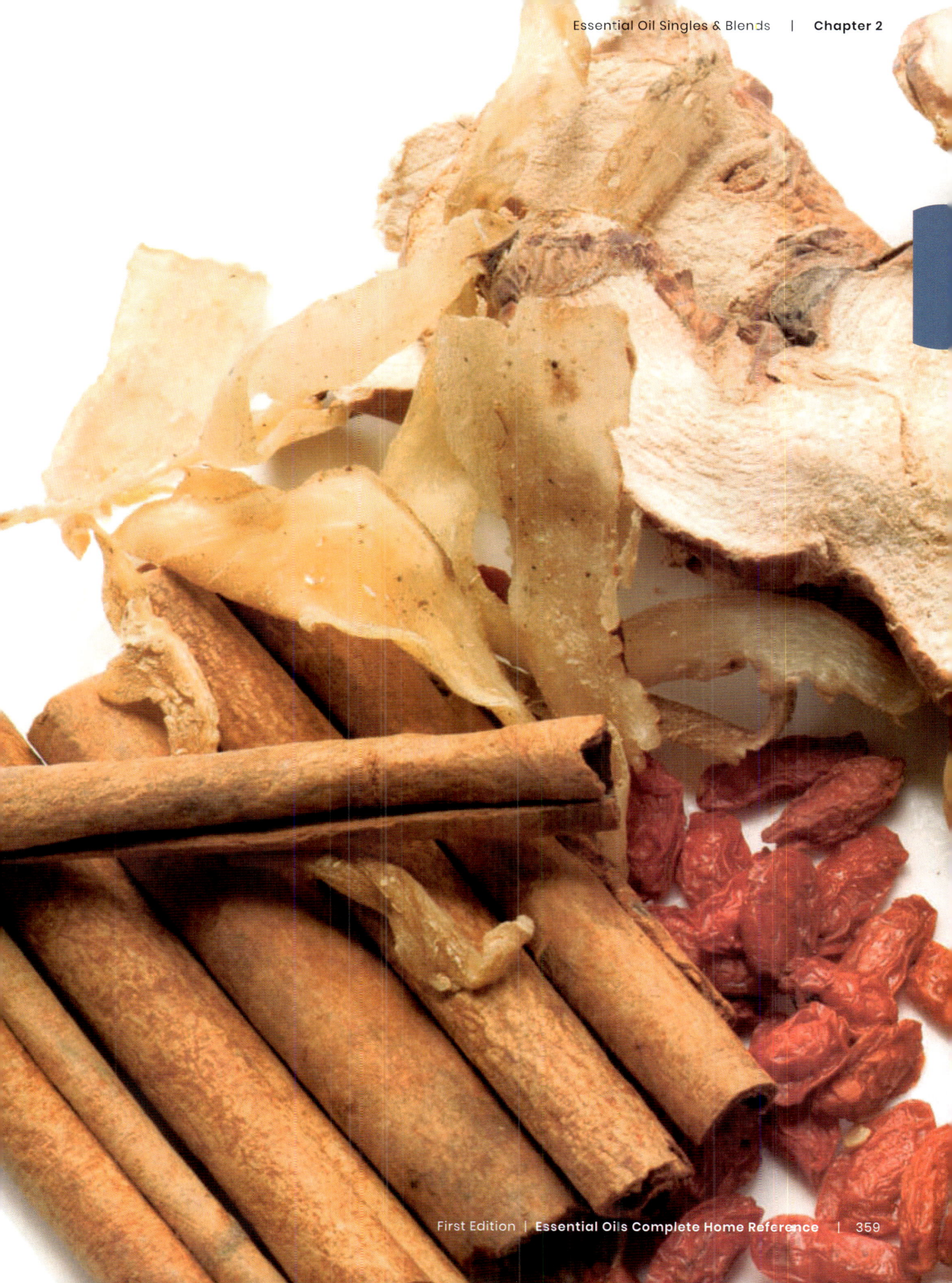

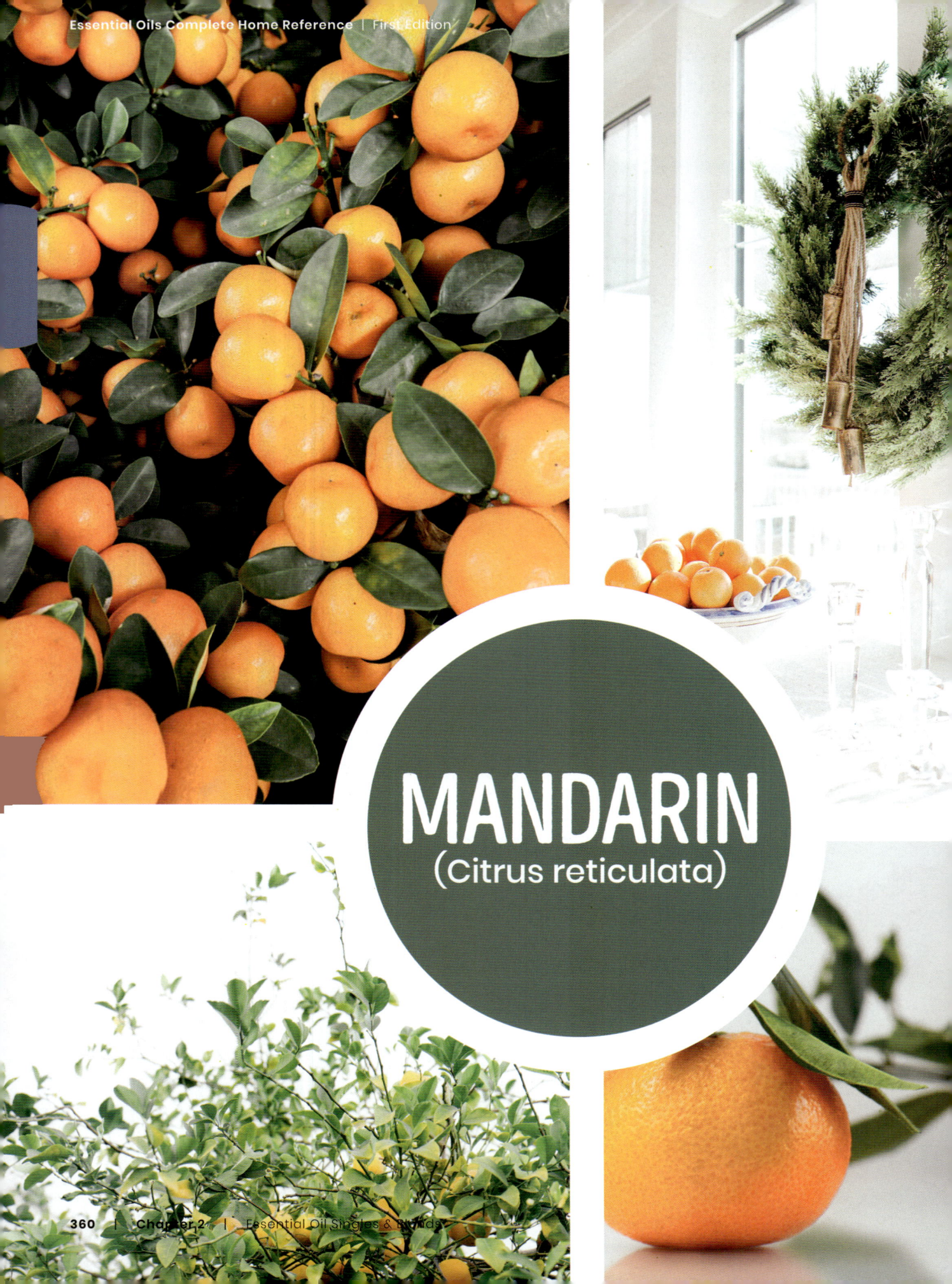

MANDARIN
(Citrus reticulata)

BOTANICAL FAMILY:
Rutaceae

PLANT ORIGIN:
Italy

EXTRACTION METHOD:
Cold pressed from rind

KEY CONSTITUENTS:
Limonene (65-75%),
Gamma-Terpinene (16-22%),
Alpha-Pinene (2-3%),
Beta-Pinene (1-2%),
Myrcene (1-2%)

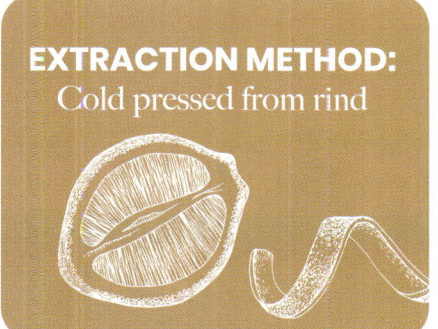

HISTORICAL DATA:
This fruit was traditionally given to Imperial Chinese officials named the Mandarins. It has a light, sweet smell enjoyed by all.

MEDICAL PROPERTIES:
Light antispasmodic, digestive tonic (digestoid), antifungal, antioxidant, stimulates the gallbladder; rich in limonene, which has been extensively studied in over 50 clinical studies for its ability to combat tumor growth.

USES:
Digestive problems, fluid retention, insomnia, anxiety, intestinal problems, skin problems (congested and oily skin, scars, acne), stretch marks (when combined with either Jasmine, Lavender, Sandalwood, and/or Frankincense)

FRAGRANT INFLUENCE:
Appeasing, gentle, promotes happiness. A Mie University study found that citrus fragrances boosted immunity, induced relaxation, and reduced depression (Komori, et al., 1995).

DIRECTIONS:
Aromatic: 60. Topical: 50-50.
Dietary: Take as a dietary supplement.

CAUTIONS:

SELECTED RESEARCH:

Wang Ym, Zang W, Ji S, Cao J, Sung C. Three Polymethoxyflavones Purified from Ougan (Citrus reticulata Cv. Suavissim) Inhibited LPS-Induced NO Elevation in the Neuroglia BV-2 Cell Line via the JAK2/STAT3 Pathway. Nurients. 2019 Apr; 11(4): 791.

Apraj VD, Pandita NS. Evaluation of skin anti-aging potential of Citrus reticulata Blanco Peel. Pharmacognosy Res. 2016 Jul-Sep;8(3):160-8.

Zhang Y, Sun Y, Xi W, Shen Y, Qiao L, Zhong L, Ye X, Zhou Z. Phenolic compositions and antioxidant capacities of Chinese wild mandarin (Citrus reticulata Blanco) fruits. Food Chem. 2014 Feb 15;145:674-80. Epub 2013 Aug 11.

El-Khadragy MF, Al-Olayan EM, Abdel Moneim AE. Neuroprotective effects of Citrus reticulata in scopolamine-induced dementia oxidative stress in rats. CNS Neurol Disord Drug Targets. 2014;13(4):684-90.

Tao N, Jia L, Zhou H. Anti-fungal activity of Citrus reticulata Blanco essential oil against Penicillium italicum and Penicillium digitatum. Food Chem. 2014 Jun 15; 53:265-71. Epub 2013 Dec 25.

Kawahata I, Yoshida M, Sun W, Nakajima A, Lai Y, Osaka N, Matsuzaki K, Yokosuka A, Mimaki Y, Naganuma A, Tomioka Y, Yamakuni T. Potent activity of nobiletin-rich Citrus reticulata peel extract to facilitate cAMP/PKA/ERK/CREB signaling associated with learning and memory in cultured hippocampal neurons: identification of the substances responsible for the pharmacological action. J Neural Transm (Vienna). 2013 Oct;120(10):1397-409. Epub 2013 Apr 16.

Manassero CA, Girotti JR, Mijailovsky S, Garcia de Bravo M, Polo M. In vitro comparative analysis of antiproliferative activity of essential oil from mandarin peel and its principle component limonene. Nat Prod Res. 2013;27(16):1475-8. Epub 2012 Sep 4.

Komori T, Fujiwara R, Tanida M, Nomura J, Yokoyama MM. Effects of citrus fragrance on immune function and depressive states. Neuroimmunomodulation. 1995 May-Jun;2(3):174-80.

BOTANICAL FAMILY:
Myrtaceae

PLANT ORIGIN:
New Zealand

EXTRACTION METHOD:
Steam distilled from leaves/flowers/branches

KEY CONSTITUENTS:
Leptospermone (8-25%),
Trans-Calamenene (9-19%),
Flavesone (up to 13%),
Cadina-3,5-diene (1-10%),
Alpha-Copaene (3-8%),
Isoleptospermone (4-8%),
Alpha-Selinene (1-7%)

MANUKA
(Leptospermum scoparium)

Similar to tea tree oil but warmer, richer, and milder, Manuka oil has long been used in the treatment of skin, foot, and hair problems. Like Tea Tree oil, it is antibacterial, antiviral, and antifungal, so it can help in eliminating a wide variety of problems. Some research suggests that Manuka essential oil may be more potent in fighting bacteria and fungi than Tea Tree oil. "Manuka" is the Maori name for the bushy tree from which the oil is produced.

MEDICAL PROPERTIES:
Antibacterial, antiviral, potential for preventing chemotherapy side effects, antifungal, antioxidant, antiphotoaging, anti-inflammatory, anti-acne. Although research is ongoing, many believe Manuka has potential in fighting antibiotic-resistant organisms such as MRSA. A leading German aromatherapist reports that the Manuka aroma is psychologically very beneficial for people who suffer from stress and anxiety. Its skin-healing properties are exceptional.

USES:
Supports appearance of healthy-looking skin, skin infections, acne, bedsores, mild sunburn, fungal infections, itching, respiratory infections, sore throats, pain relief in muscles and joints, athletes foot and ringworm, dandruff, body odor, cold sores, dermatitis, rhinitis, tonsillitis, stress relief, sleep aid

FRAGRANT INFLUENCE:
Warm, calming

DIRECTIONS:
Aromatic: 30. Topical: Neat.

CAUTIONS:

SELECTED RESEARCH:

Lin B, Daniels BJ, Middleditch MJ, Furkert DP, Brimble MA, Bong J, Stephens JM, Loomes KM. Utility of the Leptospermum scoparium Compound Lepteridine as a Chemical Marker for Manuka Honey Authenticity. ACS Omega. 2020 Apr 21; 5(15): 8858-8866. Published online Apr 8.

Orchard A, van Vuuren SF, Viljoen AM, Kamatou G. The in vitro antimicrobial evaluation of commercial essential oils and their combinations against acne. Int J Cosmet Sci. 2018 Mar 24. [Epub ahead of print].

Killeen DP, Larsen L, Dayan FE, Gordon KC, Perry NB, van Klink JW. Nortriketones: antimicrobial trimethylated acylphloroglucinols from Mānuka (Leptospermum scoparium). J Nat Prod. 2016 Mar 25;79(3):564-9. Epub 2016 Jan 5.

Hammond EN, Donkor ES. Antibacterial effect of Manuka honey on Clostridium difficile. BMC Res Notes. 2013 May 7;6:188.

Song CY, Nam EH, Park SH, Hwang CY. In vitro efficacy of the essential oil from Leptospermum scoparium (manuka) on antimicrobial susceptibility and biofilm formation in Staphylococcus pseudintermedius isolates from dogs. Vet Dermatol. 2013 Aug;24(4):404-8. Epub 2013 Jun 17.

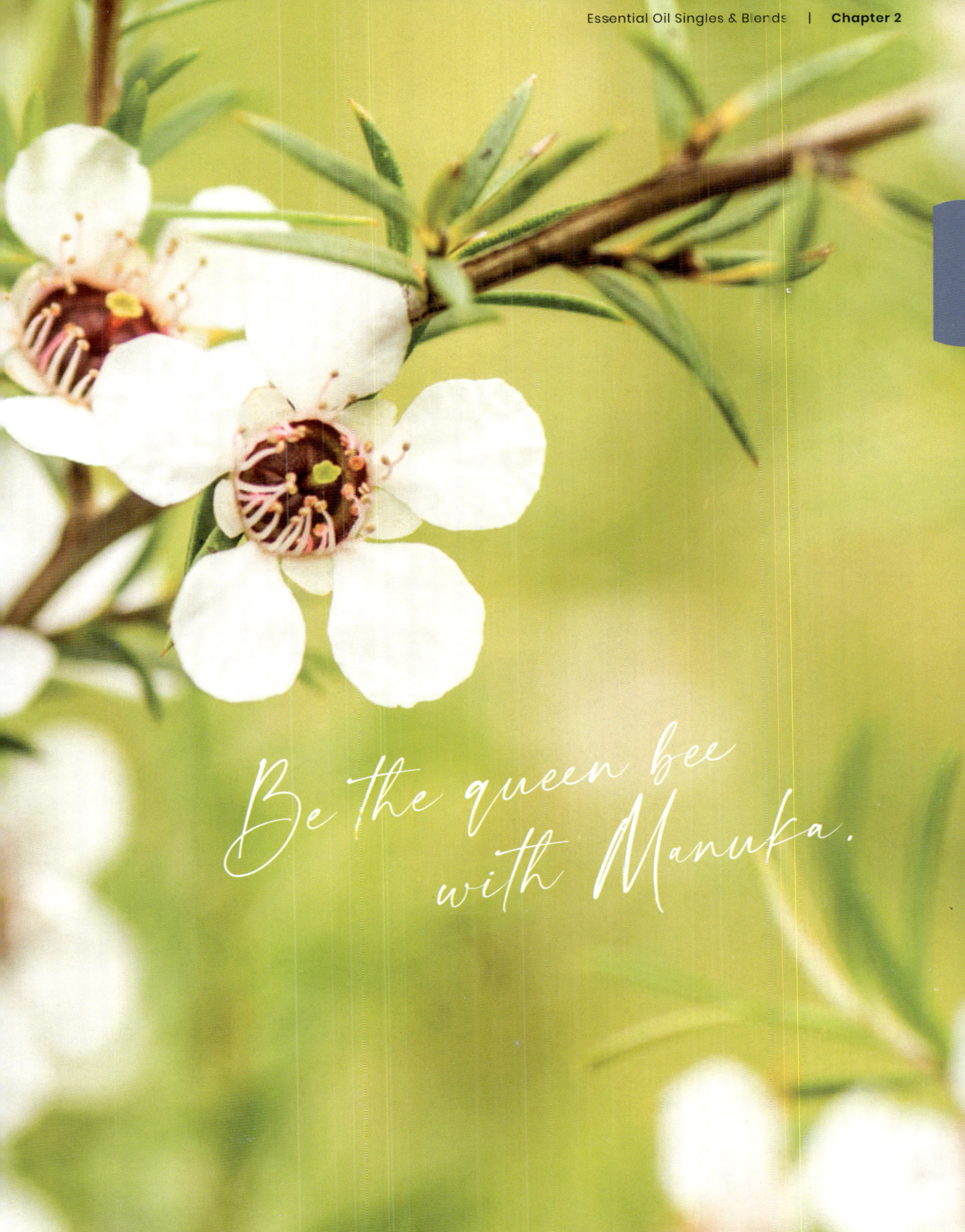

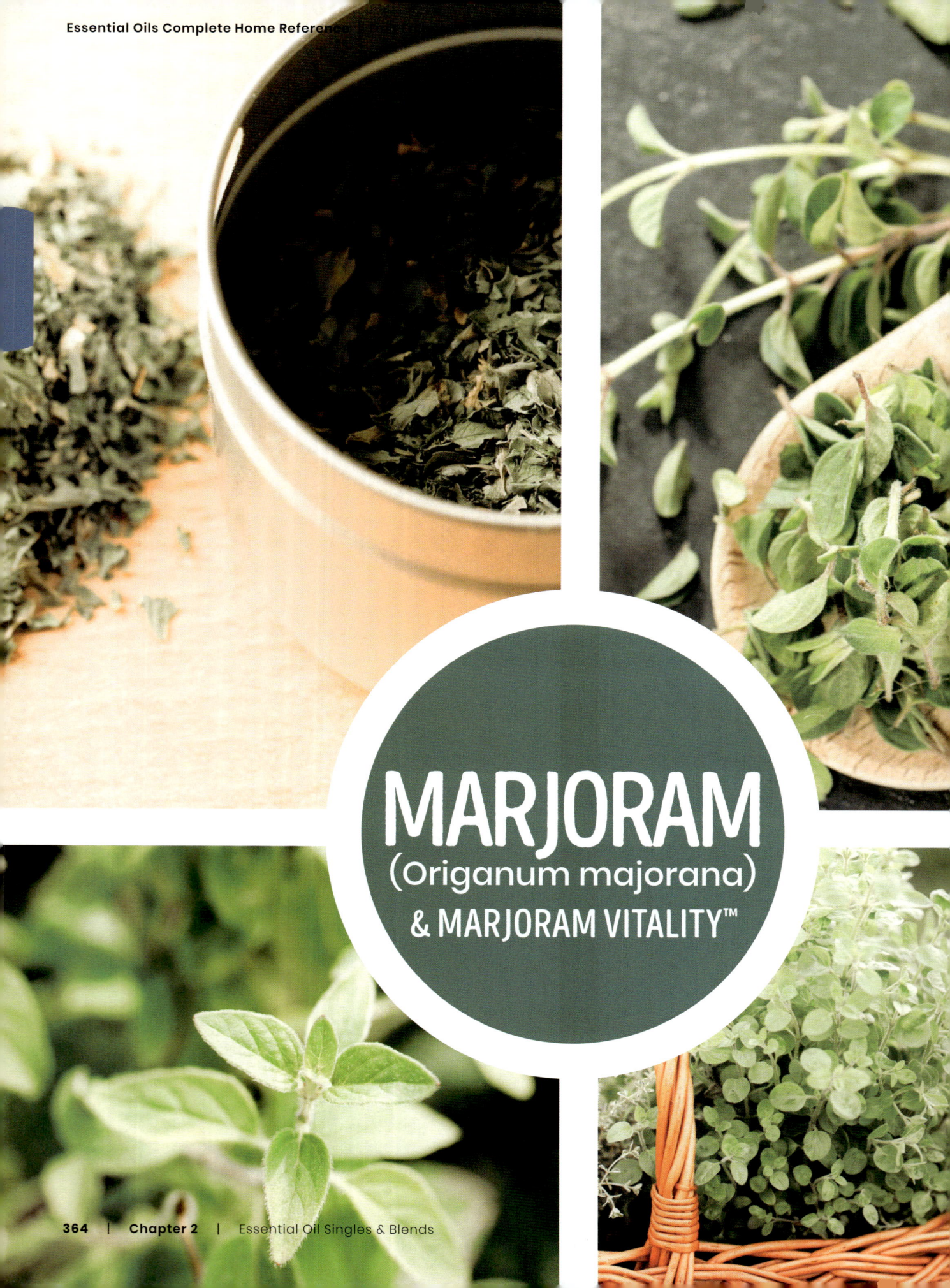

Essential Oil Singles & Blends | Chapter 2

BOTANICAL FAMILY:
Lamiaceae

PLANT ORIGIN:
Egypt

EXTRACTION METHOD:
Steam distilled from leaves

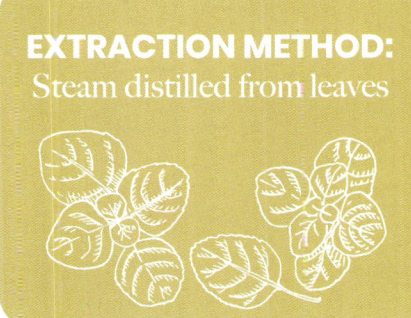

KEY CONSTITUENTS:
Terpinene-4-ol (16-29%),
Linalool + Cis-4-Thujanol (7-28%),
Gamma-Terpinene (10-16%),
Alpha-Terpinene (6-10%),
Sabinene (5-10%),
Alpha-Terpineol (2-6%),
Trans-4-Thujanol (1-6%)

HISTORICAL DATA:
Marjoram was known as the "herb of happiness" to the Romans and "joy of the mountains" to the Greeks. It was believed to increase longevity. It is listed in Dioscorides' De Materia Medica (AD 78), Europe's first authoritative guide to medicines, which became the standard reference work for herbal treatments for over 1,700 years. It was also listed in Hildegard's Medicine, a compilation of early German medicines by highly regarded Benedictine herbalist Hildegard of Bingen (1098-1179).

MEDICAL PROPERTIES:
Protective effect of gastric mucosal injury, anticancer, general relaxant, antibacterial, antifungal, vasodilator, lowers blood pressure, promotes intestinal peristalsis, expectorant, mucolytic.

USES:
Improves lung function, arthritis/rheumatism, muscle/nerve pain, headaches, circulatory disorders, respiratory infections, soothes digestive tract, menstrual problems/PMS, fungal infections, ringworm, shingles, sores, spasms, fluid retention, enhances food flavors

FRAGRANT INFLUENCE:
Herbaceous, assists in calming the nerves

DIRECTIONS:
Aromatic: 30. Topical: 50-50. Use in Raindrop Technique.
Dietary (Vitality): Dilute 1 drop with 1 drop of carrier oil. Put in a capsule and take up to 3 times daily or as needed.

CAUTIONS:

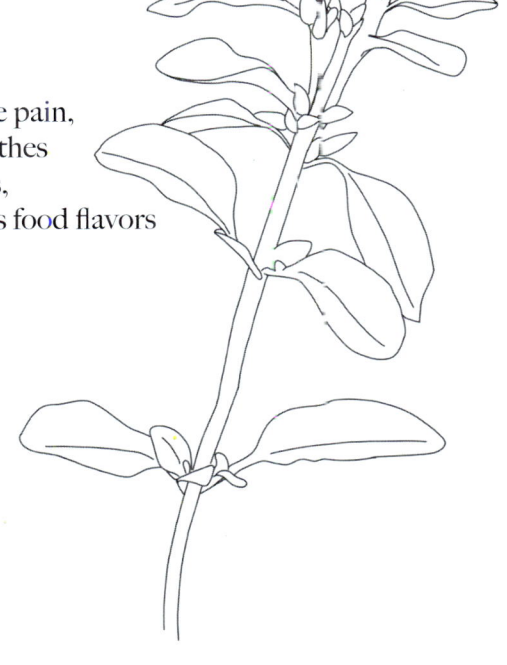

SELECTED RESEARCH:

Gomes F, Dias MI, Lima Â, Barros L, Rodrigues ME, Ferreira CFR, Henriques M. Satureja montana L. and Origanum majorana L. Decoctions: Antimicrobial Activity, Mode of Action and Phenolic Characterization. Antibiotics (Basel). 2020 June 9(6): 294. Published online 2020 May 31.

Athamneh K, Alneyadi A, Alsamri H, Alrashedi A, Palakott A, El-Tarabily K, Eid AH, Al Dhaheri Y, Iratni R. Origanum majorana Essential Oil Triggers p38 MAPK-Mediated Protective Autophagy, Apoptosis, and Caspase-Dependent Cleavage of P70S6K in Colorectal Cancer Cells. Biomolecules. 2020 Mar; 10(3): 412. Published online 2020 Mar 6.

Soliman AM, Desouky S, Marzouk M, Sayed AA. Origanum majorana attenuates nephrotoxicity of cisplatin anticancer drug through ameliorating oxidative stress. Nutrients. 2016 May 5;8(5).

Erenler R, Sen O, Aksit H, Demirtas I, Yaglioglu AS, Elmastas M, Telci I. Isolation and identification of chemical constituents from Origanum majorana and investigation of antiproliferative and antioxidant activities. J Sci Food Agric. 2016 Feb;96(3):822-36. Epub 2015 Apr 8.

Hajlaoui H, Mighri H, Aouni M, Gharsallah N, Kadri A. Chemical composition and in vitro evaluation of antioxidant, antimicrobial, cytotoxicity and anti-acetylcholinesterase properties of Tunisian Origanum majorana L. essential oil. Microbial Pathogenesis. 2015;95:86-94.

Rafaie AA, Ramadan A, Mossa AT. Oxidative damage and nephrotoxicity induced by prallethrin in rat and the protective effect of Origanum majorana essential oil. Asian Pac J Trop Med. 2014 Sep;7S1:S506-13.

Srivatstava A. Ginjupalli K, Perampalli NU, Bhat N, Ballal M. Evaluation of the properties of a tissue conditioner containing origanum oil as an antifungal additive. J Prosthet Dent. 2013 Oct;110(4):313-9.

Al Dhaheri Y, Attoub S, Arafat K, Abuqamar S, Viallet J, Saleh A, Al Agha H, Eid A, Iratni R. Antimetastatic and antitumor growth effects of Origanum majorana on highly metastatic human breast cancer cells: inhibition of NFκB signaling and reduction of nitric oxide production. PLoS One. 2013 Jul 10;8(7):e68808.

BOTANICAL FAMILY:
Verbenaceae

PLANT ORIGIN:
Ecuador

EXTRACTION METHOD:
Steam distilled from stem/leaves

KEY CONSTITUENTS:
Carvone (32-59%),
Limonene (20-40%),
Germacrene D (7-18%),
Alpha-Bourbonene (1-4%),
Beta-Caryophyllene (1-4%)

MASTRANTE
(Lippia alba)

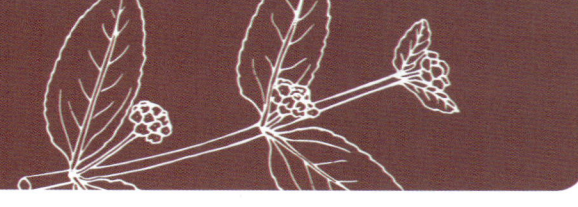

The plant Mastrante (Lippia alba) was given its botanical name by the Scottish botanist Philip Miller (1691-1771) and the British plant taxonomist N.E. Brown (1849-1934). As a result, in scientific literature it is listed as: "Lippia alba (Miller or Mill.) N.E. Brown." In Brazil, it is called erva cidreira do campo, which means "lemon balm of the field." The aromatic shrub grows in southern Texas, Mexico, the Caribbean, and Central and South America.

The leaves of Mastrante are used to flavor foods, most notably molé sauces from Oaxaca, Mexico. In folk medicine it is known as a sedative, an antidepressant, and a pain-reliever.

MEDICAL PROPERTIES:
Anticandida agent, antioxidant, analgesic, antibacterial, antiviral, antifungal, antispasmodic

USES:
Coughs, bronchitis, migraine headaches, vasorelaxant for heart disease

FRAGRANT INFLUENCE:
Grounding, calming

DIRECTIONS:
Aromatic: 30. Topical: 50-50.

CAUTIONS: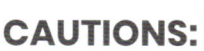

SELECTED RESEARCH:

Moreno ÉM, Leal SM, Stashenko EE, Garcia LT. Induction of programmed cell death in Trypanosoma cruzi by Lippia alba essential oils and their major and synergistic terpenes (citral, limonene and caryophyllene oxide). BMC Complement Altern Med. 2018; 18:225.

Porfirio EM, Melo HM, Pereira AMG, Cavalcante TTA, Gomes GA, de Carvalho MG, Costa RA, Catunda Júnior FEA. In Vitro Antibacterial and Antibiofilm Activity of Lippia alba Essential Oil, Citral and Carvone against Staphylococcus aureus. ScientificWorldJournal. 2017; 2017:4962707.

De Souza RC, da Costa MM, Baldisserotto B, Heinzmann BM, Schmidt D, Caron BO, Copatti CE. Antimicrobial and synergist c activity of essential oils of Aloysia triphylla and Lippia alba against Aeromonas spp. Microb Pat 1og. 2017 Dec;113:29-33. Epub 2017 Oct 14.

Olivero-Verbel J, Baretto-Maya A, Bertel-Sevilla A, Stashenko EE. Composition, anti-quorum sensing and antimicrobial activity of essential oils from Lippia alba. Braz J Microbiol. 2014; 45(3):759-767.

Machado TF, Nogueira NA, de Cássia Alves Pereira R, de Sousa CT, Batista VC. The antimicrobial efficacy of Lippia alba essential oil and its interaction with food ingredients. Braz J Microbiol. 2014 Aug 29;45(2):699-705. eCollection 2014.

Blanco MA, Colareda GA, van Baren C, Bandoni AL, Ringuelet J, Consolini AE. Antispasmodic effects and composition of the essential oils from two South American chemotypes of Lippia alba. J Ethnopharmacol. 2013 Oct 7;149(3):803-9. Epub 2013 Aug 13.

Carmona F, Angelucci MA, Sales DS, Chiaratti TM, Honorato FB, Bianchi RV, Pereira AM. Lippia alba (Miller or Mill.) N.E. Brown hydroethanolic extract of the leaves is effective in the treatment of migraine in women. Phytomedicine. 2013 Jul 15;20(10):947-50. Epub 2013 Apr 30.

Chies CE, Branco CS, Scola G, Agostini F, Gower AE, Salvador M. Antioxidant effect of Lippia alba (Miller or Mill) N.E. Brown. Antioxidants. 2013 Sep 26; 2(4):194-205.

Gómez LA, Stashenko E, Ocazionez RE. Comparative study on in vitro activities of citral, limonene and essential oils from Lippia citriodora and L. alba on yellow fever virus. Nat Prod Commun. 2013 Feb;8(2):249-52.

Heldwein CG, Silva LL, Reckziegel P, Barros FM, Bürger ME, Baldisserotto B, Mallmann CA, Schmidt D, Caron BO, Heinzmann BM. Participation of the GABAergic system in the anesthetic effect of Lippia alba (Miller or Mill.) N.E. Brown essential oil. Braz J Med Biol Res. 2012 May;45(5):436-43. Epub 2012 Apr 5.

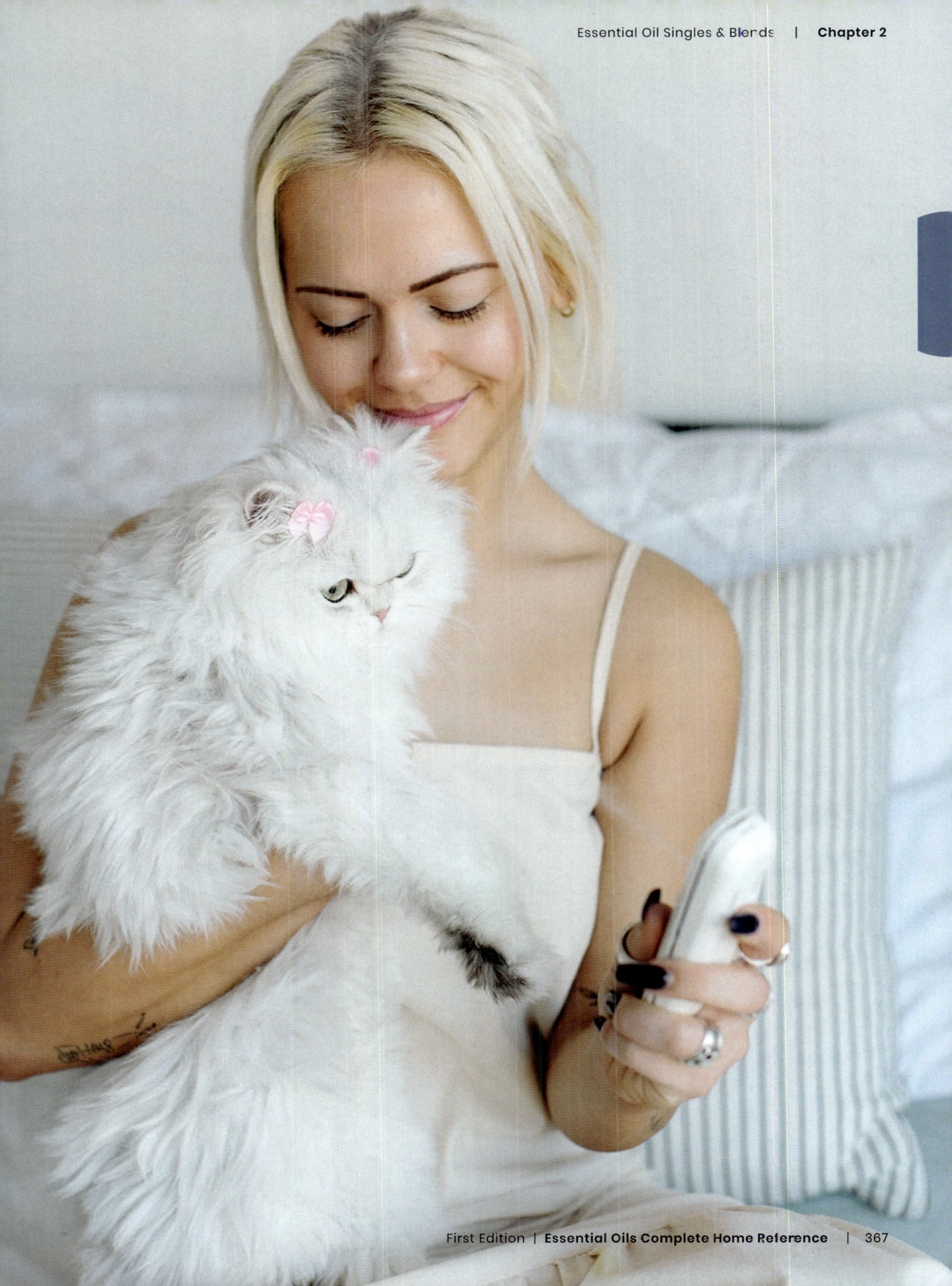

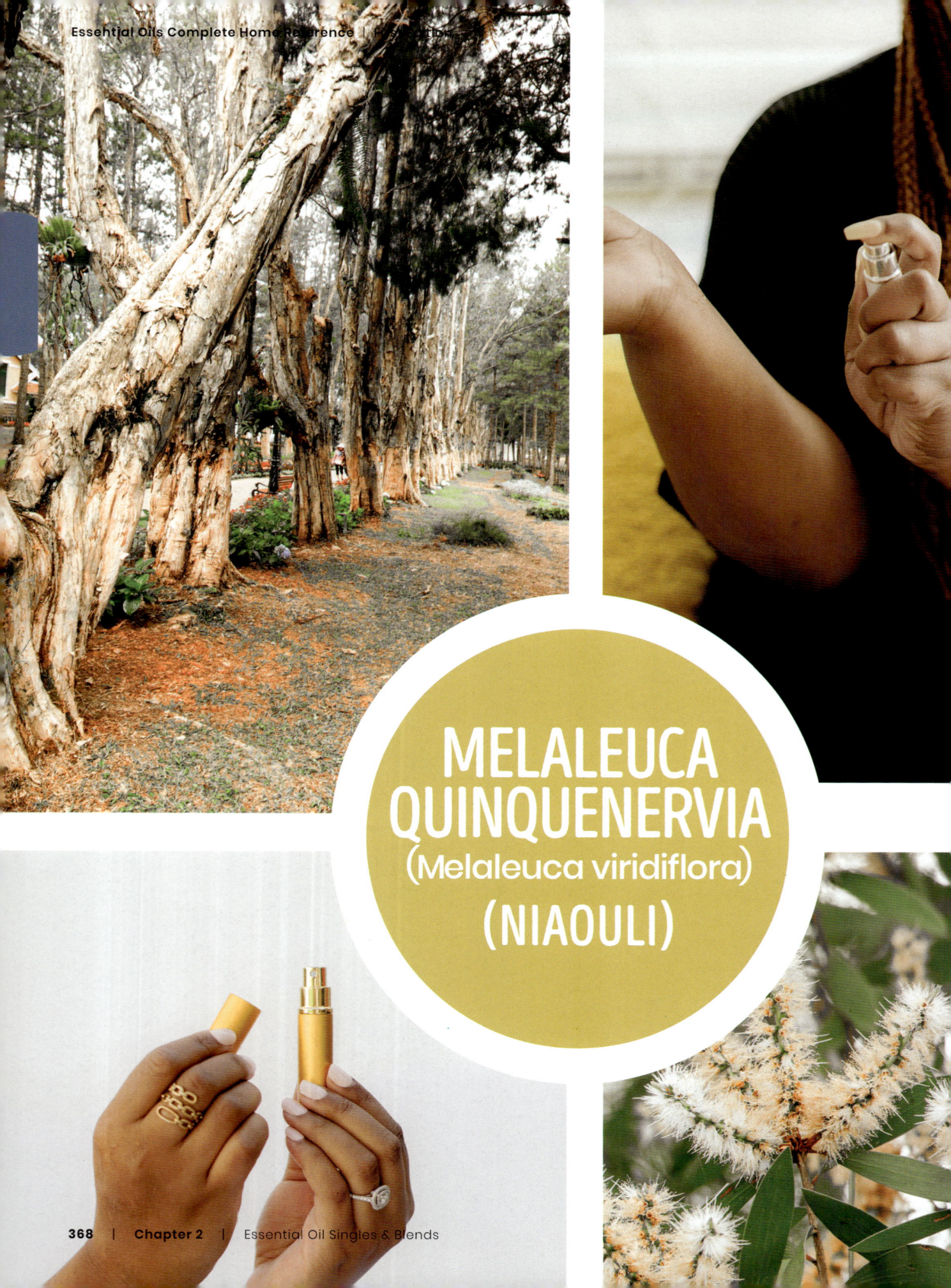

MELALEUCA QUINQUENERVIA
(Melaleuca viridiflora)
(NIAOULI)

Essential Oil Singles & Blends | Chapter 2

BOTANICAL FAMILY:
Myrtaceae

PLANT ORIGIN:
Madagascar

EXTRACTION METHOD:
Steam distilled from leaves and branches

KEY CONSTITUENTS:
Eucalyptol (52-76%),
Limonene (1-12%),
Alpha-Pinene (6-12%),
Alpha-Terpineol (3-8%),
Viridiflorol (1-6%),
Beta-Pinene (up to 4%)

HISTORICAL DATA:
A brew from the bruised leaves of Melaleuca quinquenervia was used by Aboriginal people in Australia for colds, headaches, and other sicknesses.

MEDICAL PROPERTIES:
Male hormone-like, anti-inflammatory, antibacterial, antiviral, antifungal, and antiparasitic (amoeba and parasites in the blood), vasodilating, skin penetration enhancer (hormones), antiseptic

USES:
Hypertension, urinary tract/bladder infections, respiratory/sinus infections, allergies, colds, coughs, headaches, general sickness, rheumatism, neuralgia, perfumes, honey-like food

FRAGRANT INFLUENCE:
Respiratory strengthening, calming

DIRECTIONS:
Aromatic: 30. Topical: 50-50.

CAUTIONS:

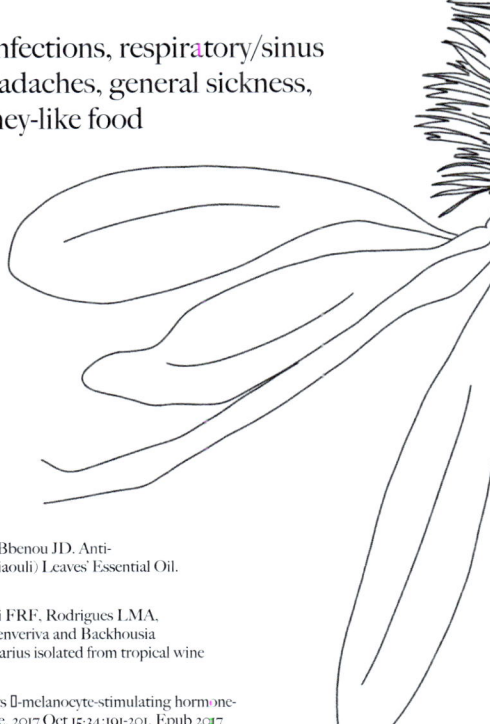

SELECTED RESEARCH:

Acha E, Aikpe JFA, Adoverlande J, Assogba MF, Agossou G, Sezan A, Dansou HP, Bbenou JD. Anti-inflammatory Properties of Melaleuca Quinquenvervia (Cav.) ST Blake Myrtaceae (Niaouli) Leaves' Essential Oil. J Chem Pharm Res. 2019; 11(1): 36-50.

de Andrade Santiago J, das Graças Cardosa M, Batista LR, Santiago WD, Passamani FRF, Rodrigues LMA, Nelson DL. Effect of the essential oils from Melaleuca alternifolica, Melaleuca quinquenveriva and Backhousia citriodora on the synthesis of ochratoxin A by Aspergillus niger and Aspergillus carbonarius isolated from tropical wine grapes. J Food Sci Technol. 2018 Jan; 55(1): 418-423.

Chao WW, Su CC, Peng HY, Chou ST. Melaleuca quinquenervia essential oil inhibits α-melanocyte-stimulating hormone-induced melanin production and oxidative stress in B16 melanoma cells. Phytomedicine. 2017 Oct 15;34:191-201. Epub 2017 Aug 24.

Leyva M, French-Pacheco L, Quintana F, Montada D, Castex M, Hernandez A, Marquetti MDS. Melaleuca quinquenervia (Cav.) S.T. Blake (Myrtales: Myrtaceae): natural alternative for mosquito control. Asian Pac J Trop Med. 2016 Oct;9(10):979-984. Epub 2016 Aug 10.

Cock IE, Winnett V, Sirdaarta J, Matthews B. The potential of selected Australian medicinal plants with anti-Proteus activity for the treatment and prevention of rheumatoid arthritis. Pharmacogn Mag. 2015 May;11(Suppl 1):S190-208.

Monti D, Tampucci S, Chetoni P, Burgalassi S, Bertoli A, Pistelli L. Niaouli oils from different sources: analysis and influence on cutaneous permeation of estradiol in vitro. Drug Deliv. 2009 Jul;16(5):237-42.

Nam SY, Chang MH, Do JS, Seo HJ, Oh HK. Essential oil of niaouli preferentially potentiates antigen-specific cellular immunity and cytokine production by macrophages. Immunopharmacol Immunotoxicol. 2008;30(3):459-74.

BOTANICAL FAMILY:
Apiaceae

PLANT ORIGIN:
Belgium, Bulgaria, Netherlands

EXTRACTION METHOD:
Steam distilled from root

KEY CONSTITUENTS:
Beta-Phellandrene (≤30%), Alpha-Phellandrene (7-28%), Alpha-Pinene (10-27%), Delta-3-Carene (8-15%), Limonene (3-13%), Sabinene (≤12%), Trans-Beta Ocimene (≤7%), Cis-Beta-Ocimene (≤4%)

MELISSA
(Melissa officinalis) (also known as Lemon Balm)

Anciently, Melissa was used for nervous disorders and many different ailments dealing with the heart or the emotions. It was also used to promote fertility. Melissa was the main ingredient in Carmelite water, distilled in France since 1611 by the Carmelite monks. The University of Maryland Medical Center writes that Melissa "was used as far back as the Middle Ages to reduce stress and anxiety, promote sleep, improve appetite, and ease pain and discomfort from indigestion." An old Arabian proverb states, "Balm makes the heart merry and joyful," which may be why Avicenna advocated the use of lemon balm in treating depression and anxiety. The life science and high technology company Sigma-Aldrich writes this about Melissa: "Studies have reported that aqueous extracts of lemon balm exhibit antiviral effects against Newcastle disease virus, Semliki forest virus, influenza virus, myxoviruses, vacciniam, and herpes simplex virus. Lemon balm extract and rosmarinic acid have demonstrated antiviral properties against HIV-1." Research in 2020 shows Melissa is antidepressive, antiviral, and anticancer. A 2019 study shows Melissa is effective against menstrual and childbirth pain, while a 2018 study shows Melissa decreased the severity of menstruation.

MEDICAL PROPERTIES:
Anti-inflammatory, antiviral, relaxant, hypotensive, antioxidative, antitumoral

USES:
Viral infections (herpes, etc.), depression, anxiety, insomnia, indigestion, nausea, immunity, healthy-looking skin

FRAGRANT INFLUENCE:
Brings out gentle characteristics within people; calming, uplifting, balances emotions; removes emotional blocks, instills a positive outlook on life

DIRECTIONS:
Aromatic: 6o. Topical: Neat. In case of sensitivity, dilute 5 drops in 15 ml of V-6. Dietary: Put 2 drops in a capsule and take 3 times daily or as needed.

CAUTIONS:

SELECTED RESEARCH:

Araj-Khodaei M, Noorbala AA, Yarani R, Emadi F, Emaratkar E, Faghihzadeh S, Parsian Z, Alijaniha F, Kamalinejad M, Naseri M. A double-blind, randomized pilot study for comparison of Melissa officinalis L. and Lavandula angustifolia Mill. with Fluoxitine for the treatment of depression. BMC Complement Med Ther. 2020; 20: 207. Published online 2020 Jul 3.

Vanti G, Ntallis SG, Panagiotidis CA, Dourdouni V, Patsoura C, Bergonzi MC, Lazari D, Bilia AR. Glycerosome of Melissa officinalis L. Essential Oil for Effective Anti-HSV Type 1. Molecules. 2020 Jul; 25(14): 3111.

Dastjerdi MN, Darooneh T, Nasiri M, Moatar F, Esmacili S, Ozgoli G. Investigating the Effect of Melissa Officinalis on After-Pains: A Randomized Single-Blind Clinical Trial. J Caring Sci. 2019 Sep; 8(3): 129-138

Mirabi P, Alamolhoda SH, Yazdkhasti M, Mojab F. The Effects of Lemon Balm on Menstrual Bleeding and the Systemic Manifestation of Dysmenorrhea. Iran J Pharm Res. 2018; 17(Suppl2): 214-223.

Asadi A, Shidfar F, Safari M, Hosseini AF, Fallah Huseini H, Heidari I, Rajab A. Efficacy of Melissa officinalis L. (lemon balm) extract on glycemic control and cardiovascular risk factors in individuals with type 2 diabetes: a randomized, double-blind, clinical trial. Phytotherapy Research. 2019;33(3):651-659.

Melissa officinalis Acidic Fraction Protects Cultured Cerebrallar Granule Neurons Against Beta Amyloid-Induced Apoptosis and Oxidative Stress. Cell J. 2017 Winter; 18(4): 556-564.

Hosseini SR, Kaka G, Joghataei MT, Hooshmandi M, Saraie SH, Yaghoobi K, Mohammadi A. Assessment of Neuroprotective Properties of Melissa officinalis In Combination With Human Umbilical Cord Blood Stem Cells After Spinal Cord Injury. ASN Neuro. 2016 Nov-Dec; 8(6): 1759091416674833.

Ozarowski M, Mikolajczak PL, Piasecka A, Kachlicki P, Kujawski R, Bogacz A, Bartkowiak-Wieczorek J, Szulc M, Kaminska E, Kujawska M, Jodynis-Libert J, Gryszczynska A, Opala B, Lowicki Z, Seremak-Mrozikiewicz A, Czerny B. Influence of the Melissa officinalis leaf extract on long-term memory in Scopolamine animal model with assessment of mechanism of activity. Evid Based Complement Alternat Med. 2016;2016:9729818. Epub 2016 Apr 28.

Pourghanbari G, Nili H, Moattari A, Mohammadi A, Iraji A. Antiviral activity of the oseltamivir and Melissa officinalis L. essential oil against avian influenza A virus (H9N2). Virusdisease. 2016 Jun;27(2):170-8. Epub 2016 May 21.

Jahanban-Esfahlan A, Modaeinama S, Abasi M, Abbasi MM, Jahanban-Esfahlan R. Anti proliferative properties of Melissa officinalis in different human cancer cells. Asian Pac J Cancer Prev. 2015;16(14):5703-7

Joukar S, Zarisfi Z, Sepehri G, Bashiri A. Efficacy of Melissa officinalis in suppressing ventricular arrhythmias following ischemia-reperfusion of the heart: a comparison with amiodarone. Med Princ Pract. 2014;23(4):340-5. Epub 2014 Jun 18.

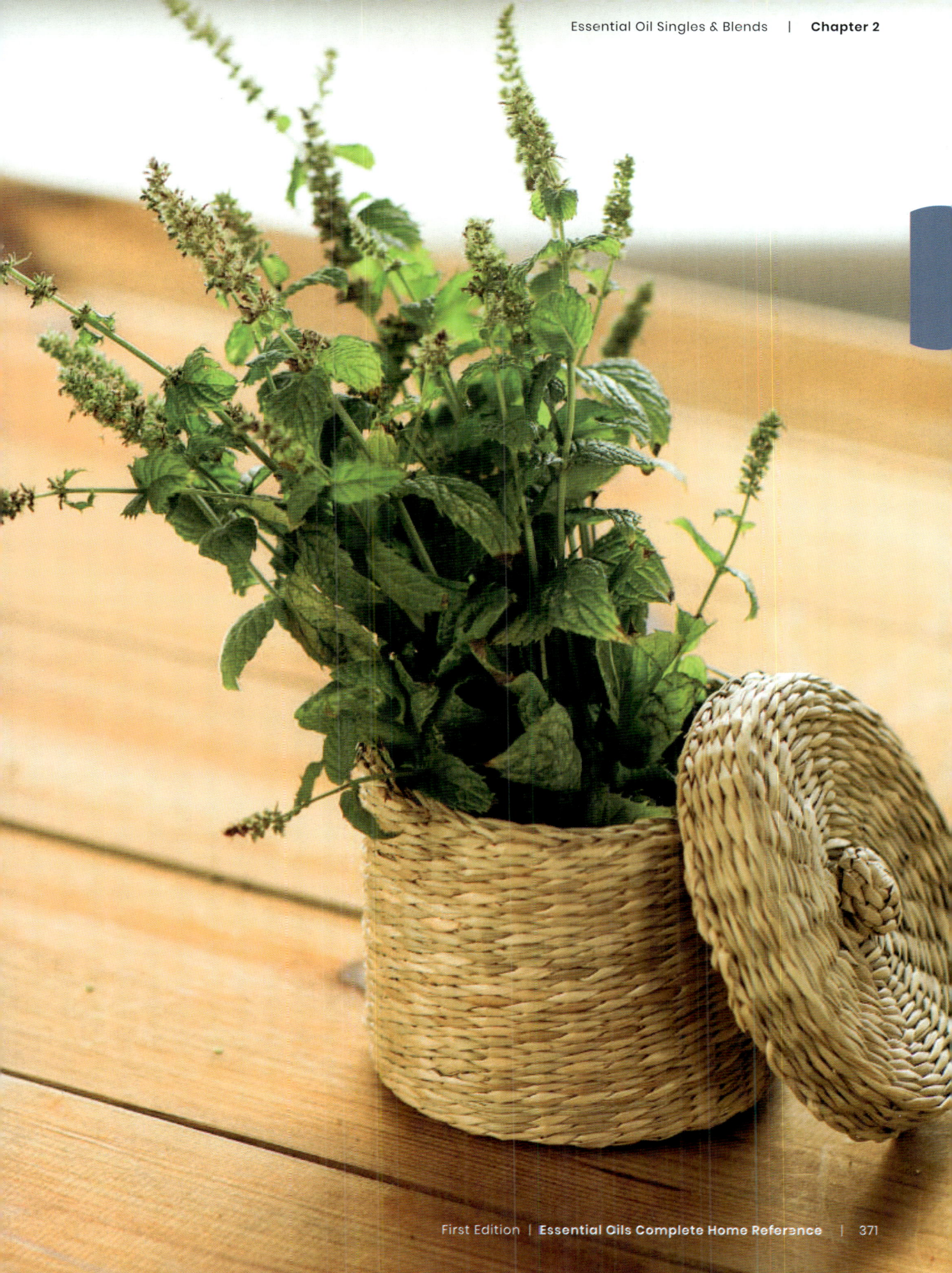

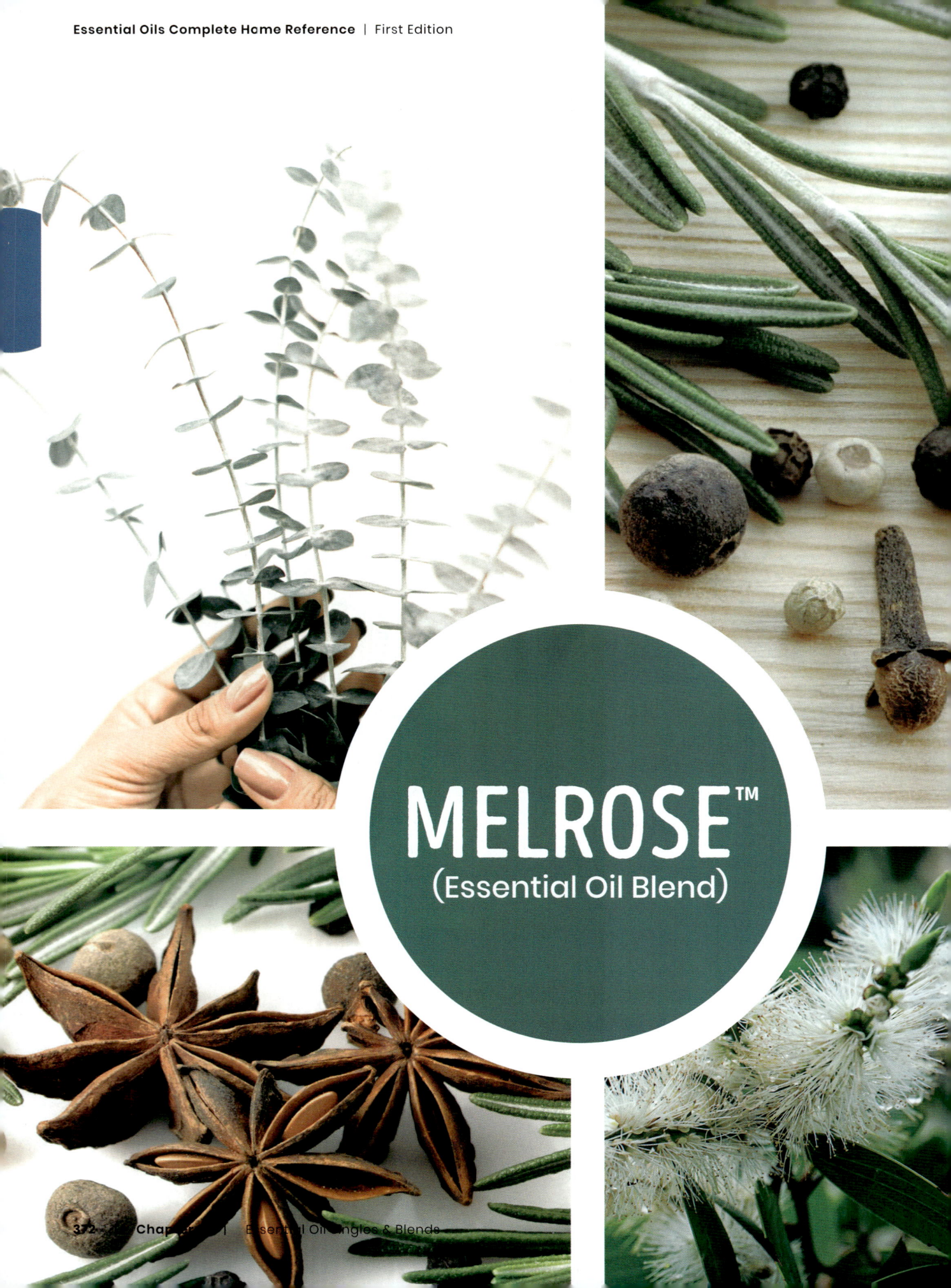

ABOUT MELROSE™:

This is a blend of four essential oils that have strong antiseptic properties to cleanse and disinfect cuts, scrapes, burns, rashes, and bruised tissue. These oils help regenerate damaged tissue and reduce inflammation. Melrose is powerful when diffused to dispel odors, purify the air, and protect against viruses and daily radiation bombardment.

MEDICAL PROPERTIES & USES:

Antiviral, antimicrobial, anti-inflammatory, antioxidative, cardiovascular supportive, organ protective, pain or swelling reducing, performance enhancing/stimulating, wellness supportive

INGREDIENTS:

Rosemary, Tea Tree, Clove, Melaleuca Quinquenervia (Niaouli)

DIRECTIONS:

Aromatic: 30. Topical: 50-50. Apply to broken skin, cuts, scrapes, burns, rashes, infection, or desired location as needed. Follow with Rose Ointment to keep oils sealed in wound. Put 1-2 drops on a piece of cotton and place in the ear for earaches. Dietary: Children over age 8: 6 drops per capsule 2 times daily or in yogurt. Adults: 20 drops per capsule, 1-2 capsules, 2 times daily or in yogurt.

CAUTIONS:

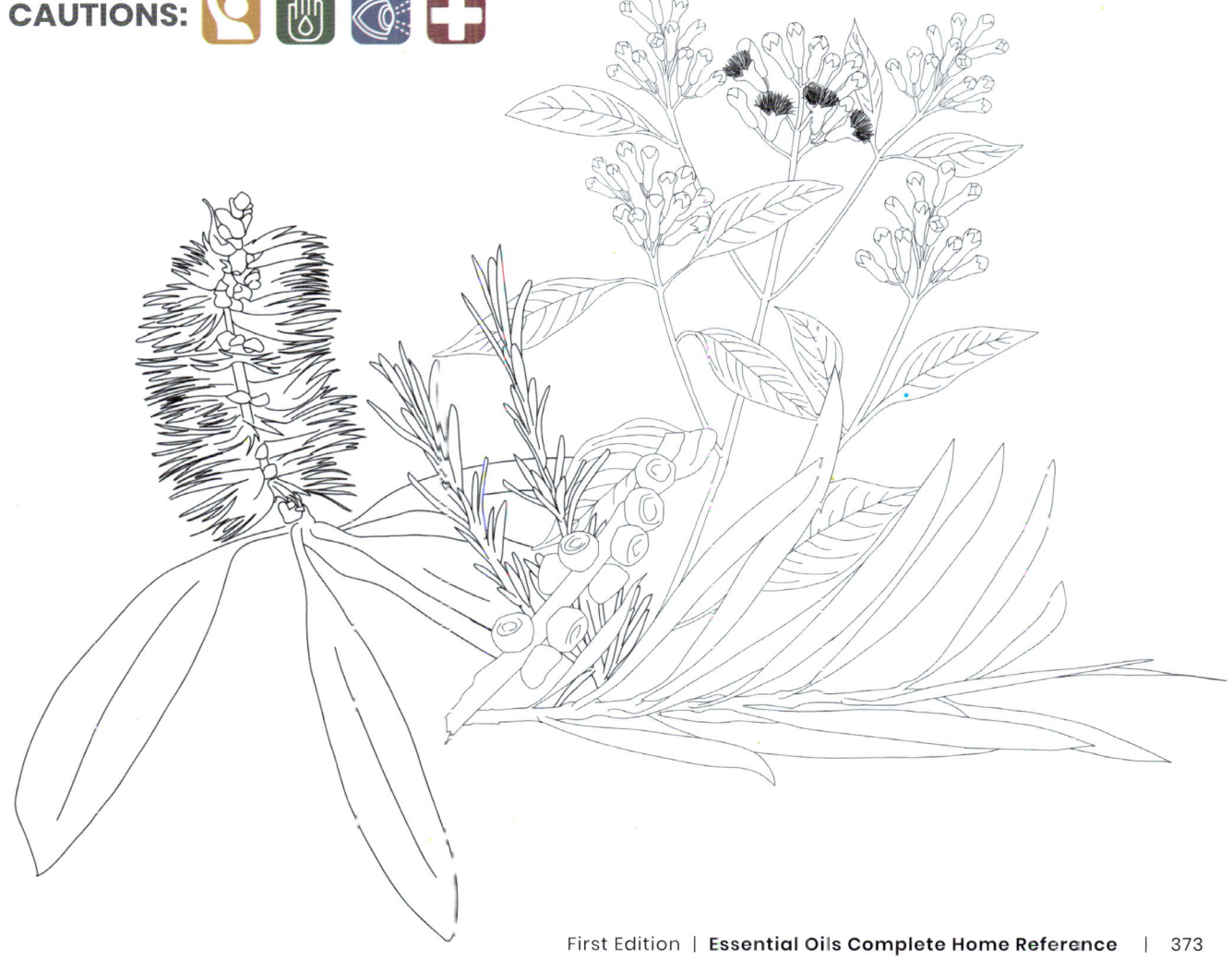

M-GRAIN™
(Essential Oil Blend)

This blend helps relieve pain from slight headaches to severe migraine headaches. It is anti-inflammatory and antispasmodic.

MEDICAL PROPERTIES & USES:
Anti-inflammatory, antimicrobial, antioxidative, calming, disease inhibitory, pain or swelling reducing, performance enhancing/stimulating

INGREDIENTS:
Basil, Marjoram, Lavender, Roman Chamomile, Peppermint, Helichrysum

DIRECTIONS:
Aromatic: 3o Topical: Neat. In case of sensitivity, dilute 2 drops in 50 ml of V-6 or other pure carrier oil.

CAUTIONS:

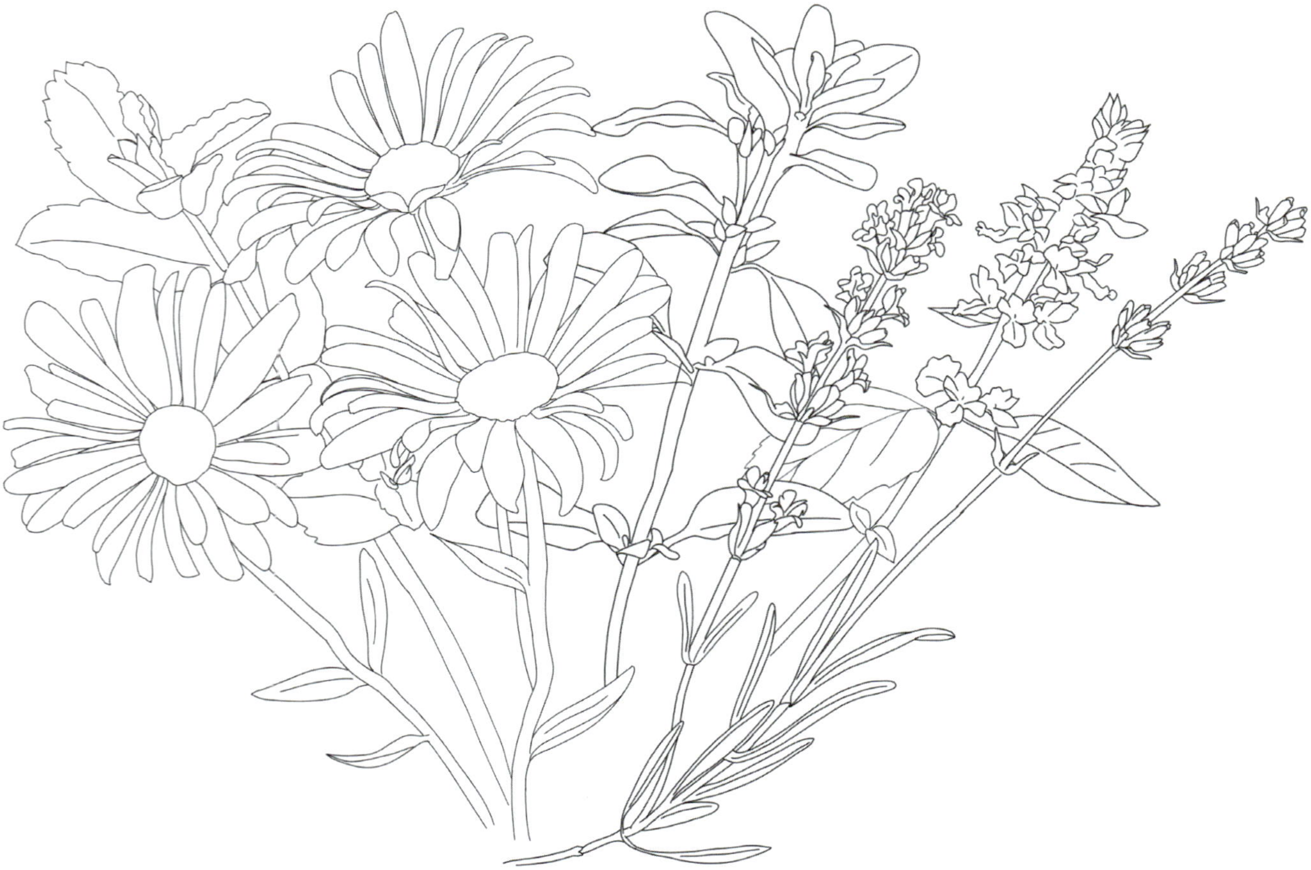

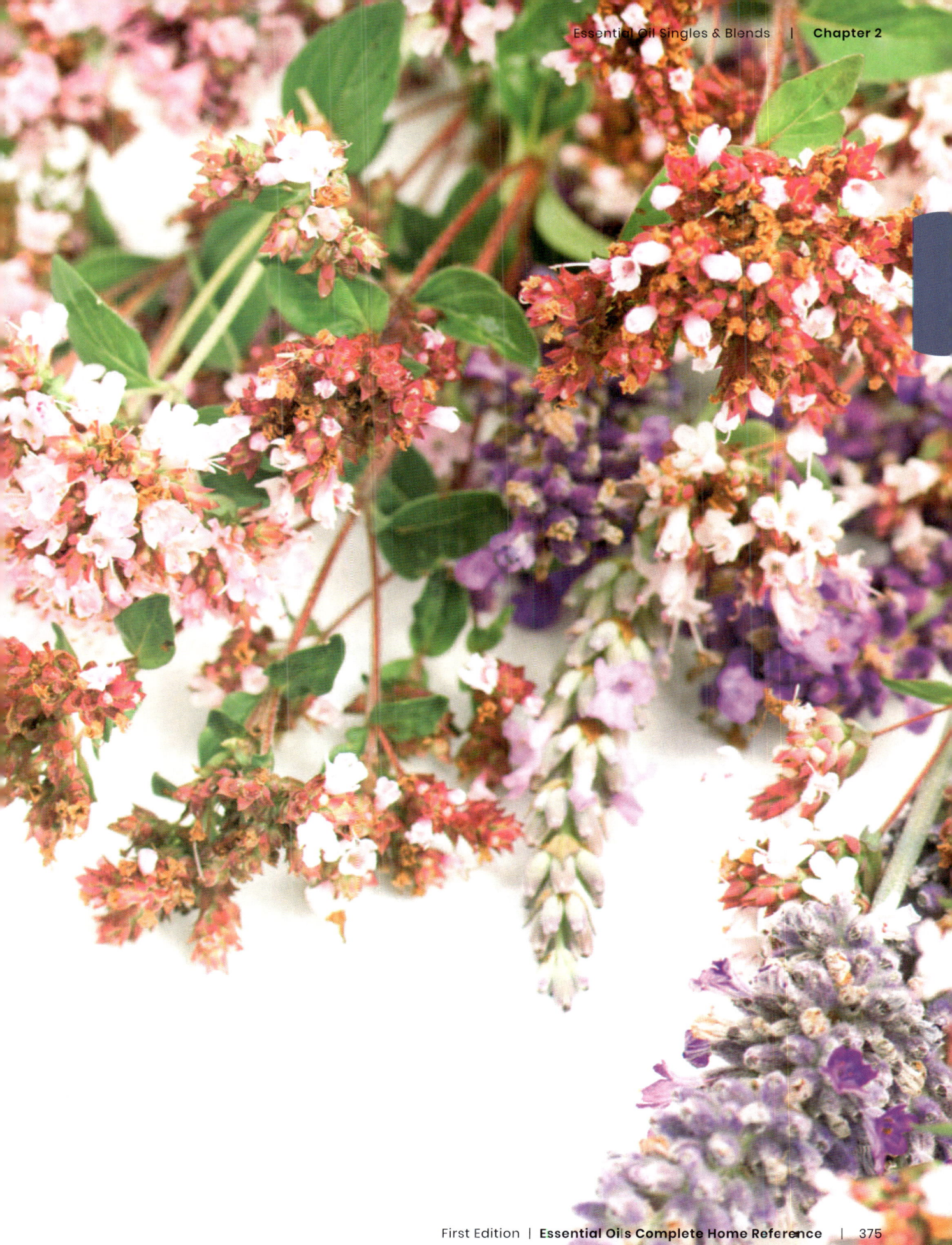

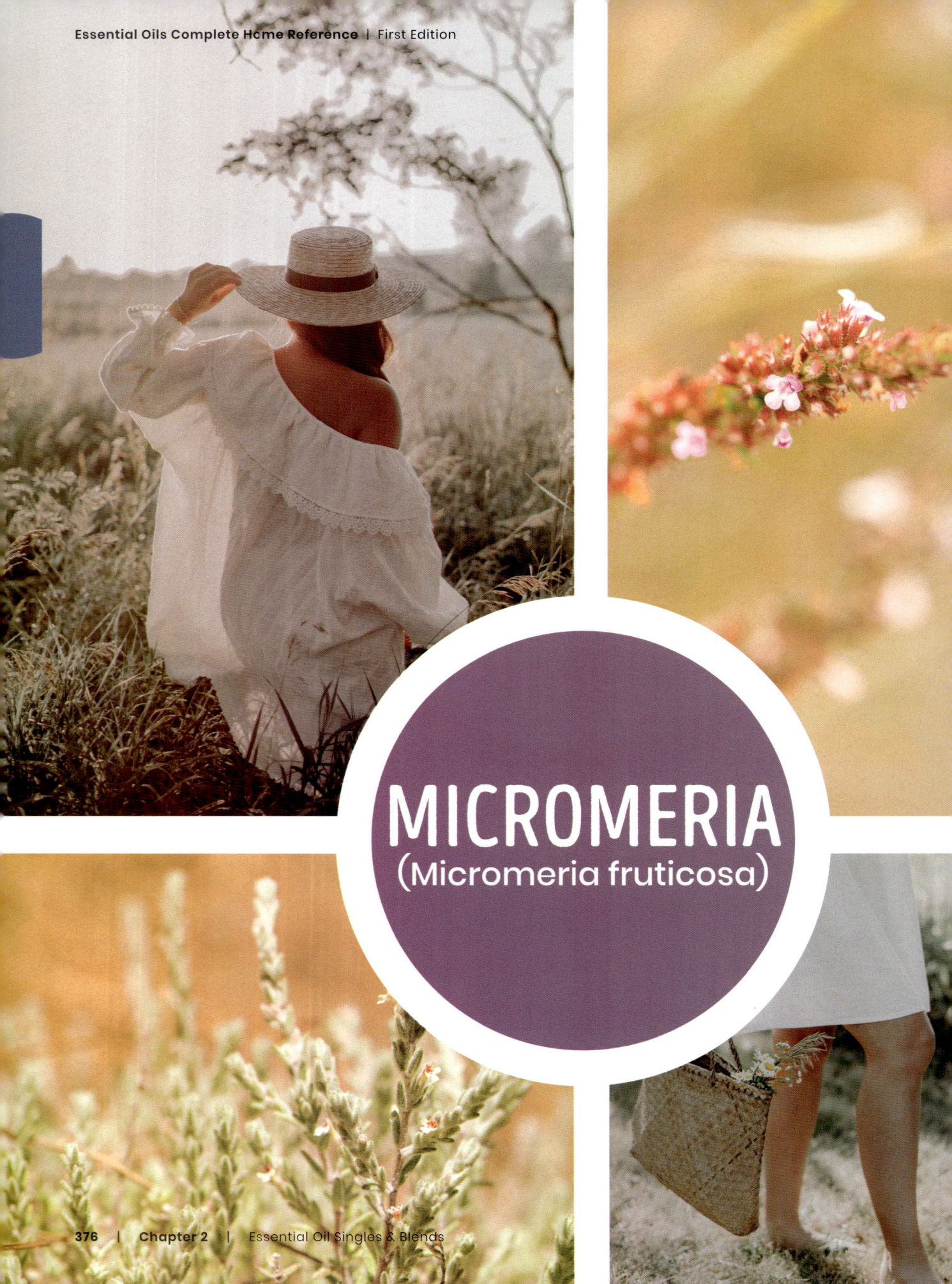

MICROMERIA
(Micromeria fruticosa)

BOTANICAL FAMILY:
Lamiaceae

PLANT ORIGIN:
Israel

EXTRACTION METHOD:
Steam distilled from leaf, stem, and flower

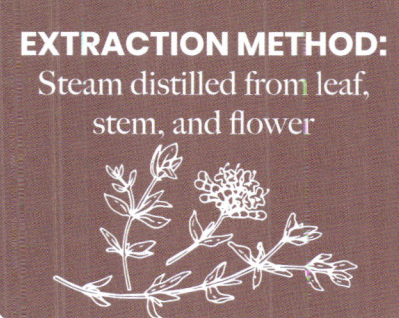

KEY CONSTITUENTS:
Pulegone (50-65%),
Menthol (7-12%),
Beta-Caryophyllene (3-9%),
Isopulegol (3-6%),
Menthone (1-5%),
Neomenthol (1-5%)

HISTORICAL DATA:
Micromeria is found in Israel and in the eastern Mediterranean. It is known in folk medicine as having anti-inflammatory properties and for digestive support.

MEDICAL PROPERTIES:
Anti-inflammatory, gastroprotective, antibacterial, antifungal, antioxidant, insecticidal, analgesic, anticonvulsant, hepatoprotective, antidepressant

USES:
Stomach upsets, hypertension, heart disorders, diarrhea, abdominal pains, colds, headaches, wounds, infections, exhaustion

FRAGRANT INFLUENCE:
Revitalizes and refreshes the mind, respiratory system, asthma, depression

DIRECTIONS:
Topical: 20-80.

CAUTIONS: Contains high levels of pulegone. Do not use if pregnant or trying to conceive.

SELECTED RESEARCH:
El-Huneidi W, Shehab NG, Bajbouj K, Vinod A, El-Serafi A, Shafarin J, Malhab LJB, Abdel-Rahman WM, Abu-Gharbieh E. Micromeria fruticose Induces Cell Cycle Arrest and Apoptosis in Breast and Colorectal Cancer Cells. Pharmaceuticals (Basel): 2020 Jun; 13(6): 115.

Salameh N, Shraim N, Jaradat N. Chemical composition and enzymatic screening of Micromeria fruticosa serpyllifolia volatile oils collected from three different regions of West Bank, Palestine. Biomed Res Int. 2018 Oct 16;2018:6536919. eCollection 2018.

Abu-Gharbieh E, Shehab NG, Khan SA. Anti-inflammatory and gastroprotective activities of the aqueous extract of Micromeria fruticosa (L.) Druce ssp Serpyllifolia in mice. Pak J Pharm Sci. 2013 Jul;26(4):799-803.

Shehab NG, Abu-Gharbieh E. Constituents and biological activity of the essential oil and the aqueous extract of Micromeria fruticosa (L.) Druce subsp. serpyllifolia. Pak J Pharm Sci. 2012 Jul;25(3):687-92.

Ali-Shtayeh MS, Jamous RM, Al-Shafie' JH, Elgharabah WA, Kherfan FA, Qarariah KH, Khdair IS, Soos IM, Musleh AA, Isa BA, Herzallah HM, Khlaid RB, Aiash SM, Swaiti GM, Abuzahra MA, Haj-Ali MM, Saifi NA, Azem HK, Nasrallah HA. Traditional knowledge of wild edible plants used in Palestine (Northern West Bank): a comparative study. J Ethnobiol Ethnomed. 2008 May 12;4:13.

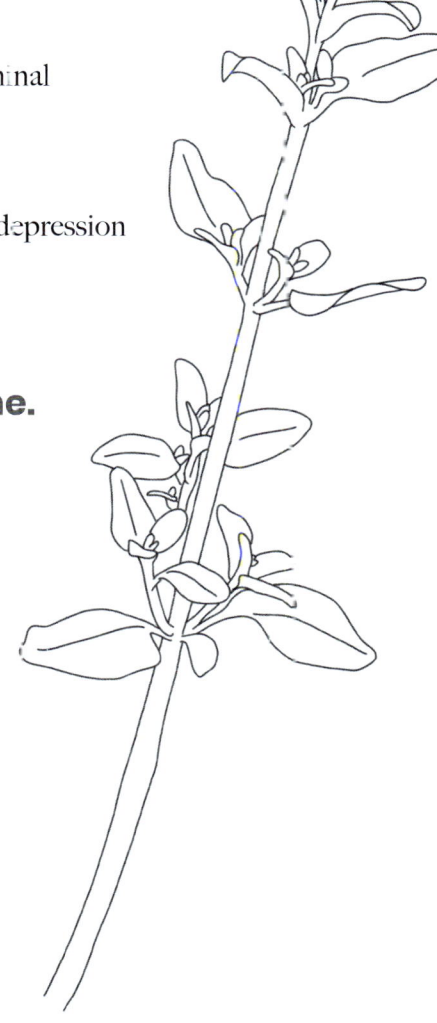

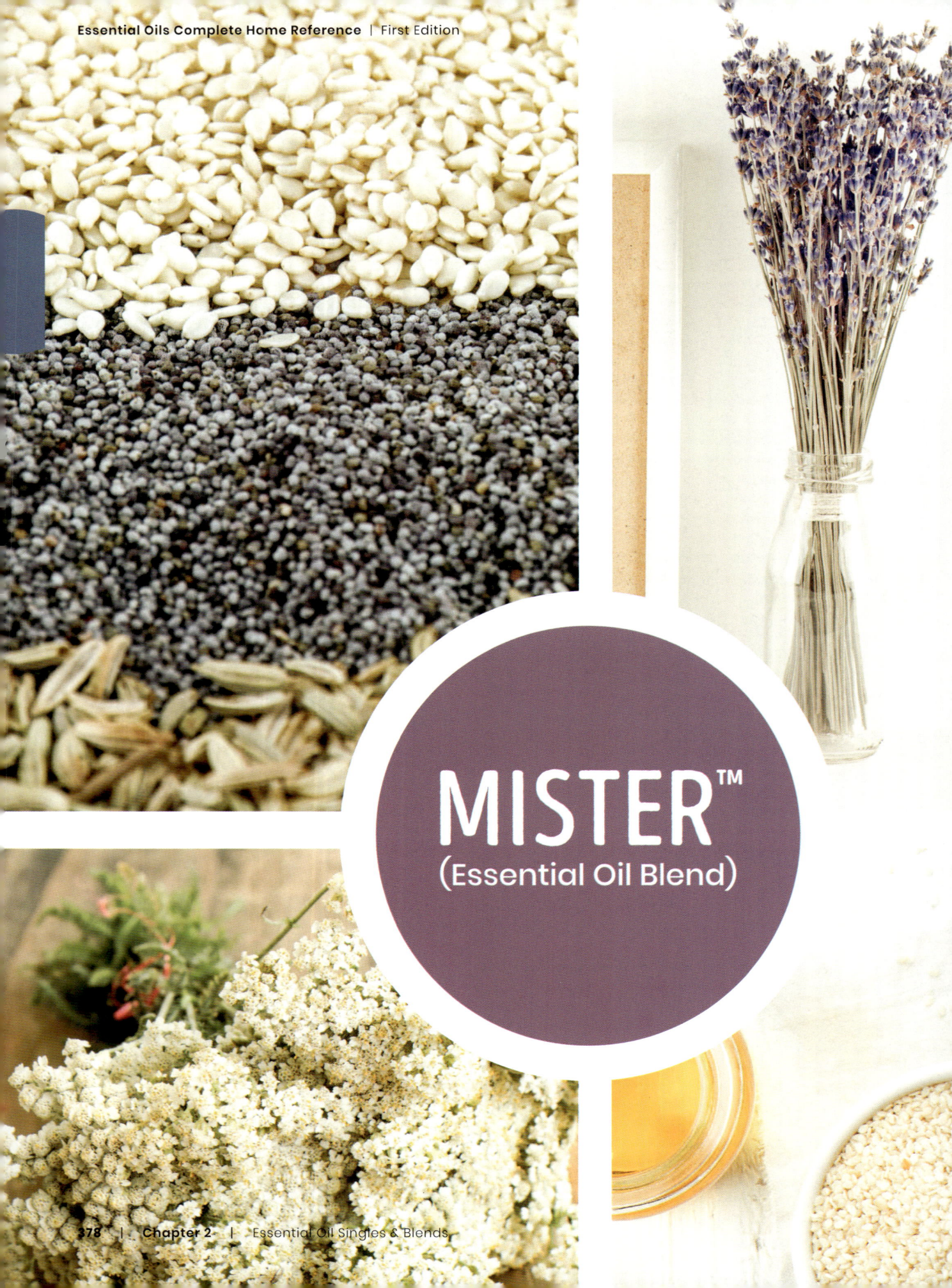

Essential Oils Complete Home Reference | First Edition

MISTER™
(Essential Oil Blend)

378 | Chapter 2 | Essential Oil Singles & Blends

ABOUT MISTER™:

This blend helps to decongest the prostate and promote greater male hormonal balance.

MEDICAL PROPERTIES & USES:

Anti-inflammatory, antimicrobial, calming, cardiovascular supportive, digestion or elimination supportive/nausea reducing, glandular/hormonal supportive, pain or swelling reducing, performance enhancing/stimulating

INGREDIENTS:

Sesame seed oil,‡ Sage, Fennel, Lavender, Myrtle, Yarrow, Peppermint

DIRECTIONS:

Aromatic: 3o. Topical: Neat. Use in a hot compress.

CAUTIONS:

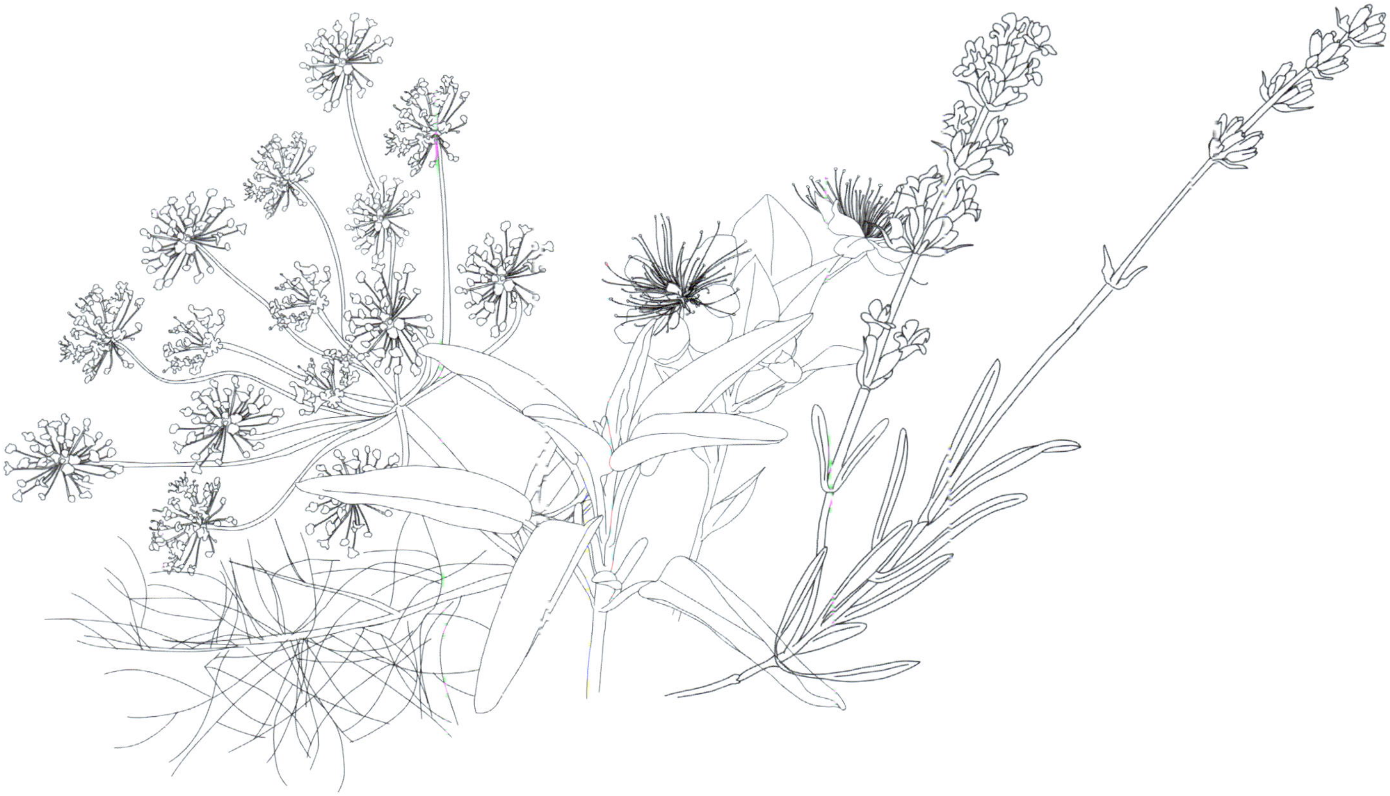

MOTIVATION™
(Essential Oil Blend)

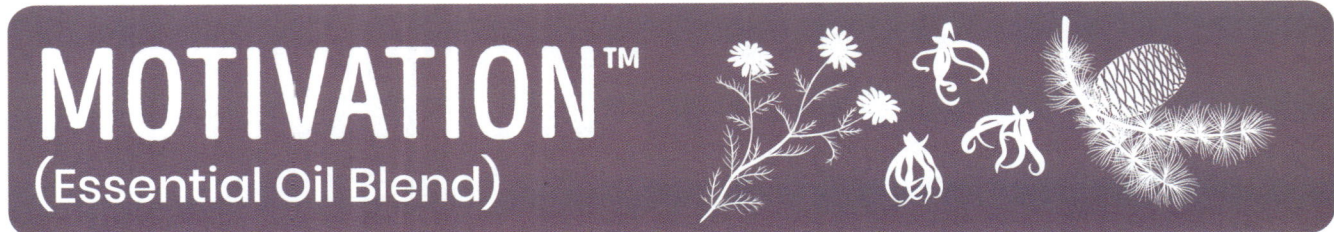

Motivation stimulates feelings of action and accomplishment, providing positive energy to help overcome feelings of fear and procrastination.

MEDICAL PROPERTIES & USES:
Anti-inflammatory, antimicrobial, antioxidative, calming

INGREDIENTS:
Roman Chamomile, Black Spruce, Ylang Ylang, Lavender

DIRECTIONS:
Aromatic: 30. Topical: 50-50.

CAUTIONS:

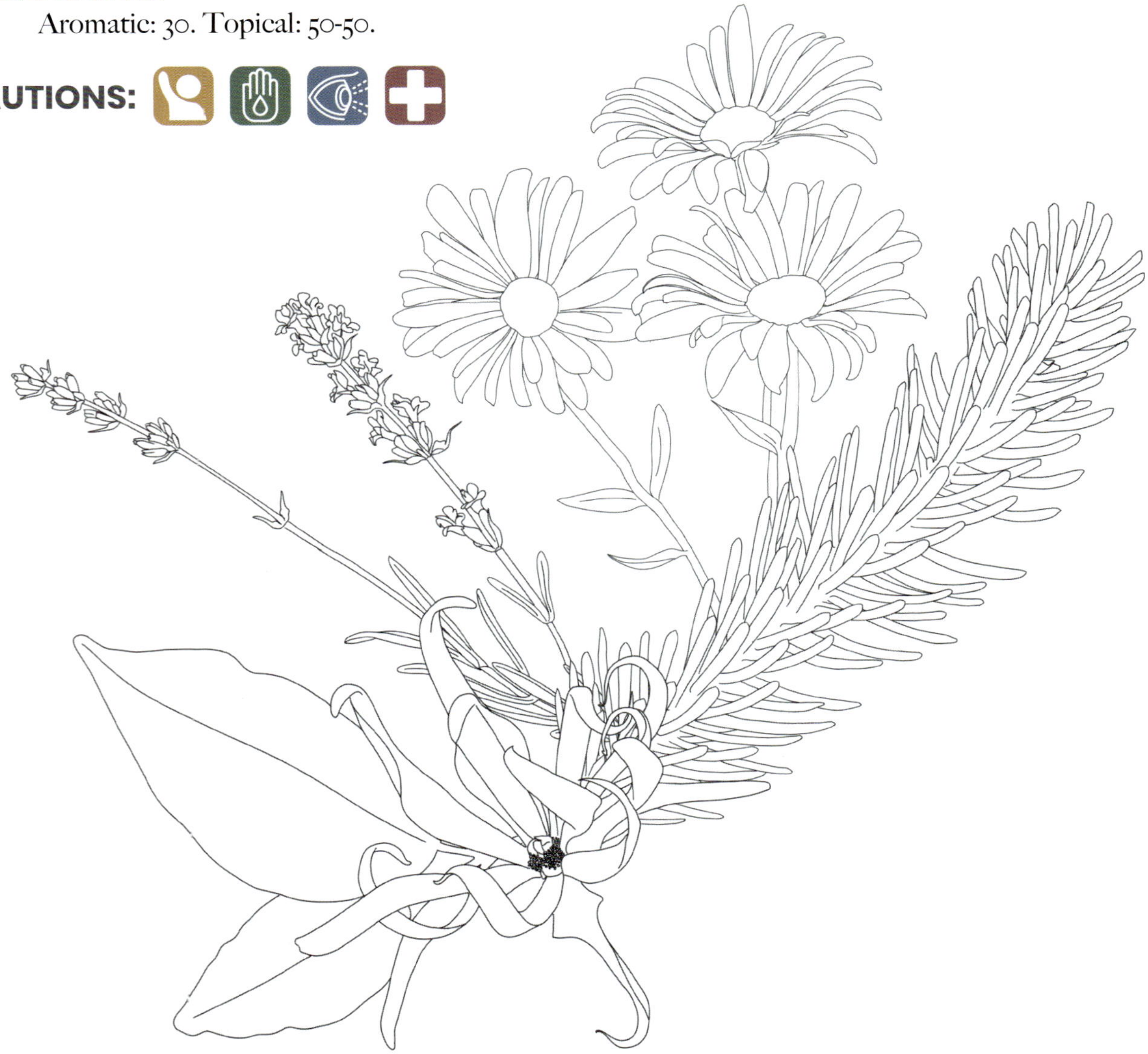

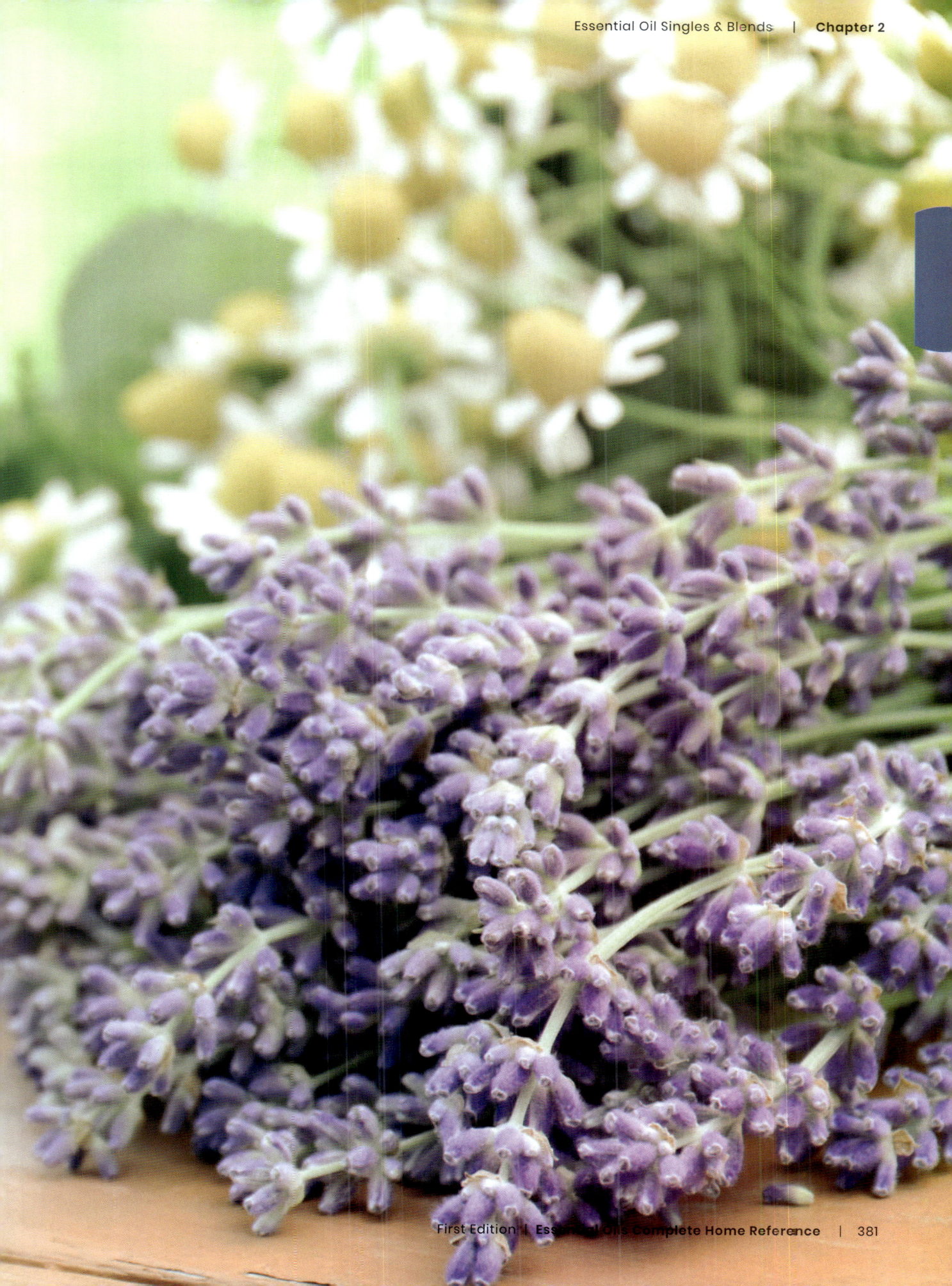

BOTANICAL FAMILY: Lamiaceae

PLANT ORIGIN: Bosnia, Herzegovina, Hungary

EXTRACTION METHOD: Steam distilled from flowering plant

KEY CONSTITUENTS: Carvacrol (10-64%), Thymol (2-30%), Para-Cymene (2-23%), Gamma-Terpinene (1-18%), Carvacrol Methyl Ether (up to 11%), T-B-Caryophyllene (1-7%), Borneol (up to 5%), Beta-Bisabolene (up to 3%), Alpha-Terpinene (up to 3%), Myrcene (1-3%)

MOUNTAIN SAVORY & MOUNTAIN SAVORY VITALITY™
(Satureja montana)

Mountain Savory has been used historically as a general tonic for the body.

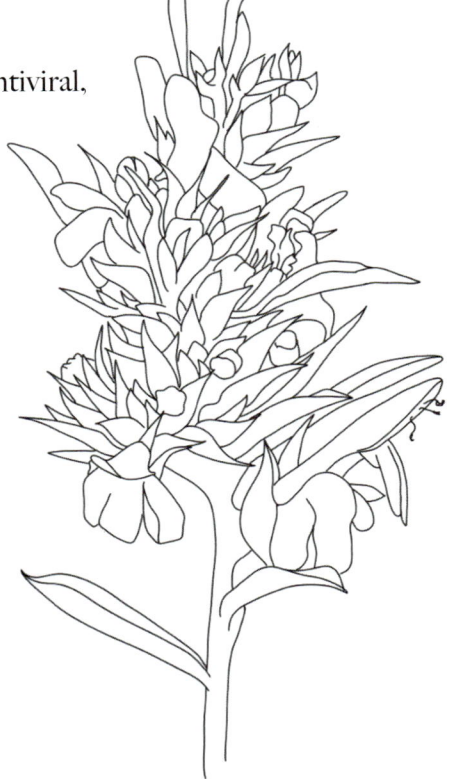

MEDICAL PROPERTIES:
Antimicrobial, antioxidative, strong antibacterial, antifungal, antiviral, antiparasitic, immune stimulant, anti-inflammatory

USES:
Viral infections (herpes, HIV, etc.), scoliosis/lumbago/back problems, improves male premature ejaculation

FRAGRANT INFLUENCE:
Revitalizes and stimulates the nervous system, powerful energizer and motivator

DIRECTIONS:
Aromatic: 10. Topical: 50-50. Dietary (Vitality): Dilute 1 drop with 4 drops of V-6 or other pure carrier oil. Put in a capsule and take 1 daily or as needed.

CAUTIONS:

SELECTED RESEARCH:

Šimunović K, Bucar F, Klančnik A, Pompei F, Paparella A, Možina SS. In Vitro Effect of the Common Culinary Herb Winter Savory (Satureja montana) against the Infamous Food Pathogenm Campylobacter jejuni. Foods. Apr; 9(4): 537.

Macelli A, Vitanza L, Imbriano A, Fraschetti C, Filippi A, Goldoni P, Maurizi L, Ammendolia MG, Crestoni ME, Fornarini S, Menghini L, Carafa M, Marianecci C, Longhi C, Rinaldi F. Satureja montana L. Essential Oils: Chemical Profiles/Phytochemical Screening, Antimicrobial Activity and O/W NanoEmulsion Formulations. Pharmaceutics. 2020 Jan; 12(1): 7.

Vitanza L, Maccelli A, Marazzato M, Seazzocchio F, Comanducci A, Fornarini S, Crestoni ME, Filippi A, Fraschetti C, Rinaldi F, Aleandri M, Goldoni P, Conte MP, Ammendolia MG, Longhi C. Satureja montana L. essential oil and it's antimicrobial activity alone or in combination with gentamicin. Microb Pathog. 2019 Jan;126:323-331. Epub 2018 Nov 17.

Miladi H, Mili D, Ben Slama R, Zouari S, Ammar E, Bakhrouf A. Antibiofilm formation and anti-adhesive property of three Mediterranean essential oils against a foodborne pathogen Salmonella strain. Microb Pathog. 2016 Apr;93:22-31. Epub 2016 Jan 21.

Kundaković T, Stanojković T, Kolundzija B, Marković S, Sukilović B, Milenković M, Lakusić B. Cytotoxicity and antimicrobial activity of the essential oil from Satureja montana subsp. pisidica (Lamiceae). Nat Prod Commun. 2014 Apr;9(4):569-72.

Marin M, Novaković M, Tešević V, Vučković I, Milojević N, Vuković-Gačić B, Marin PD. Antioxidative, antibacterial and antifungal activity of the essential oil of wild-growing Satureja montana L. from Dalmatia, Croatia. Flavour and Fragrance Journal. 2012;27(3):216-223.

Serrano C, Matos O, Teixeira B, Ramos C, Neng N, Nogueira J, Nunes ML, Marques A. Antioxidant and antimicrobial activity of Satureja montana L. extracts. J Sci Food Agric. 2011 Jul;91(9):1554-60. Epub 2011 Mar 28.

Zavatti M, Zanoli P, Benelli A, Rivasi M, Baraldi C, Baraldi M. Experimental study on Satureja montana as a treatment for premature ejaculation. J Ethnopharmacol. 2011 Jan 27;133(2):629-33. Epub 2010 Oct 30.

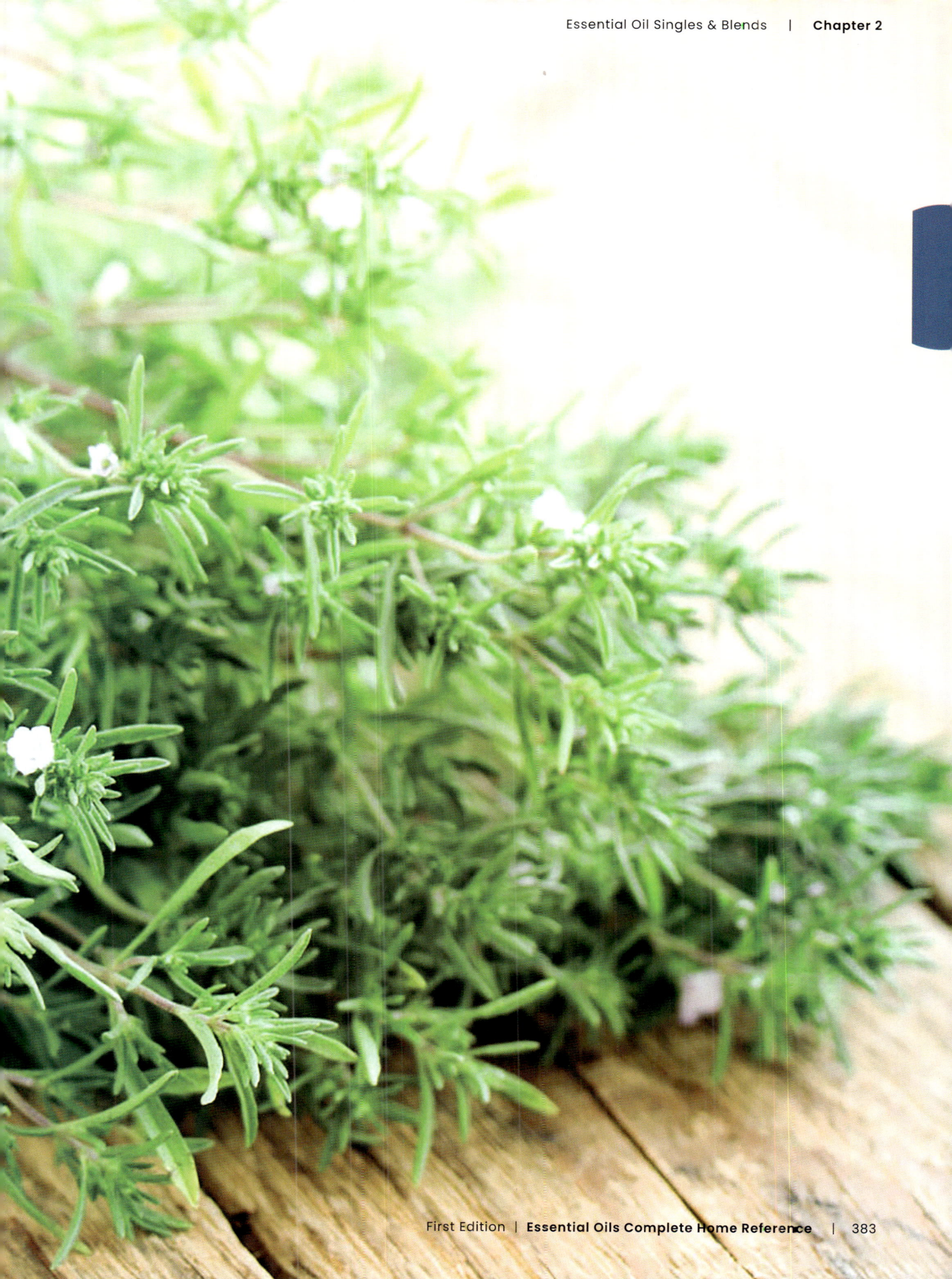

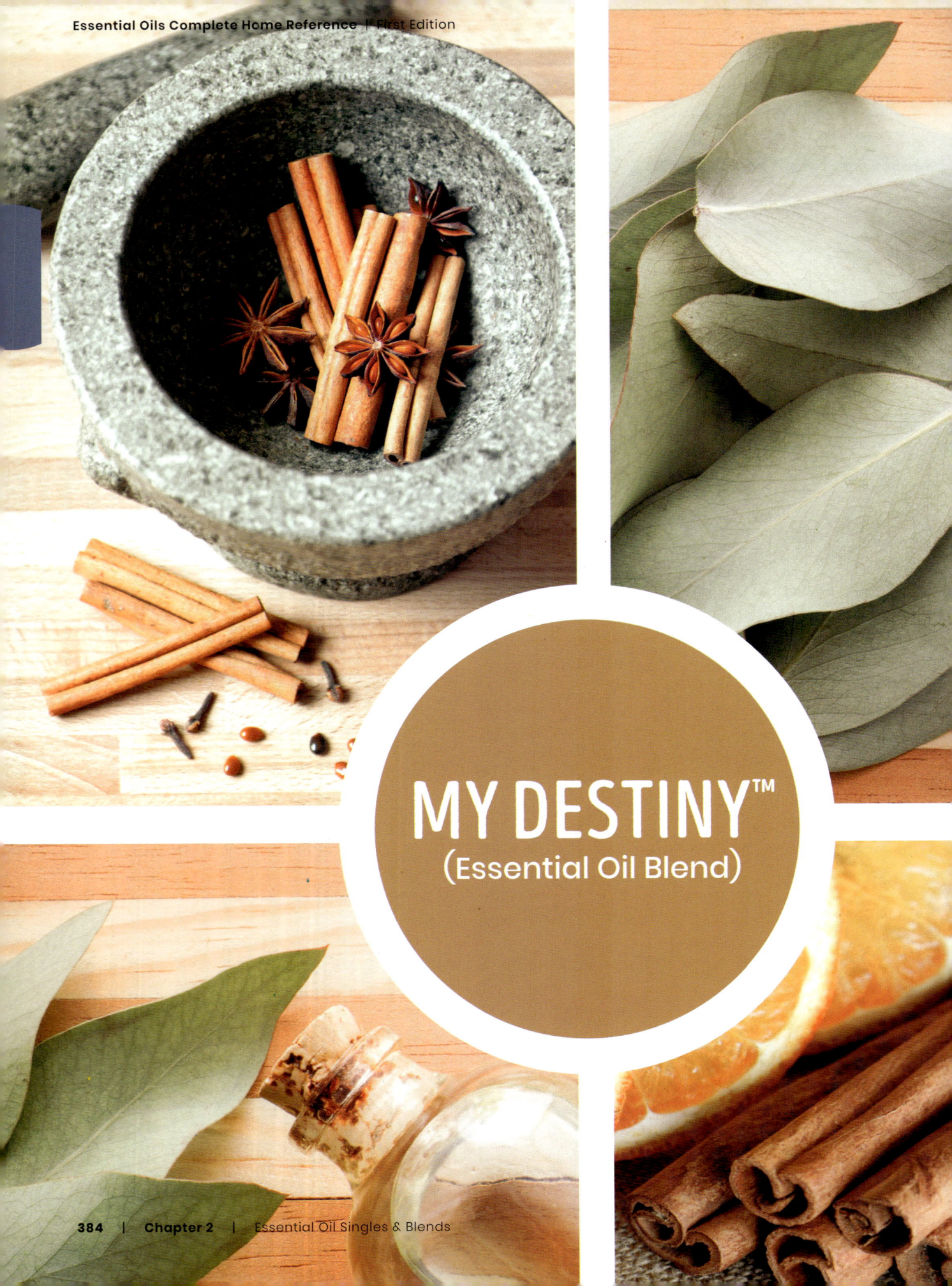
MY DESTINY™
(Essential Oil Blend)

ABOUT MY DESTINY™:

Was your destiny planned by someone else, however well-meaning? Get back in the driver's seat with the empowering scent of My Destiny, the 2017 International Grand Convention blend.

MEDICAL PROPERTIES & USES:

Antispasmodic, highly anti-inflammatory, vasodilator analgesic/anesthetic, reduces blood pressure, antiparasitic, antibacterial, antiviral, antifungal, pain relieving, appetite suppressant, nerve regeneration, hypertensive, antioxidant, anticonvulsant, improves memory, relaxation, antidepressant, muscle relaxant

INGREDIENTS:

Wintergreen, Peppermint, Helichrysum, Clove, Myrtle, Lemon, Camphor (Ravintsara), Lavender, Caprylic/capric triglyceride,† Idaho Grand Fir, Eucalyptus Globulus, Balsam Copaiba, Pine, Marjoram, Coconut oil,† Eucalyptus Radiata, Eucalyptus Citriodora, Cypress, Northern Lights Black Spruce, Vetiver, Orange, Sacred Sandalwood, Nutmeg, Ylang Ylang, Lime, Idaho Blue Spruce, Frankincense, Dorado Azul

DIRECTIONS:

Aromatic: 10. Topical: 20-80.

CAUTIONS: Intended for use by adults only.

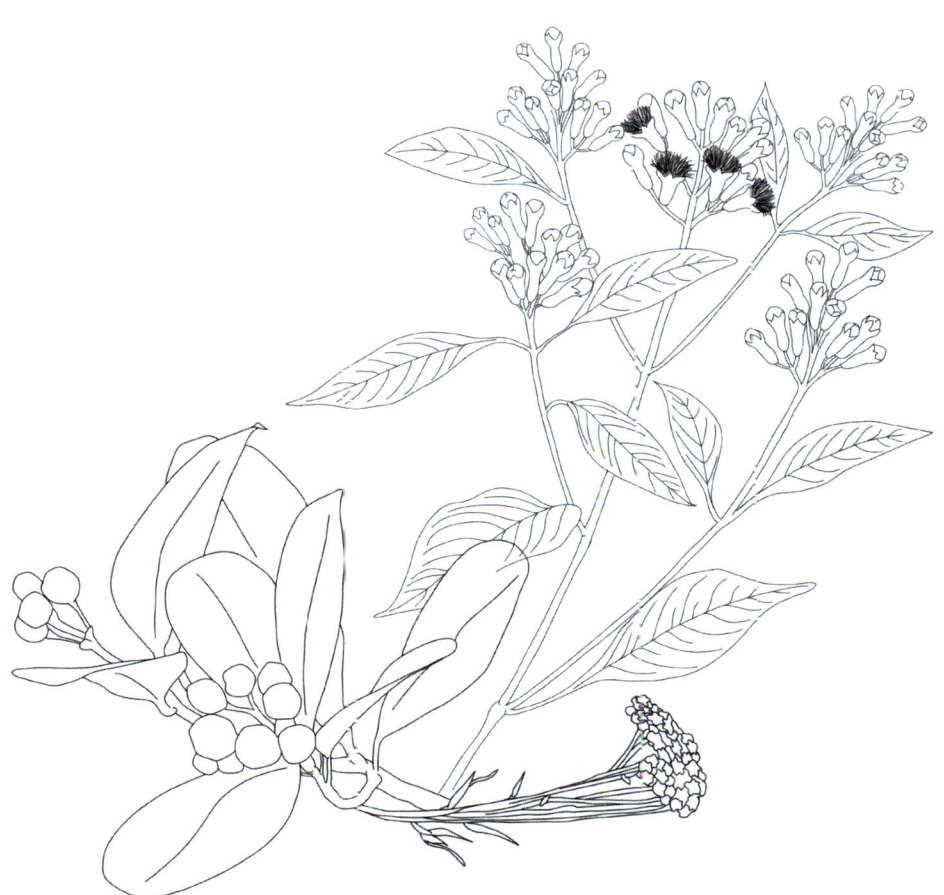

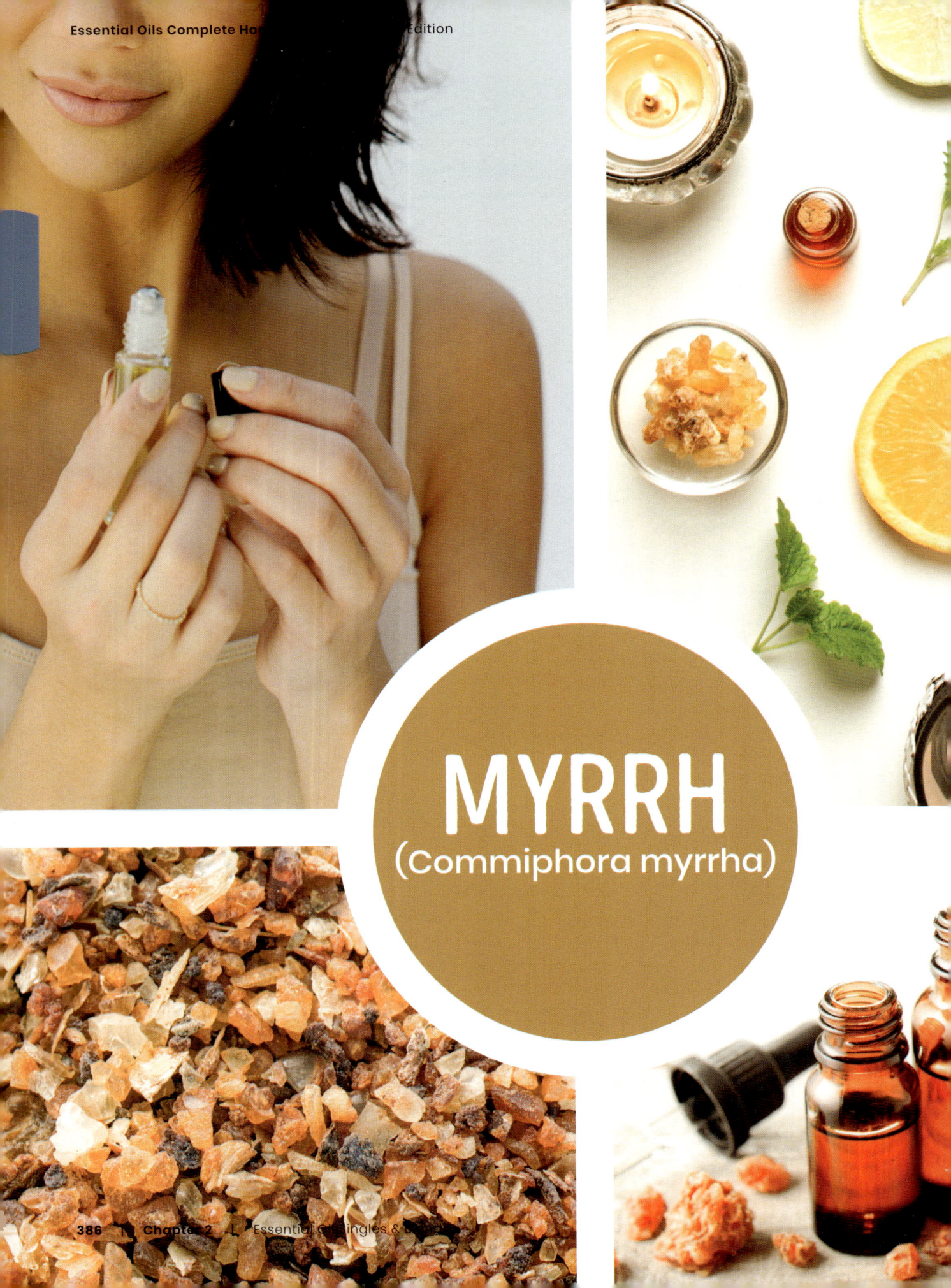

MYRRH
(Commiphora myrrha)

BOTANICAL FAMILY:
Burseraceae

PLANT ORIGIN:
Somalia

EXTRACTION METHOD:
Steam distilled gum resin exudate from stem (wounded bark)

KEY CONSTITUENTS:
Furanoeudesma-1,3-diene (22-55%), Curzerene (3-36%), Lindestrene (5-15%), 2-Methoxy Furanogermacrene (up to 9%), Beta-Elemene (up to 8%), Germacrene B (up to 5%)

HISTORICAL DATA:
Myrrh is mentioned in one of the oldest known medical records, the Ebers Papyrus (dating from 16th century BC), an ancient Egyptian list of 877 prescriptions and recipes. The Arabian people used myrrh for many skin conditions, such as chapped and cracked skin and wrinkles. It was listed in Hildegard's Medicine, a compilation of early German medicines by highly regarded Benedictine herbalist Hildegard of Bingen (1098-1179).

MEDICAL PROPERTIES:
Neuroprotective, antimicrobial, anti-inflammatory, powerful antioxidant, antitumoral, antibacterial, antiviral, antiparasitic, analgesic/anesthetic

USES:
Dental health, diabetes, cancer, hepatitis, fungal infections (candida, ringworm), tooth/gum infections, skin conditions (eczema, chapped, cracked, wrinkles, stretch marks)

FRAGRANT INFLUENCE:
Earthy, uplifting, promotes spiritual awareness. It contains sesquiterpenes, which stimulate the limbic system of the brain (the center of memory and emotions) and the hypothalamus, pineal, and pituitary glands. The hypothalamus is the master gland of the human body, producing many vital hormones, including thyroid and growth hormone.

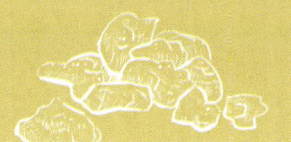

DIRECTIONS:
Aromatic: 6o. Topical: Neat.

CAUTIONS:

SELECTED RESEARCH:

Orabi SH, Al-Sabbagh ESH, Khalifa HK, El-Gaber-Mohamed MA, Elhamouly M, Gad-Allah SM, Abdel-Daim MM, Abd Eldaim MA. Commiphora myrrha Resin Alcoholic Extract Ameliorates High Fat Diet Induced Obesity via Regulation of UCP1 and Adiponectin Proteins Expression in Rats. Nutrients. 2020 Mar; 12(3): 803.

Miao X-D, Zheng L-J, Zhao Z-Z, Su S-L, Zhu Y, Guo J-M, Shang E-X, Qian D-W, Duan J-A. Protective Effect and Mechanism of Boswellic Acid and Myrrha Sesquiterpenes with Different Proportions of Compatibility on Neuroinflammation by LPS-Induced BV2 Cells Combined with Network Pharmacology. Molecules. 2019 Nov; 24(21): 3946.

Cai T, Tiscione D, Cocci A, Puglisi M, Cito G, Malossini G, Palmieri A. Hibiscus extract, vegetable proteases and Commiphora myrrha are useful to prevent symptomatic UTI episode in patients affected by recurrent uncomplicated urinary tract infections. Arch Ital Urol Androl. 2018 Sep 30;90(3):203-207.

Rosenthal R, Luettig J, Hering NA, Krug SM, Albrecht U, Fromm M, Schulzke JD. Myrrh exerts barrier-stabilising and -protective effects in HT-29/B6 and Caco-2 intestinal epithelial cells. Int J Colorectal Dis. 2017 May;32(5):623-34. Epub 2016 Dec 15.

Ahmad A, Raish M, Ganaie MA, Ahmad SR, Mohsin K, Al-Jenoobi FI, A-Mohizea AM, Alkharfy KM. Hepatoprotective effect of Commiphora myrrha against d-GalN/LPS-induced hepatic injury in a rat model through attenuation of pro inflammatory cytokines and related genes. Pharm Biol. 2015;53(12):1759-67. Epub 2015 Apr 13.

Su S, Duan J, Chen T, Huang X, Shang E, Yu L, Wei K, Zhu Y, Guo J, Guo S, Liu P, Qian D. Tang Y. Frankincense and myrrh suppress inflammation via regulation of the metabolic profiling and the MAPK signaling pathway. Sci Rep. 2015 Sep 2;5:13668.

Gao W, Su X, Dong X, Chen Y, Zhou C, Xin P, Yu C, Wei T. Cycloartan-24-ene-1α,2β,3β-triol, a cycloartane-type triterpenoid from the resinous exudates of Commiphora myrrha, induces apoptosis in human prostatic cancer PC-3 cells. Oncol Rep. 2015 Mar;33(3):1107-14. Epub 2015 Jan 15.

Chen Y, Zhou C, Ge Z, Liu Y, Liu Y, Feng W, Li S, Chen G, Wei T. Composition and potential anticancer activities of essential oils obtained from myrrh and frankincense. Oncol Lett. 2013 Oct;6(4):1140-6. Epub 2013 Aug 8.

Su S, Hua Y, Wang Y, Gu W, Zhou W, Duan JA, Jiang H, Chen T, Tang Y. Evaluation of the anti-inflammatory and analgesic properties of individual and combined extracts from Commiphora myrrha and Boswellia carterii. J Ethnopharmacol. 2012 Jan 3;139(2):649-56. Epub 2011 Dec 13.

BOTANICAL FAMILY:	EXTRACTION METHOD:	KEY CONSTITUENTS:
Myrtaceae	Steam distilled from leaves	Alpha-Pinene (48-58%), Eucalyptol (17-29%), Limonene (6-11%), Linalool (2-4%)
PLANT ORIGIN: BTunisia, Morocco		

MYRTLE
(Myrtus communis)

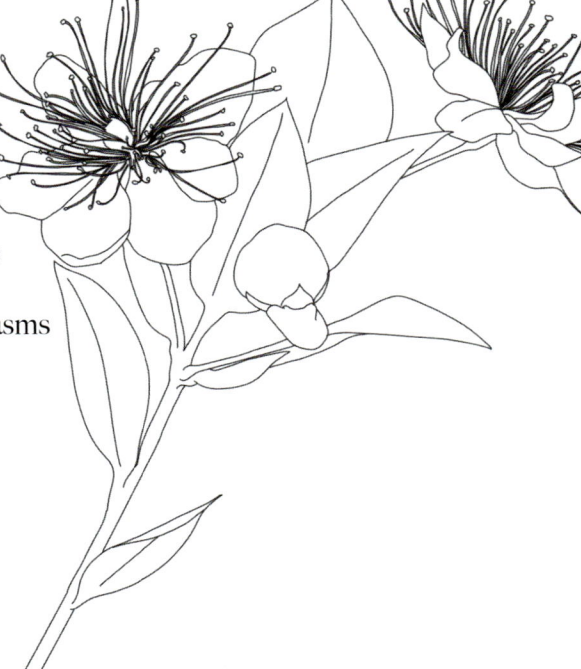

Myrtle has been researched by Dr. Daniel Pénoël for normalizing hormonal imbalances of the thyroid and ovaries, as well as balancing out hypothyroidism. It has also been researched for its soothing effects on the respiratory system.

MEDICAL PROPERTIES:
Antimutagenic, liver stimulant, prostate and thyroid stimulant, sinus/lung decongestant, antispasmodic, antihyperglycemic, anti-inflammatory, antinociceptive

USES:
Thyroid problems, throat/lung/sinus infections, prostate problems, skin irritations (blemishes, bruises, oily skin, psoriasis, etc.), promote healthy-looking skin, muscle spasms

FRAGRANT INFLUENCE:
Elevating and euphoric, respiratory system

DIRECTIONS:
Aromatic: 30. Topical: 50-50.

CAUTIONS:

SELECTED RESEARCH:

Mir MA, Bashir N, Alfaify A Oteel MDY. GC-MS analysis of Myrtus communis extract and its antibacterial activity against Gram-positive bacteria. BMC Complememt Med Ther. 2020; 20: 86.

Mahboubi M. Effectiveness of Myrtus communis in the treatment of hemorrhoids. J Integr Med. 2017 Sep;15(5):351-358.

Ebrahimabadi EH, Ghoreishi SM, Masoum S, Ebrahimabadi AH. Combination of GC/FID/Mass spectrometry fingerprints and multivariate calibration techniques for recognition of antimicrobial constituents of Myrtus communis L. essential oil. J Chromatog B Analyt Technol Biomed Life Sci. 2016 Jan 1;1008:50-57. Epub 2015 Nov 14.

Kordali S, Usanmaz A, Cakir A, Komaki A, Ercisli S. Antifungal and herbicidal effects of fruit essential oils of four Myrtus communis genotypes. Chem Biodivers. 2016 Jan;13(1):77-84.

Bouzabata A, Cabral C, Gonçalves MJ, Cruz MT, Bighelli A, Cavaleiro C, Casanova J, Tomi F, Salgueiro L. Myrtus communis L. as source of a bioactive and safe essential oil. Food Chem Toxicol. 2015 Jan;75:166-72. Epub 2014 Nov 28.

Aleksic V, Mimica-Dukic N, Simin N, Nedeljkovic NS, Knezevic P. Synergistic effect of Myrtus communis L. essential oils and conventional antibiotics against multi-drug resistant Acinetobacter baumannii wound isolates. Phytomedicine. 2014 Oct 15;21(12):1666-74. 2014.08.013 Epub 2014 Sep 15.

Ogur R. Studies with Myrtus communis L.: Anticancer properties. J Intercult Ethnopharmacol. 2014 Oct-Dec;3(4):135-7. Epub 2014 Aug 3.

Alipour G, Dashti S, Hosseinzadeh H. Review of pharmacological effects of Myrtus communis L. and active constituents. Phytother Res. 2014 Aug;28(8):1125-36. Epub 2014 Feb 4.

Janbaz KH, Nisa M, Saqib F, Imran I, Zia-Ul-Haq M, De Feo V. Bronchodilator, vasodilator and spasmolytic activities of methanolic extract of Myrtus communis L. J Physiol Pharmacol. 2013 Aug;64(4):479-84.

Messaoud C, Boussaid M. Myrtus communis berry color morphs: a comparative analysis of essential oils, fatty acids, phenolic compounds, and antioxidant activities. Chem Biodivers. 2011 Feb;8(2):300-10.

Essential Oil Singles & Blends | Chapter 2

Yes, you can actually eat myrtle berries!

No, they aren't quite the same as the essential oil from the leaves.

First Edition | **Essential Oils Complete Home Reference** | 389

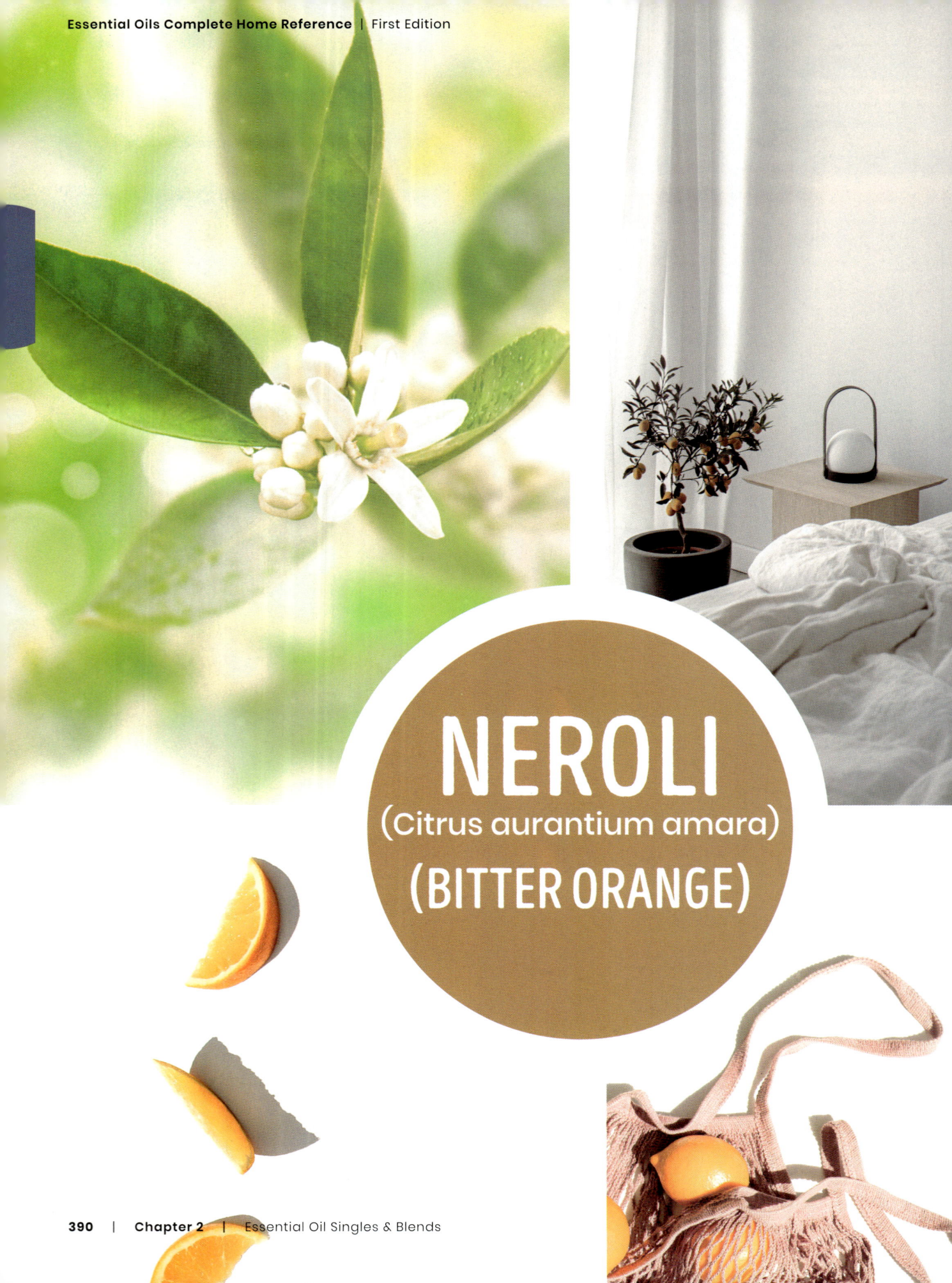

NEROLI
(Citrus aurantium amara)
(BITTER ORANGE)

BOTANICAL FAMILY:
Rutaceae

PLANT ORIGIN:
Morocco, South Africa, Tunisia

EXTRACTION METHOD:
Steam distilled from flowers

KEY CONSTITUENTS:
Linalool (26-55%), Linalyl Acetate (1-20%), Limonene (7-18%), Beta-Pinene (2-17%), Trans-Beta-Ocimene (3-9%), Alpha-Terpineol (2-8%), Neryl Acetate (up to 7%), Geranyl Acetate (1-5%), Trans-Nerolidol (up to 5%), Geraniol (1-5%), Myrcene (1-%), Trans-Trans-Farnesol (up to 4%), Alpha-Pinene (up to 2%), Nerol (up to 2%)

HISTORICAL DATA:
Highly regarded by the ancient Egyptians for ability to heal the mind, body, and spirit.

MEDICAL PROPERTIES:
Antiparasitic, digestive tonic, antidepressive, hypotensive (lowers blood pressure), antimicrobial, anifungal, antioxidant

USES:
Hypertension, anxiety, depression, hysteria, insomnia, skin conditions (acne, scars, stretch marks, thread veins, wrinkles), perfumes and body lotions, menopausal symptoms, high blood pressure, seizures, inflammation

FRAGRANT INFLUENCE:
A natural relaxant used to treat depression and anxiety. It strengthens and stabilizes the emotions and uplifts and inspires the hopeless, encouraging confidence, courage, joy, peace, and sensuality. It brings everything into focus at the moment.

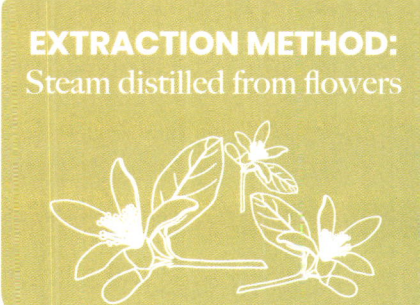

DIRECTIONS:
Aromatic: 6o. Topical: Neat. Dietary: Dilute 1 drop essential oil with 1 drop V-6 or other pure carrier oil. Put in a capsule and take up to 3 times daily or as needed.

CAUTIONS:

SELECTED RESEARCH:

Hirai M, Ito M. Sedative effects of the essential oil and headspace air of Ocimum basilicum by inhalation in mice. J Nat Med. 2019 Jan;73(1):283-288.

Kavoosi G, Amirghofran Z. Chemical composition, radical scavenging and anti-oxidant capacity of Ocimum basilicum essential oil. Journal of Essential Oil Research. 2017;29(2):189-199.

Basil (Ocimum basilicum L.) essential oil. Journal of Essential Oil Bearing Plants. 2017 Nov 02;20(6):1557-1569. Epub 2018 Jan 17.

Snoussi M, Dehmani A, Noumi E, Flamini G, Papetti A. Chemical composition and antibiofilm activity of Petroselinum crispum and Ocimum basilicum essential oils against Vibrio spp. strains. Microb Pathog. 2016 Jan;90:13-21. Epub 2015 Nov 16.

Ogaly HA, Eltablawy NA, El-Behairy AM, El-Hindi H, Abd-Elsalam RM. Hepatocyte growth factor mediates the antifibrogenic action of Ocimum basilicum essential oil against CCl4-induced liver fibrosis in rats. Molecules. 2015 Jul 23;20(8):13518-35.

Shirazi MT, Gholami H, Kavoosi G, Rowshan V, Tafsiry A. Chemical composition, antioxidant, antimicrobial and cytotoxic activities of Tagetes minuta and Ocimum basilicum essential oils. Food Sci & Nutr. 2014 Mar;2(2):146-55. Epub 2014 Jan 16.

Siddiqui BS, Bhatti HA, Begum S, Perwaiz S. Evaluation of the antimycobacterium activity of the constituents from Ocimum basilicum against Mycobacterium tuberculosis. J Ethnopharmacol. 2012 Oct 31;144(1):220-2. Epub 2012 Aug 17.

Essential Oils Complete Home Reference | First Edition

BOTANICAL FAMILY: Myristicaceae

PLANT ORIGIN: Indonesia

EXTRACTION METHOD: Steam distilled from root

KEY CONSTITUENTS: Sabinene (14-29%), Alpha-Pinene (15-28%), Beta-Pinene (12-18%), Myristicin (5-12%), Limonene (2-7%), Gamma-Terpinene (2-6%), Terpinen-4-ol (2-6%), Safrole (1-3%), Delta-3-Carene (up to 2%)

NUTMEG & NUTMEG VITALITY™
(Myristica fragrans)

Nutmeg was listed in Hildegard's Medicine, a compilation of early German medicines by highly regarded Benedictine herbalist Hildegard of Bingen (1098-1179).

MEDICAL PROPERTIES:
Antidiarrheal, antimicrobial, antidepressant, antioxidative, antidiabetic, anticonvulsant, anti-inflammatory, anticoagulant, antiseptic, antiparasitic, analgesic, liver protectant, stomach protectant (ulcers), circulatory stimulant, adrenal stimulant, muscle relaxing, increases production of growth hormone/melatonin

USES:
Memory retention, rheumatism/arthritis, cardiovascular disease, hypertension, hepatitis, ulcers, digestive disorders, parasites, nerve pain, fatigue/exhaustion, neuropathy

FRAGRANT INFLUENCE:
Warm, spicy aroma that is energizing and uplifting

DIRECTIONS:
Aromatic: 30. Topical: 50-50. Dietary (Vitality): Dilute 1 drop with 1 drop of V-6 or other pure carrier oil. Put in a capsule and take up to 3 times daily or as needed.

CAUTIONS: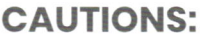

SELECTED RESEARCH:

Matulyte I, Jekabsone A, Jankauskaite L, Zavistanaviciute P, Sakiene V, Bartkiene E, Ruzauskas M, Kopustinskiene DM, Santini A, Bernatoniene J. The Essential Oil and Hydrolauts from Myristica fragrans Seeds with Magnesium Aluminometasilicate as Excipient: Antioxidant, Antibacterial, and Anti-Inflammatory Activity. Foods. 2020 Jan; 9(1): 37.

Plaingam W, Sangsuthum S, Angkhasirisap W, Tencomnao T. Kaempferia parviflora rhizome extract and Myristica fragrans volatile oil increase the levels of monoamine neurotransmitters and impact the proteomic profiles in the rat hippocampus: mechanistic insights into their neuroprotective effects. J Tradit Complement Med. 2017 Jun 15;7(4):538-552.

Muñoz Acuña U, Carcache PJ, Matthew S, Carcache de Blanco EJ. New acyclic bis phenylpropanoid and neolignans, from Myristica fragrans Houtt., exhibiting PARP-1 and NF-κB inhibitory effects. Food Chem. 2016 Jul 1;202:269-75.

Cuong TD, Hunt TM, Han HY, Roh HS, Seok JH, Lee JH, Jeong JY, Choi JS, Kim JA, Min BS. Potent acetylcholinesterase inhibitory compounds from Myristica fragrans. Nat Prod Commun. 2014 Apr;9(4):499-502.

Piaru SP, Mahmud R, Abdul Majid AM, Mahmoud Nassar ZD. Antioxidant and antiangiogenic activities of the essential oils of Myristica fragrans and Morinda citrifolia. Asian Pac J Trop Med. 2012 Apr;5(4):294-8.

Piras A, Rosa A, Marongiu B, Atzeri A, Dessi MA, Falconieri D, Porcedda S. Extraction and separation of volatile and fixed oils from seeds of Myristica fragrans by supercritical CO2: chemical composition and cytotoxic activity on Caco-2 cancer cells. J Food Sci. 2012 Apr;77(4):C448-53. Epub 2012 Mar 19.

Wahab A, Ul Haq R, Ahmed A, Khan RA, Raza M. Anticonvulsant activities of nutmeg oil of Myristica fragrans. Phytother Res. 2009 Feb;23(2):153-8.

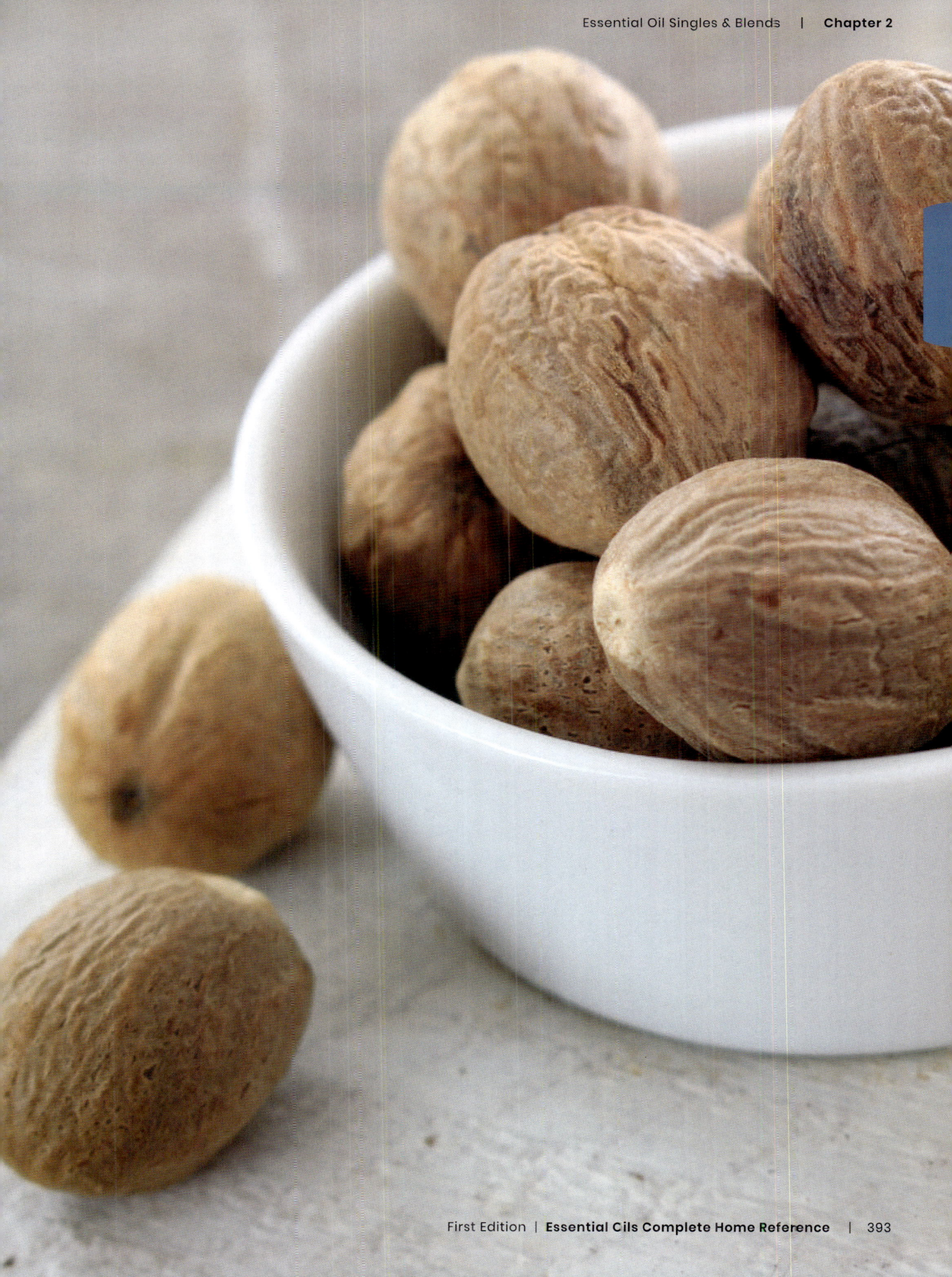

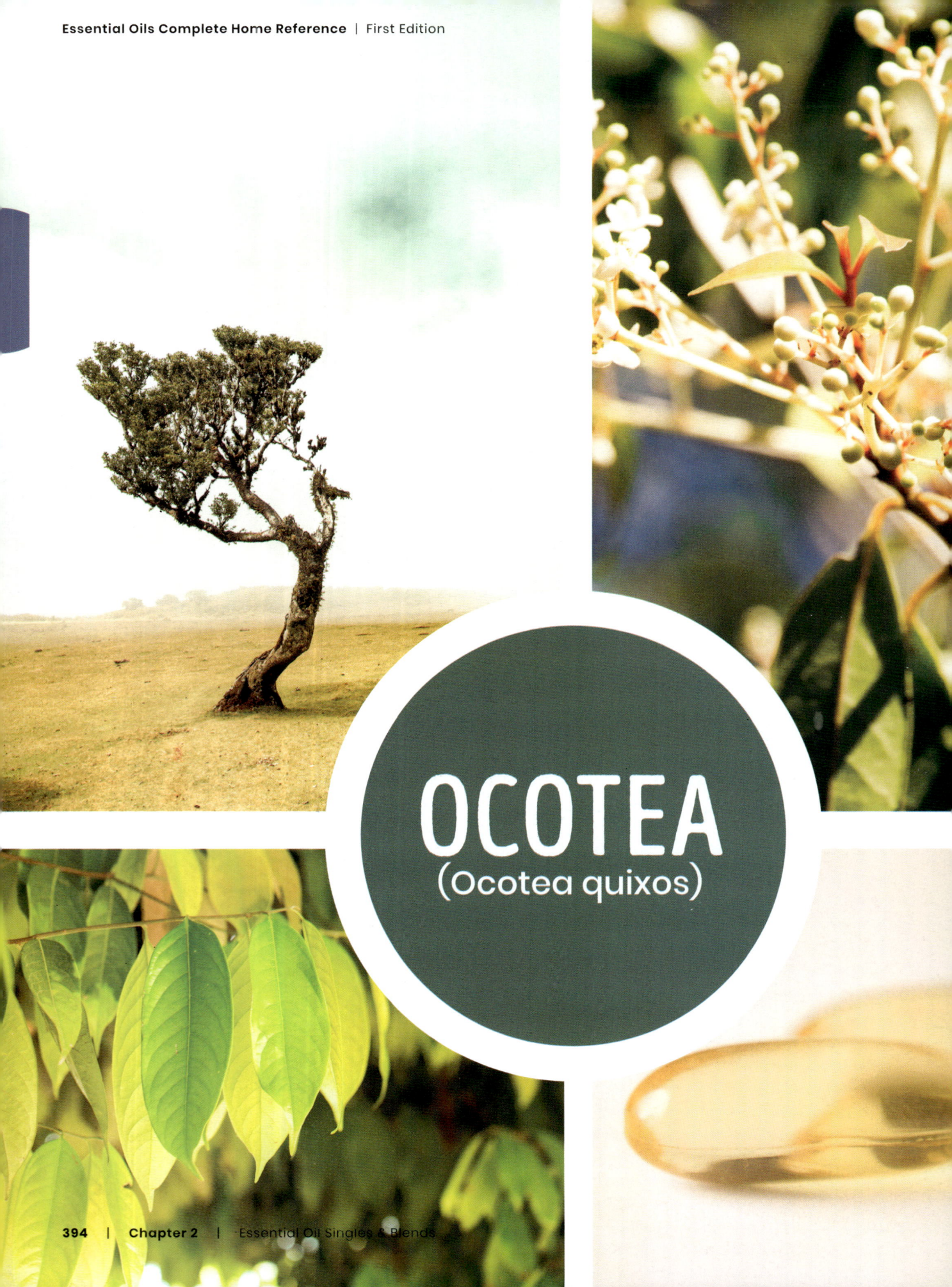

OCOTEA
(Ocotea quixos)

Essential Oil Singles & Blends | Chapter 2

BOTANICAL FAMILY:
Lauraceae

PLANT ORIGIN:
Ecuador

EXTRACTION METHOD:
Steam distilled from the leaves

KEY CONSTITUENTS:
Beta-Caryophyllene (6-34%), Methyl Cinnamate (2-27%), Cinnamyl Acetate (up to 25%), Alpha-Humulene (2-18%), Trans-Cinnamaldehyde (up to 8%)

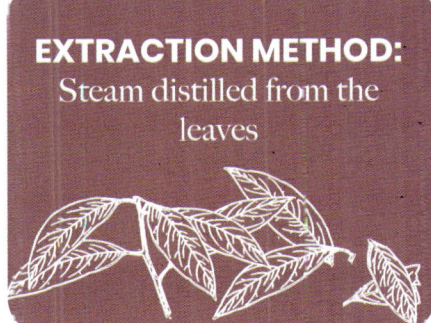

HISTORICAL DATA:
Ocotea is distilled from a tree found in the Amazon wilderness, on the ranges of the west side of the Andes Mountains. It is commonly referred to by the native people throughout Ecuador as Ishpingo and is considered to be a "false canilla" or "false cinnamon." The tree grows to a very large size, reaching up to 48 inches in diameter and over 60 feet tall, making a large canopy top. Historical use of ocotea dates back more than 500 years, when it was used to aromatize sweets and cakes.

MEDICAL PROPERTIES:
Antifungal, disinfectant, anti-inflammatory, antianxiety

USES:
Hypertension, high blood pressure, anxiety, internal irritation, may lower insulin needs for diabetics and reduce blood sugar fluctuations, infection, digestive support, purification, flavoring and spice in recipes

FRAGRANT INFLUENCE:
Complex aroma, which may increase feelings of fullness; related to the cinnamon species but has an aroma that is different from any common cinnamon; helps body minimize irritation; eases stress; cleanses and purifies the spirit

DIRECTIONS:
Aromatic: 60. Topical: 20-80. Dietary: Dilute 1 drop essential oil with 4 drops V-6 or other pure carrier oil. Put in a capsule and take 1 daily or as directed by a health care professional.

CAUTIONS: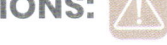

SELECTED RESEARCH:
Scalvenzi L, Radice M, Toma L, Severini F, Boccolini D, Bella A, Guerrini A, Tacchini M, Chiurato M, Romi R, D Luca M. Larvicidal activity of Ocimum campechianum, Ocotea quixos and Piper aduncum essential oils against Aedes aegypti. Parasite. 2019; 26: 23.

Ballabeni V, Tognolini M, Giorgio C, Bertoni S, Bruni R, Barocelli E. Ocotea quixos Lam. essential oil: in vitro and in vivo investigation on its anti-inflammatory properties. Fitoterapia. 2010 Jun;81(4):289-95. Epub 2009 Oct 13.

Sacchetti, G, Guerrini A, Noriega P, Bianchi A, Bruni R. Essential oil of wild Ocotea quixos (Lam.) Kosterm. (Lauraceae) leaves from Amazonian Ecuador. Flav Fragr J. 2006 Jul/Aug;21(4):674-6.

Tognolini M, Barocelli E, Ballabeni V, Bruni R, Bianchi A, Chiavarini M, Impicciatore M. Comparative screening of plant essential oils: phenylpropanoids moiety as basic core for antiplatelet activity. Life Sci. 2006 Feb 23;78(13):1419-32. Epub 2005 Nov 7.

ONE HEART™
(Essential Oil Blend)

One Heart essential oil blend was formulated to celebrate the joy of creating unity and connection in our communities by opening our hearts to love and service for others. Specifically blended to bring people together and help create awareness of The D. Gary Young, Young Living Foundation, the refreshing aroma of this balancing blend can encourage a bright outlook on life and the awareness that we are all in this together. This proprietary blend can also help you find your center and connect to your inner spirituality. Try using it during prayer or meditation for connecting with your inner self.

The beautiful One Heart label was designed by Anita Perlaza, a graduate of the Young Living Academy in rural Ecuador, who is now (in 2020) studying graphic design. Anita's mom works at Young Living's Finca Botanica Farm and Distillery in Ecuador, and her father works at the Academy. Anita said she was inspired to create the design because "I think that if all people can join and collaborate, we can do great things together."

One Heart's proprietary blend includes 100 percent pure essential oils from around the globe, produced by our Seed to Seal® quality commitment. Valor inspires strength; Northern Lights Black Spruce helps create a meditative atmosphere; and Ylang Ylang and Ocotea create a delightfully sweet, uplifting aroma characterized by sweet citrus tones.

In the spirit of this uplifting, connecting blend, 35 percent of each wholesale purchase goes to the Foundation to empower, improve, inspire, and change the lives of those in need.

MEDICAL PROPERTIES & USES:
Calming, energizing, encourages a bright outlook on life, opens your heart to love and serve others, encourages unity and connection with community, helps you find your center and connect to your inner spirituality

INGREDIENTS:
Lemon, Ylang Ylang (Ecuador), Northern Lights Black Spruce, Lime, Caprylic/capric triglyceride,‡ Roman Chamomile, Jasmine, Ocotea, Spearmint, Black Spruce, Blue Tansy, Camphor, Geranium, Frankincense

DIRECTIONS:
Aromatic: 3o. Topical: 50-50.

CAUTIONS:

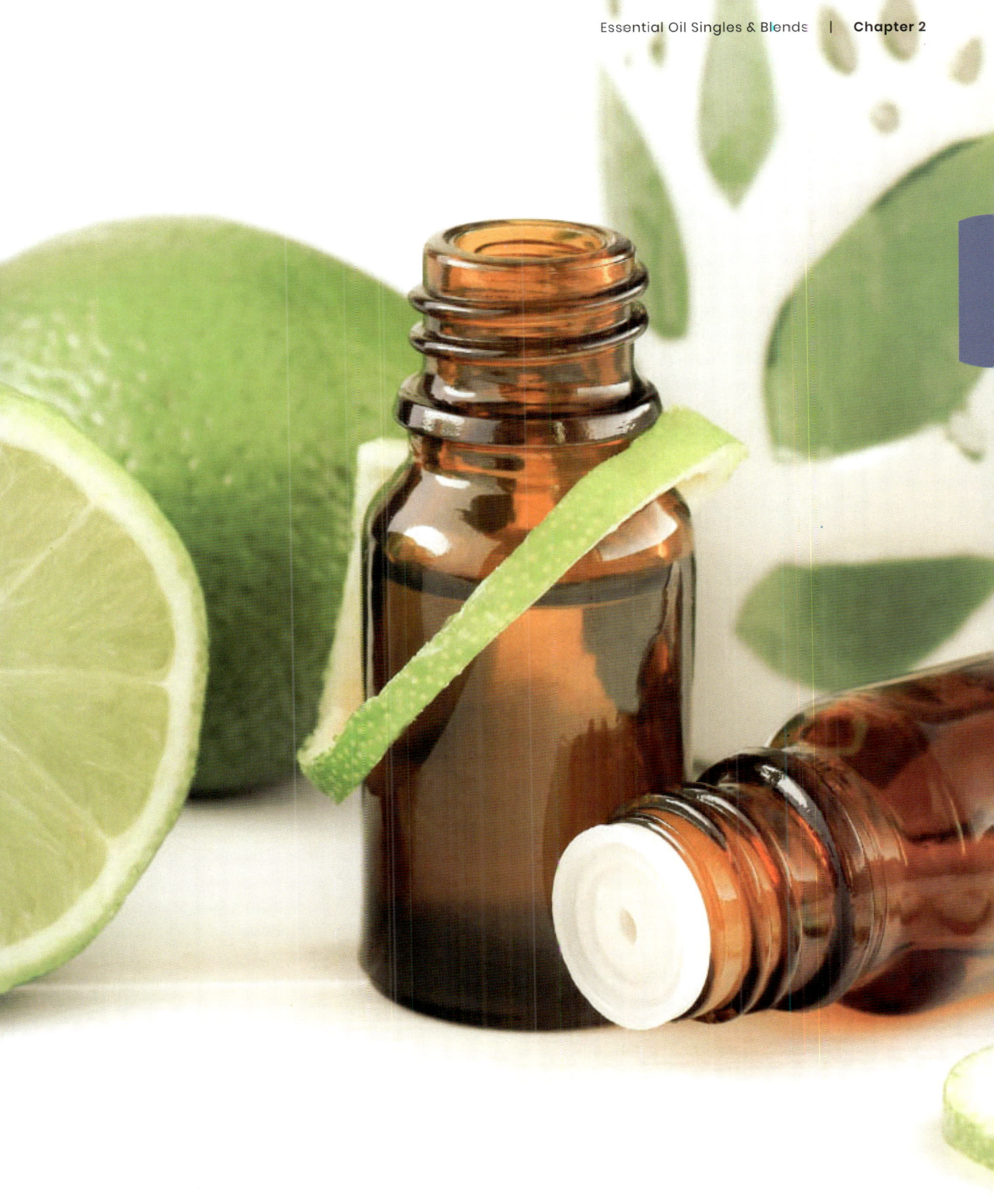

BOTANICAL FAMILY: Rutaceae

PLANT ORIGIN: Brazil, South Africa

EXTRACTION METHOD: Cold pressed from peel

KEY CONSTITUENTS: Limonene (93-96%), Myrcene (1-4%)

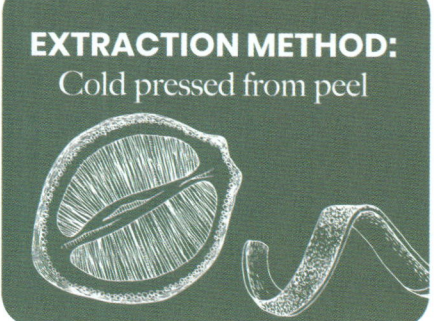

ORANGE & ORANGE VITALITY™
(Citrus sinensis)

Beloved for its clean, fresh scent, Orange essential oil was also shown to reduce anxiety in children awaiting dental treatment. Salivary cortisol levels were lowered as were pulse rates (Jafarzadeh, 2013).

MEDICAL PROPERTIES:
Antibacterial, insecticidal, relaxant, anticoagulant, circulatory stimulant. Rich in limonene, which has been extensively studied in over 50 clinical studies for its ability to combat tumor growth.

USES:
Acne, knee pain, arteriosclerosis, hypertension, cancer, insomnia, and complexion (dull and oily), fluid retention, wrinkles

FRAGRANT INFLUENCE:
Uplifting and refreshing. A Mie University study found that citrus fragrances boosted immunity, induced relaxation, and reduced depression (Komori, et al., 1995).

DIRECTIONS:
Aromatic: 6o. Topical: 50-50. Dietary (Vitality): Put 2 drops in a capsule and take 3 times daily.

CAUTIONS:

SELECTED RESEARCH:

Atolani O, Adamu N, Oguntoye OS, Zubair MF, Fabiyi OA, Oyegoke RA, Adeyemi OS, Areh ET, Tarigha DE, Kambizi L. Olatunji GA. Chemical characterization, antioxidant, cytotoxicity, Anti-Toxoplasma gondii and antimicrobial potentials of the Citrus sinensis seed oil for sustainable cosmeceutical production. Heliyon. 2020 Feb; 6(2): e03399.

Hekmatpou D, Pourandish Y, Farahani PV, Parvizrad R. The effect of aromatherapy with the essential oil of orange on pain and vital signs of patients with fractured limbs admitted to the emergency ward: a randomized clinical trial. Indian J Palliat Care. 2017 Oct-Dec;23(4):431-436.

Shetty SB, Mahin-Syed-Ismail P, Varghese S, Thomas-George B, Kandathil-Thajuraj P, Baby D, Haleem S, Sreedhar S, Devang-Divakar D. Antimicrobial effects of Citrus sinensis peel extracts against dental caries bacteria: an in vitro study. J Clin Exp Dent. 2016 Feb 1;8(1):e71-7. eCollection 2016 Feb.

Hussain KA, Tarakji B, Kandy BP, John J, Mathews J, Ramphul V, Divakar DD. Antimicrobial effects of Citrus sinensis peel extracts against periodontopathic bacteria: an in vitro study. Rocz Panstw Zakl Hig. 2015;66(2):173-8.

Hasheminia D, Kalantar Motamedi MR, Karimi Ahmadabadi H, Hashemzehi H, Haghighat A. Can ambient orange fragrance reduce patient anxiety during surgical removal of impacted mandibular third molars? J Oral Maxillofac Surg. 2014 Sep;72(9):1671-6. Epub 2014 Apr 12.

Igarashi M, Ikei H, Song C, Miyazaki Y. Effects of olfactory stimulation with rose and orange oil on prefrontal cortex activity. Complement Ther Med. 2014 Dec;22(6):1027-31. Epub 2014 Sep 28.

D'Alessio PA, Ostan R, Bisson JF, Schulzke JD, Ursini MV, Béné MC. Oral administration of d-limonene controls inflammation in rat colitis and displays anti-inflammatory properties as diet supplementation in humans. Life Sci. 2013 Jul 10;92(24-26):1151-6. Epub 2013 May 7.

Jafarzadeh M, Arman S, Pour FF. Effect of aromatherapy with orange essential oil on salivary cortisol and pulse rate in children during dental treatment: a randomized controlled clinical trial. Adv Biomed Res. 2013 Mar 6;2:10. Print 2013.

Miller JA, Lang JE, Ley M, Nagle R, Hsu CH, Thompson PA, Cordova C, Waer A, Chow HH. Human breast cancer tissue disposition and bioactivity of limonene in women with early-stage breast cancer. Cancer Prev Res (Phila). 2013 Jun;6(6):577-84. Epub 2013 Apr 3.

Komori T, Fujiwara R, Tanida M, Nomura J, Yokoyama MM. Effects of citrus fragrance on immune function and depressive states. Neuroimmunomodulation. 1995 May-Jun;2(3):174-80..

Essential Oil Singles & Blends | **Chapter 2**

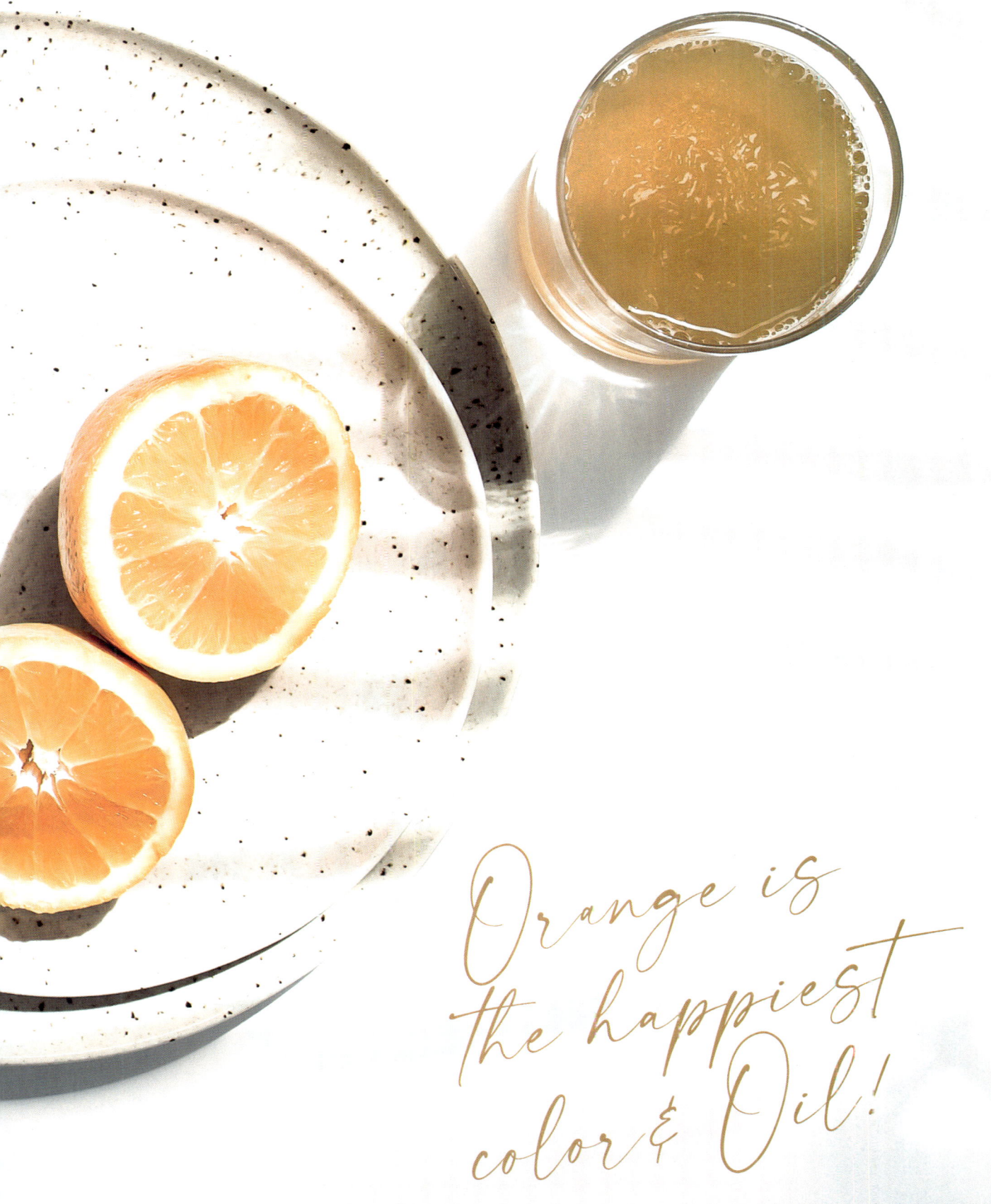

Orange is the happiest color & Oil!

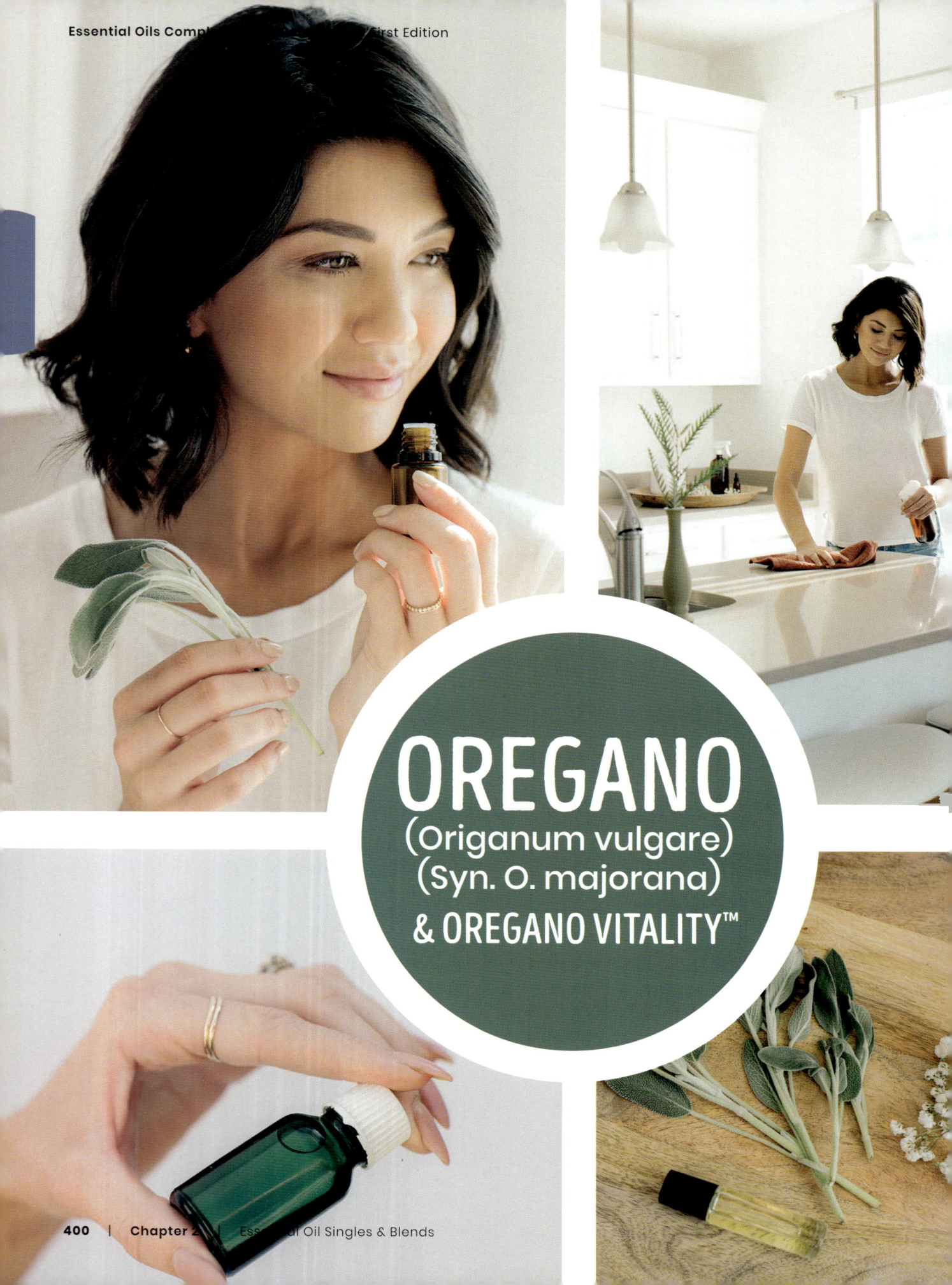

Essential Oil Singles & Blends | Chapter 2

BOTANICAL FAMILY: Lamiaceae

PLANT ORIGIN: Moldova

EXTRACTION METHOD: Steam distilled from leaves/herb/aerial parts

KEY CONSTITUENTS: Carvacrol (56-90%), Thymol (up to 12%), Gamma-Terpinene (up to 11%), Para-Cymene (2-9%), Linalool (1-8%)

HISTORICAL DATA:
Listed in Hildegard's Medicine, a compilation of early German medicines by highly regarded Benedictine herbalist Hildegard of Bingen (1098-1179).

MEDICAL PROPERTIES:
Antioxidant, antibacterial, antiaging, powerful antiviral, antimicrobial, antifungal, antiparasitic, anti-inflammatory, antioxidant, immune stimulant, antinociceptive, radioprotective, liver protectant

USES:
Arthritis, rheumatism, respiratory infectious diseases, infections, cold symptoms, tuberculosis, digestive problems, cleansing, detoxificiation, cosmetics, massage on fatigued areas, Raindrop Technique

FRAGRANT INFLUENCE:
Creates a feeling of security, purifies the air

DIRECTIONS:
Aromatic: 10. Topical: 20-80. Use in Raindrop Technique. Dietary (Vitality): Dilute 50-50. Put 2 drops in a capsule and take up to 3 times daily.

CAUTIONS: 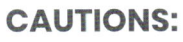   High in phenols, Oregano may irritate the nasal membranes or skin if inhaled directly from diffuser or bottle or applied neat.

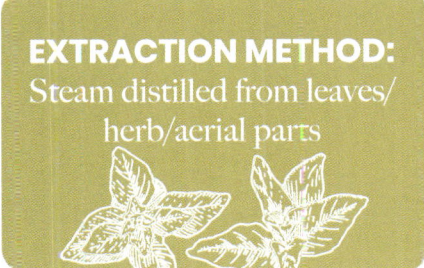

SELECTED RESEARCH:

Jan S, Rashid M, Abd Allah EF, Ahman P. Biological Efficacy of Essential Oils and Plant Extracts of Cultivated and Wild Ecotypes of Origanum vulgare L. Biomed Res Int. 2020; 2020: 8751718.

Castronovo LM, Calonico C, Ascrizzi R, Duca SD Delfino V, Chioccioli S, Vassallo A, Strozza I, De Leo M, Biffi S, Bacci G, Bogani P, Maggini V, Mengoni A, Pistelli L, Lo Nostro A, Firenzuoli F, Fani R. The Cultivable Bacterial Microbiota Associated to the Medicinal plant Oerganum vulgare L.: From Antibiotic Resistance to Growth-Inhibitory Properties. Front Microbiol. 2020; 11: 862.

Veenstra JP, Johnson JJ. Oregano (Origanum vulgare) extract for food preservation and improvement in gastrointestinal health. Int J Nutr. 2019;3(4):43-52. Epub 2019 Apr 9.

Taleb MH, Abdeltawab NF, Shamma RN, Abdelgayed SS, Mohamed SS, Farag MA, Ramadan MA. Origanum vulgare L. Essential oil as a potential anti-acne topical nanoemulsion-in vitro and in vivo study. Molecules. 2018 Sep; 23(9):2164.

Karaman M, Bogavac M, Radovanović B, Sudji J, Tešanović K, Janjušević L. Origanum vulgare essential oil affects pathogens causing vaginal infections. J Appl Microbiol. 2017 May;122(5):1177-85. Epub 2017 Apr 4.

Kubatka P, Kello M, Kajo K, Kruzliak P, Vybohová D, Mojžiš J, Adamkov M, Fialová S, Veizerová L, Zulli A, Péč M, Statelová D, Grančai D, Büsselberg D. Oregano demonstrates distinct tumour-suppressive effects in breast carcinoma model. Eur J Nutr. 2017 Apr;56(3):1303-16.

Gomes Neto NJ, Magnani M, Chueca B, Garcia-Gonzalo D, Pagán R, de Souza EL. Influence of general stress-response alternative sigma factors σ(S) (RpoS) and σ(B) (SigB) on bacterial tolerance to the essential oils from Origanum vulgare L. and Rosmarinus officinalis L. and pulsed electric fields. Int J Food Microbiol. 2015 Oct 15;211:32-7. 2015.06.030. Epub 2015 Jul 4.

Begnini KR, Nedel F, Lund RG, Carvalho PH, Rodrigues MR, Beira FT, Del-Pino FA. Composition and antiproliferative effect of essential oil of Origanum vulgare against tumor cell lines. J Med Food. 2014 Oct;17(10):1129-33. Epub 2014 Sep 17.

Afarineshe Khaki MR, Pahlavan Y, Sepehri G, Sheibani V, Pahlavan B. Antinociceptive effect of aqueous extract of Origanum vulgare L. in male rats: possible involvement of the GABAergic system. Iran J Pharm Res. 2013 Spring;12(2):407-13.

Schillaci D, Napoli EM, Cusimano MG, Vitale M, Ruberto A. Origanum vulgare subsp. hirtum essential oil prevented biofilm formation and showed antibacterial activity against planktonic and sessile bacterial cells. J Food Prod. 2013 Oct;76(10):1747-52.

BOTANICAL FAMILY:
Lamiaceae

PLANT ORIGIN:
Ecuador

EXTRACTION METHOD:
Steam distilled from leaves, herbs, and aerial parts

KEY CONSTITUENTS:
Carvacrol (28-45%),
Para-Cymene (14-26%),
Gamma-Terpinene (16-23%),
Thymol (up to 3%)

OREGANO, ECUADORIAN
(formerly called Plectranthus Oregano) (Plectranthus amboinicus)

The leaves of this plant have been used in traditional medicine for coughs, sore throats, and nasal congestion. It is also used for infections and rheumatism. Ecuadorian Oregano's flavor makes it popular for cooking, especially in soups. It can be used more easily by people who are sensitive to Oregano, which is hotter than Ecuadorian Oregano.

MEDICAL PROPERTIES:
Antitumoral, antibacterial, antioxidant, analgesic, anti-inflammatory, antihyperlipodemic, liver protectant

USES:
Infections, cancer, arthritis, diabetes, rheumatism, pain, massage, cooking

FRAGRANT INFLUENCE:
Relaxing, purifies the air

DIRECTIONS:
Aromatic: 6O. Topical: 2O-8O. May use neat in Raindrop Technique. Dietary: Dilute 50-50. Put 2 drops in a capsule and take up to 3 times daily. Use to flavor foods.

CAUTIONS:

SELECTED RESEARCH:

Hasibuan PAZ, Sumaiyah S. The Anti-Proliferative and Pro-Apoptotic Properties of Ethanol Plectranthus amboinicus (Lour.) Spreng. Leaves Ethanolic Extract Nanoparticles on T47D Cell Lines. Asian Pac J Cancer Prev. 2019; 29(3): 897-901.

Nazliniwaty N, Laila L. Formulation and Antibacterial Activity of Plectranthus amboinicus (Lour.) Spreng Leaves Ethanolic Extract as Herbal Mouthwash Against Halitotis Caused Bacteria. Open Access Maced J Med Sci. 2019 Nov 30; 7(22): 3900-3903.

Vasconcelos SECB, Melo HM, Cavalcante TTA, Júnior FEAC, de Carvalho MG, Menezes FGR, de Sousa OV, Costa RA. Plectranthus amboinicus essential oil and carvacrol bioactive against planktonic and biofilm of oxacillin- and vancomycin-resistant Staphylococcus aureus. BMC Complement Altern Med. 2017 Sep 16;17(1):462.

Arumugam G, Swamy MK, Sinniah UR. Plectranthus amboinicus (Lour.) Spreng: botanical, phytochemical, pharmacological and nutritional significance. Molecules. 2016 Mar 30;21(4):369.

Santos NO, Mariane B, Lago JH, Sartorelli P, Rosa W, Soares MG, da Silva AM, Lorenzi H, Vallim MA, Pascon RC. Assessing the chemical composition and antimicrobial activity of essential oils from Brazilian plants—Eremanthus erythropappus (Asteraceae) Plectrantus barbatus, and P. amboinicus (Lamiaceae). Molecules. 2015 May 11;20(5):8440-52.

de Oliveira FF, Torres AF, Gonçalves TB, Santiago GM, de Carvalho CB, Aguiar MB, Camar LM, Rabenhorst SH, Martins AM, Valença Junior JT, Nagao-Dias AT. Efficacy of Plectranthus amboinicus (Lour.) Spreng in a murine model of methicillin-resistant staphylococcus aureus skin abscesses. Evid Based Complement Alternat Med. 2013;2013:291592. Epub 2013 Feb 20.

Manjamalai A, Grace VM. The chemotherapeutic effect of essential oil of plectranthus amboinicus (Lour) on lung metastasis developed by B16F-10 cell line in C57BL/6 mice. Cancer Invest. 2013 Jan;31(1):74-82. Epub 2012 Dec 18.

Gonçalves TB, Braga MA, de Oliveira FF, Santiago GM, Carvalho CB, Brito e Cabral P, de Melo Santiago T, Sousa JS, Barros EB, do Nasimento RF, Nagao-Dias AT. Effect of subinhibitory and inhibitory concentrations of plectranthus amboinicus (Lour.) spreng essential oil on Klebsiella pneumoniae. Phytomedicine. 2012 Aug 15;19(11):962-8. Epub 2012 Jul 8.

Viswanathaswamy AH, Koti BC, Gore A, Thippeswamy AH, Kulkami RV. Antihyperglycemic and antihyperlipidemic activity of Plectranthus amboinicus on normal and alloxan-induced diabetic rats. Indian J Pharm Sci. 2011 Mar;73(2):139-45.

Essential Oil Singles & Blends | **Chapter 2**

Oregano is the best oil for everything... cooking, cleaning, & health.

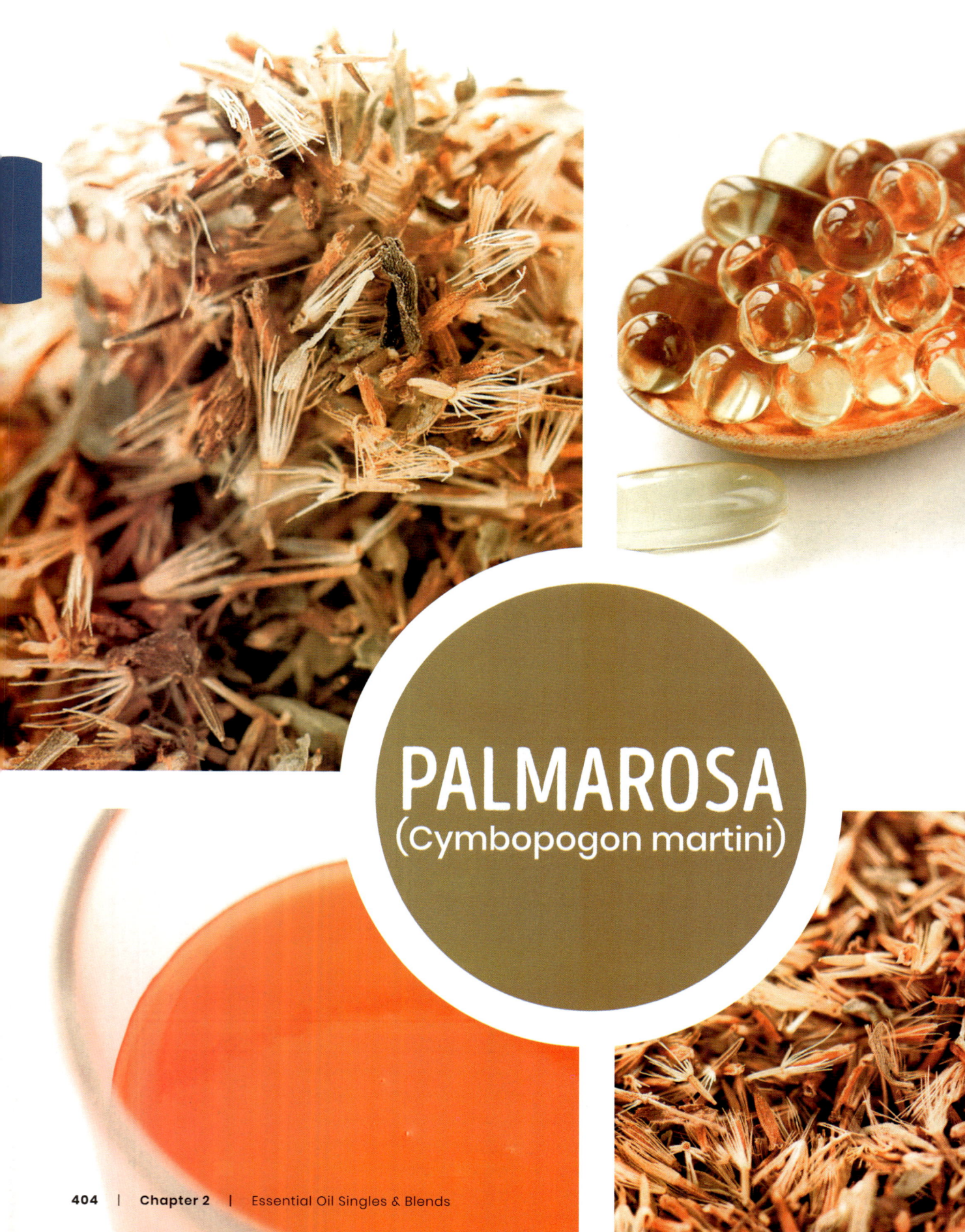

PALMAROSA
(Cymbopogon martini)

Essential Oil Singles & Blends | Chapter 2

BOTANICAL FAMILY:
Poaceae

PLANT ORIGIN:
India

EXTRACTION METHOD:
Steam distilled from leaves

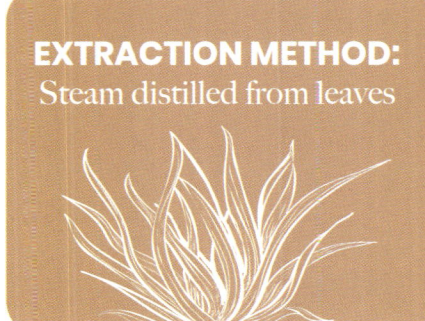

KEY CONSTITUENTS:
Geraniol (72-94%),
Geranyl Acetate (6-12%),
Linalool (1-5%)

HISTORICAL DATA:
A relative of Lemongrass, Palmarosa was used in temple incense by the ancient Egyptians.

MEDICAL PROPERTIES:
Antibacterial, antifungal, antiviral, supports heart and nervous system, reduces blood sugar fluctuations, stimulates new skin cell growth, regulates sebum production in skin

USES:
Fungal infections/candida, neuroprotective, cardiovascular/circulatory diseases, digestive problems, skin problems (acne, eczema), prevents inflammation, quells dehydration, aids in healing of cuts and bruises, helps remedy acne

FRAGRANT INFLUENCE:
Creates a feeling of security, helps to reduce stress and tension, promotes recovery from nervous exhaustion, hydrating

DIRECTIONS:
Aromatic: 6o. Topical: Neat. Dietary: Dilute 1 drop essential oil with 1 drop V-6 or other pure carrier oil, put in a capsule, and take up to 3 times daily.

CAUTIONS: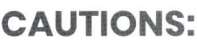

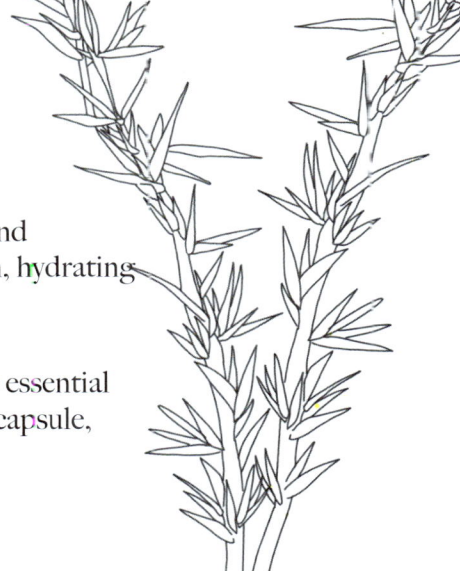

SELECTED RESEARCH:

Gemeda N, Tadele A, Lemma H, Girma B, Addis G, Tesfaye B, Abebe A, Gemechu W, Yirsaw K, Teka F, Haile C, Amano A, Woldkidan S, Geleta B, Debella A. Development, Characterization, and Evaluation of Novel Broad-Spectrum Antimicrobial Topical Formulations from Cymbopogon martini (Roxb.) W. Watson Essential Oil. Evid Based Complement Alternat Med. 2018; 2018: 9812093.

Janbaz KH, Qayyum A, Saqib F, Imran I, Zia-Ul-Haq M, de Feo V. Bronchodilator, vasodilator and spasmolytic activities of Cymbopogon martini. J Physiol Pharmacol. 2014 Dec;65(6):859-66.

Murbach Teles Andrade BF, Conti BJ, Santiago KB, Fernandex Junior A, Sforcin JM. Cymbopogon martini essential oil and geraniol at noncytotoxic concentrations exerted immunomodulatory/anti-inflammatory effects in human monocytes. J Pharm Pharmacol. 2014 Oct;66(10):1491-6. Epub 2014 Jun 16.

Buch P, Patel V, Ranpariya V, Sheth N, Parmar S. Neuroprotective activity of Cymbopogon martinii against cerebral ischemia/reperfusion-induced oxidative stress in rats. J. Ethnopharmacol. 2012 Jun 26;142(1):35-40.

Gacche RN, Shaikh RU, Chapole SM, Jadhav AD, Jadhav SG. Kinetics of inhibition of monoamine oxidase using Cymbopogon martinii (Roxb.) Wats.: a potential antidepressant herbal ingredient with antioxidant activity. Indian J Clin Biochem. 2011 Jul 26(3):303-8. Epub 2011 Mar 2.

Ghadyale V, Takalikar S, Haldavnekar V, Arvindekar A. Effective control of postprandial glucose level through inhibition of intestinal alpha glucosidase by Cymbopogon martinii (Roxb.). Evid Based Complement Alternat Med. 2012;2012:372909. Epub 2011 Jul 7.

Gacche RN, Shaikh RU, Chapole SM, Jadhav AD, Jadhav SG. Kinetics of Inhibition of Monoamine Oxidase Using Cymbopogon martinii (Roxb.) Wats.: A Potential Antidepressant Herbal Ingredient with Antioxidant Activity. Indian J Clin Biochem. 2011 Jul; 26(3): 303-308.

Sinha S, Biswas D, Mukherjee A. Antigenotoxic and antioxidant activities of palmarosa and citronella essential oils. J Ethnopharmacol. 2011 Oct 11;137(3):1521-7. Epub 2011 Aug 27.

BOTANICAL FAMILY:
Burseraceae

PLANT ORIGIN:
Ecuador

EXTRACTION METHOD:
Distilled from wood

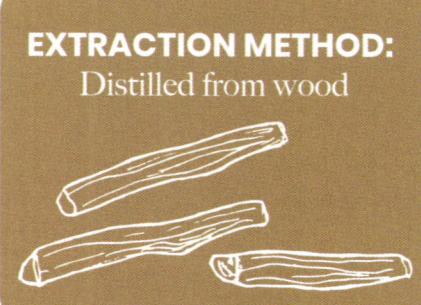

KEY CONSTITUENTS:
Limonene (46-76%), Alpha-Terpineol (5-16%), Menthofuran (up to 8%), Beta Bisabolene (up to 7%), Para Cymene (up to 6%), Fonenol up to 4%)

PALO SANTO
(Bursera graveolens)

Palo Santo comes from the same botanical family as Frankincense, although it is found in South America. Like Frankincense, Palo Santo is known as a spiritual oil, with a deep-rooted tradition in which it was used by the Incas to purify and cleanse the air of negative energies and for good luck. It is used in South America to repel mosquitoes, for fevers, infections, and skin diseases. It is currently used by shamans of the Andes in curing ceremonies. Even its Spanish name reflects how highly this oil was regarded: palo santo means "holy or sacred wood."

Note: Constituents can vary depending on whether the wood is harvested from coastal or inland areas and if the trunk is red or white.

MEDICAL PROPERTIES:
Anticancerous, antiblastic, anti-inflammatory, antibacterial, antifungal, antiviral

USES:
Inflammation, regrowth of knee cartilage, joints, arthritis, rheumatism, gout, respiratory problems, reduces airborne contaminants when diffused, colds, flu, stress, inflammation, depression, headaches, anxiety, healing during massage

FRAGRANT INFLUENCE:
Colds, flu, respiratory problems, stress, depression, anxiety

DIRECTIONS:
Aromatic: 60. Topical: 50-50. Dietary: Put 10-15 drops in a capsule and take 1 or 2 times a day. Can also put 1-6 drops under the tongue or in a glass of water.

CAUTIONS: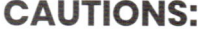

SELECTED RESEARCH:
Monzote L, Hill GM, Cuellar A, Scull R, Setzer WN. Chemical composition and anti-proliferative properties of Bursera graveolens essential oil. Nat Prod Commun. 2012 Nov;7(11):1531-4.

Young DG, Chao S, Casabianca H, Bertrand M-C, Minga D. Essential Oil of Busera graveolens (Kunth) Triana et Planch from Ecuador. J Essent. Oil Res. 19 525-526 (November/December 2007).

Nakanishi T, Inatomi Y, Murata H, Shigeta K, Iida N, Inada A, Murata J, Farrera MA, Iinuma M, Tanaka T, Tajima S, Oku N. A new and known cytotoxic aryltetralin-type lignans from stems of Bursera graveolens. Chem Pharm Bull (Tokyo). 2005 Feb;53(2):229-231.

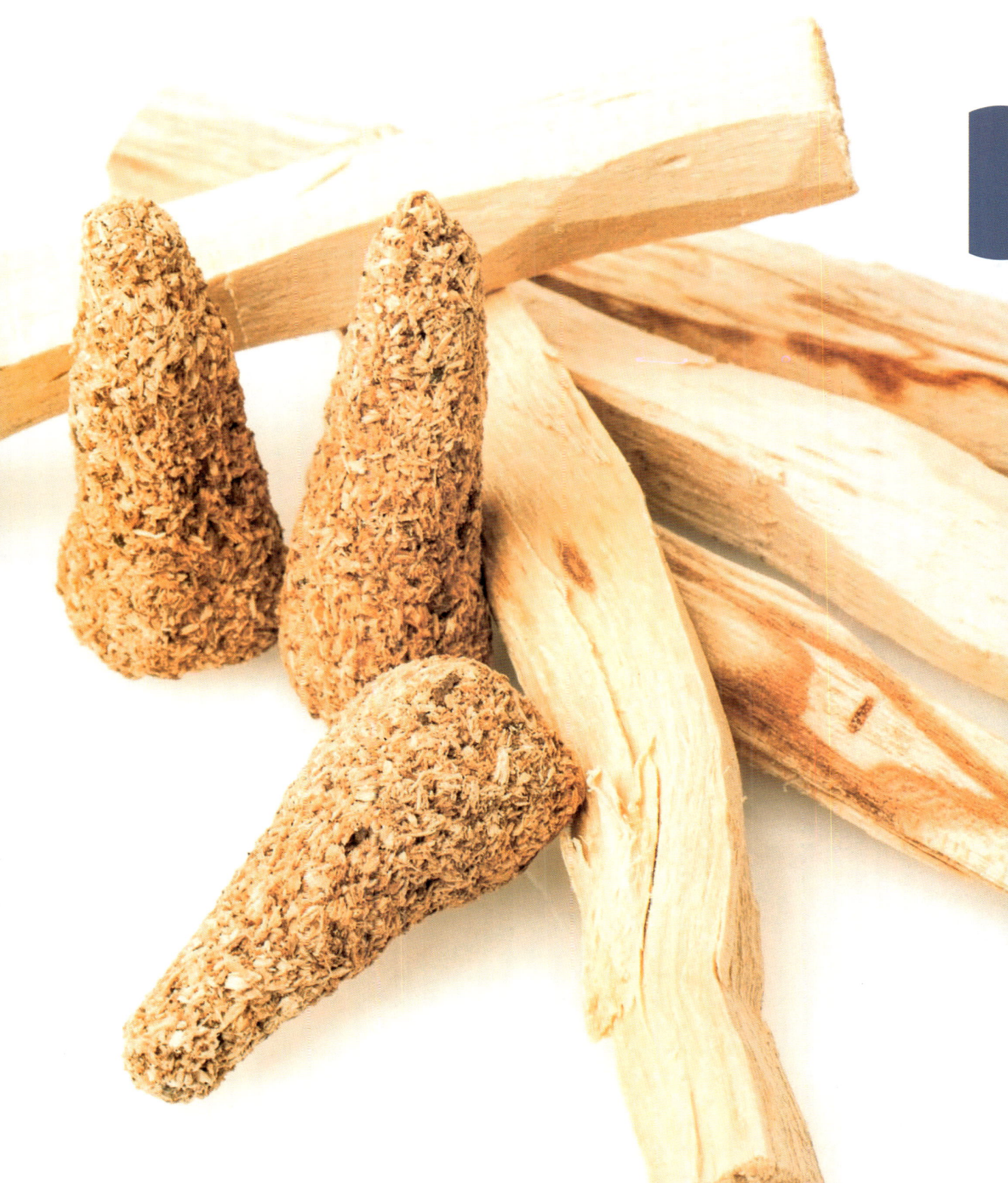

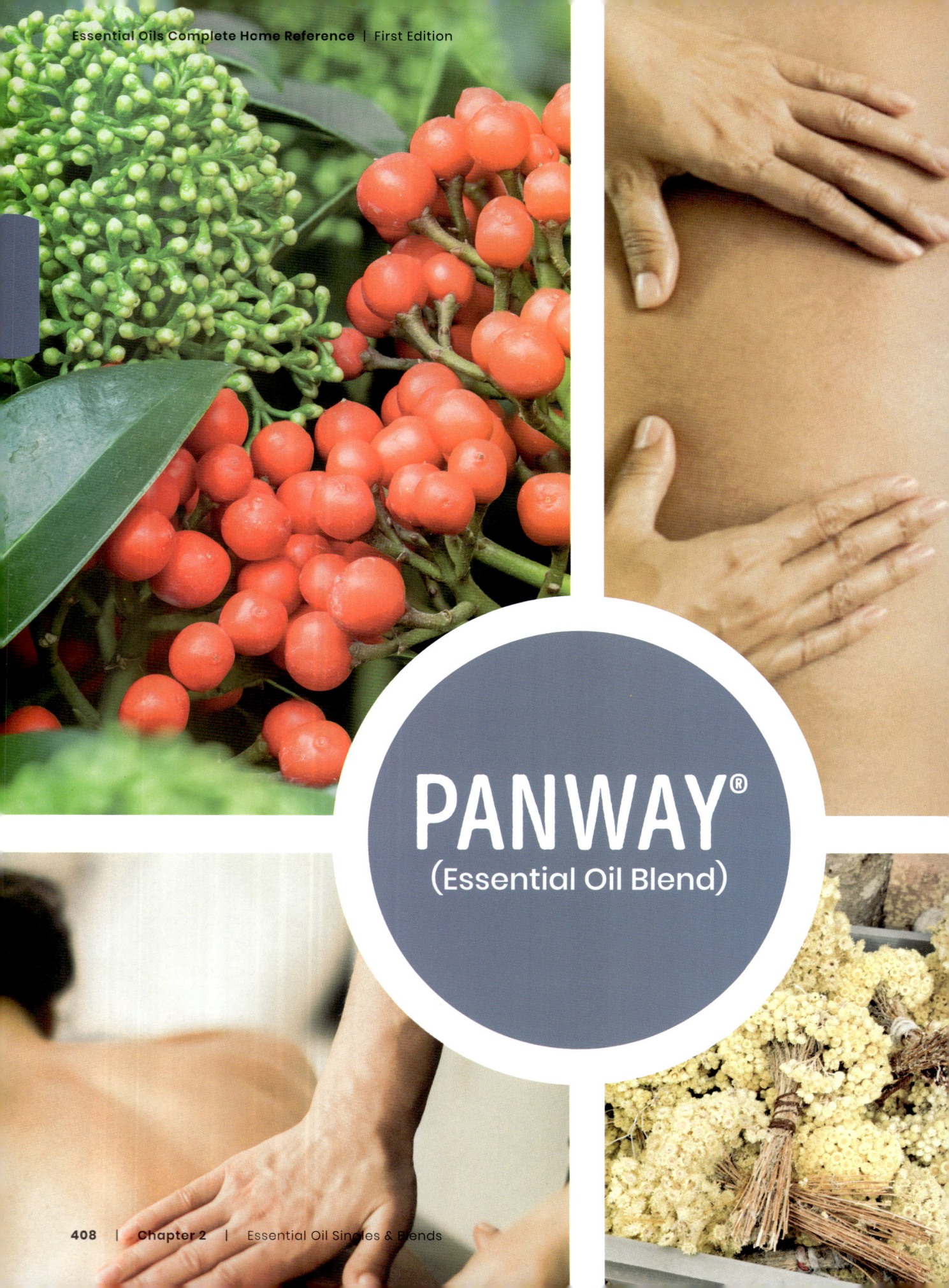

Essential Oil Singles & Blends | **Chapter 2**

ABOUT PANAWAY®:
This very popular blend reduces pain and inflammation, increases circulation, and accelerates healing. It relieves swelling and discomfort from arthritis, sprains, muscle spasms, cramps, bumps, and bruises.

MEDICAL PROPERTIES & USES:
Anti-inflammatory, antimicrobial, antioxidative, cardiovascular supportive, oral protective, pain or swelling reducing, performance enhancing/stimulating, wellness supporting

INGREDIENTS:
Wintergreen, Helichrysum, Clove, Peppermint

DIRECTIONS:
Topical: 20-80. Use as a compress or for a Raindrop Technique-style massage along the spine. Use for relief of deep tissue pain. Add additional Helichrysum to enhance the effect. When the pain is bone related, more Wintergreen may be added. May be diluted with Ortho Ease or Ortho Sport massage oils.

CAUTIONS: **Not intended for children under the age of 6 without the advice of a health care professional.**

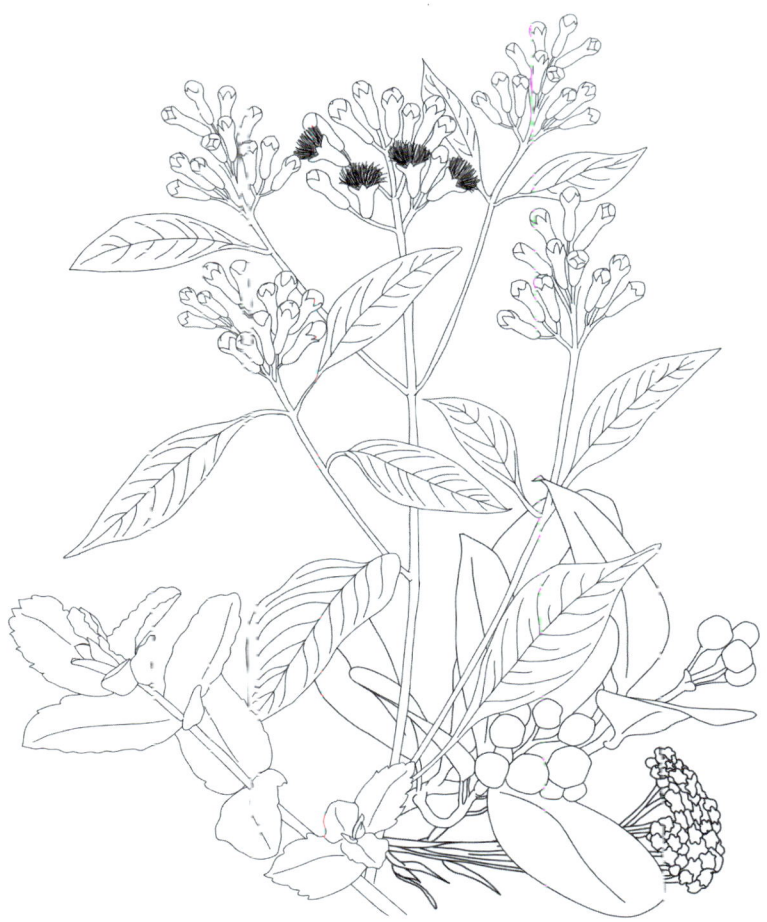

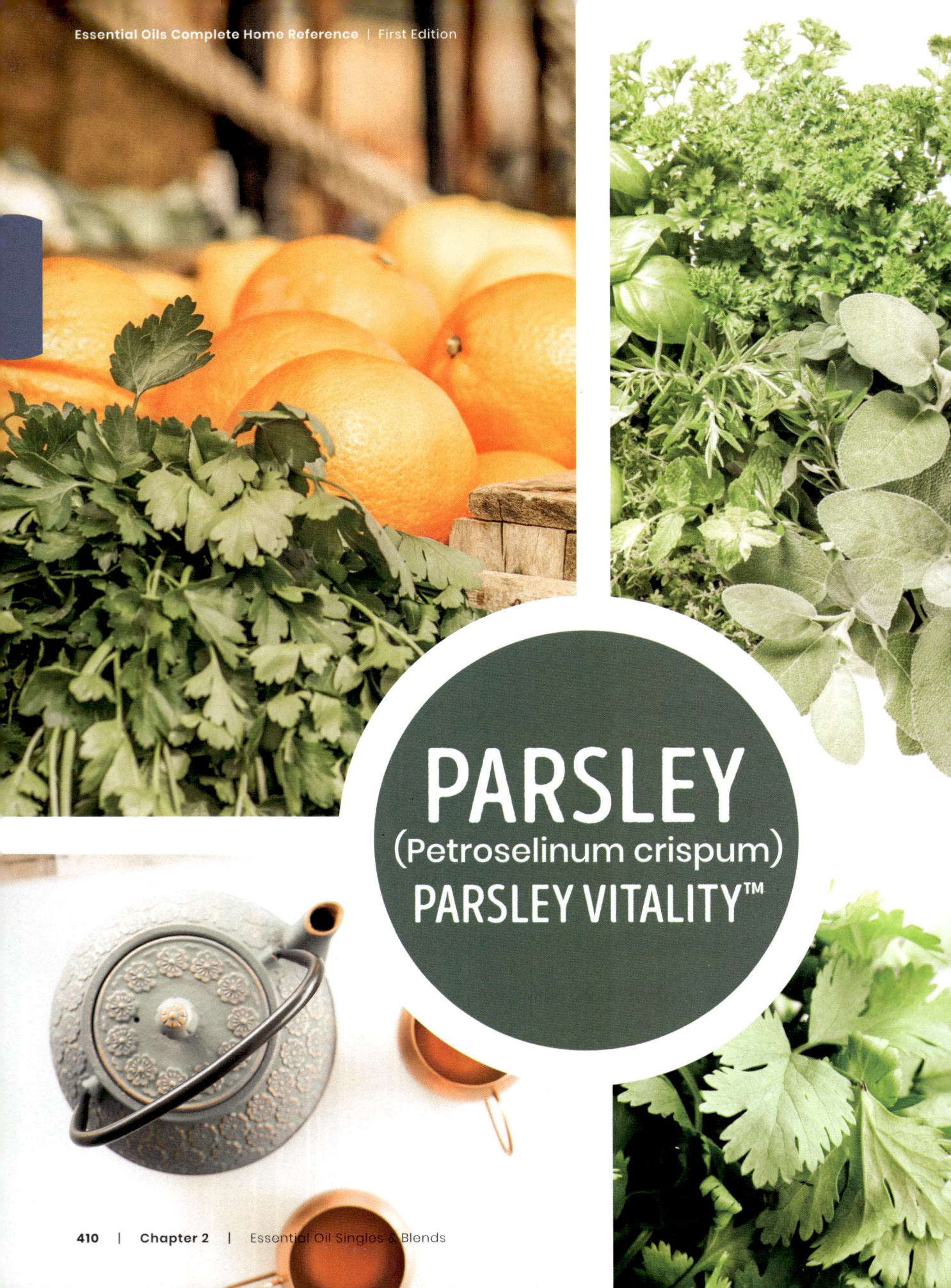

BOTANICAL FAMILY:
Lamiaceae

PLANT ORIGIN:
Vietnam

EXTRACTION METHOD:
Steam distilled from herb/leaf

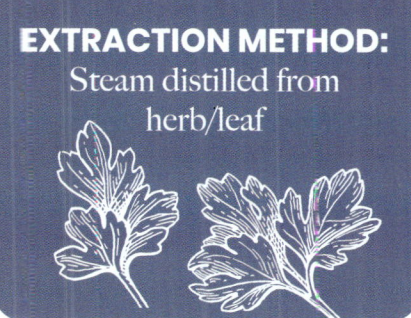

KEY CONSTITUENTS:
Myristicine (12-3?%), 1,3,8-Para-Menthatriene (10-29%), Alpha-Pinene (14-23%), Beta-Pinene (8-16%), Allyltetramethoxybenzene (up to 4%), Apiol (up to 5%), Elemicine (up to 2%)

HISTORICAL DATA:
Parsley has a strong, fresh, herbaceous aroma that can soothe and cleanse minor cuts, scrapes, and blemishes and reduce the appearance of pores and blemishes. Add Parsley Vitality to your favorite dishes for a concentrated blast of flavor.

MEDICAL PROPERTIES:
Anticancerous, antibacterial, antiarthritic, antiseptic, antioxidant, astringent, circulatory, antirheumatic, immunomodulatory

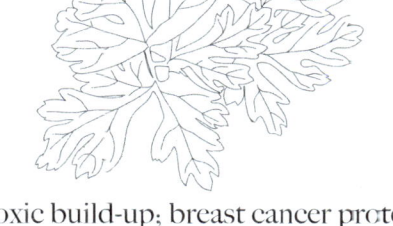

USES:
Combat staph and salmonella infections, wounds, minor skin infections, autoimmune diseases, allergies; cleanses internal organs; arthritis; bruises; indigestion; toxic build-up; breast cancer protection; inflammation; lines and wrinkles; strengthen bones; bad breath; heart trouble; bladder infections; eye problems; detoxification; diuretic; laxative; removes flatulence, nausea, vomiting

FRAGRANT INFLUENCE:
Clean, complex aroma; respiratory health

DIRECTIONS:
Aromatic: 10. Blend with other essential oils like Orange, Tea Tree, Clary Sage, and Ylang Ylang at low dilution. Topical: 50-50. Dietary (Vitality): Dilute 1 drop with 1 drop of carrier oil. Put in a capsule and take up to 3 times daily. Use in recipes that include parsley. Add 1-2 drops to water, tea, or smoothies.

CAUTIONS:
Avoid using it in the bath as it may cause skin irritation.

SELECTED RESEARCH:

Akinci A, Eşrefoğlu M, Taşlidere E, Aleş B. Petroselinum crispum is Effective in Reducing Stress-Induced Gastric Oxidative Damage. Balkan Med J. 2017 Jan; 34(1): 53-59.

Abdellatief SA, Galal AA, Farouk SM, Abdel-Daim MM. Ameliorative effect of parsley oil on cisplatin-induced hepato-cardiotoxicity: a biochemical, histopathological, and immunohistochemical study. Biomed Pharmacother. 2017 Feb;86:482-491. Epub 2016 Dec 23.

Tang EL-H, Rajarajeswaran J, Fung SY, Kanthimathi MS. Petroselinum crispum has antioxidant properties, protects against DNA damage and inhibits proliferation and migration of cancer cells. J Sci Food Agric. 2015 oct; 95(13): 2763-2771.

Linde GA, Gazim ZC, Cardoso BK, Jorge LF, Tešević V, Glamočlija J, Colauto NB. Antifungal and antibacterial activities of Petroselinum crispum essential oil. Genet Mol Res. 2016;15(3):15038538.

Mulugeta T, Unnithan CR, Tesfay D. Phytochemical screening, characterization and biological activities of petroselinum crispum (parsley) leaf oil. World Journal of Pharmacy and Pharmaceutical Sciences. 2015. 4(9) 142-151.

Yousofi A, Daneshmandi S, Soleimni N, Bagheri K, Karimi MH. Immunomodulatory effect of Parsley (Petroselinum crispum) essential oil on immune cells: mitogen-activated splenocytes and peritoneal macrophages. Immunopharmacology and Immunotoxicology. 2012;34(2):303-8.

Zhang H, Chen F, Wang X, Yao HY. Evaluation of antioxidant activity of parsley (Petroselinum crispum essential oil and identification of its antioxidant constitutents. Food research international. 2006. 39(8):833-839.

BOTANICAL FAMILY:
Lamiaceae

PLANT ORIGIN:
Indonesia

EXTRACTION METHOD:
Steam distilled from flowers

KEY CONSTITUENTS:
Patchoulol (28-37%),
Bulnesene (15-19%),
Alpha-Guaiene (11-17%),
Beta-Caryophyllene (2-6%),
Pogostol (up to 4%),
Beta-Patchoulene (1-3%),
Copaene (up to 2%)

PATCHOULI
(Pogostemon cablin)

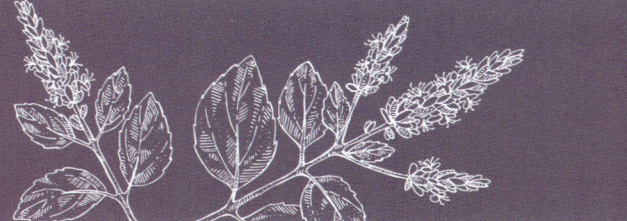

While Patchouli oil is known as an all-purpose insect repellent, it is also highly prized in the perfumery industry. Patchouli has many benefits for chapped and wrinkled skin.

MEDICAL PROPERTIES:
Analgesic, anti-allergy, relaxant, antitumoral, digestive aid that combats nausea, anti-inflammatory, antimicrobial, antifungal, insecticidal

USES:
Protects neural cell health, decreases sympathetic nervous system activity, hypertension, inflammatory bowel disease, skin conditions (eczema, acne, wrinkles, chapped), fluid retention, Listeria infection, insect repellent, colds, headaches, stomach upset, depression, dandruff, controlling appetite, itching

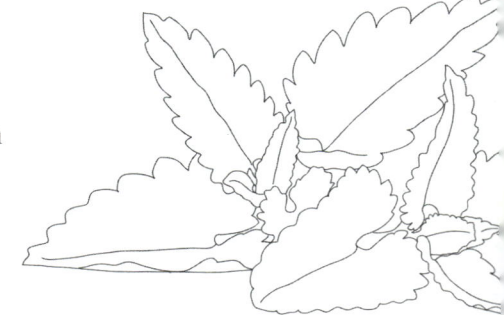

FRAGRANT INFLUENCE:
A relaxant that clarifies thoughts, allowing the discarding of jealousies, obsessions, and insecurities; calming aroma promotes feelings of relaxation and peace

DIRECTIONS:
Aromatic: 6c. Topical: Neat. Dietary: Take as a dietary supplement.

CAUTIONS:

SELECTED RESEARCH:

Hong SJ, Cho J, Boo CG, Youn MY, Pan JH, Kim JK, Shin E-C. Inhalation of Patchouli (Posgostemon Cablin Benth.) Essential Oil Improved Metabolic Parameters in Obesity-Induced Sprague Dawley Rats. Nutrients. 2020 Jul; 12 (7): 2077.

Kim EK, Kim JH, Jeon S, Choi YW, Choi HJ, Kim CY, Kim, Young-Mi. Pachypodol, a Methoxyflavonoid Isolated from Posgostemon Cablin Bentham Exerts Antioxidant and Cytoprotective Effects in HepG2 Cells: Possible Role of ERK-Dependent Nrf2 Activation. Int J Mol Sci. 2019 Sep; 20(17): 4082.

Orchard A, van Vuuren SF, Viljoen AM, Kamatou G. The in vitro antimicrobial evaluation of commercial essential oils and their combinations against acne. Int J Cosmet Sci. 2018 Mar 24. [Epub ahead of print]

Yoon SC, Je IG, Cui X, Park HR, Khang D, Park JS, Kim SH, Shin TY. Anti-allergic and anti-inflammatory effects of aqueous extract of Pogostemon cablin. Int J Mol Med. 2016 Jan;37(1):217-24. Epub 2015 Nov 3.

Swamy MK, Sinniah UR. A comprehensive review on the phytochemical constituents and pharmacological activities of Pogostemon cablin Benth.: an aromatic medicinal plant of industrial importance. Molecules. 2015 May 12;20(5):8521-47.

Lin RF, Feng XX, Li CW, Zhang XJ, Yu XT, Zhou JY, Zhang X, Xie YL, Su ZR, Zhan JY. Prevention of UV radiation-induced cutaneous photoaging in mice by topical administration of patchouli oil. J Ethnopharmacol. 2014 Jun 11;154(2):408-18.

Jeong JB, Choi J, Lou Z, Jiang X, Lee SH. Patchouli alcohol, an essential oil of Pogostemon cablin, exhibits anti-tumorigenic activity in human colorectal cancer cells. Int Immunopharmacol. 2013 Jun;16(2):184-90. Epub 2013 Apr 17.

Kocevski D, Du M, Kan J, Jing C, Lačanin I, Pavlović H. Antifungal effect of Allium tuberosum, Cinnamomum cassia, and Pogostemon cablin essential oils and their components against population of Aspergillus species. J Food Sci. 2013 May;78(5):M731-7.

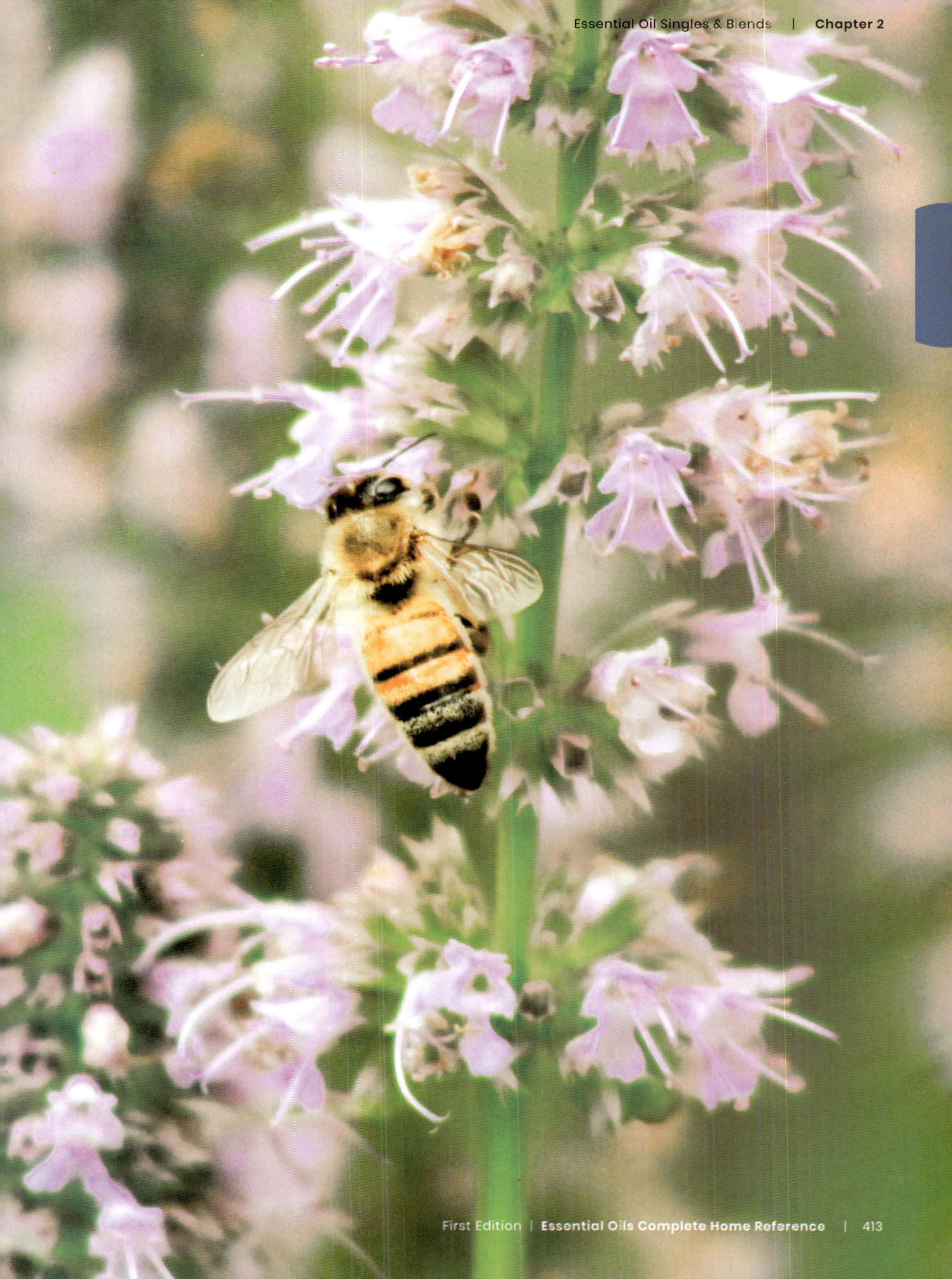

PEACE & CALMING® & PEACE & CALMING® ROLL-ON
(Essential Oil Blend)

This blend promotes relaxation and a deep sense of peace and emotional well-being, helping to dampen tensions and uplift spirits. When massaged on the bottoms of feet, it can be a wonderful prelude to a peaceful night's rest. It may calm overactive and hard-to-manage children. It also reduces depression, anxiety, stress, and insomnia. Many people use it for relief from Restless Leg Syndrome.

MEDICAL PROPERTIES & USES:
Antiallergy, anti-inflammatory, antimicrobial, calming, nervous system supportive, pain or swelling reducing, sleep inducing

INGREDIENTS:
Caprylic/capric triglyceride‡ (Roll-On only), Tangerine, Orange, Ylang Ylang, Patchouli, Blue Tansy

DIRECTIONS:
Aromatic: 6o. Topical: 50-50. Combine with Lavender for insomnia and Matricaria (German Chamomile) for calming.

CAUTIONS:

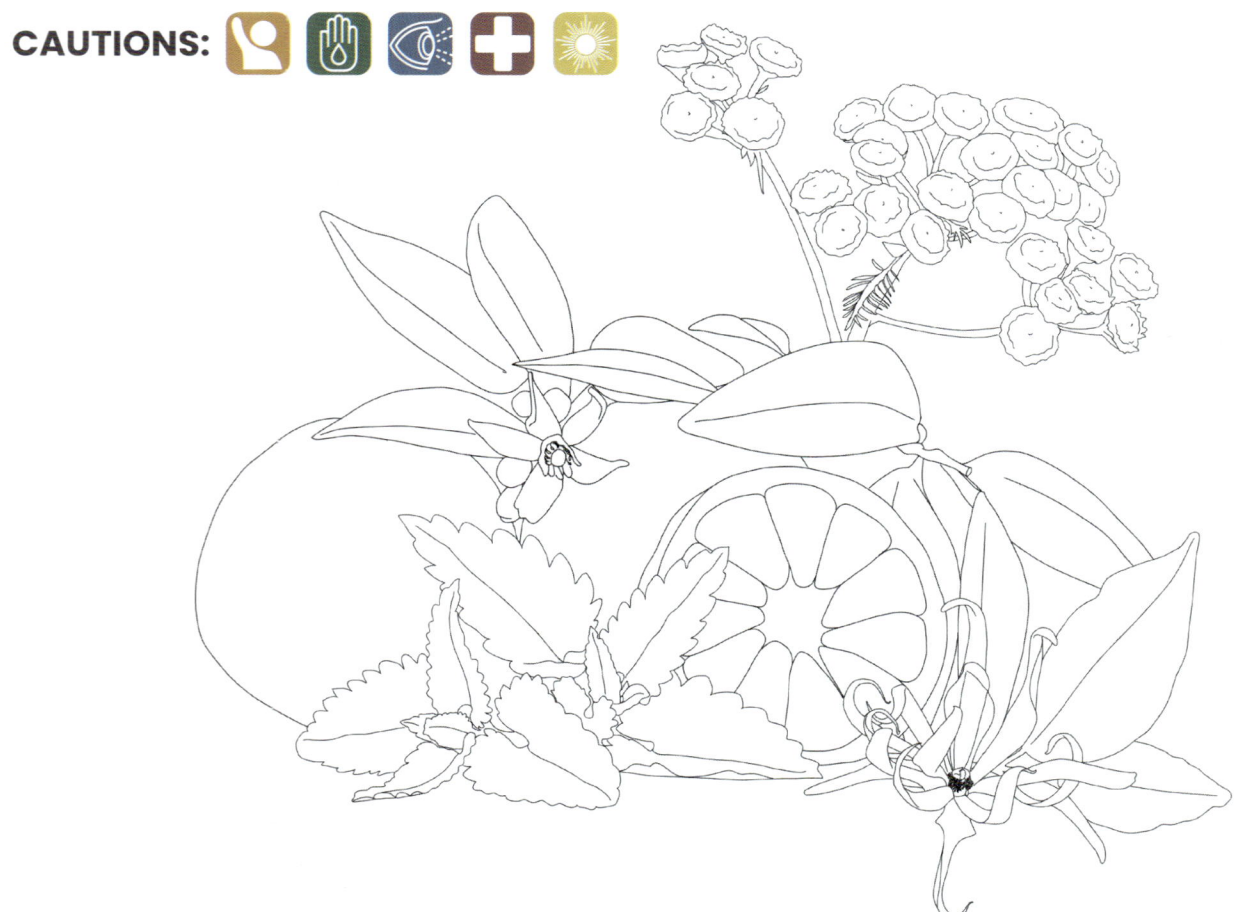

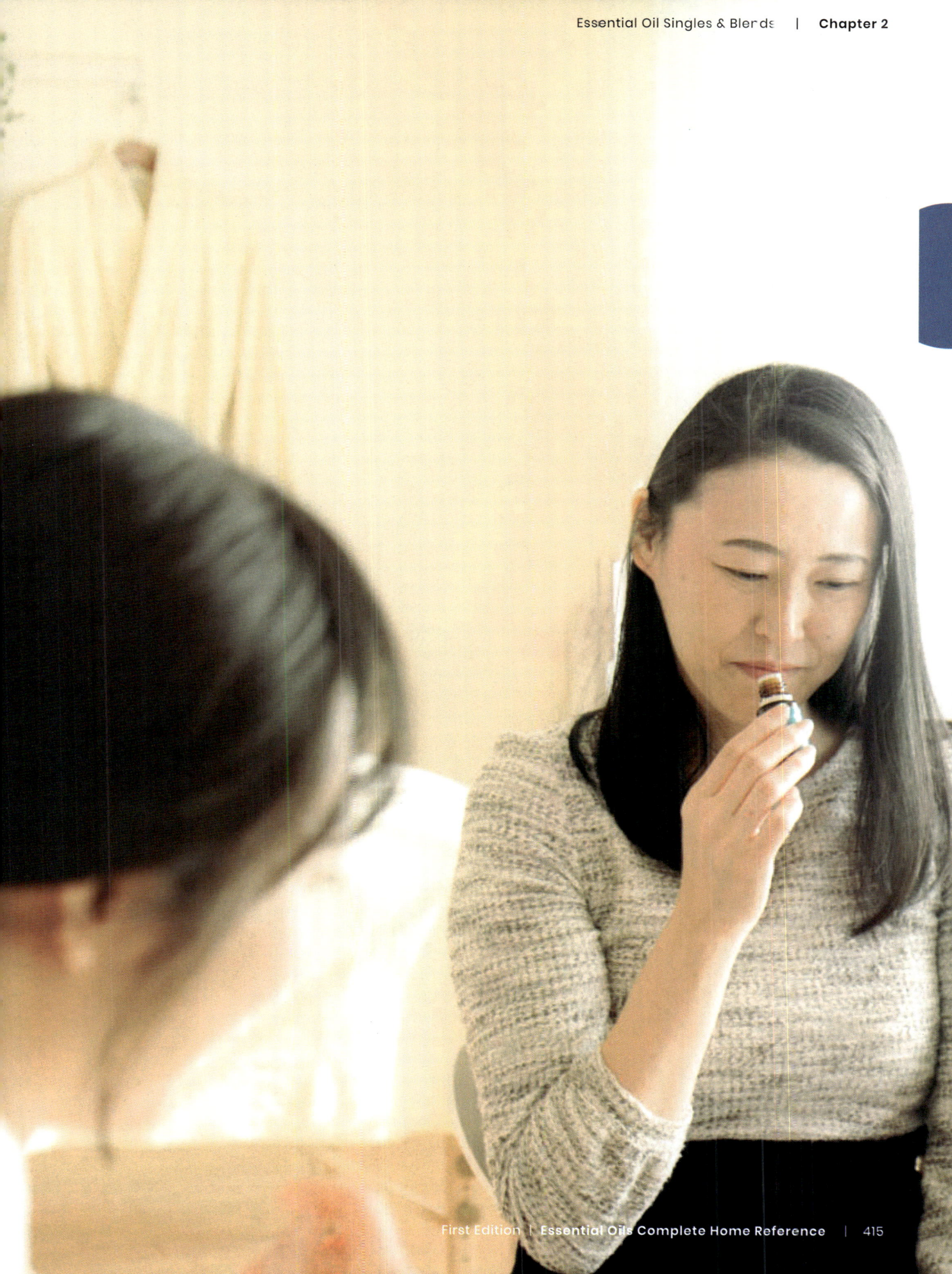

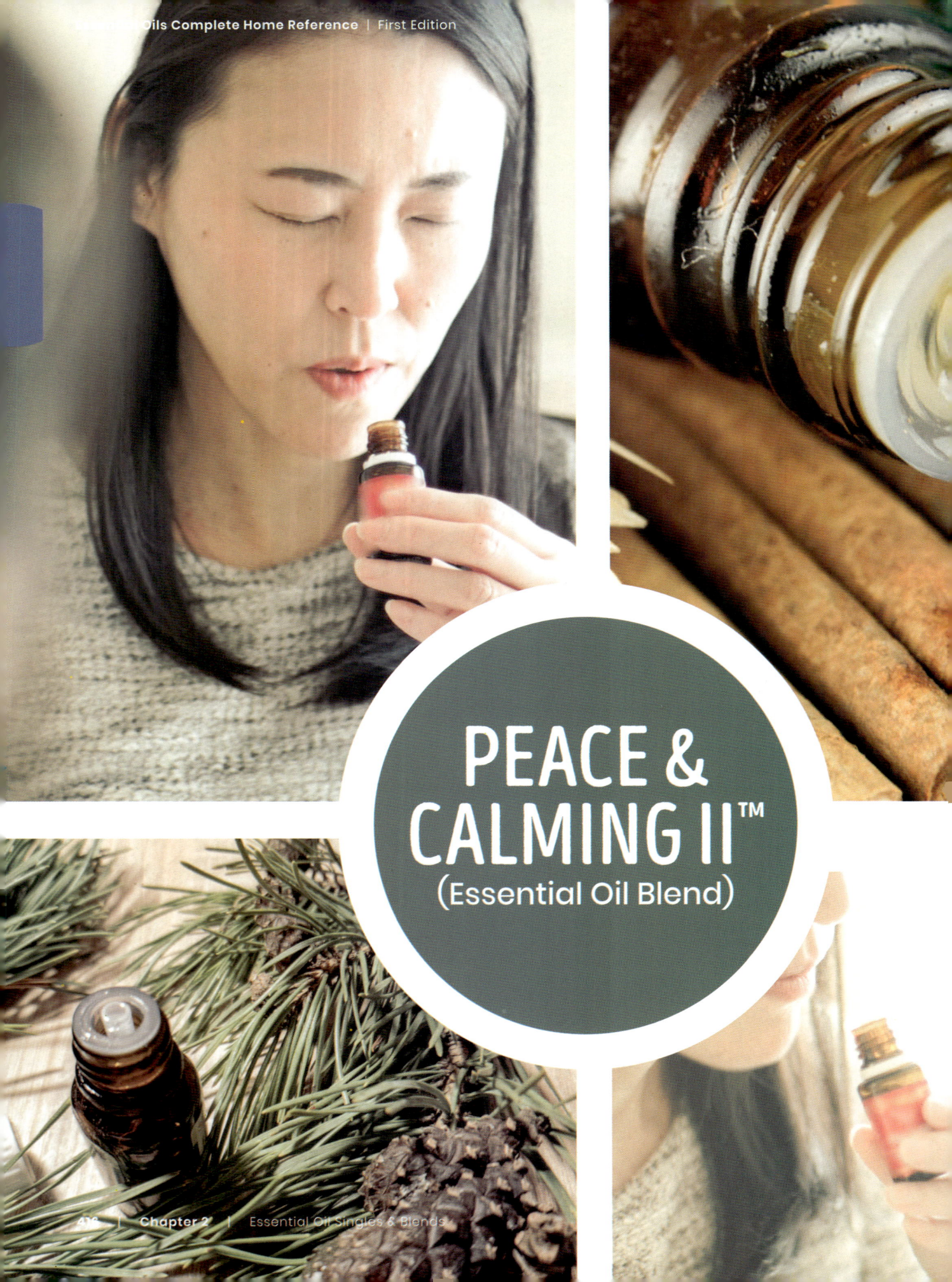

PEACE & CALMING II™
(Essential Oil Blend)

ABOUT PEACE & CALMING II™

Peace & Calming II has a relaxing and pleasant aroma that may contribute to calming the mind and giving a sense of overall well-being.

MEDICAL PROPERTIES & USES:

Antiallergy, anti-inflammatory, antimicrobial, antioxidative, calming, nervous system supportive, pain or swelling reducing, performance enhancing/stimulating, sleep inducing

INGREDIENTS:

Tangerine, Orange, Ylang Ylang, Patchouli, Northern Lights Black Spruce, Matricaria (German Chamomile), Vetiver, Cistus, Bergamot, Cassia, Davana

DIRECTIONS:

Aromatic: 60. Topical: 50-50.

CAUTIONS:

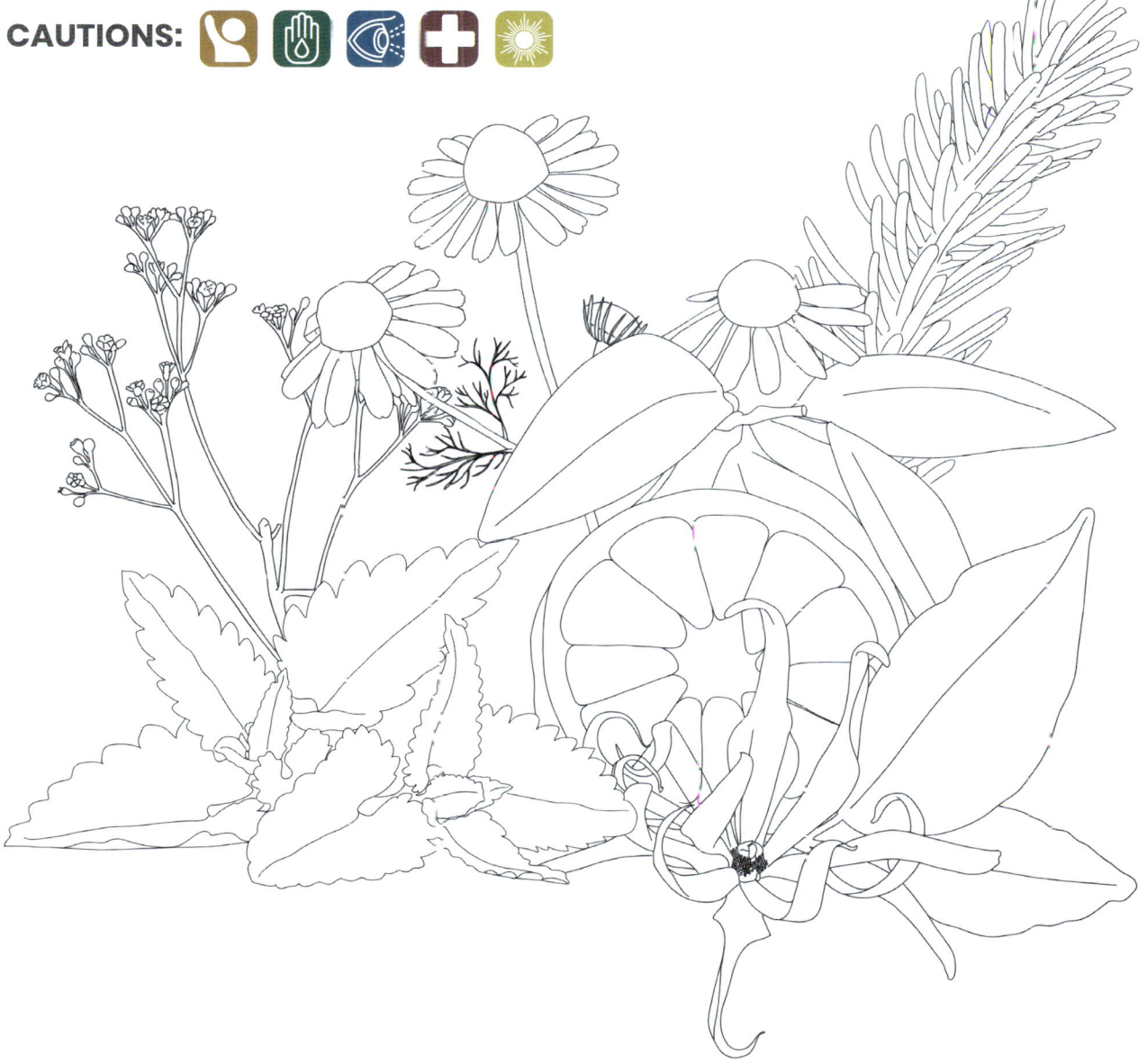

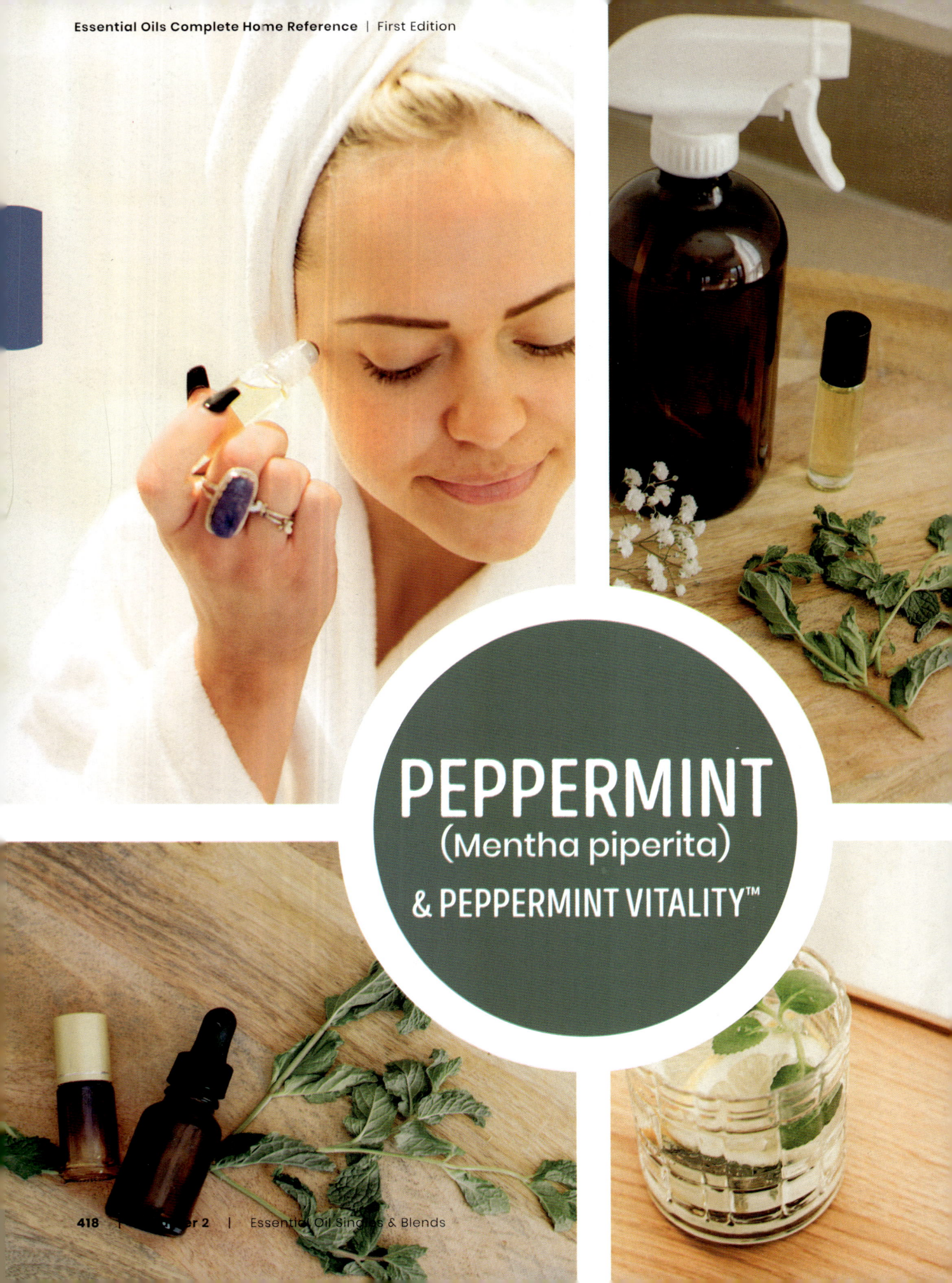

BOTANICAL FAMILY:
Lamiaceae

PLANT ORIGIN:
USA, India

EXTRACTION METHOD:
Steam distilled from aerial parts

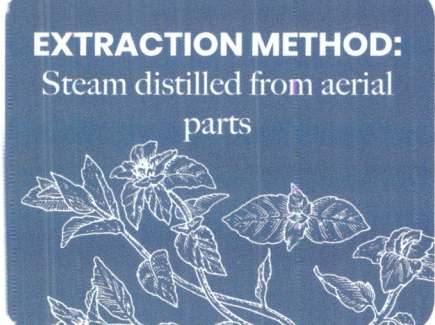

KEY CONSTITUENTS:
Menthol (32-49%), Menthone (13-28%), Eucalyptol (3-8%), Isoementhone (2-8%), Menthofuran (1-8%), Menthyl Acetate (2-8%), Neomenthol (2-6%), Beta-Caryophyllene (1-4%), Limonene (1-3%), Pulegone (up to 3%), Germacrene D (1-3%), Trans-Sabinene Hydrate (up to 3%)

HISTORICAL DATA:
Peppermint is one of the oldest and most highly regarded herbs for soothing digestion. Jean Valnet, MD, studied peppermint's effect on the liver and respiratory systems. Alan Hirsch, MD, studied peppermint's ability to directly affect the brain's satiety center (the ventromedial nucleus of the hypothalamus), which triggers a sensation of fullness after meals. A highly regarded digestive stimulant.

MEDICAL PROPERTIES:
Anti-inflammatory, antitumoral, antiparasitic (worms), antibacterial, antiviral, antifungal, gallbladder/digestive stimulant, pain relieving, appetite suppressant

USES:
Digestive system support, performance and focus enhancement, oral hygiene, rheumatism/arthritis, respiratory infections (pneumonia, tuberculosis, etc.), obesity, viral infections (herpes simplex, herpes zoster, cold sores, human papilloma virus, etc.), fungal infections/candida, digestive problems, headaches, nausea, skin conditions (itchy skin, varicose veins, eczema, psoriasis, dermatitis), scoliosis/lumbago/back problems, irritable bowel syndrome, diarrhea, migraine

FRAGRANT INFLUENCE:
Purifying and stimulating to the conscious mind. Research indicates that peppermint aroma, inhaled during mental tasks, may help attention, performance, and focus (Barker, et al., 2003). Peppermint may also be an effective appetite suppressant when inhaled (Hirsch and Gomez, 1995). University of Kiel researchers found that peppermint lessened headache pain in a double-blind, placebo-controlled, cross-over study.

DIRECTIONS:
Aromatic: 10. Inhale 5-10 times a day to curb appetite. Topical: 20-80. Rub on forehead and back of neck to relieve headaches and tiredness. Use in Raindrop Technique. Dietary (Vitality): Put 2 drops in a capsule and take 3 times daily. To improve concentration, alertness, and memory, place 1-2 drops on the tongue. Rub on back of tongue to relieve irritated throat.

CAUTIONS:
Avoid contact with eyes, mucous membranes, sensitive skin, or fresh wounds or burns. Do not apply on infants younger than 18 months of age.

SELECTED RESEARCH:

Fialová SB, Kurin E, Trajčíková E, Jánošová L, Šušaniková Ivana, Tekeľová E, Jánošová I, Tekelová D, Nagy M, Mučaji P. Molecules. 2020 Jan; 25(1): 200.

Fearrington MA, Qualls BW, Carey MG. Essential oils to reduce postoperative nausea and vomiting. J Perianesth Nurs. 2019 May 27. Epub ahead of print.

Raghavan R, Devi MPS, Varghese M, Joseph A, Madhavan SS, Sreedevi PV. Effectiveness of Mentha piperita leaf extracts against oral pathogens: an in vitro study. J Contemp Dent Pract. 2018 Sep 1;19(9):1042-6.

Haber SL, El-Ibiary SY. Peppermint oil for treatment of irritable bowel syndrome. Am J Health Syst. Pharm. 2016 Jan 15;73(2):22-31.

Husain FM, Ahmad I, Khan MS, Ahmad E, Tahseen Q, Khan MS, Alshabib NA. Sub-MICs of Mentha piperita essential oil and menthol inhibits AHL mediated quorum sensing and biofilm of gram-negative bacteria. Front Microbiol. 2015 May 13;6:420. eCollection 2015.

Meamarbashi A. Instant effects of peppermint essential oil on the physiological parameters and exercise performance. Avicenna J Phytomed. 2014 Jan;4(1):72-8.

Ferreira P, Cardoso T, Ferreira F, Fernandes-Ferreira M, Piper P, Sousa MJ. Mentha piperita essential oil induces apoptosis in yeast associated with both cytosolic and mitochondrial ROS-mediated damage. FEMS Yeast Res. 2014 Nov;14(7):1006-14. Epub 2014 Aug 26.

Rozza AL, Hiruma-Lima CA, Takahira RK, Padovani CR, Pellizzon CH. Effect of menthol in experimentally induced ulcers: pathways of gastroprotection. Chem Biol Interact. 2013 Nov 25;206(2):272-278. Epub 2013 Oct 9.

Tayarani-Najaran Z, Talasaz-Firoozi E, Nasiri R, Jalali N, Hassanzadeh M. Antiemetic activity of volatile oil from Mentha spicata and Mentha x piperita in chemotherapy-induced nausea and vomiting. Ecancermedicalscience. 2013;7:290. Epub 2013 Jan 31.

Lane BS, Cannella K, Bowen C, Copelan D, Nteff G, Barnes K, Poudevigne M, Lawson J. Examination of the effectiveness of peppermint aromatherapy on nausea in women post C-section. J Holist Nurs. 2012 Jun;30(2):90-104. quiz 105-6. Epub 2011 Oct 27.

Barker S, Grayhem P, Koon J, Perkins J, Whalen A, Raudenbush B. Improved performance on clerical tasks associated with administration of peppermint odor. Percept Mot Skills. 2003 Dec;97(3 pt 1):1007-10.

Hirsch AR, Gomez R. Weight reduction through inhalation of odorants. J Neurol Orthop Med Surg. 1995;16:28-31.

BOTANICAL FAMILY: Rutaceae

PLANT ORIGIN: Paraguay

EXTRACTION METHOD: Steam distilled from leaves and twigs

KEY CONSTITUENTS: Linalyl Acetate (32-66%), Linalool (21-28%), Alpha-Terpineol (4-7%), Geranyl Acetate (3-5%)

PETITGRAIN
(Citrus aurantium amara) (Syn. Citrus sinensis)

Petitgrain derives its name from the extraction of the oil, which at one time was from the green, unripe oranges when they were still about the size of a cherry.

MEDICAL PROPERTIES:
Antispasmodic, anti-inflammatory, antiseptic, antidepressant, deodorant, relaxant, reestablishes nerve equilibrium, sedative

USES:
Insomnia, prevents sepsis, anxiety, muscle spasms, skin and hair conditions, antitumoral, soothes nerves

FRAGRANT INFLUENCE:
Uplifting and refreshing to the senses; clears confusion, reduces mental fatigue and depression; stimulates the mind and improves memory, insomnia

DIRECTIONS:
Aromatic: 3o. Topical: Neat. Dietary: Take as a dietary supplement.

CAUTIONS:

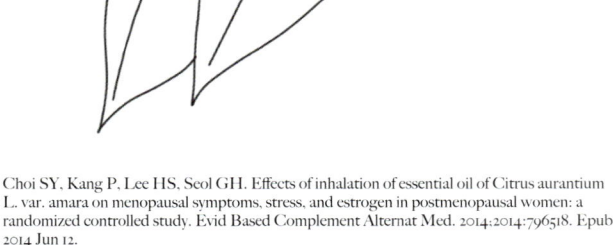

SELECTED RESEARCH:

Yu L, Chen M, Liu J, Huang X, He W, Qing Z, Zeng J. Systematic Detection and Identification of Bioactive Ingredients from Citrus aurantium L. var amara Using HLC-Q-TOF-MS Combined with a Screening Method. Molecules. 2020 Jan; 25(2): 357.

Shen CY, Jiang JG, Zhu W, Ou-Yang Q. Anti-inflammatory effect of essential oil from Citrus aurantium L. var. amara Engl. J Agric Food Chem. 2017 Oct 4;65(39):8586-8594. Epub 2017 Sep 25.

Zou Z, Xi W, Hu Y, Nie C, Zhou Z. Antioxidant activity of Citrus fruits. Food Chem. 2016 Apr 1;196:885-96. Epub 2015 Sep 21.

Metoui N, Gargouri S, Amri I, Fezzani T, Jamoussi B, Hamrouni L. Activity antifungal of the essential oils; aqueous and ethanol extracts from Citrus aurantium L. Nat Prod Res. 2015;29(23):2238-41. Epub 2015 Jul 24.

Choi SY, Kang P, Lee HS, Seol GH. Effects of inhalation of essential oil of Citrus aurantium L. var. amara on menopausal symptoms, stress, and estrogen in postmenopausal women: a randomized controlled study. Evid Based Complement Alternat Med. 2014:2014:796518. Epub 2014 Jun 12.

Soudani N, Rafrafi M, Ben Amara I, Hakim A, Troudi A, Zeghal KM, Ben Salah H, Boudawara T, Zeghal N. Oxidative stress-related lung dysfunction by chromium (VI): alleviation by Citrus aurantium L. J Physiol Biochem. 2013 Jun;69(2):239-53. doi: 10.1007/s13105-012-0207-6. Epub 2012 Sep 13.

Hawrelak JA, Cattley T, Myers SP. Essential oils in the treatment of intestinal dysbiosis: a preliminary in vitro study. Altern Med Rev. 2009 Dec;14(4):380-4.

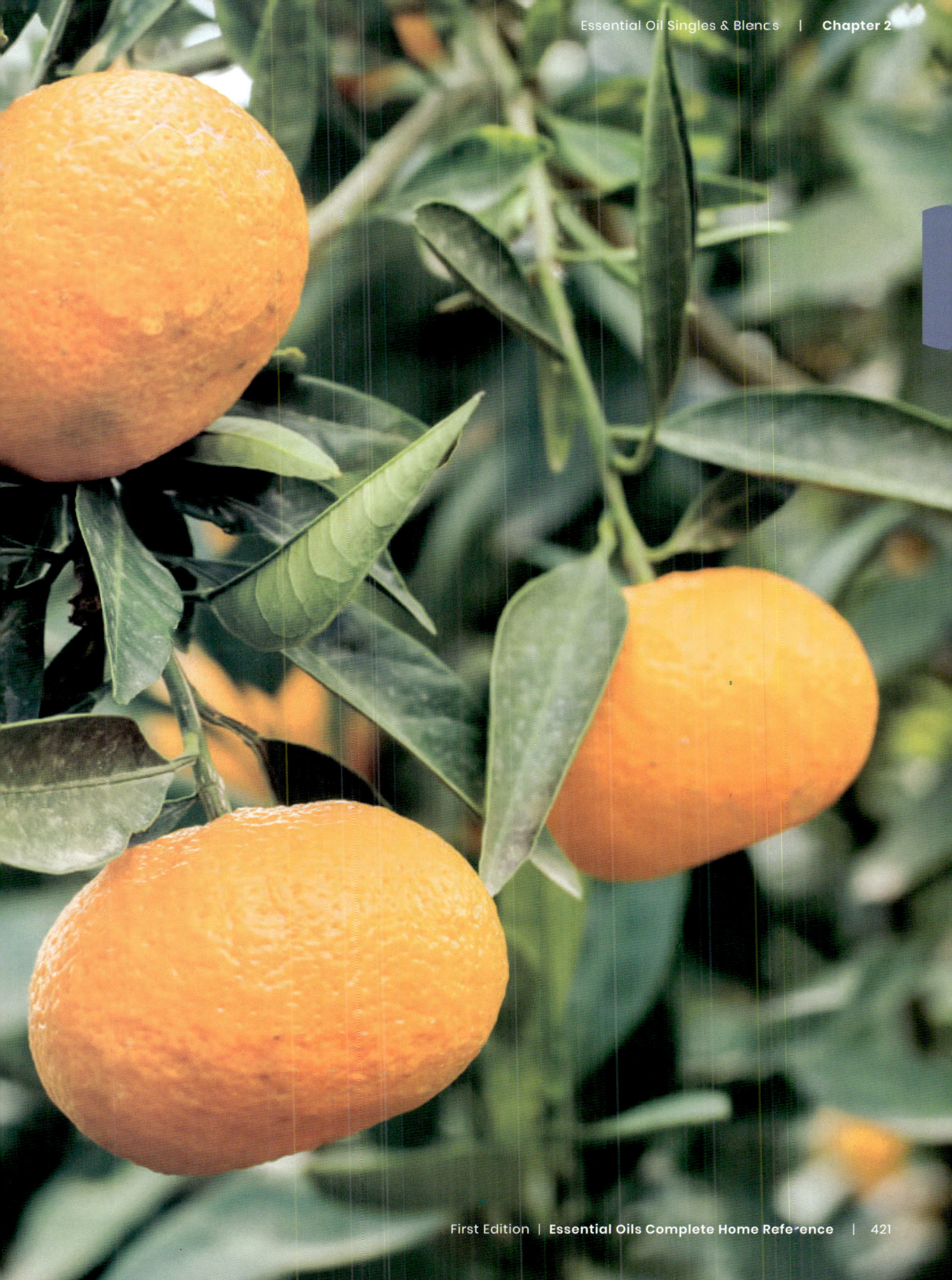

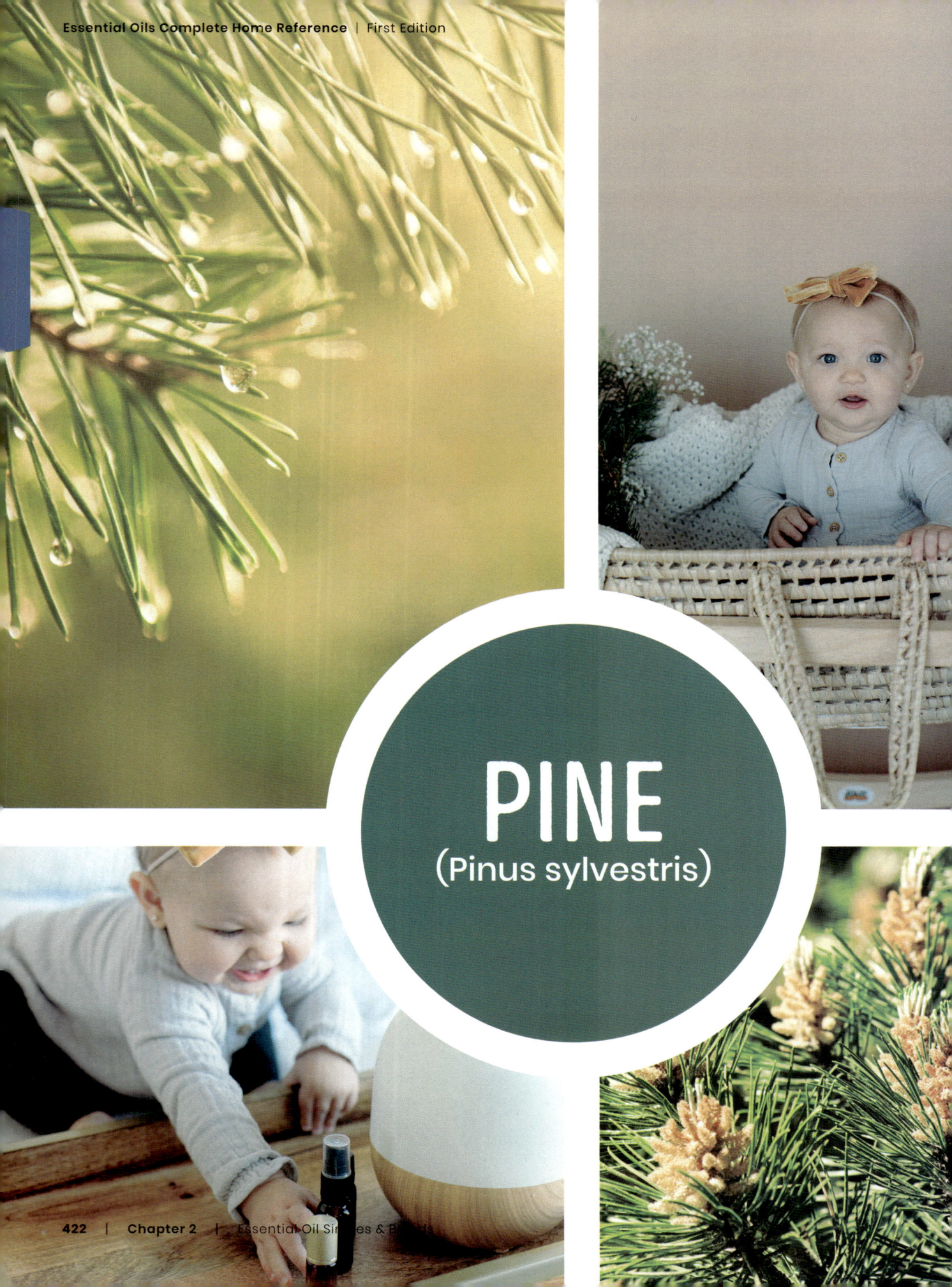

Essential Oil Singles & Blends | Chapter 2

BOTANICAL FAMILY:
Pinaceae

PLANT ORIGIN:
Austria, USA, Canada

EXTRACTION METHOD:
Steam distilled from herb/leaf

KEY CONSTITUENTS:
Alpha-Pinene (53-65%),
Beta-Pinene (4-12%),
Delta-3-Carene (6-11%),
Limonene (7-10%),
Myrcene (3-6%),
Beta-Caryophyllene (1-3%),
Para-Cymene (up to 3%),
Camphene (1-2%)

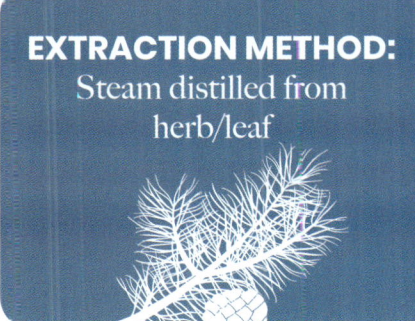

HISTORICAL DATA:

Pine was first investigated by Hippocrates, the father of Western medicine, for its benefits to the respiratory system. In 1990 Dr. Pénoël and Dr. Franchomme described pine oil's antiseptic properties in their medical textbook. Pine is also used in massage for stressed muscles and joints. It shares many of the same properties as Eucalyptus globulus, and the action of both oils is enhanced when blended. Native Americans stuffed mattresses with pine needles to repel lice and fleas. It was used to treat lung infections and even added to baths to revitalize those suffering from mental or emotional fatigue.

MEDICAL PROPERTIES:

Hormone-like, antidiabetic, cortisone-like, antiseptic, lymphatic stimulant, antibacterial, diuretic, analgesic, anti-inflammatory, antifungal

USES:

Throat/lung/sinus infections, rheumatism/arthritis, skin care, skin parasites, fleas, wrinkles, sagging skin, urinary tract infection, cancer, metabolism, food poisoning, inflammation, pain, eye health, injuries

FRAGRANT INFLUENCE:

Relieves anxiety and revitalizes mind, body, and spirit; has an empowering, yet grounding fragrance; relieves stress; respiratory health

DIRECTIONS:

Aromatic: 3o. Topical: 50-50.

CAUTIONS: 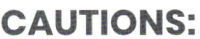   Beware of pine oils adulterated with turpentine, a low-cost, but potentially hazardous, filler.

SELECTED RESEARCH:

Scalas, D. Mandras N, Roana J, Tardugno R, Cuffini AM, Ghisetti V, Benvenuti S, Tullio V. Use of Pinus sylvestris L. (Pinaceae), Origanum vulgare L. (Lamiaceae), and Thymus vulgaris L. (Lamiaceae) essential oils and their main components to enhance itraconazole activity against azole susceptible/not-susceptible Cryptococcus neoformans strains. BMC Complementary and Alternative Medicine. 2018 May 3;18(143):13.

Hoai NT, Duc HV, Thao do T, Orav A, Raal A. Selectivity of Pinus sylvestris extract and essential oil to estrogen-insensitive breast cancer cells pinus sylvestris against cancer cells. Pharmacogn Mag. 2015 Oct;11(Suppl 2):S290-5.

Amalinei RL, Trifan A, Cioanca O, Miron SD, Mihai CT, Rotinberg P, Miron A. Polyphenol-rich extract from Pinus sylvestris L. bark—chemical and antitumor studies. Rev Med Chir Soc Med Nat Iasi. 2014 Apr-Jun;118(2):551-7.

Fayemiwo KA, Adeleke MA, Okoro OP, Awojide SH, Awoniyi IO. Larvicidal efficacies and chemical composition of essential oils of Pinus sylvestris and Syzygium aromaticum against mosquitoes. Asian Pac J Trop Biomed. 2014 Jan;4(1):30-4.

Süntar I, Tumen I, Ustün O, Keles H, Akkol EK. Appraisal on the wound healing and anti-inflammatory activities of the essential oils obtained from the cones and needles of pinus species by in vivo and in vitro experimental models. J Ethnopharmacol. 2012 Jan 31; 39(2):533-40. Epub 2011 Dec 7.

PRESENT TIME™
(Essential Oil Blend)

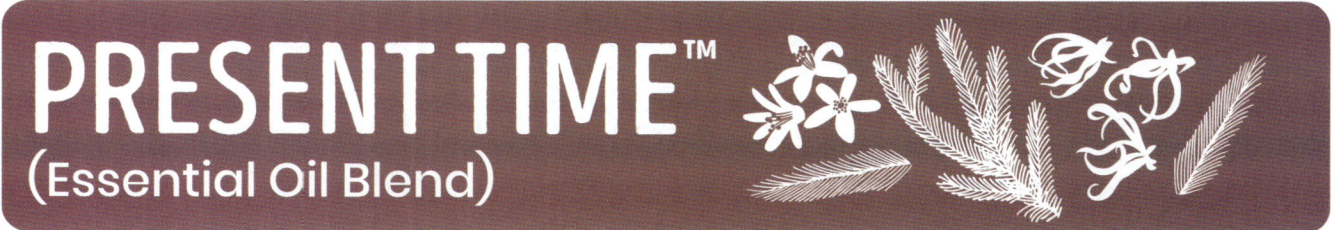

This blend is an empowering fragrance that creates a feeling of being in the moment. Disease develops when we live in the past and with regret. Being in the present time is the key to progressing and moving forward.

MEDICAL PROPERTIES & USES:
Antimicrobial, antidepressive, antiparasitic, antispasmodic, antidiabetic, lowers blood pressure, cardiovascular problems, anxiety, depression, hair loss, intestinal problems, calming

INGREDIENTS:
Sweet almond oil,‡ Bitter Orange (Neroli), Black Spruce, Ylang Ylang

DIRECTIONS:
Aromatic: 30. Topical: Neat.

CAUTIONS:

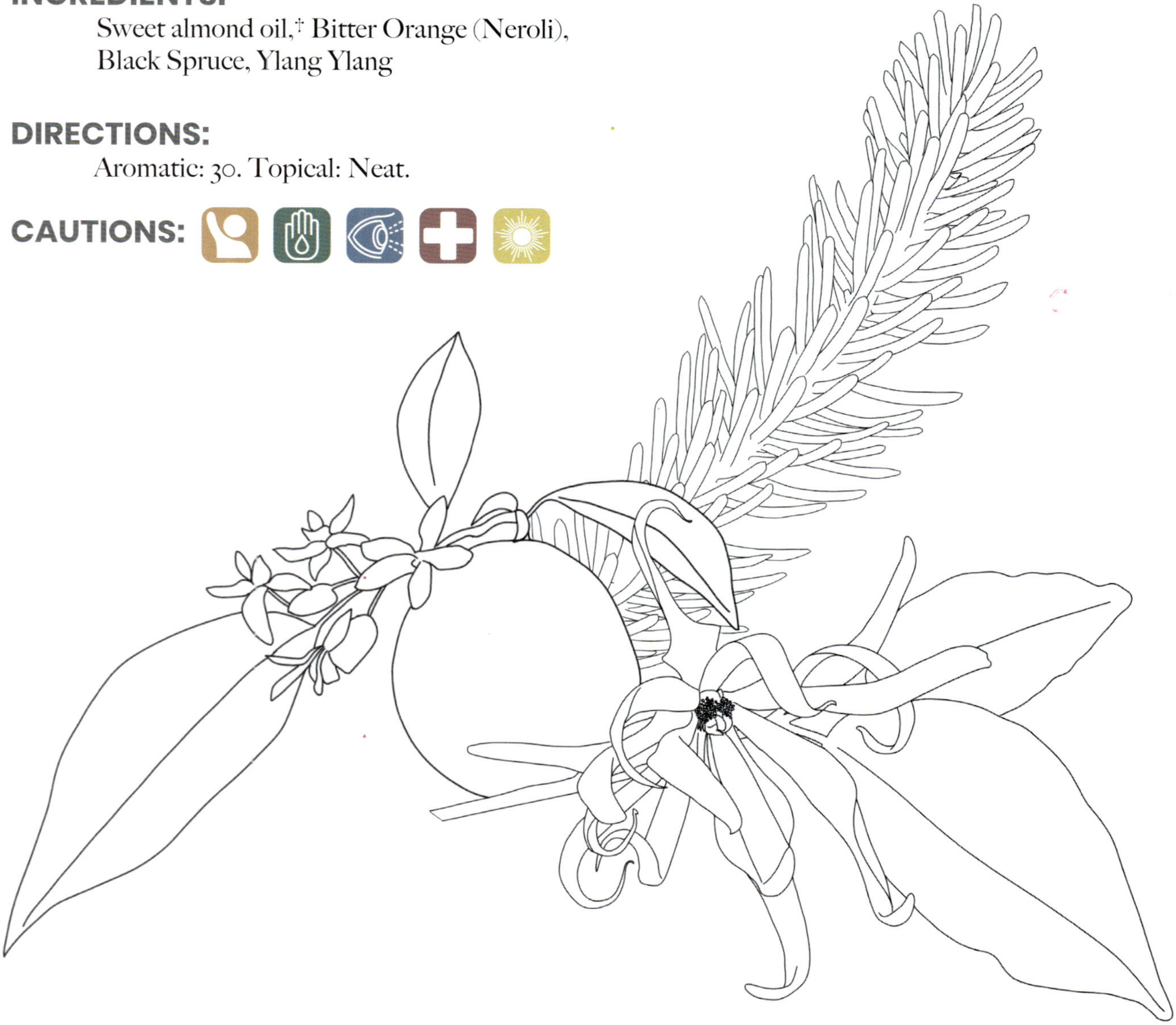

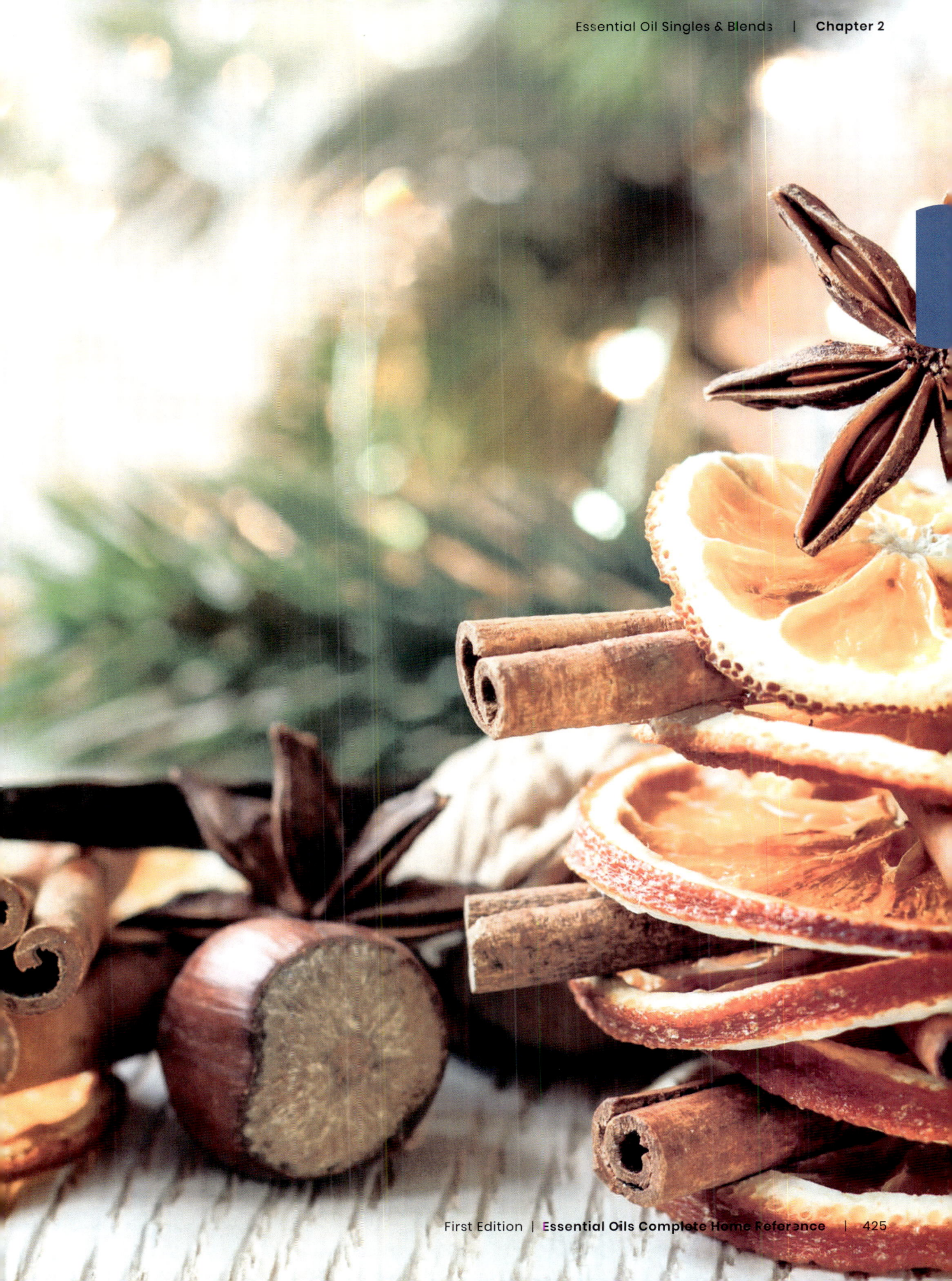

Essential Oils Complete Home Reference | First Edition

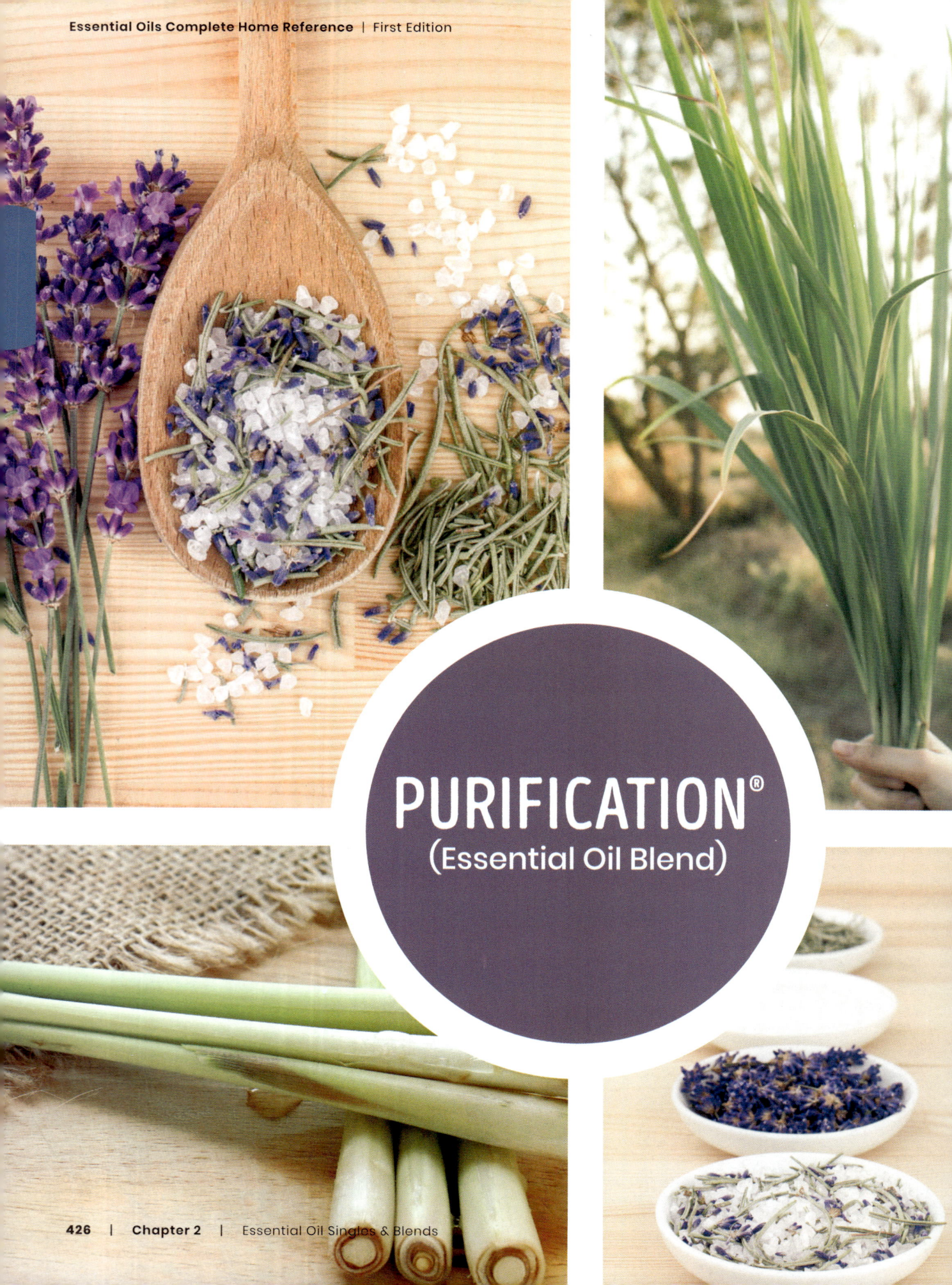

PURIFICATION®
(Essential Oil Blend)

426 | Chapter 2 | Essential Oil Singles & Blends

ABOUT PURIFICATION®:

This purifying blend cleanses and disinfects the air and neutralizes mildew, cigarette smoke, and disagreeable odors. It also disinfects and cleans cuts, scrapes, and bites from spiders, bees, hornets, and wasps.

MEDICAL PROPERTIES & USES:

Antimicrobial, antioxidative, cardiovascular supporting, disease inhibitory, insecticidal/antiparasitic, wellness supporting, antibacterial, air cleansing and disinfecting

INGREDIENTS:

Citronella, Rosemary, Lemongrass, Tea Tree, Lavandin, Myrtle

DIRECTIONS:

Aromatic: 3o. Topical: Neat.

CAUTIONS:

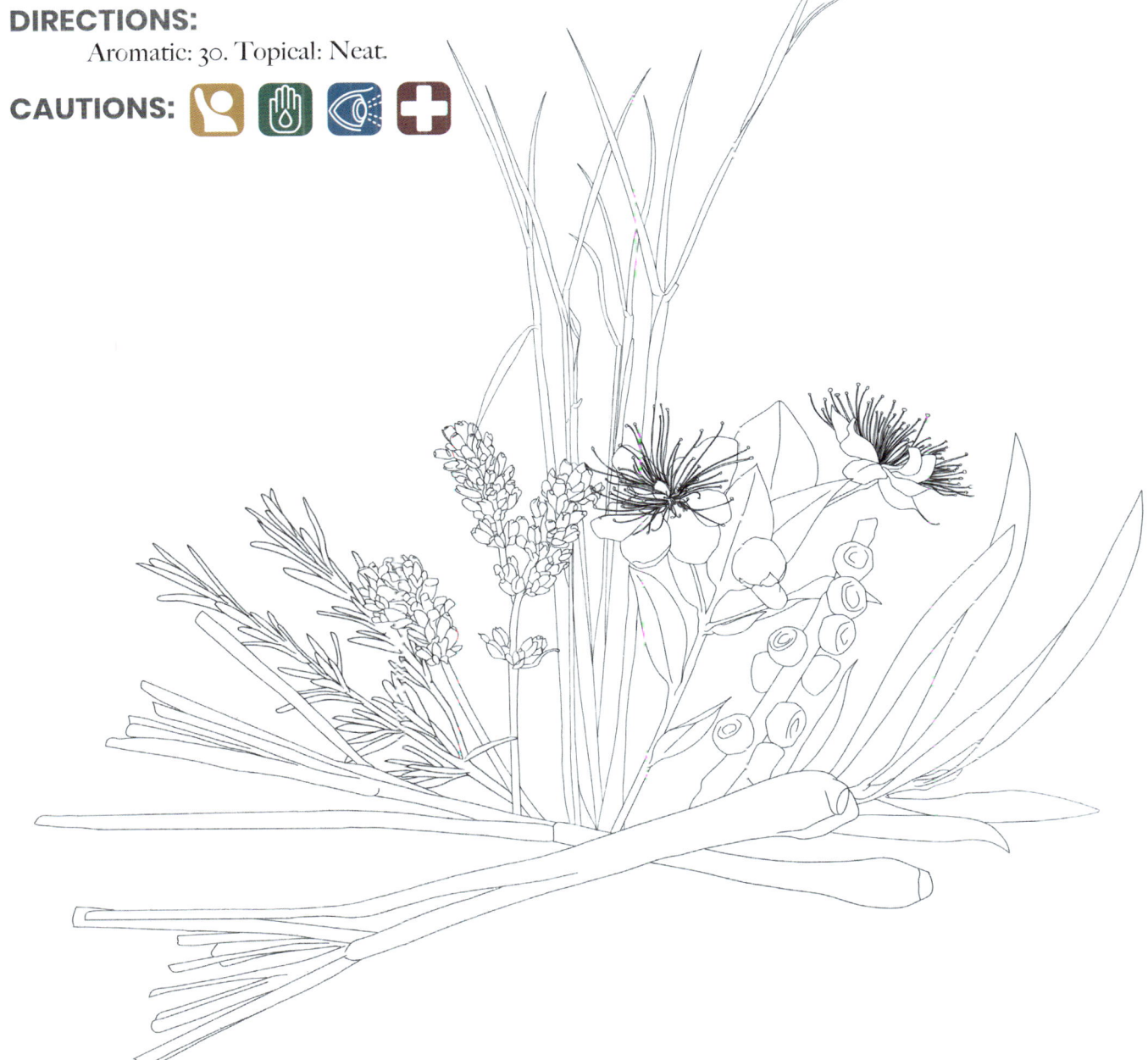

RAVEN™
(Essential Oil Blend)

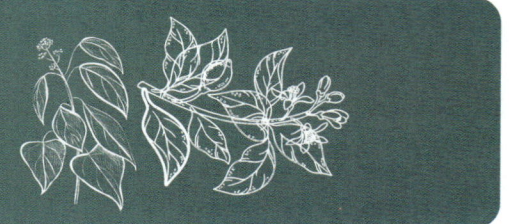

The oils of this blend fight against respiratory disease and infections such as tuberculosis, influenza, and pneumonia. It is highly antiviral and antiseptic.

MEDICAL PROPERTIES & USES:

Antiviral, antiseptic, antimicrobial, antioxidative, calming, cardiovascular supportive, digestion or elimination supportive/nausea reducing, disease inhibitory, insecticidal/antiparasitic, oral protective, organ protective, pain or swelling reducing, performance enhancing/stimulating, respiratory system supportive

INGREDIENTS:

Camphor (Ravintsara), Lemon, Wintergreen, Peppermint, Eucalyptus Radiata

DIRECTIONS:

Aromatic: 30. Topical: 50-50. Use as a hot compress over lungs or with Raindrop Technique. To use in suppository, dilute with V-6 1:10 and retain during the night.

CAUTIONS:

For external use only. Not intended for children under the age of 6 without the advice of a health care professional.

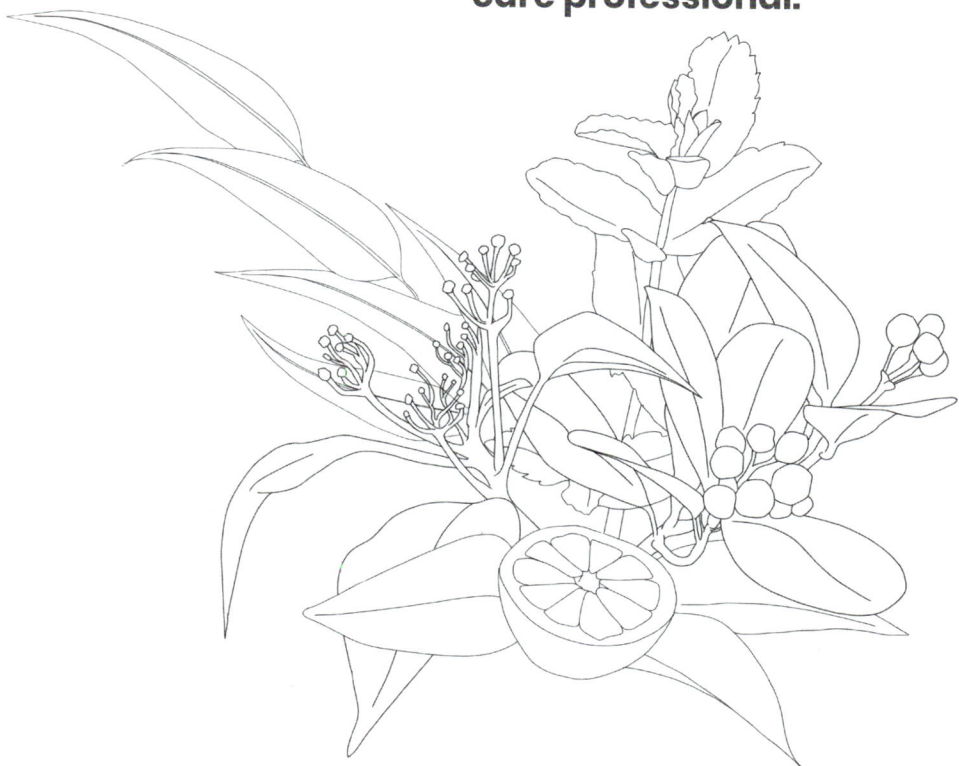

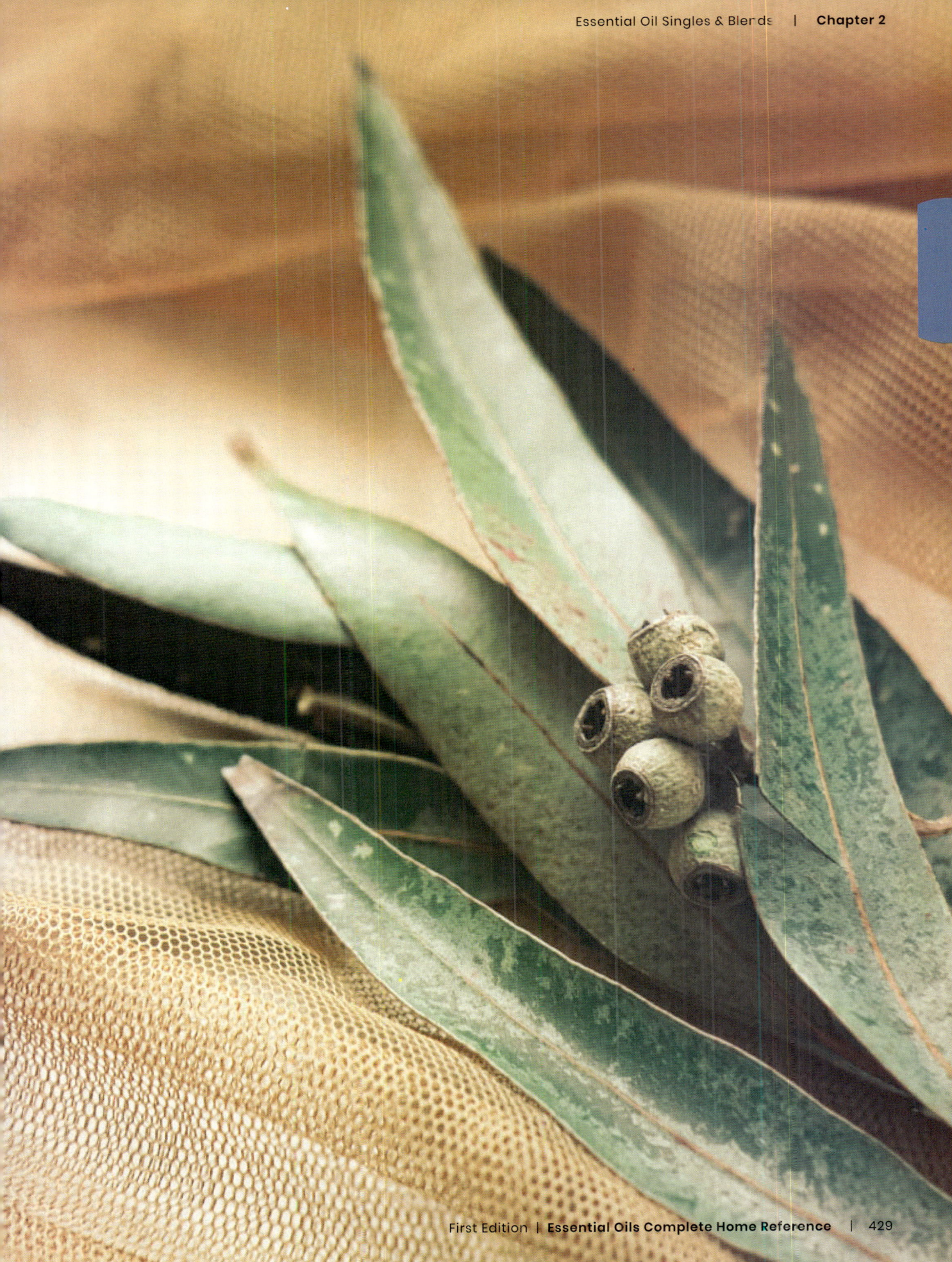

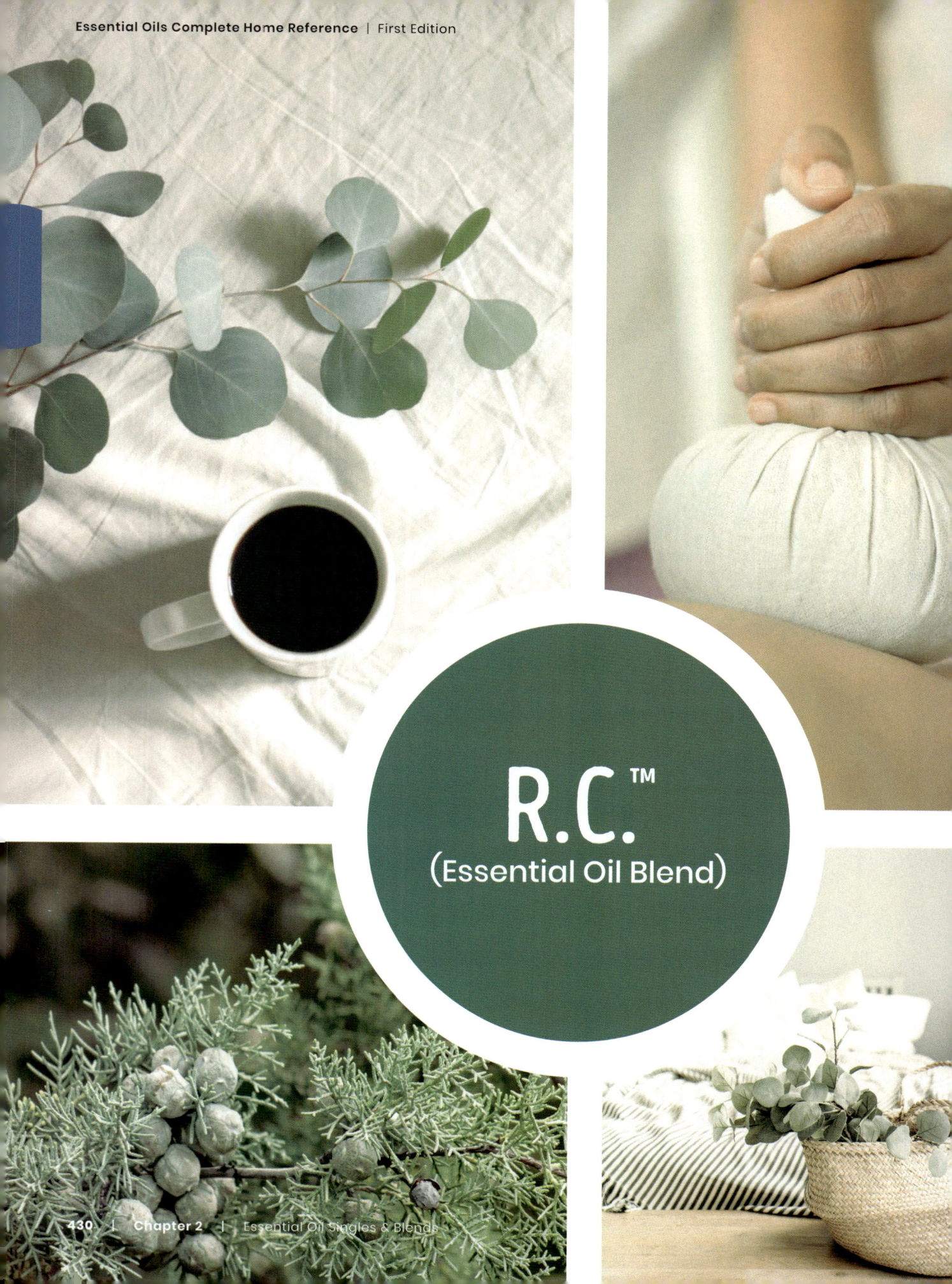

R.C.™
(Essential Oil Blend)

ABOUT R.C™:

R.C. gives relief from colds, bronchitis, sore throats, sinusitis, coughs, and respiratory congestion. It decongests sinus passages, combats lung infections, and relieves allergy symptoms.

MEDICAL PROPERTIES & USES:

Anti-inflammatory, antimicrobial, antioxidative, calming, cardiovascular supportive, digestion or elimination supportive/nausea reducing, oral protective, organ protective, pain or swelling reducing, performance enhancing/stimulating, respiratory system supportive

INGREDIENTS:

Eucalyptus Globulus, Myrtle, Marjoram, Pine, Eucalyptus Radiata, Eucalyptus Citriodora, Lavender, Cypress, Black Spruce, Peppermint

DIRECTIONS:

Aromatic: 30. To combat sinus and lung congestion, add R.C., Raven, Dorado Azul, or Eucalyptus Blue to a bowl of steaming hot water. Place a towel over your head and inhale the steam from the mixture. Combine with Raven and Thieves (alternating morning and night) to enhance effects. Topical: 50-50. Use as a hot compress or with Raindrop Technique.

CAUTIONS: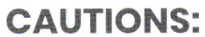

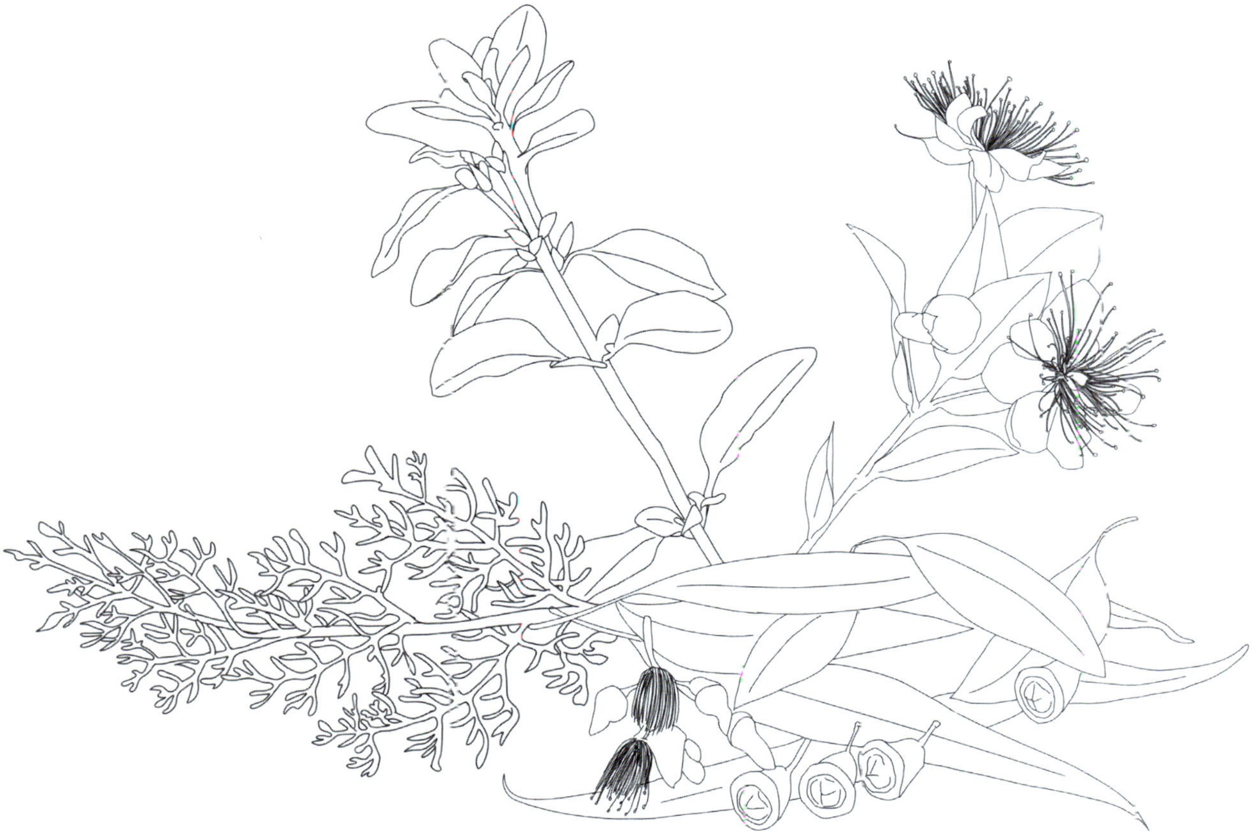

BOTANICAL FAMILY: Lauraceae

PLANT ORIGIN: Madagascar

EXTRACTION METHOD: Steam distilled from leaves

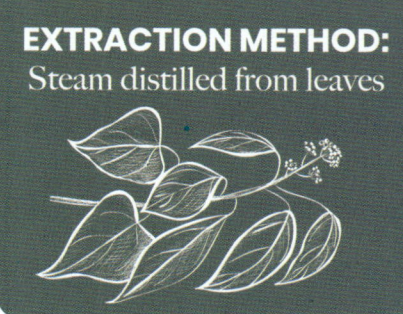

KEY CONSTITUENTS:
Eucalyptol (50-65%),
Sabinene (10-17%),
Alpha-Terpineol (5-10%),
Alpha-Pinene (3-6%)
Beta-Pinene (3-4%),
Terpinene-4-ol (1-4%)

RAVINTSARA
(Cinnamomum camphora CT cineole)

Ravintsara is referred to by the people of Madagascar as "the oil that heals." There are five commonly accepted chemotypes (cineole, linalool, camphor, isonerolidol, and safrole). Young Living uses the cineole chemotype, both as a single and in Raven.

Ravintsara is antimicrobial and supporting to the nerves and respiratory system and is known to be clarifying, stimulating, and purifying. It also helps to clear brain fog and strengthen motivation.

MEDICAL PROPERTIES:
Antitumoral, antiviral, antibacterial, anti-inflammatory

USES:
Herpes virus/viral infections (including colds, respiratory infections, coughs, whooping cough), throat/lung infections, hepatitis, shingles, pneumonia, inflammation, immune system, skin cleansing

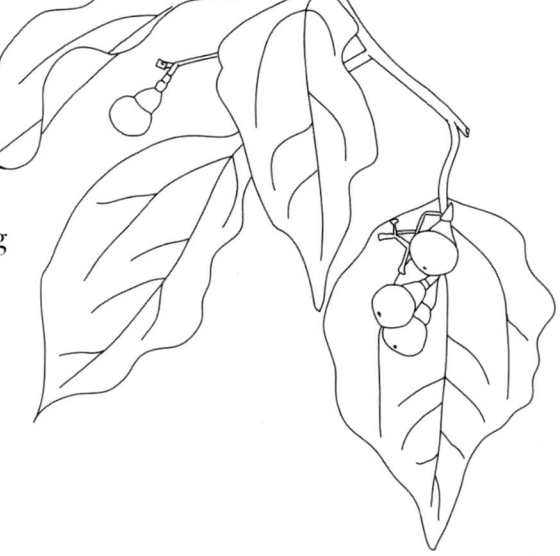

FRAGRANT INFLUENCE:
Eases breathing, meditation

DIRECTIONS:
Aromatic: 30. Topical: 50-50.

CAUTIONS:

SELECTED RESEARCH:

Wang W, Li D, Huang X, Yang H, Qui Z, Zou L, Liang Q, Shi Y, Wu Y, Wu S, Yang C, Li Y. Study on Antibacterial and Quorum-Sensing Inhibition Activities of Cinnamomum camphora Leaf Essential Oil. Molecules. 2019 Oct; 24(20): 3792.

Kang N-J, Han S-C, Yoon SH, Sim J-Y, Maeng YH, Kang H-K, Yoo E-S. Cinnamomum camphora Leaves Alleviate Allergic Skin Inflammatory Responses In Vitro and In Vivo. Toxicol Res. 2019 Jul; 35(3): 279-285.

Choi SY, Park K. Effect of inhalation of aromatherapy oil on patients with perennial allergic rhinitis: a randomized controlled trial. Evid Based Complement Alternat Med. 2016;2016:7896081. Epub 2016 Mar 13.

Fu J, Zeng C, Zeng Z, Wang B, Gong D. Cinnamomum camphora seed kernel oil ameliorates oxidative stress and inflammation in diet-induced obese rats. J Food Sci. 2016 May;81(5):H1295-300. Epub 2016 Mar 22.

Jiang H, Wang J, Song L, Cao X, Yao X, Tang F, Yue Y. GCxGC-TOFMS analysis of essential oils composition from leaves, twigs and seeds of Cinnamomum camphora L. Presl and their insecticidal and repellent activities. Molecules. 2016 Mar 28;21(4):423.

Fradelos E, Komini A. The use of essential oils as a complementary treatment for anxiety. American Journal of Nursing Science. 2015;4(1):1-5.

Marasini BP, Baral P, Aryal P, Ghimire KR, Neupane S, Dahal N, Singh A, Ghimire L, Shrestha K. Evaluation of antibacterial activity of some traditionally used medicinal plants against human pathogenic bacteria. Biomed Res Int. 2015;2015:265425. Epub 2015 Feb 9.

Yang F, Long E, Wen J, Cao L, Zhu C, Hu H, Ruan Y, Okanurak K, Hu H, Wei X, Yang X, Wang C, Zhang L, Wang X, Ji P, Zheng H, Wu Z, Lv Z. Linalool, derived from Cinnamomum camphora (L.) Presl leaf extracts, possesses molluscicidal activity against Oncomelania hupensis and inhibits infection of Schistosoma japonicum. Parasit Vectors. 2014 Aug 29;7:407.

Li H, Huang L, Zhou A, Li X, Sun J. [Study on anti-inflammatory effect of different chemotype of Cinnamomum camphora on rat arthritis model induced by Freund's adjuvant]. Zhongguo Zhong Yao Za Zhi. 2009 Dec;34(24):3251-4. Chinese.

Lee HJ, Hyun EA, Yoon WJ, Kim BH, Rhee MH, Kang HK, Cho JY, Yoo ES. In vitro anti-inflammatory and anti-oxidative effects of Cinnamomum camphora extracts. J Ethnopharmacol. 2006 Jan 16;103(2):208-216. Epub 2005 Sep 22.

Essential Oil Singles & Blends | **Chapter 2**

Ravintsara is known for its amazing healing powers & amazing smell.

RECONNECT™
(Essential Oil Blend)

(found only in the Reconnect Collection)
Apply Reconnect to help the mind to react positively and to help you reconnect to your surroundings.

MEDICAL PROPERTIES & USES:
Antimicrobial, anti-inflammatory, antinociceptive (analgesic; reduces sensitivity to pain), antioxidative, antibacterial, antimicrobial, relaxant, sedative, antidepressant, antiseptic, antifungal, antiviral, antitumoral, anticonvulsant

INGREDIENTS:
Caprylic/capric triglyceride,† Sacred Frankincense, Lavender, Blue Cypress, Cedarwood, Melissa, Idaho Blue Spruce, Palo Santo, Northern Lights Black Spruce, Sweet almond oil,‡ Bergamot, Myrrh, Vetiver, Geranium, Royal Hawaiian Sandalwood, Ylang Ylang, Hyssop, Coriander, Rose

DIRECTIONS:
Aromatic: (6o). Topical: Neat. To be applied only by a trusted adult or under adult supervision.

CAUTIONS:

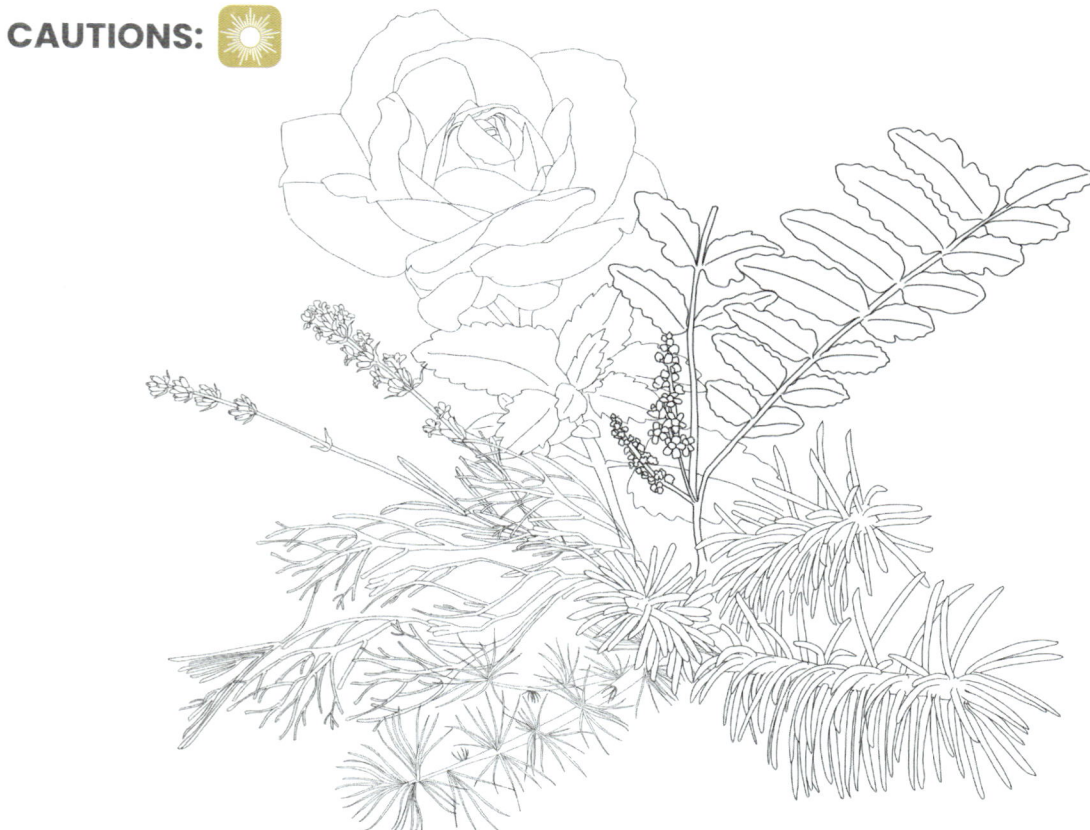

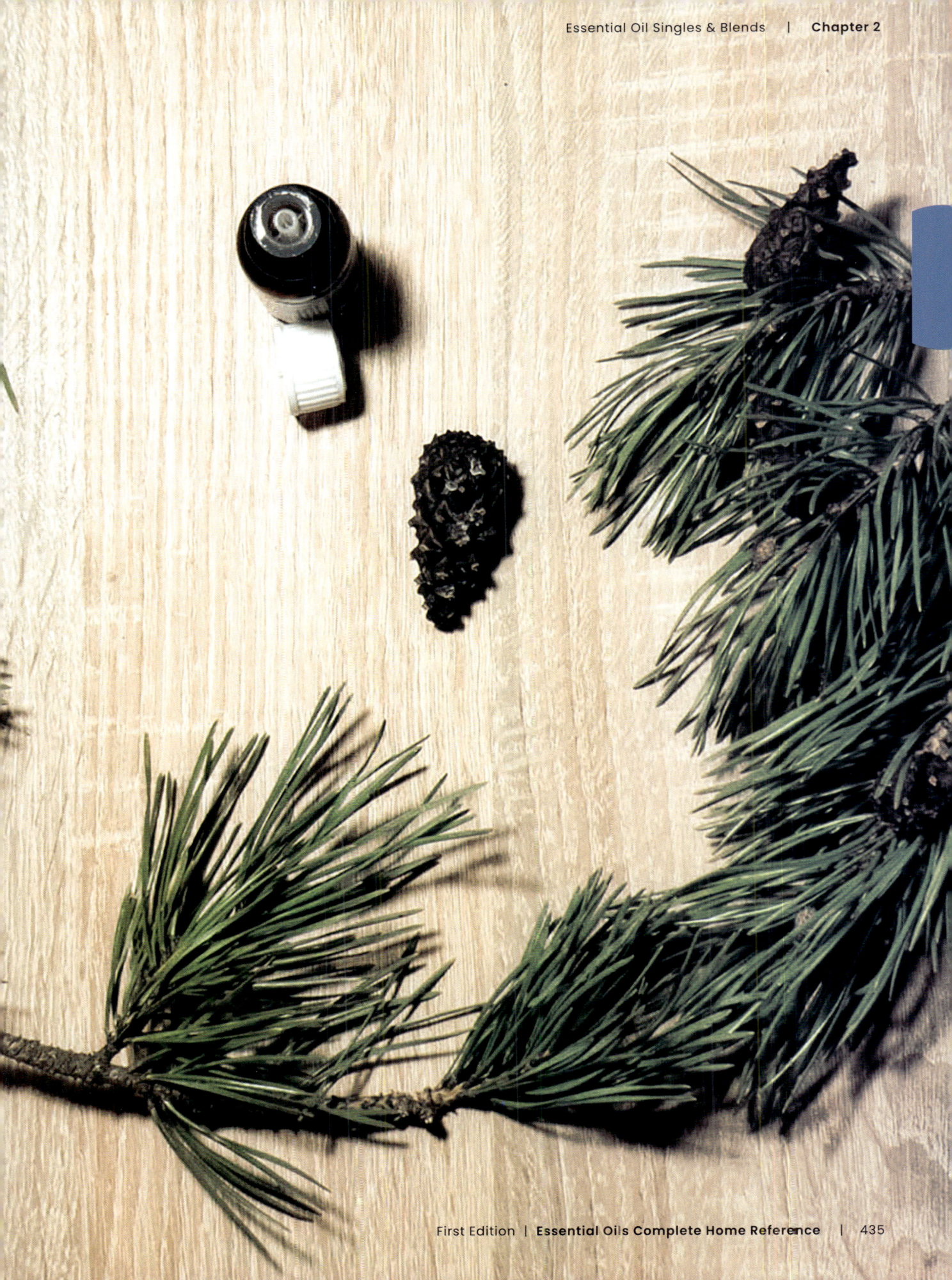

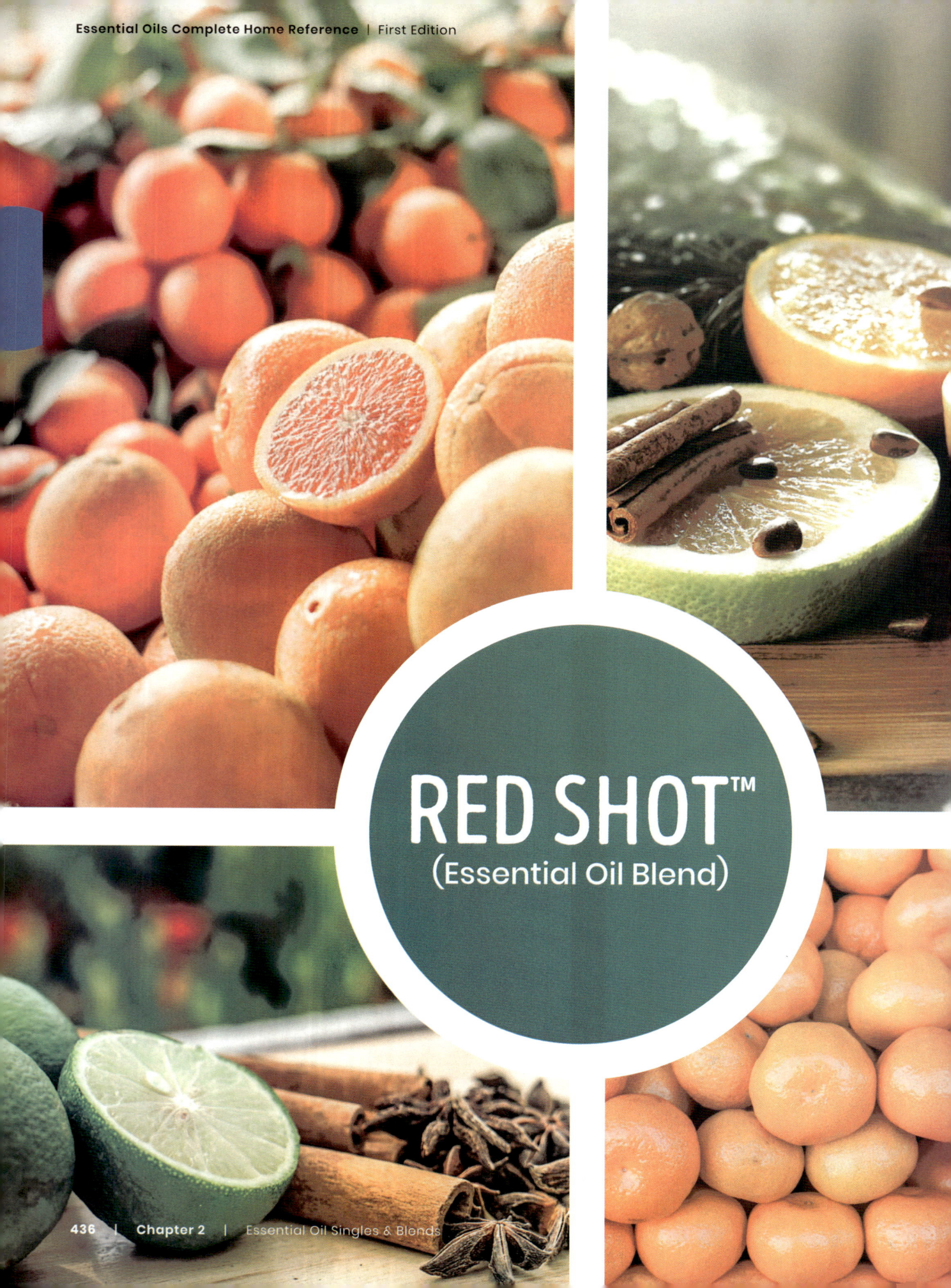

ABOUT RED SHOT™:

Red Shot is a limited-time-only blend that adds a delicious variation to NingXia Red.

MEDICAL PROPERTIES & USES:
Digestive support, weight loss, insomnia, irritability, lung health, learning and memory support, antiviral, antibacterial, decongest the lymphatic system, refreshing and uplifting

INGREDIENTS:
Tangerine, Mandarin, Lime, Grapefruit, Cassia, Spearmint

DIRECTIONS:
Add 1-2 drops to 2 ounces of NingXia Red or put 2 drops in a capsule and take 3 times daily or as needed.

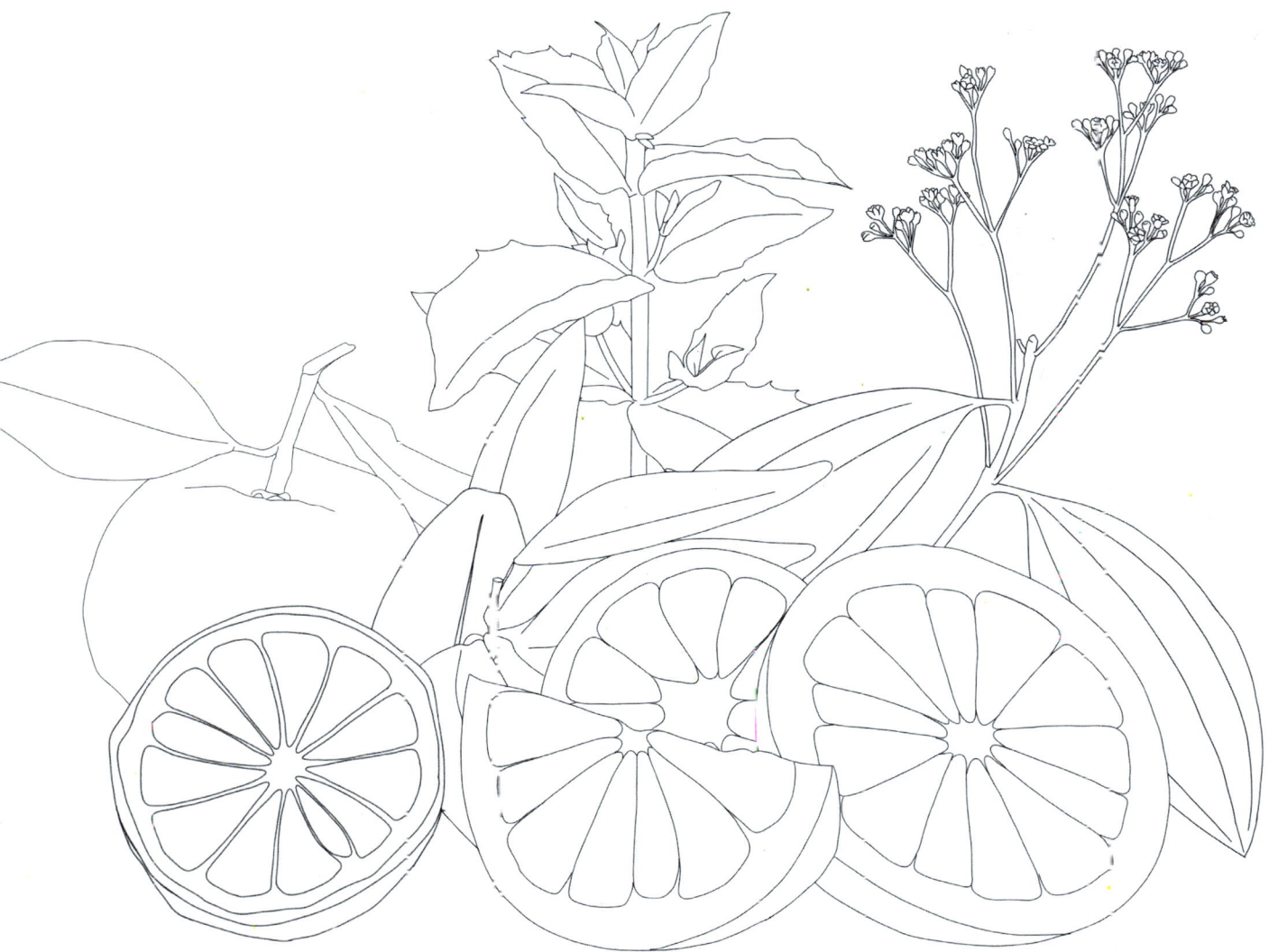

RELEASE™
(Essential Oil Blend)

This is a helpful blend to release anger and memory trauma from the liver in order to create emotional well-being. It helps open the subconscious mind through pineal stimulation to release deep-seated trauma. It is one of the most powerful of the emotionally supporting essential oil blends.

MEDICAL PROPERTIES & USES:
Emotionally supportive, anti-inflammatory, antimicrobial, antioxidative, calming, disease inhibitory, organ protective, pain or swelling reducing, wellness supportive

INGREDIENTS:
Ylang Ylang, Olive oil,‡ Lavandin, Geranium, Royal Hawaiian Sandalwood, Grapefruit, Tangerine, Spearmint, Lemon, Blue Cypress, Davana, Kaffir Lime, Ocotea, Jasmine, Matricaria (German Chamomile), Blue Tansy, Rose

DIRECTIONS:
Aromatic: 6o. Topical: Neat. Apply over liver, anywhere trauma has occurred, or use as a compress. Massage on bottoms of feet and behind ears as needed.

CAUTIONS:

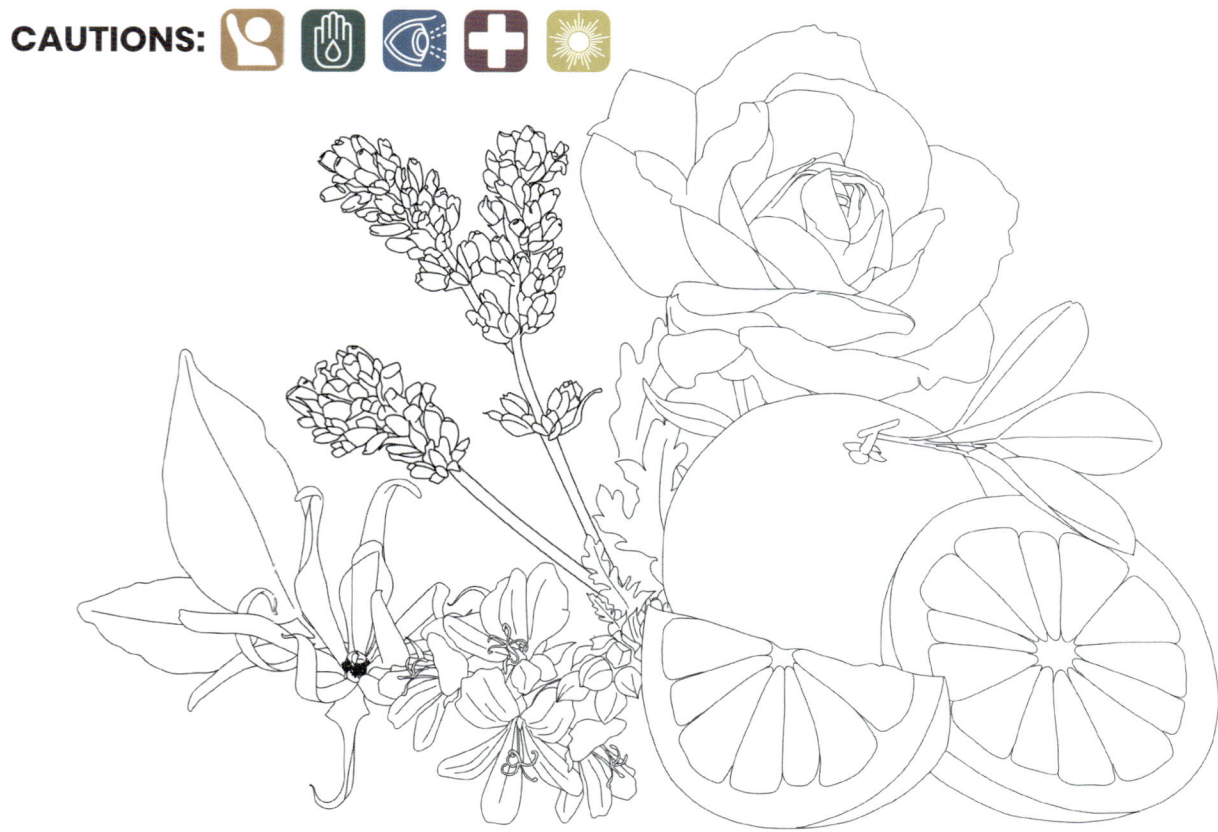

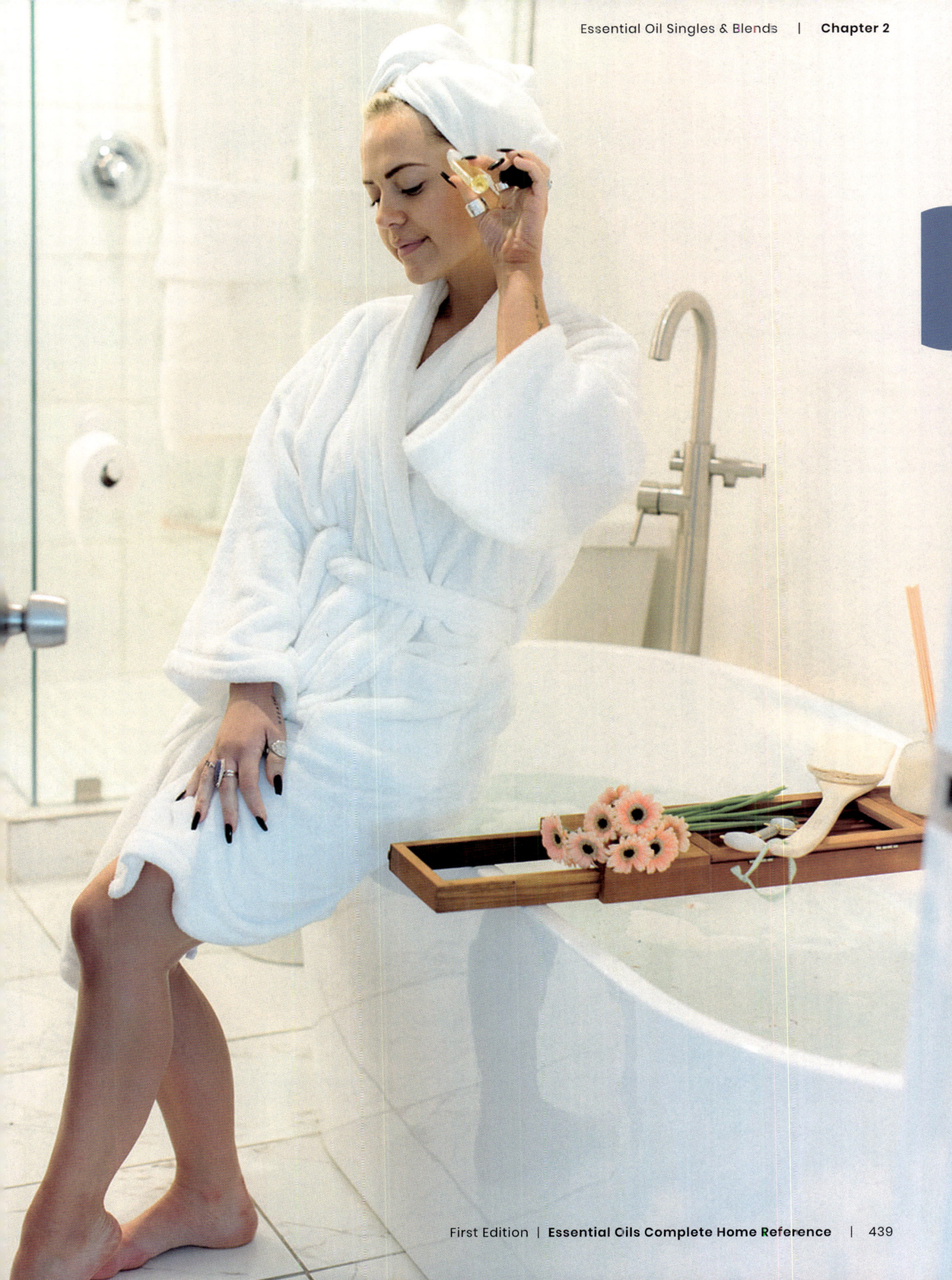

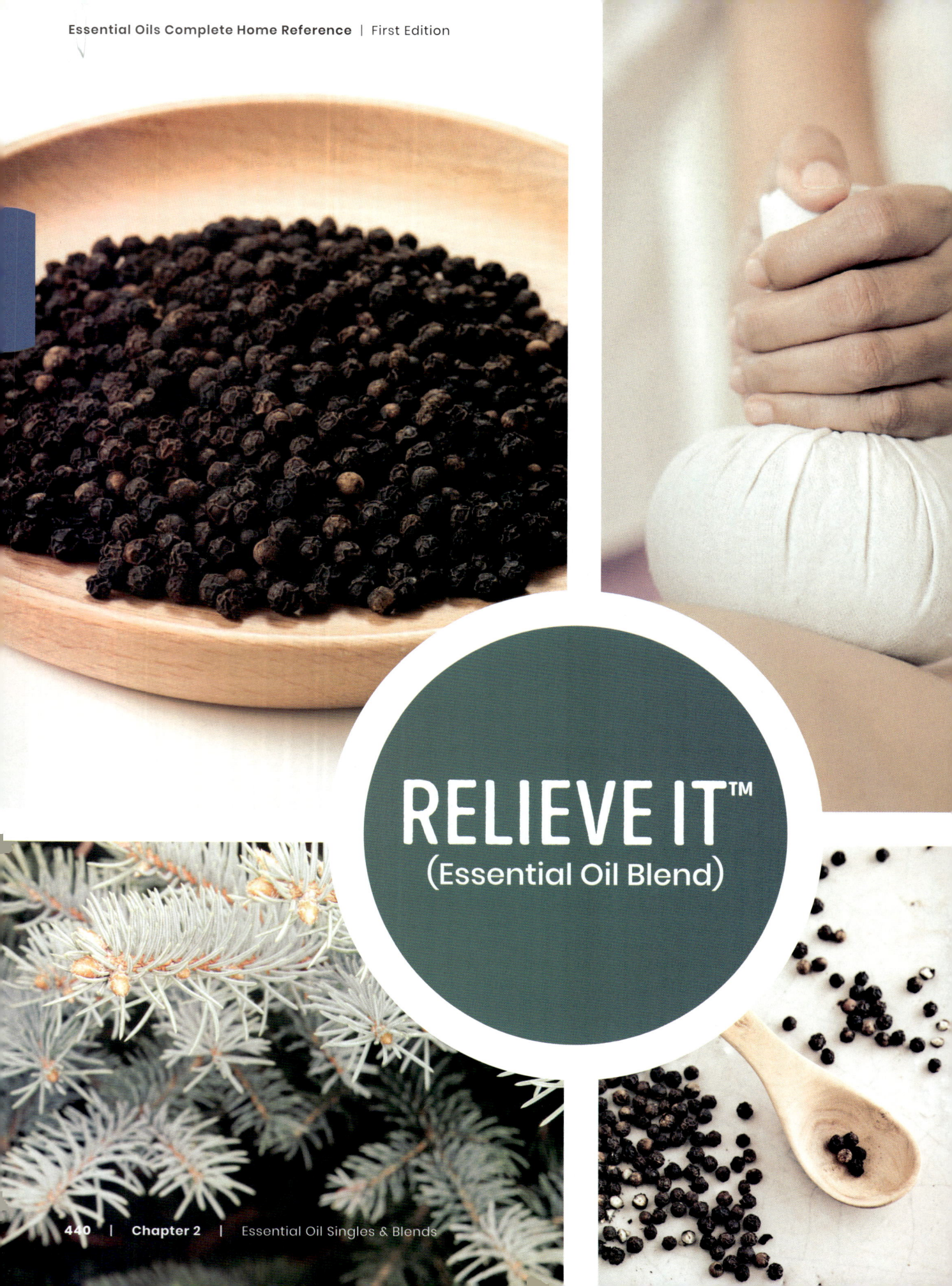

Essential Oil Singles & Blends | **Chapter 2**

ABOUT RELIEVE IT™:
This blend is high in anti-inflammatory compounds that relieve deep tissue pain and muscle soreness.

MEDICAL PROPERTIES & USES:
Pain or swelling reducing, anti-inflammatory, oral protective, performance enhancing/stimulating

INGREDIENTS:
Black Spruce, Black Pepper, Hyssop, Peppermint

DIRECTIONS:
Aromatic: 10. Topical: 50-50. Use as a cold or hot compress.

CAUTIONS:

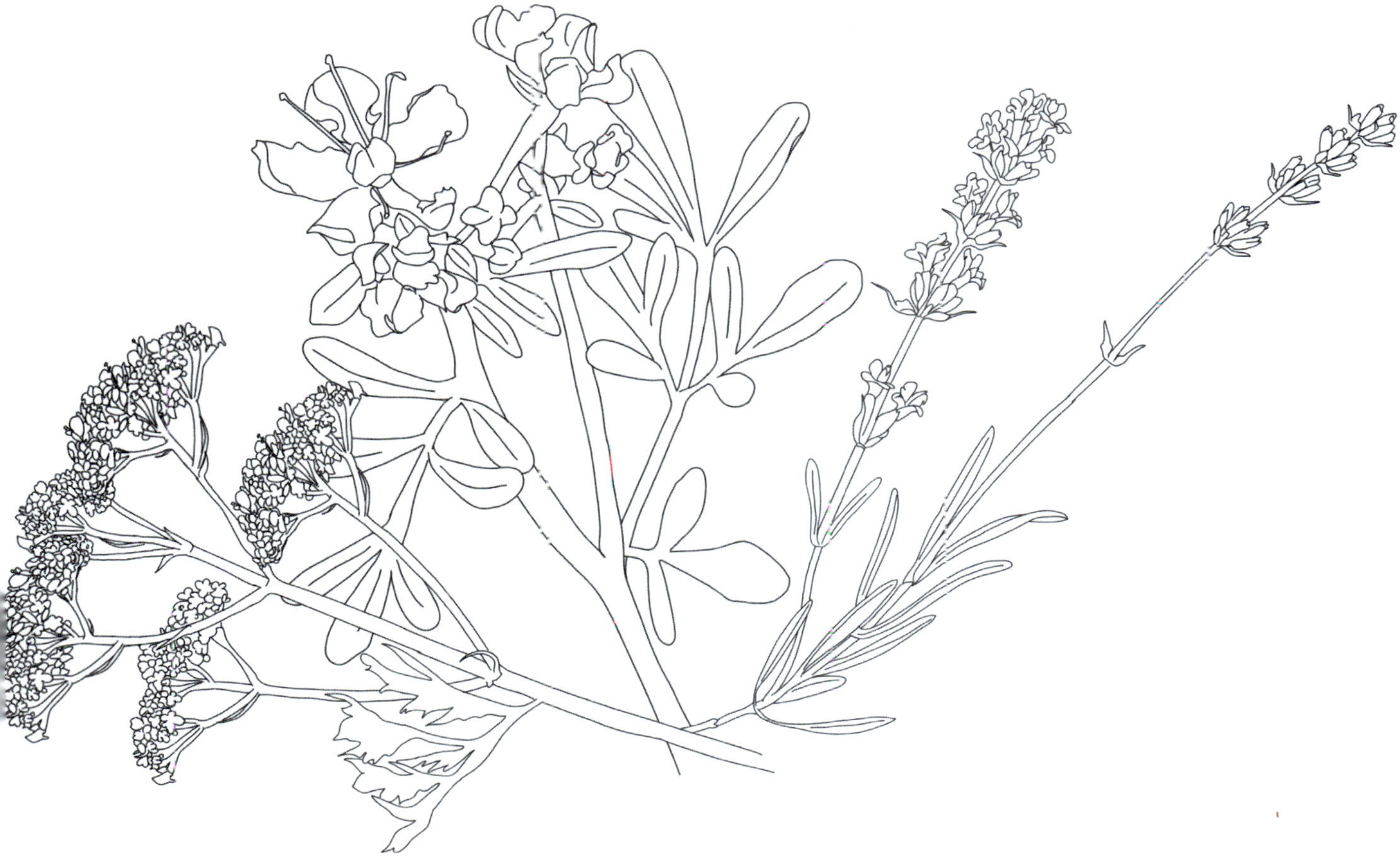

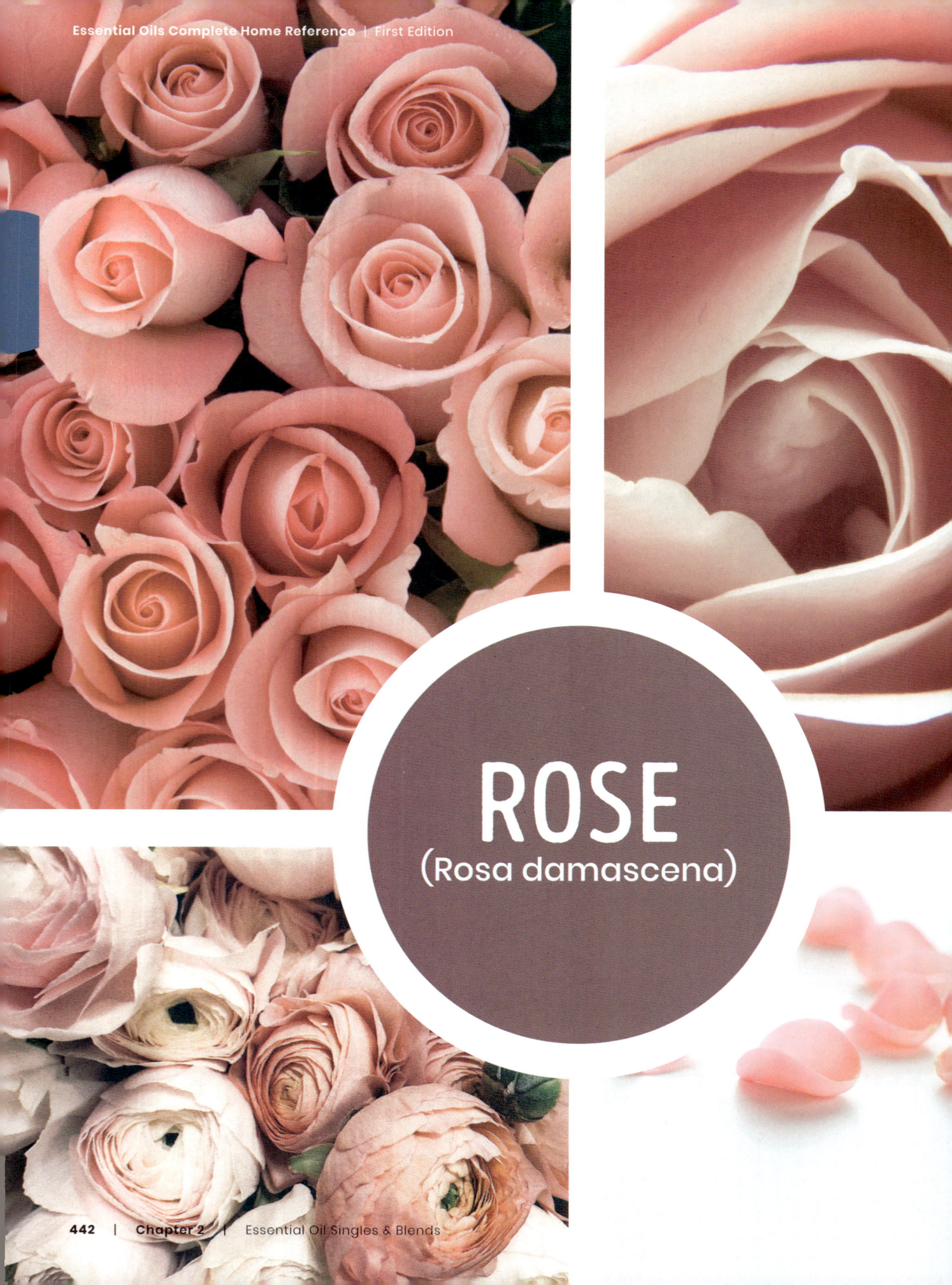

ROSE
(Rosa damascena)

BOTANICAL FAMILY:
Rosaceae

PLANT ORIGIN:
Bulgaria

EXTRACTION METHOD:
Two-part steam distilled from flowers and petals

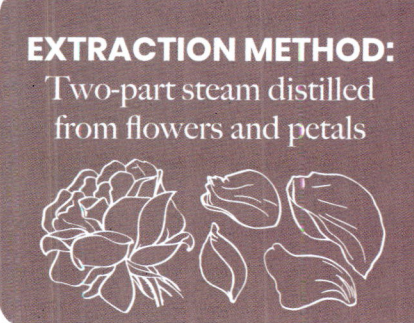

KEY CONSTITUENTS:
Citronellol (20-50%),
Geraniol (6-29%),
Paraffin C19 (6-16%),
Nerol (3-13%),
Ethanol (up to 7%),
Paraffin C21 (1-6%),
Paraffin C17 (up to 4%),
Beta-Phenylethanol (up to 4%)

HISTORICAL DATA:
Rose has been used for the skin for thousands of years. The Arab physician Avicenna was responsible for first distilling rose oil, eventually authoring an entire book on the healing attributes of the rose water derived from the distillation of rose. Throughout much of ancient history, the oil was produced by enfleurage, a process of pressing the petals along with a vegetable oil to extract the essence. Today, however, almost all rose oils are solvent extracted.
Note: The Bulgarian Rosa damascena (high in citronellol) is very different from Moroccan Rosa centifolia (high in phenyl ethanol). They have different colors, aromas, and therapeutic actions.

MEDICAL PROPERTIES:
Anti-inflammatory, anti-HIV, antioxidant, anxiolytic, hepatoprotective, relaxant, reduces scarring, antiulcer, immunomodulating, cancer chemopreventive, DNA damage prevention, analgesic

USES:
Anxiety, possible therapeutic for depression, hypertension, heart strengthening, anxiety, viral infections (herpes simplex), skin conditions (scarring, wrinkles, acne), ulcers

FRAGRANT INFLUENCE:
Its beautiful fragrance is intoxicating and aphrodisiac-like. It helps bring balance and harmony, allowing one to overcome insecurities. The effect of rose on the heart brings good cheer with calming and a lightness of spirit.

DIRECTIONS:
Aromatic: 60. Topical: Neat. Dietary: Take as a dietary supplement.

CAUTIONS: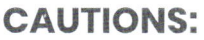

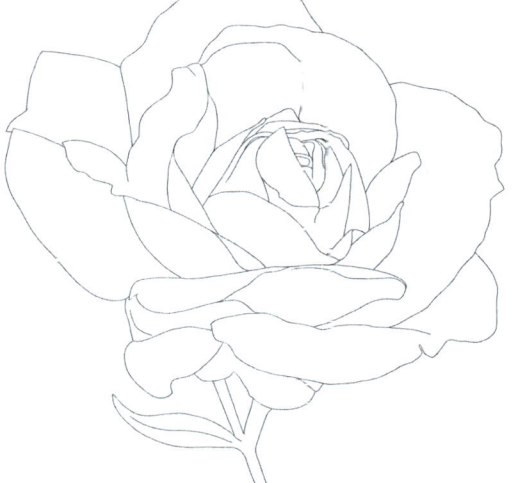

SELECTED RESEARCH:
Fatemi F, Golbodagh A, Hojihosseini R, Dadkhah A, Akbarzadeh K, Din S, Malayeri MRM. Anti-inflammatory Effects of Deuterium-Depleted Water Plus Rosa damascena Mill. Essential Oil Via Cyclooxygenase-2 Pathway in Rats. Turk J Pharm Sci. 2020 Feb; 7(1): 99-107.

Davoodi I, Rahimi R, Abdollahi M, Farzaei F, Farzaei MH, Memariani Z, Najafi F. Promising effect of Rosa damascena extract on high-fat diet-induced nonalchoholic fatty liver. J Tradit Complement Med. 2017 Oct; 7(4): 508-514.

Zhu S, Li H, Dong J, Yang W, Liu T, Wang Y, Wang X, Wan M, Zhi D. Rose essential oil delayed Alzheimer's Disease-like symptoms by SKN-1 pathway in C. elegans. J Agric Food Chem. 2017 Oct 11;65(40):8855-8865. Epub 2017 Sep 27.

Niazi M, Hashempur MH, Taghizadeh M, Heydari M, Shariat A. Efficacy of topical Rose (Rosa damascena Mill.) oil for migraine headache: a randomized double-blinded placebo-controlled cross-over trial. Complement Ther Med. 2017 Oct;34:35-41. Epub 2017 Jul 25.

Uysal M, Doğru HY, Sapmaz E, Tas U, Çakmak B, Ozsoy AZ, Sahin F, Ayan S, Esen M. Investigating the effect of rose essential oil in patients with primary dysmenorrhea. Complement Ther Clin Pract. 2016 Aug;24:45-9. Epub 2016 May 7.

Esfandiary E, Karimipour M, Mardani M, Ghanadian M, Alaei HA, Mohammadnejad D, Esmaeili A. Neuroprotective effects of Rosa damascena extract on learning and memory in a rat model of amyloid-β-induced Alzheimer's disease. Adv Biomed Res. 2015 Ju 27;4:131. eCollection 2015.

Mahboubi M. Rosa damascena as holy ancient herb with novel applications. J Tradit Complement Med. 2015 Oct 30;6(1):10-6. eCollection 2016 Jan.

Mohammadpour T, Hosseini M, Naderi A, Karami R, Sadeghnia HR, Soukhtanloo M, Vafaee F. Protection against brain tissues oxidative damage as a possible mechanism for the beneficial effects of Rosa damascena hydroalcoholic extract on scopolamine induced memory impairment in rats. Nutr Neurosci. 2015 Oct;18(7):329-36. Epub 2014 Jun 29.

Bani S, Hasanpour S, Mousavi Z, Mostafa Garehbaghi P, Gojazadeh M. The effect of Rosa damascena extract on primary dysmenorrhea: a double-blind cross-over clinical trial. Iran Red Crescent Med J. 2014 Jan;16(1):e14643. Epub 2014 Jan 5.

Hongratanaworakit T. Relaxing effect of rose oil on humans. Nat Prod Commun. 2009 Feb;4(2):291-6.

BOTANICAL FAMILY:
Lamiaceae

PLANT ORIGIN:
Morocco

EXTRACTION METHOD:
Steam distilled from leaves, herbs, and aerial parts

KEY CONSTITUENTS:
Eucalyptol (3-55%), Camphor (5-15%), Alpha-Pinene (8-15%), Beta-Pinene (4-9%), Camphene (2-6%), Borneol (1-5%), Limonene (1-4%), Para-Cymene (up to 3%), Alpha-Terpineol (1-3%), Myrcene (1-2%), Linalool (up to 2%), Bornyl Acetate (up to 2%)

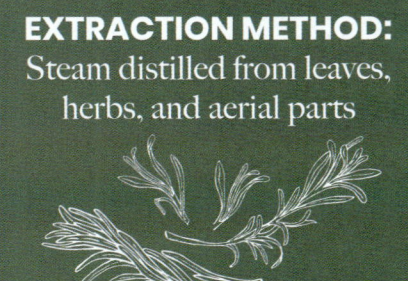

ROSEMARY & ROSEMARY VITALITY™
(Rosmarinus officinalis)

Rosemary was part of the "Marseilles Vinegar" or "Four Thieves Vinegar" that bandits who robbed the dead and dying used to protect themselves during the 15th century plague. The name of the oil is derived from the Latin words for dew of the sea (ros + marinus). According to folklore history, rosemary originally had white flowers; however, they turned red after the Virgin Mary laid her cloak on the bush. At the time of ancient Greece (about 1,000 BC), rosemary was burned as incense. Later cultures believed that it warded off devils, a practice that eventually became adopted by the sick, who then burned rosemary to protect against infection. It was listed in Hildegard's Medicine, a compilation of early German medicines by highly regarded Benedictine herbalist Hildegard of Bingen (1098-1179). Until recently, French hospitals used rosemary to disinfect the air.

MEDICAL PROPERTIES:
Anticancerous, antioxidant, antimicrobial, liver-protecting, anti-inflammatory, antitumoral, antifungal, antibacterial, antidepressant

USES:
Maintains normal cell health, increases locomotor activity, helps support healthy brain function, emotionally stimulating, helps support healthy blood and blood pressure, infectious disease, liver conditions/hepatitis, throat/lung infections, hair loss (alopecia areata), acne, impaired memory/Alzheimer's, enhances mental clarity and concentration, weight loss

FRAGRANT INFLUENCE:
Helps overcome mental fatigue and improves mental clarity and focus. Freshens the air. University of Miami scientists found that inhaling rosemary boosted alertness, eased anxiety, and amplified analytic and mental ability.

DIRECTIONS:
Aromatic: 10. Topical: 20-80. In case of sensitivity, dilute 2 drops in 15 ml of V-6 or other pure carrier oil.
Dietary (Vitality): Dilute 1 drop with 4 drops of V-6 or other pure carrier oil. Put in a capsule and take 1 daily.

CAUTIONS: Do not use on children under 4 years of age. Do not use Rosemary for high blood pressure if already taking ACE inhibitor prescription drugs.

SELECTED RESEARCH:

Al-Megrin WA, AlSadhan NA, Metwally DM, Al-Talhi RA, El-Khadragy MF, Abdel-Hafez LJM. Potential antiviral agents of Rosmarinus officinalis extract against herpes viruses 1 and 2. Biosci Rep. 2020 Jun 26; 40(6): BSR20200992.

Allegra A, Tonacci A, Pioggia G, Musolino C, Gangemi S. Anticancer Activity of Rosmarinus officinalis L.: Mechanisms of Action and Therapeutic Potentials. Nutrients. 2020 Jun; 12(6): 1739.

Chraibi M, Farah A, Elamin O, Iraqui HM, Fikri-Benbrahim K. Characterization, antioxidant, antimycobacterial, antimicrobial effects of Moroccan rosemary essential oil, and its synergistic antimicrobial potential with carvacrol. J Adv Pharm Technol Res. 2020 Jan-Mar; 11(1): 25-29.

Manilal A, sabu KR, Shewangizaw M, Aklilu A, Seid M, Merdikios B, Tsegaye B. In vitro antibacterial activity of medicinal plants against biofilm-forming methicillin-resistant Staphylococcus aureus: efficacy of Moringa stenopetala and Rosmarinus officinalis extracts. Heliyon. 2020 Jan; 6(1): e03303.

Khezri K, Farahpour MR, Mounesi Rad S. Accelerated infected wound healing by topical application of encapsulated Rosemary essential oil into nanostructured lipid carriers. Artif Cells Nanomed Biotechnol. 2019 Mar 11; 47(1): 980-988.

El-Naggar SA, Abdel-Farid IB, Germoush MO, Elgebaly HA, Alm-Eldeen AA. Efficacy of Rosmarinus officinalis leaves extract against cyclophosphamide-induced hepatotoxicity. Pharm Biol. 2016 Oct; 54(10): 2007-16. Epub 2016 Feb 1.

Sebai H, Selmi S, Rtibi K, Gharbi N, Sakly M. Protective effect of Lavandula stoechas and Rosmarinus officinalis essential oils against reproductive damage and oxidative stress in alloxan-induced diabetic rats. J Med Food. 2015 Feb; 18(2): 241-9. Epub 2014 Aug 8.

Gauch LM, Silveira-Gomes F, Esteves RA, Pedrosa SS, Gurgel ES, Arruda AC, Marques-da-Silva SH. Effects of Rosmarinus officinalis essential oil on germ tube formation by Candida albicans isolated from denture wearers. Rev Soc Bras Med Trop. 2014 May-Jun; 47(3): 389-91.

Rašković A, Milanović I, Pavlović N, Ćebović T, Vukmirović S, Mikov M. Antioxidant activity of rosemary (Rosmarinus officinalis L.) essential oil and its hepatoprotective potential. BMC Complement Altern Med. 2014 Jul 7; 14: 225.

Petrolini FV, Lucarini R, de Souza MG, Pires RH, Cunha WR, Martins CH. Evaluation of the antibacterial potential of Petroselinum crispin and Rosmarinus officinalis against bacteria that cause urinary tract infections. Braz J Microbiol. 2013 Dec 17; 44(3): 829-34. eCollection 2013.

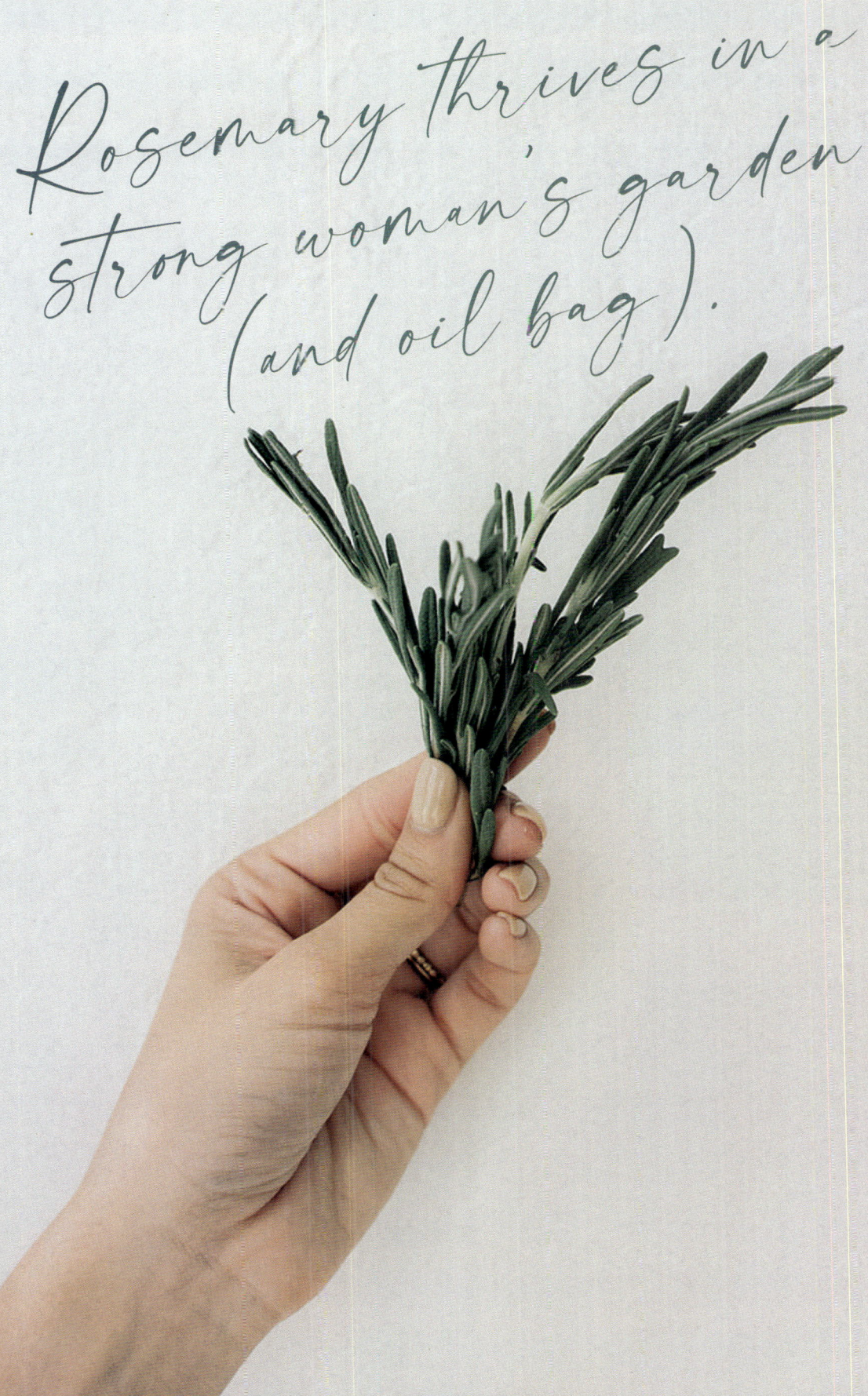

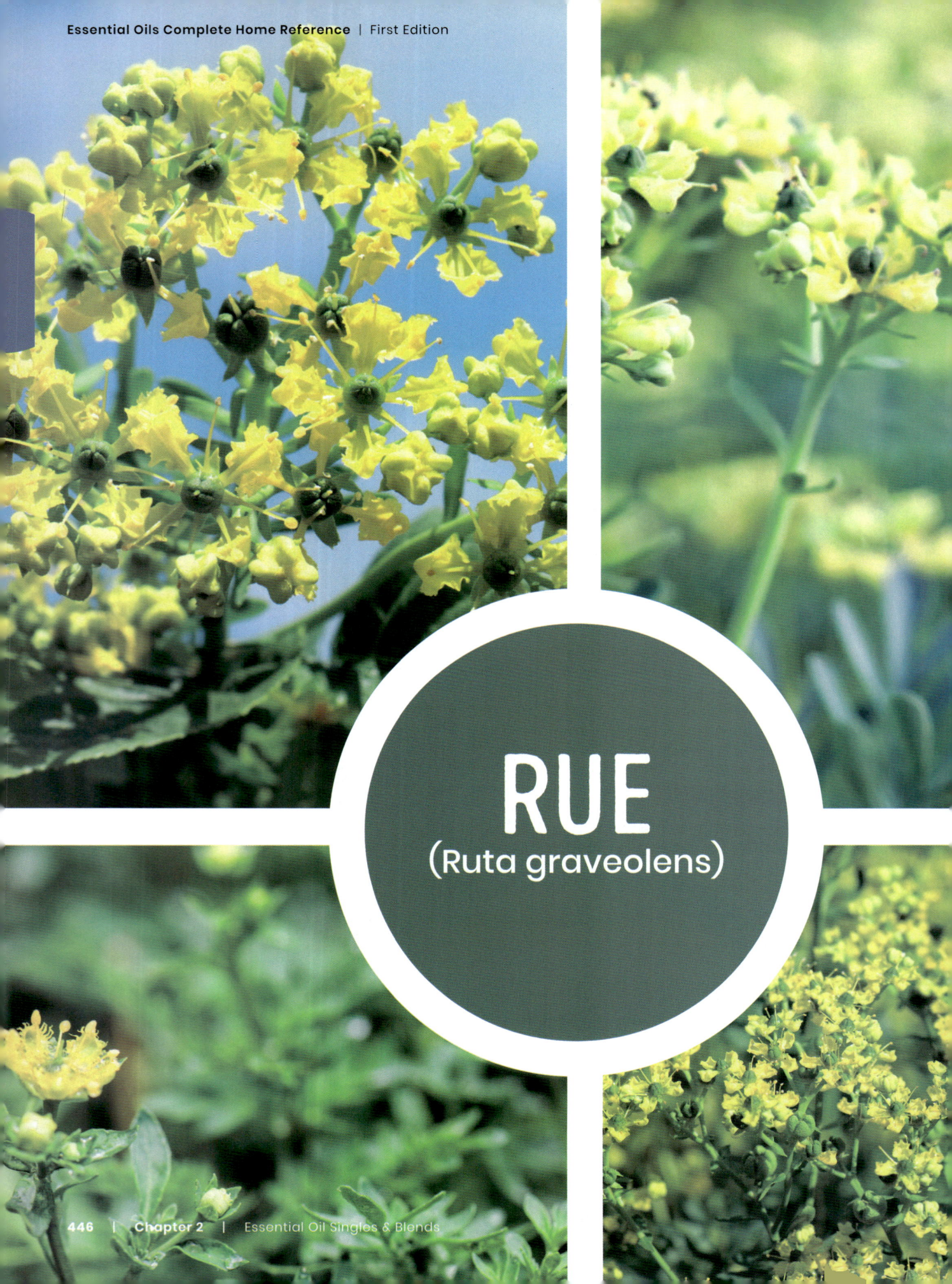

RUE
(Ruta graveolens)

Essential Oil Singles & Blends | **Chapter 2**

BOTANICAL FAMILY:
Rutaceae

PLANT ORIGIN:
Ecuador

EXTRACTION METHOD:
Steam distilled from herb/aerial parts/flowering plant

KEY CONSTITUENTS:
2-Nonanone (35-55%),
2-Undecanone (33-52%),
Geijerene (up to 3%)

HISTORICAL DATA:
In traditional medicine, rue was used as a magic herb and a protection against evil. It was used to treat nervous afflictions, digestive problems, hysterics, and as an abortifacient. Formerly, it was used to treat menstrual disorders and hysteria. Anecdotal reports suggest it has sleep-inducing properties.

MEDICAL PROPERTIES:
Anti-inflammatory, antidiabetic, antimicrobial, hypotensive, anxiolytic, sleep promoting, antispasmodic, antifungal, antioxidant

USES:
Hysteria, stress, nervousness, digestion, stiff neck, headache, dizziness, inner ear problems, antidote for poisons, cuts, cholic, skin inflammation, menstrual problems, nervousness, circulatory issues, coughing, muscle spasms, insect repellent

FRAGRANT INFLUENCE:
Calming and relaxing, grounding, peaceful energy, breathing problems

DIRECTIONS:
Aromatic: 60. Topical: 50-50.

CAUTIONS:

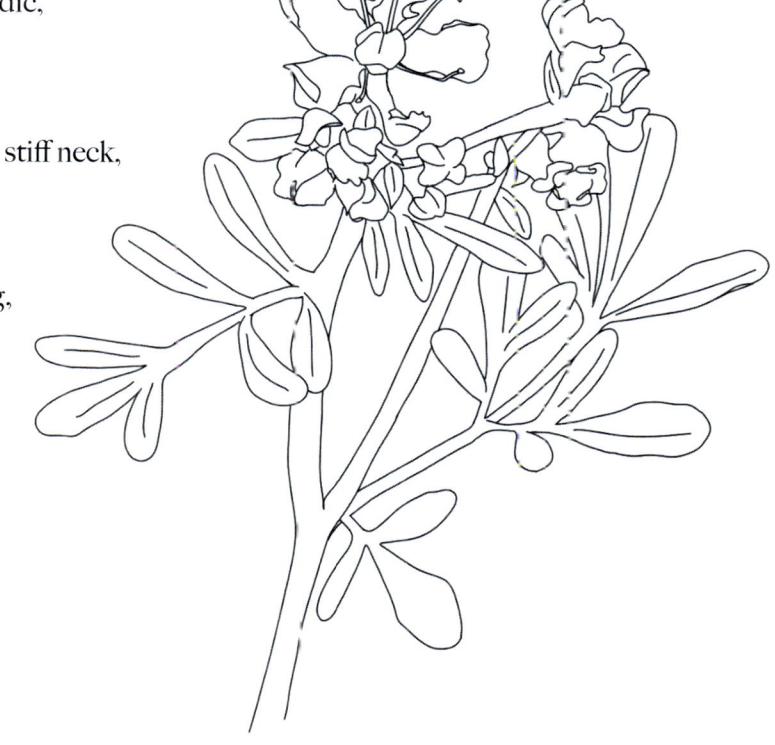

SELECTED RESEARCH:

Asgharian S, Hojjait MR, Ahari M, Bijad E, Deris F, Lorigooini Z. Ruta graveolens and rutin, as its major compound; investigating their effect on spatial memory and passive avoidance memory in rats. Pharm Biol. 2020; 58(1): 447-453.

Schelz Z, Ocsovszki I, Bozsity N, Hohmann J, Zupkó I. Antiproliferative effects of various furanoacridones isolated from Ruta graveolens on human breast cancer cell lines. Anticancer Res. 2016 Jun;36(6):2751-8.

Karp JC, Sanchez C, Guilbert P, Mina W, Demonceaux A, Curé H. Treatment with Ruta graveolens 5CH and Rhus toxicodendron 9CH may reduce joint pain and stiffness linked to aromatase inhibitors in women with early breast cancer: results of a pilot observational study. Homeopathy. 2016 Nov;105(4):299-308. Epub 2016 Aug 9.

Arora S, Tandon S. DNA fragmentation and cell cycle arrest: a hallmark of apoptosis induced by Ruta graveolens in human colon cancer cells. Homeopathy. 2015 Jan;104(1):36-47. Epub 2014 Nov 29.

Sivakamavalli J, Deepa O, Vaseeharan B. Discrete nanoparticles of Ruta graveolens induces the bacterial and fungal biofilm inhibition. Cell Commun Adhes. 2014 Aug;21(4):229-38.

Ghosh S, Bishayee K, Khuda-Bukhsh AR. Graveoline isolated from ethanolic extract of Ruta graveolens triggers apoptosis and autophagy in skin melanoma cells: a novel apoptosis independent autophagic signaling pathway. Phytother Res. 2014 Aug;28(8):1153-62. Epub 2013 Dec 17.

Ratheesh M, Helen A. Oral administration of alkaloid fraction from Ruta graveolens inhibits oxidative stress and inflammation in hypercholesterolemic rabbits. Pharm Biol. 2013 Dec;51(12):1552-8. Epub 2013 Sep 13.

Ivanova A, Mikhova B, Najdenski H, Tsvetkova I, Kostova I. Antimicrobial and cytotoxic activities of Ruta graveolens. Fitoterapia. 2005 Jun;76(3-4):344-7. Epub 2005 May 14.

RUTAVALA™ & RUTAVALA™ ROLL-ON
(Essential Oil Blend)

RutaVaLa is a proprietary blend of Ruta graveolens (Rue), Lavender, and Valerian essential oils that promotes relaxation of the body and mind, soothes stressed nerves, and induces sleep. Rue has long been used in South America to promote the relaxation of body and mind, relieve and soothe stressed nerves, and revitalize passion.

MEDICAL PROPERTIES & USES:
Anti-inflammatory, antimicrobial, calming and relaxing, glandular/hormonal supportive, performance enhancing, sleep improving

INGREDIENTS:
Caprylic/capric triglyceride‡ (Roll-On only), Lavender, Valerian, Rue

DIRECTIONS:
Aromatic: 3O. Topical: 50-50.

CAUTIONS:

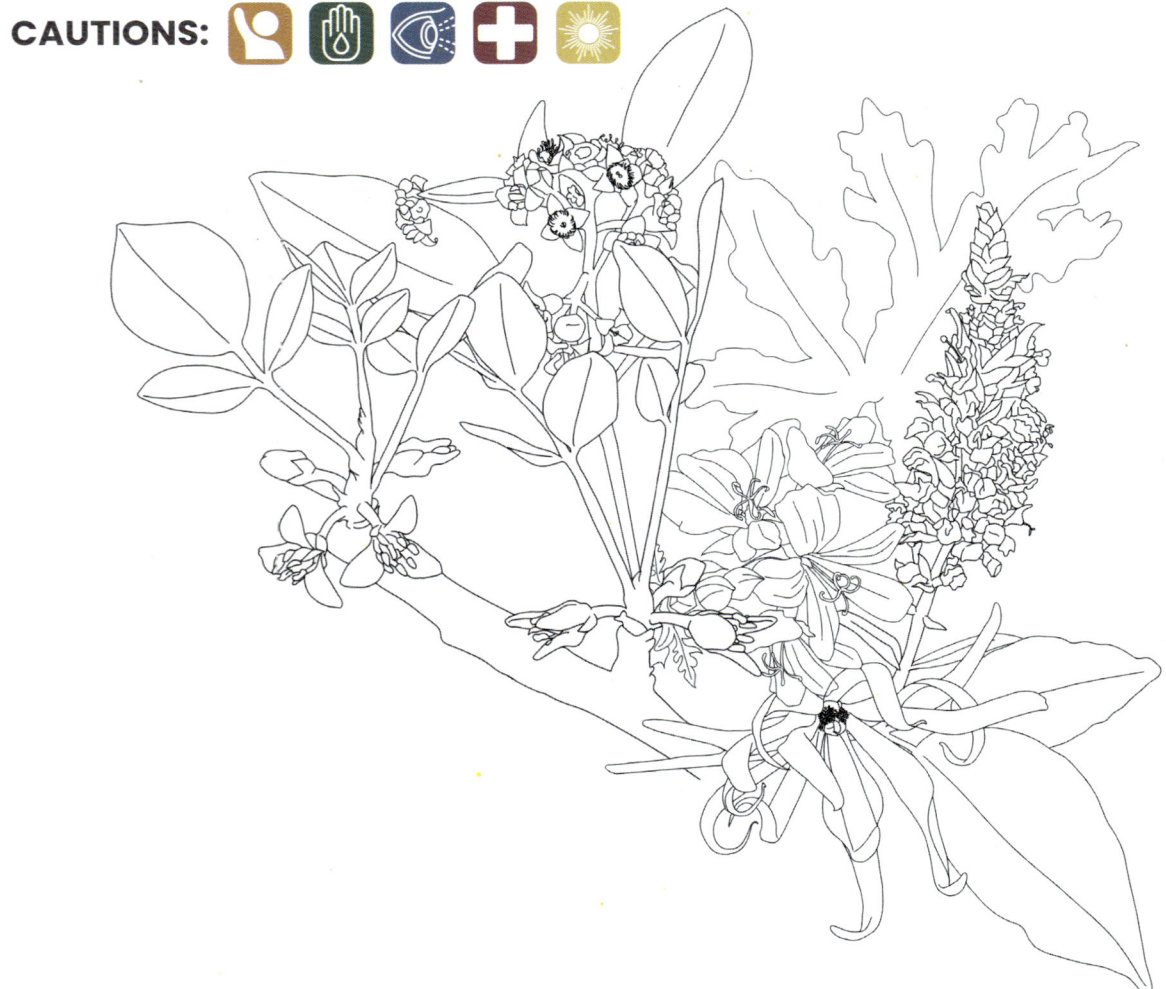

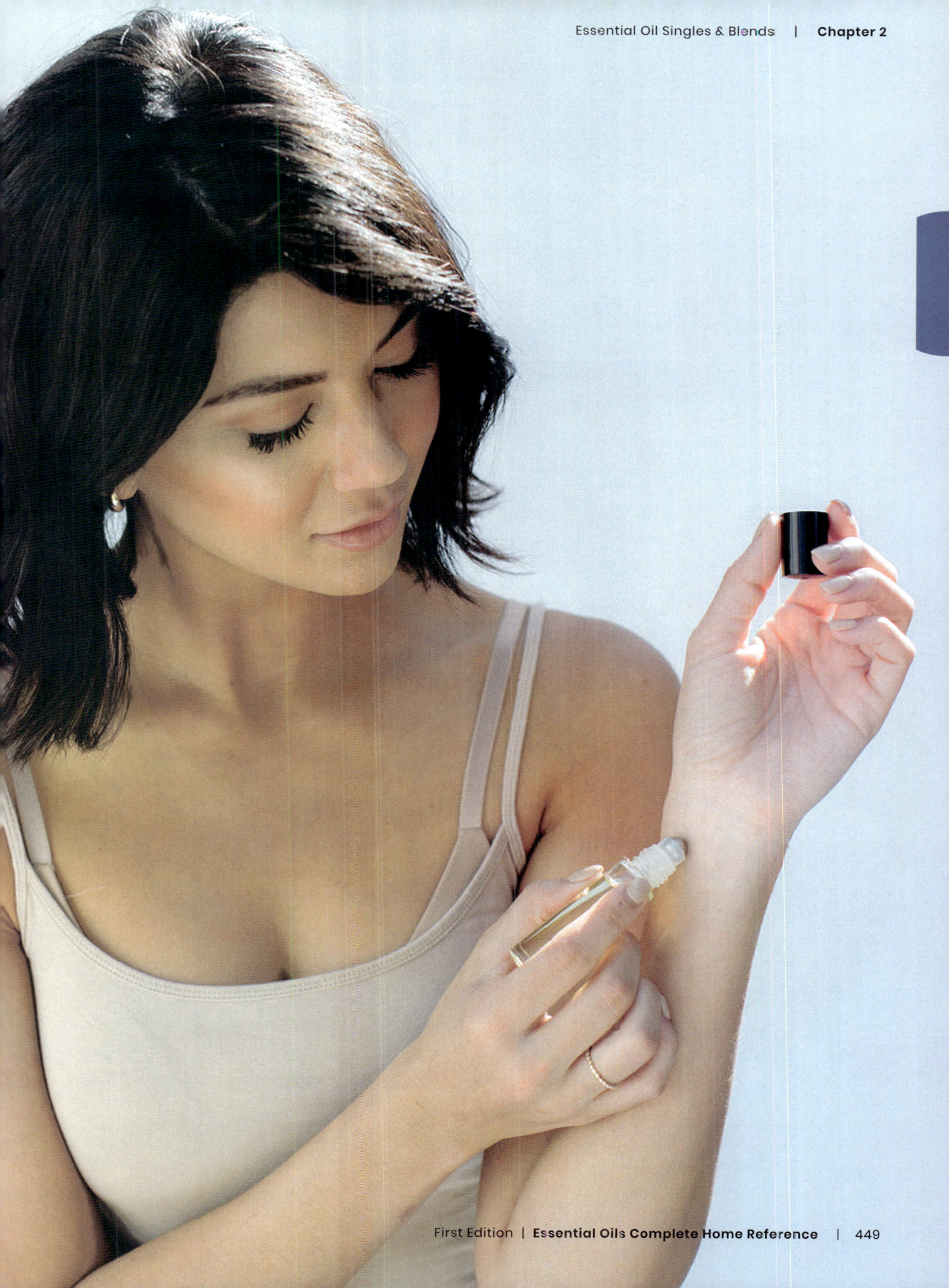

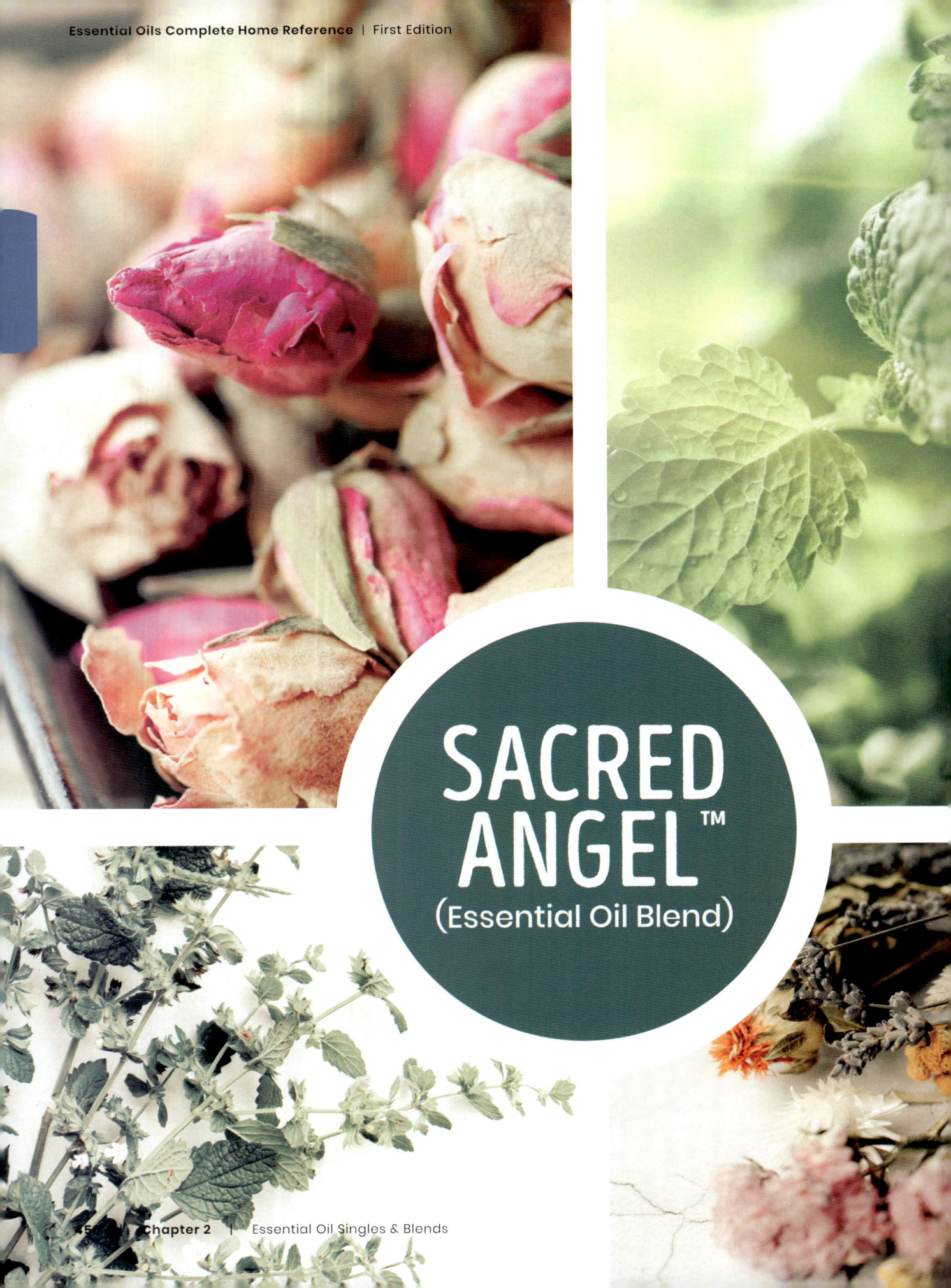

ABOUT SACRED ANGEL™:

Sacred Angel is a limited-edition blend of essential oils that can help align positive, feminine energies and provide spiritual grounding. It contains Angelica essential oil, which the Europeans traditionally called "holy spirit root" or "oil of angels." Angelica's history of healing powers was so strong that it was believed to be of divine origin.

MEDICAL PROPERTIES & USES:

Antimicrobial, neuroprotective, anti-inflammatory, antioxidant, antibacterial, antiviral, antiparasitic, analgesic/anesthetic, sedative, antianxiety, antidepressant, decongestant, aphrodisiac, enhance feelings of spirituality, open and release emotional blocks, balance, well-being, elevates the mind, grounding, prayer and meditation

INGREDIENTS:

Myrrh, Ylang Ylang, Caprylic/capric glyceride, Hyssop, Sacred Sandalwood, Geranium, Black Spruce, Coriander, Camphor (Ho Wood), Melissa, Rose, Angelica

DIRECTIONS:

Aromatic: 3O. Topical: Neat.

CAUTIONS:

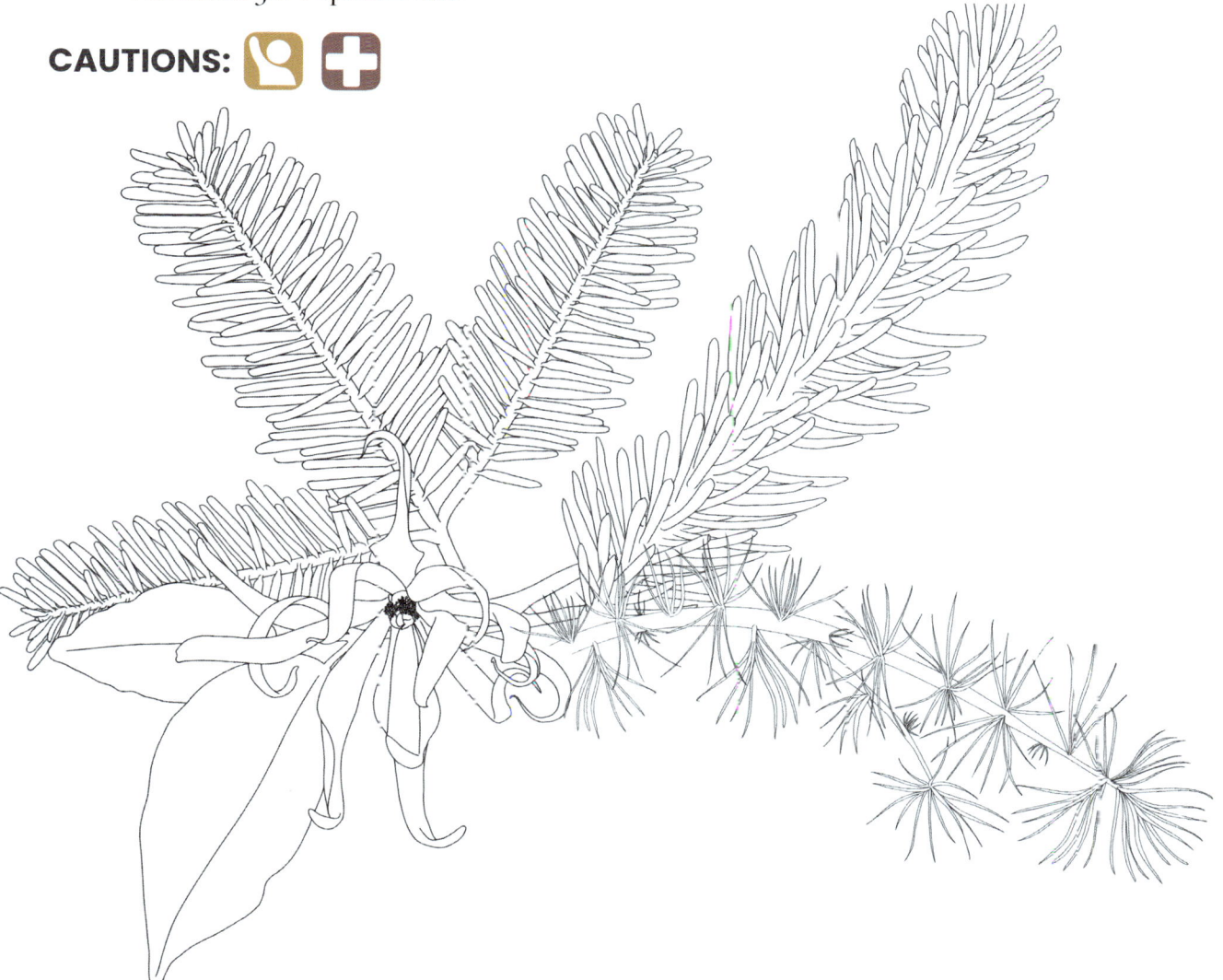

SACRED MOUNTAIN™
(Essential Oil Blend)

Mountain aromas instill strength, empowerment, grounding, and protection with the spiritual feeling of being in a sacred environment.

MEDICAL PROPERTIES & USES:
Antispasmodic, cardiovascular problems, antidiabetic, anti-inflammatory, anxiety, hypertension, depression, intestinal problems, calming, disease inhibitory, lymphatic stimulant, fatigue

INGREDIENTS:
Black Spruce, Ylang Ylang, Idaho Grand Fir, Cedarwood

DIRECTIONS:
Aromatic: 30. Topical: 50-50.

CAUTIONS:

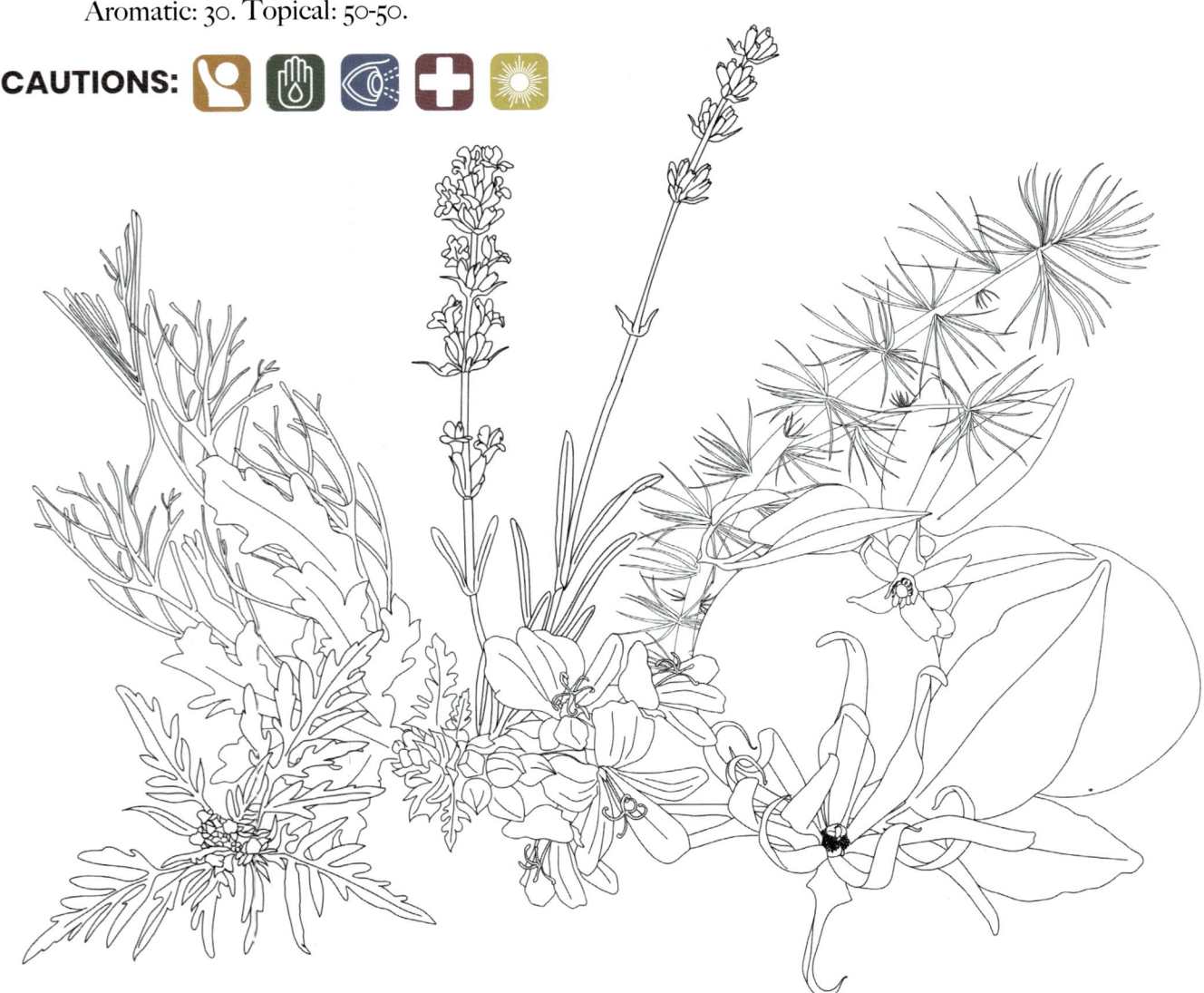

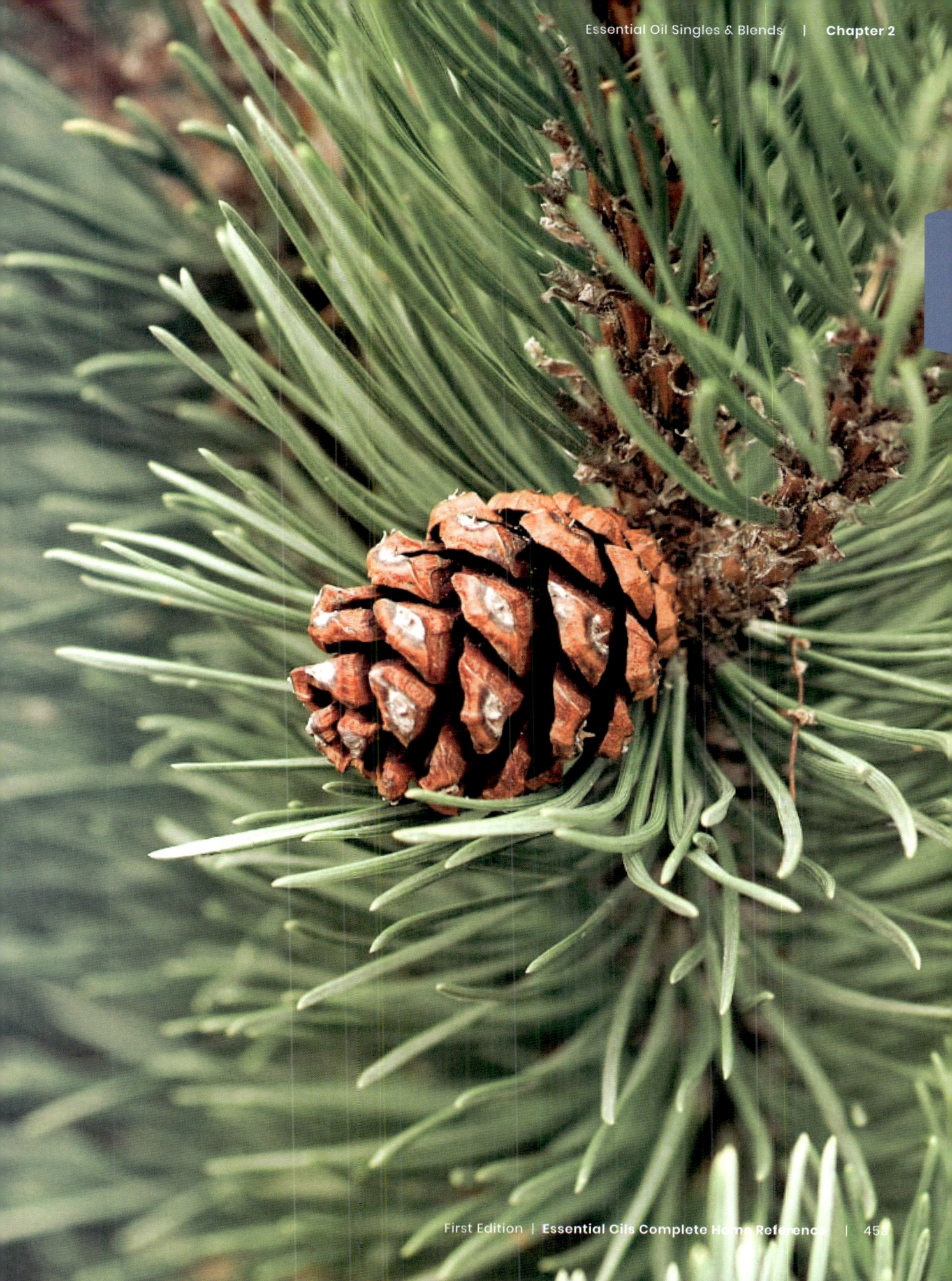

BOTANICAL FAMILY: Lamiaceae

PLANT ORIGIN: Albania, France, Montenegro, United Kingdom

EXTRACTION METHOD: Steam distilled from aerial parts and flowering plants

KEY CONSTITUENTS: Alpha-Thujone (18-43%), Camphor (4-25%), Eucalyptol (5-13%), Alpha-Humulene (up to 12%), Beta-Thujone (3-9%), Camphene (1-7%), Alpha-Pinene (1-7%), Limonene (up to 3%), Bornyl Acetate (up to 3%)

SAGE & SAGE VITALITY™
(Angelica archangelica)

Known as "herba sacra" or sacred herb by the ancient Romans, sage's name, Salvia, is derived from the word for "salvation." Sage has been used in Europe for oral infections and skin conditions. It has been recognized for its benefits of strengthening the vital centers and supporting metabolism.

MEDICAL PROPERTIES:
Antimicrobial, insecticide, anticell proliferation, antibacterial, antifungal, antioxidant, antitumoral, anti-inflammatory, anxiolytic, hormone regulating, estrogen-like, antiviral, circulatory stimulant, gallbladder stimulant

USES:
Hot flashes, supports wellness, menstrual problems/PMS, estrogen, progesterone, and testosterone deficiencies, liver problems

FRAGRANT INFLUENCE:
Mentally stimulating, anxiety-reducing, and helps combat despair and mental fatigue; strengthens the vital centers of the body, balancing the root (pelvic) chakra, where negative emotions from denial and abuse are stored.

DIRECTIONS:
Aromatic: 3O. Topical: 2O-8O. Dietary (Vitality): Dilute 1 drop with 4 drops of V-6 or other pure carrier oil. Put in a capsule and take 1 daily.

CAUTIONS: Avoid if epileptic. Avoid use on persons with high blood pressure.

SELECTED RESEARCH:

Zeidabadi A, Yazdanpanahi Z, Dabbaghmanesh MH, Sasani MR, Emamghoreishi M, Akbarzadeh M. The effect of Salvia officinalis on symptoms of flushing, night sweat, sleep disorders, and score of forgetfulness in postmenopausal women. J Familyu Med Prim Care. 2020 Feb; 9(2): 1086-1092.

Choukairi Z, Hazzaz T, LkhiderM, Ferrandez JM, Fechtali T. Effect of Salvia Officinalis L. and Rosmarinus Officinalis L. leaves extracts on anxiety and neural activity. Bioinformation. 2019; 15(3): 172-178.

Kolac UK, Ustuner MC, Tekin N, Ustuner D, Colak E, Entok E. The anti-inflammatory and antioxidant effects of Salvia officinalis on Lipopolysaccharide-induced inflammation in rats. J Med Food. 2017 Dec;20(12):1193-1200. Epub 2017 Nov 13.

Garcia CS, Menti C, Lambert AP, Barcellos T, Moura S, Calloni C, Branco CS, Salvador M, Roesch-Ely M, Henriques JA. Pharmacological perspectives from Brazilian Salvia officinalis (Lamiaceae): antioxidant, and antitumor in mammalian cells. An Acad Bras Cienc. 2016 Mar;88(1):281-92. Epub 2016 Feb 2.

Chovanová R, Mezovská J, Vaverková Š, Mikulášová M. The inhibition of the Tet(K) efflux pump of tetracycline resistant Staphylococcus epidermis by essential oils from three Salvia species. Lett Appl Microbiol. 2015 Jul;61(1):58-62. Epub 2015 May 1.

Martins N, Barros L, Santos-Buelga C, Henriques M, Silva S, Ferreira IC. Evaluation of bioactive properties and phenolic compounds in different extracts prepared from Salvia officinalis L. Food Chem. 2015 Mar 1;170:378-85. Epub 2014 Aug 29.

Miroddi M, Navarra M, Quattropani MC, Calapai F, Gangemi S, Calapai G. Systematic review of clinical trials assessing pharmacological properties of Salvia species on memory, cognitive impairment and Alzheimer's disease. CNS Neurosci Ther. 2014 Jun;20(6):485-95. Epub 2014 Apr 10.

Shahneh FZ, Valiyari S, Baradaran B, Abdolalizadeh J, Bandehagh A, Azadmehr A, Hajiaghaee R. Inhibitory and cytotoxic activities of Salvia officinalis L. extract on human lymphoma and leukemia cells by induction of apoptosis. Adv Pharm Bull. 2013;3(1):51-5. Epub 2013 Feb 7.

Kozies K, Klusová V, Srančikova A, Mučaji P, Slameňová D, Hunáková L, Kusznierewicz B, Horváthová E. Effects of Salvia officinalis and Thymus vulgaris on oxidant-induced DNA damage and antioxidant status in HepG2 cells. Food Chem. 2013 Dec 1;141(3):2198-206. Epub 2013 May 9.

Fellah S, Diouf PN, Petrissans M, Perrin D, Romdhane M, Abderrabba M. Chemical composition and antioxidant properties of salvia officinalis L. oil from two culture sites in Tunisia. Journal of Essential Oil Research. 2006 Sept 1;18(5):553-556.

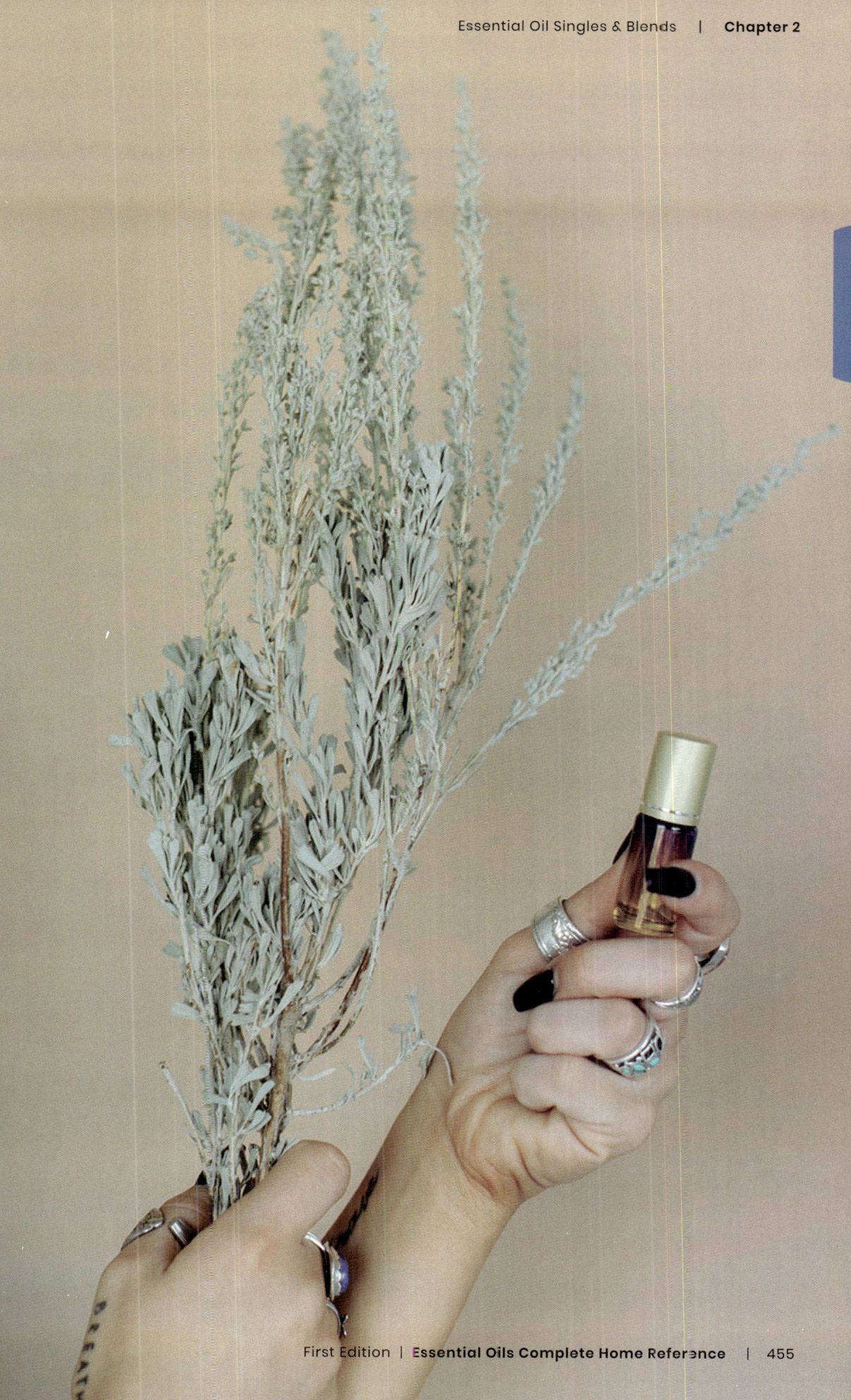

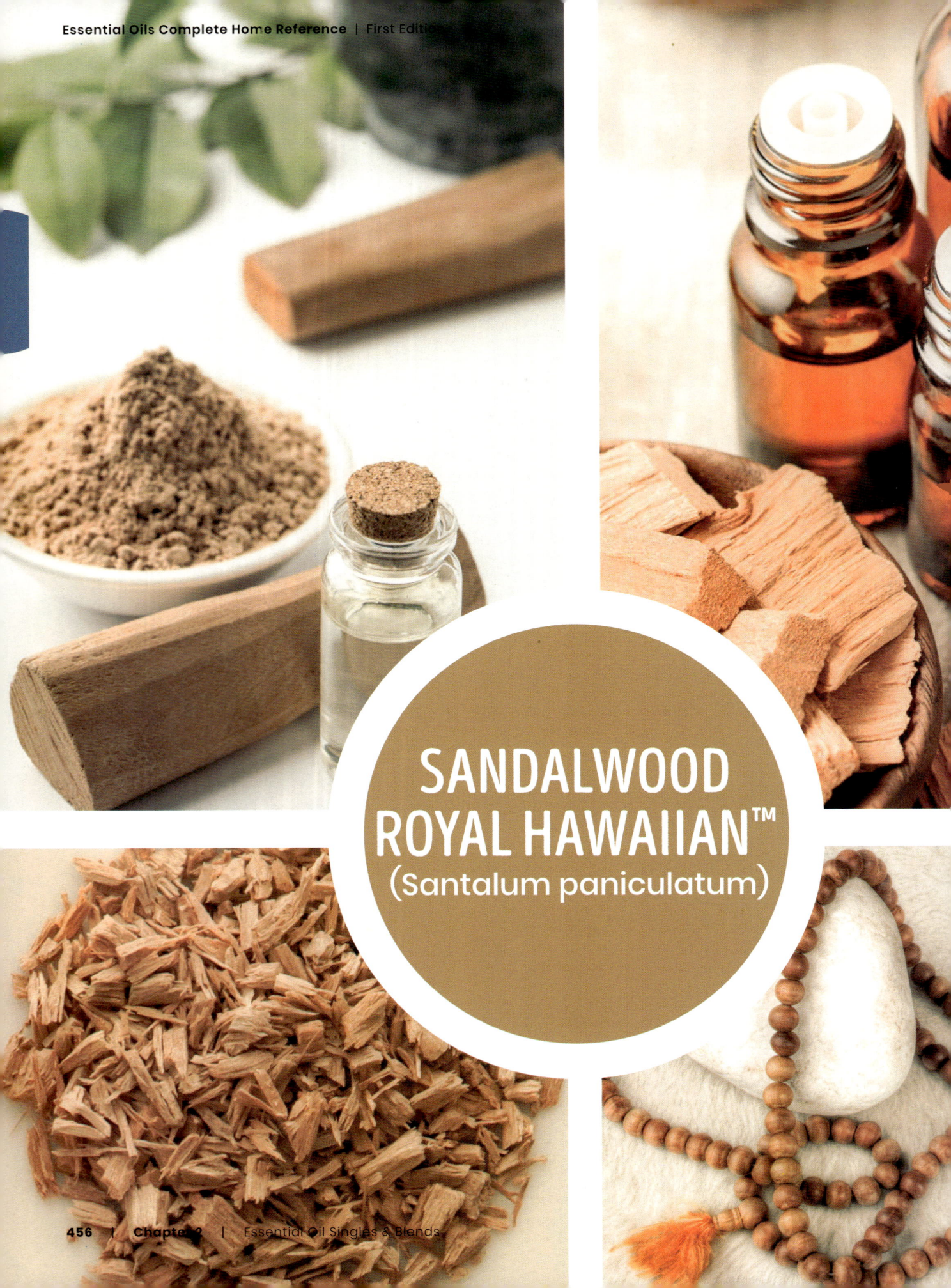

SANDALWOOD ROYAL HAWAIIAN™
(Santalum paniculatum)

BOTANICAL FAMILY:
Santalaceae

PLANT ORIGIN:
USA (Hawaii)

EXTRACTION METHOD:
Steam distilled from wood

KEY CONSTITUENTS:
Cis-Alpha-Santalol (30-56%),
Cis-Beta-Santalol (16-21%)

HISTORICAL DATA:
Sandalwood has been used for centuries in Ayurvedic medicine for skin revitalization, yoga, and meditation. Listed in Dioscorides' De Materia Medica (AD 78), Europe's first authoritative guide to medicines, which became the standard reference work for herbal treatments for over 1,700 years.

Research at Brigham Young University in Provo, Utah, documented Sandalwood's ability to inhibit several types of cancerous cells (Stevens).

MEDICAL PROPERTIES:
Antitumoral, antibacterial, antiviral, immune stimulant

USES:
Cancer, viral infections (herpes simplex, herpes zoster, cold sores, human papilloma virus, etc.), skin conditions (acne, wrinkles, scars, etc.), colds, digestive problems, hemorrhoids, muscle problems

FRAGRANT INFLUENCE:
Woodsy, soft, nurturing aroma; enhances deep sleep and may help remove negative programming from the cells. It is high in sesquiterpenes that stimulate the pineal gland and the limbic region of the brain, the center of emotions. The pineal gland is responsible for releasing melatonin, a powerful immune stimulant and antitumoral agent. It can be grounding and stabilizing.

DIRECTIONS:
Aromatic: 6o. Topical: Neat. Dietary: Take as a dietary supplement.

CAUTIONS:

SELECTED RESEARCH:
Teixeira da Silva JA, Kher MM, Soner D, Page T, Zhang X, Nataraj M, Ma G. Sandalwood: basic biology, tissue culture, and genetic transformation. Planta. 2016 Apr;243(4):847-87. Epub 2016 Jan 8.

Dozmorov MG, Yang Q, Wu W, Wren J, Suhail MM, Woolley CL, Young DG, Fung KM, Lin HK. Differential effects of selective frankincense (Ru Xiang) essential oil versus non-selective sandalwood (Tan Xiang) essential oil on cultured bladder cancer cells: a microarray and bioinformatics study. Chin Med. 2014 Jul 2;9:18. eCollection 2014.

Kulkarni CR, Joglekar MM, Patil SB, Arvindekar AU. Antihyperglycemic and antihyperlipidemic effect of Santalum album in streptozotocin induced diabetic rats. Pharm Biol. 2012 Mar;50(3):360-5. Epub 2011 Dec 1.

*Royal Hawaiian Sandalwood™ is a trademark of Jawmin, LLC.

BOTANICAL FAMILY:
Apiaceae

PLANT ORIGIN:
Belgium, Bulgaria, Netherlands

EXTRACTION METHOD:
Steam distilled from root

KEY CONSTITUENTS:
Beta-Phellandrene (≤30%), Alpha-Phellandrene (7-28%), Alpha-Pinene (10-27%), Delta-3-Carene (8-15%), Limonene (3-13%), Sabinene (≤12%), Trans-Beta Ocimene (≤7%), Cis-Beta-Ocimene (≤4%)

SANDALWOOD, SACRED
(Santalum album)

Sandalwood has been used for centuries in Ayurvedic medicine for skin revitalization, yoga, and meditation. It is listed in Dioscorides' De Materia Medica (AD 78), Europe's first authoritative guide to medicines, which became the standard reference work for herbal treatments for over 1,700 years. A 2017 study showed a powdered mixture of Arnica montana, Calendula officinalis, Mentha arvensis, and Santalum album was effective in palliative (end-of-life) wound care. At the conclusion of the study, 95 percent of caregivers recommended the mixture for this population. Also, research at Brigham Young University documented the ability of sandalwood essential oil to inhibit several types of cancerous cells (Stevens).

MEDICAL PROPERTIES:
Antioxidant, antimicrobial, antitumoral, antibacterial, antiviral, immune stimulating, anti-inflammatory

USES:
Cancer, viral infections (herpes simplex, herpes zoster, cold sores, human papilloma virus, etc.), skin conditions (acne, wrinkles, scars, etc.), colds, digestive problems, hemorrhoids, skin problems, muscle problems

FRAGRANT INFLUENCE:
Rich, woodsy, slightly sweet aroma; enhances deep sleep and may help remove negative programming from the cells. It is high in sesquiterpenes that stimulate the pineal gland and the limbic region of the brain, the center of emotions. The pineal gland is responsible for releasing melatonin, a powerful immune stimulant and antitumoral agent. Can be grounding and stabilizing.before trauma or anger was experienced

DIRECTIONS:
Aromatic: 60. Topical: Neat. Dietary: Take as a dietary supplement.

CAUTIONS:

SELECTED RESEARCH:

Mohankumar A, Shanmugam G, Kalaiselvi D, Levenson C, Nivitha S, Thiruppathi G, Sundararaj P. East Indian sandalwood (Santalum album L.) oil confers neuroprotection and geroprotection in Caenorhabditis elegans via activating SKN-1/Nrf2 signaling pathways. RSC Adv. 2018 Oct. 3; 8(58): 33753-33774.

Madisetti M, Kelechi TJ, Mueller M, Amella EJ, Prentice MA. Feasibility, acceptability, and tolerability of RGN107 in the palliative wound care management of chronic wound symptoms. J Wound Care. 2017 Jan 2;26(Sup1):S25-S34.

Moy RL, Levenson C. Sandalwood album oil as a botanical therapeutic in dermatology. J Clin Aesthet Dermatol. 2017 Oct;10(10):34-9. Epub 2017 Oct 1.

Teixeira da Silva JA, Kher MM, Soner D, Page T, Zhang X, Nataraj M, Ma G. Sandalwood: basic biology, tissue culture, and genetic transformation. Planta. 2016 Apr;243(4):847-87. Epub 2016 Jan 8.

Santha S, Dwivedi C. Anticancer effects of Sandalwood (Santalum album). Anticancer Res. 2015 Jun;35(6):3137-45.

Dozmorov MG, Yang Q, Wu W, Wren J, Suhail MM, Woolley CL, Young DG, Fung KM, Lin HK. Differential effects of selective frankincense (Ru Xiang) essential oil versus non-selective sandalwood (Tan Xiang) essential oil on cultured bladder cancer cells: a microarray and bioinformatics study. Chin Med. 2014 Jul 2;9:18. eCollection 2014.

Kulkarni CR, Joglekar MM, Patil SB, Arvindekar AU. Antihyperglycemic and antihyperlipidemic effect of Santalum album in streptozotocin induced diabetic rats. Pharm Biol. 2012 Mar;50(3):360-5. Epub 2011 Dec 1.

Essential Oil Singles & Blends | **Chapter 2**

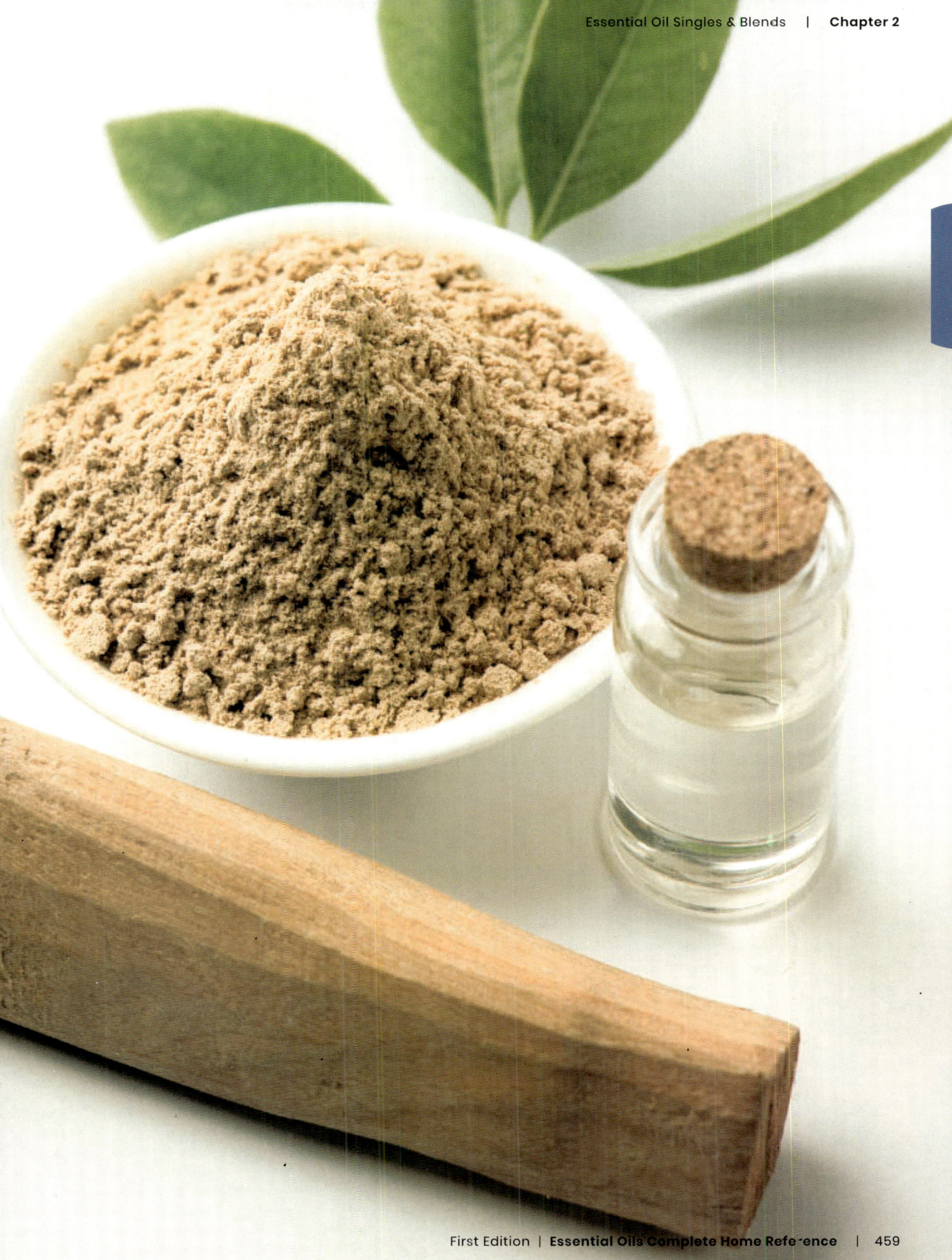

First Edition | **Essential Oils Complete Home Reference** | 459

Essential Oils Complete Home Reference | First Edition

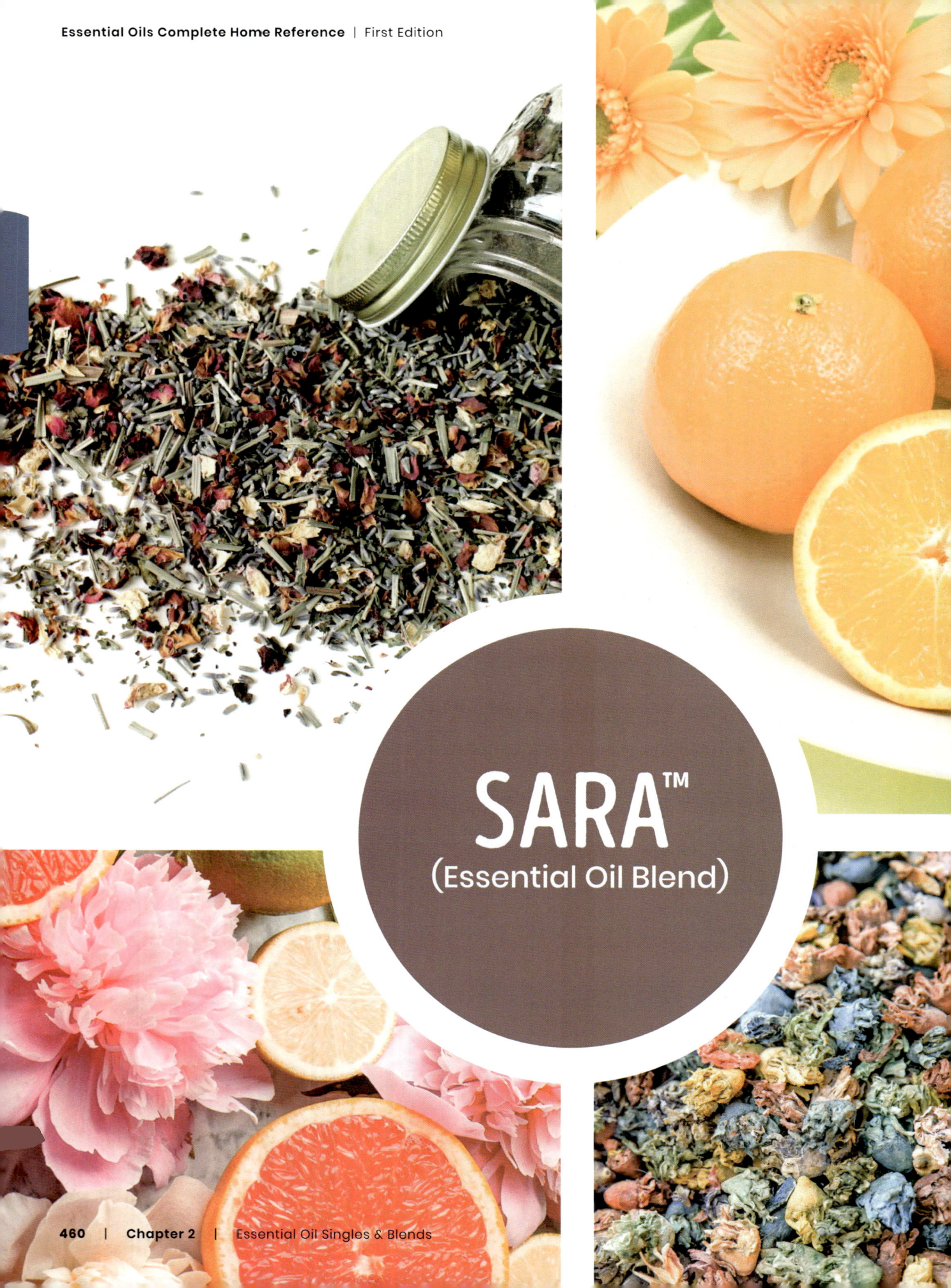

SARA™
(Essential Oil Blend)

460 | Chapter 2 | Essential Oil Singles & Blends

Essential Oil Singles & Blends | **Chapter 2**

ABOUT SARA™:

This very specific blend enables one to relax into a mental state that facilitates the release of trauma from sexual and/or ritual abuse. SARA also helps unlock other traumatic experiences such as physical and emotional abuse.

MEDICAL PROPERTIES & USES:

Anti-inflammatory, antimicrobial, antioxidative, emotional supportive, calming, cardiovascular supportive, disease inhibitory, organ protective, pain or swelling reducing, performance enhancing/stimulating, wellness supportive

INGREDIENTS:

Sweet almond oil, Ylang Ylang, Geranium, Lavender, Orange, Cedarwood, Blue Cypress, Davana, Citrus Hystrix, Jasmine, Rose, Matricaria (German Chamomile), Blue Tansy, Grapefruit, Tangerine, Spearmint, Lemon, Ocotea, White Lotus

DIRECTIONS:

Aromatic: 3o. Topical: 20-8o.

CAUTIONS: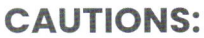

First Edition | **Essential Oils Complete Home Reference** | 461

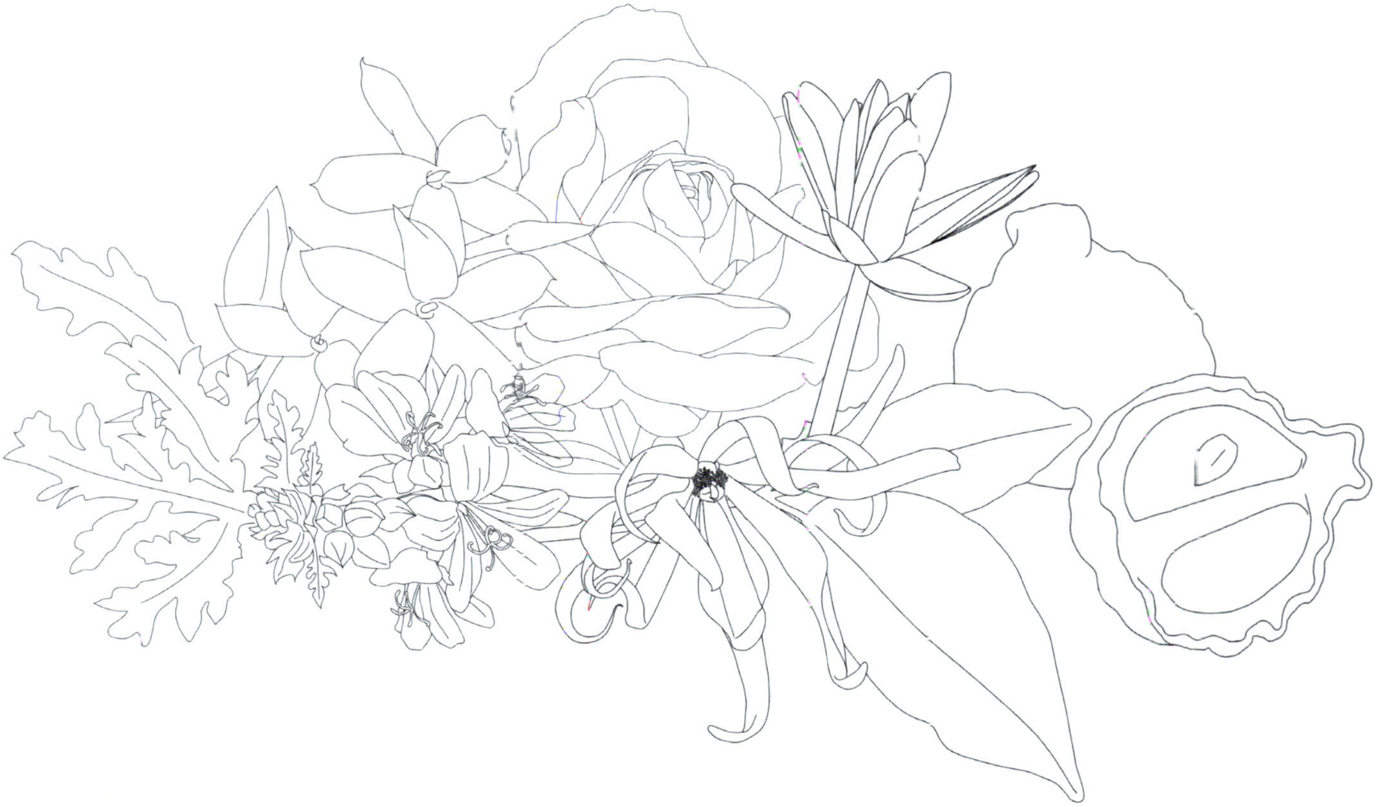

SCLARESSENCE™ & SCLARESSENCE VITALITY™
(Essential Oil Blend)

This blend balances hormones naturally using essential oil phytoestrogens. It helps to increase estrogen levels by supporting the body's own production of hormones. It combines the soothing effects of Peppermint with the balancing power of Fennel and Clary Sage and the calming action of Spanish Sage for an extraordinary topical and aromatic blend and Vitality dietary supplement.

MEDICAL PROPERTIES & USES:
Antimicrobial, antioxidative, calming, digestion or elimination supportive/nausea reducing, oral protective, pain or swelling reducing, performance enhancing/stimulating, respiratory system supportive, hormone supportive

INGREDIENTS:
Clary Sage, Peppermint, Spanish Sage, Fennel

DIRECTIONS:
Aromatic: 30. Topical: 50-50. Dietary (Vitality): Dilute 1 drop with 1 drop of V-6 or other pure carrier oil. Put in a capsule and take up to 3 times daily or as needed.

CAUTIONS: **Do not use in conjunction with any other hormone products.**

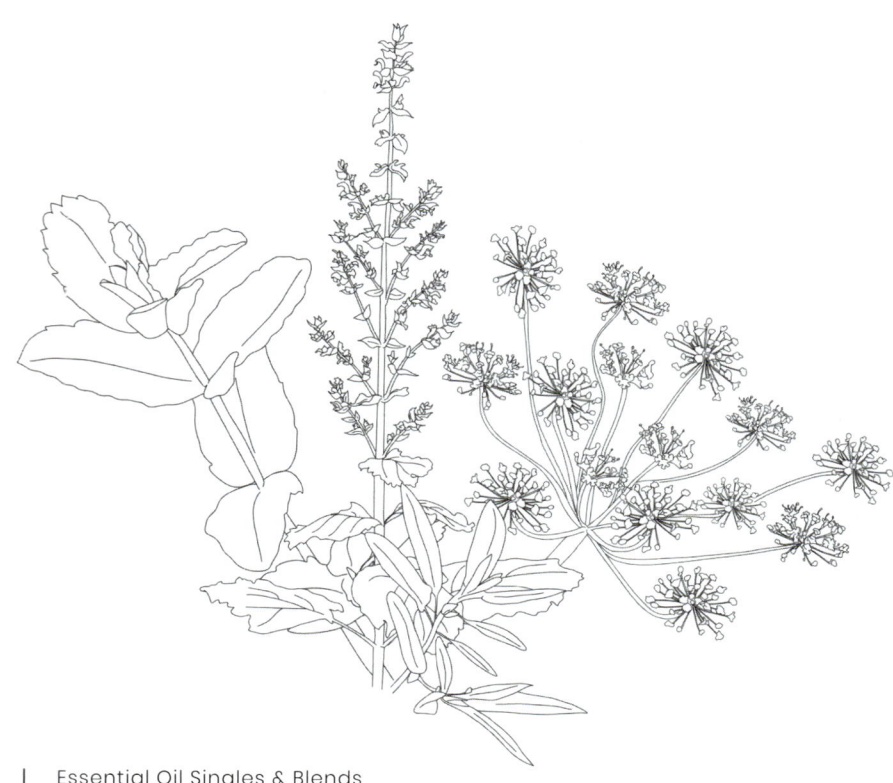

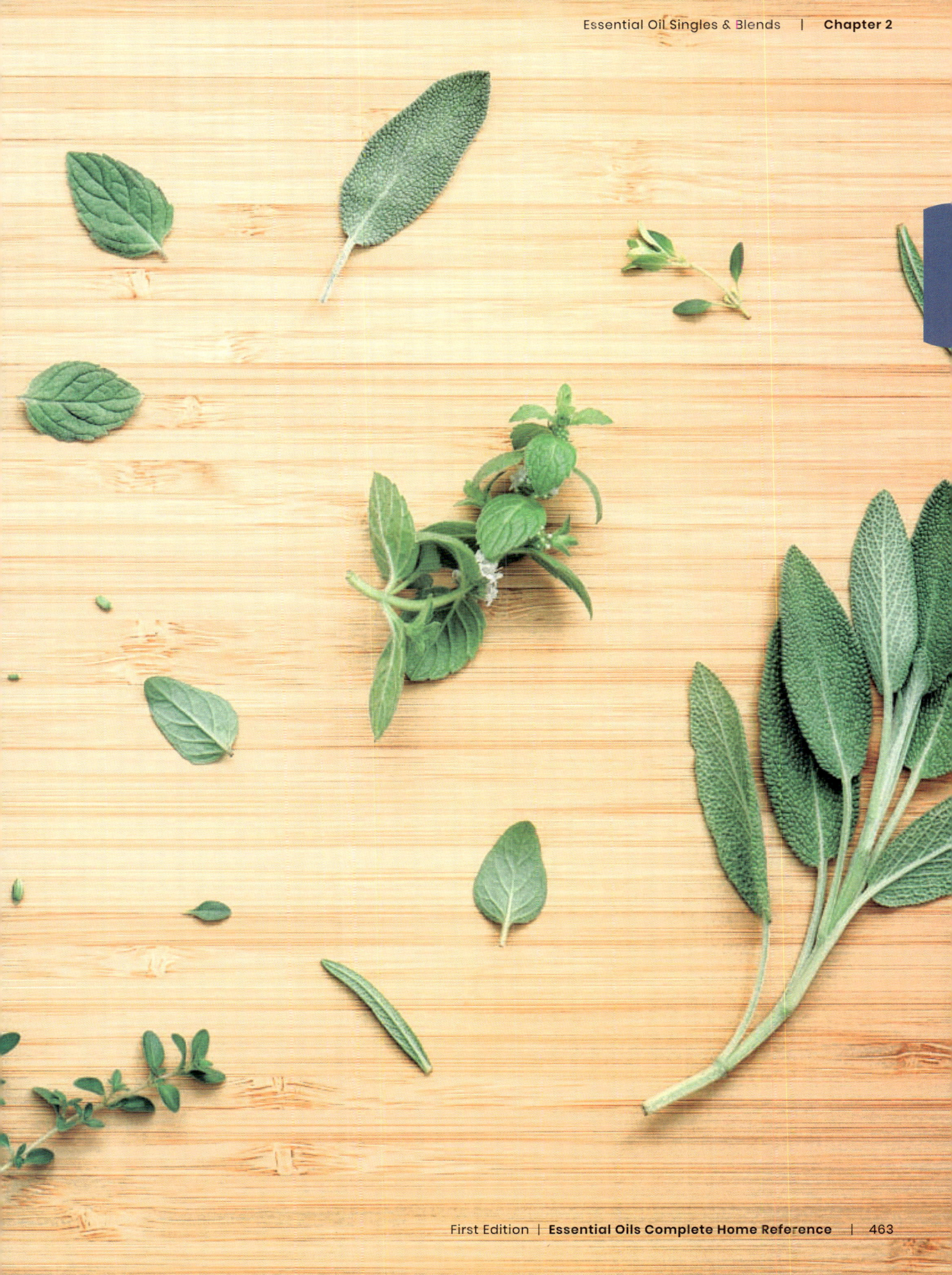

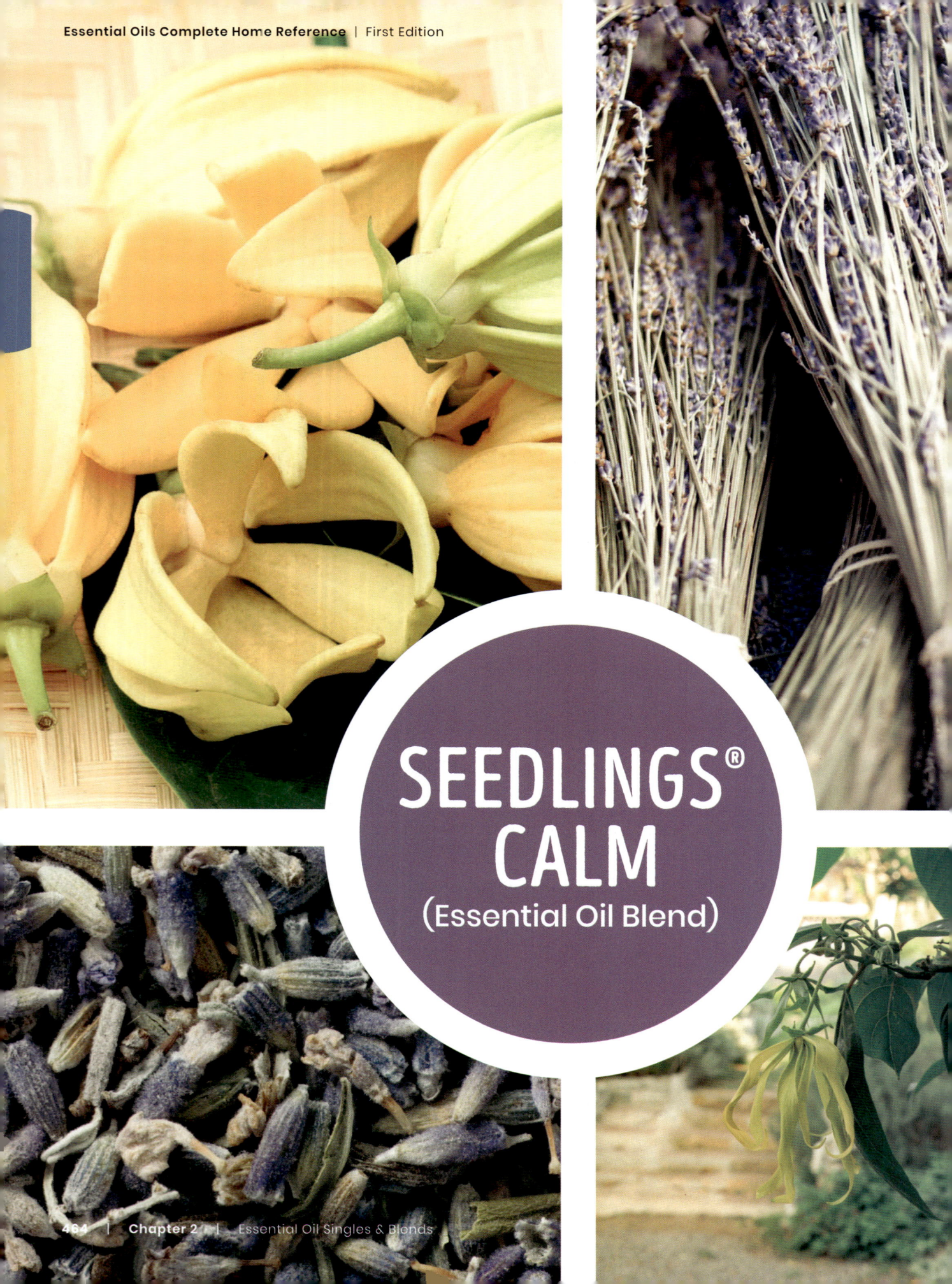

ABOUT SEEDLINGS® CALM:

This soothing, gentle blend is formulated for children, with its soft, relaxing, floral notes. A great way to spread the scent of your favorite Seedlings products around your child's room or the whole house.

MEDICAL PROPERTIES & USES:
Anti-inflammatory, antimicrobial, antioxidative, calming, relaxing, disease inhibitory, organ protective, pain or swelling reducing

INGREDIENTS:
Lavender, Caprylic/capric triglyceride, Coriander, Bergamot, Ylang Ylang, Geranium

DIRECTIONS:
Aromatic: 30

CAUTIONS: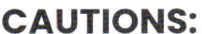
To be handled only by a trusted adult or under adult supervision For aromatic use only. Clean the diffuser thoroughly after each use.

ALLERGEN WARNING:
Contains coconut product.

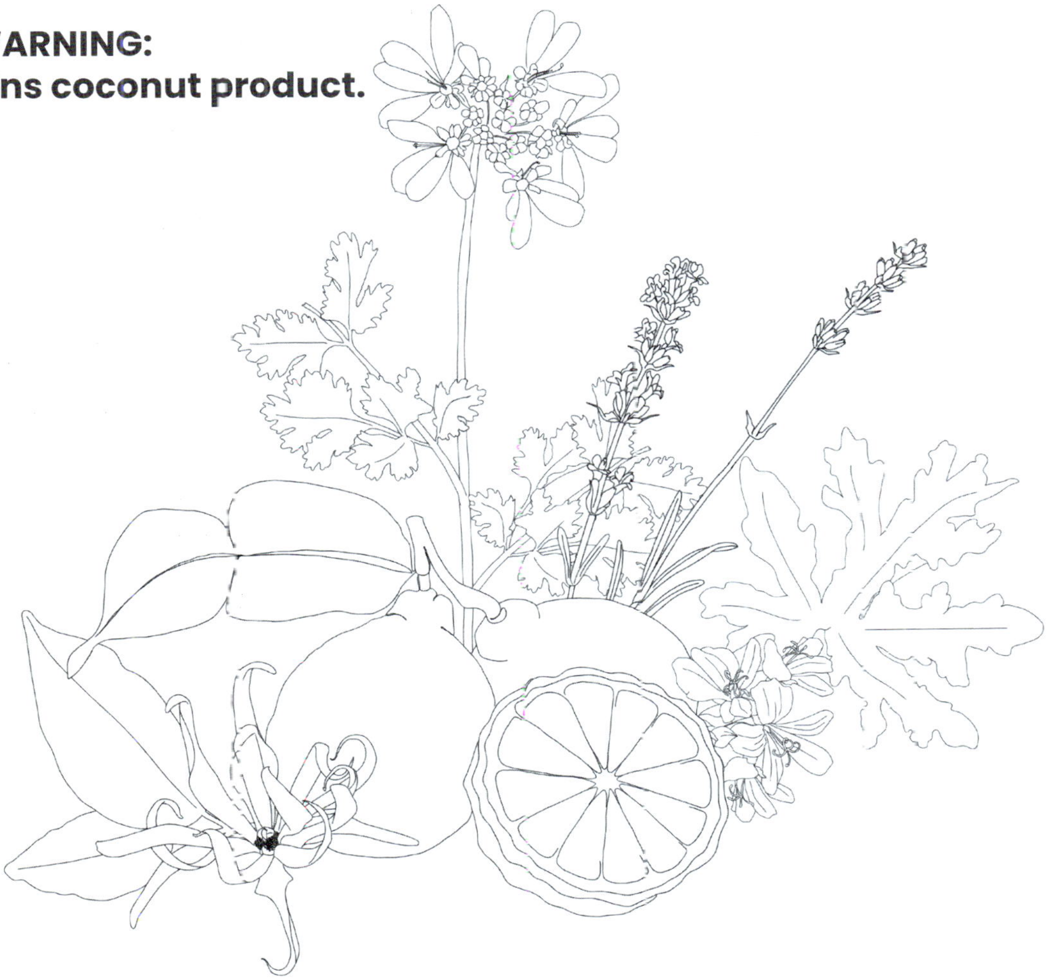

SENSATION™
(Essential Oil Blend)

This beautiful smell is profoundly romantic, refreshing, and arousing. It amplifies the excitement of experiencing new heights of self-expression and awareness. Sensation is also nourishing and hydrating for the skin and is beneficial for many skin problems.

MEDICAL PROPERTIES & USES:
Anti-inflammatory, antimicrobial, antioxidative, emotion supportive, calming, disease inhibitory, organ protective, pain or swelling reducing, skin improving

INGREDIENTS:
Coriander, Ylang Ylang, Bergamot (Furocoumarin-free), Jasmine, Geranium

DIRECTIONS:
Aromatic: 6o. Topical: Neat. Use as a compress over abdomen.

CAUTIONS:

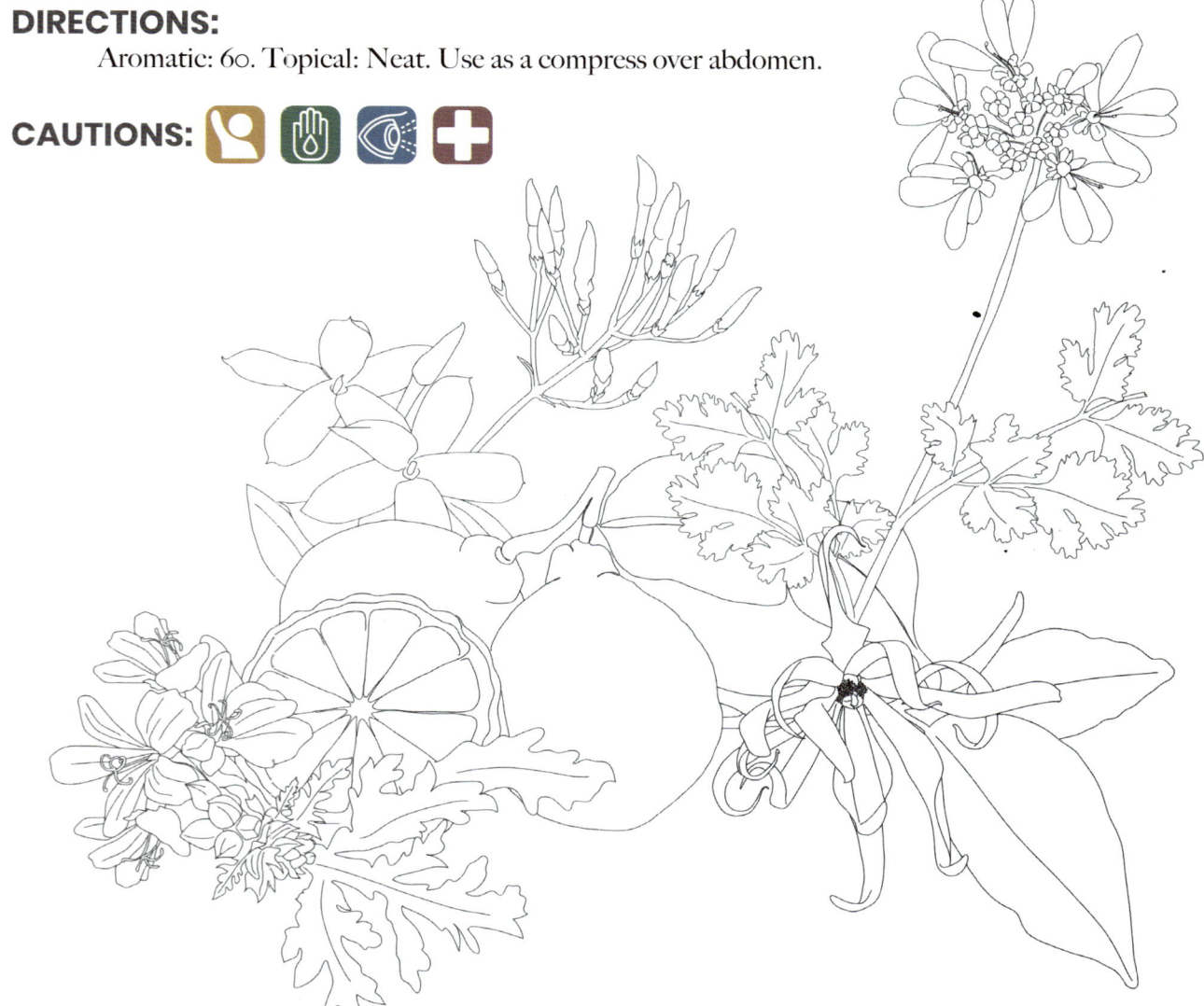

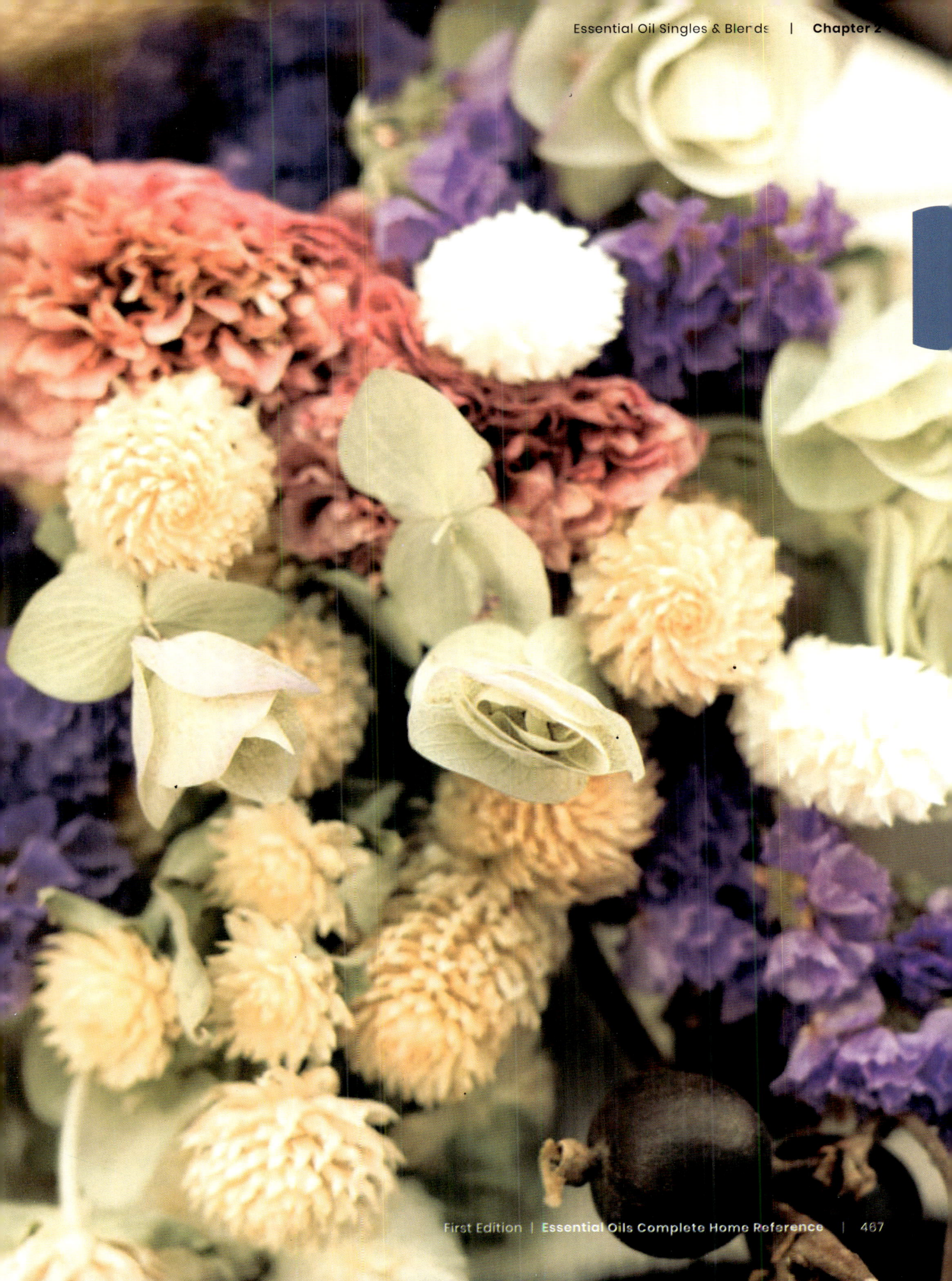

Essential Oils Complete Home Reference | First Edition

SHUTRAN™
(Essential Oil Blend)

468 | Chapter 2 | Essential Oil Singles & Blends

ABOUT SHUTRAN™:

Shutran is an empowering essential oil blend that is specifically designed for men to boost feelings of masculinity and confidence.

MEDICAL PROPERTIES & USES:

Anti-inflammatory, antimicrobial, antioxidative, emotion supportive, calming, cardiovascular supportive, digestion or elimination supportive/nausea reducing, disease inhibitory, organ protective, pain or swelling reducing, skin and hair improving

INGREDIENTS:

Idaho Blue Spruce, Ylang Ylang, Ocotea, Hinoki, Davana, Cedarwood, Lavender, Coriander, Lemon, Northern Lights Black Spruce

DIRECTIONS:

Topical: Neat. In case of sensitivity, dilute 15 drops in 10 ml of V-6.

CAUTIONS:

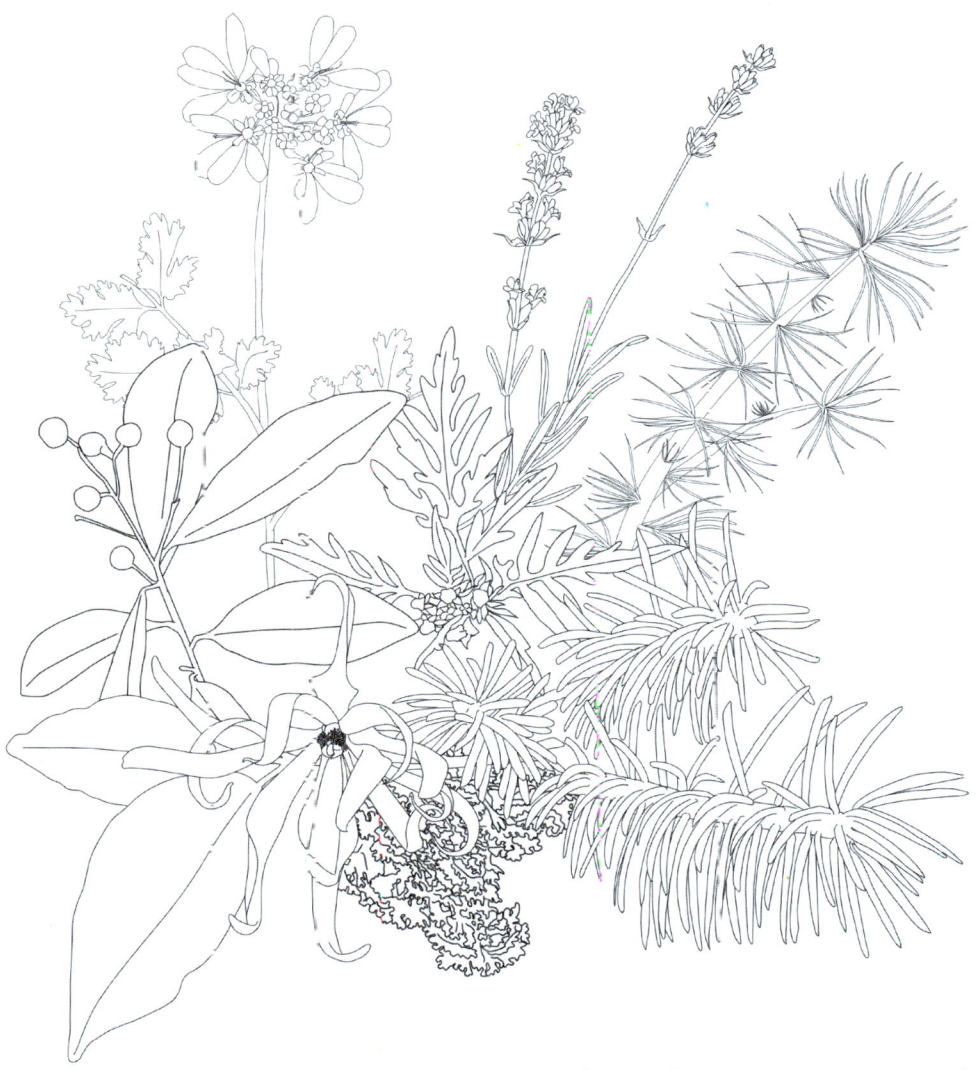

SLIQUE™ ESSENCE
(Essential Oil Blend)

Slique Essence combines powerful essential oils and stevia extract to support healthy weight-management goals. It suppresses food cravings, especially when used in conjunction with Slique Tea or any of the Slique products. The oils in this blend add a flavorful and uplifting element to any day, with the added support of Spearmint to aid proper digestion. Ocotea essential oil was chosen for its irresistible cinnamon-esque aroma, which can help trigger feelings of fullness and reduce the number of unexpected cravings. Slique Essence is antibacterial, antifungal, a lipid regulator, and a glucose regulator.

Stevia is added as an all-natural sweetener that provides a pleasant, sweet taste with no added calories.

MEDICAL PROPERTIES & USES:
Antimicrobial, antibacterial, antifungal, antioxidative, calming, cardiovascular supportive, dietary, digestion or elimination supportive/nausea reducing, cravings reducing, glucose regulator, disease inhibitory, pain or swelling reducing, wellness supportive

INGREDIENTS:
Grapefruit, Tangerine, Spearmint, Lemon, Ocotea, Stevia extract

DIRECTIONS:
Aromatic: Direct inhalation preferred. Note: The stevia extract in this formula may impede diffuser performance. Topical: Neat. Dilution not required, except for the most sensitive skin. Shake well and apply liberally to temples, back of neck, or wrists as needed. Dietary: Shake vigorously before use. Add 2-4 drops to 4-6 oz. of your favorite beverage, Slique Tea, or water. Use between and during meals regularly throughout the day whenever hunger feelings occur.

CAUTIONS:

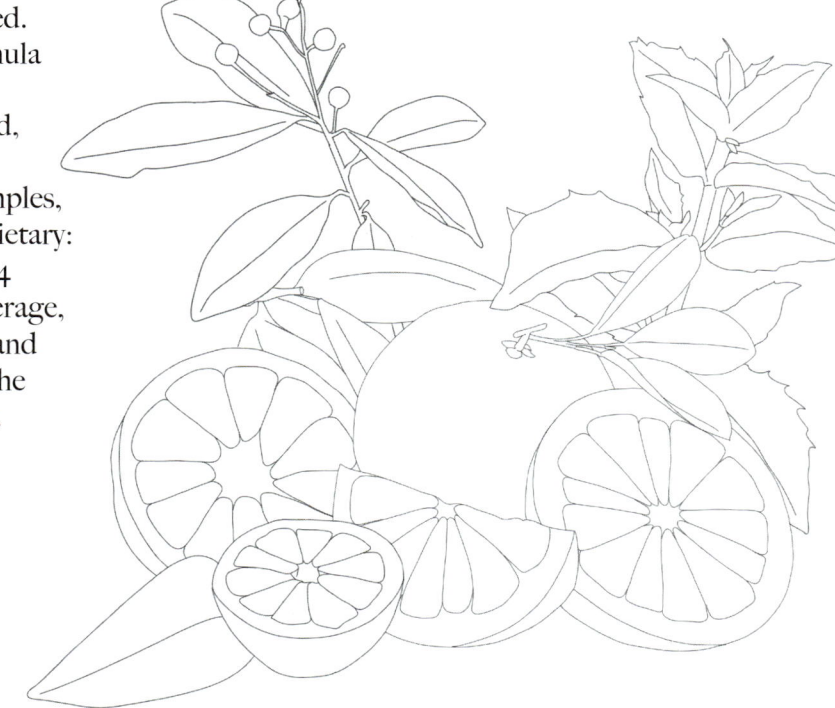

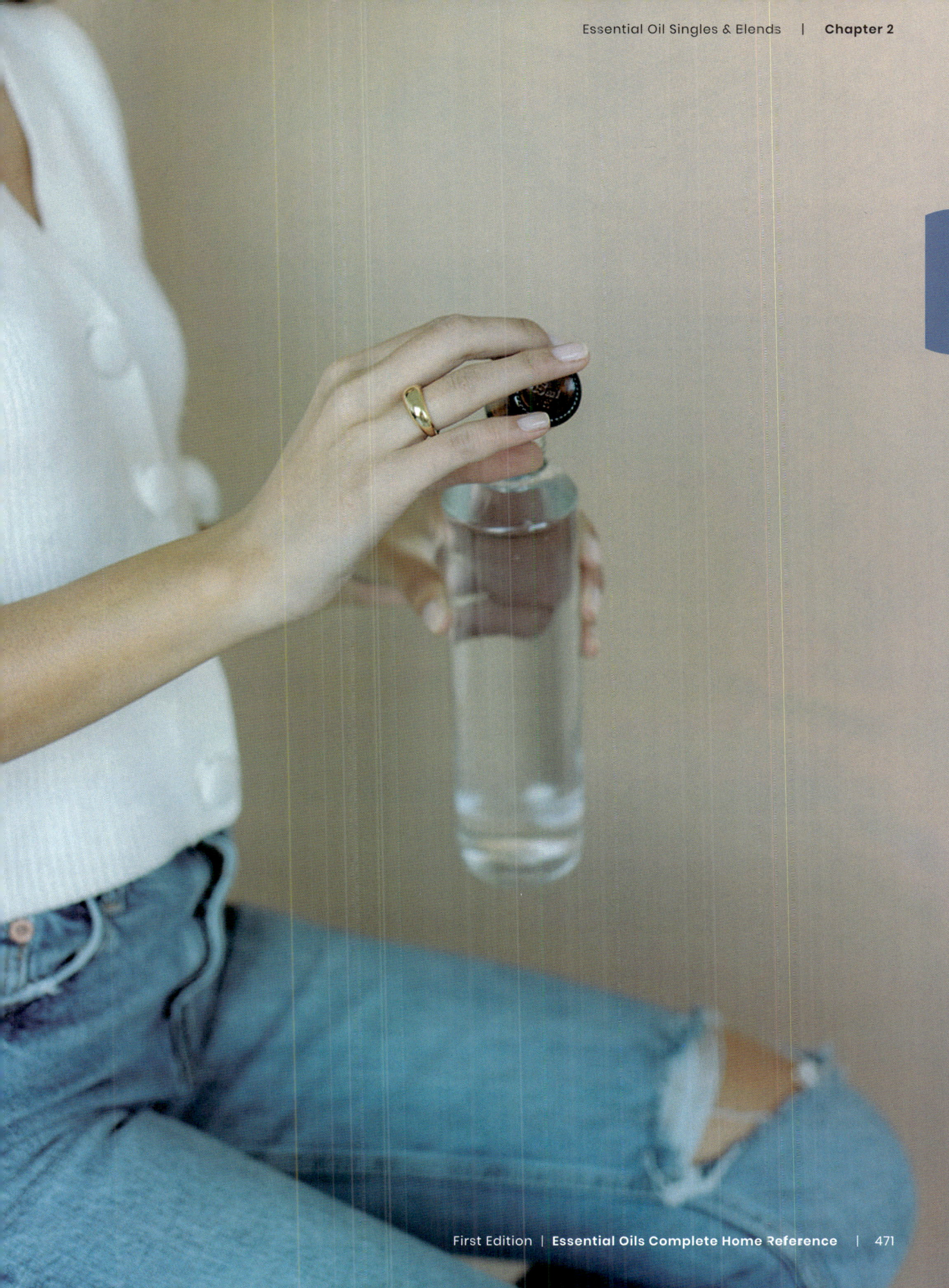

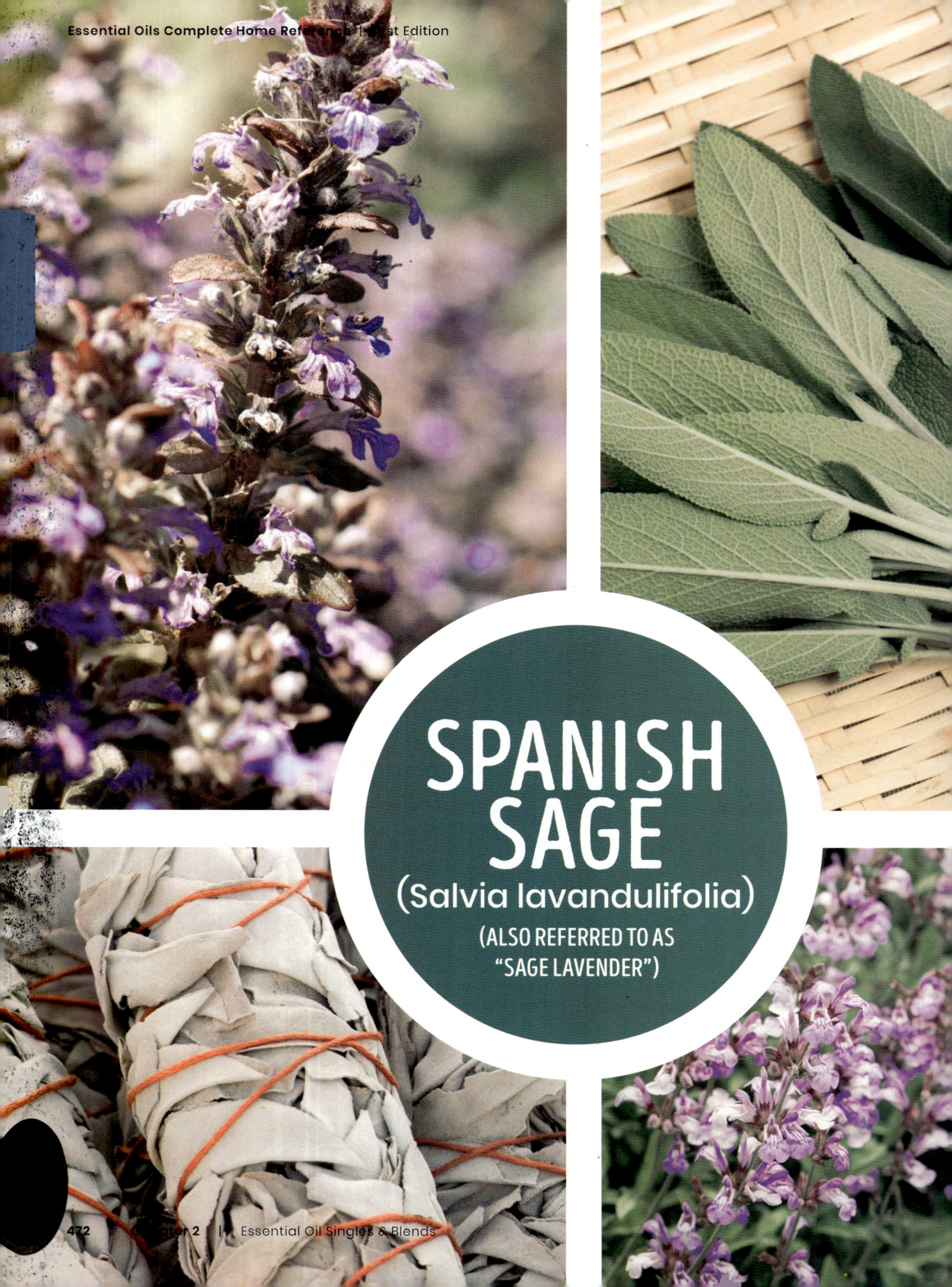

SPANISH SAGE
(Salvia lavandulifolia)
(ALSO REFERRED TO AS "SAGE LAVENDER")

Essential Oil Singles & Blends | **Chapter 2**

BOTANICAL FAMILY:
Lamiaceae

PLANT ORIGIN:
Spain

EXTRACTION METHOD:
Steam distilled from aerial parts of flowering plants

KEY CONSTITUENTS:
Camphor (20-42%),
Eucalyptol (17-35%),
Alpha-Pinene (4-11%),
Alpha-Terpinyl Acetate (up to 8%),
Limonene (3-7%),
Linalyl Acetate (up to 5%),
Linalol (up to 4%)

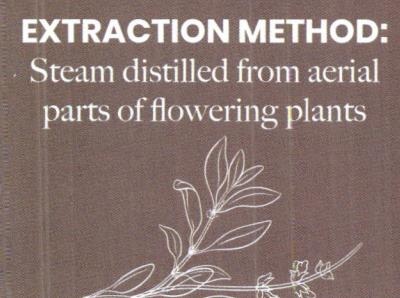

HISTORICAL DATA:
The sage plant has been highly praised throughout history for its powers of longevity and healing. Pliny the Elder said that sage (called "salvia" by the Romans) was used as a local anesthetic for the skin and as a diuretic, in addition to other uses. It was considered a sacred herb to the Romans and was harvested by a person wearing a white tunic who had well-washed, bare feet. During the Middle Ages, the plant was prized throughout Europe because of its exceptional healing effects and was used in a mixture with other herbs designed to ward off the plague. In Spain, Spanish sage is used in cooking. It has a stronger aroma and flavor than common sage (S. officinalis).

MEDICAL PROPERTIES:
Antiseptic, astringent, chemopreventive, expectorant, reduces mucous, reduces fevers, purifies the blood, eliminates toxins, aids digestion, lowers blood sugar levels without affecting insulin levels, acts as a tonic to improve general health

USES:
Age-related memory loss, cuts, acne, arthritis, dandruff, colds, flu, eczema, hair loss, sweating, anxiety, headaches, asthma, laryngitis, coughs, muscular aches and pains, depression, epilepsy, soothing agent, menstrual disorders, digestive disorders. In food it is used as a spice; in manufacturing it is used as a fragrance component in soaps and cosmetics.

FRAGRANT INFLUENCE:
Camphoraceous, herbaceous, similar to Rosemary

DIRECTIONS
Aromatic: 6o. Topical: 5o-5o.
Dietary: Take as a dietary supplement.

CAUTIONS:
Avoid if epileptic. Avoid use on persons with high blood pressure.

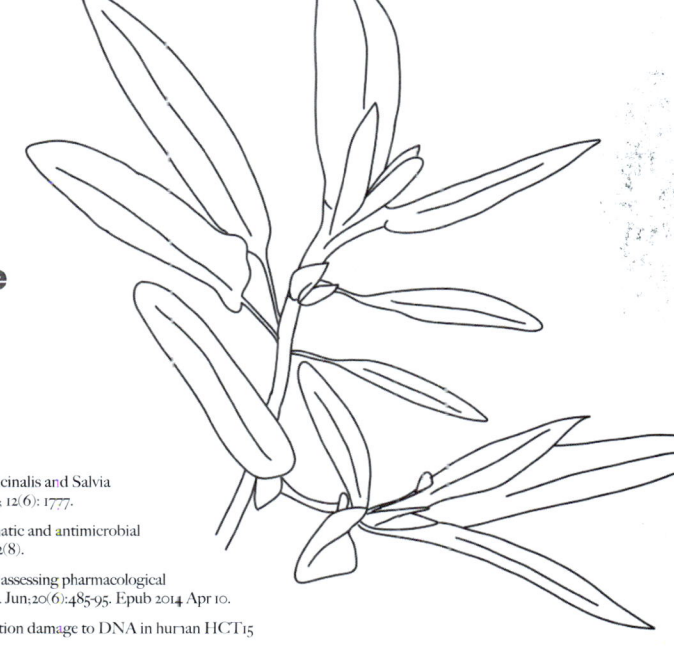

SELECTED RESEARCH:
Dinel A-L, Lucas C, Gillemet D, Layé S, Pallet V, Joffre C. Chronic Supplementation with a mix of Salvia officinalis and Salvia lavandulaefolia Improves Morris Water Maze Learning in Normal Adult C57Bl/6J Mice. Nutrients. 2020 Jun; 12(6): 1777.

Cutillas AB, Carrasco A, Martinez-Gutierrez R, Tomas V, Tudela J. Composition and antioxidant, antienzymatic and antimicrobial activities of volatile molecules from Spanish Salvia lavandulifolia (Vahl) essential oils. Molecules. 2017 Aug 21;22(8).

Miroddi M, Navarra M, Quattropani MC, Calapai F, Gangemi S, Calapai G. Systematic review of clinical trials assessing pharmacological properties of Salvia species on memory, cognitive impairment and Alzheimer's disease. CNS Neurosci Ther. 2014 Jun;20(6):485-95. Epub 2014 Apr 10.

Ramos AA, Pedro D, Collins AR, Pereira-Wilson C. Protection by Salvia extracts against oxidative and alkylation damage to DNA in human HCT15 and CO115 cells. J Toxicol Environ Health A. 2012;75(13-15):765-75.

Kennedy DO, Dodd FL, Robertson BC, Okello EJ, Reay JL, Scholey AB, Haskell CF. Monoterpenoid extract of sage (Salvia lavandulaefolia) with cholinesterase inhibiting properties improves cognitive performance and mood in healthy adults. J Psychopharmacol. 2011 Aug;25(8):1088-100. Epub 2010 Oct 11.

BOTANICAL FAMILY: Lamiaceae

PLANT ORIGIN: USA

EXTRACTION METHOD: Steam distilled from leaves

KEY CONSTITUENTS: Carvone (up to 50%), Limonene (up to 39%), Cis-Dihydrocarvone (up to 10%), Menthone (up to 3%)

SPEARMINT & SPEARMINT VITALITY™
(Mentha spicata)

Spearmint is gentler than Peppermint yet is beneficial for headaches and migraines, fatigue, nervous disorders, and digestive problems.

MEDICAL PROPERTIES:
Increases metabolism, antibacterial, antispasmodic, anti-inflammatory, antiseptic, mucolytic, gallbladder stimulant, digestive aid, antitumoral

USES:
Obesity, intestinal/digestive disorders, nausea, hepatitis

FRAGRANT INFLUENCE:
Opens and releases emotional blocks and brings about a feeling of balance and a lasting sense of well-being

DIRECTIONS:
Aromatic: 30. Topical: 50-50. Dietary (Vitality): Dilute 1 drop with 1 drop of V-6 or other pure carrier oil. Put in a capsule and take up to 3 times daily.

CAUTIONS:

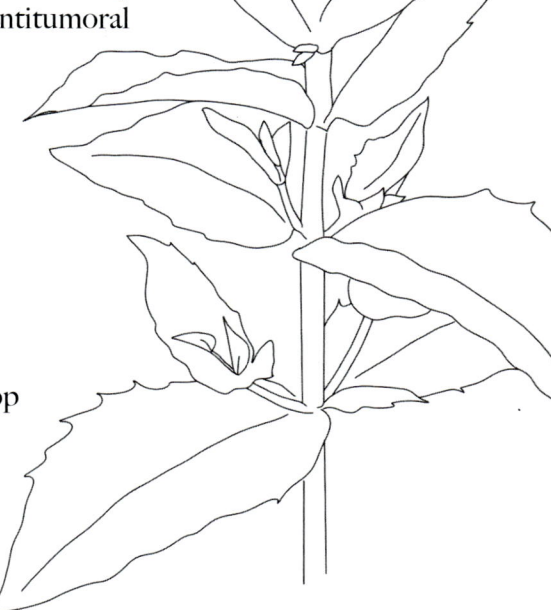

SELECTED RESEARCH:

Ali-Shtayeh MS, Jamous RM, Abu-Zaitoun SY, Khasati AI, Kalbouneh SR. Biological Properties and Bioactive Components of Mentha spicata L. Esssential Oil: Focus on Potential Benefits in the Treatment of Obesity, Alzheimer's Diseasem, Dermotophytosis, and Drug-Resistant Infections. Evid Based Complement Alternat Med. 2019; 2019: 3834265. Published online 2019 Oct 20.

Bardaweel SK, Backhiche B, Al Salamat HA, Rezzoug M, Gherib A, Flamini G. Chemical composition, antioxidant, antimicrobial and antiproliferative activities of essential oil of Mentha spicata L. (Lamiaceae) from Algerian Saharan atlas. BMC Complement Altern Med. 2018 Jul 3;18(1):201.

Ben Saad A, Rjeibi I, Alimi H, Ncib S, Bouhamda T, Zouari N. Protective effects of Mentha spicata against nicotine-induced toxicity in liver and erythrocytes of Wistar rats. Appl Physiol Nutr Metab. 2018 Jan;43(1):77-83. Epub 2017 Sep 11.

Mahboubi M. Mentha spicata as natural analgesia for treatment of pain in osteoarthritis patients. Complement Ther Clin Pract. 2017 Feb;26:1-4.

Nogoceke FP, Barcaro IM, de Sousa DP, Andreatini R. Antimanic-like effects of (R)-(-)-carvone and (S)-(+)-carvone in mice. Neurosci Lett. 2016 Apr 21;619:43-8. Epub 2016 Mar 10.

Snoussi M, Noumi E, Trabelsi N, Flamini G, Papetti A, De Feo V. Mentha spicata essential oil: chemical composition, antioxidant and antibacterial activities against planktonic and biofilm cultures of Vibrio pp. strains. Molecules. 2015 Aug 7;20(8):14402-24.

Shahbazi Y. Chemical composition and in vitro antibacterial activity of Mentha spicata essential oil against common food-borne pathegenic bacteria. J Pathog. 2015;2015:916305. Epub 2015 Aug 16.

Tayarani-Najaran Z, Talasaz-Firoozi E, Nasiri R, Jalali N, Hassanzadeh M. Antiemetic activity of volatile oil from Mentha spicata and Mentha x piperita in chemotherapy-induced nausea and vomiting. Ecancermedicalscience. 2013;7:290. Epub 2013 Jan 31.

Mousavi NS, Mousavi Nadoshan S, Owlia P, Moein Najafabadi L, Rasooli I, Saderi H, Salari MH. Effects of subinhibitory concentrations of essential oils of Mentha spicata and Cuminum cyminum on virulence factors of Pseudomonas aeruginosa. J Med Plants. 2010 Winter;9(6):124-30.

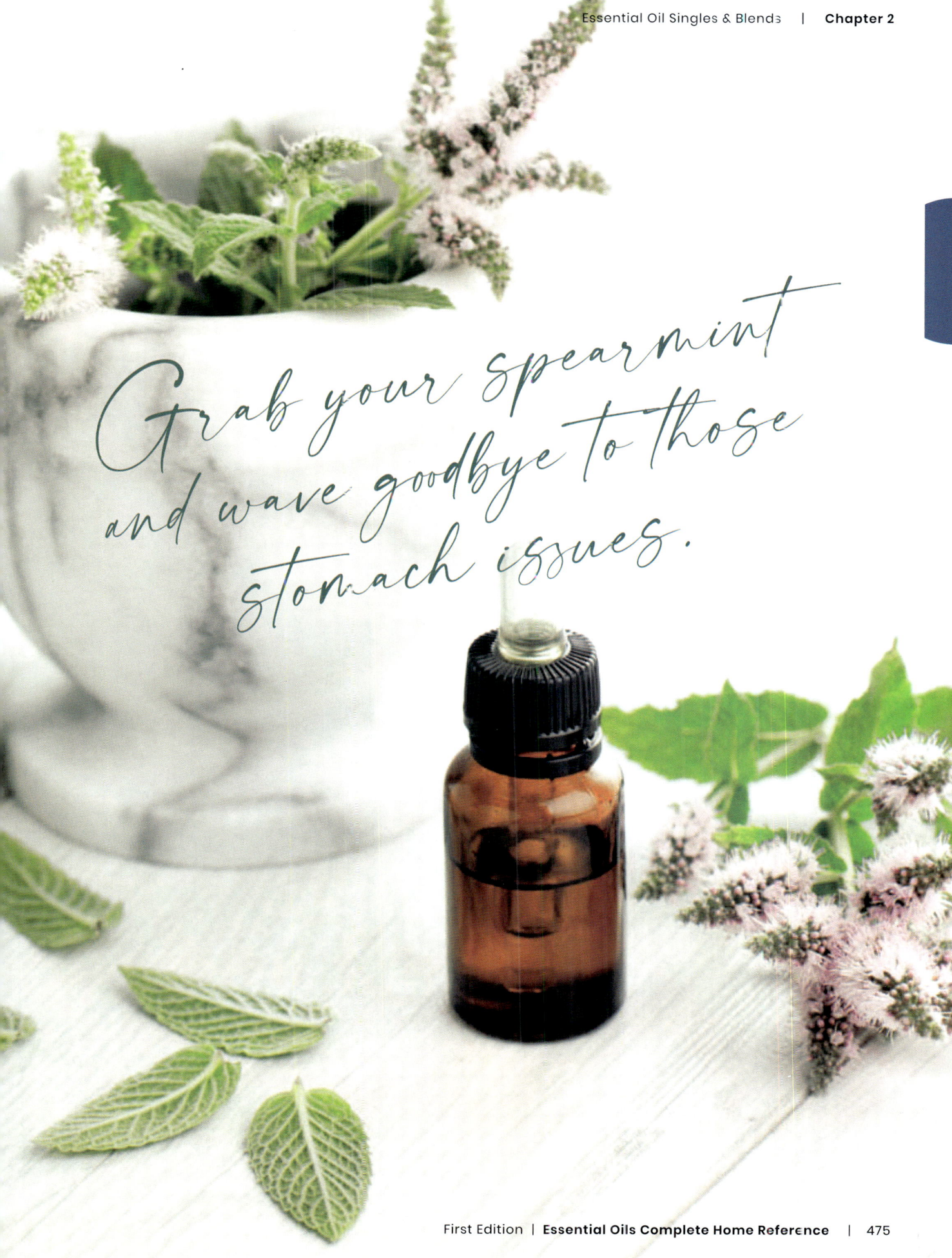

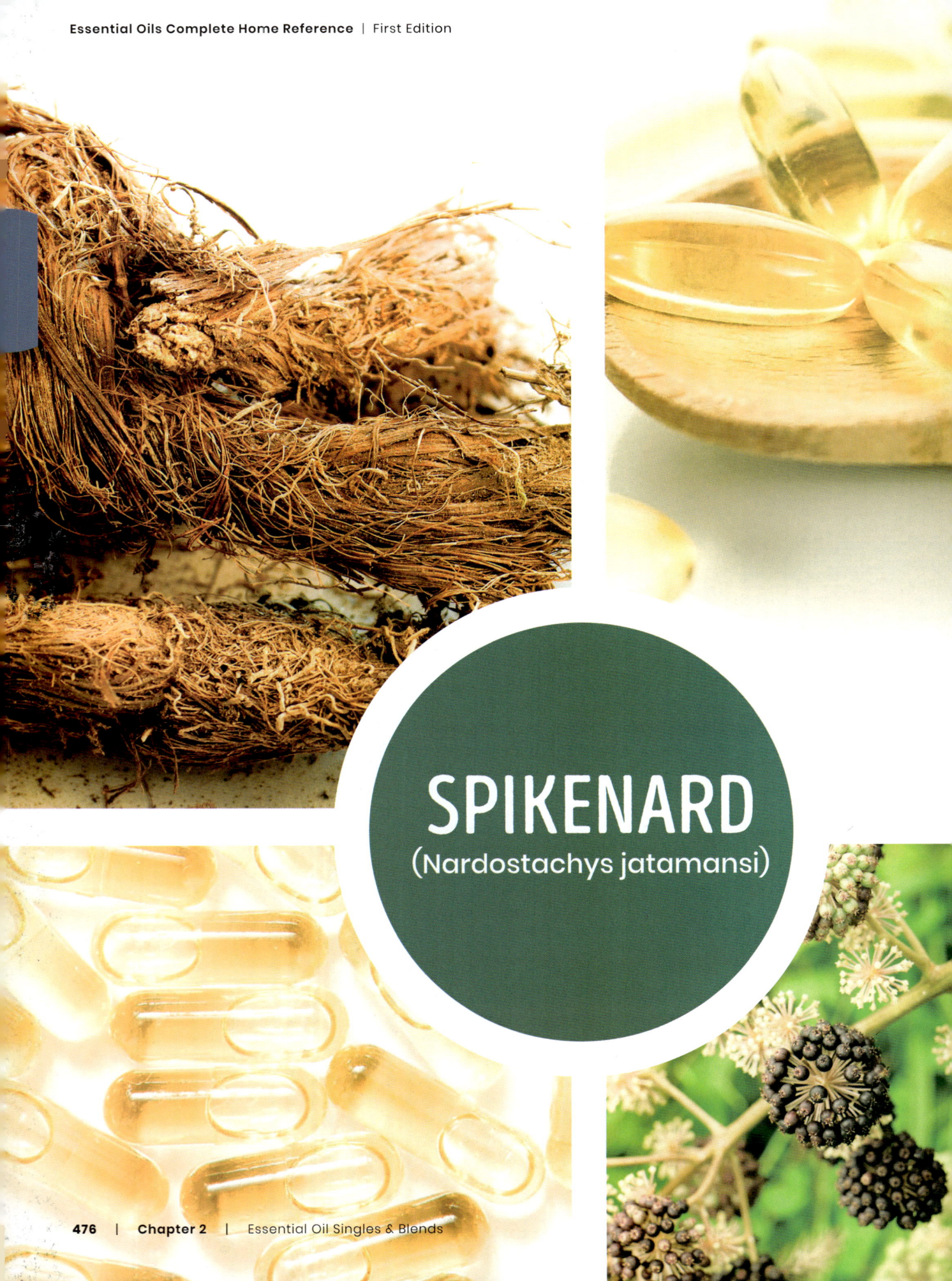

SPIKENARD
(Nardostachys jatamansi)

BOTANICAL FAMILY:
Valerianaceae

PLANT ORIGIN:
India

EXTRACTION METHOD:
Steam distilled from roots

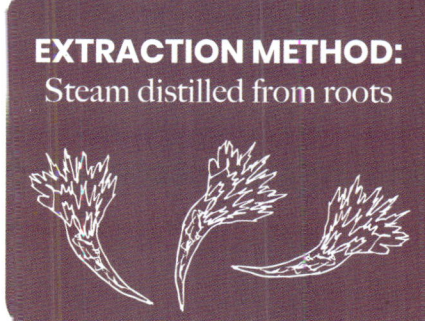

KEY CONSTITUENTS:
Calarene (10-35%),
Beta-Maaliene (4-13%),
Alpha-Copaene (5-14%),
Aristolene (2-9%),
Seychellene (1-5%),
Patchouli Alcohol (2-7%),
9-Aristolen-1-ol (1-5%)

HISTORICAL DATA:
Highly regarded in India as a medicinal herb. It was the one of the most precious oils in ancient times, used only by priests, kings, or high initiates. References in the New Testament describe how Mary of Bethany used spikenard oil to anoint the feet of Jesus before the Last Supper (John 12:3). Current research shows interest in Spikenard's neuroprotective mechanisms in cognitive disorders with sesquiterpenes that are anti-neuroinflammatory. Breast cancer, hyperglycemia, and hypertension are also investigated.

MEDICAL PROPERTIES:
Antibacterial, antifungal, anticancer, anti-inflammatory, antioxidant, antidepressant, neuroprotectant, anxiolytic, immune stimulant

USES:
Insomnia, menstrual problems/PMS, heart arrhythmias, nervous tension, anxiety, depression, stress, healthy skin, uplifting, athlete's foot, joint pain, migraine, constipation

FRAGRANT INFLUENCE:
Relaxing, soothing, helps nourish and regenerate the skin

DIRECTIONS:
Aromatic: 6o. Topical: Neat. Dilution not required except for the most sensitive skin. Dietary: Take as a dietary supplement.

CAUTIONS: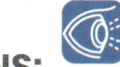

SELECTED RESEARCH:
Cornara L, Ambu G, Trombetta D, Denaro M, Alloisio S, Frigero J, Labra M, Ghimire G, Valussi M, Smeriglio A. Comparative and Functional Screening of Three Species Traditionally used as Antidepressants: Valeriana officinalis L., Valeriana jatamansi Jones ex Roxb. and Nardostachys jatamansi (D. Don) DC. Plants (Basel). 2020 Aug 5;9(8):E924.

Bose B, Tripathy D, Chatterjee A, Tandon P, Kumaria S. Secondary metabolite profiling, cytotoxicity, anti-inflammatory potential and in vitro inhibitory activities of Nardostachys jatamansi on key enzymes linked to hyperglycemia, hypertension and cognitive disorders. Phytomedicine 2019 Mar 1;55:58-69.

Yoon C-S, Kim D-C, Park J-S, Kim K-W, Kim Y-C, Oh H. Isolation of Novel Sesquiterpenoids and Anti-neuroinflammatory Metabolites from Nardostachys jatamansi. Molecules. 2018 Sep 17;23(9): 2367.

Liu QF, Jeon Y, Sung Y-w, Lee JH, Jeong H, Kim Y-M, Yun HS, Chin Y-W, Jeon S, Cho KS, Koo B-S. Nardostachys jatamansi Ethanol Extract Ameliorates Aβ42 Cytotoxicity. Biol Pharm Bull. 2018 41, 470-477.

Jalali S, Zarrinhaghighi A, Sadraei S, Ghasemi Y, Sakhteman A, Faridi P. A System Pharmacology Study for Deciphering Anti Depression Activity of Nardostachys jatamani. Curr Drug Metab. 2018;19(5):469-476.

Razack S, Kandikattu HK, Venuprasad MP, Amruta N, Khanum F, Chuttani K, Mishra AK. Anxiolytic actions of Nardostachys jatamansi via GABA benzodiazepine channel complex mechanism and its biodistribution studies. Metab Brain Dis. 2018 Oct;33(5): 1533-1549.

Chaudhary S, Chandrashekar KS, Pai KSR, Setty MM, Devkar RA, Reddy ND, Shoja MH. Evaluation of antioxidant and anticancer activity of extract and fractions of Nardostachys jatamansi DC in breast carcinoma. BMC Complement Altern Med. 2015; 15: 50.

Bae GS, Bae GS, Heo KH, Choi SB, Jo IJ, Kim DG, Shin JY, Seo SH, Park KC, Lee DS, Oh H, Kim YC, Song HJ, Shin BC, Park SJ. Beneficial effects of fractions of Nardostacys jatamansi on lipopolysaccharide-induced inflammatory response. Evid Based Complement Alternat Med. 2014;2014:837835.

Dhuna K, Dhuna V, Bhatia G, Singh J, Kamboj SS. Cytoprotective effect of methanolic extract of Nardostachys jatamansi against hydrogen peroxide induced oxidative damage I C6 glioma cells. Acta Biochem Pol. 2013;60(1):21-31. Epub 2013 Mar 20.

Lyle N, Bhattacharyya D, Sur TK, Munshi S, Paul S, Chatterjee S, Gomes A. Stress modulating antioxidant effect of Nardostachys jatamansi. Indian J Biochem Biophys. 2009 Feb;46(1):93-8.

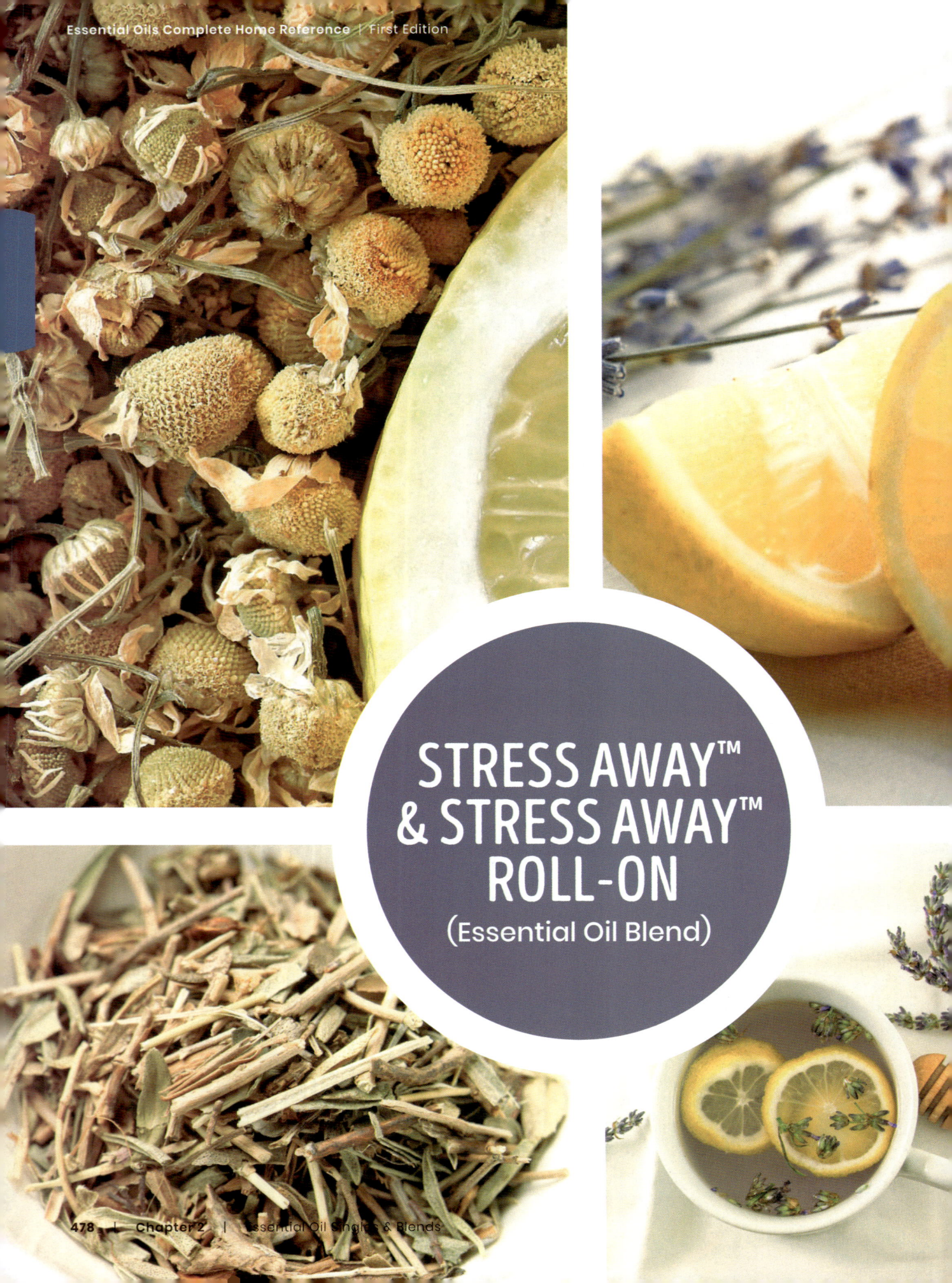

ABOUT STRESS AWAY™ & STRESS AWAY™ ROLL-ON:

This is a gentle, fragrant blend that brings feelings of peace and tranquility to both children and adults and helps relieve daily stress and nervous tension. It helps with normal, everyday stress, improves mental response, restores equilibrium, promotes relaxation, and lowers hypertension.

MEDICAL PROPERTIES & USES:
Anti-inflammatory, antimicrobial, emotion supporting, calming, cardiovascular supportive, disease inhibitory, insecticidal/antiparasitic, pain or swelling reducing

INGREDIENTS:
Balsam Copaiba, Lime, Cedarwood, Vanilla, Ocotea, Lavender

DIRECTIONS:
Aromatic: (30). Topical: Neat. Shake well and apply liberally to temples, back of neck, or wrists as needed.

CAUTIONS: 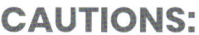   In case of sensitivity, dilute 10 drops in 10 ml of V-6.

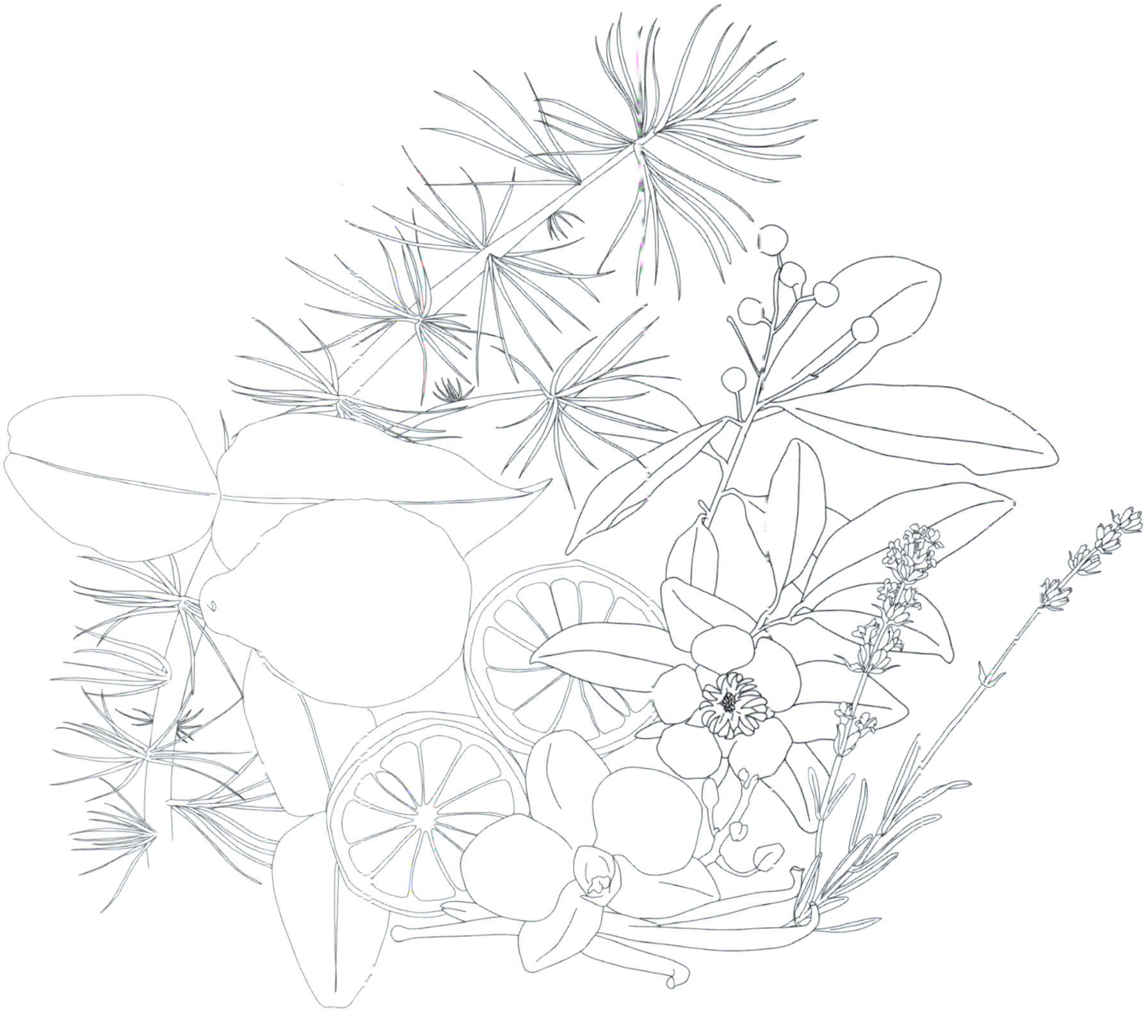

SURRENDER™
(Essential Oil Blend)

This inviting oil blend helps one surrender aggression and a controlling attitude. Stress and tension are released quickly when we surrender willfulness.

MEDICAL PROPERTIES & USES:
Anti-inflammatory, antimicrobial, antioxidative, emotion supporting, calming, cardiovascular supportive, disease inhibitory, organ protective, pain or swelling reducing, performance enhancing/stimulating, skin and hair improving

INGREDIENTS:
Lavender, Lemon, Black Spruce, Roman Chamomile, Angelica, Mountain Savory, Matricaria (German Chamomile)

DIRECTIONS:
Aromatic: 6o. Topical: Neat.

CAUTIONS:

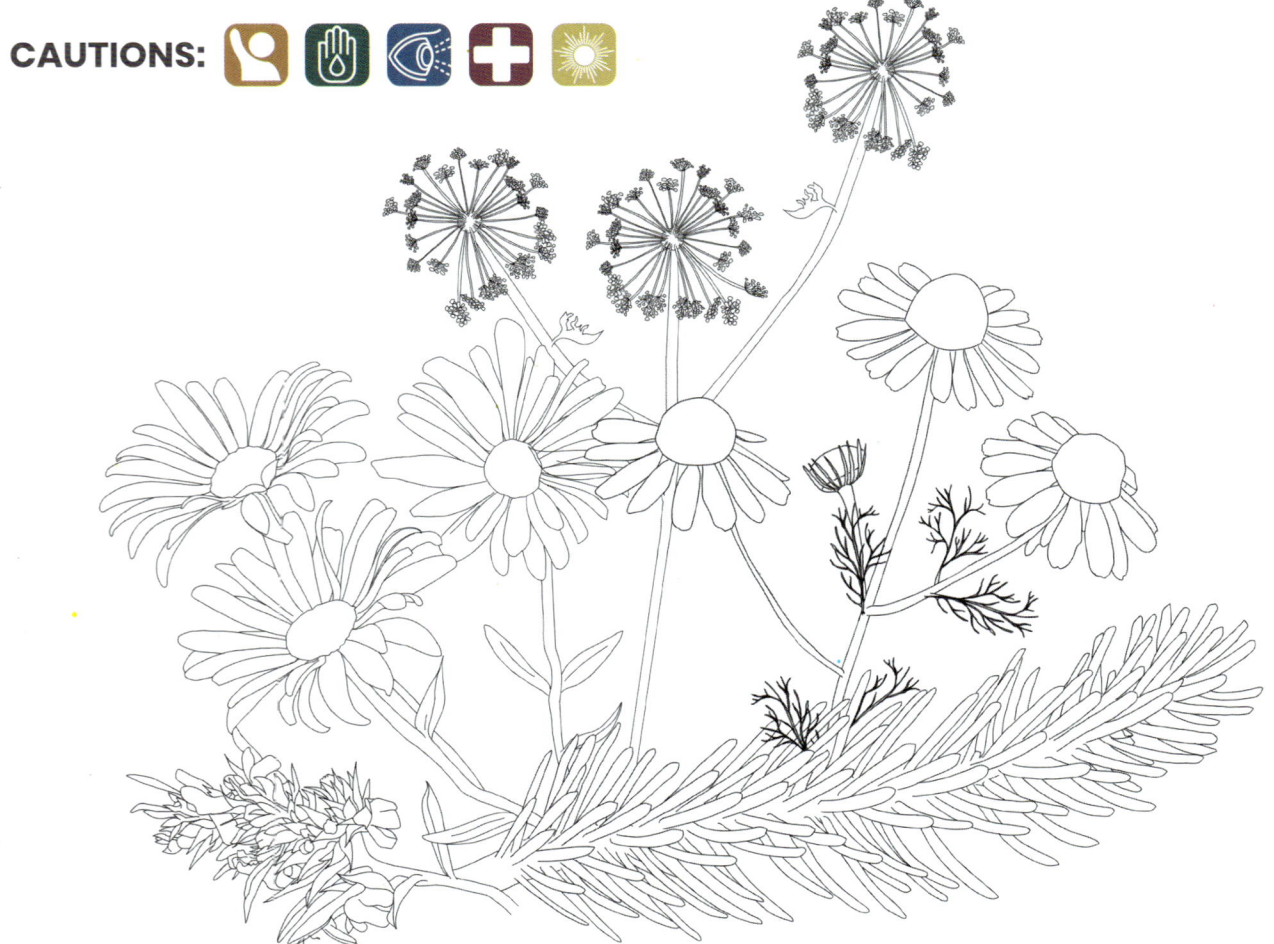

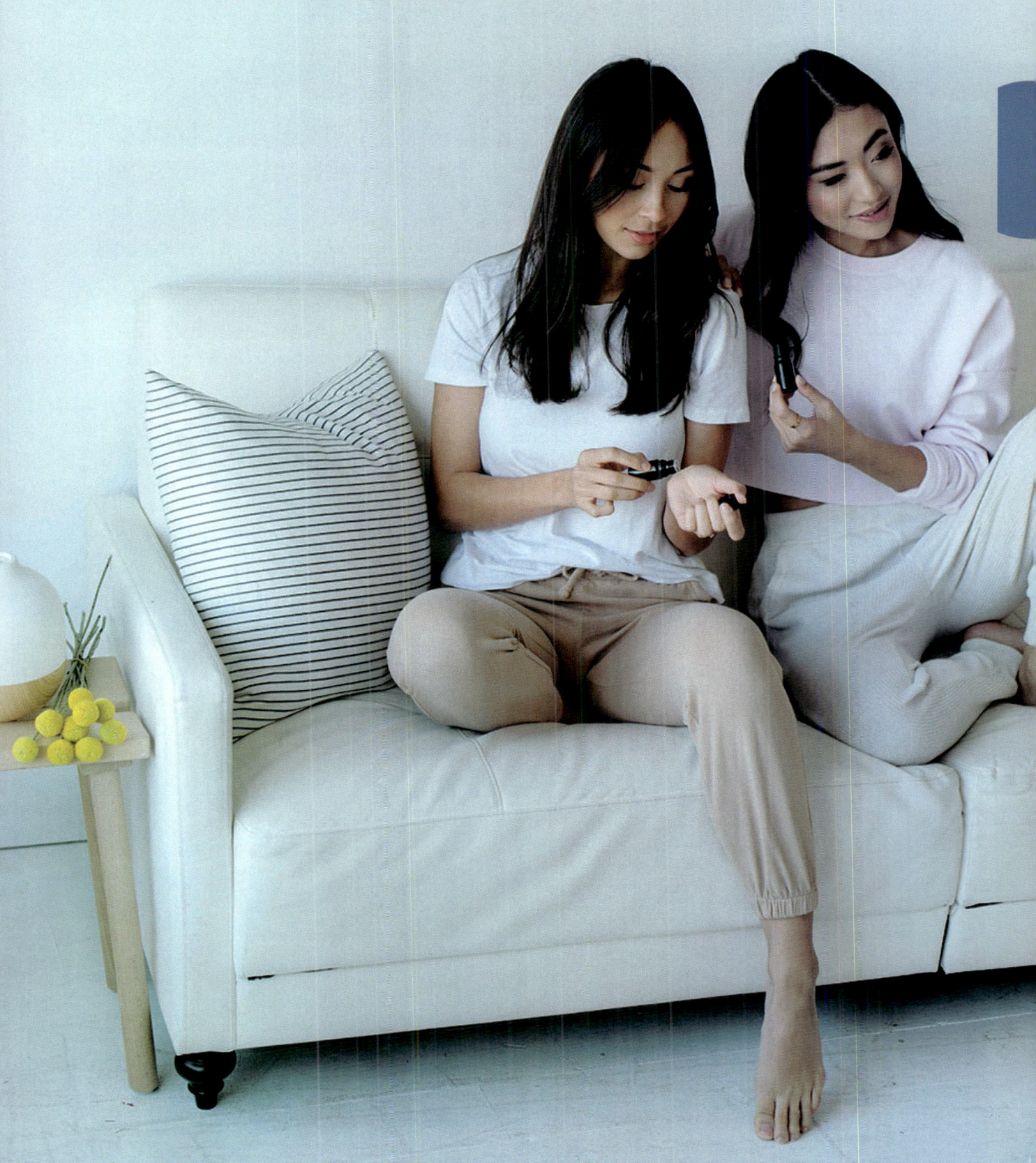

BOTANICAL FAMILY: Rutaceae

PLANT ORIGIN: Mexico

EXTRACTION METHOD: Cold pressed from rind

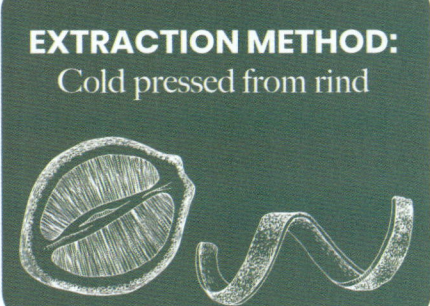

KEY CONSTITUENTS: Limonene (88-99%), Gamma-Terpinene (up to 5%), Myrcene (1-3

TANGERINE & TANGERINE VITALITY™
(Citrus reticulata)

Because of Tangerine essential oil's high limonene content, it is a great booster for the immune system.

MEDICAL PROPERTIES:
Antifungal, anticancerous, antimicrobial, antitumoral, relaxant, antispasmodic, digestive aid, and circulatory enhancer; immune supporting; rich in limonene, which has been extensively studied in over 50 clinical studies for its ability to combat tumor growth.

USES:
Obesity, anxiety, insomnia, irritability, lung health, learning and memory support, Alzheimer's, liver problems, digestive problems, blood purification, metabolism, parasites, fluid retention, skin care: anti-aging

FRAGRANT INFLUENCE:
Fresh, clean aroma; promotes happiness; calming; helps with anxiety and nervousness. A Mie University study found that citrus fragrances boosted immunity, induced relaxation, and reduced depression.

DIRECTIONS:
Aromatic: 6o. Topical: 50-50. Dietary (Vitality): Put 2 drops in a capsule and take 3 times daily.

CAUTIONS: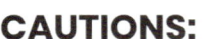

SELECTED RESEARCH:

Wang F, Chen L, Chen H, Chen S, Liu Y. Analysiss of Flavonoid Metabolites in Citruts Peels (Citrus reticulata "Dahongpao") Using UPLC-ESI-MS/MS. Molecules. 2019 Aug; 24(15): 2680.

Wang Y, Qian J, Cao J, Wang D, Liu C, Yang R, Li X, Sun C. Antioxidant capacity, anticancer ability and flavonoids composition of 35 Citrus (Citrus reticulata Blanco) varieties. Molecules. 2017 Jul 5;22(7).

Apraj VD, Pandia NS. Evaluation of Skin Anti-aging Potential of Citrus reticulata Blanco Peel. Pharmacognosy Res. 2016 Jul-Sep; 8(3) :160-168.

Fomani M, Ngeufa Happi E, Nouga Bisoue A, Ndom JC, Kamdem Waffo AF, Sewald N, Wansi JD. Oxidative burst inhibition, cytotoxicity and antibacterial acriquinoline alkaloids from Citrus reticulata (Blanco). Bioorg Med Chem Lett. 2016 Jan 15;26(2):306-9. Epub 2015 Dec 11.

Javed S, Javaid A, Nawaz S, Saeed MK. Mahmood Z, Siddiqui SZ, Ahmad R. GC-MS analysis, antioxidant and antimicrobial potential of essential oil from five citrus species. Phytochemistry. 2014;6(3):201.

Zhang Y, Sun Y, Xi W, Shen Y, Qiao L. Zhong L, Ye X, Zhou Z. Phenolic compositions and antioxidant capacities of Chinese wild mandarin (Citrus reticulata Blanco) fruits. Food Chem. 2014 Feb 15;145:674-80. Epub 2013 Aug 11.

Tao N, Jia L, Zhou H. Anti-fungal activity of Citrus reticulata Blanco essential oil against Penicillium italicum and Penicillium digitatum. Food Chem. 2014 Jun 15;153:265-71. Epub 2013 Dec 25.

Seki T, Kamiya T, Furukawa K, Azumi M, Ishizuka S, Takayama S, Nagase S, Arai H, Yamakuni T, Yaegashi N. Nobiletin-rich Citrus reticulata peels, a kampo medicine for Alzheimer's disease: a case series. Geriatr Gerontol Int. 2013 Jan;13(1):236-8.

Kawahata I, Yoshida M, Sun W, Nakajima A, Lai Y, Osaka N, Matsuzaki K, Yokosuka A, Mimaki Y, Naganuma A, Tomioka Y, Yamakuni T. Potent activity of nobiletin-rich Citrus reticulata peel extract to facilitate cAMP/PKA/ERK/CREB-signaling associated with learning and memory in cultured hippocampal neurons: identification of the substances responsible for pharmacological action. J Neural Transm (Vienna). 2013 Oct;120(10):1397-409. Epub 2013 Apr 16.

Kim MJ, Park HJ, Hong MS, Park HJ, Kim MS, Leem KH, Kim JB, Kim YJ, Kim HK. Citrus reticulata Blanco induces apoptosis in human gastric cancer cells SNU-668. Nutr Cancer. 2005;51(1):78-82.

Komori T, Fujiwara R, Tanida M, Nomura J, Yokoyama MM. Effects of citrus fragrance on immune function and depressive states. Neuroimmunomodulation. 1995 May-Jun;2(3):174-80.

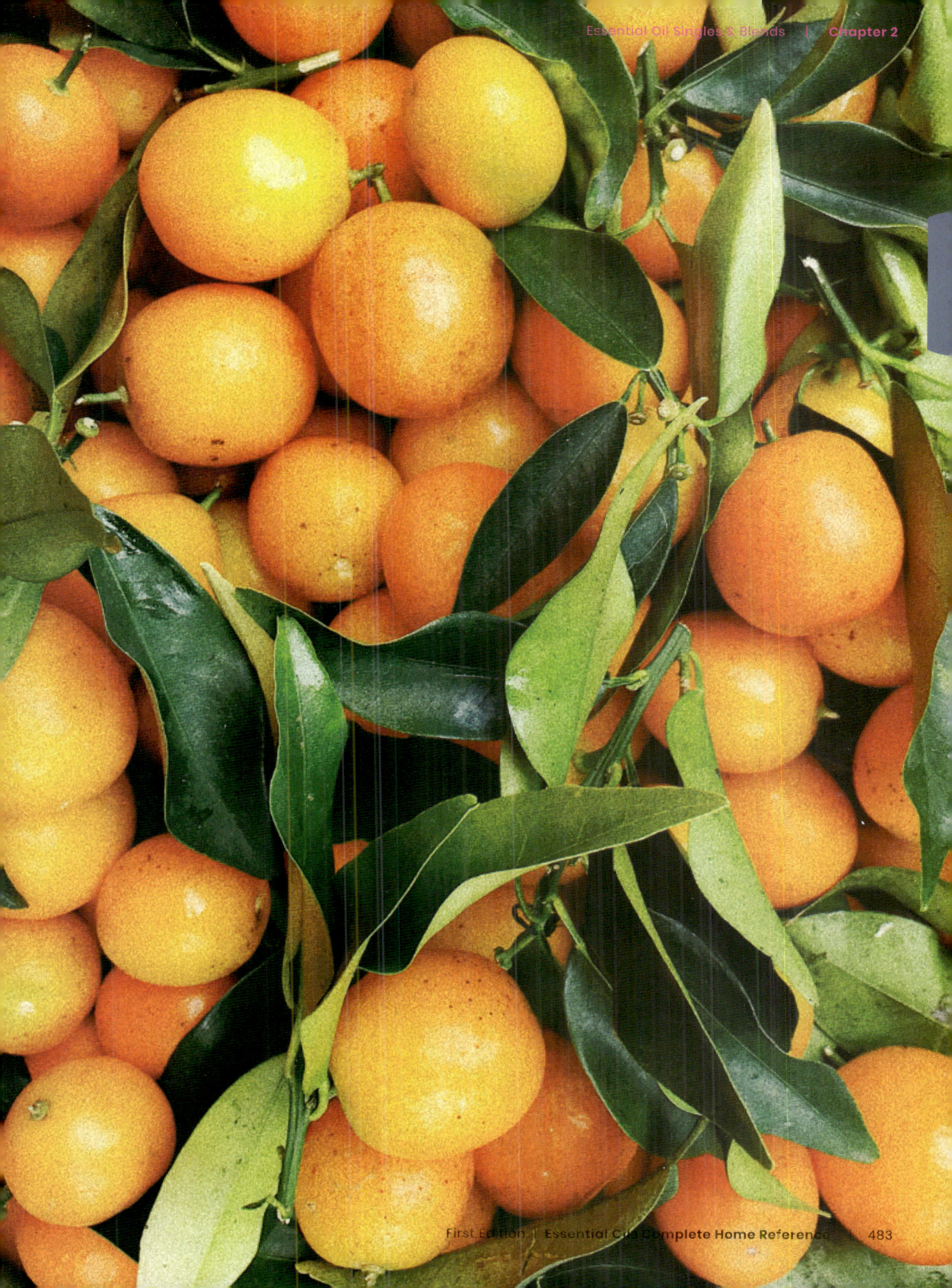

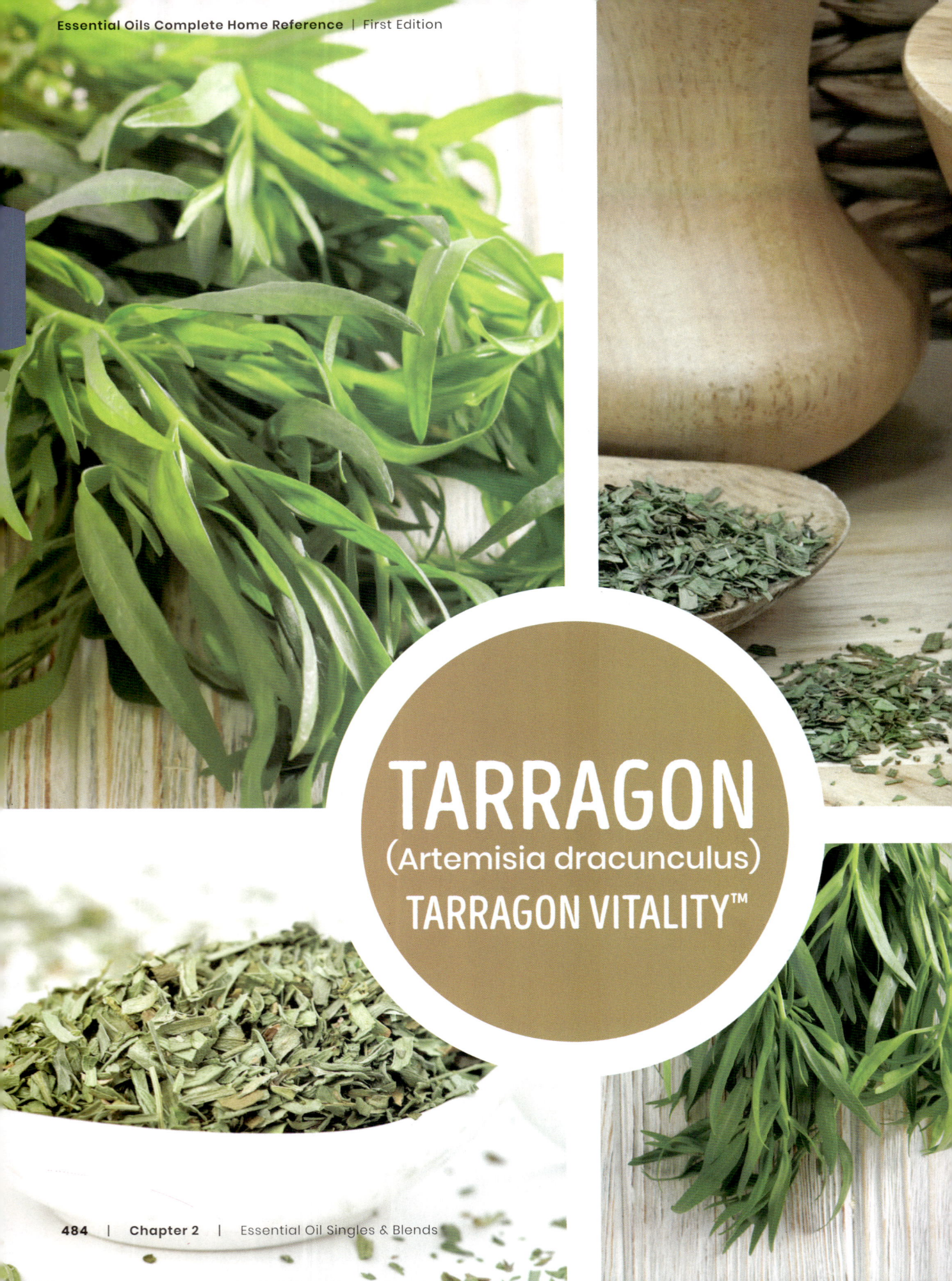

Essential Oil Singles & Blends | Chapter 2

BOTANICAL FAMILY:
Asteraceae

PLANT ORIGIN:
Hungary

EXTRACTION METHOD:
Steam distilled from leaves

KEY CONSTITUENTS:
Methyl Chavicol (68-84%),
Cis-Beta-Ocimene (5-13%),
Trans-Beta-Ocimene (6-12%),
Limonene (2-7%),
Alpha-Pinene (up to 2%),
Methyl Eugenol (up to 1%)

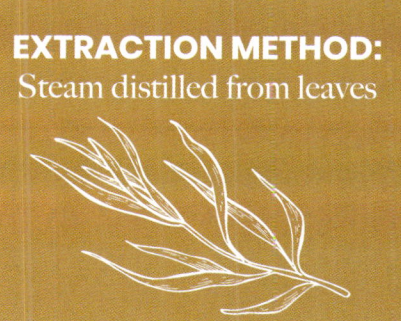

HISTORICAL DATA:
Tarragon's botanical name is from the Greek and Latin. Artemisia is for the Greek goddess Artemis, and dracunculus is derived from the Latin for "little dragon." However intimidating the name, tarragon was recommended by the Arab healer Avicenna for bad digestion. Tarragon may have been introduced to Europe by the Crusaders returning from the Middle East.

MEDICAL PROPERTIES:
Analgesic, antibacterial, anticonvulsant, sedative, antispasmodic, anti-inflammatory, antiparasitic, digestive aid, enhances insulin sensitivity

USES:
May counter diabetic symptoms, increases sympathetic nervous system activity, intestinal disorders, urinary tract infection, nausea, menstrual problems/PMS, strong, herbaceous flavor

FRAGRANT INFLUENCE:
May help alleviate deep depression

DIRECTIONS:
Aromatic: 30. Topical: 50-50. Dietary (Vitality): Dilute 1 drop with 4 drops of carrier oil. Put in a capsule and take 1 daily or as needed.

CAUTIONS: Avoid use if epileptic

SELECTED RESEARCH:

RezaeiR, Hazrati Tappeh K, Seyyedi S, Mikaili P, The Anti-leishmania Efficacy of Artemisia dracunculus Ethanolic Extract in Vitro and Its Effects on IFN-Y and IL-4 Response. Iran J Parasitol. 207 Jul-Sep; 12(3): 398-407.

Méndez-Del Villar M1, Puebla-Pérez AM, Sánchez-Peña MJ, González-Ortiz LJ, Martinez-Abundis E, González-Ortiz M. Effect of Artemisia dracunculus administration on glycemic control, insulin sensitivity, and insulin secretion in patients with impaired glucose tolerance. J Med Food. 2016 May;19(5):481-5. Epub 2016 Apr 20.

Mohammad Reza S, Hamideh M, Zahra S. The nociceptive and anti-inflammatory effects of Artemisia dracunculus L. aqueous extract on fructose fed male rats. Evid Based Complement Alternat Med. 2015;2015:895417. Epub 2015 Jun 11.

Hong L, Ying SH. Ethanol extract and isolated constituents from Artemsia dracunculus inhibit esophageal squamous cell carcinoma and induce apoptotic cell death. Drug Res (Stuttg). 2015 Feb 65(2):101-6. Epub 2014 Jul 30.

Maham M, Moslemzadeh H, Jalilzadeh-Amin G. Antinociceptive effect of the essential oil of tarragon (Artemisia dracunculus). Pharm Biol. 2014 Feb;52(2):208-12. Epub 2013 Sep 30.

Obanda DN, Ribnicky DM, Raskin I, Cefalu WT. Bioactives of Artemisia dracunculus L. enhance insulin sensitivity by modulation of ceramide metabolism in rat skeletal muscle cells. Nutrition. 2014 Jul-Aug;30(7-8 Suppl):S59-66. Epub 2014 Mar 19.

Sayyah M, Nadjafnia L, Kamalinejad M. Anticonvulsant activity and chemical composition of Artemisia dracunculus L. essential oil. Journal of Ethnopharmacology. 2004 Oct;94(2-3):283-7.

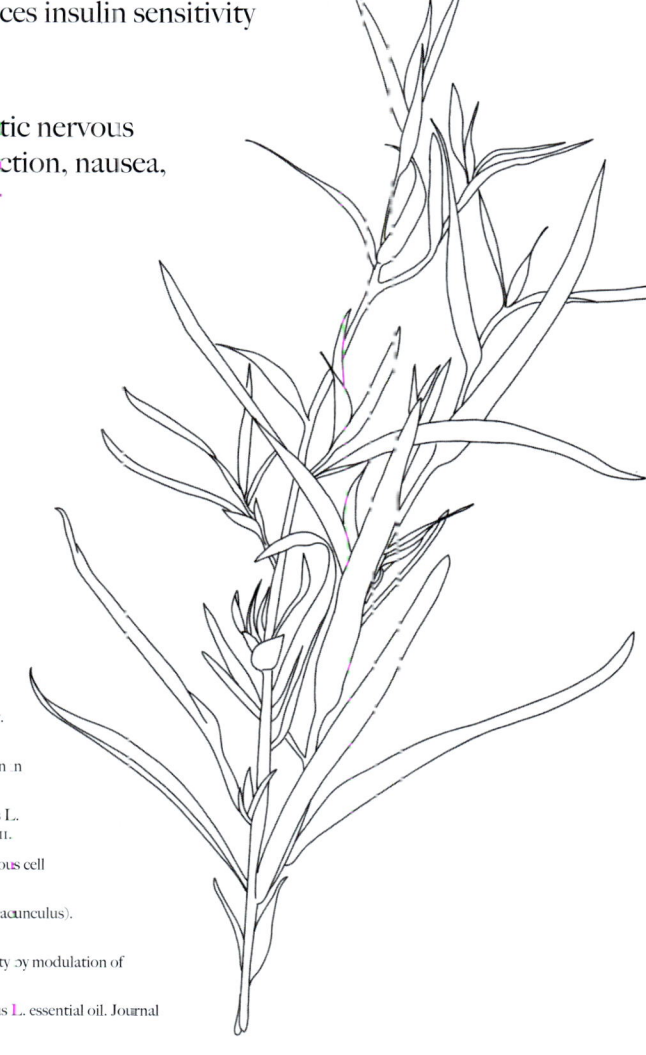

BOTANICAL FAMILY: Myrtaceae

PLANT ORIGIN: Australia, South Africa

EXTRACTION METHOD: Steam distilled from leaves

KEY CONSTITUENTS: Terpinen-4-ol (30-48%), Gamma-Terpinene (10-28%), Eucalyptol + Beta-Phellandrene (up to 15%), Alpha-Terpinene (5-13%), Para-Cymene (up to 8%), Alpha-Terpineol (1-8%), Alpha-Pinene (1-6%), Terpinolene (1-5%), Sabinene (up to 4%), Aromadendrene (up to 3%), Ledene (syn. Viridiflorene) (up to 3%), Delta-Cadinene (up to 3%), Limonene (up to 2%)

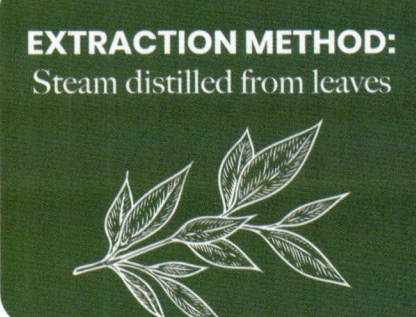

TEA TREE
(Melaleuca alternifolia)

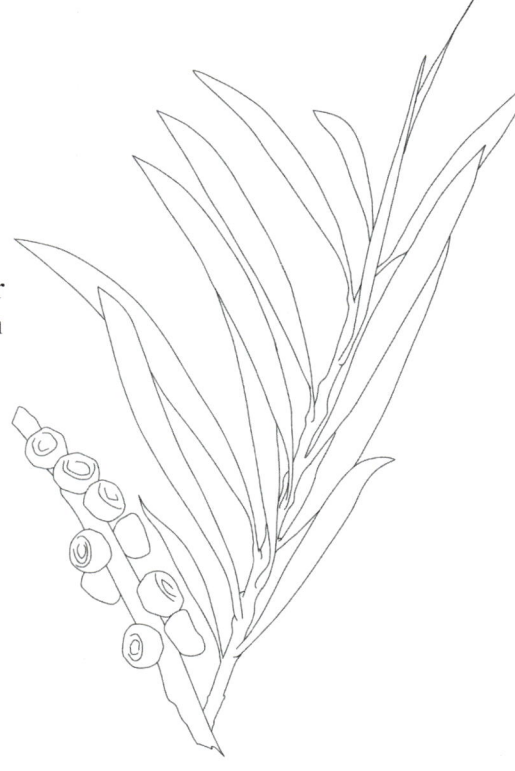

Highly regarded as an antimicrobial and antiseptic essential oil. It has high levels of terpinen-4-ol.

MEDICAL PROPERTIES:
Powerful antibacterial, antifungal, anti-infectious, antiviral, antiparasitic, anti-inflammatory action

USES:
Gingivitis, acne, psoriasis, dandruff, Athlete's foot, onychomycosis, fungal infections (candida, ringworm), sinus/lung infections, insect bites, tooth/gum disease, water retention/hypertension, inflammation, lice, nail fungus, skin conditions (eczema, acne, sores, dry, oily, itchy), infections, hair and scalp issues

FRAGRANT INFLUENCE:
Promotes cleansing and purity

DIRECTIONS:
Aromatic: 3o. Topical: Neat.

CAUTIONS:

SELECTED RESEARCH:

Cordeiro L, Figueiredo P, Souza G, Sousa A, Andrade-Júnior F, Medeiros D, Nóbrega J, Silva D, Martins E, Barbosa-Filho J, Lima E. Terpinen-4-ol as an Antibacterial Agent Against Staphylococcus aureus. Int J Mol Sci. 2020 Jun; 21(12): 4531.

Oliva A, Costantini S, De Angelis M, Garzoli S, Gožović M, Mascellino MT, Vullo V, Ragno R. High potency of Melaleuca alternifolia essential oil against multi-drug resistant gram-negative bacteria and methicillin-resistant Staphylococcus aureus. Molecules. 2018 Oct 9;23(10).

Felipe LO, Júnior WFDS, Araújo KC, Fabrino DL. Lactoferrin, chitosan and Melaleuca alternifolia-natural products that show promise in candidiasis treatment. Braz J Microbiol. 2018 Apr - Jun;49(2):212-219. Epub 2017 Nov 11.

Li M, Zhu L, Liu B, Du L, Jia X, Han L, Jin Y. Tea tree oil nanoemulsions for inhalation therapies of bacterial and fungal pneumonia. Colloids Surf B Biointerfaces. 2016 May 1;141:408-416. doi: 10.1016/j.colsurfb.2016.02.017. Epub 2016 Feb 9.

Comin VM, Lopes LQ, Quatrin PM, de Souza ME, Bonez PC, Pintos FG, Raffin RP, Vaucher Rde A, Martinez DS, Santos RC. Influence of Melaleuca alternifolia oil nanoparticles on aspects of Pseudomonas aeruginosa biofilm. Microb Pathog. 2016 Apr;93:120-5. Epub 2016 Jan 25.

Hammer KA. Treatment of acne with tea tree oil (Melaleuca) products: a review of efficacy, tolerability and potential modes of action. Int J Antimicrob Agents. 2015 Feb;45(2):106-10. Epub 2014 Nov 13.

Mertas A, Garbusińska A, Szliszka E, Jureczko A, Kowalska M, Król W. The influence of tea tree oil (Melaleuca alternifolia) on fluconazole activity against fluconazole-resistant Candida albicans. Biomed Res Int. 2015;2015:590470. Epub 2015 Feb 4.

Li X, Duan S, Chu C, Xu J, Zeng G, Lam AK, Zhou J, Yin Y, Fang D, Reynolds MJ, Gu H, Jiang L. Melaleuca alternifolia concentrate inhibits in vitro entry of influenza virus into host cells. Molecules. 2013 Aug 9;18(8):9550-66.

Chin KB, Cordell B. The effect of tea tree oil (Melaleuca alternifolia) on wound healing using a dressing model. J Altern Complement Med. 2013 Dec;19(12):942-5. Epub 2013 Jul 13.

Cuaron JA, Dulal S, Song Y, Singh AK, Montelongo CE, Yu W, Nagarajan V, Jayaswal RK, Wilkinson BJ, Gustafson JE. Tea tree oil-induced transcriptional alterations in Staphylococcus aureus. Phytother Res. 2013 Mar;27(3):390-6. Epub 2012 May 23.

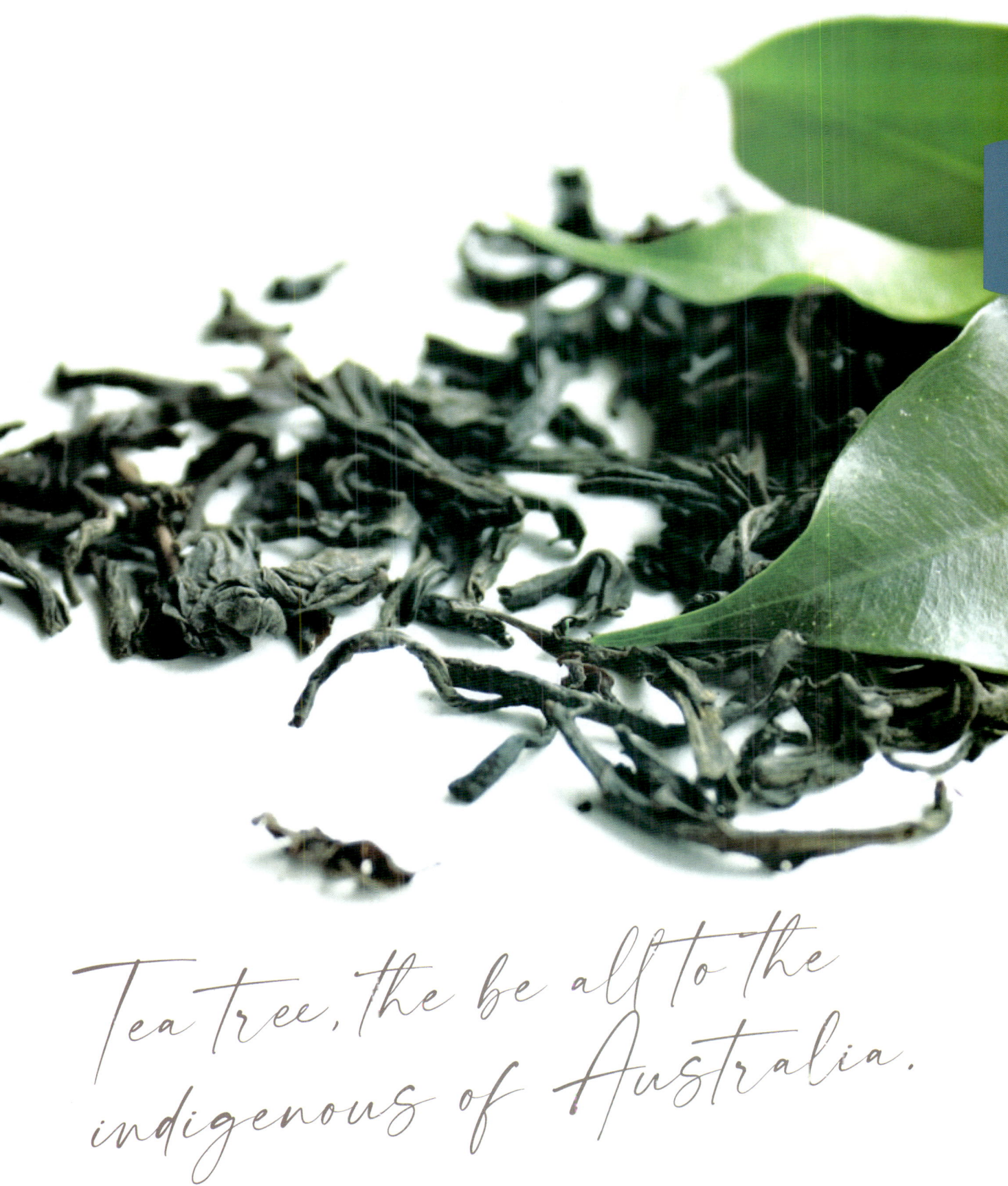

Tea tree, the be all to the indigenous of Australia.

Essential Oils Complete Home Reference | First Edition

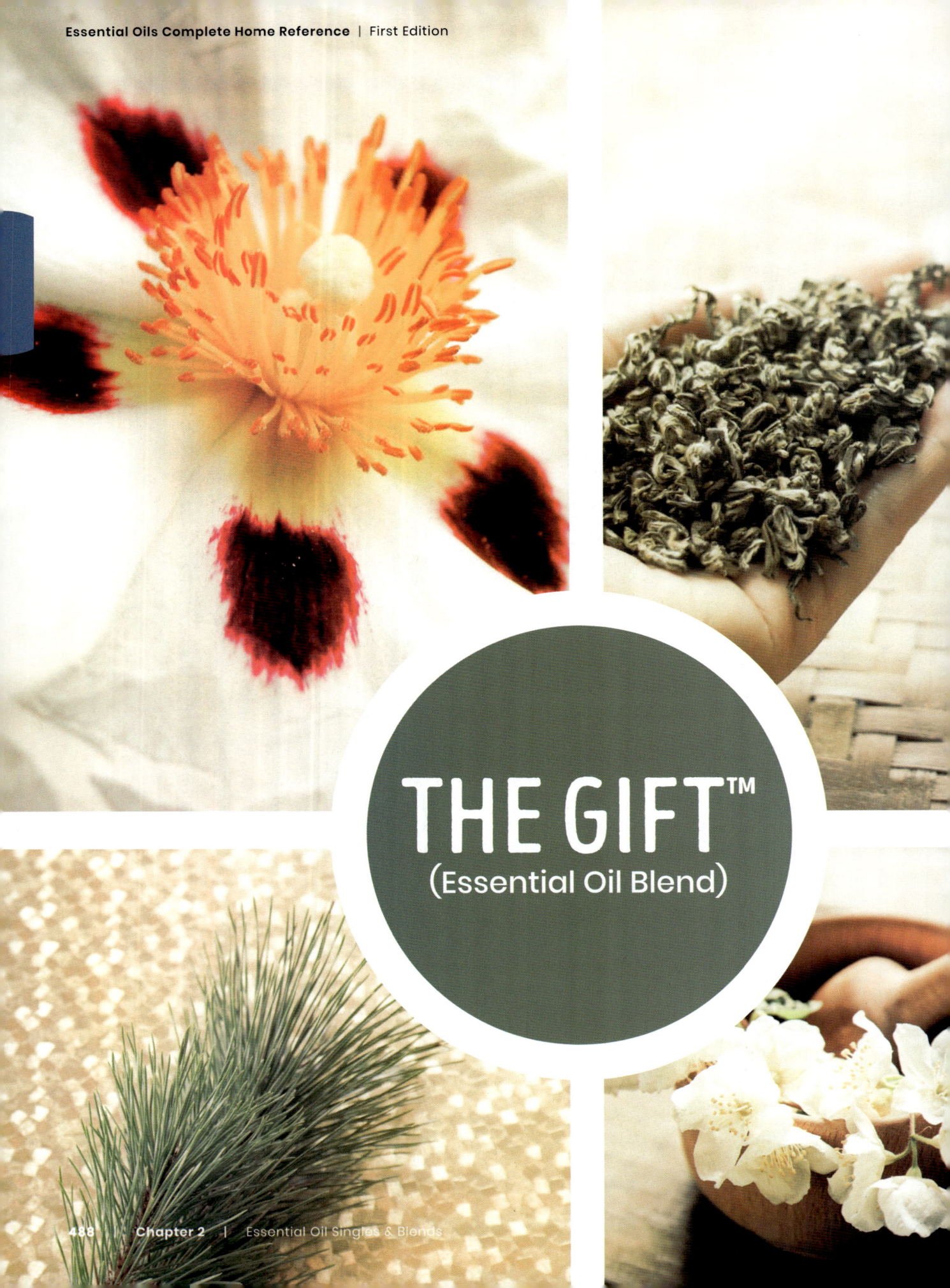

THE GIFT™
(Essential Oil Blend)

488 | Chapter 2 | Essential Oil Singles & Blends

ABOUT THE GIFT:

The Gift is the very "essence of Arabia," blending the oils of antiquity into a most unique and exotic fragrance. It combines seven ancient therapeutic oils to capture the spirit of Arabia. This oil blend represents Mary's gift to Gary in honor of Shutran's noble journey through the book The One Gift, a historical novel depicting the wit, intrigue, sorrow, and romance of the ancient frankincense and myrrh caravans.

Out of the writings and legends of antiquity, healing mysteries unfold as we discover powerful uses for herbs and oils in healing the injuries of war, accidents, scorpion stings, and snakebites and in sacred rituals for attaining greater spiritual attunement for healing and protecting the body.

Present-day science is now documenting the properties of these oils that augment the immune system, stimulate healing, and overcome depression. Myrrh and Frankincense are being touted for their anticancerous, anti-infectious, antibacterial, and antiviral abilities, as well as for being topical anesthetics and having the ability to regenerate bone and cartilage. They are the oldest-known substances to ever come out of the ancient world for their immune-stimulating and healing powers.

MEDICAL PROPERTIES & USES:

Anti-inflammatory, antimicrobial, antioxidative, antiviral, antibacterial, emotion supporting, calming, immune stimulating, disease inhibitory, insecticidal/antiparasitic, oral protective, organ protective, bone and cartilage regenerating, pain or swelling reducing, performance enhancing/stimulating

INGREDIENTS:

Idaho Grand Fir, Sacred Frankincense, Jasmine, Northern Lights Black Spruce, Myrrh, Vetiver, Cistus

DIRECTIONS:

Aromatic: 30. Topical: 50-50.
Wear as a fragrance. Massage on the bottoms of feet.

CAUTIONS:

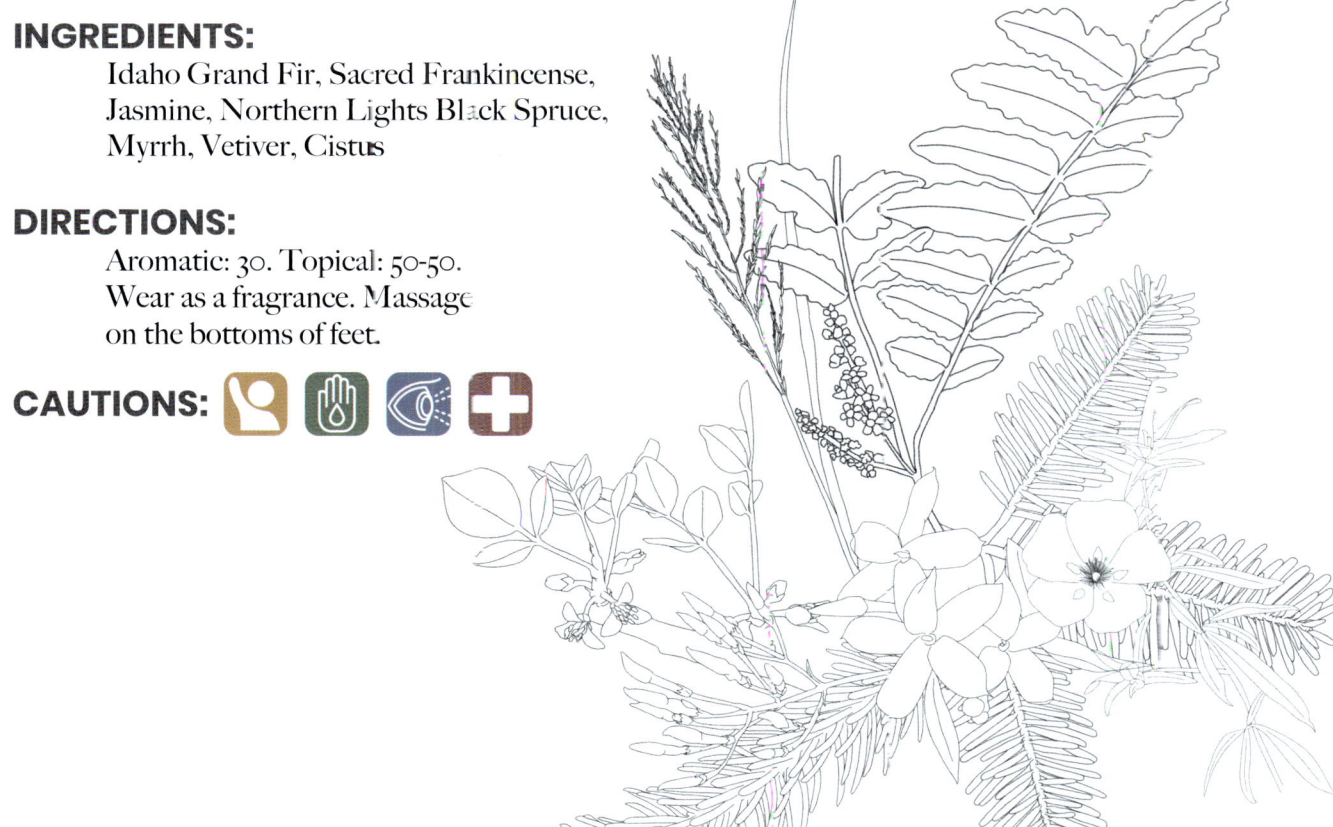

THIEVES®, THIEVES® ROLL-ON, & THIEVES® VITALITY®
(Essential Oil Blend)

This is a most amazing blend of highly antiviral, antiseptic, antibacterial, antifungal, and anti-infectious essential oils.

It was created from research based on legends about a group of 15th-century thieves who rubbed botanicals on themselves to avoid contracting the plague while they robbed the bodies of the dead and dying. When apprehended, the thieves were forced to tell what their secret was and disclosed the formula of the herbs, spices, and oils they used to protect themselves in exchange for more lenient punishment.

Studies conducted at Weber State University (Ogden, UT) in 1997 demonstrated the killing power of these amazing oils against airborne microorganisms. The analysis showed that after 10 minutes of Thieves diffusion in the air, there was an 82 percent reduction in the gram-positive Micrococcus luteus organism bioaerosol, a 96 percent reduction in gram-negative Pseudomonas aeruginosa organism bioaerosol, and a 44 percent reduction in S. aureus bioaerosol.

A 2000 study by Sue Chao and Gary Young found antifungal properties for Cinnamon Bark, Lemon, Rosemary, and Eucalyptus Radiata oils, four of the five oils in Thieves blend.

A 2015 study found Clove essential oil (Cinnamomum zeylanicum syn. Cinnamomum aromaticum) to be antifungal as well as antibacterial. Gary Young personally used Thieves blend to eliminate black mold.

Essential oil expert Kurt Schnaubelt has written that essential oils do not kill beneficial bacteria. He explains that phenylpropanoids such as cinnamic aldehyde, eugenol, and carvacrol are antimicrobial. However, they are also unique in the way that beneficial probiotic bacteria can harmlessly metabolize them.

MEDICAL PROPERTIES & USES:
Anti-inflammatory, antiviral, antibacterial, antimicrobial, antioxidative, calming, cardiovascular supportive, dietary, digestion or elimination supportive/nausea reducing, disease inhibitory, muscle relaxant/bone-joint preservative, oral protective, organ protective, pain or swelling reducing, performance enhancing/stimulating, respiratory system supportive, wellness supportive

INGREDIENTS:
Clove, Lemon, Cinnamon Bark, Eucalyptus Radiata, Rosemary, Fractionated coconut oil (Roll-On only)

DIRECTIONS:
Aromatic: 10 Topical: 20-80. For headaches, put 1 drop on tongue and push against roof of mouth. Apply neat to bottoms of feet. Dietary (Vitality): Dilute 1 drop with 4 drops of V-6 or other pure carrier oil. Put in a capsule and take 1 daily.

CAUTIONS:

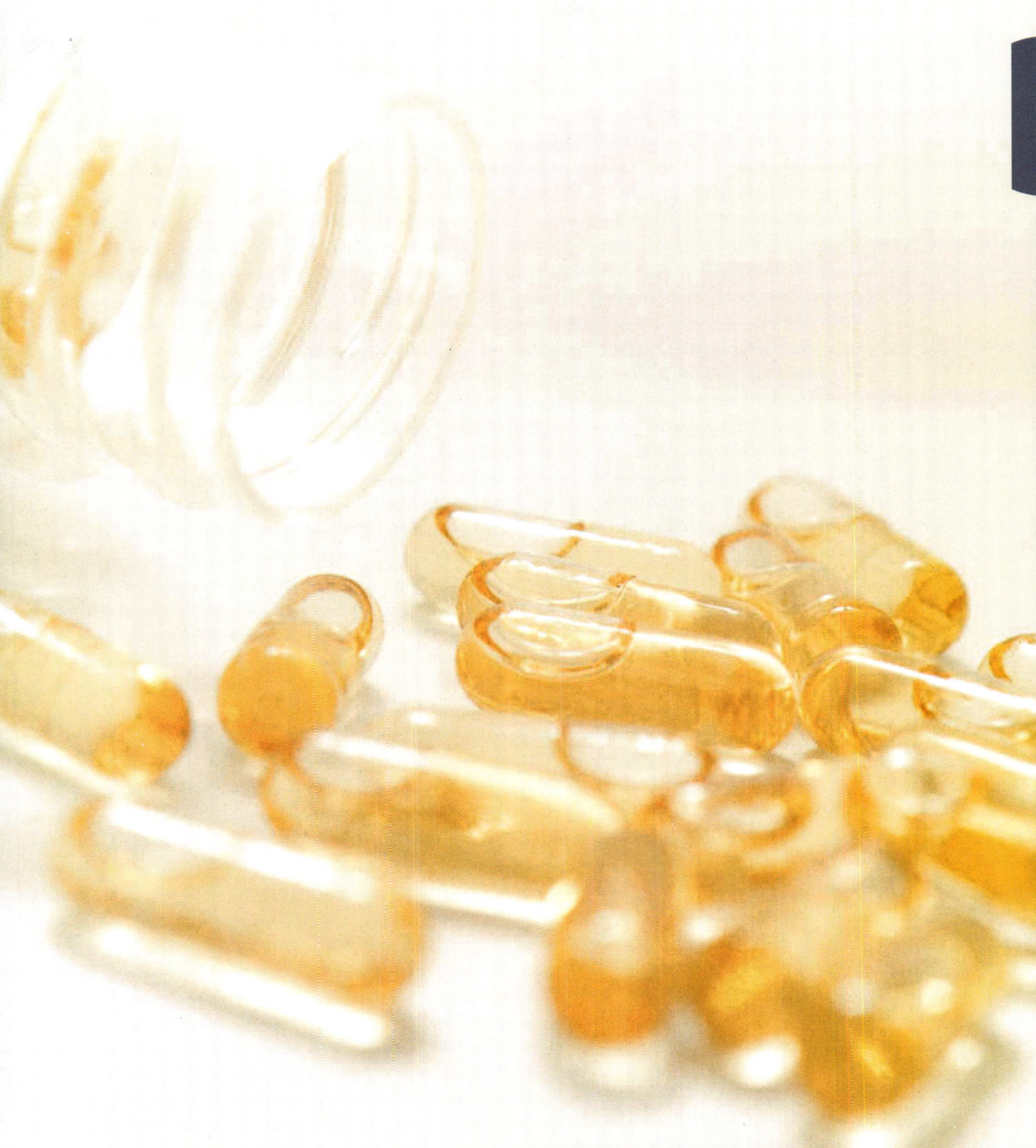

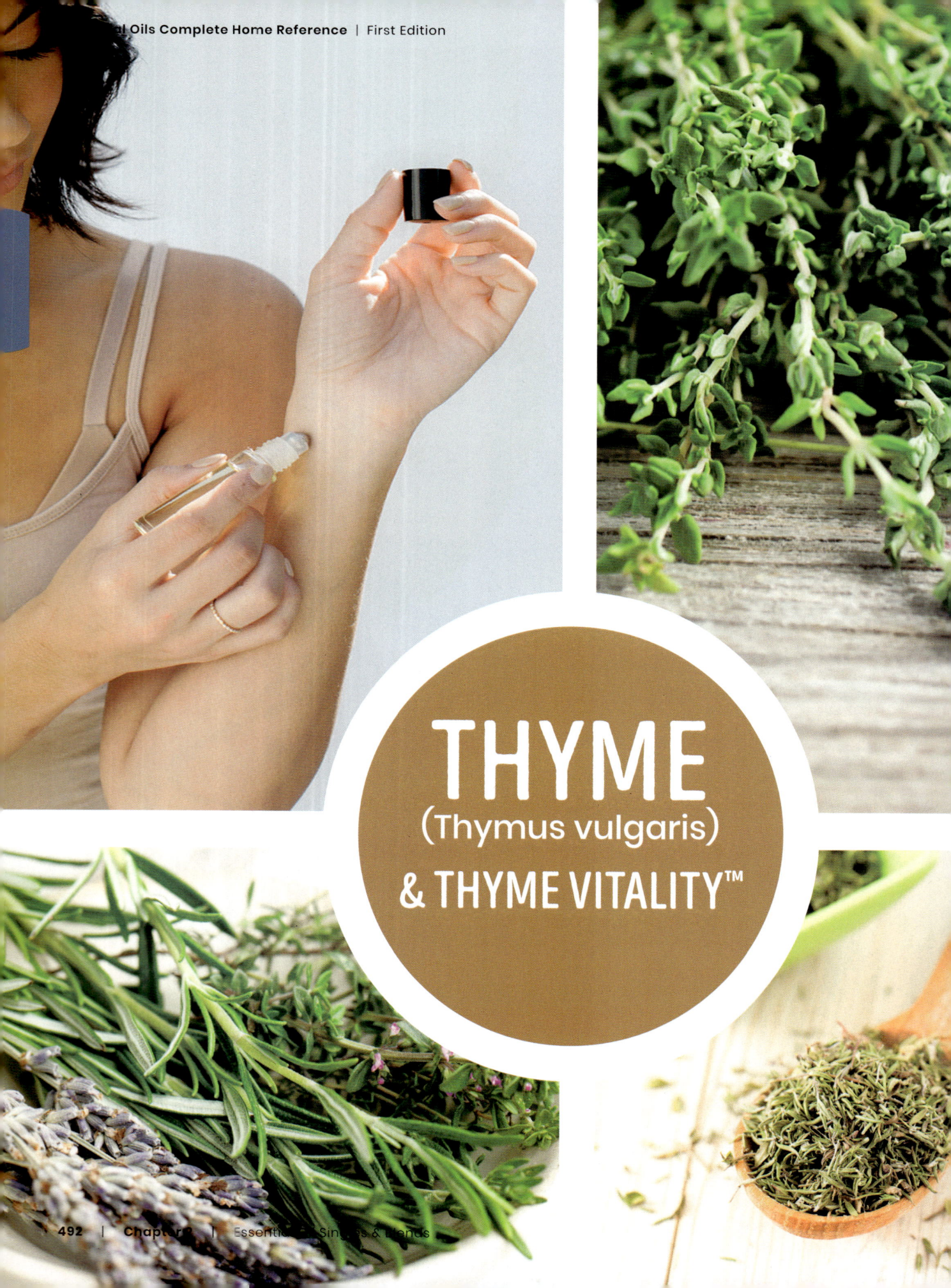
THYME
(Thymus vulgaris)
& THYME VITALITY™

Essential Oil Singles & Blends | Chapter 2

BOTANICAL FAMILY:
Lamiaceae

PLANT ORIGIN:
Egypt, Spain

EXTRACTION METHOD:
Steam distilled from herbs and aerial parts

KEY CONSTITUENTS:
Thymol (37-55%), Para-Cymene (14-28%), Gamma-Terpinene (4-11%), Linalool (3-7%), Carvacrol (up to 6%), Myrcene (1-3%), Alpha-Terpinene (up to 3%), Alpha-Pinene (up to 3%), Terpinen-4-ol (up to 3%), Beta-Caryophyllene (up to 2%), Alpha-Thujene (up to 2%), Carvacrol Methyl Ether (up to 2%)

HISTORICAL DATA:

Also known as Red Thyme. It is mentioned in one of the oldest known medical records, the Ebers Papyrus (dating from 16th century BC), an ancient Egyptian list of 877 prescriptions and recipes. The Egyptians used thyme for embalming. It is listed in Dioscorides' De Materia Medica (AD 78), Europe's first authoritative guide to medicines, which became the standard reference work for herbal treatments for over 1,700 years. Thyme was also listed in Hildegard's Medicine, a compilation of early German medicines by highly regarded Benedictine herbalist Hildegard of Bingen (1098-1179).

MEDICAL PROPERTIES:

Antiaging, antioxidant, anti-inflammatory, antispasmodic, highly antimicrobial, antifungal, antiviral, antiparasitic. A solution of thyme's most active ingredient, thymol, is used in many over-the-counter products such as mouthwash and vapor rubs because of its purifying agents.

USES:

Infectious diseases, cardiovascular disease, Alzheimer's disease, colds, coughs, hair loss, hepatitis, preservative, yeast infections, insect repellent

FRAGRANT INFLUENCE:

It may be beneficial in helping to overcome fatigue and exhaustion after illness.

DIRECTIONS:

Aromatic: 10. Topical: 20-80. Test for sensitivity on a small area of skin on the underside of arm and apply to desired area as needed. Use in Raindrop Technique. Dietary (Vitality): Dilute 1 drop with 1 drop of V-6 or other pure carrier oil. Put in a capsule and take up to 3 times daily.

CAUTIONS: 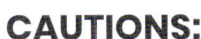   May irritate the nasal membranes or skin if inhaled directly from diffuser or bottle or applied neat.

SELECTED RESEARCH:

Zeng Q, Che Y, Zhang Y, Chen M, Guo Q, Zhang W. Thymol isolated from Thymus vulgaris L. Inhibits Colorectal Cancer Cell Growth and Metastasis by Suppressing the Wnt/β-Catenin Pathway. Drug Des Devel Ther. 2020: 14: 2535-2547.

Gedikoğlu A, Sökman M, Çivit A. Evaluation of Thymus vulgaris and Thymbra spicata essential oils and plant extracts for chemical composition, antioxidant, and antimicrobial properties. Food Sci Nutr. 2019 Apr 2;7(5):1704-1714. eCollection 2019 May.

Ben Jabeur M, Somai-Jemmali L, Hamada W. Thyme essential oil as an alternative mechanism: biofungicide-causing sensitivity of Mycosphaerella graminicola. J Appl Microbiol. 2017 Apr;122(4):932-939.

Rudolph K, Parthier C, Egerer-Sieber C, Geiger W, Muller YA, Kreis W, Müller-Uri F. Expression, crystallization and structure elucidation of β-terpinene synthase from Thymus vulgaris. Acta Crystallogr F Struct Biol Commun. 2016 Jan;72(Pt 1):16-23. Epub 2016 Jan 1.

Perina FJ, Amaral DC, Fernandes RS, Labory CR, Teixeira GA, Alves E. Thymus vulgaris essential oil and thymol against Alternaria alternata (Fr.) Keissler: effects on growth, viability, early infection and cellular mode of action. Pest Manag Sci. 2015 Oct;71(10):1371-8. Epub 2014 Dec 4.

Ahmad A, van Vuuren S, Viljoen A. Unraveling the complex antimicrobial interactions of essential oils—the case of Thymus vulgaris (thyme). Molecules. 2014 Mar 6;19(3):2896-910.

Grespan R, Aguiar RP, Giubilei FN, Fuso RR, Damião MJ, Silva EL, Mikcha JG, Hernandes L, Bersani Amado C, Cuman RK. Hepatoprotective effect of pretreatment with Thymus vulgaris essential oil experimental model of acetaminophen-induced injury. Evid Based Complement Alternat Med. 2014;2014:954136. Epub 2014 Feb 4.

Salmalian H, Saghebi R, Moghadamnia AA, Bijani A, Faramarzi M, Nasiri Amiri F, Bakouei F, Behmanesh F, Bekhradi R. Comparative effect of Thymus vulgaris and ibuprofen on primary dysmenorrhea: a triple-blind clinical study. Caspian J Intern Med. 2014 Spring;5(2):82-8.

Fachini-Queiroz FC, Kummer R, Estevão-Silva CF, Carvalho MD, Cunha JM, Grespan R, Bersani-Amado CA, Cuman RK. Effects of thymol and carvacrol, constituents of Thymus vulgaris L. essential oil, on the inflammatory response. Evid Based Complement Alternat Med. 2012;2012:657026. Epub 2012 Jul 5.

Šipailienė A, Venskutonis PR, Baranauskienė R, Šarkinas A. Antimicrobial activity of commercial samples of Thyme and Marjoram oils. Journal of Essential Oil Research. 2012 Oct 16;18(6):698-703.

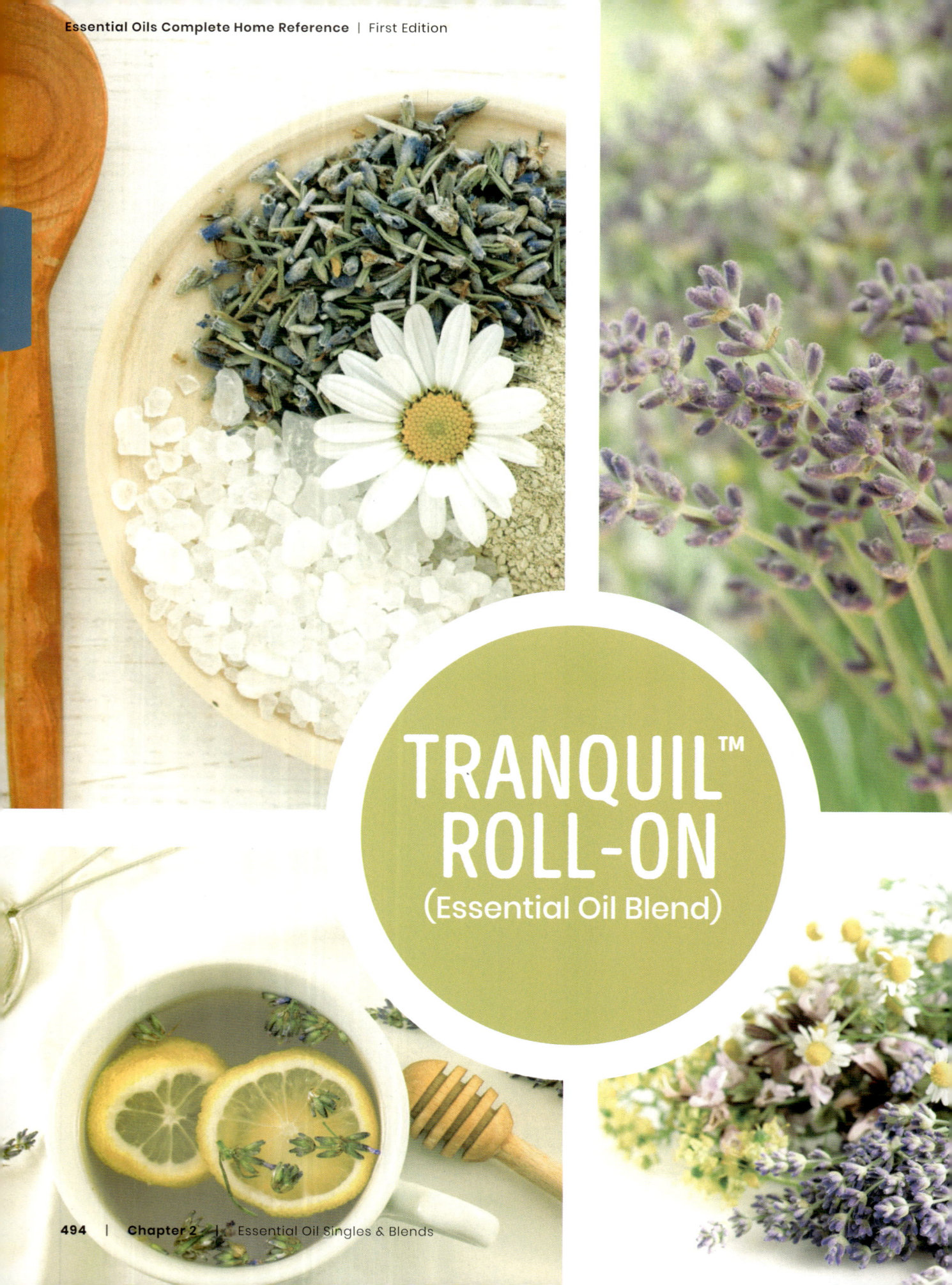

ABOUT TRANQUIL™ ROLL-ON:

This proprietary blend of Lavender, Cedarwood, and Roman Chamomile essential oils, packaged in a roll-on applicator, provides convenient and portable relaxation and stress relief. All three of these oils have been well documented as being effective in reducing restlessness, decreasing anxiety, and inducing a calming feeling to mind and body. Their combined effect is uplifting as well as relaxing and can be useful in promoting sleep as well as reducing stress.

MEDICAL PROPERTIES & USES:
Anti-inflammatory, antimicrobial, antioxidative, calming, disease inhibitory, skin and hair improving, emotion supporting, relaxation

INGREDIENTS:
Lavender, Cedarwood, Caprylic/capric triglyceride, Roman Chamomile, Coconut oil

DIRECTIONS:
Topical: Neat.

CAUTIONS:

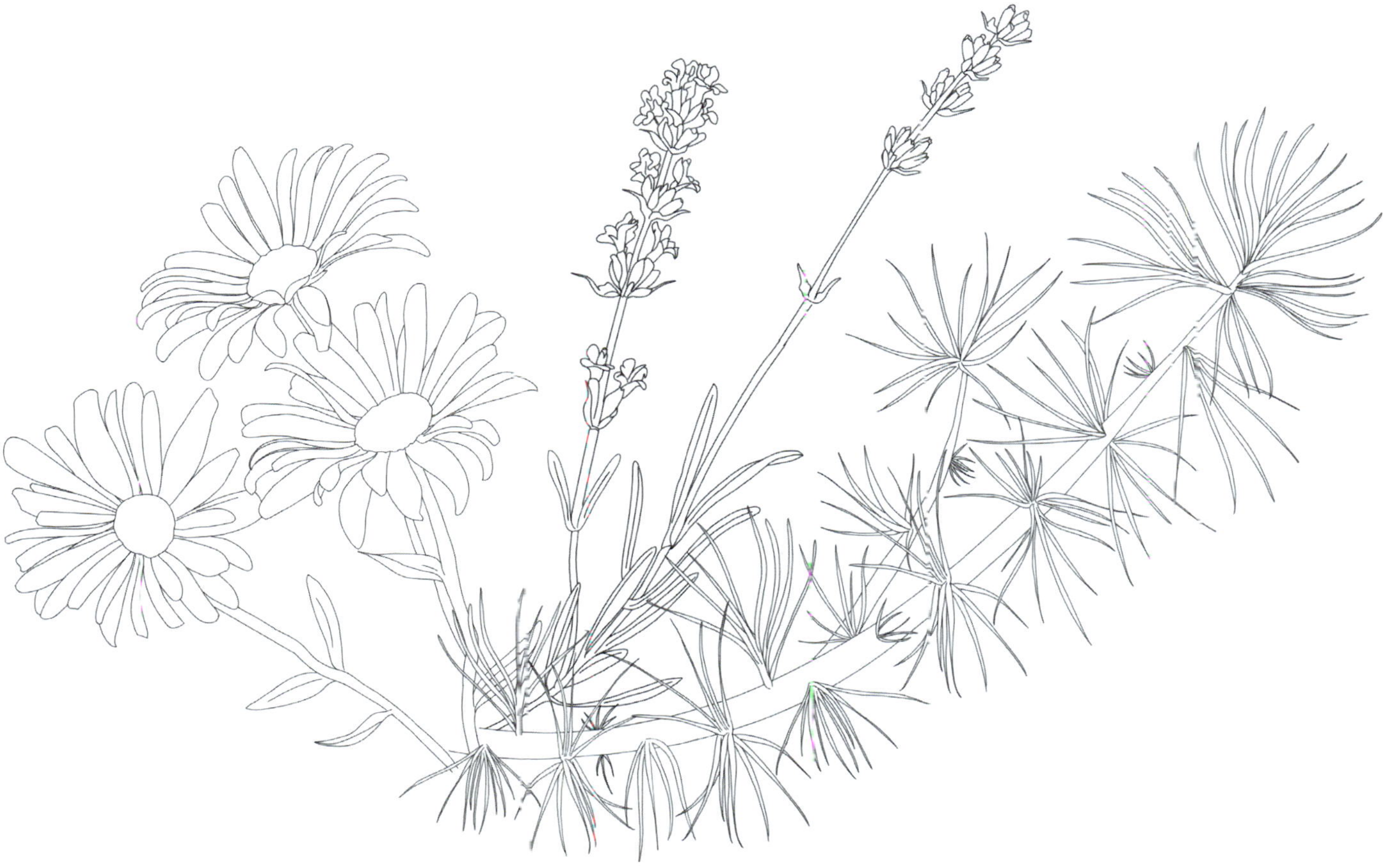

TRANSFORMATION™
(Essential Oil Blend)

Repressed trauma and tragedy from the past may be out of sight, but they are definitely not out of mind. Memories are imprinted in our cells for better or worse. Stored negative emotions need to be released and replaced with joy, hope, courage, and other positive emotions. Transformation blend radiates with the purifying oils of Lemon and Peppermint, along with the revitalizing power of sesquiterpenes from Sandalwood and Frankincense. Idaho Blue Spruce anchors new mental programming.

Reaching into the deepest recesses of memory, Transformation empowers and upholds the changes you want to make in your belief system. Positive, uplifting beliefs are foundational for the transformation of behavior.

MEDICAL PROPERTIES & USES:
Anti-inflammatory, antimicrobial, antioxidative, emotion supporting, calming, cardiovascular supportive, digestion or elimination supportive/nausea reducing, disease inhibitory, organ protective, pain or swelling reducing, performance enhancing/stimulating, wellness supportive

INGREDIENTS:
Lemon, Peppermint, Royal Hawaiian Sandalwood, Clary Sage, Sacred Frankincense, Idaho Blue Spruce, Cardamom, Ocotea, Palo Santo

DIRECTIONS:
Aromatic: 6o. Topical: 50-50.

CAUTIONS:

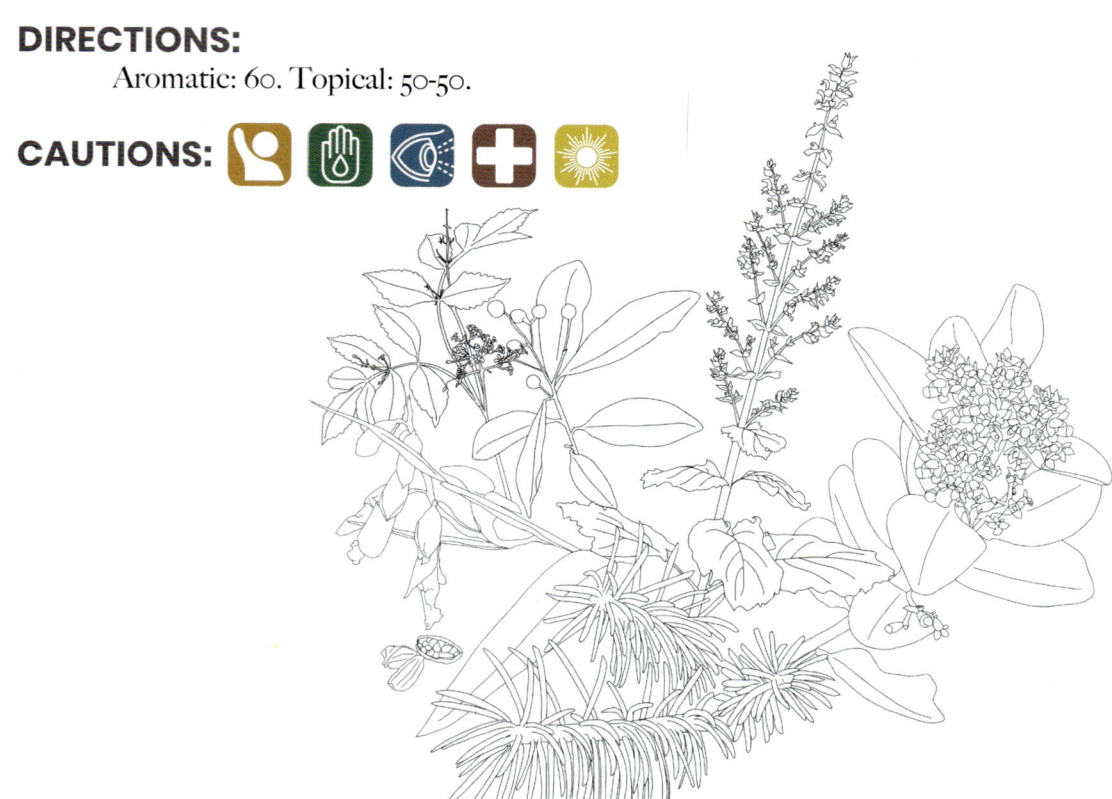

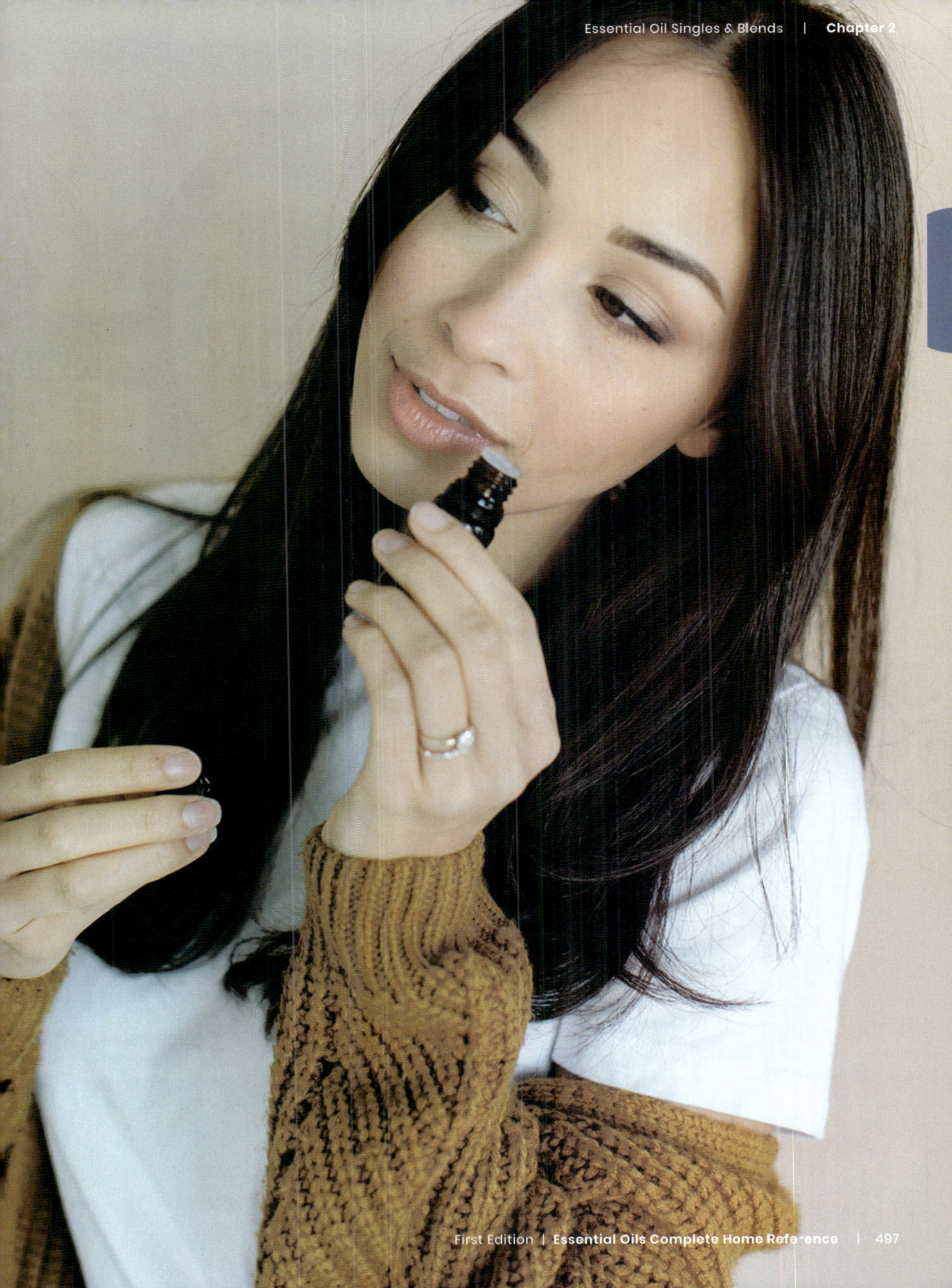

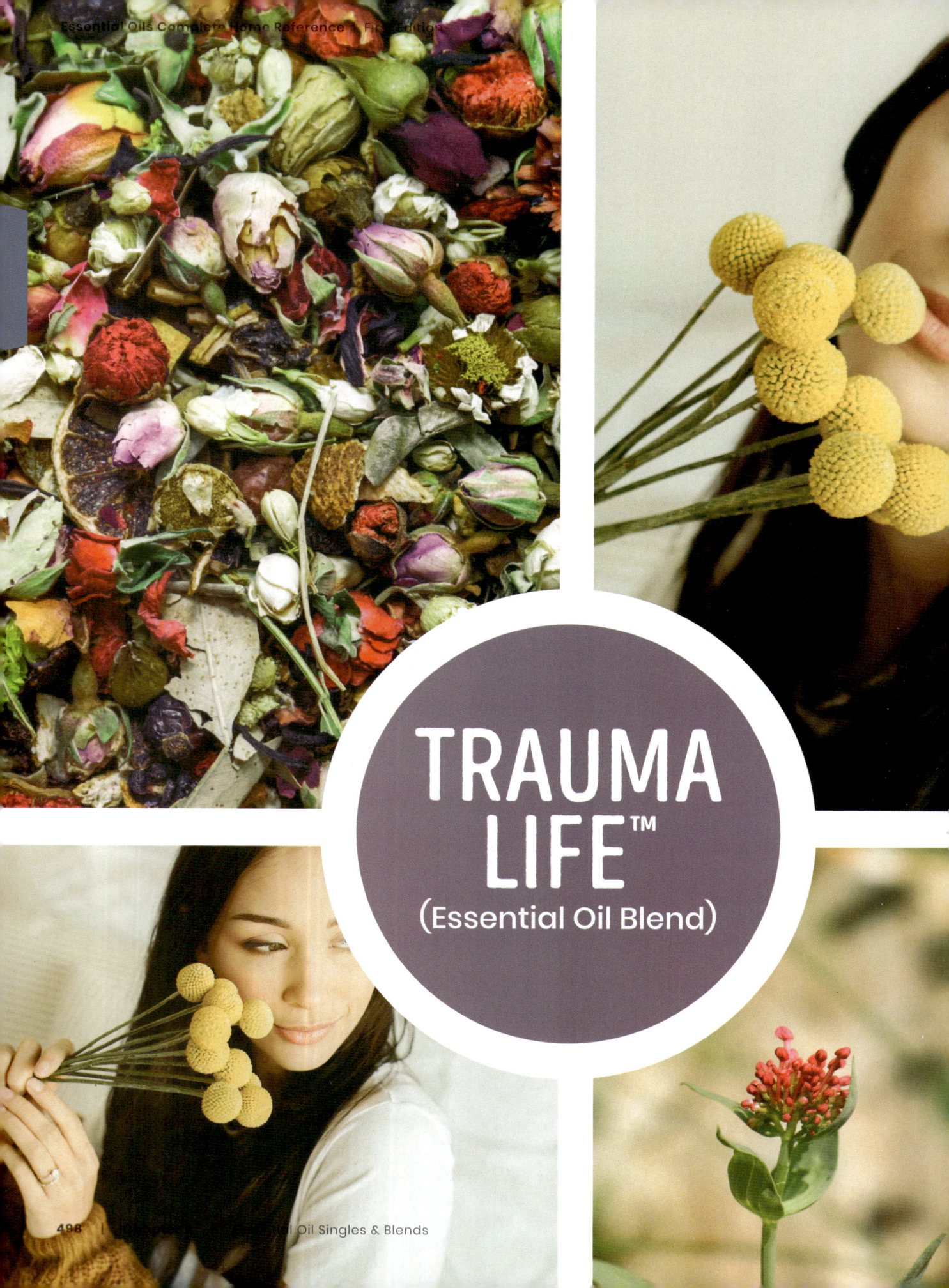

TRAUMA LIFE™
(Essential Oil Blend)

ABOUT TRAUMA LIFE™:

The emotional trauma from accidents, death of loved ones, assault, abuse, etc., can implant its devastation deep within the hidden recesses of the mind, causing lifelong problems that seem endless.

Being able to release such burdens can bring about a new "lease on life" with a return to motivation and vitality.

This blend combats stress and uproots trauma that cause insomnia, anger, restlessness, and a weakened immune response.

MEDICAL PROPERTIES & USES:

Anti-inflammatory, immune stimulating, antimicrobial, antioxidative, emotion supporting, calming, disease inhibitory, glandular/hormonal supportive, organ protective, pain or swelling reducing, performance enhancing/stimulating, sleep improving

INGREDIENTS:

Royal Hawaiian Sandalwood, Frankincense, Valerian, Black Spruce, Davana, Lavender, Geranium, Helichrysum, Citrus Hystrix, Rose

DIRECTIONS:

Aromatic: 6o. Topical: 50-50.

CAUTIONS:

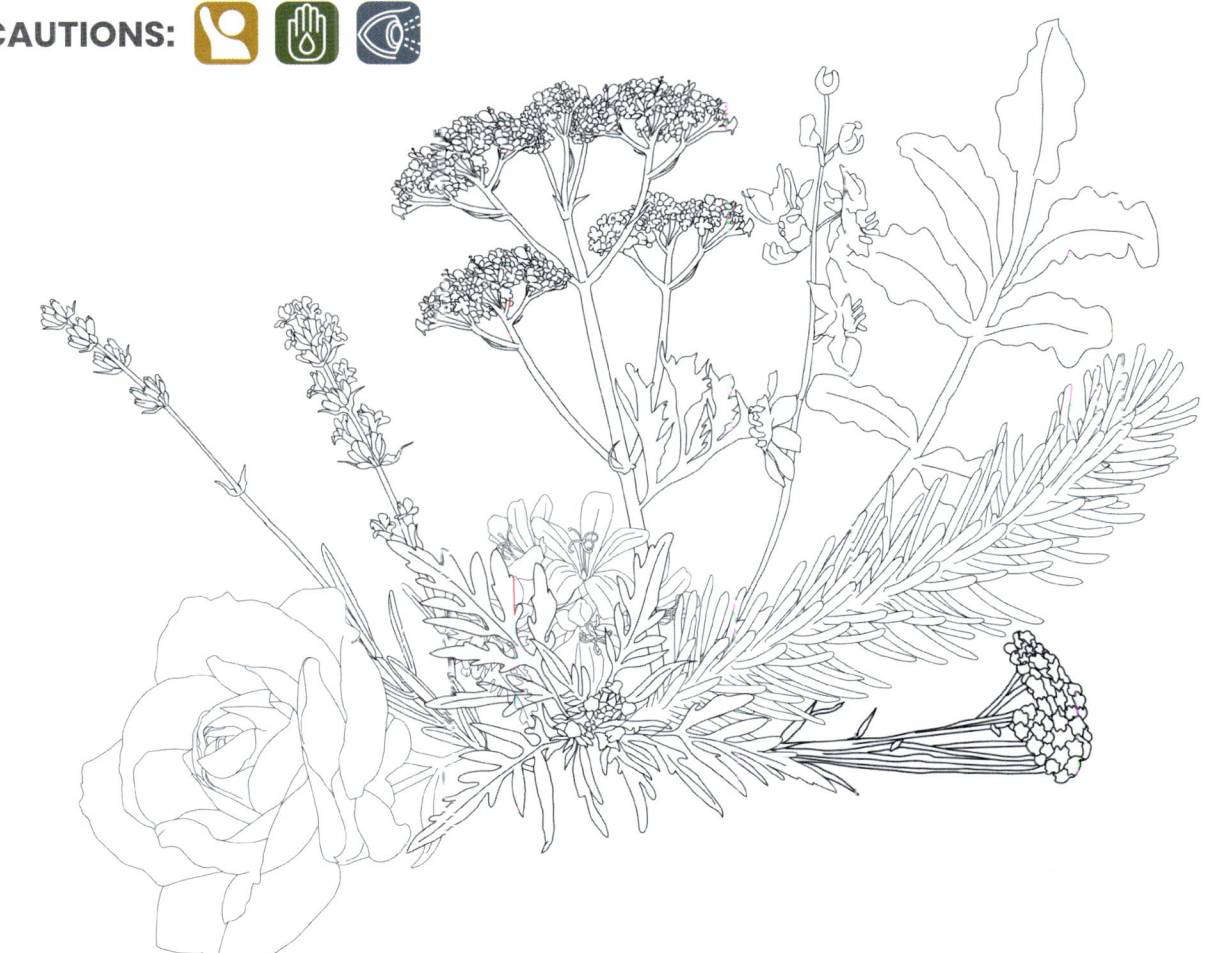

T.R. CARE™
(Essential Oil Blend)

This unique blend is designed to restore confidence and uplift emotions by reducing stress and calming the mind, body, and spirit

MEDICAL PROPERTIES & USES:
Antioxidant, anti-inflammatory, antimicrobial, antiparasitic, antibacterial, anesthetic, antifungal, anticancerous, antitumoral, antiseptic, emotion supporting, anxiety, ADHD, depression, insomnia, relaxant, muscle relaxant, sedative, antispasmodic, digestive aid, circulatory enhancer, high blood pressure, burns, immune supporting, respiratory infections, skin and hair conditions

INGREDIENTS:
Roman Chamomile, Tangerine, Lavender, Bergamot, Ylang Ylang, Frankincense, Valerian, Blue Cypress, Orange, Royal Hawaiian Sandalwood, Sacred Sandalwood, Geranium, Black Spruce, Davana, Rue, Jasmine, Angelica, Cedarwood, Helichrysum, Hyssop, Spanish Sage, Patchouli, Citrus Hystrix, Northern Lights Black Spruce, White Fir, Blue Tansy, Vetiver, Coriander, Bergamot (Furocoumarin-free), Rose, Lemon, Cinnamon Bark, Palmarosa, Matricaria (German Chamomile), Grapefruit, Spearmint, Ocotea

DIRECTIONS:
Aromatic: (30). Topical: Neat.

CAUTIONS:

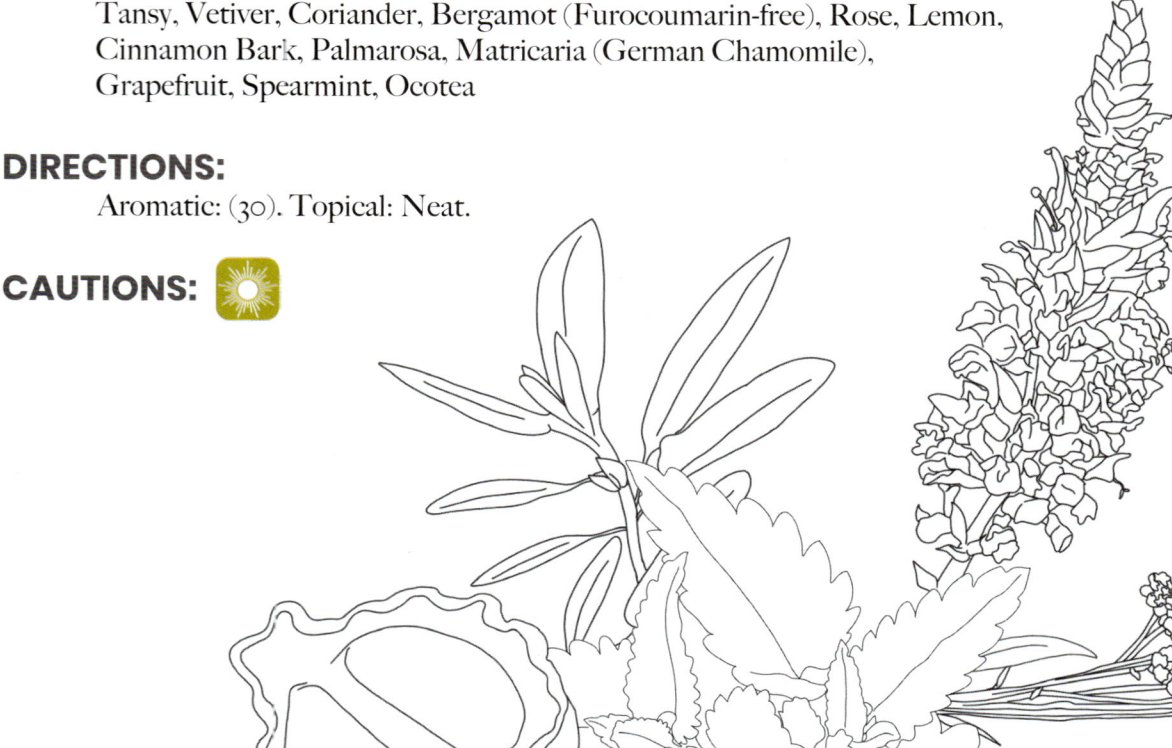

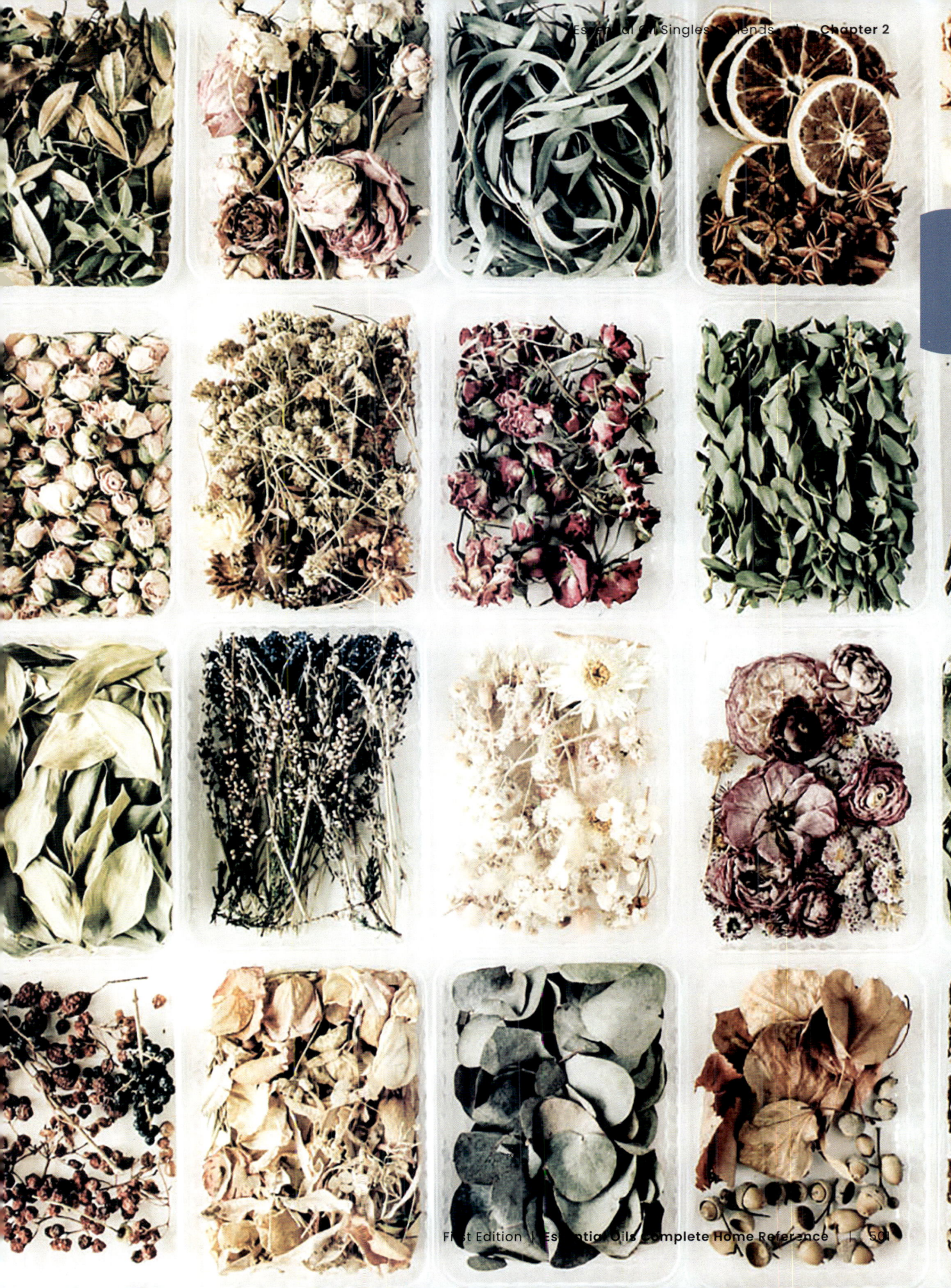

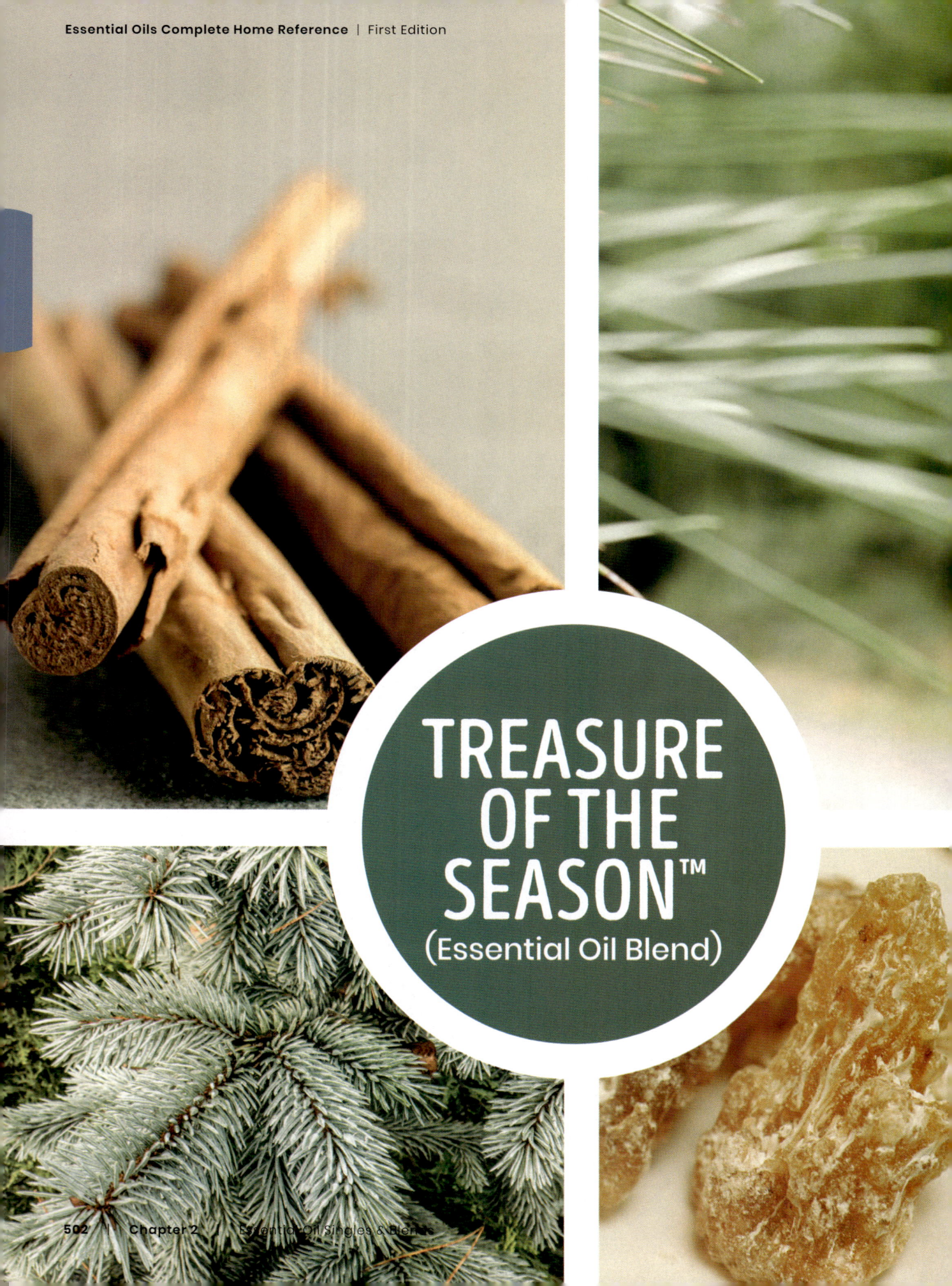

ABOUT TREASURE OF THE SEASON™:

Young Living's limited-release blend Treasure of the Season delights the senses with the rich fragrance of Frankincense and Frereana Frankincense. The addition of spicy Cinnamon Bark and the fresh scent of Idaho Grand Fir captures the essence of the holiday season.

MEDICAL PROPERTIES & USES:

Antitumoral, immuno-stimulant, emotion supporting, antidepressant, calming, muscle relaxing, antifungal, anti-inflammatory, anticancerous, antibacterial, antispasmodic, analgesic, antiviral, anticoagulant, antiparasitic, circulatory stimulant

INGREDIENTS:

Frankincense, Frereana Frankincense, Cinnamon Bark, Idaho Grand Fir

DIRECTIONS:

Aromatic: 3o. Topical: 5o-5c. Apply around ear for earache. Use in Raindrop Technique. Dietary (Vitality): Dilute 1 drop with 4 drops of carrier oil. Put in a capsule and take 1 daily.

CAUTIONS:

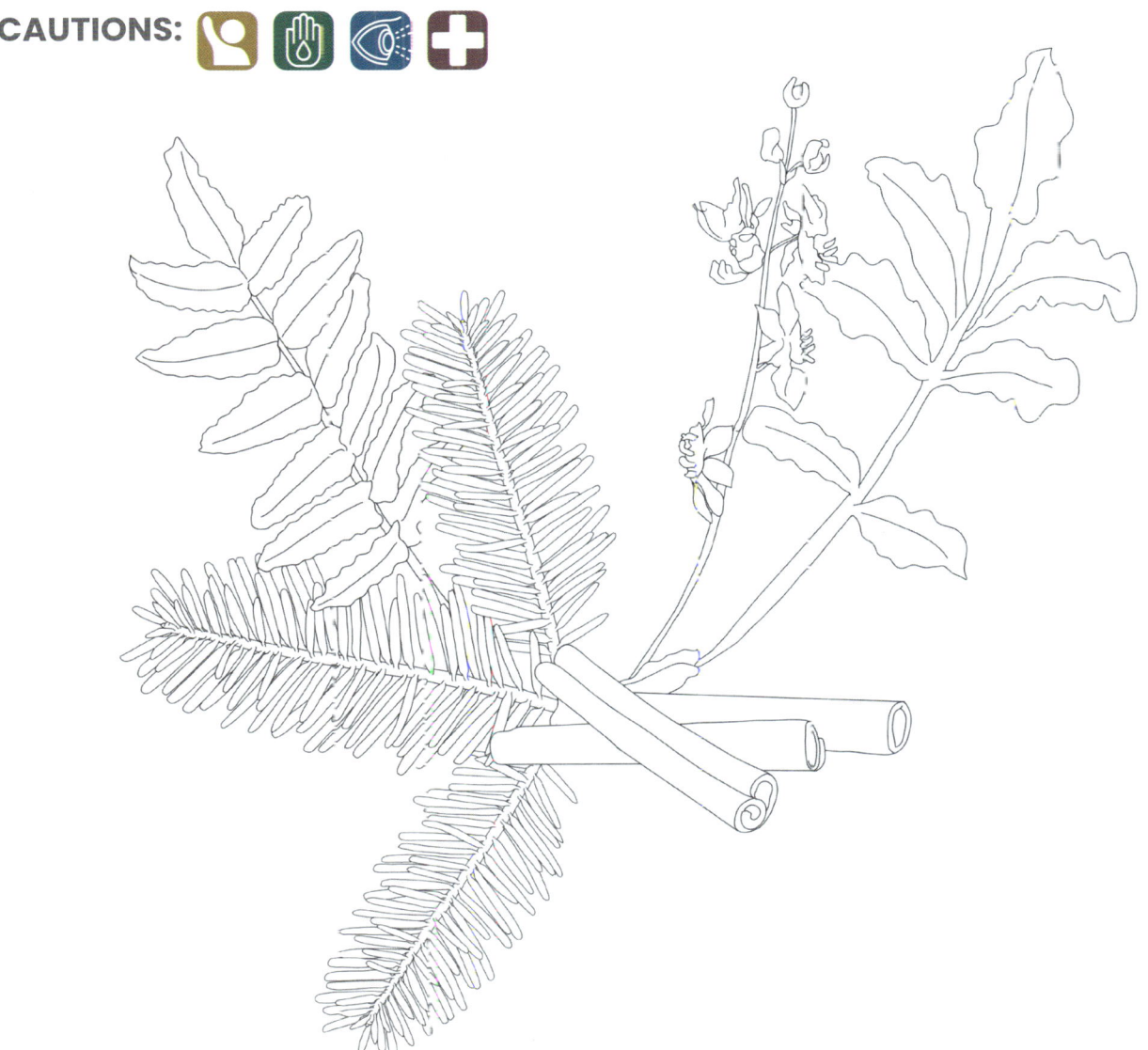

BOTANICAL FAMILY:
Pinaceae

PLANT ORIGIN:
Canada

EXTRACTION METHOD:
Steam distilled from needles, twigs, and branches

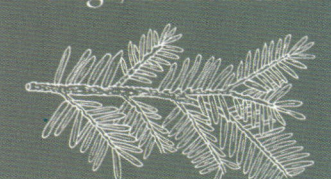

KEY CONSTITUENTS:
Bornyl Acetate (26-43%),
Alpha-Pinene (16-25%),
Camphene (13-19%),
Tricyclene (4-9%),
Limonene (3-5%),
Myrcene (1-5%),
Beta-Pinene (1-3%)

TSUGA
(Tsuga canadensis)

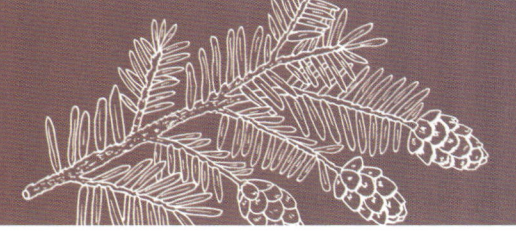

Several North American Indian tribes, including the Cherokees, used Tsuga for a number of complaints. To this day, it is used in modern herbalism for its antiseptic and astringent properties. Diarrhea, colitis, cystitis, and diverticulitis are treated by a tsuga tea; it can also be used as a poultice to cleanse wounds.

MEDICAL PROPERTIES:
Analgesic, antirheumatic, blood cleanser, stimulant, cell regenerating

USES:
Respiratory conditions, coughs, flu, colds, bronchitis, kidney/urinary infections, skin conditions, venereal diseases, anxiety, muscle aches, acne

FRAGRANT INFLUENCE:
Spiritually uplifting, stress

DIRECTIONS:
Aromatic: 30. Topical: 50-50.

CAUTIONS: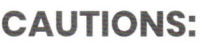

SELECTED RESEARCH:
Setzer WN. The Phytochemistry of Cherokee Aromatic Medicinal Plants. Medicines (Basel) 2018 Dec; 5(4):121.

Saikat S, Raja C. The role of antioxidants in human health. Oxidative Stress: Diagnostics, Prevention, and Therapy. Washington, DC: American Chemical Society; 2011. 1083. p 1-37.

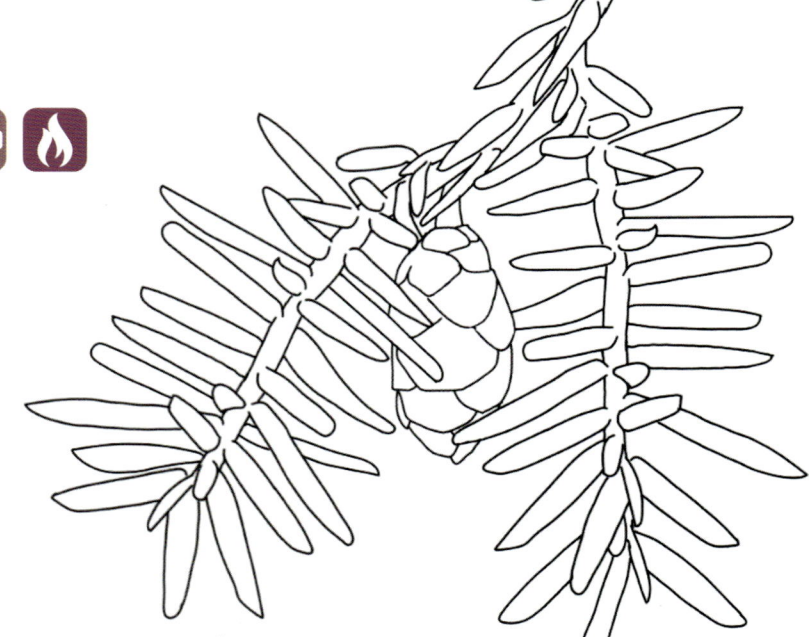

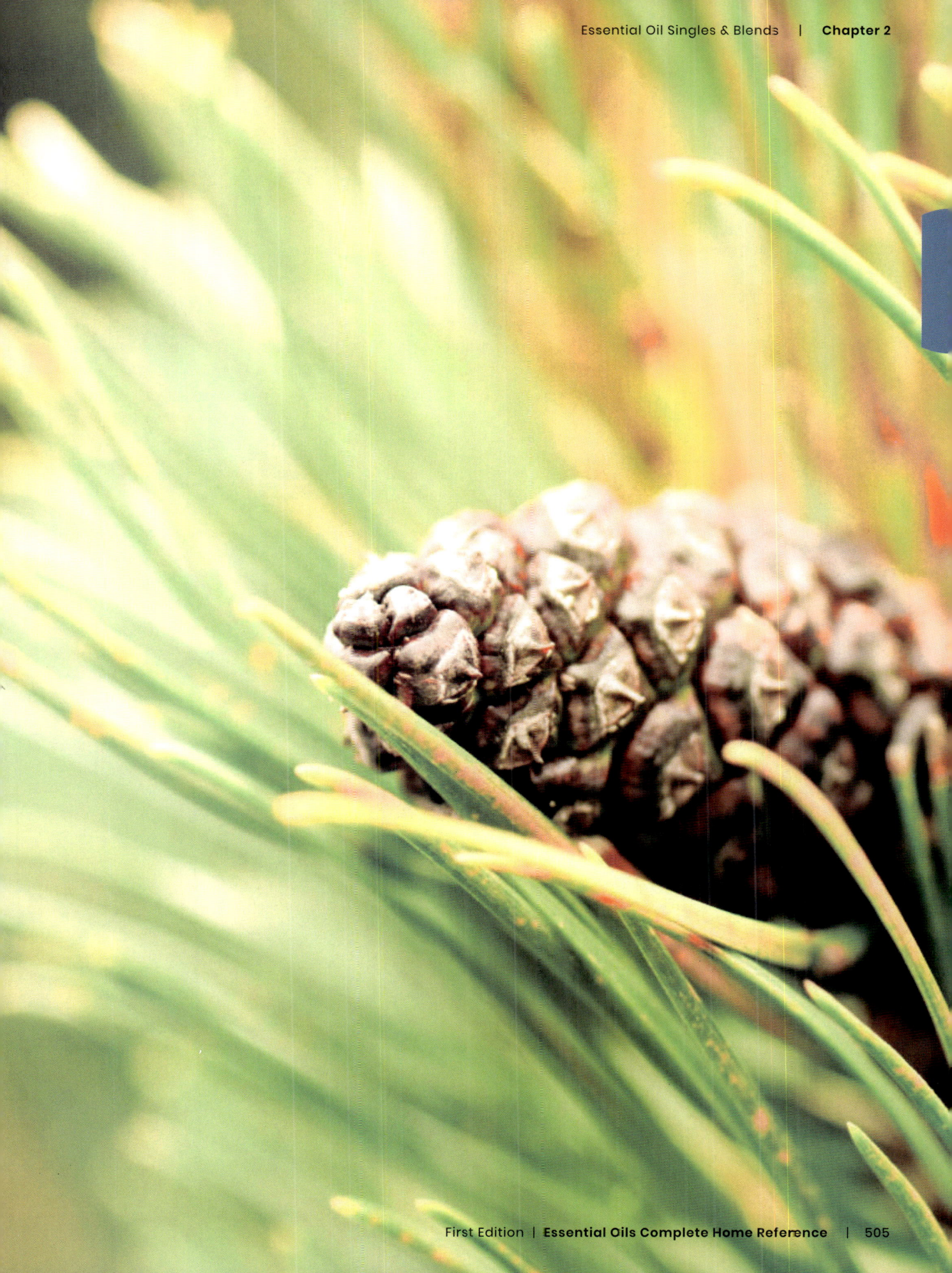

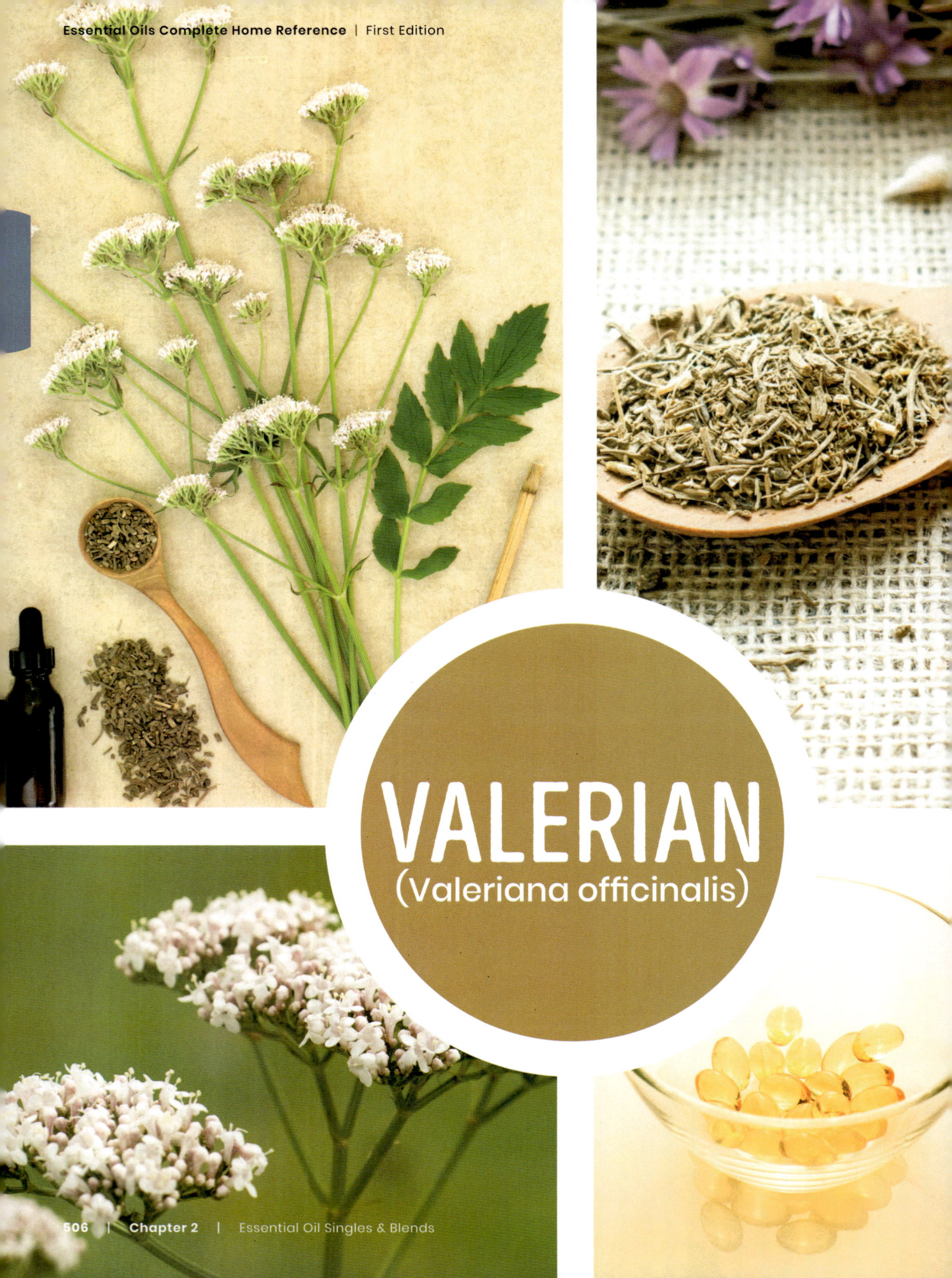

VALERIAN
(Valeriana officinalis)

Essential Oil Singles & Blends | Chapter 2

BOTANICAL FAMILY:
Caprifoliaceae

PLANT ORIGIN:
Belgium, Bulgaria, China

EXTRACTION METHOD:
Steam distilled from root

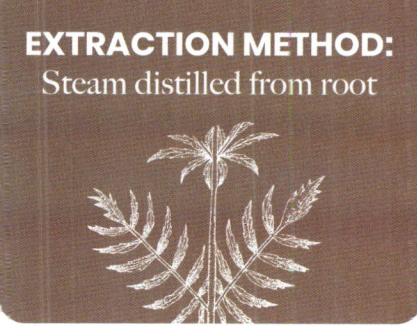

KEY CONSTITUENTS:
Bornyl Acetate (34-42%),
Camphene (24-30%),
Alpha-Pinene (6-8%),
Valerenal (2-7%),
Beta-Pinene (4-5%),
Myrtenyl Acetate (3-5%),
Borneol (up to 3%),
Limonene (1-3%)

HISTORICAL DATA:
During the last three decades, valerian has been clinically investigated for its tranquilizing properties. Researchers have pinpointed the sesquiterpenes valerenic acid and valerone as the active constituents that exert a calming effect on the central nervous system. The German Commission E has pronounced Valerian to be an effective treatment for restlessness and for sleep disturbances resulting from nervous conditions.

MEDICAL PROPERTIES:
Sedative and tranquilizing to the central nervous system, antispasmodic

USES:
Insomnia, restlessness, focus problems, hot flashes, anxiety, dysmenorrhea

FRAGRANT INFLUENCE:
Nurturing, soothing aroma, calming, relaxing, grounding, emotionally balancing

DIRECTIONS:
Aromatic: 30. Topical: Neat. Dietary: Put 2 drops in a capsule and take 3 times daily or as needed.

CAUTIONS:

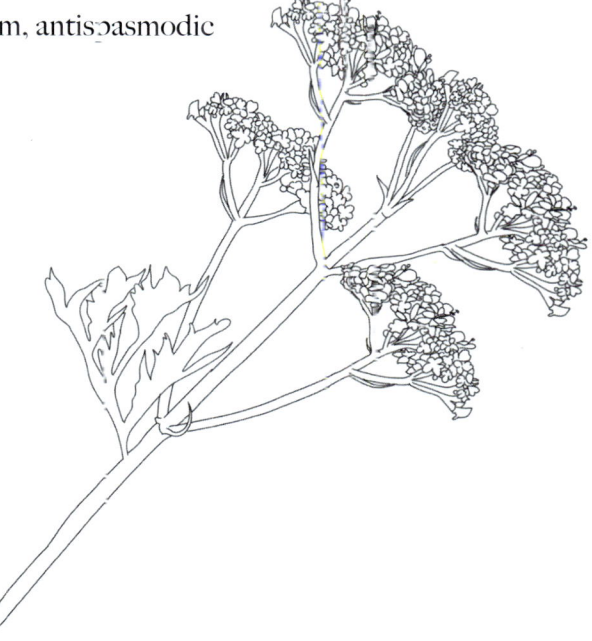

SELECTED RESEARCH:

Azizi H, Shojaii A, Hashem-Dabaghian F, Noras M, Boroumand A, Haghani BE, Ghods R. Effects of Valeriana officinalis (Valerian) on tension-type headache: A randomized, placebo-controlled, double-blind clinical trial. Avicenna J Phytomed. 2020 May-Jun; 10(3): 297-304.

Abdelllah SA, Berlin A, Blondeau C, Guinobert I, Guilbot A, Beck M, Duforez F. A combination of Eschscholtzia California Cham. And Valeriana officinalis L. extracts for adjustment insomnia: A prospective observational study. J Tradit Complement Med. 2020 Mar; 10(2): 116-123.

Samaei A, Nobahar M, Hydarinia-Naieni Z, Ebrahimian AA, Tammadon MR, Ghorbani R, Vafaei A. Effect of valerian on cognitive disorders and electroencephalography in hemodialysis patients: a randomized, cross over, double-blind clinical study. BMC Nephrol. 2018; 19: 379.

Ahmadi M, Khalili H, Abbasian L, Ghaeli P. Effect of Valerian in preventing neuropsychiatric adverse effects of Efavirenz in HIV-positive patients: a pilot randomized, placebo-controlled clinical trial. Ann Pharmacother. 2017 Jun;51(6):457-464. Epub 2017 Feb 1.

Hassani S, Alipour A, Darvishi Khezri H, Firouzian A, Emami Zeydi A, Gholipour Baradari A, Ghafari R, Habibi WA, Tahmasebi H, Alipour F, Ebrahim Zadeh P. Can Valeriana officinalis root extract prevent early postoperative cognitive dysfunction after CABG [coronary artery bypass graft] surgery? A randomized, double-blind, placebo-controlled study. Psychopharmacology (Berl). 2015 Mar;232(5):843-50. Epub 2014 Aug 31.

Jung HY, Yoo DY, Nam SM, Kim JW, Choi JH, Yoo M, Lee S, Yoon YS, Hwang IK. Valerenic acid protects against physical and psychological stress by reducing the turnover of serotonin and norepinephrine in mouse hippocampus-amygdala region. J Med Food. 2015 Dec;18(12):1333-9. Epub 2015 Jul 15.

Becker A, Felgentreff F, Schröder H, Meier B, Brattström A. The anxiolytic effects of a Valerian extract is based on valerenic acid. BMC Complement Altern Med. 2014 Jul 28;14:267.

Gromball J, Beschorner F, Wantzen C, Paulsen U, Burkart M. Hyperactivity, concentration difficulties and impulsiveness improve during seven weeks' treatment with valerian root and lemon balm extracts in primary school children. Phytomedicine. 2014 Jul-Aug;21(8-9):1098-103. Epub 2014 May 15.

VALOR® & VALOR® ROLL-ON
(Essential Oil Blend)

Valor Essential Oil Blend is an empowering combination of therapeutic-grade essential oils that works with both the physical and spiritual aspects of the body to increase feelings of strength, courage, and self-esteem in the face of adversity. Renowned for its strengthening qualities, Valor enhances an individual's internal resources. It helps the body self-correct its balance and alignment.

This is a very popular blend and is also offered in a portable, convenient, roll-on application.

MEDICAL PROPERTIES & USES:
Anti-inflammatory, antimicrobial, antioxidative, emotion supporting, calming, disease inhibitory, muscle and bone supporting, organ protective, pain or swelling reducing, skin and hair improving

INGREDIENTS:
Fractionated coconut oil, Black Spruce, Camphor (Ho Wood), Blue Tansy, Frankincense, Geranium

DIRECTIONS:
Aromatic: 6o. Topical: Neat. When using a series of oils, apply Valor first and wait 5 to 10 minutes before applying other oils. Use in Raindrop Technique. Wear as a fragrance.

CAUTIONS:

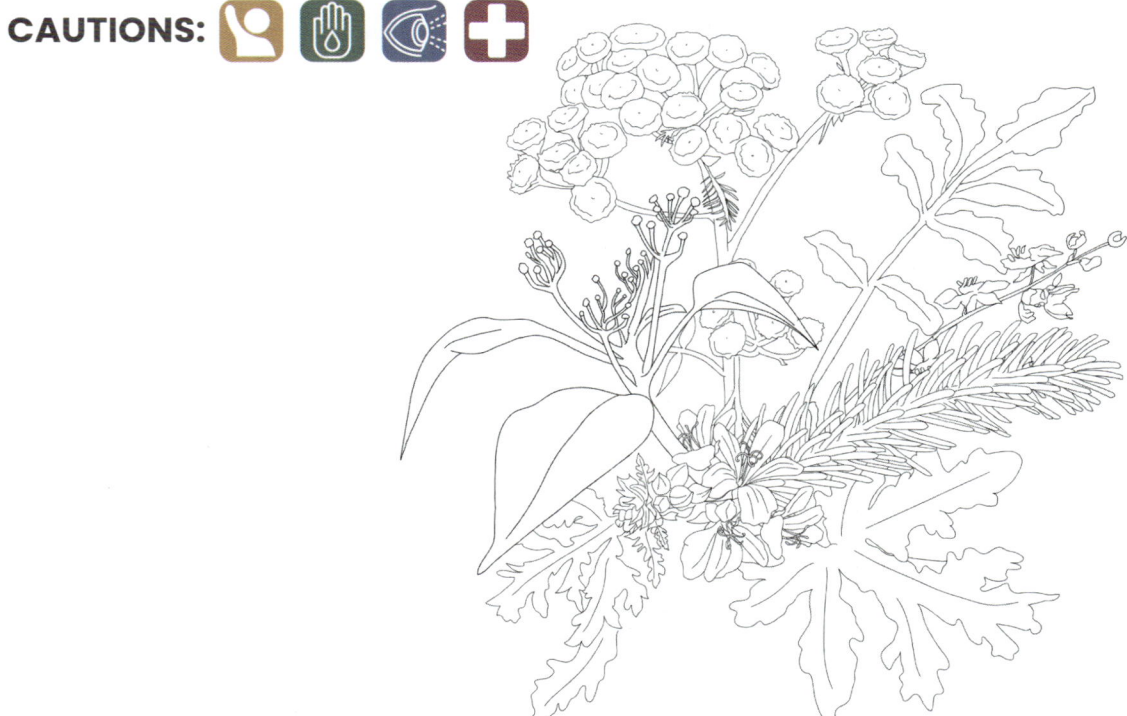

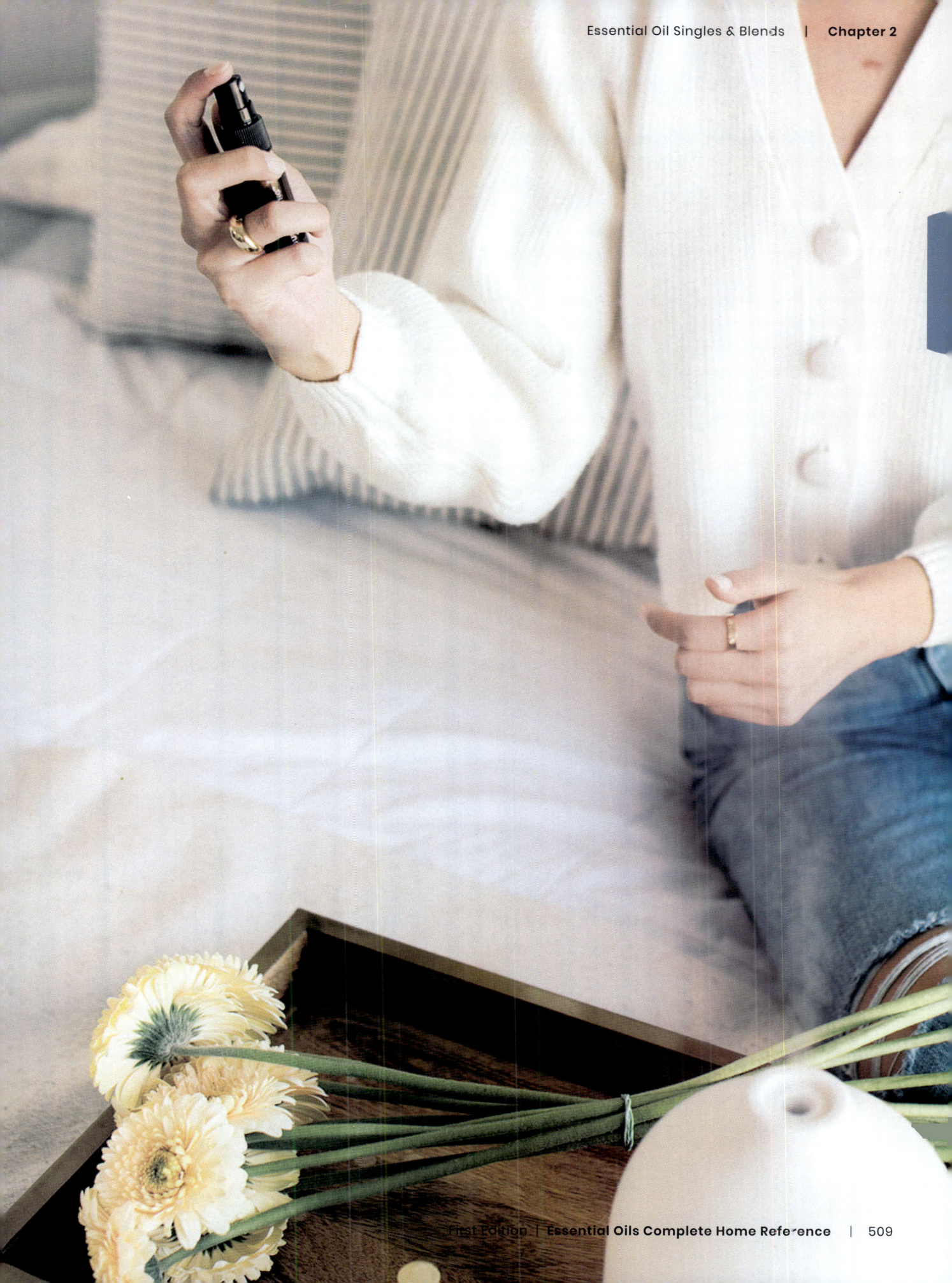

BOTANICAL FAMILY:
Orchidaceae

PLANT ORIGIN:
Madagascar

EXTRACTION METHOD:
Proprietary vacuum distillation

KEY CONSTITUENTS:
Vanillin (85-95%)

VANILLA
(Vanilla planifolia)

HISTORICAL DATA:

Young Living's Vanilla is an oleoresin, not an essential oil. It is also not an extract or an absolute; these types of vanillas contain mostly alcohol and do not blend well with other essential oils. Young Living scientists wanted to find a vanilla that would not only follow our Seed to Seal process but would also be compatible with our essential oils. They searched for more than a year to find the right product, and with a first-of-its-kind extraction method using Vanilla oleoresin and fractionated coconut oil, Young Living's Vanilla is not only 100 percent pure, but it is also perfect for diffusing and blending with other essential oils.

Vanilla oleoresin, created for the first time by Young Living Essential Oils, is the highest known oil in vanillin, which is similar in chemical structure to the aromatic compound eugenol, found in cloves. Recent tests conducted at independent laboratories found that the vanilla content of this vanilla oil is over 10 times higher than commercially available super-concentrated vanilla extracts. The same way that eugenol in clove oil numbs dental tissue, vanillin numbs stress and food cravings.

The importance of vanillin is now being investigated by scientists who are researching the ways in which activating vanilloid-type brain receptors can enhance well-being and combat depression.
Vanilla is produced from an orchid called Vanilla planifolia that grows long, green vanilla bean pods. The process of obtaining Vanilla is very extensive. It can take up to 4 years for the vine to mature from the time the seed is planted. The vine produces orchid blossoms that last only 24 hours and must be pollinated by hand within 8 to 12 hours, otherwise the vanilla bean will not grow. The entire process from growing and pollinating to drying, curing, and preparing for export takes about one year.

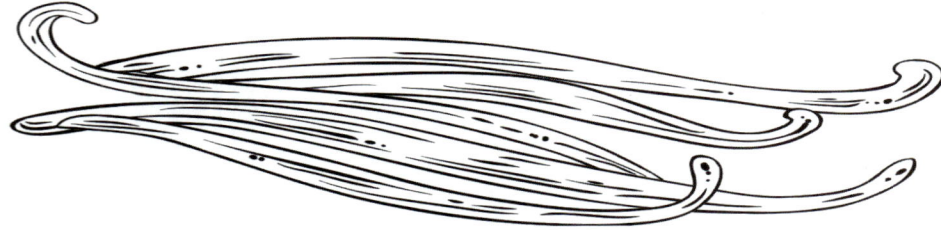

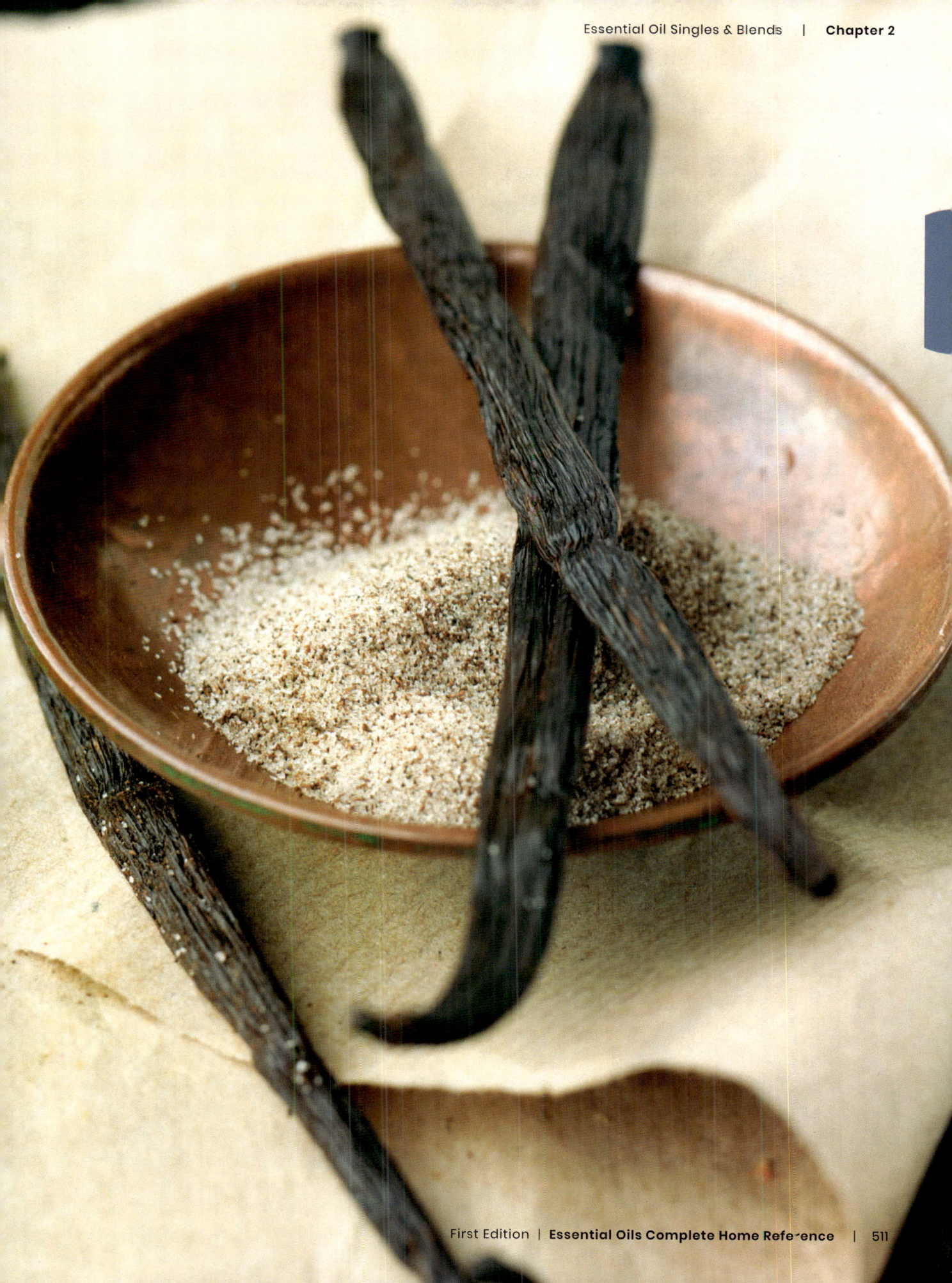

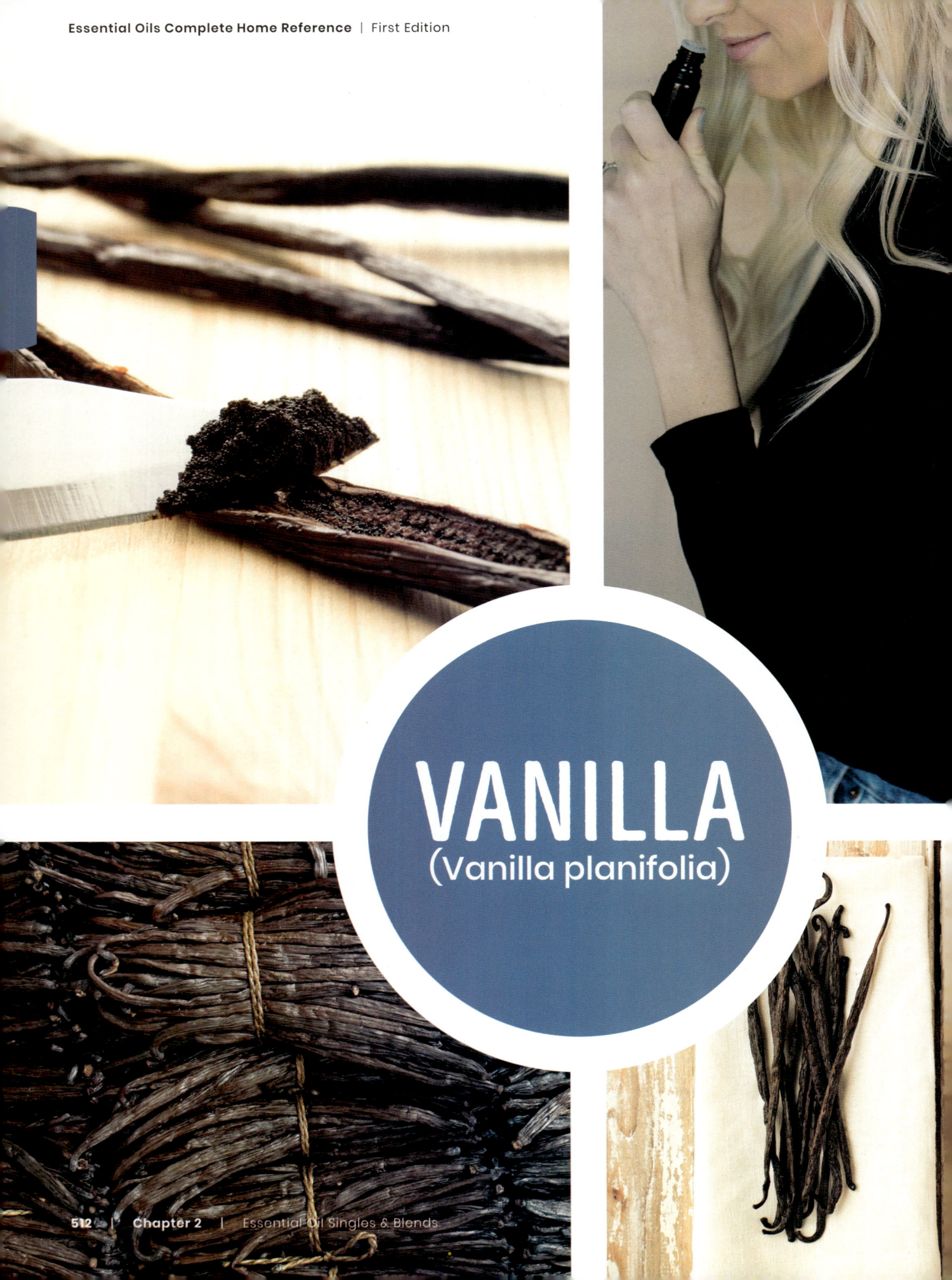

VANILLA
(Vanilla planifolia)

Essential Oil Singles & Blends | **Chapter 2**

BOTANICAL FAMILY:
Orchidaceae

PLANT ORIGIN:
Madagascar

EXTRACTION METHOD:
Proprietary vacuum distillation

KEY CONSTITUENTS:
Vanillin (85-95%)

MEDICAL PROPERTIES:
Mood elevating; weakens or numbs stress and food cravings, antimutagenic, antidepressant, tranquilizing, sedative, antioxidant, anti-inflammatory

USES:
Appetite control, depression, skin irritation, blood pressure, PMS symptoms, skin and hair conditioning and moisturizing

FRAGRANT INFLUENCE:
Uplifts mood through vanilloid receptor action in brain; warm, sweet aroma; balancing aroma that helps relax the body and mind; calming, mood-boosting scent; creates a comforting, welcoming atmosphere when diffused

INGREDIENTS:
Vanilla planifolia (Vanilla) fruit extract (100 percent pure), Caprylic/capric triglyceride (Fractionated coconut oil)

DIRECTIONS:
Aromatic: 30. Topical: 50/50. Dietary: Not for use as flavoring in cooking.

CAUTIONS:

SELECTED RESEARCH:

Srinual S, Chanvorachote P, Pongrakhananon V. Suppression of cancer stem-like phenotypes in NCI-H460 lung cancer cells by vanillin through an Akt-dependent pathway. Int J Oncol. 2017 Apr;50(4):1341-1351. Epub 2017 Feb 17.

Bilcu M, Grumezescu AM, Oprea AE, Popescu RC, Mogoșanu GD, Hristu R, Stanciu GA, Mihailescu DF, Lazar V, Bezirtzoglou E, Chifiriuc MC. Efficiency of vanilla, patchouli and ylang ylang essential oils stabilized by iron oxide@C14 nanostructures against bacterial adherence and biofilms formed by Staphylococcus aureus and Klebsiella pneumoniae clinical strains. Molecules. 2014 Nov 4;19(11):17943-56.

Kundu A, Mitra A. Flavoring extracts of Hemidesmus indicus roots and Vanilla planifolia pods exhibit in vitro acetylcholinesterase inhibitory activities. Plant Foods Hum Nutr. 2013 Sep;68(3):247-53.

Widiez T, Hartman TG, Dudai N, Yan Q, Lawton M, Havkin-Frenkel D, Belanger FC. Functional characterization of two new members of the caffeoyl CoA O-methyltransferase-like gene family from Vanilla planifolia reveals a new class of plastid-localized O-methyltransferase. Plant Mol Biol. 2011 Aug;76(6):475-88. Epub 2011 Apr 5.

Moussaieff A, Rimmerman N, Bregman T, Straiker A, Felder CC, Shoham S, Kashman Y, Huang SM, Lee H, Shohami E, Mackie K, Caterina MJ, Walker JM, Fride E, Mechoulam R. Incensole acetate, an incense component, elicits psychoactivity by activating TRPV3 channels in the brain. FASEB J. 2008 Aug;22(8):3024-34. Epub 2008 May 20.

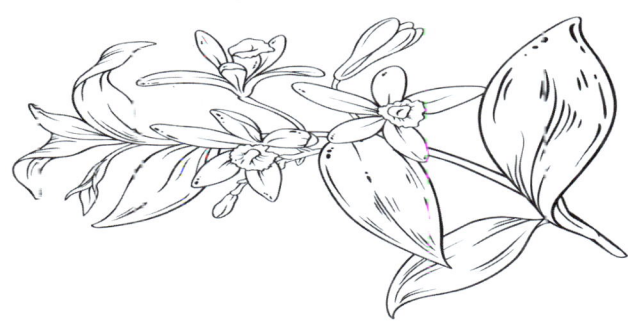

BOTANICAL FAMILY:
Poaceae

PLANT ORIGIN:
Haiti

EXTRACTION METHOD:
Steam distilled from root

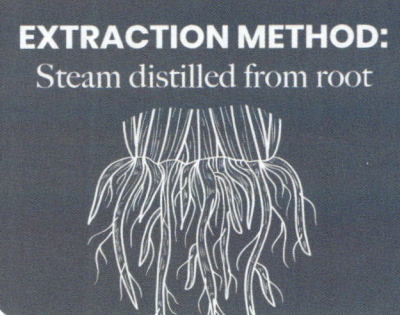

KEY CONSTITUENTS:
Khusimol (5-18%),
Isovalencenol (1-18%),
Beta-Vetivenene (up to 9%),
Alpha-Vetivone (1-8%),
Beta-Vetivone (1-7%)

VETIVER
(Vetiveria zizanoides) (Syn. V. zizanioides)

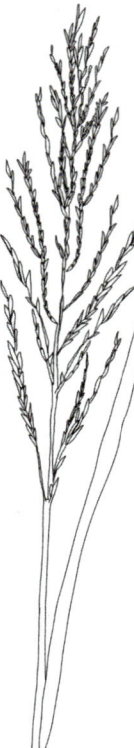

Vetiver is well known for its anti-inflammatory properties and is traditionally used for arthritic symptoms.

MEDICAL PROPERTIES:
Antioxidant, sedative, larvicidal/insecticidal, antiseptic, antispasmodic, relaxant, circulatory stimulant

USES:
ADHD, anxiety, rheumatism/arthritis, depression (including postpartum), insomnia, skin care (oily, aging, acne, wrinkles), perfumes, massage therapy, calming

FRAGRANT INFLUENCE:
Earthy, balancing aroma. Psychologically grounding, calming, and stabilizing. It helps us cope with stress and recover from emotional trauma. Terry Friedmann, MD, found in preliminary clinical tests that Vetiver may be successful in the treatment of ADD and ADHD (attention deficit disorders) in children.

DIRECTIONS:
Aromatic: 6O. Topical: Neat. Dietary: Take as a dietary supplement.

CAUTIONS: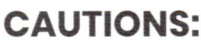

SELECTED RESEARCH:

Seshadri VD, Vijayaraghavan P, Kim Y-O, Kim H-J, Al-Ghamdi AA, Elshikh MS, A;-Dosary MA, Alsubaie QD. In vitro antioxidant and cytotoxic activities of polyherbal extracts from Vetiver zizanioides, Trichosanthese cucumerina, and Molluga Cerviana on HeLa and MCF-7 cell lines. Saudi J Biol Sci. 2020 Jun; 27(6): 1475-1481.

Lavanya P, Ramaiah S, Anbarasu A. Ethyl 4-(4-methylphenyl)-4 pentenoate from Vetiver zizanioides inhibits dengue NS2B-NS3 protease and prevents viral assembly: a computational molecular dynamics and docking study. Cell Biochem Biophys. 2016 Sep;74(3):337-51. Epub 2016 Jun 21.

Saiyudthong S, Pongmayteegul S, Marsden CA, Phansuwan-Pujito P. Anxiety-like behaviour and c-fos expression in rats that inhaled vetiver essential oil. Nat Prod Res. 2015;29(22):2141-7. Epub 2015 Jan 2.

Peng HY, Lai CC, Lin CC, Chou ST. Effect of Vetiveria zizanioides essential oil on melanogenesis in melanoma cells: downregulation of tyrosinase expression and suppression of oxidative stress. ScientificWorldJournal. 2014 Mar 19;2014:213013. eCollection 2014.

Dwivedi GR. Gupta S, Roy S, Kalani K, Pal A, Thakur JP, Saikia D, Sharma A, Darmwal NS, Darokar MP, Srivastava SK. Tricyclic sesquiterpenes from Vetiveria zizanioides (L.) Nash as antimycobacterial agents. Chem Biol Drug Des. 2013 Nov;82(5):587-94. Epub 2013 Aug 21.

Gupta R, Sharma KK, Afzal M, Damanhouri ZA, Ali B, Kaur R, Kazmi I, Anwar F. Anticonvulsant activity of ethanol extracts of Vetiveria zizanioides roots in experimental mice. Pharm Biol. 2013 Dec;51(12):1521-4. Epub 2013 Jul 18.

Matsubara E, Shimizu K, Fukagawa M, Ishizi Y, Kakoi C. Hatayama T, Nagano J, Okamoto T, Ohnuki K, Kondo R. Volatiles emitted from the roots of Vetiveria zizanioides suppress the decline in attention during a visual display task. Biomed Res. 2012;33(5):299-308.

Friedmann T. Attention deficit and hyperactivity disorder (ADHD). 2002. (Unpublished study) http://files.meetup.com/1481956/ADHD%20Research%20by%20Dr.%20Terry%20Friedmann.pdf.

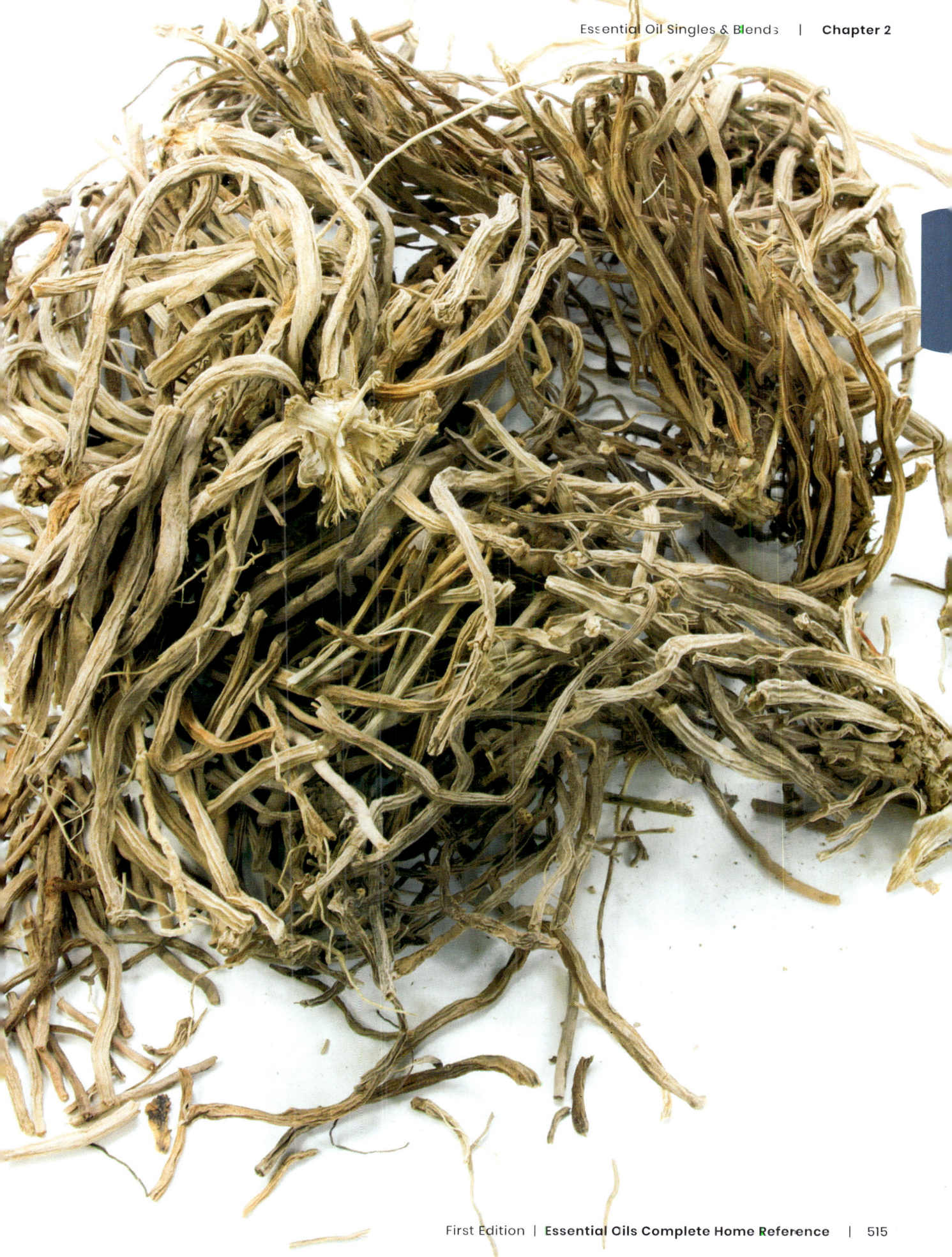

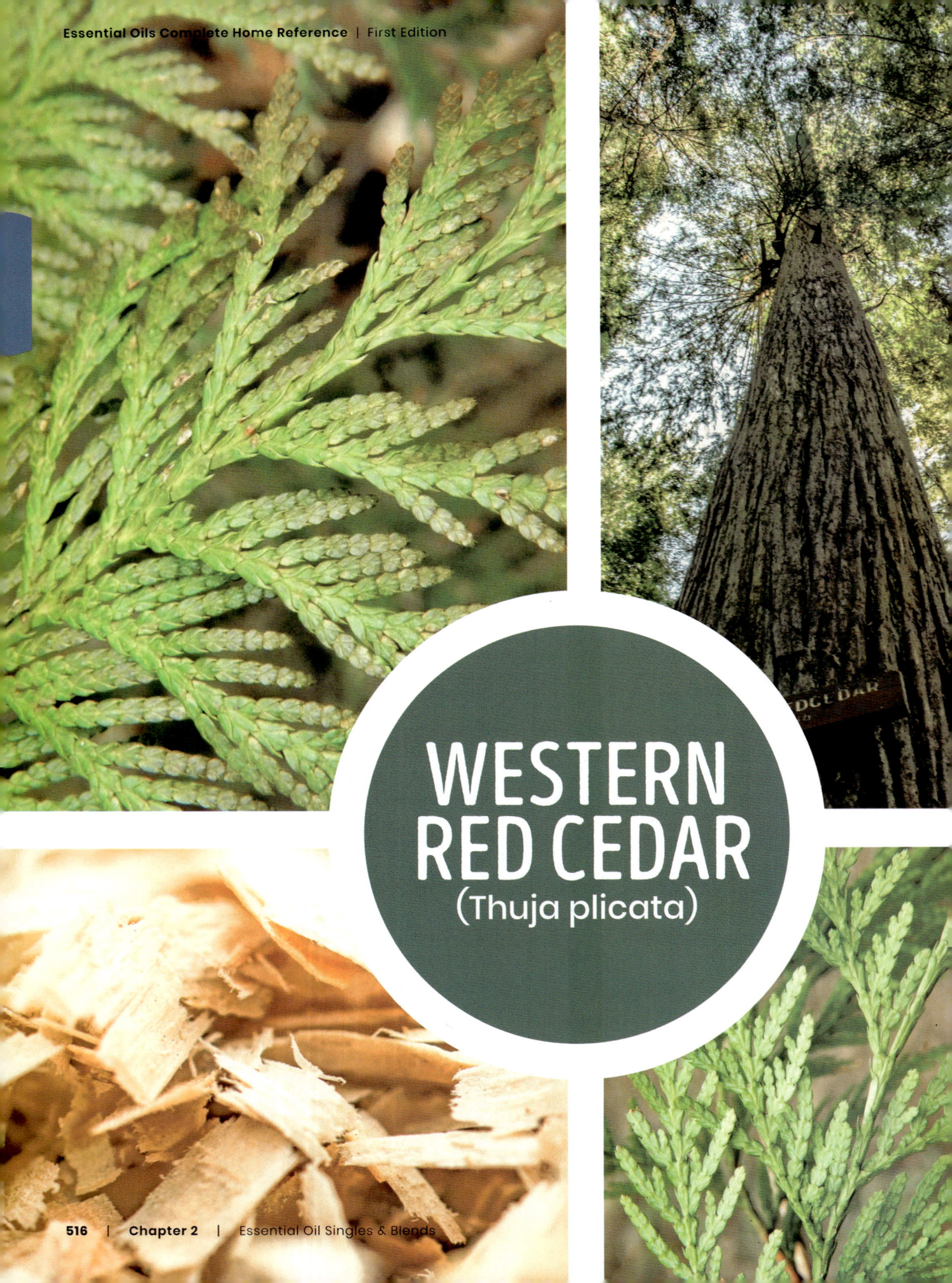

BOTANICAL FAMILY:
Cupressaceae

PLANT ORIGIN:
Utah, Idaho, Canada

EXTRACTION METHOD:
Steam distilled from needles and branches

KEY CONSTITUENTS:
Alpha-Thujone (60-80%), Beta-Thujone (4-7%), Alpha-Pinene (2-20%), Sabinene (2-4%)

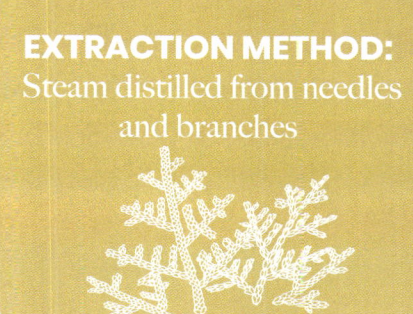

HISTORICAL DATA:
This oil is different from Canadian Red Cedar, which is distilled from the bark of the same plant, Thuja plicata. This oil is not red in color, because it is derived from needles and branches.

MEDICAL PROPERTIES:
Antiseptic, antimicrobial, antirheumatic, astringent, diuretic

USES:
Throat/lung infections, urinary tract infections, kidney problems, water retention, foot fungus, rheumatism, oral care, cough, clearing mucous

FRAGRANT INFLUENCE:
Recognized for its calming, purifying properties and helping a person cope with stress and emotional traumas, air purifying, insect spray, seasonal allergies

DIRECTIONS:
Aromatic: 60. Topical: 50-50. Other: Add to woodchips and place in closets and dressers to repel insects.

CAUTIONS: Do not use if pregnant.

SELECTED RESEARCH:
Han X, Parker TL. Aborvitae (Thuja plicata) essential oil significantly inhibited critical inflammation- and tissue remodeling-relatred proteins and genes in human dermal fibroblasts. Biochim Open. 2017 Jun; 4: 56-60.

Foster AJ, Hall DE, Mortimer L, Abercromby S, Gries R, Gries G, Bohmann J, Russell J, Mattsson J. Identification of genes in Thuja plicata foliar terpenoid defenses. Plant Physiol. 2013 Apr;161(4):1993-2004. Epub 2013 Feb 6.

Hudson J, Kuo M, Vimalanathan S. The antimicrobial properties of cedar leaf (Thuja plicata) oil: a safe and efficient decontamination agent for buildings. Int J Environ Res Public Health. 2011 Dec;8(12):4477-87. Epub 2011 Nov 30.

Tsiri D, Graikou K, Pobłocka-Olech L, Krauze-Baranowska M, Spyropoulos C, Chinou I. Chemosystematic value of the essential oil composition of Thuja species cultivated in Poland—antimicrobial activity. Molecules. 2009 Nov 19;14(11):4707-15.

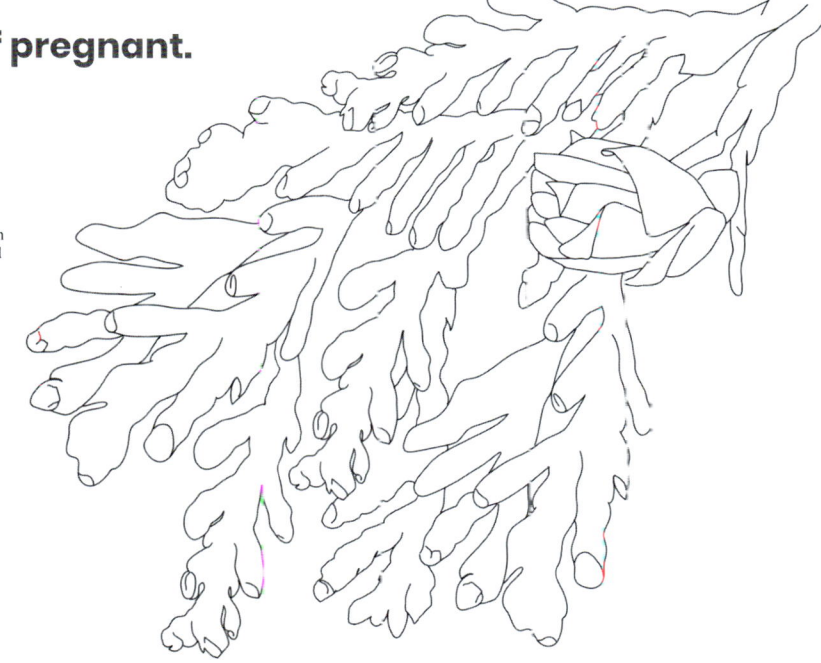

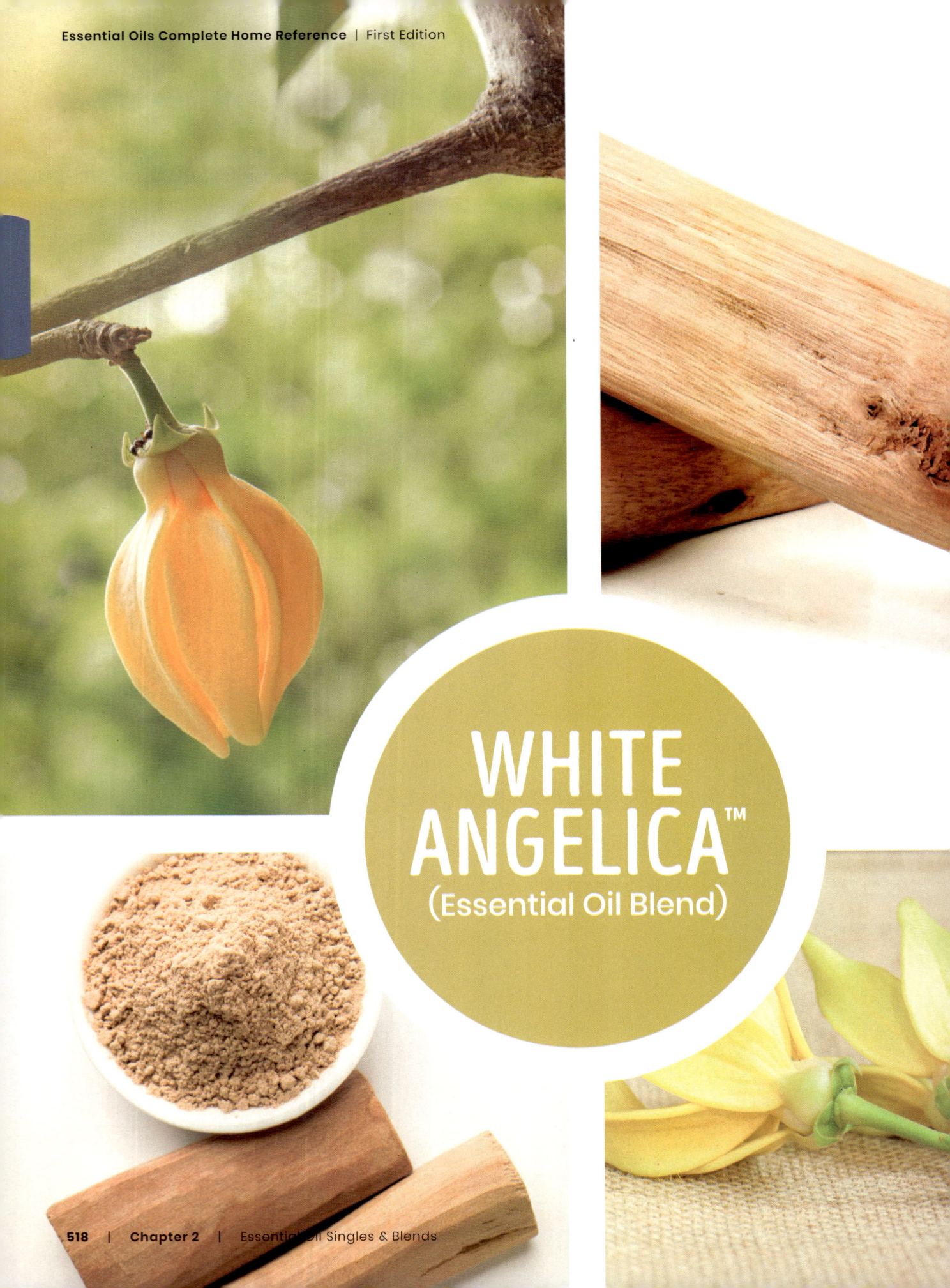

ABOUT WHITE ANGELICA™:

Increases and strengthens the aura around the body to bring a renewed sense of strength and protection, creating a feeling of wholeness in the realm of one's own spirituality. Its frequency neutralizes negative energy and gives a feeling of security.

MEDICAL PROPERTIES & USES:

Calming, hormonal supportive, emotion supporting, antibacterial, antidepressant, antioxidant, antitumoral, anti-inflammatory, antiviral, antidiabetic, analgesic/anesthetic, immune stimulant, relaxant.

INGREDIENTS:

Sweet almond oil, Bergamot, Myrrh, Geranium, Sacred Sandalwood, Ylang Ylang, Coriander, Black Spruce, Melissa, Hyssop, Rose

DIRECTIONS:

Aromatic: 30. Topical: Neat. Use in Raindrop Technique.

CAUTIONS:

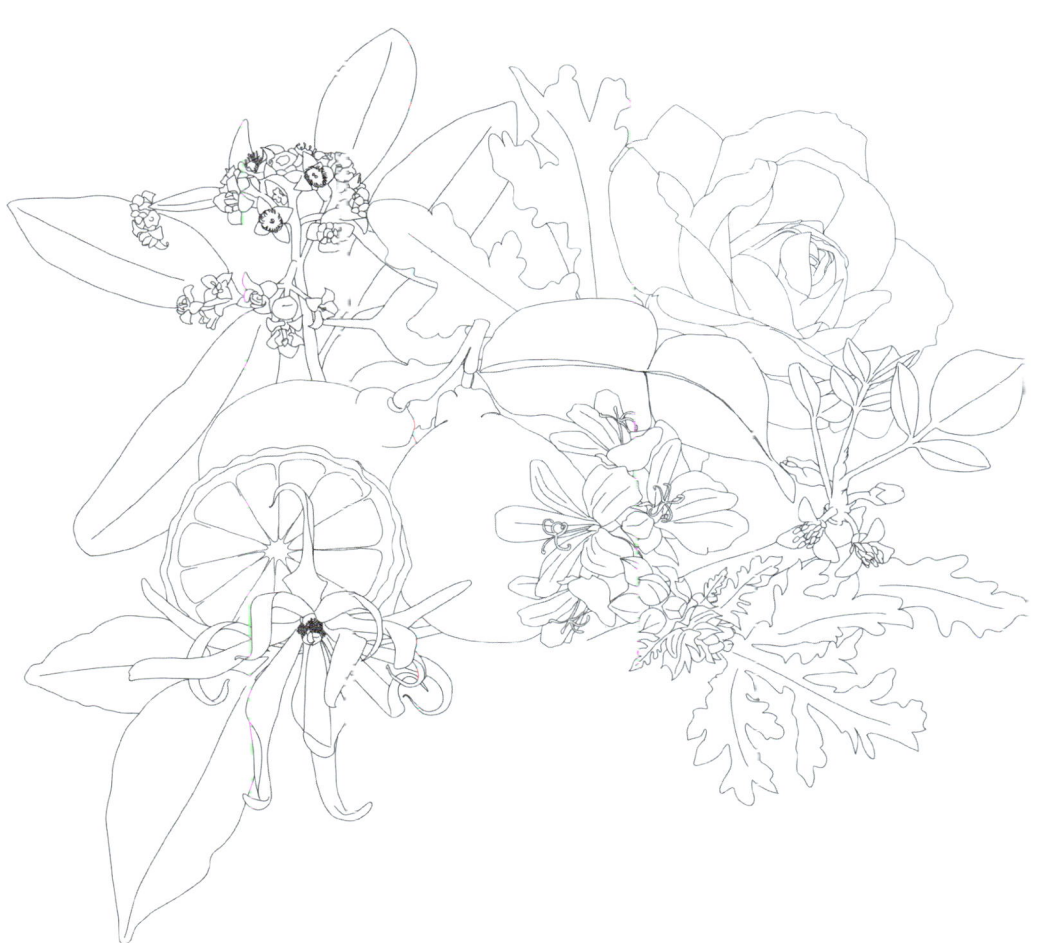

BOTANICAL FAMILY:
Pinaceae

PLANT ORIGIN:
USA

EXTRACTION METHOD:
Steam distilled from twigs and needles

KEY CONSTITUENTS:
Beta-Pinene (21-30%),
Bornyl Acetate (9-20%),
Beta-Phellandrene (8-17%),
Camphene (10-14%),
Alpha-Pinene (5-11%),
Limonene (1-6%),
Delta Cadinene (2-6%)

WHITE FIR
(Abies concolor)

A white fir infusion of the needles was used as a bath by the Acoma and Laguna Indians to help with rheumatism. The Tewa Indians used the sap from the main stem and larger branches for cuts. A 2017 study of Abies concolor seeds and cones reported: "essential oils from these conifers may be a valuable addition to medicines and cosmetics with a gentle antibacterial action."

MEDICAL PROPERTIES:
Antitumoral, anticancerous, antioxidant, anti-infectious, antimicrobial, antifungal

USES:
Respiratory infections, stress, skin conditions, pain, low energy, immune system, metabolism, body odor, wounds, bruising, sore muscles, obesity, heart conditions, inflammation, massage

FRAGRANT INFLUENCE:
Calming, energizing

DIRECTIONS:
Aromatic: 60. Topical: Neat. Dietary: Put 2 drops in a capsule and take 3 times daily or as needed.

CAUTIONS:

SELECTED RESEARCH:
Wajs-Bonikowska A, Szoka L, Karna E, Wiktorowska-Owczarek A, Sienkiewicz M. Abies Concolor Seeds and Cones as a New Source of Essential Oils—Composition and Biological Activity. Molecules. 2017 Nov; 22(11): 1880.

Bağci E, Diğrak M. Antimicrobial activity of essential oils from some Abies (Fir) species from Turkey. Flavour Fragr J. 1996 Jul/Aug;11(4):251-56.

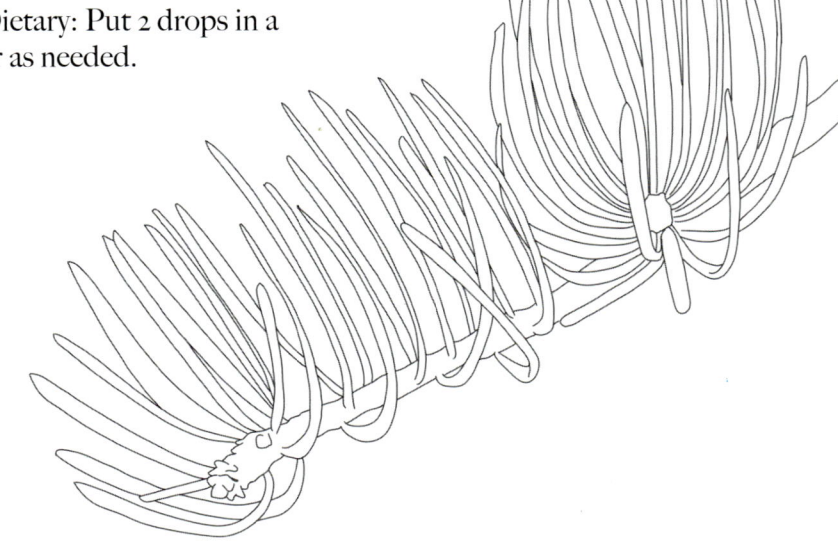

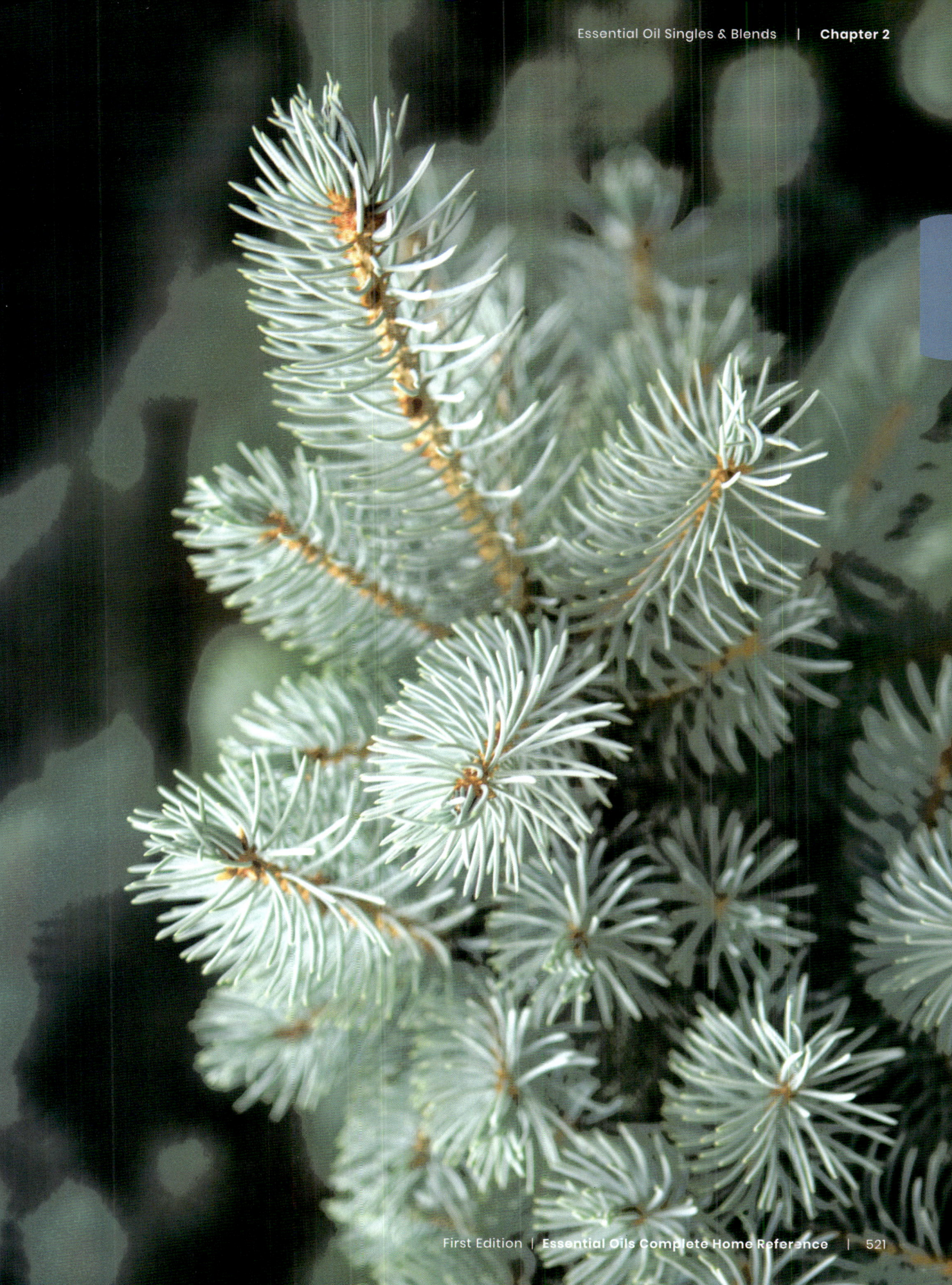

WHITE LIGHT™
(Essential Oil Blend)

White Light is a balancing essential oil blend meant to elevate the mind, awaken the senses, boost confidence, and promote harmony with nature. These four white conifers from Canada and our Highland Flats Tree Farm in Idaho symbolize light, new beginnings, cleanliness, and purity. Traditionally, Native Americans used the conifers in this blend for ceremonies, food, medicines, and building materials.

MEDICAL PROPERTIES & USES:
Uplifting, balancing, higher consciousness and awareness, empowering, arthritis, muscular aches and pains, rheumatism, bronchitis, coughs, sinusitis, colds, fever, flu, asthma, neuralgia, rheumatic pain, anti-inflammatory, antioxidant, antiseptic, antibacterial, analgesic, antinociceptive, psoriasis, angina, stomachache, sores and cuts, skin rashes, blood poisoning, boils, surface cleanser, prayer, meditation, yoga

INGREDIENTS:
White Fir, White Cedar, White Pine, White Spruce

DIRECTIONS:
Aromatic: 30. Topical: 50-50.

CAUTIONS:

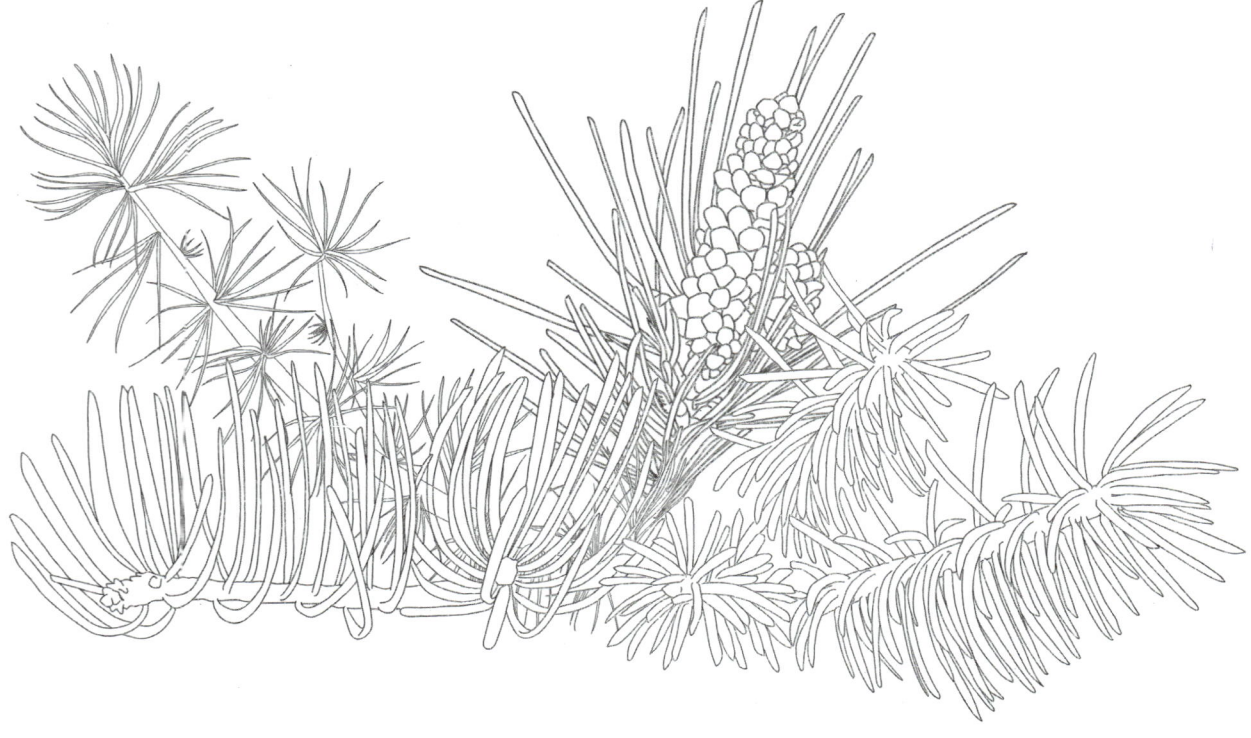

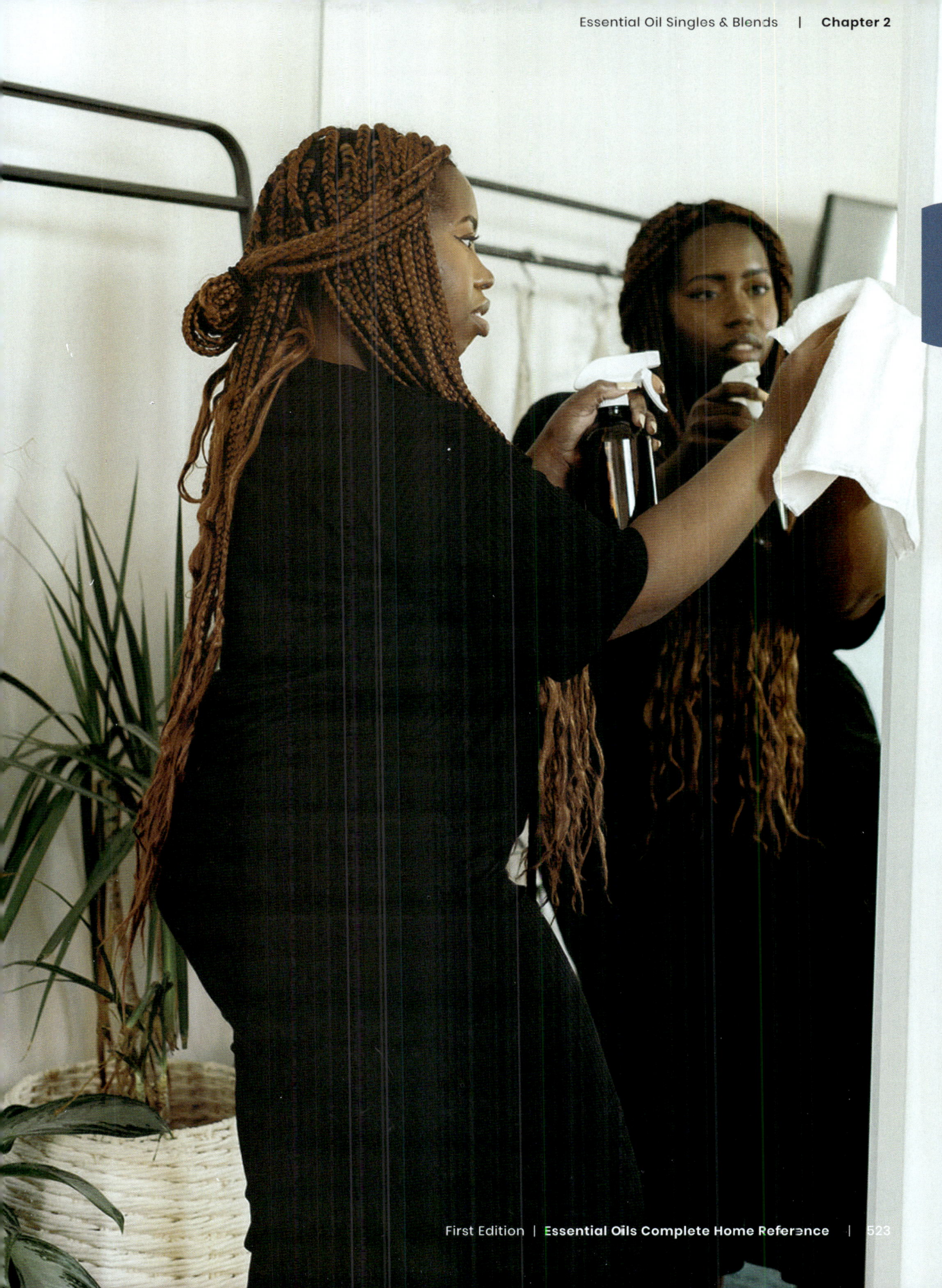

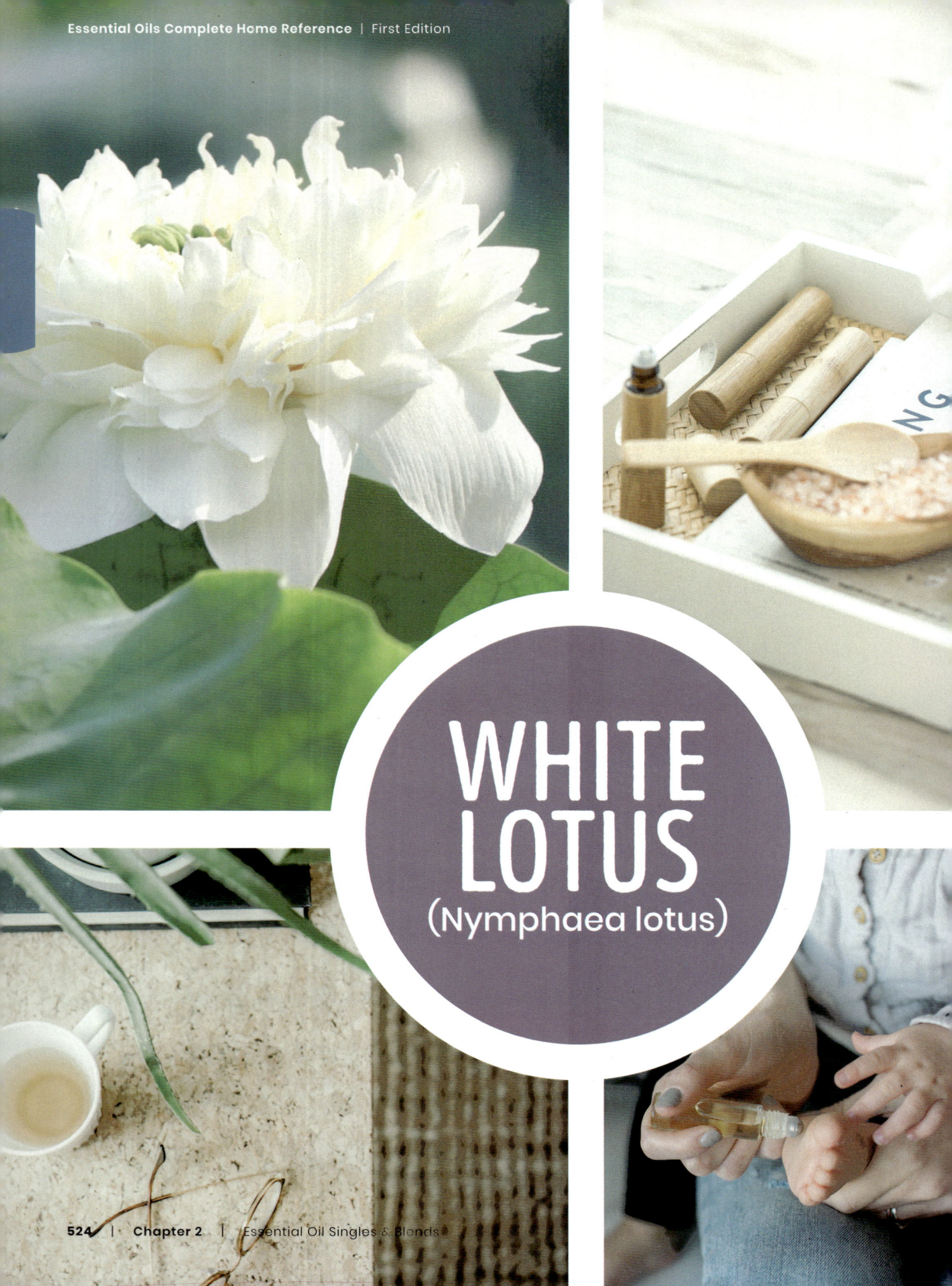

WHITE LOTUS
(Nymphaea lotus)

BOTANICAL FAMILY:
Nymphaeaceae

PLANT ORIGIN:
Egypt

EXTRACTION METHOD:
Absolute from flowers

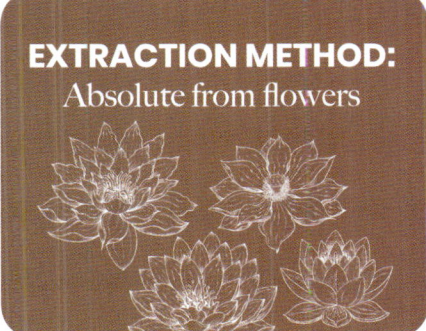

KEY CONSTITUENTS:
Tetradecanol (2-5%), 1,4 Demitoxy Benzene (1-4\%), Benzyl Benzoate (up to 3%), Linalool (up to 2%)

HISTORICAL DATA:
In ancient Egypt the lotus was used widely as a religious and ceremonial icon. In 400 AD, the Christian church of Ephesus designated Mary as "The Bearer of God." The numerous churches dedicated to Mary that were built thereafter incorporated the image of the lotus, including one image of lotus leaves, flowers, and fruits surrounding a golden cross.

MEDICAL PROPERTIES:
Anticancerous, anti-inflammatory, immune supporting

USES:
Inflamed eyes, jaundice, kidneys, liver spots, menstruation (promotes), palpitations, rheumatism, sciatica, sprains, sunburn, toothaches, tuberculosis, vomiting, skin texture, astringent, antiaging, appetite, high blood pressure, concentration

FRAGRANT INFLUENCE:
Stimulates a positive attitude and a general feeling of well-being; enhances concentration, peace and clarity

DIRECTIONS:
Topical: 50-50.

CAUTIONS:

SELECTED RESEARCH:
Fajemiroye JO, Adam K, Zjawiony JK, Alves CE, Aderoju AA. Evaluation of Anxiolytic and Antidepressant-like Activity of Aqueous Leaf Extract of Nymphaea lotus Linn. in mice. Iran j Pharm Res. 2018 Spring; 17(2): 613-626.

Bello FH, Maiha BB, Anuka JA. The effect of methanol rhizome extract on Nymphaea lotus Linn. (Nymphaeaceae) in animal modes of diarrhoea. J Ethnopharmacol. 2016 Aug 22;190:13-21. Epub 2016 May 20.

Debnath S, Ghosh S, Hazra B. Inhibitory effect of Nymphaea pubescens Willd. [syn. Nymphaea lotus L.] flower extract on carrageenan-induced inflammation and CCl-induced hepatoxicity in rats. Food Chem Toxicol. 2013 Sep;59:485-91. Epub 2013 Jul 1.

Zhu M, Zheng X, Shu Q, Li H, Zhong P, Zhang H, Xu Y, Wang L, Wang L. Relationship between the composition of flavonoids and flower colors variation in tropical water lily (Nymphaea) cultivars. PLoS One. 2012;7(4):e34335. Epub 2012 Apr 2.

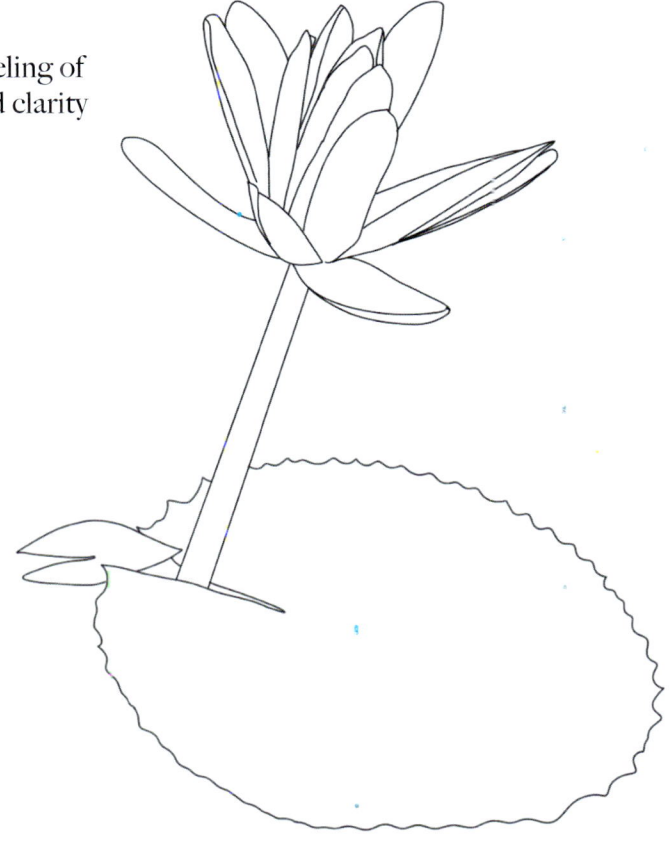

BOTANICAL FAMILY:
Ericaceae

PLANT ORIGIN:
China

EXTRACTION METHOD:
Steam distilled from leaves, herbs, and aerial parts

KEY CONSTITUENTS:
Methyl Salicylate (98-100%)

WINTERGREEN
(Gaultheria procumbens)

Gualtheria procumbens leaves have been chewed to increase respiratory capacity by Native Americans when running long distances and performing difficult labor. Settlers in early America had their children chew the leaves for several weeks each spring to prevent tooth decay. Wintergreen was used as a substitute for black tea during the Revolutionary War.

MEDICAL PROPERTIES:
Anticoagulant, antispasmodic, highly anti-inflammatory, vasodilator, analgesic/anesthetic, antimicrobial, antifungal, insecticidal

USES:
Arthritis/rheumatism, reduces blood pressure and all types of pain, muscle/nerve pain, hypertension, arteriosclerosis, hepatitis/fatty liver. Methyl salicylate, the principal constituent of wintergreen oil, has been incorporated into numerous liniments and ointments for musculoskeletal problems. The oil is also used as a flavoring agent in candies and chewing gums.

FRAGRANT INFLUENCE:
Minty, sweet aroma; it stimulates and increases awareness in all levels of the sensory system.

DIRECTIONS:
Aromatic: 10. Topical: 20-80. Use in Raindrop Technique. Dietary: Take as a dietary supplement.

CAUTIONS: Avoid use if epileptic. Anticoagulant properties can be enhanced when used with aspirin.

SELECTED RESEARCH:

Piotr M, Granica S, Magiera A, Rosińsk K, Jurek M, Poraj L, Olszewska MA. Salicylate and Procyanidin-Rich Stem Extracts of Gaultheria procumbens L. Inhibit Pro-Infammatory Enzmes and Suppress Pro-Inflammatory and Pro-Oxidant Functions of Human Neutrophils Ex Vivo. Int J Mol Sci. 2019 Apr; 20(7): 1753.

Piotr M, Owczarek A, Matczak M, Kosno M, Szymański P, Mikiciuk-Olasik E, Kilanowicz A, Wesołowski W Olszewska MA. Metabolic Profiling of Eastern Teaberry (Gaultheria procumbens L.) Lipophilic Leaf Extracts with Hyaluronidase and Lipoxygenase Inhibitory Activity. Molecules. 2017 Mar; 22(3): 412. Published online 2017 Mar 6.

Michel P, Dobrowolska A, Kicel A. Owczarek A, Bazylko A, Granica S, Piwowarski JP, Olszewska MA. Polyphenolic profile, antioxidant and anti-inflammatory activity of eastern teaberry (Gaultheria procumbens L.) leaf extracts. Molecules. 2014 Dec 8;19(2):20498-20520.

Salleh FM, Anuar TS, Yasin AM, Moktar N. Wintergreen oil: a novel method in Wheatley's trichrome staining technique. J Microbiol Methods. 2012 Oct;91(1):174-8. Epub 2012 Aug 17.

Tanen DA. Danish DC, Reardon JM, Chisholm CB, Matteucci MJ, Riffenburgh RH. Comparison of oral aspirin versus topical applied methyl salicylate for platelet inhibition. Ann Pharmacother. 2008 Oct;42(10):1396-1401. Epub 2008 Aug 12.

Charles CH, Vincent JW, Borycheski L, Amatnieks Y, Sarina M, Qaqish J, Proskin HM. Effect of an essential oil-containing dentifrice on dental plaque microbial composition. Am J Dent. 2000 Sep;13(Spec No):26C-30C.

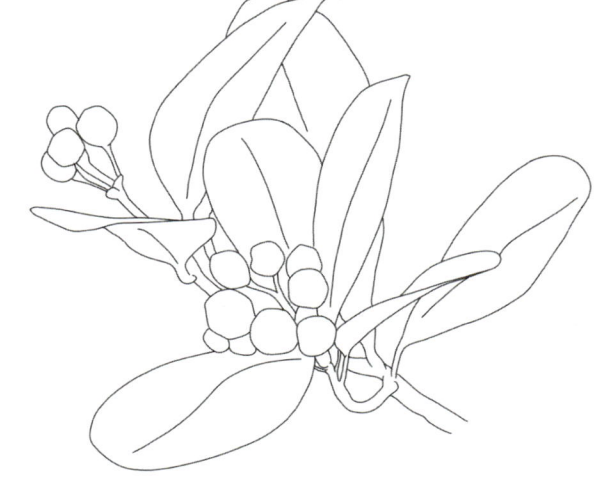

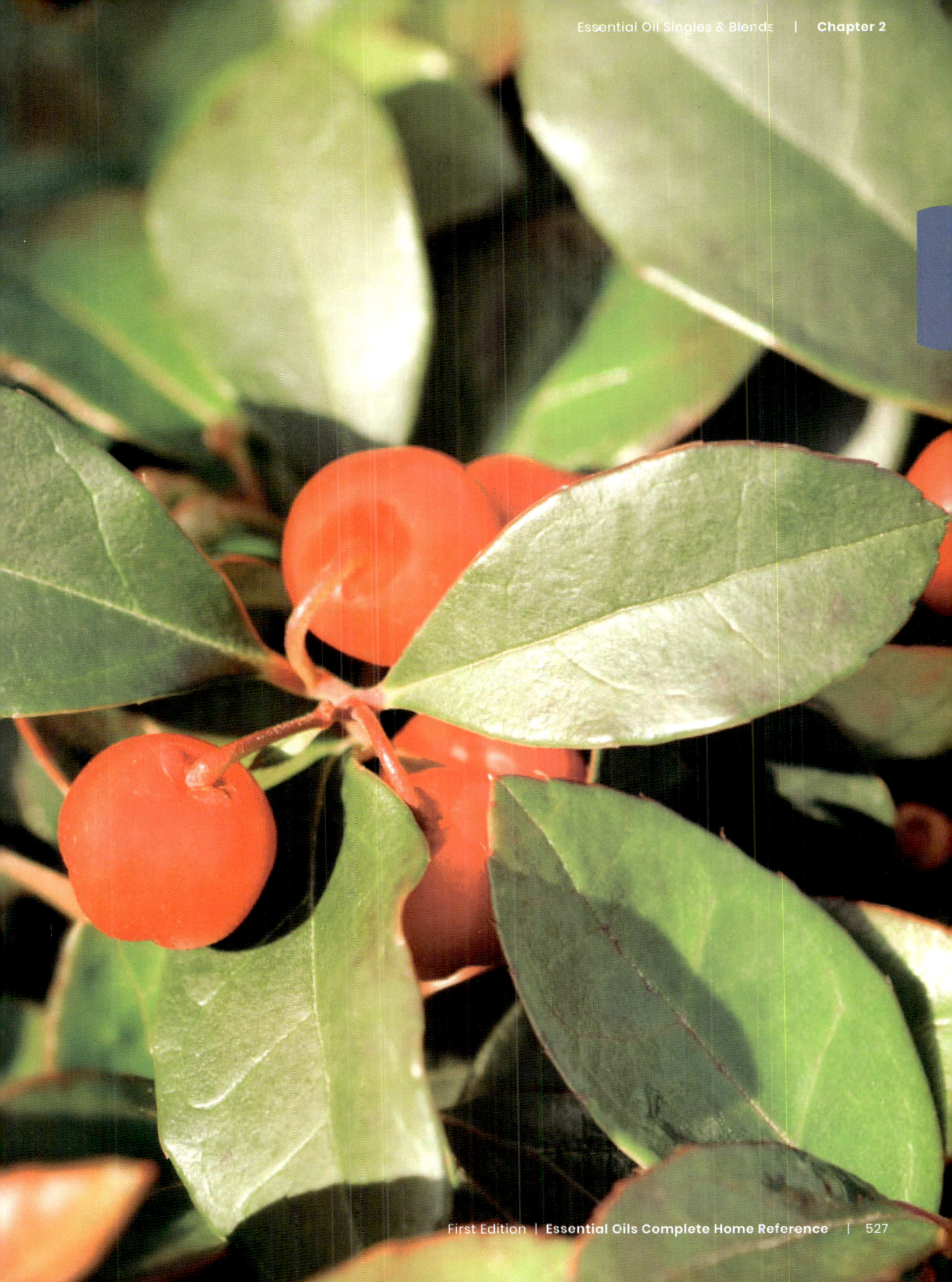

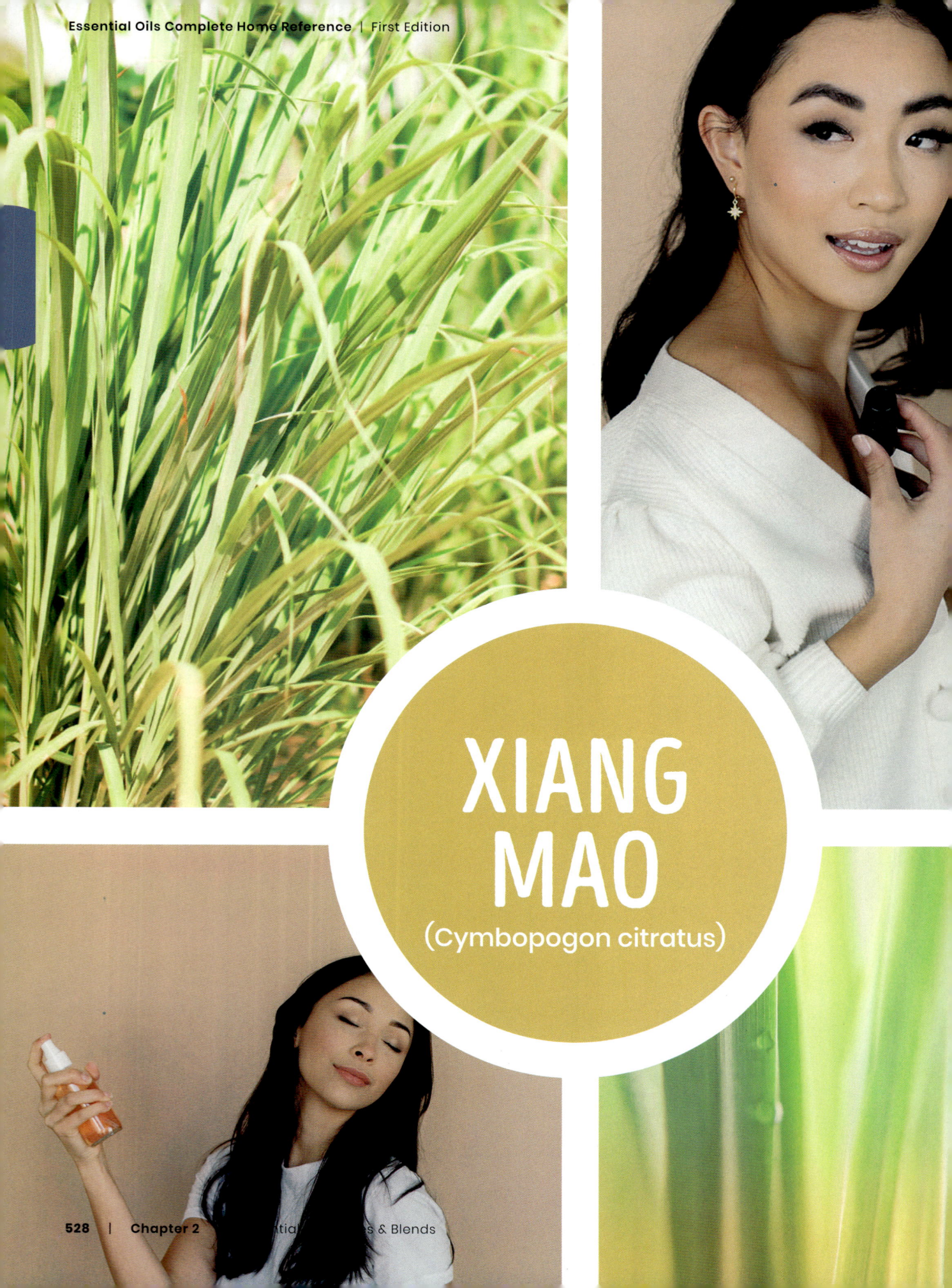

XIANG MAO
(Cymbopogon citratus)

Chapter 2 | Essential Oil Singles & Blends

BOTANICAL FAMILY:
Poaceae

PLANT ORIGIN:
Taiwan

EXTRACTION METHOD:
Steam distilled from leaves

KEY CONSTITUENTS:
Citronellal (38-59%),
Geraniol (13-21%),
Citronellol (12-19%),
Limonene (4-7%),
Germacrene-D (2-4%),
Alpha-Elemol (1-2%)

HISTORICAL DATA:
This aromatic grass is sometimes called "red lemongrass" or "lemongrass" and has been used in folk medicine as a calming agent. Traditionally, it was used to freshen household air, enlighten the mind, and moisten the skin.

MEDICAL PROPERTIES:
Chemopreventive, antimicrobial, anxiolytic, renal protective, gastroprotective, antifungal, antiparasitic, cholesterol reducer

USES:
Bladder infection, respiratory/sinus infection, digestive problems, parasites, torn ligaments/muscles, fluid retention, varicose veins, Salmonella, Candida albicans

FRAGRANT INFLUENCE:
Like its close cousin, Cymbopogon flexuosus, this lemongrass species sharpens awareness and is a purifier.

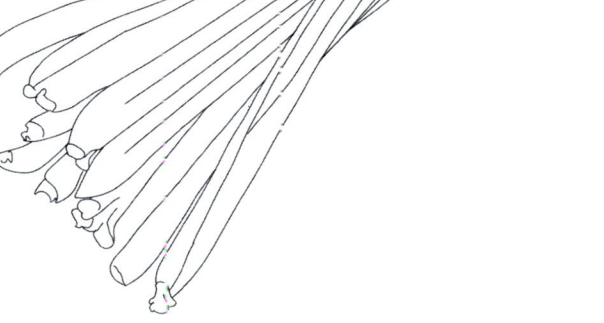

DIRECTIONS:
Aromatic: 6o. Topical: Neat.

CAUTIONS:

SELECTED RESEARCH:

Cherian T, Ali K, Saquib Q, Faisal M, Wahab R, Musarrat J. Cymbopogon Ctratus Functionalized Green Synthesis of CuO-Nanoparticles: Novel Prospects as Antibacterial and Antibiofilm Agents. Biomolecules. 2020 Feb; 10(2): 169.

Oliveira MAC, Borges AC, Brighenti FL, Salvador MJ, Gontijo AVL, Koga-Ito CY. Cymbopogon citratus essential oil: effect on polymicrobial caries-related biofilm with low cytotoxicity. Braz Oral Res. 2017 Nov 6;31:e89.

Leite CJ, de Sousa JP, Medeiros JA, da Conceição ML, dos Santos Falcão-Silva V, de Souza EL. Inactivation of Escherichia coli, Listeria monocytogenes, and Salmonella enteritidis by Cymbopogn citratus D.C. Stapf. essential oil in pineapple juice. J Food Prot. 2016 Feb;79(2):213-9.

Goes TC, Ursulino FR, Almeida-Souza TH, Alves PB, Teixeira-Silva F. Effect of lemongrass aroma on experimental anxiety in humans. J Altern Complement Med. 2015 Dec;21(12):766-73. Epub 2015 Sep 14.

Sagradas J, Costa G, Figueirinha A, Castel-Branco MM, Silvério Cabrita AM, Figueiredo IV, Batista MT. Gastroprotective effect of Cymbopogon citratus infusion on acute ethanol-induced gastric lesions in rats. J Ethnopharmacol. 2015 Sep 15;173:134-8. Epub 2015 Jul 6.

Bao XL, Yuan HH, Wang CZ, Fan W, Lan MB. Polysaccharides from Cymbopogon citratus with antitumor and immunomodulatory activity. Pharm Biol. 2015 Jan;53( ):117-24. Epub 2014 Sep 26.

Boukhatem MN, Ferhat MA, Kameli A, Saidi F, Kebir HT. Lemongrass (Cymbopogon citratus) essential oil as a potent anti-inflammatory and antifungal drug. Libyan J Med. 2014 Sep 19;9:25431. eCollection 2014.

Korenblum E, Regina de Vasconcelos Goulart F, de Almeida Rodrigues I, Abreu F, Lins U, Alves PB, Blank AF, Valoni E, Sebastián GV, Alviano DS, Alviano CS, Seldin L. Antimicrobial action and anti-corrosion effect against sulfate reducing bacteria by lemongrass (Cymbopogon citratus) essential oil and its major component, the citral. AMB Express. 2013 Aug 10;3(1):44.

BOTANICAL FAMILY: Annonaceae

PLANT ORIGIN: Ecuador, Comoros, Madagascar

EXTRACTION METHOD: Steam distilled from flowers

KEY CONSTITUENTS: Germacrene D (13-28%), (E,E)-Alpha-Farnesene (4-23%), B-Caryophyllene (4-18%), Linalool (2-12%), Geranyl Acetate (2-10%), Benzyl Benzoate (5-8%), Benzyl Acetate (up to 7%), p-Cresyl Methyl Ether (up to 7%), E-Cinnamyl Acetate (up to 5%), E,E-Farnesyl Acetate (1-5%), Benzyl Salicylate (1-5%), Methyl Benzoate (up to 4%)

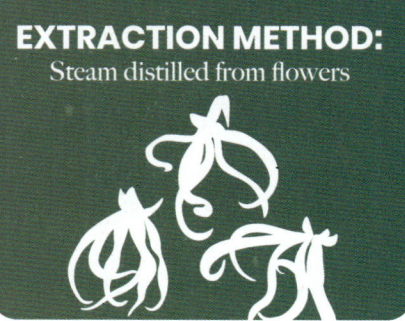

YLANG YLANG & AMAZONIAN ECUADORIAN YLANG YLANG
(Cananga odorata Equitoriana)(Cananga odorata)

Ylang ylang means "flower of flowers." The flowers have been used to cover the beds of newlywed couples on their wedding night. Traditionally used in hair formulas to promote thick, shiny, lustrous hair. Flowers are picked early in the morning to maximize oil yield. The highest quality oil is drawn from the first distillation and is known as ylang ylang complete. Gary Young translocated trees to the Young Living farm in Ecuador, where the aromatic flowers from thousands of trees are picked every day.

MEDICAL PROPERTIES:
Antibacterial, insecticidal, relaxant, sedative, anti-inflammatory, antianxiety, analgesic, antidepressant, antifungal, antiviral, antimicrobial, decongestant, disinfectant, antiseborrheic

USES:
Cardiac arrhythmia, cardiac problems, anxiety, wounds, hypertension, blood pressure, depression, hair loss, inflammation, circulation, aphrodisiac, intestinal problems. While renowned for its calming effect, several studies show it brings relief for the depressed and stressed, while it increases attentiveness and alertness, causing researches to say it is "harmonizing."

FRAGRANT INFLUENCE:
Rich, sweet floral aroma that evokes calming, relaxing, and comforting properties; balances male-female energies, enhances spiritual attunement, combats anger and low self-esteem, increases focus of thought, filters out negative energy, restores confidence and peace, energizing, uplifting

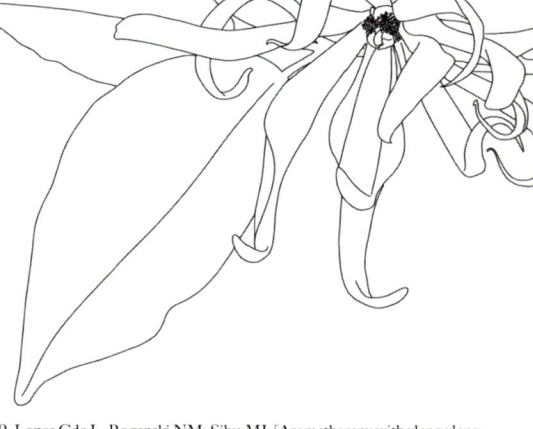

DIRECTIONS:
Aromatic: 6o. Topical: Neat.

CAUTIONS:

SELECTED RESEARCH:
Indrasetiawan P, Aoki-Utsubo C, Hanafi M, Hartati S, Wahyuni TS, Kameoka M, Yano Y, Hotta H, Hayashi Y. Antiviral Activity of Cananga odorata against Hepatitis B Virus. Kobe J Med Sci. 2019; 65(2):E71-E79. Published online 2019 Nov. 12.

Zhang N, Zhang L, Feng L, Yao L. Cananga odorata essential oil reverses the anxiety induced by the 1-(3-chlorophenyl) piperazine through regulating the MAPK pathway and serotonin system in mice. J Ethnopharmacol. 2018 Jun 12; 219:23-30. Epub 2018 Mar 12.

Soonwera M. Efficacy of essential oil from Cananga odorata (Lamk.) Hook.f. & Thomson (Annonaceae) against three mosquito species Aedes aegypti (L.), Anapheles dirus (Peyton and Harrisoh), and Culex quinquefasciatus (Say). Parasitol Res. 2015 Dec;114(12):4531-43. Epub 2015 Sep 4.

Tan LT, Lee LH, Yin WF, Chan CK, Abdul Kadir H, Chan KG, Goh BH. Traditional uses, phytochemistry, and bioactives of Cananga odorata (Ylang-Ylang). Evid Based Complement Alternat Med. 2015;2015:896314. Epub 2015 Jul 30.

Gnatta JR, Piason PP, Lopes Cde L, Rogenski NM, Silva MJ. [Aromatherapy with ylang ylang for anxiety and self-esteem: a pilot study.] Rev Esc Eferm USP. 2014 Jun;48(3):492-9. Portuguese.

Moss M, Hewitt S, Moss L, Wesnes K. Modulation of cognitive performance and mood by aromas of peppermint and ylang ylang. Int J Neurosci. 2008 Jan;118(1):59-77.

Hongratanaworakit T, Buchbauer G. Relaxing effect of ylang ylang oil on humans after transdermal absorption. Phytother Res. 2006 Sep;20(9):758-763.

Hongratanaworakit T, Buchbauer G. Evaluation of the harmonizing effect of ylang-ylang oil on humans after inhalation. Planta Med. 2004 Jul;70(7):632-6.

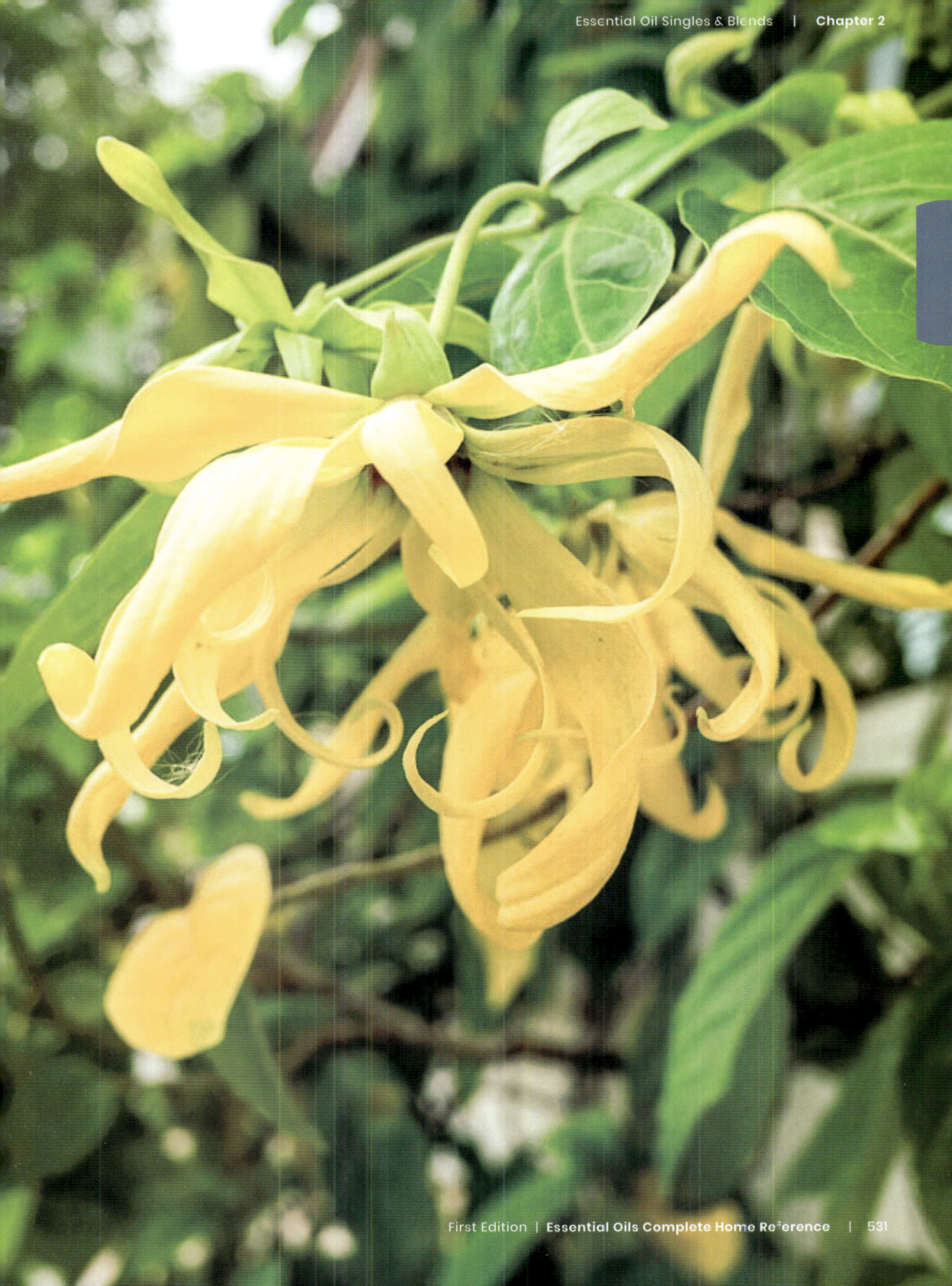

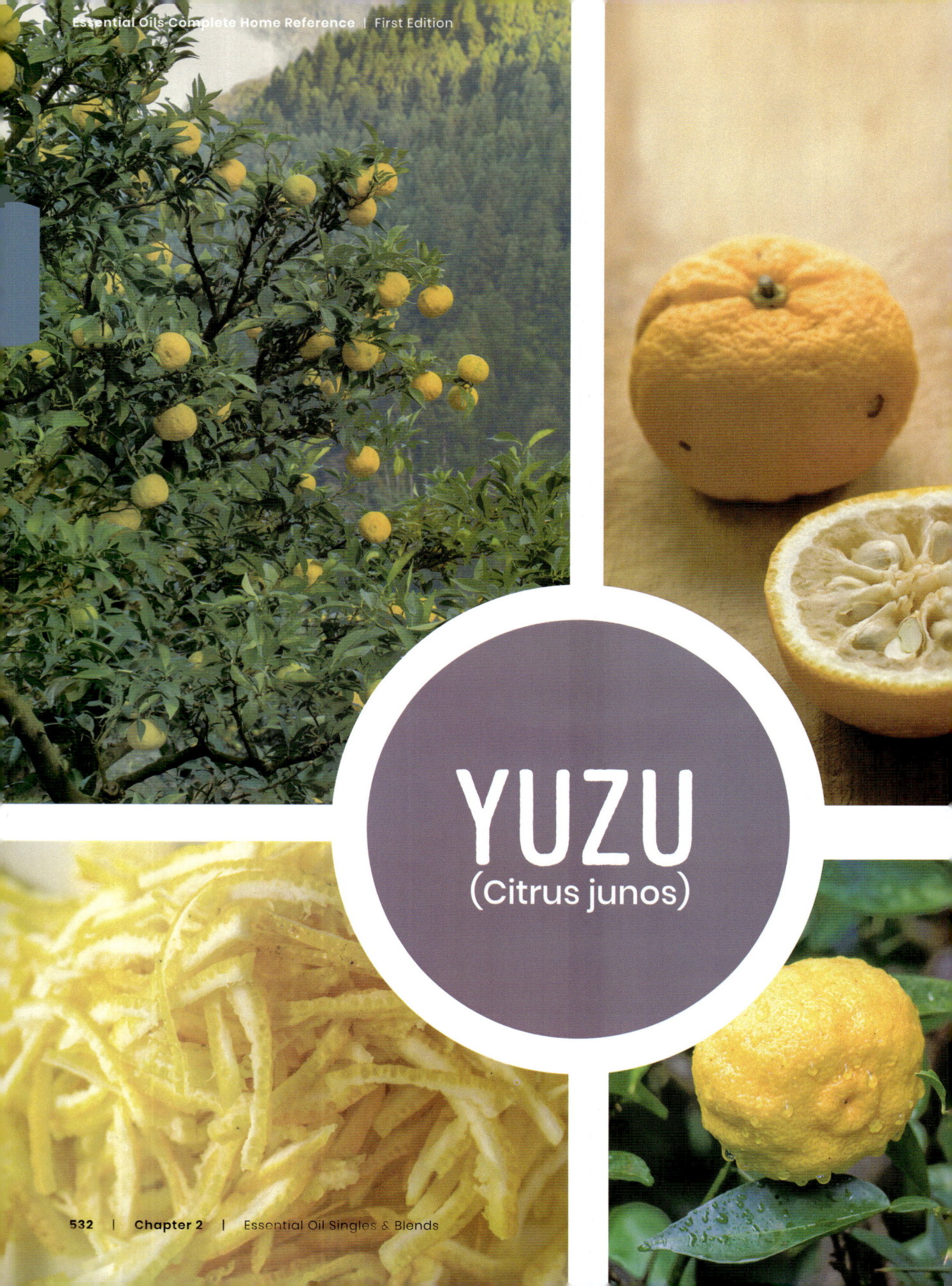

YUZU
(Citrus junos)

BOTANICAL FAMILY:
Rutaceae

PLANT ORIGIN:
Japan

EXTRACTION METHOD:
Hydrodistilled from peel

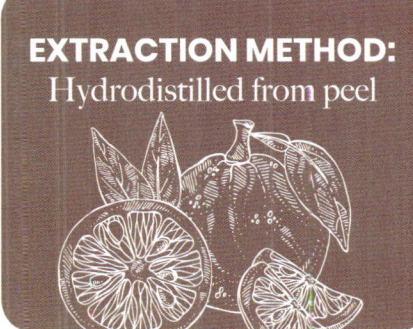

KEY CONSTITUENTS:
Limonene (70-87%),
Gamma Terpinene (7-11%),
Beta Phellandrene (2-4%),
Myrcene (1-3%)

HISTORICAL DATA:
Thought to be a hybrid between Ichang papeda and Satsuma mandarin, Yuzu is commonly used in cooking and for enhancing flavors due to the fragrant rind. There are a few reports on the use of Yuzu essential oil for cosmetics and aromatherapy.

MEDICAL PROPERTIES:
Anti-inflammatory, anticancerous, antidiabetic, asthma

USES:
Flavorant, inflammation, brain protection, stress, anxiety, tension, depression, sleep, skin issues, immune system, cold, flu

FRAGRANT INFLUENCE:
High levels of limonene positively affect mood and heighten senses, reduces negative emotional stress, promotes restful sleep

DIRECTIONS:
Aromatic: 30. Topical: Neat. Dietary: Put 2 drops in a capsule and take 3 times daily or as needed.

CAUTIONS: 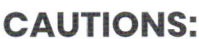   Do not use on small children or if pregnant or breastfeeding.

SELECTED RESEARCH:

Sharma K, Adhikari D, Kim HJ, Oh SH, Oak MH, Yi E. Citrus junos fruit extract facilitates anti-adipogenic activity of Garcinia cambogia extract in 3T3-L1 adipocytes by reducing oxidative stress. J Nanosci Nanotechnol. 2019 Feb 1;19(2):915-921.

Yoo KM, Moon B. Comparative carotenoid compositions during maturation and their antioxidant capacities of three citrus varieties. Food Chem. 2016 Apr 1;196:544-09. Epub 2015 Sep 25.

Matsumoto T, Kimura T, Hayashi T. Aromatic effects of a Japanese citrus fruit—yuzu (Citrus junos Sieb. ex Tanaka—on psychoemotional states and autonomic nervous system activity during the menstrual cycle: a single-blind randomized controlled crossover study. Biopsychosoc Med. 2016; 10/11.

Kim TH, Kim HM, Park SW, Jung YS. Inhibitory effects of yuzu and its components on human platelet aggregation. Biomol Ther (Seoul). 2015 Mar;23(2):149-55. Epub 2015 Mar 1.

Matsumoto T, Asakura H, Hayashi T. Effects of olfactory stimulation from the fragrance of the Japanese citrus fruit yuzu (Citrus junos Sieb. ex Tanaka) on mood states and salivary chromogranin A as an endocrinologic stress marker. J Altern Complement Med. 2014 Jun;20(6):500-6 Epub 2014 Apr 17.

Yang HJ, Hwang JT, Kwon DY, Kim MJ, Kang S, Moon NR, Park S. Yuzu extract prevents cognitive decline and impaired glucose homeostasis in β-amyloid-infused rats. J Nutr. 2013 Jul;143(7):1093-9. Epub 2013 May 29.

Kim SH, Hur HJ, Yang HJ, Kim HJ, Kim MJ, Park JH, Sung MJ, Kim MS, Kwon DY, Hwang JT. Citrus junos tanaka peel extract exerts antidiabetic effects via AMPK and PPAR-γ both in vitro and in vivo in mice fed a high-fat diet. Evid Based Complement Alternat Med. 2013;2013:921012. Epub 2013 May 22.

Hirota R, Roger NN, Nakamura H, Song HS, Sawamura M, Suganuma N. Anti-inflammatory effects on limonene from Yuzu (Citrus junos Tanaka) essential oil on eosinophils. J Food Sci. 2010 Apr;75(3):H87-92.

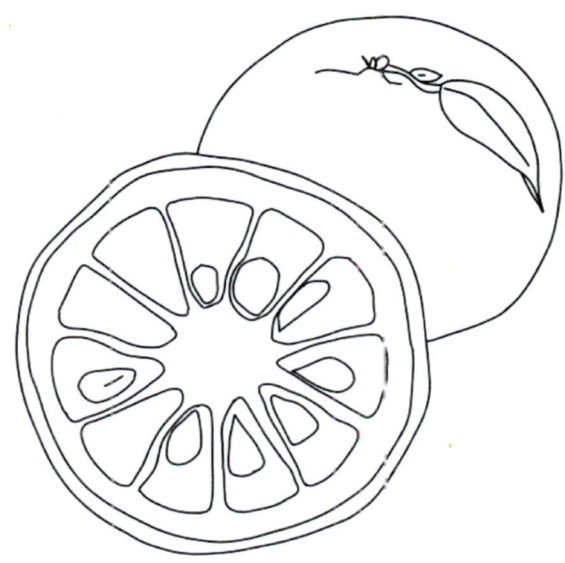

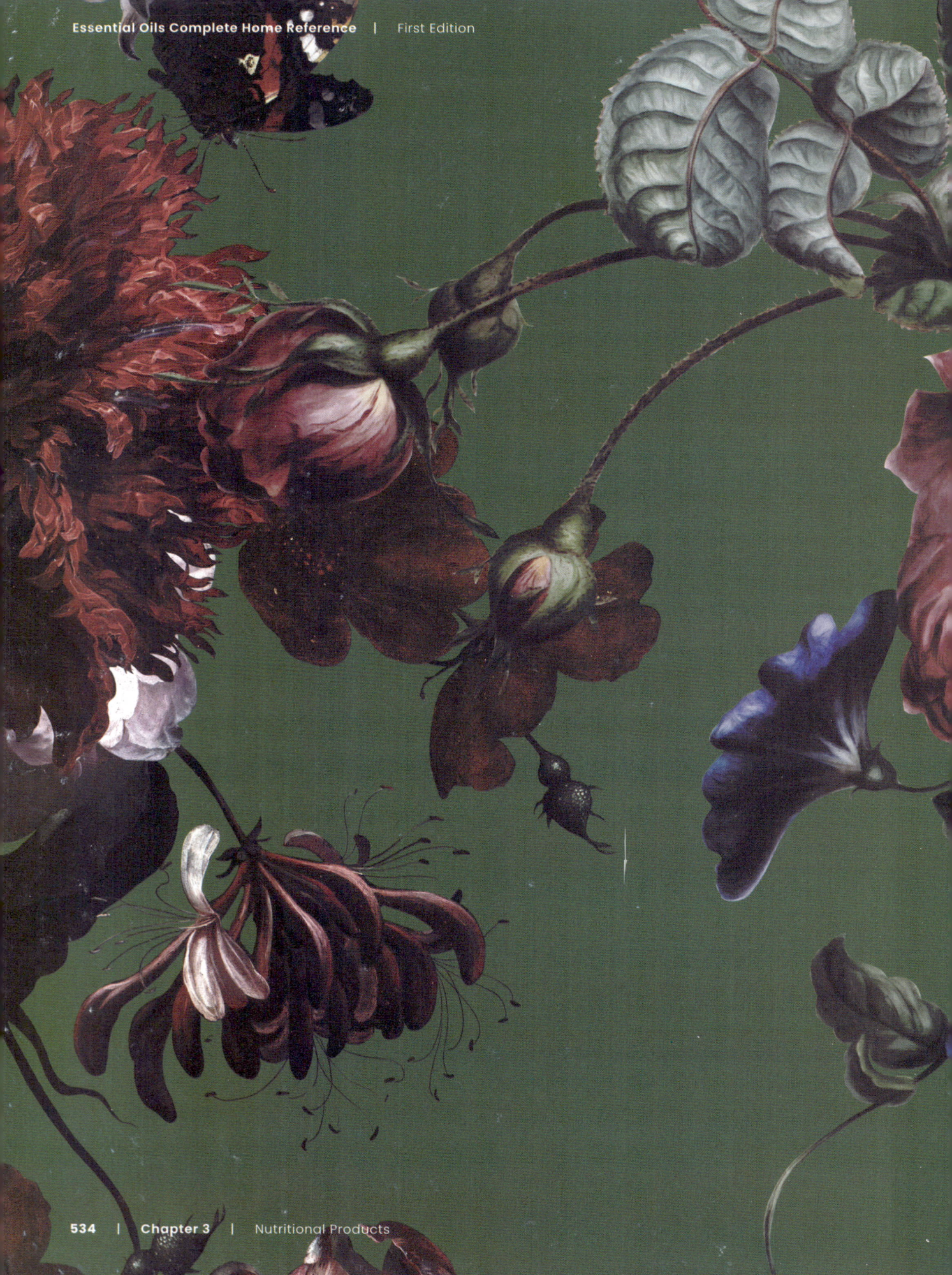

Nutritional Products | Chapter 3

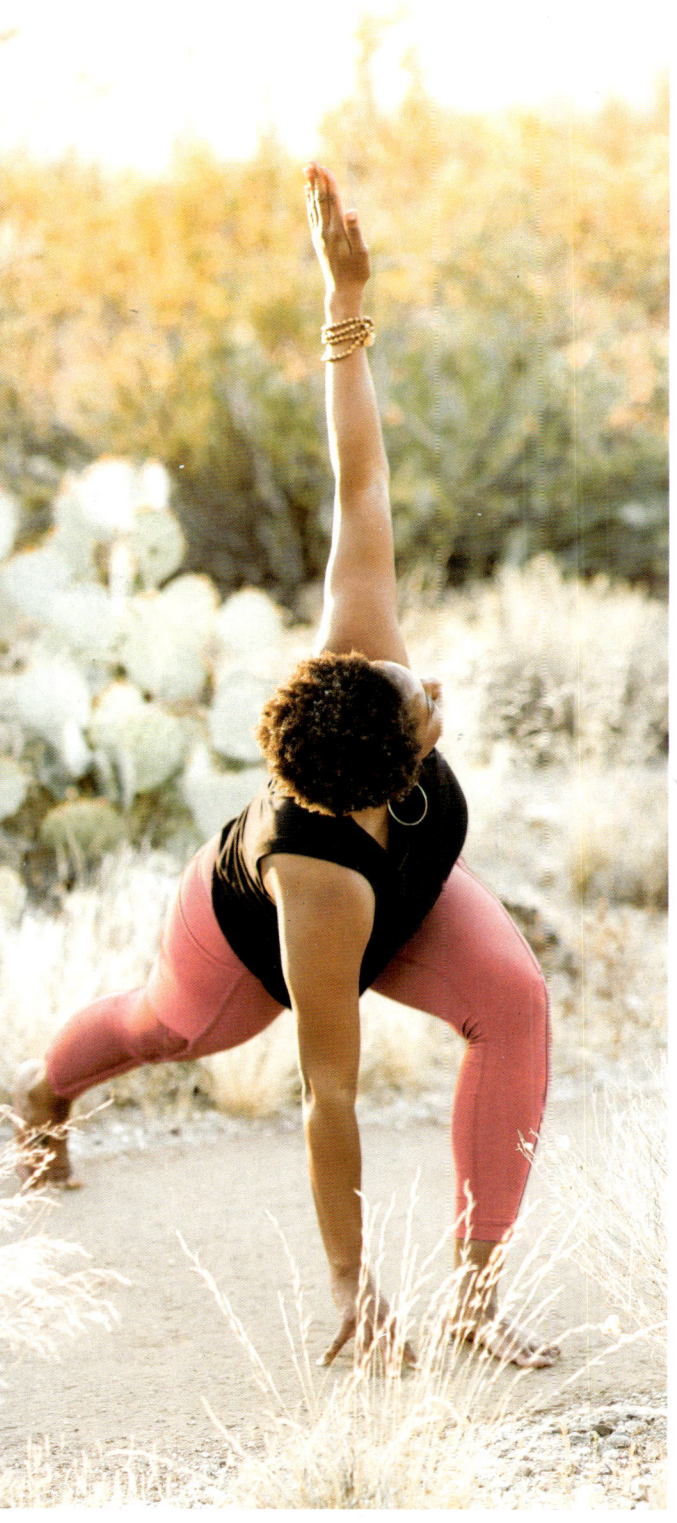

Nutritional Products

Nutritional supplementation is a great blessing that modern technology has provided for our world today, but the value is determined by quality, quantity, and frequency. With those in place, you are certain to achieve great benefits to your health in our very busy world today.

AGILEASE®

Perfect for an active lifestyle, AgilEase supports the body's response to acute inflammation in healthy individuals, promotes healthy joint flexibility and mobility, and supports cartilage health.

Ingredients: Frankincense resin powder, Calcium fructoborate (froilicon dioxide, Potassium chloride)

Essential Oils: Wintergreen, Copaiba, Clove, Northern Lights Black Spruce

Directions: Take 2 capsules daily.

Cautions: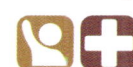

ALKALIME® and AlkaLime Stick Packs

This specially designed alkaline mineral powder contains an array of high-alkaline salts and other yeast- and fungus-fighting elements, such as citric acid and essential oils. This precisely balanced, acid-neutralizing mineral formulation helps preserve the body's proper pH balance, the cornerstone of health. By boosting blood alkalinity, yeast and fungus are deprived of the acidic terrain they require to flourish. When the blood and tissues of the body are already alkaline balanced, the effectiveness of the essential oils and other nutrients is even greater.

AlkaLime may help reduce the following signs of acid-based yeast and fungus dominance:

- Fatigue/low energy
- Irritability/mood swings
- Unexplained aches
- Indigestion and pains
- Colitis/ulcers

First Edition | Essential Oils Complete Home Reference | 535

- Overweight conditions
- Diarrhea/constipation
- Low resistance to illness
- Urinary tract infections
- Allergies
- Rectal/vaginal itch
- Headaches
- Candida

Ingredients: Sodium (as sodium bicarbonate, sodium phosphate, sodium sulfate), Calcium (as calcium carbonate, di-calcium phosphate, calcium sulfate), Potassium (as potassium bicarbonate, potassium phosphate, potassium sulfate, potassium chloride), Lemon fruit powder, Lemon peel oil, Lime peel oil, Tartaric acid, Citric acid, Stevia leaf extract, Magnesium phosphate

Essential Oils: Lemon, Lime

Directions: Add 1 level teaspoon to 4-6 ounces of distilled or purified water; let sit for 20-25 seconds. Gently stir until thoroughly mixed and then drink immediately. Mix only with water. Take 1-3 times daily, 1 hour before meals or before retiring to bed to support optimal pH balance in the stomach. As an antacid and an aid in alkalizing, AlkaLime may be taken as needed.

Cautions: Not recommended for sodium-restricted diets or for individuals with high blood pressure.

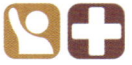

ALLERZYME®

Allerzyme is a vegetarian complex blend of enzymes, complementary botanicals, Ginger, Peppermint, and other essential oils that support proper digestion, waste elimination, and nutrient utilization. This potent enzyme complex is formulated to combat allergies, gas, fermentation, fatigue, and irritable bowel syndrome (IBS). It also contains a powerful combination of sugar- and starch-splitting enzymes, as well as small amounts of fat- and protein-digesting enzymes.

Ingredients: Allerzyme Blend: [Plantain leaf, Amylase, Bromelain, Peptidase, Protease, Invertase, Phytase, Barley grass, Lipase, Lactase, Cellulase, Alpha-galactosidase, Diastase], Allerzyme Oil Blend: [Tarragon leaf oil, Ginger root oil, Peppermint leaf oil, Juniper leaf oil, Fennel seed oil, Lemongrass leaf oil, Anise fruit oil, Patchouli flower oil], Hypromellose, Water, Silica

Essential Oils: Tarragon, Ginger, Peppermint, Juniper, Fennel, Lemongrass, Anise, Patchouli

Directions: Take 1 capsule, 3 times daily just prior to meals or as needed.

Cautions: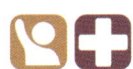

AMINOWISE™

AminoWise is your personal workout booster. Containing amino acids and antioxidants, AminoWise targets muscle recovery while enhancing performance. It aids in muscle building and repair and helps to reduce muscle fatigue, while replenishing minerals lost during workout and exercise. It is also a good source of vitamin E and zinc and helps support the production of nitric oxide, which can improve blood flow. Flavored with Lemon and Lime essential oils, it contains no preservatives, synthetic colors or flavors, and no added sugar or artificial sweeteners.

Ingredients: Calcium, Potassium, Sodium, Vitamin E, Magnesium, Zinc; Muscle Performance Blend: [Branched chain amino acids (2:1:1 leucine, isoleucine, valine), L-citrulline, L-glutamine, Beta-alanine, L-arginine, L-taurine], Recovery Blend: [Ningxia wolfberry powder, Lime fruit powder, Polyphenols extract, d-alpha Tocopherol acetate, Zinc gluconate, Lemon peel oil, Lime rind oil], Hydration Mineral Blend: [Sodium citrate, Potassium citrate, Calcium citrate, Magnesium citrate], Fructooligosaccharides, Tapioca maltodextrin, Citric acid, Natural flavors, Calcium silicate, Stevia leaf extract, Silica, Tapioca starch

Essential Oils: Lemon, Lime

Directions: Mix 1 scoop with 8 ounces of water and consume during or after exercise.

Cautions: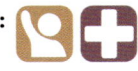

BALANCE COMPLETE™

Balance Complete is a super-food meal replacement that is high in fiber and protein, consisting of good fats, enzymes, vitamins, and minerals needed to form a nutritious, great-tasting protein drink that satisfies the appetite. It is a powerful nutritive energizer and a cleanser, which helps to improve digestion and support colon health. The high antioxidant benefits of the Ningxia wolfberry (Lycium barbarum) powder, in combination with brown rice bran, barley grass, aloe vera, cinnamon powder, and whey protein blend, create the building blocks for strengthening the immune system and bringing back feelings of energy and vitality.

Ingredients: Proprietary V-Fiber™ Blend: [Larch polysaccharides, Ningxia wolfberry fruit, Brown rice bran, Guar gum, Konjac, Xanthan gum, Chicory root fiber extract (FOS), Sodium alginate], Whey protein concentrate, Natural flavors, Nonfat dry milk, Medium-chain triglycerides. Fructose, Lecithin, Calcium (Tricalcium phosphate), Proprietary Enzyme Complex: [Lactase, Lipase, Bromelain, Papain, Amylase], Xylitol. Magnesium oxide, Barley grass, Neohesperidin derivative (flavor from natural citrus), Cinnamon bark, Mixed carotenoids (Vitamin A), Lo han kuo fruit extract, Barley grass juice, Aloe vera leaf, Vitamin C (ascorbic acid), Mixed tocopherols (Vitamin E), Vitamin B3 (Niacinamide), Zinc oxide, Selenium (Selenomethionine), Beta-carotene, Molybdenum citrate, Vitamin B5 (Pantothenic acid from calcium pantothenate), Vitamin B6 (Pyridoxine HCl), Chromium amino nicotinate, Vitamin B1 (Thiamine HCl), Vitamin B2 (Riboflavin), Vitamin D3 (Cholecalciferol), Vitamin B12 (Methylcobalamin), Folic acid, Orange peel oil, Biotin, Iodine (Potassium iodide)

Essential Oils: Orange

Directions: Add 2 scoops of Balance Complete to 8 ounces of cold water. May be mixed with rice, almond, or other milk. Shake, stir, or blend until smooth. For added flavor, add fruit or other essential oils.

Tip: For a delicious nutritional drink, mix 1-2 scoops of Balance Complete with ½ cup carrot juice, ½ cup coconut milk, 1 drop Orange oil, and ¼ cup water (or equivalent amount of ice). Blend and enjoy nutrition at its best!

Tip: For a five-day cleanse, replace all three daily meals with Balance Complete and follow the recommended schedule. For daily cleansing, use V-Fiber™. As part of a low-calorie diet, replace two daily meals with Balance Complete.

Allergen Warning: Contains ingredients derived from milk and soy.

Cautions: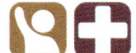

BLM™ (Bones, Ligaments, and Muscles)

BLM supports normal bone and joint health. This formula combines powerful, natural ingredients, such as Type II collagen, MSM, glucosamine sulfate, and manganese citrate, with the anti-inflammatory and pain-relieving essential oils of Idaho Grand Fir, Wintergreen, and Clove.

These ingredients support healthy cell function and encourage joint health and fluid movement.

This product is a highly effective arthritis treatment for building bones, ligaments, and muscles. The exclusive collagen and hyaluronic acid blend strengthens and rebuilds damaged joints and cartilage as it combats arthritis inflammation and bone pain.

Ingredients (Capsules): BLM Blend: Glucosamine sulfate, Type II collagen (chicken sternum extract), MSM (methylsulfonylmethane), Idaho Grand Fir leaf/branch oil, Wintergreen leaf oil, Manganese citrate, Clove flower bud oil, Rice flour, Gelatin, Magnesium stearate, Silicon dioxide

Essential Oils (Capsules): Idaho Grand Fir, Wintergreen. Clove

Directions (Capsules): Take 1 capsule 3 times daily if you weigh less than 120 pounds. Take 1 capsule 4 times daily if you weigh between 120 and 200 pounds. Take 1 capsule 5 times daily if you weigh over 200 pounds. Allow 4-8 weeks of daily use before expecting noticeable results.

Ingredients (Powder): BLM Powder Blend: [Glucosamine sulfate, Type II collagen (chicken sternum extract), Xylitol, MSM (methylsulfonylmethane)], Clove flower bud oil, Peppermint leaf oil, Idaho Grand Fir leaf/branch oil, Wintergreen leaf oil, Manganese citrate, Potassium chloride, Rice bran

Essential Oils (Powder): Clove, Peppermint, Idaho Grand Fir, Wintergreen

Directions (Powder): Take ¼ teaspoon 3 times daily if you weigh less than 120 pounds. Take ¼ teaspoon 4 times daily if you weigh between 120 and 200 pounds. Take ¼ teaspoon 5 times daily if you weigh over 200 pounds. Powder can be taken with water, soy, or rice milk. Allow 4-8 weeks of daily use before expecting noticeable results.

Allergen Warning (Capsules and Powder): Contains ingredients derived from shellfish (crab and shrimp).

Cautions (Capsules and Powder):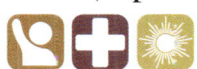

CBD (Cannabidiol)

(see CBD in Chapter 2, Singles & Blends)

CARDIOGIZE™

The perfect combination of heart health and circulation support is found in CardioGize, with vital CoQ10, selenium, vitamin K2, and other supportive herbals. The deodorized garlic and CoQ10 have antioxidant properties. Astragalus and dong quai have been used traditionally in China for cardiovascular support because of their synergistic properties.

Ingredients: Healthy Heart Blend: Garlic bulb extract, CoQ10 (as ubiquinone), Astragalus root powder, Dong quai root powder, Motherwort herb powder, Cat's claw bark powder, Hawthorn berry powder, Cactus cladode powder, Cardamom seed powder, CardioGize Essential Oil Blend: [Angelica root oil, Cardamom seed oil, Cypress leaf/nut/stem oil, Lavender oil, Helichrysum flower oil, Rosemary leaf oil, Cinnamon bark oil], Hypromellose, Water, Silica

Essential Oils: Angelica, Cardamom, Cypress, Lavender, Helichrysum, Rosemary, Cinnamon Bark

Directions: Take 2 capsules daily.

Cautions: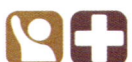

COMFORTONE®

ComforTone is an effective combination of herbs and essential oils that supports the health of the digestive system by eliminating residues from the colon and enhancing its natural ability to function optimally. Because it supports normal peristalsis (the wave-like contractions that move food through the intestines), ComforTone is ideal for strengthening the system that delivers nutrients to the rest of the body. This herbal formulation is combined with powerful essential oils that are antiparasitic, anti-inflammatory, and that can ease intestinal cramps, help soothe discomforts of the digestive tract, and aid in the elimination process.

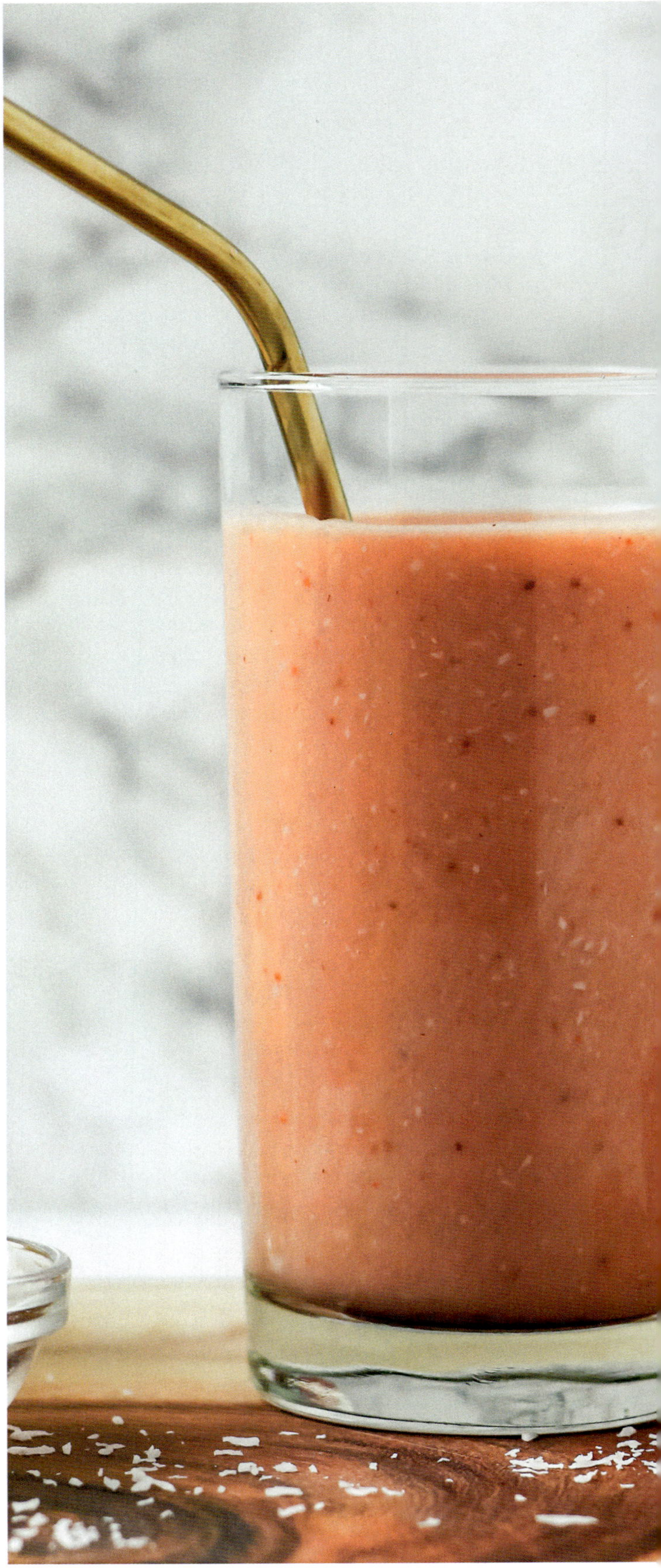

The unique essential oil of Ocotea, produced from a plant that grows in the Amazon, is extremely powerful in combating candida, which is the foundation for many health concerns. The other essential oils in this complex

formulation truly make it the overall best product for cleansing the colon while benefiting the liver, gallbladder, and overall process of digestion.

Ingredients: Cascara sagrada bark, Psyllium seed, Barberry bark, Burdock root, Fennel seed, Garlic bulb, Echinacea root, Bentonite, Diatomaceous earth, Ginger root, German Chamomile flower extract, Apple pectin, Licorice root, Cayenne fruit, Tarragon leaf oil, Ginger root oil, Tangerine rind oil, Rosemary leaf oil, Anise seed oil, Peppermint leaf oil, Ocotea leaf oil, German Chamomile flower oil, Gelatin, Water, Silicon dioxide

Essential Oils: Tarragon, Ginger, Tangerine, Rosemary, Anise, Peppermint, Ocotea, German Chamomile

Directions: Take 1 capsule 3 times daily. Drink at least 64 ounces of water throughout the day for best results.

Cautions: This product contains cascara sagrada bark. Read and follow directions carefully. Do not use if you have or develop diarrhea, loose stools, or abdominal pain. Do not exceed recommended dosage. Not for long-term use; do not exceed two weeks. Not to be used as a weight-loss product.

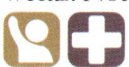

CORTISTOP®

CortiStop is a dietary supplement designed to help the body maintain its natural balance and harmony. When under stress, the body produces cortisol. When too much cortisol is produced, it can have negative health consequences, such as feelings of fatigue, difficulty maintaining healthy weight, and difficulty maintaining optimal health of cardiovascular systems. CortiStop supports the glandular systems of women.

Ingredients: CortiStop Blend: [Pregnenolone, L-a-phosphatidylserine, L-a-phosphatidylcholine, Black cohosh root extract, DHEA (derived from wild yam root), Clary Sage flowering top oil, Canadian Fleabane flowering top oil, Fennel seed oil, Frankincense gum/resin oil, Peppermint aerial parts oil], Rice flour, Silica, Gelatin

Essential Oils: Clary Sage, Canadian Fleabane, Fennel, Frankincense, Peppermint

Directions: Take 2 capsules in the morning before breakfast. If desired, for extra benefits, take 2 more capsules before bedtime. Use daily for 8 weeks. Discontinue for 2-4 weeks before resuming.

Cautions: For adult use only.

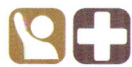

DETOXZYME®

Detoxzyme combines powerful and effective essential oils with a myriad of fast-acting enzymes that assist in the complete digestive process, helping to detoxify and promote cleansing, which is essential for maintaining and building health.

The enzymes in this product are designed to digest starches, sugars, proteins, and fats and, along with trace minerals, help the body detoxify, thus reducing cholesterol and triglycerides. Detoxzyme helps in opening the gallbladder duct and cleansing the liver, preventing candida and yeast overgrowth while promoting detoxification and parasite cleansing.

Detoxzyme also contains phytase, an enzyme essential for unlocking the mineral content of many grains, nuts, seeds, and other foods that contain high levels of essential minerals that are unavailable to the human body because they are bound up in insoluble, indigestible phytate complexes. Thus, the phytase in Detoxzyme results in a huge boost in mineral absorption from diets high in nuts, seeds, and whole grains.

This important enzyme formula facilitates remarkable absorption of nutrients from foods and supplements, thus providing increased energy levels and optimal health.

Ingredients: Amylase, Cumin seed powder, Invertase, Protease 4.5, Glucoamylase, Bromelain, Phytase, Lipase, Cellulase, Alpha-galactosidase, Lactase, Cumin seed oil, Anise seed oil, Fennel seed oil, Rice Bran, Silica, Magnesium Stearate, Hypromellose, Water

Essential Oils: Cumin, Anise, Fennel

Directions: Take 1-2 capsules 3 times daily between meals or as needed. This product may be used in conjunction with a detoxifying program.

Cautions: Not for children under 12 years of age except under the supervision of a health care professional. If discomfort persists, discontinue use and consult your physician.

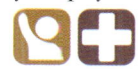

DIGEST & CLEANSE™

Digest & Cleanse is formulated with clinically proven and time-tested essential oils that work synergistically to help soothe gastrointestinal upset, prevent gas, and stimulate stomach secretions, supporting healthy digestion.

Essential oils are distilled from large amounts of fresh and/or dried herbs, plants, and trees. It often takes many pounds of plant material to make 1 ounce of an essential oil. Because the oils are so potent, it takes only a few drops of oil to achieve the desired digestive and cleansing effects. Thus, only one Digest & Cleanse softgel taken one to three times daily provides potent and optimal release in the intestines, the targeted area for optimal absorption.

Good health begins with a healthy bowel. Stress, overeating, and toxins can irritate the gastrointestinal system and cause cramps, gas, and nausea that interfere with the body's natural digestive and detoxification functions. Supplementing with Digest & Cleanse will soothe the bowel, prevent gas, and stimulate the liver, gallbladder, and stomach secretions, thus aiding digestion and absorption that is imperative for good health.

Ingredients: Peppermint aerial parts oil, Fractionated coconut fruit oil, Caraway fruit oil, Virgin coconut fruit oil, Lemon peel oil, Ginger root oil, Anise seed oil, Fennel seed oil, Gelatin, Water, Glycerin, Ethyl cellulose, Sodium alginate, Ammonium hydroxide, Medium-chain triglycerides, Oleic acid, Stearic acid

Essential Oils: Peppermint, Caraway, Lemon, Ginger, Anise, Fennel

Directions: Take 1 softgel 1-3 times daily with water 30-60 minutes prior to meals.

Cautions: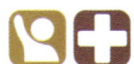

ECUADORIAN DARK CHOCOLESSENCE™

Ecuadorian Dark Chocolessence is a delicacy packed with cacao's nutritional goodness. The result is. Complex, slightly acidic, and luxuriously dark, the small-batch Ecuadorian chocolate brings together a mosaic of pure Young Living essential oils combined with the distinctive cacao flavors of exclusively sourced Ecuadorian cacao beans. It is crafted with the expertise of an award-winning chocolatier for the richest experience possible.

Cacao has been sought throughout history for its rich flavor and high amounts of beneficial flavonoids and antioxidants. It was so precious that it was saved for royalty and the elite. Today cacao is considered one of the world's premier superfoods.

Ecuadorian Dark Chocolessence is in a class by itself. The health benefits include cardiovascular support, mood support, skin support, immune support, weight-management support, and oral care support.

Ecuadorian Dark Chocolessence with Cinnamon Bark, Nutmeg, and Clove

Ingredients: Ecuadorian cacao beans, Cane sugar, Cocoa butter, Cinnamon bark oil, Nutmeg kernel oil, Clove bud oil

Essential Oils: Cinnamon Bark Vitality, Nutmeg Vitality, Clove Vitality

Ecuadorian Dark Chocolessence with Peppermint and Almond

Ingredients: Cacao beans, Cane sugar, Almonds, Cocoa butter, Peppermint leaf oil

Essential Oils: Peppermint Vitality

Ecuadorian Dark Chocolessence with Tangerine and Ginger

Ingredients: Ecuadorian cacao beans, Cane sugar, Cocoa butter, Tangerine peel oil, Ginger root oil

Essential Oils: Tangerine Vitality, Ginger Vitality

Ecuadorian Dark Chocolessence Wolfberry Truffle

Ingredients: Ecuadorian cacao beans, Cane sugar, Coconut oil, Cocoa butter, Wolfberry powder

Cautions: Contains tree nuts (coconut)

Directions: Consume as desired.

EINKORN GRAIN (Wheat)

(see Gary's True Grit Einkorn Products)

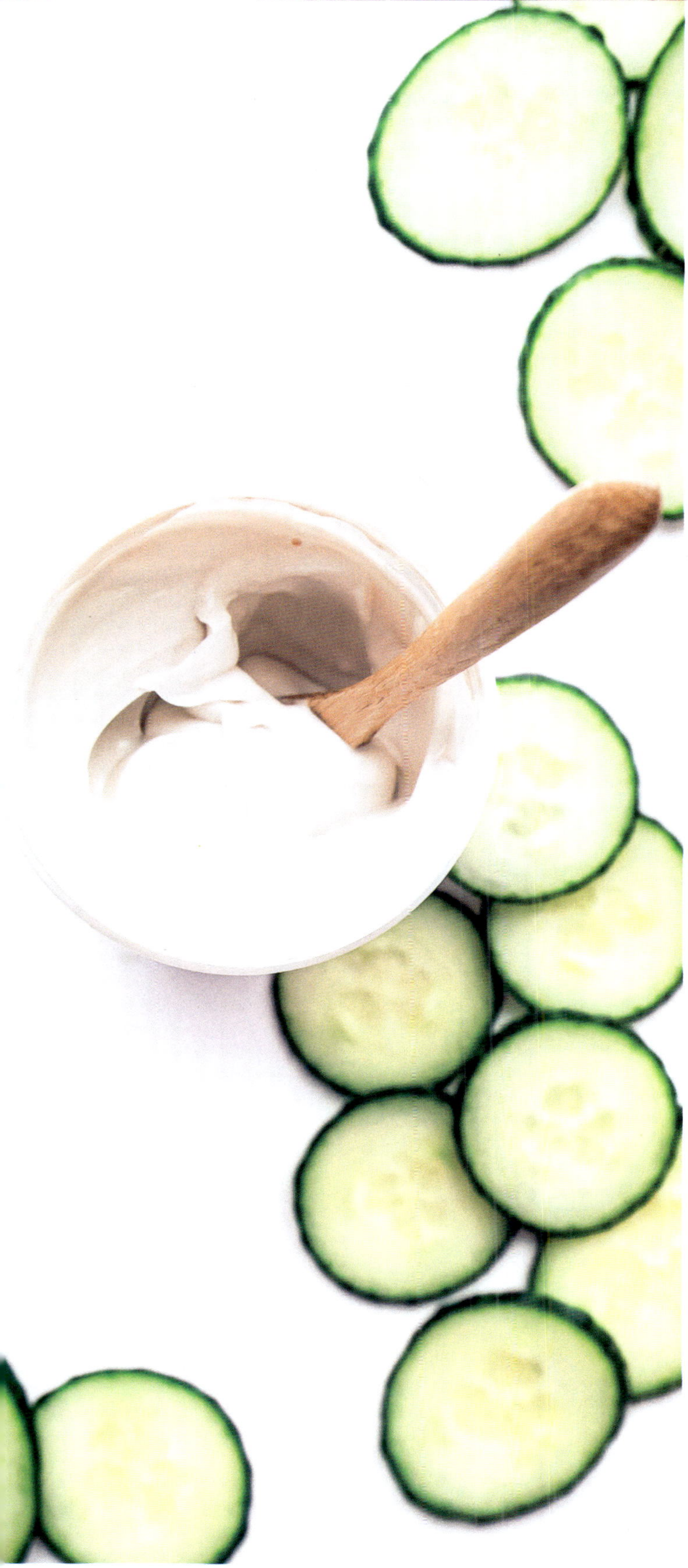

ENDOGIZE™

EndoGize helps women maintain a healthy endocrine system. With everyday worries and poor nutritional practices, their bodies become stressed and out of balance. This can increase cortisol levels and decrease estrogen or testosterone, which can lead to a diminished libido and imbalanced metabolism that further leads to a decrease in energy and an increase in food consumption.

For a woman's body to maintain health and vitality, it is critical for her to maintain a healthy endocrine system, which regulates several body systems by releasing hormones into the bloodstream. Once in the bloodstream, hormones travel to specific body systems, such as the adrenals, pituitary, hypothalamus, thyroid, and ovaries. When the endocrine system is not balanced, each of these body systems is unable to function properly and can put undue stress on other systems within the body.

Ingredients: EndoGize Blend: [Ashwagandha root powder, Muira puama bark, L-arginine, Epimedium aerial parts, Tribulus fruit extract, Phosphatidylcholine, Lecithin (soy), DHEA (dehydroepiandrosterone), Black pepper fruit extract, Glucoamylase, Acid stable protease, Longjack root extract, Amylase, Cellulase], EndoGize Oil Blend: [Ginger root oil, Myrrh gum/resin oil, Cassia branch/leaf oil, Clary Sage flowering top oil, Canadian Fleabane flowering top oil], Rice flour, Gelatin

Essential Oils: Ginger, Myrrh, Cassia, Clary Sage, Canadian Fleabane

Directions: Take 1 capsule 2 times daily for 4 weeks. Discontinue use for 2 weeks before resuming.

Allergen Warning: Contains soy.

Cautions: Do not use if you are pregnant or lactating. Intended for adult use only.

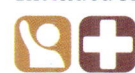

ESSENTIALZYME®

Essentialzyme is an advanced, multienzyme complex that promotes digestion and assists in the assimilation of nutrients. Enzyme supplementation is particularly important for people suffering from chronic pancreatitis, cystic fibrosis, or any condition where the pancreatic duct or common bile duct is blocked, thereby preventing enzymes from reaching the intestines.

Essentialzyme is a bilayer, Peppermint-coated caplet that combines pure essential oils, herbs, and pancreatic- and plant-derived enzymes to support overall digestion. Its dual time-release technology increases its effectiveness during digestion.

Essentialzyme helps re-establish proper enzyme balance in the digestive system and throughout the body, improves intestinal flora, and may also help retard the aging process. This is a high-quality, complex enzyme formula created to help improve and aid digestion and elimination of toxic waste from the body, which in turn means more energy and vitality.

Ingredients: Proprietary Blend (Light): [Pancrealipase, Pancreatin, Trypsin], Proprietary Blend (Dark): [Betaine HCl, Bromelain, Thyme leaf powder, Carrot root powder, Alfalfa sprout powder, Alfalfa leaf powder, Papain, Cumin seed powder, Anise seed oil, Fennel seed oil, Peppermint leaf oil, Tarragon aerial parts oil, Clove bud oil], Microcrystalline cellulose, Dicalcium phosphate, Hydroxypropylcellulose, Hydroxypropylmethylcellulose, Stearic acid, Croscarmellose sodium, Silicon dioxide, Peppermint leaf oil, Sodium citrate, Sodium carboxymethyl cellulose, Dextrin, Lecithin, Dextrose

Essential Oils: Anise, Fennel, Peppermint, Tarragon, Clove

Directions: Take 1 caplet before meals for best results.

Cautions: Do not expose to excessive heat or sunlight.

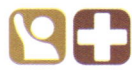

NingXia Wolfberry

CHINESE WOLFBERRY COMES TO THE MODERN WORLD

Wolfberry legends and records of ancient Chinese medicine reach back 5,000 years. Ben Zao Gen Mo, a physician's handbook written during the Ming Dynasty (1468-1664 AD), documents the ancient use of wolfberry.

The Ningxia wolfberry is still included in a number of Chinese herbal pharmacopoeias and is prescribed for patients with liver and kidney deficiencies, as well as with diabetes and vision problems.

For most of their long history, the people of the west elbow plateau of the Yellow River where the Ningxia wolfberry grows have been relatively isolated from the rest of civilization by deserts, mountains, and the enormous landmass of central China, which shielded them from outside influences and cultures.

This geographical isolation, in addition to China's political isolation, has contributed to the late discovery of this Chinese superfood by the West.

Nutritional Profile

In the mid-1980's when biochemists at the Ningxia Institute of Nutrition analyzed the Ningxia wolfberry, they found that it is 15.6 percent protein (dry weight) and contains at least 21 essential minerals, as well as significant levels of vitamins such as thiamin (vitamin B1), niacin (vitamin B3), and vitamin C. In fact, the Ningxia wolfberry is one of the richest known whole-food sources of natural vitamin B1 or thiamin, which is essential for proper energy production, carbohydrate metabolism, and thyroid function.[1,2]

Protein

With a total of 15.6 percent protein (dry weight), the Ningxia wolfberry contains as much protein as raw oats, one of the richest known sources of plant protein.[1,2] Just as important as the total protein content are the amino acids that are present, as amino acids are the building blocks of proteins. The wolfberry is rich in the essential amino acid leucine, as well as in the semi-essential amino acid L-arginine.

Protein is a vital building block of white blood cells and antibodies, which are some of the most prolifically reproducing cells in the body.

Protein also helps maintain a healthy thymus gland, which is vital for optimum cell-mediated immunity.

Leucine

Since it is not possible for the body to synthesize leucine, it is critical that foods containing leucine be included in one's diet. Leucine is the only dietary protein that has the capacity to cause the growth of muscle tissue and as a dietary supplement has shown to slow muscle atrophy in aged mice.[3]

Arginine

A semi-essential amino acid, L-arginine is considered an important nutrient for healthy immunity. L-arginine's ability to ramp up non-inflammatory immunity may be due to its use in the production of nitric oxide, which is used by the body to kill pathogens.[4,5] L-arginine also plays a key role in cell division, tissue regeneration, and wound healing. For that reason, many hospitals add it to enteral and parenteral tube feedings for burn and trauma patients.

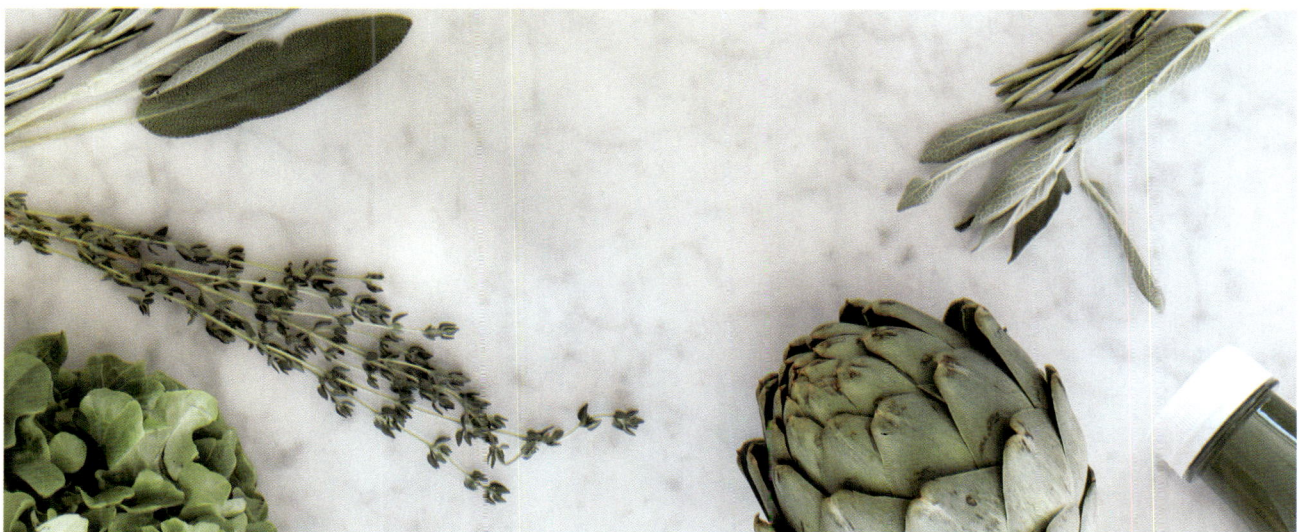

Nutrients in 100 Grams of Ningxia Wolfberry

Nutrient	Amount	% RDA
Protein	15.6 g	31.2
Fiber	21 g	84
Fat	0.45 g	<1
Sugar	42 g	N/A
Vitamin A	12,600 iu	250
Vitamin B-1	27 mg	1800
Vitamin B-3	88 mg	440
Vitamin B-5	88 mg	440
Vitamin C	148 mg	246
Biotin	28 μg	9
Calcium	110 mg	11
Chromium	79 mg	65
Copper	1.1 mg	55
Iron	11 mg	61
Magnesium	130 mg	32.5
Manganese	1.3 mg	65
Potassium	1,600 mg	102
Zinc	1.8 mg	12

Source: Preliminary data from dried fruit of Ningxia wolfberry (Lycium barbarum) stored 1-3 years.

Synergy of Arginine and Glutamine

L-arginine's stimulation of healthy immunity may be amplified when combined with another amino acid found in the Ningxia wolfberry: L-glutamine.

A medical group at Shanghai Medical University in China researched the use of an arginine and glutamine solution for tube feeding in gastrointestinal cancer patients, where adequate nutrition and amplified immunity is of life-or-death importance.

In this double-blind clinical trial, 48 patients were randomized into a control group with a standard diet and a treatment group supplemented with arginine and glutamine. The study lasted eight days.

Tolerance of both diets was excellent, according to the researchers, but with big differences in immune and inflammatory responses between the two groups.

Patients who received these two amino acids showed greater immunity and less inflammation than the control group.

The supplemented group had much higher levels of nitric oxide, total lymphocytes, T-lymphocytes, T-helper cells, and NK cells. They also exhibited lower levels of C-reactive protein, a marker for inflammation and heart disease.6

Location, Location, Location: Silt Water and Minerals

The location where the Ningxia wolfberry crop is grown is a large, contributing factor to the rich mineral profile of the Ningxia wolfberry.

The Yellow River flood plain, where the Ningxia wolfberry crop is concentrated, derives its water from the foothills of the Bayan Har Mountains of the Himalayan range in Qinghai Provence.

As this water flows down through mountain gorges and valleys, it becomes charged with minerals. By the time it reaches the Ningxia province of Northern China, it is mineral-rich silt water. The silt concentration in the river is so high that the Yellow River is named for the coloration these minerals impart to the water.

Vitamins and Minerals: Key to Long Life

Vitamins and minerals often work in pairs, such that many minerals cannot be assimilated into the body without the presence of a specific vitamin. It is interesting to note that the Ningxia wolfberry contains many of these vitamin-mineral pairs.

Some of the many functions that minerals perform in the body include electrolyte balance of our cells, nerve conduction for muscle contraction, bone and teeth formation, and enzyme activation. Minerals are so important that every process of the body depends on them.

Potassium

The Ningxia wolfberry is one of the highest whole-food sources of potassium.

Potassium is an essential mineral micronutrient in human nutrition. The body does not make it; so, therefore, it must be found through dietary sources.

Potassium cations are important in neuron function (brain and nerve) and in influencing osmotic balance between cells.

The potassium ion channels modulate the release of GABA in the brain.7 Researchers have found that the age-related decline in higher brain functions is due, in large part, to a lack of the inhibitory neurotransmitter GABA. Higher brain functions, such as visual recognition and language comprehension, decline as people get older. This decline appears to be due to a reduction of GABA, which results in neurons with specific tasks being more easily fired by some other types of stimulus, slowing down processing of information in the brain.8

Zinc

The Ningxia wolfberry is a rich vegetarian source of zinc, a mineral critical for healthy immunity. The dried berry has five times as much zinc as Brussels sprouts and more zinc than raw eggs.1,2

Zinc plays an essential role in the production of natural killer cells, IgG, gamma interferon, and tumor necrosis factor alpha. Zinc also enhances the microbe-killing activity of macrophages and increases levels of CD4 cytotoxic lymphocytes while lowering levels of CD8 immune-suppressing lymphocytes.9

According to Lothar Rink, an immunologist at the University of Lubeck School of Medicine in Germany, "The important role of zinc as an essential trace element for immune function has already been well established." He cited over 100 studies in support of this.10

Zinc deficiencies have been shown in both animal and human models to produce a variety of immune deficits, including T-lymphocyte depletion in the spleen and lymph nodes, impaired antibody response, shrinking of the thymus gland, and lower populations of cells associated with both humoral and cell-mediated immunity.11

Even more disconcerting is the fact that zinc deficiencies become more pronounced with advancing age as stomach acid declines, making it more difficult for the body to absorb zinc.

A Wayne State University study discovered that among a group of 180 randomly selected elderly subjects, the mean dietary intake of zinc was only 9 mg per day, which is 40 percent less than the recommended dietary allowance of 15 mg per day set by the Food and Nutrition Board.

Moreover, 36 percent of this group had depleted levels of zinc in two types of immune cells, granulocytes and lymphocytes, which correlated with depleted interleukin-1 (IL-1) production. Following zinc supplementation in a selected group, IL-1 jumped and lymphocyte activity surged.12

A September 2004 Case Western Reserve University review strongly indicates that zinc is effective for treating the common cold caused by the rhinovirus. "Clinical trial data support the value of zinc in reducing the duration and severity of symptoms of the common cold when administered within 24 hours of the onset of common cold symptoms," states Hulisz in the Journal of the American Pharmaceutical Association.13

The value of zinc was confirmed by a 2015 common cold study that showed "zinc acetate lozenges shortened the duration of nasal discharges by 34%, sneezing by 22%, scratchy throat by 33%, sore throat by 18%, hoarseness by 43%, and cough by 46%. Zinc lozenges shortened the duration of muscle ache by 54%, but there was no difference in the duration of headache and fever."14

Minerals such as zinc also constitute central components of some of the most powerful antioxidant compounds in the body. For instance, the mineral zinc is instrumental in the formation of superoxide dismutase (SOD), a key enzymatic antioxidant that declines with age. Antioxidants are discussed in further detail later.

Fiber

With over 21 percent fiber by weight, the Ningxia wolfberry has more fiber than oat bran and double the fiber of buckwheat. In fact, the Ningxia wolfberry has one of the highest percentages of fiber of any whole food.1,2

The Ningxia wolfberry is also rich in soluble fiber, which is highly efficient in removing triglycerides and cholesterol from the blood and lowering the risk of heart disease. Numerous studies have linked a high intake of soluble fiber with lowered blood pressure and improved cardiovascular health.15-18

Cholesterol is one of the few compounds in the body that cannot be broken down into smaller components and excreted. The only mechanism by which cholesterol can be flushed from the body is through bile acids. However, if feces lack sufficient fiber, cholesterol is not sufficiently

Amino Acids in 100 Grams of Ningxia Wolfberry

Alanine .... 720 mg	Glycine .... 430 mg
Lysine .... 390 mg	Serine .... 640 mg
Arginine .... 930 mg	Histidine .... 270 mg
Methionine ..... 148 mg	Threonine ...... 460 mg
Aspartate ..... 2,100 mg	Isoleucine .... 350 mg
Phenylalanine . 380 mg	Tyrosine .... 160 mg
Glutamine .... 1,400 mg	Leucine .... 630 mg
Proline .... 1,030 mg	Valine .... 1,040 mg

Source: Data from the dried fruit of Ningxia wolfberry (Lycium barbarum) stored 1-3 years.

excreted, forcing the remainder to be recirculated in the gall bladder.

Besides lowering cholesterol, a diet high in fiber has been directly linked to a lower risk of cancer, increased stability of blood sugar levels, and a lowered risk of heart disease.

More than Vitamins, Minerals, and Amino Acids

The Ningxia wolfberry is more than just a whole food high in minerals and vitamins; it also contains many unique phytonutrients that have been shown to protect the liver, eyes, heart, and cellular DNA from age-related degeneration and disease.

Carotenoids

During the past five years, food scientists working for the state government in Germany have identified a number of carotenoids that can stimulate immunity without provoking inflammation that can worsen the symptoms of arthritis. Chief among these is beta cryptoxanthin, but other carotenoids have also been identified, including alpha carotene and lutein.

As one of the richest sources of carotenoids, the Ningxia wolfberry can provide significant immune-boosting potential.[19-20]

Some of these carotenoids are zeaxanthin, lutein, and beta-cryptoxanthin.

Zeaxanthin is a pigment concentrated in the eye.

Both zeaxanthin and lutein have been shown to protect against skin cancer and protect the eyes against diseases such as age-related macular degeneration, the most common cause of blindness in older people.[21] One study found that "lutein and zeaxanthin and foods rich in these carotenoids may decrease the risk of cataracts severe enough to require extractions."[22]

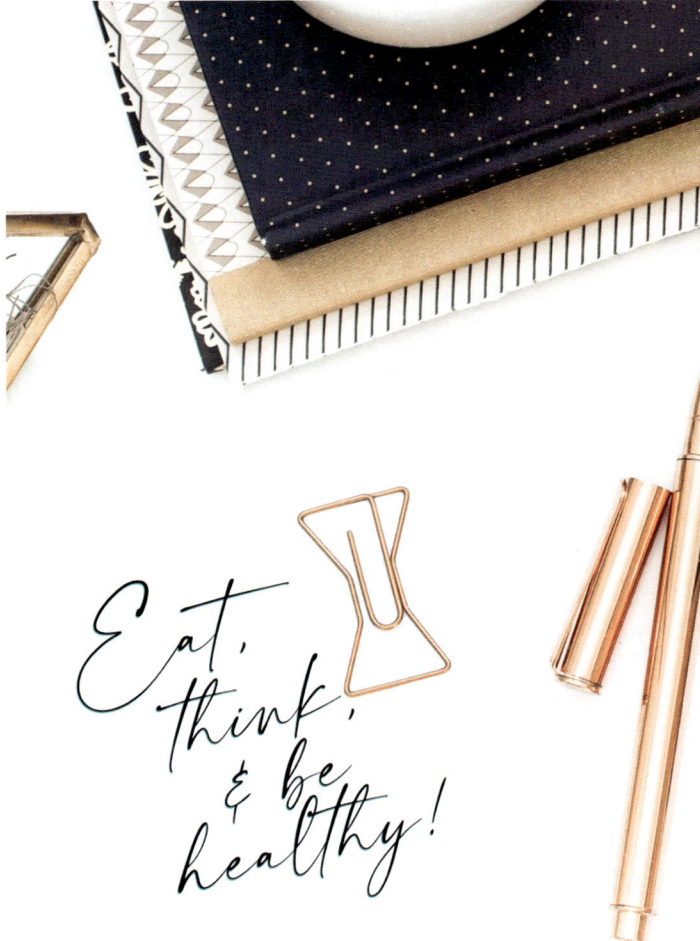

Carotenoid (Xanthophyl) Content of 100 Grams of Ningxia Wolfberry

Alpha carotene	101 µg
Beta carotene	23 µg
Lutein	2.1 µg
Zeaxanthin	278 µg
Beta cryptoxanthin	32 µg

Source: Preliminary data from dried fruit of Ningxia wolfberry (Lycium barbarum) stored 1-3 years. Analysis by Eurofins Scientific, Petaluma, CA

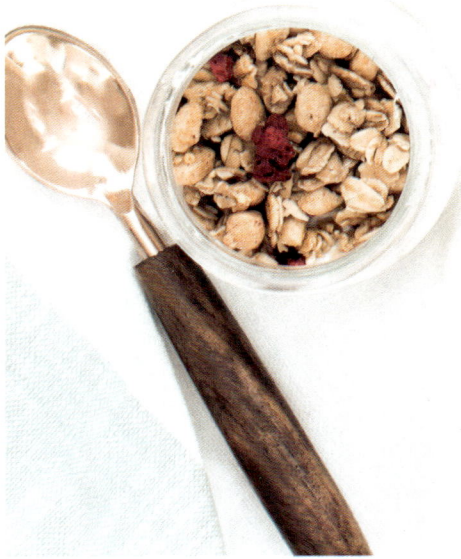
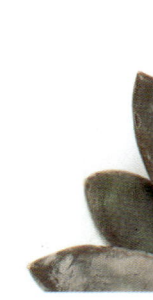

Beta-cryptoxanthin has been shown to inhibit cancer. It has also been researched for stimulating bone growth.23-28

Cerebrosides and Pyrroles

In 1998 Korean researchers discovered special compounds in wolfberries that afford powerful protection for the most important organ in the human body: the liver.

Known as pyrroles and cerobrosides, these nutrients have been shown to protect against liver damage caused by both toxins and hepatitis.29-31

Polysaccharides

The Ningxia wolfberry ranks high in a protein-sugar complex known as a polysaccharide. During the last 15 years, a number of studies have documented the cardioprotective, anticancerous, and immune-stimulating properties of the wolfberry polysaccharide. Studies show that polysaccharides in the Ningxia wolfberry positively affect natural killer cell function, which helps fight cancer.32-34

The first wolfberry polysaccharide was identified in 1994 when Chinese biochemists extracted a protein-carbohydrate complex (also known as a glycoprotein) from the wolfberry.35

Dubbing it "Lycium barbarum polysaccharide," researchers began learning that this low-glycemic, long-chain molecule could be responsible for many of the wolfberry's strong immune-boosting, anticancer, and cardiovascular protective benefits.

Lycium barbarum polysaccharide is a very large sugar-protein complex that occurs only in wolfberries. Of all the wolfberry species, Lycium barbarum L. contains the highest concentrations of Lycium barbarum polysaccharide.

The high polysaccharide and fiber content of the Ningxia wolfberry can promote the growth of beneficial bacteria in the gastrointestinal system. Diets high in protective, vegetable fibers, such as those in the wolfberry, result in higher levels of health-giving lactobacilli cultures and reduced populations of damaging cultures like Clostridium perfringens.

Beneficial bacteria may block cancer by producing short-chain fatty acids in the colon, which acidify the terrain.36 This reduced pH in the colon is strongly associated with lower colon cancer risk.37

Clinical Studies on Wolfberry Extracts

The Ningxia wolfberry's immune-boosting effect seems to be combined with an anti-inflammatory effect.38 This means that the immune-supporting action of Ningxia wolfberry is less likely to trigger worsening of arthritis or other autoimmune diseases that are inflammatory in nature.

- A 2003 Institute of Medicinal Biotechnology study at the Peking Union Medical College in Beijing, China, found that Ningxia wolfberry polysaccharide stimulated production of interleukin-2, a non-inflammatory part of immunity that protects against cancer cells and microbial invasion.39

- A March 2003 study published in the European Journal of Pharmacology showed in vitro data that Ningxia wolfberry polysaccharide dramatically expanded output of interleukin-2 and tumor necrosis factor alpha from specialized human immune cells known as peripheral mononuclear cells (PMC).

  The surges in both interleukin-2 and tumor necrosis factor alpha hit a peak after 4 to 12 hours and remained well above baseline for 24 hours.32

- A 2014 Chinese study showed Lycium barbarum polysaccharides protect the epithelial cells in the human eye.40

- An August 2001 study by the State Key Laboratory of Bio-Organic Chemistry in Shanghai showed that the Ningxia wolfberry polysaccharide had an unusual combination of "good immunoactivity and antioxidative activity."

  The polysaccharide markedly spurred phagocyte immune cell activity and promoted lymphocyte upregulation.41

- A 2004 study at the Huazhong University of Science and Technology in Wuhan, China, documented the ability of wolfberry polysaccharide to enhance the proliferation of lymphocyte immune cells in the spleen.42

- A 2015 study in the journal Food Nutrition Research found that Lycium barbarum polysaccharides cause human hepatoma (malignant tumor of the liver) cells to self-destruct (induce apoptosis).43

- A 2004 Huazhong University of Science and Technology study found that mice treated with 10 mg/kg of wolfberry polysaccharide for 10 days showed improved macrophage phagocytosis, spleen lymphocyte proliferation, cytotoxic T-lymphocyte (CTL) activity, and interleukin-2 (IL-2) expression. Polysaccharide-fed animals could also resist the growth of transplanted cancer tumor cells (sarcoma S180).44

All Sugars Are Not Equal

The dried wolfberries used extensively by the Ningxia people have been shown to have a very low glycemic index. A glycemic index is a measure of the impact a food has on blood sugar levels two hours after ingestion. The lower the rise in blood sugar levels, the lower the glycemic index.

The consumption of low glycemic foods is very important for minimizing the insidious degenerative damage caused by long-term, elevated blood sugar levels, which are strenuous to the heart, kidneys, pancreas, and circulatory system. Over time, the injury can become cumulative, shaving years off one's life.

Synergy: 1 + 1 = 3

Ultimately, the synergy of all of these nutrients may be responsible for the Ningxia wolfberry's ability to support so many different functions of the body.

According to Cornell University biochemist Riu Liu, PhD, "The additive and synergistic effects of phytochemicals in fruits and vegetables are responsible for their potent antioxidant and anticancer activities. This partially explains why no single antioxidant can replace the combination of natural phytochemicals in fruits and vegetables in achieving the health benefits."[45]

Protecting Cells from Oxidation

Each of the 3 trillion cells of the human body has a cell membrane composed primarily of fats that is susceptible to oxidative damage. The cell's energy is produced in mitochondria, where carbohydrates and oxygen are combined.

As this reaction takes place, free radical "sparks" shoot off that can damage the cell. Some of this damage occurs to the fats (lipids) that form the outer structure of both the mitochondria and the cell itself.

When these fats become oxidized or "rancid," malondialdehyde (MDA) starts to build up. The more of these "lipid peroxides" and MDA that form, the more brittle the cell membrane becomes, and the poorer the cell functions until eventually it self-destructs.

Protecting these fats from oxidative damage (or rancidity) is crucial for slowing down the damage that occurs with aging and keeping the machinery humming normally.

Oxidative stress to the body has been linked to diseases ranging from cancer to heart disease. This is why antioxidants are so important to the body. The simplest way to maximize antioxidant levels is with a diet high in antioxidant foods.

Other Bioactive Components of Ningxia Wolfberry

Alpha carotene[1,2]	Cerobrosides[6]	Monomenthyl succinate[9]	Scopoletin[4,12]
Beta-D-Glucopyranosyl ascorbate[3]	Cyclic diterpene glycosides[7]	Monoterpene glycosides[9]	Taurine[13]
Betaine[4,5]	Cyclic peptides[7]	P-coumaric acid[4]	Vanillic acid[12]
Beta cryptoxanthin[1,2]	Daucosterol[4]	Polyphenols[8]	Withanolides[14]
Beta sitosterol[4]	Ellagic Acid[8]	Polysaccharides[6,11]	Zeaxanthin dipalmitate[4,7,8,15]
	Lutein[1,2]	Pyrrole alkaloids[16]	

1. Li Z, Peng G, Zhang S. [Separation and determination of carotenoids in Fructus lycii by isocratic non-aqueous reversed-phase liquid chromatography]. Se Pu. 1998 Jul;16(4):341-3. Chinese.
2. Analysis by Eurofins Scientific, Petaluma, CA.
3. Toyoda-Ono Y, Maeda M, Nakao M, Yoshimura M, Sugiura-Tomimori N, Fukami H. 2-O-(beta-D-Glucopyranosyl) ascorbic acid, a novel ascorbic acid analogue isolated from Lycium fruit. J Agric Food Chem. 2004 Apr 7;52(7):2092-6.
4. Xie C, Xu LZ, Li XM, Li KM, Zhao BH, Yang SL. [Studies on chemical constituents in fruit of Lycium barbarum L]. Zhongguo Zhong Yao Za Zhi. 2001 May;26(5):323-4. Chinese.
5. Shin YG, Cho KH, Kim JM, Park MK, Park JH. Determination of betaine in Lycium chinense fruits by liquid chromatography-electrospray ionization mass spectrometry. J Chromatogr A. 1999 Oct 1;857(1-2):331-5.
6. Kim SY, Lee EJ, Kim HP, Lee HS, Kim YC. LCC, a cerebroside from Lycium chinense, protects primary cultured rat hepatocytes exposed to galactosamine. Phytother Res. 2000 Sep;14(6):448-51.
7. Yahara S, Shigeyama C, Ura T, Wakamatsu K, Yasuhara T, Nohara T. Cyclic peptides, acyclic diterpene glycosides and other compounds from Lycium chinense Mill. Chem Pharm Bull (Tokyo). 1993 Apr;41(4):703-9.
8. Brunswick Laboratories, Wareham, MA 2005.
9. Hiserodt RD, Adedeji J, John TV, Dewis ML. Identification of monomenthyl succinate, monomenthyl glutarate, and dimenthyl glutarate in nature by high perfor- mance liquid chromatography-tandem mass spectrometry. J Agric Food Chem. 2004 Jun 2;52(11):3536-41.
10. Huang LJ, Tian GY, Ji GZ. Structure elucidation of glycan of glycoconjugate LbGp3 isolated from the fruit of Lycium barbarum L. J Asian Nat Prod Res. 1999;1(4):259-67.
11. Peng X, Tian G. Structural characterization of the glycan part of glycoconjugate LbGp2 from Lycium barbarum L. Carbohydr Res. 2001 Mar 9;331(1):95-9.
12. Hansel R, Huang JT. Lycium chinense, III: isolation of scopoletin and vanillic acid. Arch Pharm (Weinheim). 1977 Jan;310(1):38-40.
13. Xie H, Zhang S. Determination of taurine in Lycium barbarum L. by high performance liquid chromatography with OPA-urea pre-column derivatization. Se Pu. 1997 Jan;15(1):54-6.
14. Hansel R, Huang JT, Rosenberg D. Two withanolides from Lycium chinense. Arch Pharm (Weinheim). 1975 Aug;308(8):653-4.
15. Weller P, Breithaupt DE. Identification and quantification of zeaxanthin esters in plants using liquid chromatography-mass spectrometry. J Agric Food Chem. 2003 Nov 19;51(24):7044-9.
16. Li J (et al or) Pan L, Naman CB, Deng Y, Chai H, Keller WJ, Kinghorn AD. Pyrrole alkaloids with potential cancer chemopreventive activity isolated from a goji berry-[containing] commercial sample of African mango. J Agri Food Chem. 2014 Jun 4;62(22):5054-60.

ORAC Test Measures Antioxidant Levels of Common Foods

In 1994 Tufts University developed a powerful, new method of assaying the antioxidant capacity of common foods called the Oxygen Radical Absorbance Capacity assay (ORAC). A food's ORAC score is a measure of its free-radical fighting capacity.

The ORAC assay is currently the most sensitive and reliable method used for calculating a food's antioxidant potential against the free radical peroxyl. The peroxyl radical is the second most common in the human body.

Sugars Found in Ningxia Wolfberry

Rhamnose	1.03%
Mannose	14.8%
Galactose	4.3%
Xylose	13.3%
Glucose	62.7%

Source: Huang L, et al. Isolation, purification and physico-chemical properties of immunoactive constituents from the fruit of Lycium barbarum L. Yao Xue Xue Bao. 1998 Jul;33(7):512-6.

Glycemic Index* of Selected Foods

Glucose	100
Brown Rice	66
Millet	72
Buckwheat	54
Ningxia Wolfberry	29

*Measures the speed with which a food raises blood sugar levels.

An Astounding Antioxidant

In 2000 Young Living Essential Oils commissioned an ORAC assay on the Ningxia wolfberry. The results were astonishing and showed that dried Ningxia wolfberries had 5 times the antioxidant capacity of prunes, 10 times that of oranges, 12 times that of raisins, and 55 times that of cauliflower. In fact, according to the published ORAC data, dried Ningxia wolfberries had one of the highest known ORAC scores of any whole food (303 μmTE/g).46

Protecting Against Superoxide and Other Free Radicals

While the peroxyl radical is the second most prevalent antioxidant in the body, the most prevalent and most damaging in the body is superoxide. A test has been developed that measures the superoxide-scavenging capacity of a food.

Animal Studies on Reversing Aging

Other studies have confirmed that Ningxia wolfberry has strong activity against the superoxide radical. A 2003 investigation by the Chinese Academy of Science tested the ability of Ningxia wolfberry polysaccharide (LBP) to reverse the effects of aging in three-month-old female mice who were dosed with a chemical that vastly accelerates the aging process, D-galactose.39

D-galactose was used because it mimics the type of damage typically seen in the elderly and diabetics.

To measure the animals' ability to resist aging, lead researcher Hong-Bin Deng used a number of tests, including an immunological assay, a memory test, and an AGE (advanced glycosylated end products) test. He also assayed serum levels of superoxide dismutase (SOD), which is the most important free-radical deactivator, due to its function of quenching deadly superoxide radicals.

Hong-Bin Deng found that the wolfberry polysaccharide restored SOD levels in aging animals to that of more youthful levels. The polysaccharide also blunted the damaging effects of D-galactose on mental function and AGE levels in the tissues. In short, the wolfberry appeared to reverse aging in animals subjected to a chemical that hastened the onset of old age.

Top Antioxidant Foods[1]

Food	ORAC[2] (μmTE/g)	Food	ORAC[2] (μmTE/g)
Ningxia Wolfberry (Lycium barbarum), dried[3]	303	Kale	18
Chinese wolfberry (Lycium chinense)	202	Raspberry	16
Acai, fresh	184	Apple	14
Black Raspberry	164	Peach	13
Pomegranate	105	Spinach	12
Ningxia Wolfberry (Lycium barbarum), fresh[4]	95	Red Grape	11
Prune	57	Brussels Sprouts	9
Blackberry	51	Alfalfa Sprouts	9
Boysenberry	35	Broccoli Florets	9
Blueberry	32	Kiwi	9
Plum	28	Beet	8
Red Raspberry	27	Onion	4
Strawberry	26	Cauliflower	4
Orange	24	Mango	3
Cherry	21	Cabbage	3
Raisin	21	Banana	3
Garlic	19	Apple	3
		Tomato	2
		Carrot	2

1 All foods are fresh unless otherwise noted as "dried."

2 Oxygen Radical Absorbance Capacity

3 Data from dried fruit stored 1-3 years. Analysis performed by Brunswick Labs, Wareham, MA.

4 Analysis performed by Brunswick Labs, Wareham, MA.

Ningxia Wolfberry vs. High-altitude Stress

A related study at the Faculty of Preventive Medicine at Ningxia Medicine College in Yinchuan tested SOD and catalase activity in a group of 56 mice that were subjected to oxidative stress caused by lack of oxygen. These "hypoxic" conditions were similar to what you would find at high altitudes.

In a subgroup fed Ningxia wolfberry, both SOD and catalase activity jumped significantly compared with the control group.

The simultaneous elevation of both of these antioxidant enzymes is important because the two depend on each other to maximize their effectiveness. While SOD deactivates superoxide free radicals, catalase mops up hydrogen peroxide free radicals.

The combination of the two working together is vital because SOD actually produces hydrogen peroxide as a byproduct of defusing superoxide. Catalase is one of the few enzymes capable of neutralizing hydrogen peroxide.47

Ningxia Wolfberry Extends Cell Life

Gerontologists at the Department of Cell Biology and Genetics at Peking University discovered that including a vanishingly small amount of wolfberry (0.025 percent) in the culture medium could extend the number of times human lung cells could divide from 49 times to 61 times.

Each time a cell divides, the chance of error creeps in, as well as the cumulative burden of oxidative damage. Using wolfberry in the nutrient broth, researchers effectively increased the lifespan of the lung tissue by 22 percent.48

An October 2002 study at the Department of Histology and Embryology at the Ningxia Medical College in Yinchuan tested the ability of Ningxia wolfberry to help sperm-producing cells resist damage from excess cold (hypothermic conditions) and ultraviolet sunlight radiation.

According to the lead researcher, Wang, "We found that fructus lycii polysaccharide (FLPS) is a potent inhibitor of both of these reactions. Together, these results demonstrate the protective effect of FLPS on time and hyperthermia induced testicular degeneration in vitro."49

This study is significant not only because of its implications for increased fertility (yes, it is true that Ningxia wolfberry extracts have been used for centuries to boost reproductive success) but also as it pertains to the antioxidant protection that Ningxia wolfberry affords to cells that are most vulnerable to oxidative damage: testicle cells.

Reproductive cells are very easily damaged by cold stresses and UV radiation, so the ability of Ningxia wolfberry to effectively defend against these types of attacks helps to show the true measure of the berry's antioxidant potential.

Healthy Immunity and Antiaging

As mentioned previously, the Ningxia wolfberry contains a polysaccharide that has been shown to positively affect natural killer cell function.34

During the past two decades, a number of clinical studies have shown a direct link between cancer, accelerated aging, and poor immune function. In particular, a key weapon in our nonspecific immunity called a "natural killer" cell is very adept at automatically destroying suspicious-looking cancer cells without requiring "education" in the immune glands of the body (e.g., thymus).50-55

A 2002 study at the University of Milan documented a direct link between stress and inflammation and lowered natural killer cell activity and poorer outcomes in cancer cases.56

An earlier study published in the International Journal of Cancer showed that animals with higher levels of NK (natural killer) activity were able to suppress metastatic cancer growth by up to 7-fold in comparison with normal mice.57

Researchers at the Mount Sinai Medical Center in New York also showed a link between low immunity (natural killer cell activity) and poor outcomes in cancer survival.

After analyzing the survival data from 102 colorectal cancer patients, Tartter and Steinberg found that having a preoperative low NK cell function triggered a frightening jump in the danger of cancer recurrence.58

Similarly, a 2002 Chiba University study on 140 patients with colorectal cancer found that lowered NK cell activity was linked to a 50 percent risk of cancer colonization and spread compared to patients with normal or better NK cell function.

Lead researcher Eisuke Kondo stated that "the patient's own anticancer immunity, as well as the potent malignancy of the tumor, may play a role in the development of recurrence following curative surgery. . . . Preliminary data showed that among several immunological parameters examined . . . , preoperative natural killer (NK) cell activity was the only one associated with . . . distant metastasis following curative surgery for colorectal cancer."59

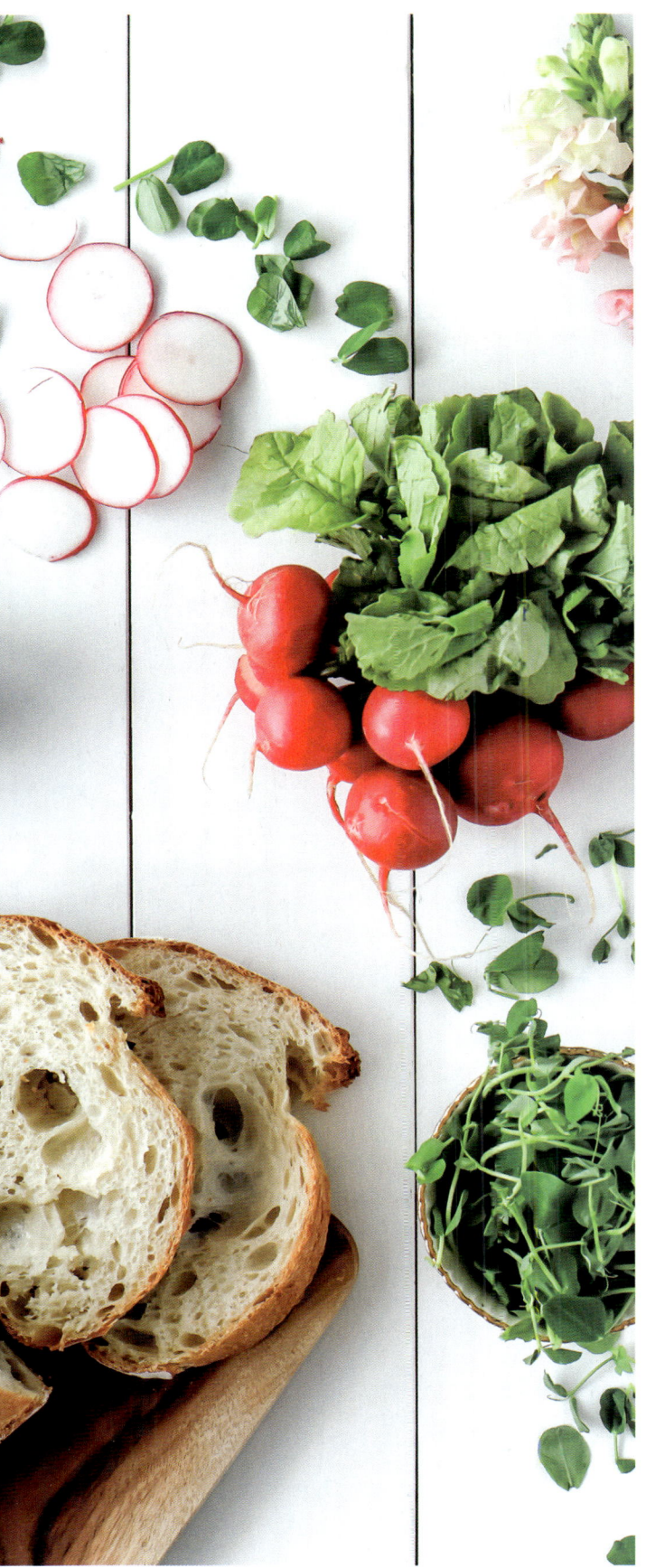

Whole Wolfberry Clinical Trials

The first study conducted on the power of the wolfberry to protect against superoxide measured the ability of the body to produce the free-radical, enzymatic, antioxidant superoxide dismutase (SOD). SOD is the body's frontline defense against superoxide, and it is this enzymatic antioxidant that is so important in neutralizing the free radical superoxide.

In 1982 the following study was conducted in China. Fifty persons aged 64-80 were given 50 grams of wolfberries for 10 days.

Blood samples were taken before the study began and after 10 days of consuming a diet that included wolfberries. The blood samples at the end of 10 days showed that levels of SOD had increased by 48 percent. In addition, lipid peroxides had dropped by 65 percent.60

Another study published in December 2004 by Kaohsiung Medical University in Taiwan indicates that the Ningxia wolfberry may indeed have strong superoxide-neutralizing activity.

Researchers found that depending on its concentration, a water extract of wolfberry scavenged from 28.8 percent to 82.2 percent of superoxide radicals. The concentrations of wolfberry that inhibited 50 percent of the superoxide activity were tiny, ranging from 0.77 to 2.55 parts per million. This works out to 0.000077 and 0.00025 percent.

The minute concentrations used are indicative of the Ningxia wolfberry's exceptional superoxide-neutralizing power.61

For further reading, please see: Young DG, Lawrence R, Schreuder M. Discovery of the Ultimate Superfood. Lehi, UT: Life Science Publishing, 2005.

NUTRITIONAL PRODUCTS WITH NINGXIA WOLFBERRY

(see Chapter 3, "Nutritional Products," for more information)

The Ningxia wolfberry is a fabulous source of nutrients for nutritional products.

All of the following products contain Ningxia wolfberry (Lycium barbarum), which is the highest antioxidant food known, making it an excellent whole food with 18 amino acids; 21 trace minerals; vitamins B1, B2, B6, C, E; polyphenols; carotenoids; magnesium; and potassium.

Balance Complete™ Vanilla Cream Meal Replacement

Balance Complete is a super-food meal replacement that is high in fiber and protein, with the good fats, enzymes, vitamins, and minerals needed to form a nutritious, great tasting protein drink that satisfies the appetite. It is a powerful nutritive energizer and cleanser, which helps to improve digestion and support colon health.

The high antioxidant benefits of the Ningxia wolfberry powder, brown rice bran, barley grass, aloe vera, cinnamon powder, and whey protein blend create the building blocks for strengthening the immune system and bringing back the renewed feelings of energy and vitality.

Gary's True Grit™ Chocolate-Coated Wolfberry Crisp™ Bars

The Chocolate-Coated Wolfberry Crisp bars are delicious, convenient, whole-food, low-glycemic, super-nutrient bars, each containing 6 grams of protein and are delightfully coated in chocolate. They are rich in antioxidants and phytonutrients and do not significantly raise blood sugar levels. They are a great all-natural snack for when you're on the go, at work, at school, or even when you want a meal replacement.

Gary's True Grit™ Einkorn Granola

The tasty combination of naturally sourced grains, nuts, berries, and seeds provides both simple and complex carbs to keep you going throughout the day. The crunchy clusters are mixed with Organic Dried Ningxia Wolfberries, cranberries, cacao nibs, coconut sugar, sunflower seeds, almonds, walnuts, and pecans, with just the right amount of sea salt.

Gary's True Grit™ NingXia Berry Syrup

This premium all-purpose syrup combines natural, delicious ingredients, including wolfberry seed oil, with pure Orange and Lemon essential oils to create the perfect complement to Gary's True Grit Einkorn Pancake and Waffle Mix or your favorite dessert.

ImmuPro™

ImmuPro chewable tablets are packed with some of the most powerful immune stimulants known, including wolfberry polysaccharide and beta glucan (a polysaccharide from reishi, maitake, and Agaricus blazei mushrooms).

Numerous studies have documented the ability of these botanicals to reverse cancer and stimulate both cell-mediated and humoral immunity, dramatically boosting levels of macrophages, neutrophils, phagocytes, B-cells, T-cells, natural killer cells, interleukins, and interferons.

ImmuPro combines complex and potent, immune-boosting minerals such as zinc, copper, and selenium. It also contains melatonin, one of the most powerful immune stimulants known, shown to clinically reverse tumor growth. Melatonin levels steadily decrease with age and are a factor that contributes to accelerated aging.

KidScents® MightyVites™

KidScents MightyVites is a whole-food multinutrient that contains wolfberry fruit and other super fruits, plants, and vegetables that deliver the full spectrum of vitamins, minerals, antioxidants, and phytonutrients, specifically designed for children's developing bodies.

Children's diets often need to bridge between what they are eating and what they should be eating. To fuel growth and normal activity levels, a child's diet must provide plenty of vitamins and minerals as well as store nutrients in preparation for the accelerated growth spurts of the teenage years.

This super enriched, chewable vitamin is perfect for children to energize, build their bodies, and protect their entire system the way Mother Nature intended.

Master Formula™

Master Formula is a full-spectrum, premium multinutrient supplement that contains wolfberry fruit powder, providing vitamins, minerals, and food-based nutriment to support general health and well-being for men and women.

By using a Synergistic Suspension Isolation process (SSI Technology), ingredients are delivered in three distinct forms. Collectively, these ingredients provide a premium, synergistic complex to support your body.

NingXia Nitro™

NingXia Nitro is an all-natural way to increase cognitive alertness, enhance mental fitness, and support overall performance. It contains a wide range of powerful cognitive enhancers, including wolfberry seed oil and a proprietary blend of pure Black Pepper, Nutmeg, Vanilla, Chocolate, Yerba Mate, Spearmint, and Peppermint essential oils.

NingXia Nitro contains Bioenergy Ribose®, a form of D-Ribose that has been clinically tested for its ability to increase energy, endurance, and aerobic activity and is

Ningxia Red® Recipes

The Holy Cow
- 1 drop Peppermint
- 2 drops Frankincense
- 1 drop Lemon

To Your Health
- 1 drop Orange
- 2 drops Tangerine
- 1 drop Thieves blend

Oh, My Gosh
- 1 drop Ocotea
- 4 drops Peppermint
- 3 drops Tangerine
- 3 drops Lemon

Oh, My Gosh, for Your Digestion
- 2 drops Tangerine
- 1 drop Frankincense
- 1 drop Fennel
- 1 drop Peppermint

The Nuclear Explosion
- 1 drop Peppermint
- 1 drop Lavender
- 1 drop Frankincense
- 1 drop Lemon
- 1 drop Tangerine
- 1 drop Orange

Who Let the Dogs Out?
- 1 drop Lemon
- 2 drops Tangerine
- 1 drop Frankincense
- 1 drop Cinnamon Bark

(Take the shot; then go "woof, woof, woof, woof, woof.")

Variation: Put 1 drop Cassia on the back of your hand and lick it off just before consuming the drink.

---

currently used by the Olympic athletes. This ingredient improves physical performance, speeds up recovery, and increases overall energy reserves.

Other supportive ingredients in NingXia Nitro, such as B vitamins, green tea extract, choline, and Korean ginseng, sharpen the mind and invigorate the senses.

NingXia Red®

NingXia Red is a powerful antioxidant supplement drink made from wolfberry juice, blueberry juice, pomegranate juice, apricot juice, raspberry juice, and Lemon and Orange essential oils.

NingXia Red supports immune function, liver function, and eye health and is reported to increase energy.

It is the highest known protection against the dangerous superoxide free radicals, as documented in the S-ORAC test conducted by Brunswick Laboratories. It is rich in ellagic acid, polyphenols, flavonoids, vitamins, and minerals. In addition, it has 18 amino acids, 21 trace minerals, beta-carotene, and vitamins B1, B2, B6, and E.

It is an excellent whole-food source of nutrients that gives energy and strength to the body without harmful stimulants. It also has an amazing low glycemic index of 11 that does not spike the blood sugar levels.

Ningxia Wolfberries (Organic Dried)

The Ningxia wolfberry is one of earth's most powerful antioxidant fruits. It is rich in polysaccharides, with more vitamin C than oranges, more beta-carotene than carrots, and more calcium than broccoli.

These little, red Ningxia wolfberries are delicious and make a great, healthy snack. They can be used in cooking, salads, desserts, etc.

NingXia Zyng™

NingXia Zyng is a light, sparkling beverage that delivers a splash of hydrating energy. Zyng is fueled by a proprietary blend of pure Black Pepper and Lime essential oils, wolfberry puree, and white tea extract, coupled with a blend of vitamins to create a unique and refreshing experience. Containing just 35 calories, 8.4 ounces of NingXia Zyng will invigorate your senses with no artificial flavors, colors, sweeteners, or preservatives.

Slique® Bars—Tropical Berry Crunch

Slique Bars are safe, innovative weight-management tools that utilize a dual-target approach to help manage satiety. First, Slique Bars are loaded with exotic baru nuts and wholesome almonds that promote satiation when combined with protein and high levels of fiber.

Second, Slique bars contain clinical amounts of Slendesta®, an all-natural ingredient derived from potato skin extract that when ingested triggers the release of cholecystokinin in the body, increasing the duration of feelings of fullness.

Slique Bars also deliver essential nutrients and antioxidants through the addition of pure Cinnamon Bark, Vanilla, and Orange essential oils; a dried-fruit blend featuring goldenberries and wolfberries; and D. Gary Young's exclusive dehydrated cacao nibs. Slique Bars' dual-targeted satiety approach and medley of exotic fruits, nuts, and science creates the perfect stimulant-free nutritious snack to help you feel fuller longer.

Slique® Bars—Chocolate-Coated

Chocolate-Coated Slique Bars are a safe, delicious weight-management snack loaded with exotic baru nuts and wholesome almonds. Slique Bars deliver essential nutrients from a unique superfruit blend of goldenberries and wolfberries, plus Cinnamon, Vanilla, and Orange essential oils.

Slique® Shake

Slique Shake is a complete meal replacement that provides quick, satisfying, and delicious nutrition. It is sweetened with stevia, organic coconut palm sugar, wolfberries, and strawberries and uses pea protein, quinoa, wolfberry, pumpkin seed protein, and alfalfa grass juice, making it an excellent source of protein and dietary fiber. In a convenient single-serving size packet, it's great to take with you for a quick and easy meal.

Sulfurzyme® Capsules and Powder

Sulfurzyme is a unique combination of MSM, the protein-building compound found in breast milk, fresh fruits and vegetables, and Ningxia wolfberry. Together, they create a new concept in balancing the immune system and supporting almost every major function of the body.

Of particular importance is the ability of MSM to equalize water pressure inside the cells, a considerable benefit for those plagued with bursitis, arthritis, or tendonitis.

Ningxia wolfberry supplies nutrients to enhance the proper assimilation and metabolism of sulfur.

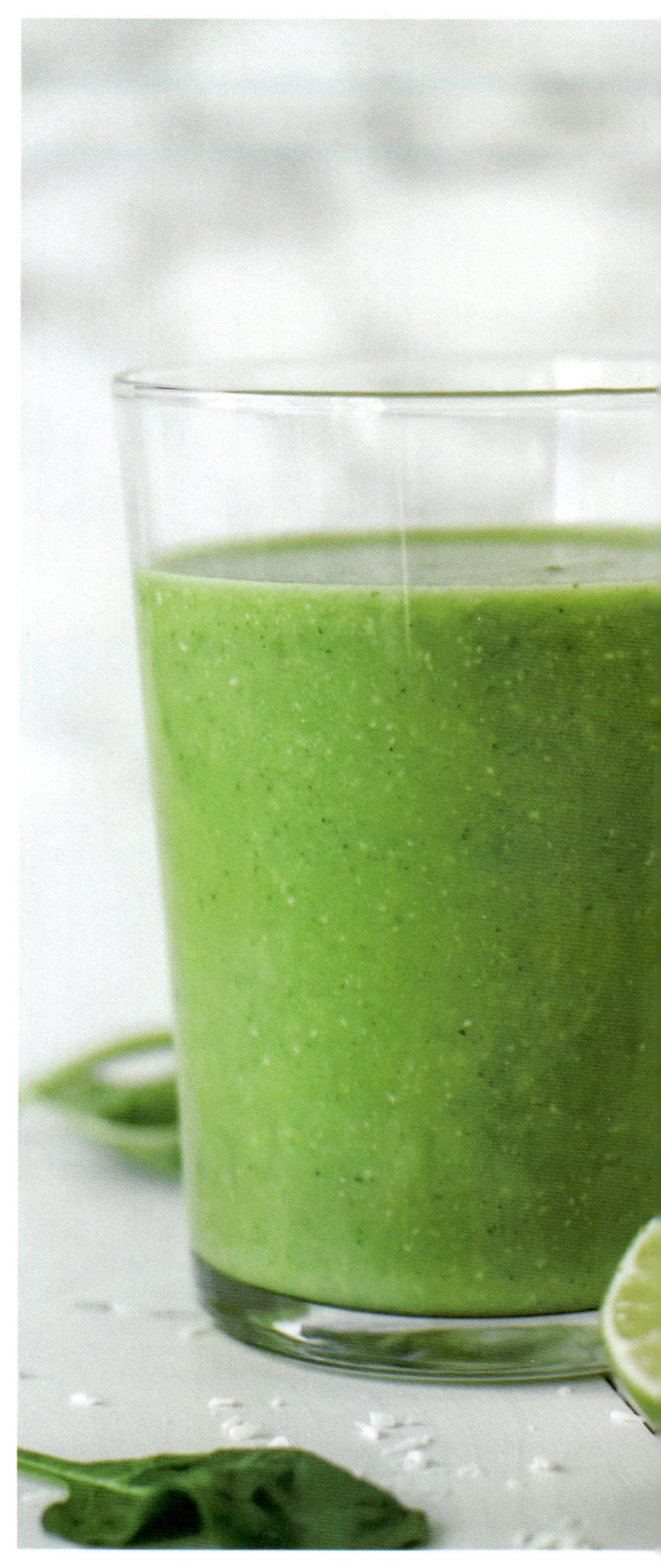

Wolfberry Crisp™

Wolfberry Crisp is a delicious, convenient, whole-food, low-glycemic, super-nutrient bar, containing 16 grams of protein.

It is rich in antioxidants and phytonutrients and does not significantly raise blood sugar levels. It also contains soy and whey protein complex, organic blue agave nectar, wolfberry fruit, pumpkin seeds, cashews, walnuts, carob chips, vanilla bean extract, and natural banana flavoring.

It is a delicious meal replacement that is all natural and certified kosher.

Wolfberry Crisp™ Bars, Chocolate Coated

(see Gary's True Grit™ Chocolate-Coated Wolfberry Crisp™ Bars)

PERSONAL CARE PRODUCTS WITH NINGXIA WOLFBERRY

(see Chapter 11, "Personal Body Care," for more information)

For centuries, the Chinese living in Inner Mongolia have been using a very unusual oil with exceptional benefits for the skin: wolfberry seed oil.

This rare and expensive oil from Inner Mongolia is painstakingly extracted from the seeds of the Ningxia wolfberry. Not only is the oil rich in vitamin E and linoleic and linolenic acids, but it also has an unusual chemistry that makes it ideal for nourishing and hydrating the skin.

"The wolfberry seed oil is one of the best oils for the skin," according to researcher Sue Chao. "It is sought after throughout Asia and has some very unusual regenerative properties such as protecting aging skin and adding luster to skin."

All of the following personal body care products contain Ningxia wolfberry.

Boswellia Wrinkle Cream™

Boswellia Wrinkle Cream contains the pure essential oils of Frankincense, Sandalwood, Myrrh, Ylang Ylang, and Geranium that moisturize while minimizing shine, relaxing facial tension, and reducing the effects of sun damage.

This wrinkle cream also contains wolfberry seed oil, which helps build collagen and when used daily will help minimize and prevent wrinkles.

Copaiba Vanilla Moisturizing Conditioner

Plant-based, safe, and environmentally responsible, Copaiba Vanilla Moisturizing Conditioner is a rich, hydrating conditioner for dry or damaged hair.

Formulated with botanical extracts; vitamins; silk proteins; wolfberry fruit extract and berries; pure Copaiba, Lavender, Geranium, and Lime essential oils; and vanilla absolute, this gentle conditioner protects and conditions for a soothing, revitalizing experience.

Copaiba Vanilla Moisturizing Shampoo

Copaiba Vanilla Moisturizing Shampoo calms and moisturizes dry, irritated scalps and is a natural sealant that can help tame "flyaway" hair and lock in moisture.

Plant-based, safe, and environmentally responsible, this shampoo contains wolfberry fruit extract and berries and the essential oils of Copaiba, Lavender, Geranium, Lime, plus vanilla absolute and is a rich, hydrating cleanser for dry or damaged hair.

Essential Beauty™ Serum (Dry)

Essential oils provide wonderful benefits when used on the skin. Lavender, Blue Cypress, and Royal Hawaiian Sandalwood™ are known for their ability to restore the skin's natural moisture balance. The fine lipid structure of essential oils enables them to penetrate deep into skin tissues, carrying many active ingredients that renew, balance, and build skin health.

This serum has a wonderful skin-conditioning base of coconut, avocado, jojoba, rosehip seed, and wolfberry seed oils. Vitamin E and lecithin are added for a greater softening effect.

Lavender Bath & Shower Gel

Infused with pure Lavender oil, Lavender Bath & Shower Gel will cleanse and rejuvenate your skin while it soothes and relaxes your mind.

It is free of chemicals and synthetic preservatives and contains plant-based ingredients like wolfberry fruit extract and berries and the essential oils of Lavender, Lemon, Myrrh, and Davana.

Lavender Hand & Body Lotion

Infused with wolfberry seed oil; Lavender, Myrrh, Lemon, and Davana essential oils; and other plant-based ingredients, Lavender Hand & Body Lotion moisturizes and protects skin from overexposure for long-lasting hydration.

This formula is certified eco-friendly and all natural.

Lavender Mint Invigorating Conditioner

Plant-based, safe, and environmentally responsible, Lavender Mint Invigorating Conditioner is an invigorating daily moisture blend suitable for all hair types.

Containing botanical extracts, vitamins, silk protein, wolfberry fruit extract and berries, and pure Lavender and Peppermint essential oils, this conditioner provides a rejuvenating and invigorating experience suitable for all hair types.

Lavender Mint Invigorating Shampoo

Lavender Mint Invigorating Shampoo contains wolfberry fruit extract and berries and Lavender essential oil to soothe the scalp and calm unmanageable hair and Peppermint essential oil to stimulate the blood flow to the hair follicle—allowing hair to better absorb nutrients.

Plant-based, safe, and environmentally responsible, this shampoo is an invigorating, daily cleansing blend suitable for all hair types.

Lip Balm, Cinnamint™

This balm moisturizes and protects your lips by combining the nutritious wolfberry seed oil with MSM and pure Cinnamon Bark, Peppermint, Spearmint, and Orange essential oils. Cinnamint Lip Balm helps prevent skin dehydration for soft, smooth lips.

Lip Balm, Grapefruit

This balm is infused with Grapefruit essential oil, wolfberry seed oil, and antioxidants that seal in moisture to prevent dehydration for smooth, supple lips.

Lip Balm, Lavender

This balm soothes dry, chapped lips with gentle, protective Lavender essential oil and the moisturizing benefits of wolfberry seed oil, jojoba oil, and vitamin E.

Orange Blossom Facial Wash™

This gentle, soap-free facial wash cleanses the skin without stripping natural oils. In addition to wolfberry seed oil, it contains MSM for softening, kelp to improve elasticity, and Lavender essential oil to soothe skin prone to acne and other problems.

Prenolone® + Body Cream

Prenolone Plus Body Cream contains pregnenolone; DHEA; wolfberry seed oil; blue and black cohosh; and Ylang Ylang, Clary Sage, and other essential oils to nourish the skin and help maintain healthy estrogen levels.

Regenolone Moisturizing Cream™

Regenolone is a natural moisturizer formulated to support proper estrogen levels in women.

In addition to wolfberry seed oil, it contains wild yam; black and blue cohosh; and Peppermint, Wintergreen, and other essential oils to invigorate the skin and enhance absorption.

Sandalwood Moisture Cream™

Sandalwood Moisture Cream is an ultra-hydrating moisturizer infused with wolfberry seed oil and the pure essential oils of Myrrh, Lavender, Sandalwood, and Rosemary. In addition, MSM—a naturally occurring, plant-based chemical—softens skin and promotes elasticity.

When used daily after cleansing and toning, this moisture cream promotes younger, healthier skin.

Wolfberry Eye Cream™

Wolfberry Eye Cream is a natural, water-based moisturizer. Containing the anti-aging properties of wolfberry seed oil and the essential oils of Lavender, Roman Chamomile, Frankincense, and Geranium. This cream soothes tired eyes and minimizes the appearance of bags, circles, and fine lines. Use in the morning and before bed.

ENDNOTES

1. Young G, Lawrence R, Schreuder M. Ningxia wolfberry: Ultimate superfood: how the Ningxia wolfberry and four other foods help combat heart disease, cancer, chronic fatigue, depression, diabetes and more. Lehi: Life Science Publishing, 2006. 266 p.

2. U.S. Department of Agriculture, Agricultural Research Service [Internet]. 2011. USDA Nutrient Database for Standard Reference, Release 24. Nutrient Data Laboratory Home Page. Available from: http://www.ars.usda.gov/ba/bhnrc/ndl.

3. Combaret L, Dardevet D, Rieu I, Pouch MN, Béchet D, Taillandier D, Grizard J, Attaix D. A leucine-supplemented diet restores the defective post prandial inhibition of proteasome-dependent proteolysis in aged rat skeletal muscle. J physiol. 2005;569(2):489-499.

4. Bogdan C, Röllinghoff M, Diefenbach A. The role of nitric oxide in innate immunity. Immunol Rev. 2000 Feb;173:17-26.

5. Jyothi MD, Khar A. Induction of nitric oxide production by natural killer cells: its role in tumor cell death. Nitric Oxide. 1999 Oct;3(5):409-418.

6. Wu GH, Zhang YW, Wu ZH. Modulation of postoperative immune and inflammatory response by immune-enhancing enteral diet in gastrointestinal cancer patients. World J Gastroenterol. 2001 Jun;7(3):357-362.

7. Chan O, Lawson M, Zhu W, Beverly JL, Sherwin RS. ATP-sensitive K(+) channels regulate the release of GABA in the ventromedial hypothalamus during hypoglycemia. Diabetes. 2007;56(4):1120-1126.

8. Leventhal AG, Wang Y, Pu M, Zhou Y, Ma Y. GABA and its agonists improved visual cortical function in senescent monkeys. Science. 2003;300(5620):812.

9. Shankar AH, Prasad AS. Zinc and immune function: the biological basis of altered resistance to infection. Am J Clin Nutr. 1998 Aug;68(2 Suppl):447S-463S.

10. Rink L, Kirchner H. Zinc-altered immune function and cytokine production. J Nutr. 2000 May;130(5S Suppl):1407S-1411S.

11. Shankar AH, Prasad AS. Zinc and immune function: the biological basis of altered resistance to infection. Am J Clin Nutr. 1998 Aug;68(2 Suppl):447S-463S.

12. Prasad AS, Fitzgerald JT, Hess JW, Kaplan J, Pelen F, Dardenne M. Zinc deficiency in elderly patients. Nutrition. 1993 May-Jun;9(3):218-24.

13. Hulisz D. Efficacy of zinc against common cold viruses: an overview. J Am Pharm Assoc. 2004 Sep-Oct;44(5):594-603

14. Hemilä H, Chalker E. The effectiveness of high dose zinc acetate lozenges on various common cold symptoms: a meta-analysis. BMC Fam Prac. 2015 Feb 25;16:24.

15. Brown L, Rosner B, Willett WW, Sacks FM. Cholesterol-lowering effects of dietary fiber: a meta-analysis. Am J Clin Nutr. 1999;69(1)30-42.

16. Romero AL, Romero JE, Galaviz S, Fernandez ML. Cookies enriched with psyllium or oat bran lower plasma LDL cholesterol in normal and hypercholesterolemic men from Northern Mexico. J Am Coll Nutr. 1998;17(6):601-608.

17. Mekki N, Dubois C, Charbonnier M, Cara L, Senft M, Pauli AM, Portugal H, Gassin AL, Lafont H, Lairon D. Effects of lowering fat and increasing dietary fiber on fasting and postprandial plasma lipids in hypercholesterolemic subjects consuming a mixed Mediterranean-Western diet. Am J Clin Nutr. 1997;66(6):1443-1451.

18. Ullrich IH. Evaluation of a high-fiber diet in hyperlipidemia: a review. J Am Coll Nutr. 1987;6(1):19-25.

19. Watzl B, Bub A, Briviba K, Rechkemmer G. Supplementation of a low-carotenoid diet with tomato or carrot juice modulates immune functions in healthy men. Ann Nutr Metab. 2003;47(6):255-261.

20. Watzl B, Bub A, Brandstetter BR, Reehkemmer G. Modulation of human T-lymphocyte functions by the consumption of carotenoid-rich vegetables. Br J Nutr. 1999 Nov;82(5):383-389.

21. Gale CR, Hall NF, Phillips DI, Martyn CN. Lutein and zeaxanthin status and risk of age-related macular degeneration. Invest Opthalmol Vis Sci. 2003 Jun;44(6):2461-2465.

22. Chasen-Taber L, Willett WC, Seddor JM, Stampfer MJ, Rosner B, Colditz GA, Speizer FE, Hankinson SE. A prospective study of carotenoid and vitamin A intakes and risk of cataract extraction in US women. Am J Clin Nutr. 1999 Oct;70(4):509-516.

23. Noguchi S, Sumida T, Ogawa H, Tada M, Takahata K. Effects of oxygenated carotenoid beta-cryptoxanthin on morphological differentiation and apoptosis in Neuro2a neuroblastoma cells. Biosci Biotechnol Biochem. 2003 Nov;67(11):2467-2469.

24. Donaldson MS. Nutrition and cancer: a review of the evidence for an anti-cancer diet. Nutr J. 2004 Oct 20;3(1):19.

25. Nomura AM, Lee J, Stemmermann GN, Franke AA. Serum vitamins and the subsequent risk of bladder cancer. J Urol. 2003 Oct;170(4 Pt 1):1146-1150.

26. Uchiyama S, Yamaguchi M. beta-Cryptoxanthin stimulates cell proliferation and transcriptional activity in osteoblastic MC3T3-E1 cells. Int J Mol Med. 2005 Apr;15(4):675-681.

27. Yamaguchi M, Uchiyama S. beta-Cryptoxanthin stimulates bone formation and inhibits bone resorption in tissue culture in vitro. Mol Cell Biochem. 2004 Mar;258(1-2):137-144.

28. Uchiyama S, Sumida T, Yamaguchi M. Oral administration of beta-cryptoxanthin induces anabolic effects on bone components in the femoral tissues of rats in vivo. Biol Pharm Bull. 2004 Feb;27(2):232-235.

29. Kim SY, Choi YH, Huh H, Kim J, Kim YC, Lee HS. New antihepatotoxic cerebroside from Lycium chinense fruits. J Nat Prod. 1997 Mar;60(3):274-276.

30. Chin YW, Lim SW, Kim SH, Shin DY, Suh YG, Kim YB, Kim YC, Kim J. Hepatoprotective pyrrole derivatives of Lycium chinense fruits. Bioorg Med Chem Lett. 2003 Jan 6;13(1):79-81.

31. Kim HP, Choi YH, Huh H, Kim J, Kim YC, Lee HS. Zeaxanthin dipalmitate from Lycium chinense fruit reduces experimentally induced hepatic fibrosis in rats. Biol Pharm Bull. 2002 Mar;25(3):390-392.

32. Gan L, Zhang SH, Liu Q, Xu HB. A polysaccharide-protein complex from Lycium barbarum upregulates cytokine expression in human peripheral blood mononuclear cells. Eur J Pharmacol. 2003 Jun 27;471(3):217-222.

33. Jia YX, Dong JW, Wu XX, Ma TM, Shi AY. [The effect of Lycium barbarum polysaccharide on vascular tension in two-kidney, one clip model of hypertension]. Sheng Li Xue Bao. 1998 Jun;50(3):309-314. Chinese.

34. Hu Q, Jia BL, Gao TS, E ZE, Gao YJ, Huo LM. A study on the anti-cancer effect of ningxia wolfberry. J Tradit Chin Med. 1989 Jun;9(2):117-124.

35. Tian G-Y, Wang C. [Structure elucidation of a high MW glycan of a glycoprotein isolated from the fruit of Lycium barbarum L]. Acta Bioch Bioph Sin. 1995;05. Chinese.

36. Goldin BR, Gorbach SL. The effect of milk and lactobacillus feeding on human intestinal bacterial enzyme activity. Am J Clin Nutr. 1984;39(5):756-761.

37. Aso Y, Akazan H. Prophylactic effect of a Lactobacillus casei preparation on the recurrence of superficial bladder cancer. BLP Study Group. Urol Int. 1992;49(3):125-129.

38. Xu Y, He L, Xu L, Liu Y. [Advances in immunopharmacological study of Lycium barbarum L]. Zhong Yao Cai. 2000 May;23(5):295-298. Chinese.

39. Deng HB, Cui DP, Jiang JM, Feng YC, Cai NS, Li DD. Inhibiting effects of Achyranthes bidentata polysaccharide and Lycium barbarum polysaccharide on nonenzyme glycation in D-galactose induced mouse aging model. Biomed Environ Sci.

2003 Sep;16(3):267-275.

40. Qi B, Ji Q, Wen Y, Liu L, Guo X, Hou G, Wang G, Zhong J. Lycium barbarum polysaccharides protect human lens epithelial cells against oxidative stress-induced apoptosis and senescence. PLoS One. 2014 Oct 15;9(10):e110275.

41. Peng XM, Wang ZF, Tian GY. [Physico-chemical properties and activity of glycoconjugate LbGp2 from Lycium barbarum L]. Yao Xue Bao. 2001 Aug;36(8):599-602. Chinese.

42. Du G, Liu L, Fang J. Experimental study on the enhancement of murine splenic lymphocyte proliferation by Lycium barbarum glycopeptide. J Huazhong Univ Sci Technolog Med Sci. 2004;24(5):518-20, 527.

43. Zhang Q, Lv X, Wu T, Ma Q, Teng A, Zhang Y, Zhang M. Composition of Lycium barbarum polysaccharides and their apoptosis-inducing effect on human hepatoma SMMC-7721 cells. Food Nutr Res. 2015 Nov 11;59:28696.

44. Gan L, Hua Zhang S, Liang Yang X, Bi Xu H. Immunomodulation and antitumor activity by a polysaccharide-protein complex from Lycium barbarum. Int Immunopharmacol. 2004 Apr;4(4):563-569.

45. Liu RH. Health benefits of fruit and vegetables are from additive and synergistic combinations of phytochemicals. Am J Clin Nutr. 2003 Sep;78(3 Suppl):517S-520S.

46. Data from dried fruit stored 1-3 years. Analysis performed by Brunswick Laboratories, Wareham, MA.

47. Li G, Yang J, Ren B, Wang Z. [Effect of Lycium barbarum L on defending free radicals of mice caused by hypoxia]. Wei Sheng Yan Jiu. 2002 Feb;31(1):30-31. Chinese.

48. Wu BY, Zou JH, Meng SC. [Effect of wolfberry fruit and epimedium on DNA synthesis of the aging-youth 2BS fusion cells]. Zhongguo Zhong Xi Yi Jie He Za Zhi. 2003 Dec;23(12):926-928. Chinese.

49. Wang Y, Zhao H, Sheng X, Gambino PE, Costello B, Bojanowski K. Protective effect of Fructus lycii polysaccharides against time and hyperthermia-induced damage in cultured seminiferous epithelium. J Ethnopharmacol. 2002 Oct;82(2-3):169-175.

50. Krtolica A, Parrinello S, Lockett S, Desprez PY, Campisi J. Senescent fibroblasts promote epithelial cell growth and tumorgenesis: a link between cancer and aging. Proc Natl Acad Sci U S A. 2001 Oct;98(21):12072-12077.

51. Talmadge J, Meyers KM, Prieur DJ, Starkey JR. Role of NK cells in tumour growth and metastasis in beige mice. Nature. 1980 Apr;284(5757):622-624.

52. Wu J, Lanier LL. Natural killer cells and cancer. Adv Cancer Res. 2003;90:127-156.

53. Herberman RB, Ortaldo JR. Natural killer cells: their roles in defenses against disease. Science. 1981 Oct;214(4516):24-30.

54. Levy SM, Herberman RB, Maluish AM, Schlien B, Lippman M. Prognostic risk assessment in primary breast cancer by behavioral and immunological parameters. Health Psychol. 1985;4(2):99-113.

55. Schantz SP, Brown BW, Lira E, Taylor DL, Beddingfield N. Evidence for the role of natural immunity in the control of metastatic spread of head and neck cancer. Cancer Immunol Immunother. 1987;25(2):141-148.

56. Gaspani L, Bianchi M, Limiroli E, Panerai AE, Sacerdote P. The analgesic drug tramadol prevents the effect of surgery on natural killer cell activity and metastatic colonization in rats. J Neuroimmunol. 2002 Aug;129(1-2):18-24.

57. Gorelik E, Wiltrout RH, Okumura K, Habu S, Herberman RB. Role of NK cells in the control of metastatic spread and growth of tumor cells in mice. Int J Cancer. 1982 Jul 15;30(1):107-112.

58. Tartter PI, Steinberg B, Barron DM, Martinelli G. The prognostic significance of natural killer cytotoxicity in patients with colorectal cancer. Arch Surg. 1987 Nov;122(11):1264-1268.

59. Kondo E, Koda K, Takiguchi N, Oda K, Seike K, Ishizuka M, Miyazaki M. Preoperative natural killer cell activity as a prognostic factor for distant metastasis following surgery for colon cancer. Dig Surg. 2003;20(5):445-451.

60. Li Xueru, et al. Clinical Experiment on Lycium. Bulletin on Achievements in Scientific and Technological Research, Serial 84, No. 4, 1988.

61. Wu SJ, Ng LT, Lin CC. Antioxidant activities of some common ingredients of traditional Chinese medicine, Angelica sinensis, Lycium barbarum and Poria cocos. Phytother Res. 2004 Dec;18(12):1008-1012.

Understanding Hormone Health

Hormones are critical to maintaining vibrant health because they regulate numerous activities in the body. The pituitary gland sends hormone messages to your other glands and other areas of the body to signal them into action. Hormones help control blood pressure, fight against eye degeneration, and work to overcome or reduce various cancers.

Estrogen and progesterone need to be balanced to work together as counterparts. Together, they are responsible for balance in blood clotting and the storage or use of fat in the body. But the estrogen and progesterone balance can be upset, disrupting a positive attitude and normal feelings of well-being. Xenoestrogens (literally, "foreign" estrogens) are chemically manufactured hormones that are used in pesticides and animal growth hormones. They are increasingly found in food and cause an overbalance of estrogen in the body with many adverse effects.

Progesterone and testosterone increase physical desire. Testosterone helps build muscle and decrease fat, while both estrogen and testosterone convert the bad cholesterol (LDL) to good cholesterol (HDL). Hormones help with good brain function in maintaining optimal body functions, and most important, they work to help keep us young.

Hormonal Testing

Before starting any type of natural progesterone, pregnenolone, or DHEA program that targets the hormone system of the body, it is important to have your hormone levels tested by requesting a blood hormone panel taken in your doctor's office, hospital, clinic, or qualified laboratory. After the analysis is evaluated by your doctor or health care professional, you may ask for his or her help in determining the best program for you.

In order to have the most accurate type of testing, you have to be prepared to spend some money, and perhaps more than you were planning to spend; however, because of the complexity of hormone therapy, any deficiencies must be correctly identified before supplementation begins.

A good hormone panel will cost between $350 and $450, as costs will vary from clinic to clinic. It is also much better to ask for a specialist, not just a general practitioner, who might tell you that your hormones are just fine for your age. Unfortunately, most health care practitioners know very little about hormone analysis, ranges, subsequent causes and effects, and solutions. To be able to determine your needs, you should have your hormone panel taken every week for four weeks to cover the complete cycle, thereby giving you the best results. Otherwise, you may have a single panel taken at the time when your estrogen is high and be told all is well, even when you may think and feel differently.

Other types of analyses—such as saliva testing or hair analysis—are available that determine hormone levels, but they are unreliable and are not recommended. Naturopath D. Gary Young found, in 25 years of research, that hormones and enzymes are two of the most critical needs of the human body and are among the least understood. Bringing balance takes a lot more than just taking natural progesterone.

The body ages faster when we do not eat live foods that are rich in natural enzymes and hormones. Our world today is a world of processed and prepackaged foods treated with all kinds of chemicals, sugars, and salts. Fruits and vegetables are sprayed with pesticides, insecticides, herbicides, and other growth and beautifying chemicals for our consumption. Animals are given synthetic growth hormones, which displace women's natural hormones. Our air is polluted and the water we drink is often contaminated or treated with chemicals for purification. Then we wonder why hormones start to decline at age 25, and strange, unexpected maladies start to show up in children and young adults. More men and women are becoming victims of sterility as young as 20 years of age. In addition, never in history have we seen young women between the ages of 25 and 30 experiencing bone density loss, which leads them into osteoporosis.

Why is this happening? Why are there more cancers, more cases of heart disease, diabetes, respiratory failure, viruses, mutations of bacteria, and fungus? Why is there such increased disease and body dysfunction, not only in older people but in children and young adults as well? Why are so many babies being born with birth defects and diseases that seem unexplainable?

Lack of proper nutrients, hormone imbalance, and insufficient enzymes are key factors in the cause of overall diminishing health leading to a state of disease and malfunction of the body. Balancing hormones is one of the secrets to maintaining good health, and without proper enzymes, no hormone therapy program will be as effective as it could be for either women or men.

Natural estrogens are called steroid hormones and passively enter into the cells, where they bind to and activate the estrogen receptors. It is important to understand that there are different types of estrogens—three major hormones that the body naturally produces in women: estrone (E1), which is produced during menopause; estradiol (E2), which is predominant in nonpregnant females; and estriol (E3), which is predominant in pregnancy. All three are produced from androgens through enzymatic activity, which produces testosterone. The conversion of testosterone to estradiol and androstenedione to estrone is performed by the enzyme aromatase.

More than 50 percent of the body's estrogen is in the form of estrone, which is manufactured and stored as estrone sulphate in the fat cells and ovaries so that the body can call for it when needed, so it can be converted as the body dictates. However, estrone sulphate is a chemical compound that attracts breast cancer cells when too much is produced.

Oncologists for years have warned about estrogen therapy and its tendency to cause cancer, for which reason they tell women to stay away from products containing estrogen or products that stimulate estrogen production. Unfortunately, doctors do not tell you that there are two forms of estrone, which are good or bad depending on the biological activity, or potency, of the estrogen. Estrogens are important in many cellular activities, including growth, strength, mental clarity, etc. in various target cells. This is normal and beneficial, but too much estrogenic stimulation can have a negative effect. Therefore, proper metabolism and excretion of estrogens is crucial.

Estradiol converts to either 2-hydroxyestrone, a good estrone metabolite that prevents cancer, or 16-alpha-hydroxyestrone, a bad one that feeds cancer cells. If these estrogens are metabolized into the 2-hydroxylated estrone and estradiol, they lose much of their estrogenic activity and cell proliferation and are termed "good" estrogen metabolites. Studies show that when the production of 2-hydroxyestrone increases, the body resists cancer; and when 2-hydroxyestrone decreases, cancer risk increases.[1]

Research indicates that women who metabolize more estrogens down the C-16 pathway, as opposed to the C-2 pathway, have elevated breast cancer risk.[2]

Follow four simple rules to maintain good hormone production:

1. Keep the liver clean.
2. Consume enzyme-rich foods or add good quality, active, complex enzymes such as Essentialzyme and Essentialzymes-4 to give your digestive system a natural boost. Children who start early by consuming the supplement MightyZyme will have a head start on maintaining hormone balance and healthy body function as they grow older.
3. Eat a fiber-rich diet supplemented with ICP and JuvaPower.
4. Avoid processed foods, foods grown with chemicals, body and hair care products formulated with damaging chemicals, and the use of synthetic chemicals in all forms.

Declining Hormones Signal Old Age

As we age, hormone imbalances can contribute to accelerated aging and heightened risk of cancer and other chronic diseases. Hormone replacement therapy using natural hormones (not synthetic compounds or look-alikes) in a cream application for transdermal absorption is one of the most common ways to address hormone imbalances. Natural hormone therapy is often very beneficial for combating a number of health problems such as sleep disturbance, depression, anxiety, and obesity, as well as reducing the risk of cancer and helping to fight chronic diseases such as osteoporosis.

In the specific case of progesterone, Harvard University researcher John R. Lee, MD, found that natural progesterone is very well absorbed through the skin 20 to 40 times more efficiently than if taken by mouth.[3] Topical hormone creams with essential oils have a greater ability to penetrate through the skin and enter into the blood much more quickly than other hormone creams that do not have essential oils.

The 16-alpha-hydroxyestrone, or bad estrone, is deemed carcinogenic and increases the risk with estrogen-sensitive cancers. All inorganic estrogen compounds will manufacture 16-alpha-hydroxyestrone.

Natural, organic compounds will metabolize to 2-hydroxyestrone, or good anticancer estrone, unless the liver is toxic and/or enzyme deficient.

Hormones such as DHEA, melatonin, testosterone, and progesterone decrease with age. Estrogen (estradiol) also drops with age, although not as quickly as progesterone; but as progesterone drops, an estrogen-dominant condition is created that is common in women over 40.

Melatonin: The Hormone of Dark

Melatonin is a natural hormone that regulates sleep. During daylight, the pineal gland in the brain produces an important neurotransmitter called serotonin. A neurotransmitter is a chemical that relays messages between nerve cells.

At night, however, the pineal gland stops producing serotonin and instead makes melatonin, which, when released, causes drowsiness and lowers body temperature, inducing sleep. Your body produces melatonin when it's dark. The darker your sleeping environment, the more melatonin your body will produce. If you happen to sleep with a night light on, your body will produce less melatonin, which might account for why some people have difficulty falling asleep.

Children sleep far better in a completely dark room than with a light on somewhere to help them find the bathroom in the middle of the night or to ease their fears about the dark or being alone. With good melatonin production, children and adults alike will awake in the morning refreshed and positive for a new day.

Melatonin's benefits extend beyond sleep health, though. Sufficient melatonin helps to reduce irritable bowel syndrome, anxiety, elevated blood pressure at night, and cluster headaches. Melatonin supplements appear to be helpful for people whose natural sleep cycle has been disturbed, such as travelers suffering from jet lag.

It has been suggested that melatonin might work through the nervous system to help in the digestive tract. A preliminary, double-blind study suggests that melatonin may decrease nocturnal seizure frequency for children with epilepsy, perhaps by improving sleep and reducing the side effects of medication.4 One double-blind study suggests that topical application of melatonin may increase hair growth in women with thinning hair, for undiscovered reasons.5 Additional research helps us to further understand the influence of melatonin on hair physiology.6,7 Melatonin might also be helpful to individuals trying to quit using sleeping pills.

Melatonin has been used with conventional cancer therapy in more than a dozen clinical studies. Preliminary results have been surprisingly good. A double-blind study was conducted on 30 people with advanced brain tumors who had received standard radiation treatment. It was suggested that melatonin might prolong life and also improve the quality of life. These 30 participants were divided into two groups. One group received 20 mg daily of melatonin, and the other did not. After one year, 6 of 14 individuals in the melatonin group were still alive, but just 1 of 16 from the control group was alive.8 The melatonin group also had fewer side effects from the radiation treatment—a notable improvement in their quality of life.9

Melatonin also works as a very powerful antioxidant at night while we are sleeping. It crosses through cell membranes and the blood-brain barrier working as a free radical scavenger. Interestingly enough, melatonin is sometimes referred to as a "suicidal antioxidant" because of its tremendous free-radical absorbent capacity. When melatonin reacts with free radicals, it oxidizes and cannot convert back to its former state because it forms several stable end products and can no longer function as an antioxidant.

Melatonin has shown remarkable benefits in preventing gallstones by converting cholesterol to bile and increasing the production of aromatase or increasing the mobility of stones and moving them out of the gallbladder. Aromatase is an enzyme found in the adrenal glands, brain, and many other tissues of the body. Its main function is to convert androstenedione to estrone and testosterone to estradiol, which is an important part of sexual development.

Recent research demonstrates the ability of melatonin to prevent DNA damage by some carcinogens and stops the mechanism by which cancer begins.10 Melatonin appears to work by increasing levels of the body's own tumor-fighting proteins, which are known as cytokines.

Recent research shows that melatonin enhances the effectiveness of standard therapy for breast cancer, prostate cancers, and glioblastoma multiforme (GBM), which is the most common and aggressive type of primary brain tumor in humans.11 Although it is the most prevalent, GBMs occur in only 2-3 cases per 100,000 people in Europe and North America. Glioblastomas are a common type of brain tumor of the canine species, and research is ongoing to use this as a model for developing treatments in humans. Melatonin definitely shows possible benefits not only for humans but for animals as well in the fight against this terrible affliction.

Melatonin is helpful in regulating metabolism and increasing thermogenesis, as well as in increasing energy during the wake cycle, which could explain the weight loss in several case studies. Research has greatly increased since 2008 and will continue to help discover more benefits for the human body with this special hormone.

At one time, it was thought that melatonin levels declined with age; however, newer evidence suggests that melatonin levels do not decline with age after all. A decline of melatonin is most likely caused by foods devoid of sufficient nutrients and enzymes.

Low melatonin levels seem to be directly linked to lowered immunity, resulting in disturbed sleep cycles, anxiousness, heightened cancer risk, etc. Some evidence suggests that individuals with cluster headaches have lower-than-average levels of the hormone melatonin. The discussion is still ongoing.

DHEA: Vibrant Health

The most common hormone in the body is 5-Dehydroepiandrosterone (5-DHEA). It is the most abundantly circulating natural steroid hormone produced in the bodies of both men and women because it is the precursor to over 50 other hormones in the body. It is manufactured by enzymes from cholesterol and secreted by the adrenal glands, the gonads, adipose tissue, and the brain.

DHEA is converted by enzymes to pregnenolone and then to 17O-Hydroxypregnenolone, which helps regulate steroid hormones and directs them down their final metabolic pathway for further conversion to proper male and female hormones for normal body function.

DHEA has a broad range of biological effects in humans and other mammals. It acts on the androgen receptor both directly and through its metabolites, which include androstenediol and androstenedione, which further convert to the production of the male sex hormone androgen, which converts to testosterone and the female estrogens to estrone and estradiol.

Although DHEA is manufactured naturally in the body, it is also produced as a supplement, which can be made in a laboratory from a substance called diosgenin, found in soybeans and wild yam. Wild yam cream and supplements are a natural source of DHEA, but the body cannot convert wild yam to DHEA on its own. The conversion must be done in a laboratory.

Dehydroepiandrosterone sulfate (DHEAS) is the sulfate version of DHEA, which is primarily converted in the adrenals, liver, and small intestine. In the blood, most DHEA is found as DHEAS, with levels that are about 300 times higher than those of free DHEA. Orally ingested DHEA is converted to its sulfate form when passing through intestines and liver. DHEA levels naturally reach their peak in the early morning hours, but DHEAS levels show no variation throughout the day. DHEAS may be viewed as a storage reservoir for the body to produce sex hormones on demand when needed to maintain normal body functions.

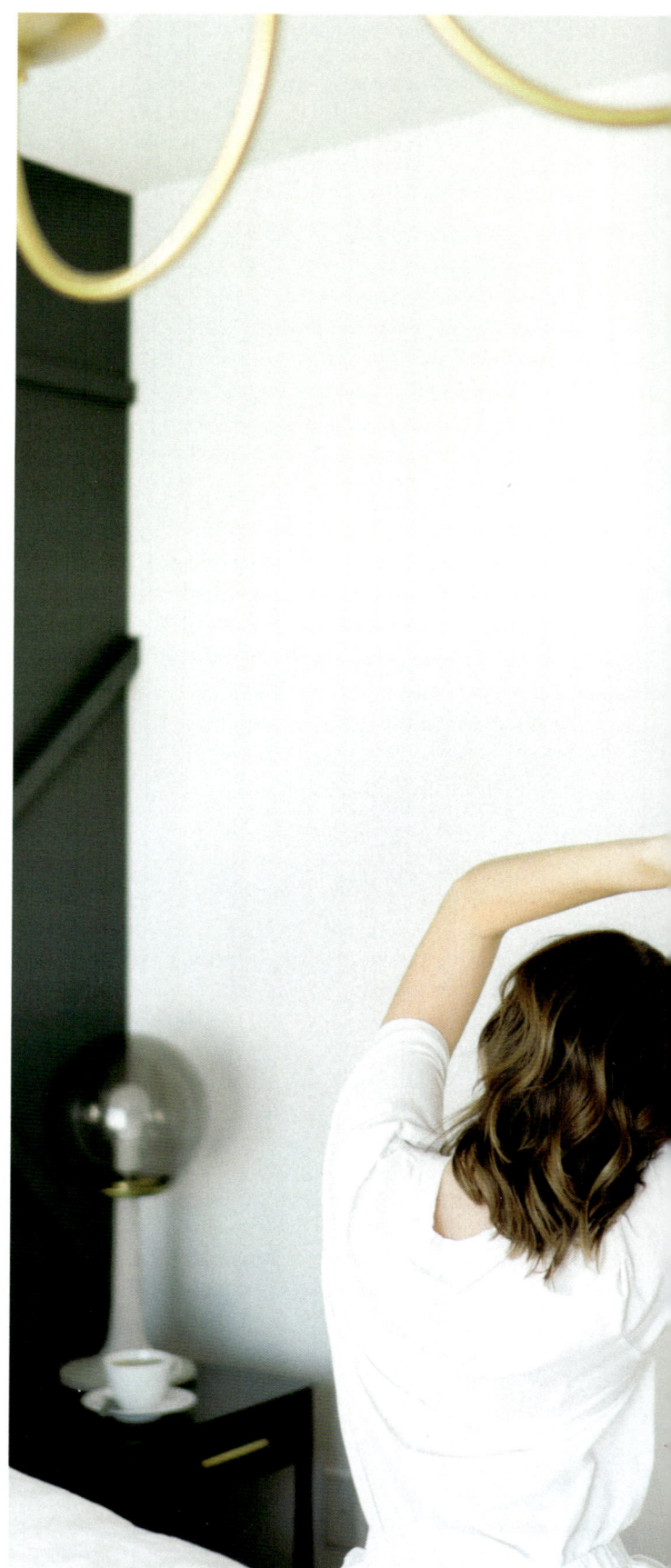

A decline in DHEA is directly correlated with obesity and lower energy. The greater the production and proper balance with DHEA, the better the sex life, energy, weight balance, normal sleep patterns, and feelings of well-being an individual enjoys. DHEA also strengthens the neurons in the brain for better memory retention with sharp, clear thinking.

Another benefit of DHEA is that it keeps cortisol levels in balance, which helps the immune system operate at an optimal level. This in turn helps to reduce the risk of Alzheimer's disease and premature aging, which are always associated with bone density loss.

DHEA produces hormones responsible for burning fat and converting fat to muscle. Instead of losing weight because of muscle breakdown and fluid loss, it actually helps build lean muscle tissue. It appears that DHEA blocks G6PD (glucose-6-phosphate-dehyrogenase), the major enzyme that produces fat tissue and cancer cells. G6PD redirects excess glucose from anabolic (growth) fat production into catabolic (breakdown) energy metabolism. This would seem to make man dependent upon diet for weight control.

The following shows the chain of conversion from cholesterol to estrogen.

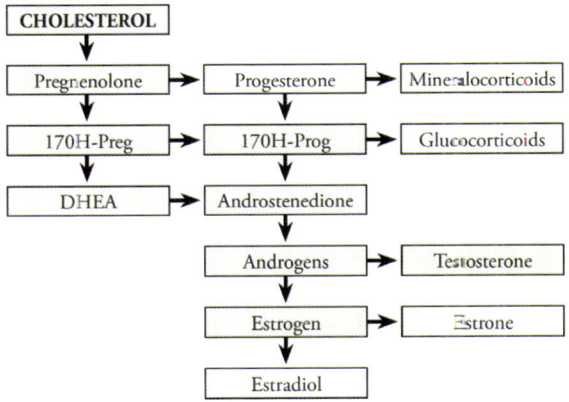

DHEA seems to have many benefits to the well-being of the mind and body. It seems to have a positive effect on the mind, helping memory, decreasing mood swings, and protecting against degenerative diseases such as Alzheimer's, various cancers, immune dysfunction, heart disease, blood platelet abnormality, weight gain, and more. This is a hormone that is well worth studying, as its value to the human body seems immense. There is much yet for research to discover and science to substantiate.

Cortisol: The Death Hormone

Cortisol helps you handle ongoing and difficult stress situations. When stress levels continue, cortisol levels go up, which can lead to adrenal fatigue and burnout. Cortisol is important for normal functioning of the brain, immune system, muscle tone and strength, blood circulation, and sugar levels.

Although cortisol is a valuable hormone, levels that are too high or too low can be dangerous and even fatal. Cortisol is known not only as the "death hormone" but also as the "stress hormone" and the "fight-or-flight hormone." Cortisol seems to increase with age, contributing to a number of problems such as high blood pressure, obesity, and blood sugar imbalances. Lowering cortisol levels not only decreases immunity but also increases insulin sensitivity and enhances fat metabolism.

Cortisol is manufactured in the adrenal glands and secreted through the adrenal cortex when the body reacts to stress, triggering an immunological response to heighten the survival instincts. It gives us that burst of energy in the morning when we need to "jump start" the heart after a night of sleep-inducing melatonin. Cortisol also reduces sensitivity to pain, suppresses the immune system by stopping overproduction of white blood cells, aids in the breakdown of fat and protein to help metabolize and convert glucose in the liver to increase blood sugar, and stops the release of inflammatory substances in the body.

However, low cortisol levels can be risky and, therefore, need to be understood. Adrenal exhaustion can lead to dangerously low levels of cortisol that could bring on cardiac arrest or failure to wake up the heart in the morning. Keeping cortisol levels in balance is critical to life. High cortisol can lead to rapid weight gain and obesity. Low cortisol can cause chronic fatigue, low sex drive, and depression. It can also decrease thyroid function, which results in mental fatigue, digestive problems, lowered immune resistance, increased blood pressure, and muscle wasting. Cortisol increases because of stress and excessive acid in the body. Coffee and other caffeine-containing drinks stimulate the production of cortisol.

A major key to healthy levels of cortisol is to keep the hormone system balanced. Higher levels of DHEA will lower cortisol levels as well as many other aspects of body functions. However, the foundation for a healthy body and balanced hormones is to eat live, unprocessed, nutritious foods; get enough rest and exercise; and maintain a balanced lifestyle that supports the needs of work, home, and family.

If your cortisol is too high or you are just concerned about having good balance, then the product CortiStop would be a supplement to add to your daily regimen.

DANGERS OF SYNTHETIC HORMONES

Recent research has discredited many of the supposed benefits of synthetic hormones, such as those made with horse urine, estrogens, medroxyprogesterone acetate, and other synthetic progestins. These patented synthetic hormones are very different biochemically from the natural hormones found in plants and human bodies, and their effects can be hazardous to health. Long-term use of these synthetic hormones has been linked with dramatically higher risks of heart disease, stroke, ovarian cancer, breast cancer, and osteoporosis.

Natural hormones cannot be patented, which makes them unpopular with companies making synthetic products. Natural hormones found in the human body are some of the safest natural compounds used to prevent heart disease and cancer. It is interesting that when a woman reaches the later stage of pregnancy, her levels of progesterone rise to over 300 times that of normal, and both mother and child thrive. Obviously, the body knows what it needs, and the body's production of natural progesterone is totally safe and healthy. When the body receives the right tools, or natural substances, it usually knows what to do.

Osteoporosis and Prostate Cancer

Natural progesterone has been used to successfully treat osteoporosis, heart disease, and breast cancer in women. Research by John R. Lee, MD, has shown that progesterone can be used to effectively treat prostate cancer and Benign Prostate Hyperplasia (BPH) in men.[12]

Lowering Cancer Risk Naturally

As women grow older and approach menopause, between the ages of 40 and 50, they become increasingly susceptible to estrogen dominance, due to an increased frequency of ovulation and dramatically lowered production of progesterone. This shortage of progesterone can lead to osteoporosis, mood swings, depression, weight gain, and increased risk of breast, endometrial, cervical, and uterine cancers.

Premenopausal women can also suffer from an estrogen deficiency, which can markedly increase their risk of heart disease. This is one reason why heart disease in women reaches the equivalent of men after age 40. A simultaneous estrogen and progesterone deficiency is one of the most common and insidious conditions afflicting women over age 40 and can result in significant detrimental effects on both physical and mental health.

Transdermal hormone creams have revolutionized the way women can manage hormone control. Because natural progesterone, pregnenolone, and DHEA are readily absorbed through the skin and into the tissues, they are rapidly becoming the standard for convenient and economical hormone replacement therapy in the United States. Many transdermal hormone creams are available to balance progesterone, estrogen, and DHEA deficiencies in women. Women who are primarily progesterone deficient and estrogen dominant need progesterone support, and women who are deficient in both estrogen and progesterone need both pregnenolone and progesterone hormones. The body will convert pregnenolone into the amount of estrogen the body needs.

Andropause: Menopause in Men

A cream containing DHEA and pregnenolone is a first line of defense for men with declining testosterone and DHEA. Men over 40 often begin to see various symptoms manifest that could indicate the beginning of a possible hormone imbalance. Symptoms such as those listed would suggest further investigation and the beginning of a preventative program before conditions worsen:

- Loss of sexual desire
- Less strength and shrinking muscles
- Reduced energy
- Depression
- Increased anxiety
- Thinning hair
- Wrinkles and aging
- Prostate problems: restricted urine flow, declining sexual performance, etc.

Essential Oils: Enhanced Hormone Penetration of the Skin

A number of clinical studies have shown that essential oils greatly enhance the ability of hormones and other medical products to penetrate the skin and enter the blood stream. Studies conducted at Pisa University in 2002 found that essential oils such as cajuput, cardamom, melissa, myrtle, niaouli, and orange, containing essential oil chemical constituents such as 1,8-cineole, alpha-pinene, alpha-terpineol, and d-limonene, boosted estradiol hormone penetration through the skin and into the blood and body tissues.[13] A study at the China Pharmaceutical University in Nanjing also found a dramatic increase in drug absorption using formulations with eucalyptus and peppermint essential oils.[14]

PRODUCTS FOR HORMONE SUPPORT

CAUTIONS

Note which cautions are applicable to which oil under each oil's listing. Not all cautions apply to all oils.

 Keep out of reach of children.

 For external use only.

 Avoid contact with eyes and mucous membranes.

 If you are pregnant, nursing, taking medication, or have a medical condition, consult a health professional prior to use.

 Flammable. Keep away from fire, heat, or sparks. Do not store above room temperature.

 PH = Photosensitizing. Avoid direct sunlight or UV rays (e.g., sunlamps, tanning beds, etc.) for up to 12 hours after applying oil. Sunlight should be avoided for 24 hours after applying some oils, shown as (24).

 May stain some surfaces, skin, or clothing.

 Some oils might cause a stinging, burning sensation, rash, redness, pain, blisters, inflammation, swelling, itching, or darkening of the skin. Test for sensitivity on a small area of skin on the underside of your arm and apply as needed.

These statements have not been evaluated by the Food and Drug Administration. These products are not intended to diagnose, treat, cure, or prevent any disease. Consult individual product labels for safety information.

Bolded ingredients are essential oils.

All Young Living Vitality™ essential oils are Non-GMO Project Verified! To receive this certification, all Vitality oils passed through third-party verification, auditing, and testing.

CortiStop®

This capsule contains natural progesterone and hormone precursors, which help support the female glandular system and balance cortisol production in the body.

Ingredients: CortiStop Blend: [Pregnenolone, L-a-phosphatidylserine, L-a-phosphatidylcholine, Black cohosh root extract], DHEA (derived from wild yam root), **Clary Sage flowering top oil, Canadian Fleabane flowering top oil, Fennel seed oil, Frankincense gum/resin oil, Peppermint aerial parts oil**, Rice flour, Silica, Gelatin

Essential Oils: Clary Sage, Canadian Fleabane, Fennel, Frankincense, Peppermint

Directions: Take 2 capsules in the morning before breakfast. If desired, take another 2 capsules before bedtime. Use daily for 8 weeks. Discontinue use for 2-4 weeks before resuming.

Cautions: For adult use only.

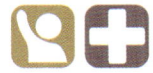

EndoGize™

This daily supplement was formulated to support and maintain a healthy and balanced endocrine system. Women can benefit greatly with strong support to the hormone activity of the body.

Ingredients: Vitamin B6 (as pyridoxine HCl); Zinc (as z. aspartate), EndoGize Blend: [Ashwagandha root powder, Muira puama bark, L-arginine, Epimedium aerial parts, Tribulus terrestris fruit extract, Phosphatidylcholine, Lecithin (soy), DHEA, Black pepper fruit extract, Glucoamylase, Acid Stable Protease, Longjack root extract, Amylase, Cellulase], **EndoGize Oil Blend: [Ginger root oil, Myrrh gum/resin oil, Cassia branch/leaf oil, Clary Sage flowering top oil, Canadian Fleabane flowering top oil]**, Rice flour, Gelatin

Essential Oils: Ginger, Myrrh, Cassia, Clary Sage, Canadian Fleabane

Directions: Take 1 capsule 2 times daily for 4 weeks. Discontinue for 2 weeks before resuming.

Cautions: For adult use only. Do not use if you are pregnant or lactating.

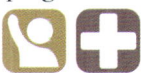

Allergen Warning: Contains soy.

FemiGen™

A good product to support a woman's reproductive system is always helpful in maintaining balance as a woman transitions into menopause.

Ingredients: Magnesium, FemiGen Blend: [Damiana leaf, Epimedium aerial plant, Wild yam root, Dong quai root, Muira puama root, American ginseng root, Licorice root extract, Black cohosh root, L-carnitine, Dimethylglycine HCl, Cramp bark, Squaw vine aerial parts, L-phenylalanine, L-cystine, L-cysteine HCl, Fennel seed oil, Clary Sage flowering top oil, Sage leaf oil, Ylang Ylang flower oil], Gelatin, Silica

Essential Oils: Fennel, Clary Sage, Sage, Ylang Ylang

Directions: Take 2 capsules with breakfast and 2 capsules with midday meal.

Cautions: Accidental overdose of iron-containing products is a leading cause of fatal poisoning in children under 6. Keep this product out of reach of children. In case of accidental overdose, call a doctor or poison control center immediately.

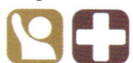

ImmuPro™

This tasty tablet boosts melatonin and T-lymphocyte immune cells. It is designed for people who have difficulty sleeping, shortened sleep cycles, low immunity, or high risk of cancer. It is a powerful antioxidant that provides energy and immune support. It is also helpful for children who are restless at night and have trouble getting to sleep. Chewing one-half of a tablet is often sufficient for children.

Ingredients: Calcium (as c. carbonate), Zinc (as z. citrate), Selenium (as selenium glycinate chelate), Copper (as c. bisglycinate chelate), ImmuPro Blend: [Strawberry fruit powder, Wolfberry fruit polysaccharides, Raspberry fruit powder, Reishi whole mushroom powder, Maitake mushroom mycelia powder, Arabinogalactan (from larch tree wood extract), Mushroom mycelia powder, Orange peel oil], Melatonin, Dextrose, Hydroxypropyl cellulose, Stevia, Silicon dioxide, Magnesium stearate, Maltodextrin (non-GMO)

Essential Oil: Orange

Directions: Take 1-2 chewable tablets daily as needed, at bedtime. Do not exceed 2 tablets per day.

Cautions: Consult a health care professional prior to use with children. ImmuPro contains melatonin, which may cause drowsiness. Do not drive or operate machinery when taking melatonin.

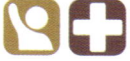

PD 80/20™

Easy to take in a capsule, this product is designed to give natural, overall hormone support.

Ingredients: Pregnenolone, DHEA, Rice flour, Gelatin

Directions: Take 1 capsule daily.

Cautions: Not for use by individuals under the age of 18 years. Consult a physician or licensed qualified health care professional before using this product if you have, or have a family history of, breast cancer, prostate cancer, prostate enlargement, heart disease, low "good" cholesterol (HDL), a medical condition, or if you are using any other dietary supplement, prescription drug, or over-the-counter drug. Do not exceed recommended serving. Exceeding recommended serving may cause serious adverse health effects. Possible side effects include acne, hair loss, hair growth on the face (in women), aggressiveness, irritability, and increased levels of estrogen. Discontinue use and call a physician or licensed qualified health care professional immediately if you experience rapid heartbeat, dizziness, blurred vision, or other similar symptoms.

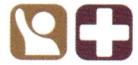

Prenolone® Plus Body Cream

This triple hormone cream contains pure pregnenolone derived from soy and DHEA derived from wild yam. Pregnenolone is the precursor hormone from which the body creates all other sex and adrenal hormones, including progesterone, estradiol, estrone, estriol, testosterone, DHEA, and aldosterone. Soy-derived progesterone works the same way as progesterone naturally produced in the human body and is easily absorbed and used by the body.

This cream is a broad-spectrum hormone supplement that helps boost levels of estrogen and progesterone in both men and women. It is formulated to help with symptoms of estrogen dominance, which include osteoporosis, depression, bloating, mood swings, weight gain, PMS, hot flashes, menstrual irregularity, cramps, increased risk of breast and endometrial cancer, and heart disease.

Studies have shown that topical application of progesterone creams has far better results than hormones taken orally.3 Essential oils also increase the absorption of hormones through the skin into the blood stream. John Lee, MD, discusses in detail the benefits of topically applied progesterone in his book What Your Doctor May Not Tell You About Menopause.

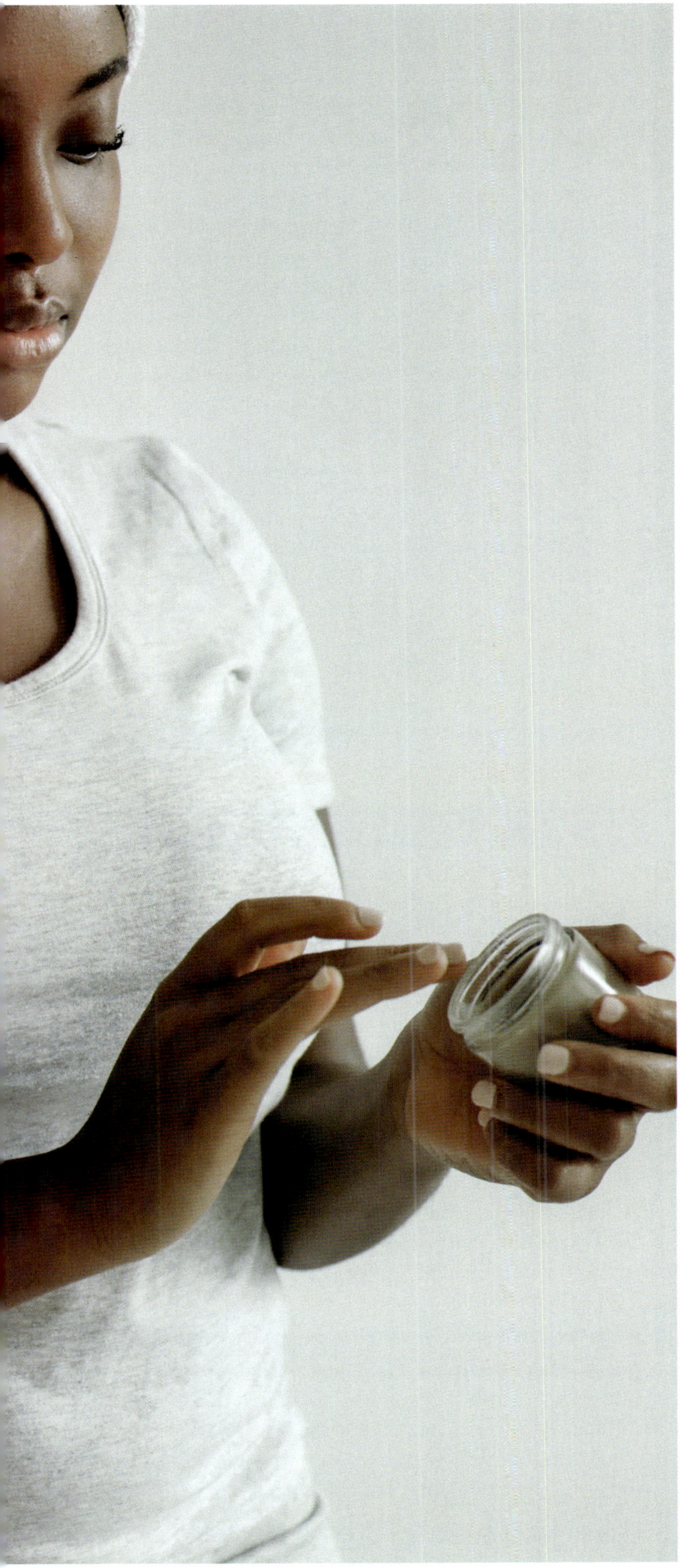

According to Dr. Lee, progesterone can actually reverse bone loss in older women as well as reduce the need for hormone replacement in women lacking ovaries or not ovulating.12

Ingredients: Water, Dimethyl sulfone (MSM), Caprylic/capric triglyceride, Sorbitol, Lecithin, Pregnenolone, acetate, Shea butter, Wolfberry seed oil, Glyceryl stearate, Aloe vera leaf juice, Sodium PCA, Stearic Acid, English marigold flower extract, Roman chamomile flower extract, Rosebud flower extract, Green tea leaf extract, St. John's wort extract, Gingko biloba leaf extract, Grape seed extract, Algae extract, Prasterone (DHEA), Tocopheryl acetate, Hydrolyzed wheat protein, Locust bean gum, Sea salt, Flax seed oil, Wheat germ oil, Ylang Ylang flower oil, Allantoin, Wild yam root extract, Eleuthero root extra, Clary Sage oil, Kelp extract, Retinyl palmitate, Tocopheryl linoleate, Black cohosh root, Blue cohosh root, Geranium flower oil, Bergamot peel oil, Fennel seed oil, Sage oil, Blue Yarrow oil, Ascorbic acid

Essential Oils: Ylang Ylang, Clary Sage, Geranium, Bergamot, Fennel, Sage, Blue Yarrow

Directions: Begin using one day after menstrual cycle ends or as desired. Apply $\frac{1}{4}$-$\frac{1}{2}$ teaspoon 1-2 times daily for 21 consecutive days. Discontinue use for 7 days, then repeat. Massage cream thoroughly into soft tissue areas of the body, such as arms, thighs, abdomen, neck, etc., until absorbed. Individual needs may vary. Apply for three weeks, rest for one week, and then start again.

Cautions: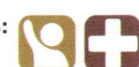

Allergen Warning: Contains wheat.

Progessence® Plus™

With this first-ever pure progesterone serum to enter the market, many women are reporting excellent results in balancing and normalizing hormone levels. As women age, hormone levels drop, causing all kinds of maladies such as sleep and mood disorders and eventually the possibility of more critical ailments. This product was formulated by Dan Purser, MD, and D. Gary Young, ND, to balance and enhance the natural effects of progesterone. Pure, USP-grade, super-micronized progesterone from wild yam is infused into pure, therapeutic-grade essential oils, creating a smooth, revitalizing serum that is easily absorbed into the skin. Another great benefit is that there is no need to change application sites like progesterone creams. The serum is a clear, smooth liquid that easily penetrates the skin. It does not have a cream base.

Ingredients: Balsam Copaiba resin oil, Sacred Frankincense resin/gum oil, Cedarwood bark oil, Caprylic/capric triglyceride, Mixed tocopherols, Bergamot peel oil (Furocoumarin-free), Peppermint leaf oil, USP-grade progesterone (from wild yam extract), Clove bud oil

Essential Oils: Copaiba, Sacred Frankincense, Cedarwood, Bergamot (Furocoumarin-free), Peppermint, Clove

Directions: Apply 2-4 drops to the stomach, feet, or inner thighs each day, rotating application sites to avoid applying to the same area 2 days in a row. For added effect, 1-2 extra drops may be applied. Do not exceed 2 applications per day.

Cautions:

Prostate Health™

Contains high-powered herbal extracts such as saw palmetto that improve prostate function. It slows the body's production of DHT, a hormone that creates abnormal cell proliferation in the prostate. BPH (benign prostate hyperplasia), common in men over age 40, can eventually lead to prostate cancer, one of the most common forms of cancer in the United States. BPH symptoms include incontinence, restricted urine flow, and impotence.

Ingredients: Saw palmetto fruit extract, Pumpkin seed oil, Geranium flower/leaf oil, Fennel seed oil, Lavender flowering top oil, Myrtle leaf oil, Peppermint aerial parts oil, Porcine gelatin, Water, Silica

Essential Oils: Geranium, Fennel, Lavender, Myrtle, Peppermint

Directions: Take 1 softgel capsule 2 times daily.

Cautions:

Regenolone™ Moisturizing Cream

This muscle and joint pain cream is designed for people who suffer severe pain from inflammation or stiffness from arthritis, rheumatism, or other muscle and joint conditions. Formulated with pregnenolone, wolfberry seed oil, progesterone, MSM, plant and herb extracts, and essential oils, this product provides unmatched relief from all types of arthritic, muscle, and skeletal pain.

Ingredients: Water, Dimethyl sulfone (MSM), Caprylic/capric triglyceride, Sorbitol, Lecithin, Pregnenolone acetate, Wintergreen leaf oil, Shea butter, Wolfberry seed oil, Glyceryl stearate, Aloe vera leaf juice, Chamomile flower extract, English marigold flower extract, Green tea leaf extract, Gingko biloba leaf extract, St. John's wort flower/leaf/stem extract, Dog rose flower extract, Sodium PCA, Stearic acid, Grape seed extract, Peppermint leaf oil, Algae extract, Balsam Canada needle oil, Oregano oil, Hydrolyzed wheat protein, Tocopherol acetate, Carob gum, Trace minerals, Linseed seed oil, Wheat germ oil, Allantoin, Wild yam root extract, Eleuthero root extract, Kelp extract, Retinyl palmitate, Tocopherol linoleate, Blue cohosh rhizome/root, Black cohosh root, Ascorbic acid

Essential Oils: Wintergreen, Peppermint, Balsam Canada, Oregano

Directions: Apply a dime-size amount ($1/8$-$1/4$ teaspoon) directly on dry skin as needed 3 times a day to combat pain associated with arthritis, sciatica, back pain, and carpal tunnel syndrome. Do not exceed 5 applications per day.

Cautions:

Allergen Warning: Contains wheat product.

ESSENTIAL OIL HORMONE SUPPORT

Many women over the age of 40 have found that essential oils effectively combat PMS and menopause problems. Oils with estrogen-like activity include Fennel, Anise, Clary Sage, and Sage. These oils may be combined in equal proportions in a double oo size capsule and ingested. Take 2 to 8 capsules daily to raise estrogen levels according to need.

It is recommended that you find an endocrinologist who can monitor your estrogen levels through blood testing every 30 days until you have reached optimal levels. Research conducted at the Young Life Research Clinic in Springville, Utah, showed that ingestion of these oils, up to 8 capsules per day, did not cause any side effects or toxicity in the human body.

ESSENTIAL OIL BLENDS

Dragon Time™ contains natural phytoestrogens, which help to balance emotions, especially during the monthly cycle. It may be used by both young and mature women, depending on desire and need.

Essential Oils: Fennel, Clary, Marjoram, Lavender, Yarrow, Jasmine

Directions: Aromatic: 30. Topical: Dilute 1 drop with 1 drop V-6 or other pure carrier oil and apply to desired area as needed.

Cautions:

Joy™ and Transformation™ are two essential oil blends that are both uplifting and calming at the same time. They may help to replace negative thoughts with positive and motivating thoughts that may help change your general attitude, emotional well-being, and behavior. They are both great for a relaxing massage.

Essential Oils in Joy: Bergamot (Furocoumarin-free), Ylang Ylang, Geranium, Lemon, Coriander, Tangerine, Jasmine, Roman Chamomile, Palmarosa, Rose

Directions: Aromatic: 60. Topical: Apply 2-4 drops directly to desired area. Dilution not required, except for the most sensitive skin. Use as needed.

Cautions:

Essential Oils in Transformation: Lemon, Peppermint, Royal Hawaiian Sandalwood, Clary Sage, Sacred Frankincense, Idaho Blue Spruce, Cardamom, Ocotea, Palo Santo

Directions: Aromatic: 60. Topical: Dilute 1 drop with 1 drop of V-6 or other pure carrier oil and apply to desired areas as needed.

Cautions: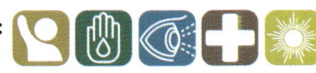

Lady Sclareol™ helps balance emotions, promotes mental clarity, and supports the endocrine system while menstruating.

Essential Oils: Geranium, Coriander, Vetiver, Orange, Clary Sage, Bergamot (Furocoumarin-free), Ylang Ylang, Royal Hawaiian Sandalwood, Spanish Sage, Jasmine, Idaho Blue Spruce, Spearmint

Directions: Aromatic: 60 Topical: Apply 2-4 drops directly on desired area, especially on hips and navel areas. Dilution not required, except for the most sensitive skin.

Cautions:

Mister™ is an essential oil blend for men that helps balance emotions and promotes mental stability during times of stress for men of all ages. This essential oil blend supports the male reproductive system.

Essential Oils: Sage, Fennel, Lavender, Myrtle, Blue Yarrow, Peppermint

Directions: Aromatic: 30. Topical: Apply 2-4 drops to desired area as needed. Use as needed. Dilution not required, except for the most sensitive skin. Dietary: Put 3-10 drops under tongue 2-3 times daily or 10-20 drops in water or in a capsule 2 times daily. Use for 7 days and then rest the body for 4 days. Massage on the Vita Flex points between scrotum and rectum.

Cautions:

SclarEssence™ contains properties that may support the overall emotional health of women, bringing about a peaceful attitude with daily activities and accomplishments.

Essential Oils: Clary Sage, Peppermint, Spanish Sage, Fennel

Directions: Aromatic: 30 Topical: Dilute 1 drop with 1 drop of V-6 or other pure carrier oil and apply to desired area as needed. Dietary: Put 2-3 drops in water and take as needed.

Cautions:

For more information on the many regenerative abilities of pregnenolone, please refer to the publication *Pregnenolone: A Radical New Approach to Health, Long Life, and Emotional Well-Being* by D. Gary Young, ND

ENDNOTES

1. Bradlow H, Telang N, Sepkovic D, Osborne M. 2-hydroxyestrone: the 'good' estrogen. Journal of Endocrinology. 1996 Sept;150 Suppl:259-65.
2. Muti P. Estrogen metabolism and risk of breast cancer: a prospective study of the 2:16α-hydroxyestrone ratio in premenopausal and postmenopausal women. Epidemiology. 2000 Nov;11(6):635-40.
3. Lee J. Topical progesterone. Menopause. 2003 Jul-Aug;10(4):374-79.
4. Fauteck J-D, Schmidt H, Lerchl A, Kurlemann G, Wittkowski W. Melatonin in epilepsy: first results of replacement therapy and first clinical results. Neurosignals. 1999;8(1-2):105-10.
5. Fischer TW, Burmeister G, Schmidt HW, Elsner P. Melatonin increases anagen hair rate in women with androgenetic alopecia or diffuse alopecia: results of a pilot randomized controlled trial. British Journal of Dermatology. 2004;150(2):341-45.
6. Fischer, TW, Slominski A, Tobin DJ, Paus R. Melatonin and the hair follicle. Journal of Pineal Research. 2008 Jan;44(1):1-15.
7. Fischer, TW. The influence of melatonin on hair physiology. Hautarzt. 2009 Dec;60(12):962-72.
8. Lissoni P, Meregalli S, Nosetto L, Barni S, Tancini G, Fossati V, Maestroni G. Increased survival time in brain glioblastomas by a radioneuroendocrine strategy with radiotherapy plus melatonin compared to radiotherapy alone. Oncology. 1996;53(1):43-46.
9. Lissoni P, Brivio F, Fumagalli L, Messina G, Vigoré L, Parolini D, Colciago M, Rovelli F. Neuroimmunomodulation in medical oncology: application of psychoneuroimmunology with subcutaneous low-dose IL-2 and the pineal hormone melatonin in

patients with untreatable metastatic solid tumors. Anticancer Res. 2008 Mar-Apr;28(2B):1377-81.

10. Jung B, Ahmad N. Melatonin in cancer management: progress and promise. Cancer Research. 2006;66(20):9789-793.

11. Sánchez-Hidalgo M, Guerrero M J, Villegas I, Packham G, De La Lastra C. Melatonin, a natural programmed cell death inducer in cancer. Current Medicinal Chemistry. 2012;19(22):3805-821.

12. Lee JR, Hopkins V. What your doctor may not tell you about menopause: the breakthrough book on natural progesterone. New York (NY): Grand Central Publishing; c2004. 534 p.

13. Monti D, Chetoni P, Burgalassi S, Najarro M, Saettone MF, Boldrini E. Effect of different terpene-containing essential oils on permeation of estradiol through hairless mouse skin. International Journal of Pharmaceutics. 2002;237(1-2):209-14.

14. Abdullah D. Enhancing effect of essential oils on the penetration of 5-fluorouracil through rat skin. Yao Xue Bao. 1996;31(3):214-21.

Safe, Natural Products

Being conscious of what you put in your body is very important. However, since your skin is your largest organ, being careful what you put on it is equally important. You will find our personal care products—including shower gels, moisturizers, soaps, oral care, skin care, and deodorant products—free from chemicals, sulfates, toxins, synthetic colorants, dyes, artificial flavors, and preservatives.

You can feel safe using these high quality, essential oil-infused products.

CAUTIONS

Note which cautions are applicable to which oil under each oil's listing. Not all cautions apply to all oils.

 Keep out of reach of children.

 For external use only.

 Avoid contact with eyes and mucous membranes.

 If you are pregnant, nursing, taking medication, or have a medical condition, consult a health professional prior to use.

 Flammable. Keep away from fire, heat, or sparks. Do not store above room temperature.

 PH = Photosensitizing. Avoid direct sunlight or UV rays (e.g., sunlamps, tanning beds, etc.) for up to 12 hours after applying oil. Sunlight should be avoided for 24 hours after applying some oils, shown as (24).

 May stain some surfaces, skin, or clothing.

 Some oils might cause a stinging, burning sensation, rash, redness, pain, blisters, inflammation, swelling, itching, or darkening of the skin. Test for sensitivity on a small area of skin on the underside of your arm and apply as needed.

These statements have not been evaluated by the Food and Drug Administration. These products are not intended to diagnose, treat, cure, or prevent any disease. Consult individual product labels for safety information.

Bolded ingredients are essential oils.

All Young Living Vitality™ essential oils are Non-GMO Project Verified! To receive this certification, all Vitality oils passed through third-party verification, auditing, and testing.

BATH & SHOWER GELS

Bath & Shower Gel Base

Bath & Shower Gel Base is the perfect way to create a customized aromatherapy bath. Add a few drops of a favorite essential oil single or blend for a fragrant and luxurious experience. Bath & Shower Gel Base contains only natural botanical ingredients that are perfect for cleansing the pores.

Ingredients: Water, Decyl glucoside, Coco-betaine, Lauryl glucoside, Coco-glucoside, Glycerin, Glyceryl oleate, Xanthan gum, Inulin, Sodium anisate, Sodium phytate

Directions: Add 5-15 drops of one or more essential oils to 8 ounces of gel base. More than one oil may be added at a time. Mix well. Apply liberally to the body during bath or shower.

Cautions: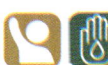

Evening Peace™ Bath & Shower Gel

Evening Peace Bath & Shower Gel refreshes the skin and calms the mind. Designed to relax tired, fatigued muscles and help soothe away stress and tension at the end of the day, this shower gel invokes feelings of serenity and relaxation while nourishing the skin naturally.

Ingredients: Water, Decyl glucoside, Coco-betaine, Lauryl glucoside, Coco-glucoside, Glycerin, Glyceryl oleate, Xanthan gum, Inulin, Sodium levulinate, Citric acid, Sodium anisate, **Ylang Ylang** flower oil, **Royal Hawaiian Sandalwood** wood oil, **Coriander** seed oil, **Bergamot** peel oil (Furocoumarin-free), Sodium phytate, **Blue Tansy** flower oil, **Geranium** flower oil, **Clary Sage** oil, **Lemon** peel oil, **Jasmine** oil, **Roman Chamomile** flower oil, **Palmarosa** oil

Essential Oils: Ylang Ylang, Royal Hawaiian Sandalwood, Coriander, Bergamot (Furocoumarin-free), Blue Tansy, Geranium, Clary Sage, Lemon, Jasmine, Roman Chamomile, Palmarosa

Directions: Apply liberally to the body during bath or shower.

Cautions:

Lavender Bath & Shower Gel

Infused with pure Lavender oil, Lavender Bath & Shower Gel will cleanse and rejuvenate your skin while it soothes and relaxes your mind. It is free of chemicals and synthetic preservatives and contains plant-based ingredients, not animal-derived ingredients.

Ingredients: Water, Sodium chloride, Sodium methyl cocoyl taurate, Sodium lauroamphoacetate, Lauramidopropyl betaine, Hydroxypropyl methylcellulose, Lavender oil, Glycerin, Sodium levulinate, Myristamidopropyl betaine, Citric acid, Potassium sorbate, Sodium astrocaryum murumuruate, Sodium anisate, Lemon peel oil, Sodium phytate, Rosemary leaf oil, Davana flower oil, Myrrh oil, Leuconostoc/radish root ferment filtrate, Disodium EDTA, Alcohol, Magnesium carbonate

Essential Oils: Lavender, Lemon, Rosemary, Davana, Myrrh

Directions: Lather. Wash. Rinse.

Cautions:

Morning Start® Bath & Shower Gel

Morning Start Bath & Shower Gel is an invigorating gel full of naturally cleansing and moisturizing botanicals to jumpstart your day with vigor and energy.

Peppermint, Lemongrass, and Rosemary essential oils uplift and energize the body and mind, while Juniper purifies and cleanses the skin.

Ingredients: Water, Decyl glucoside, Coco-betaine, Lauryl glucoside, Coco-glucoside, Glycerin, Glyceryl oleate, Xanthan gum, Inulin, Sodium levulinate, Lemongrass oil, Citric acid, Sodium anisate, Rosemary leaf oil, Juniper oil, Peppermint oil, Sodium phytate

Essential Oils: Lemongrass, Rosemary, Juniper, Peppermint

Directions: Apply liberally to the body during bath or shower.

Cautions: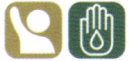

Sensation™ Bath & Shower Gel

Sensation Bath & Shower Gel combines an enchantingly fragrant mix of oils purportedly used by Cleopatra to enhance love and increase desire. Containing the finest natural ingredients, this shower gel nourishes and refreshes the skin.

Ingredients: Water, Decyl glucoside, Coco-betaine, Lauryl glucoside, Coco-glucoside, Glycerin, Glyceryl oleate, Inulin, Xanthan gum, Sodium levulinate, Coriander seed oil, Ylang Ylang flower oil, Citric acid, Sodium anisate, Bergamot peel oil (Furocoumarin-free), Jasmine oil, Sodium phytate, Geranium flower oil

Essential Oils: Coriander, Ylang Ylang, Bergamot (Furocoumarin-free), Jasmine, Geranium

Directions: Lather. Wash. Rinse.

Cautions:

BATH BOMBS

Lavender Calming Bath Bombs

A tranquil bathing experience is yours with Lavender Calming Bath Bombs that soothe with Lavender essential oil and skin-nourishing sweet almond and coconut oils.

Ingredients: Sodium bicarbonate, Citric acid, Sucrose, Lavender oil, Coconut oil, Sweet almond oil, Maltodextrin

Essential Oils: Lavender

Directions: Drop 1 bath bomb into tub filled with warm water, then enjoy a fragrant bathing experience.

Cautions: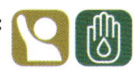

Stress Away™ Relaxing Bath Bombs

With the relaxing and calming effects of Young Living's Stress Away blend, bathing with this skin-softening, relaxing bath bomb is a true spa experience.

Ingredients: Sodium bicarbonate, Citric acid, Sucrose, Coconut oil, Balsam copaiba resin, Sweet almond oil, Lime oil, Cedarwood bark oil, Vanilla fruit extract, Maltodextrin, Ocotea leaf oil, Lavender oil

Essential Oils: Copaiba, Lime, Cedarwood, Ocotea, Lavender

Directions: Drop 1 bath bomb into tub filled with warm water to enjoy a relaxing, calming bath.

Cautions: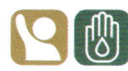

BODY LOTIONS

Coconut-Lime Replenishing Body Butter

This all plant- and oil-based body butter is non-greasy and will moisturize and soothe your skin. The crisp, clean scent of Lime essential oil (among others) will leave you feeling refreshed and invigorated.

Ingredients: Mango seed butter, Sunflower seed oil, Caprylic/capric triglycerides, Cupuacu seed butter, Jojoba seed oil, Rose hips fruit oil, Coconut oil, Aloe vera leaf extract, Rice bran oil, Tocopherol, Lime oil, Lemon Myrtle leaf oil, Orange peel oil, Tangerine peel oil, Grapefruit peel oil, Lemon peel oil, Mandarin peel oil, Spearmint leaf extract

Essential Oils: Lime, Lemon Myrtle, Orange, Tangerine, Grapefruit, Lemon, Mandarin, Spearmint

Directions: Apply liberally all over body, taking extra care on elbows, knees, or other dry spots.

Cautions: Discontinue use if skin irritation occurs.

Allergen Warning: Contains coconut/palm ingredients

Genesis™ Hand & Body Lotion

Genesis Hand & Body Lotion is an ultra-moisturizing cream containing sweet almond oil and other natural botanicals to soothe and nourish dry, dehydrated skin.

Geranium, Jasmine, and other pure essential oils are included for their therapeutic skin care benefits.

Ingredients: Water, Dimethyl sulfone (MSM), Glyceryl stearate, Stearic acid, Glycerin, Grape seed extract, Sodium hyaluronate, Sorbitol, Rose hips seed oil, Shea butter, Mango seed butter, Wheat germ oil, Kukui seed oil, Lecithin, Safflower seed oil, Apricot seed oil, Sweet almond oil, Tocopheryl acetate, Retinyl palmitate, Jojoba seed oil, Sesame seed oil, English marigold flower extract, Matricaria extract, Green tea leaf extract, St. John's wort flower/leaf/stem extract, Fucus vesiculosus extract, Aloe vera leaf juice, Ascorbic acid, Ginkgo Biloba leaf extract, Palmarosa oil, Coriander seed oil, Bergamot peel oil (Furocoumarin-free), Geranium flower oil, Jasmine oil, Lemon peel oil, Ylang Ylang flower oil, Roman Chamomile flower oil

Essential Oils: Palmarosa, Coriander, Bergamot (Furocoumarin-free), Geranium, Jasmine, Lemon, Ylang Ylang, Roman Chamomile

Directions: Use as needed to moisturize dehydrated skin.

Cautions: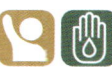

Allergen Warning: Contains wheat product.

Lavender Hand & Body Lotion

Infused with Lavender essential oil and other plant-based ingredients, Lavender Hand & Body Lotion moisturizes and protects skin from overexposure to the elements for long-lasting hydration. This formula is certified eco-friendly and all natural.

Ingredients: Water, Glyceryl oleate citrate, Caprylic/capric triglyceride, Glycerin, Barley extract, Glyceryl stearate, Cetearyl alcohol, Lavender oil, Phellodendron amurense bark extract, Sandalwood extract, Sodium stearoyl lactylate, Sodium levulinate, Xanthan gum, Sodium anisate, Laminaria digitata extract, Sorbic acid, Hydrolyzed silk, Tocopherol, Astrocaryum murumuru seed butter, Wolfberry seed oil, Olive fruit unsaponifiables, Lemon peel oil, Sodium phytate, Rosemary extract, Davana flower oil, Myrrh oil, Alcohol

Essential Oils: Lavender, Lemon, Davana, Myrrh

Directions: Use as needed to moisturize dehydrated skin.

Cautions:

Allergen Warning: Contains coconut product.

Sensation™ Hand & Body Lotion

Sensation Hand & Body Lotion is an ultra-moisturizing cream that contains several pure essential oils purportedly revered by Cleopatra for enhancing feelings of love and romance. Ylang Ylang encourages relaxation, Jasmine balances female energy, and Geranium nourishes and refreshes the skin. This lotion leaves the skin soft and moist while protecting it from harsh weather, chemicals, and dry air.

Ingredients: Water, Dimethyl sulfone (MSM), Glyceryl stearate, Stearic acid, Glycerine, Grape seed extract, Sodium hyaluronate, Sorbitol, Rose hip seed oil, Shea butter, Mango seed butter, Wheat germ oil, Kukui seed oil, Lecithin, Safflower seed oil, Apricot kernel oil, Sweet almond oil, Tocopheryl acetate, Retinyl palmitate, Jojoba seed oil, Sesame seed oil, Calendula extract, Chamomile extract, Green tea leaf extract, St. John's wort extract, Algae extract, Aloe vera gel, Ascorbic acid, Gingko biloba leaf extract, Ylang Ylang flower oil, Coriander seed oil, Bergamot (Furocoumarin-free) peel oil, Jasmine oil, Geranium flower oil

Essential Oils: Ylang Ylang, Coriander, Bergamot (Furocoumarin-free), Jasmine, Geranium

Directions: Apply all over body to moisturize skin. Use daily.

Allergen Warning: Contains wheat product.

Essential Beauty™ Serum (Dry Skin)

Wonderful benefits are seen when essential oils are used on the skin. The fine lipid structure of essential oils enables them to penetrate deep into skin tissues, carrying many active ingredients that renew, balance, and build skin health. Essential Beauty Serum for dry skin contains essential oils like Blue Cypress and Lavender, known for their ability to restore the skin's natural moisture balance.

Ingredients: Cedarwood bark oil, Coconut oil, Avocado oil, Blue Cypress wood oil, Rose hip seed extract, Jojoba seed oil, Lavender oil, Myrrh oil, Clove bud oil, Tocopherol, Wolfberry seed oil, Lecithin, Royal Hawaiian Sandalwood wood oil

Essential Oils: Cedarwood, Blue Cypress, Lavender, Myrrh, Clove, Royal Hawaiian Sandalwood

Directions: Add 3-5 drops to daily moisturizer and apply gently over face and neck. For spot treatment, apply serum directly onto desired areas on the face and rub gently into skin as needed.

Cautions: Discontinue use if irritation occurs.

Allergen Warning: Contains coconut product.

COUGH AND CONGESTION RELIEF
Thieves™ Chest Rub

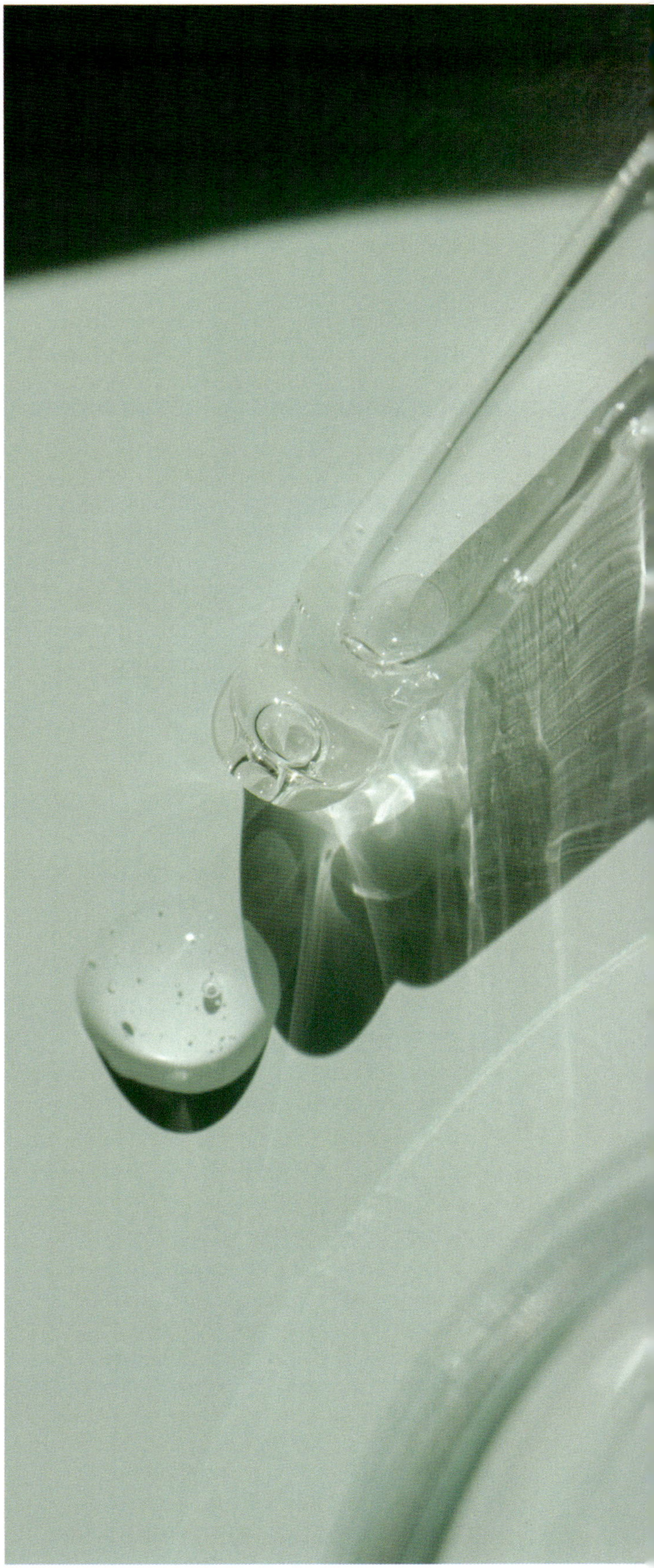

Thieves Chest Rub is an essential oil-infused, topical analgesic, and cough suppressant ointment. Its vapors soothe nasal passages with natural menthol. It

temporarily relieves stuffiness, cough, and congestion due to minor throat and bronchial irritation associated with the common cold.

Active Ingredients: Camphor, Menthol, Eucalyptus

Inactive Ingredients: Sunflower oil, Safflower oil, Castor oil, Grape seed oil, Toxicodendron succedaneum whole, Helianthus annuus seed wax, Olive oil, Tocopherol, Ascorbyl palmitate, Clove oil, Glyceryl linolenate, Lemon oil, Beta-sitoserol, Cinnamon Bark oil, Squaline, Rosemary oil, Eucalyptus Radiata leaf oil

Essential Oils: Thieves blend: Clove, Lemon, Cinnamon Bark, Rosemary, Eucalyptus Radiata

Directions: For cough suppression, rub a thick layer on throat and chest. Use up to 3 times daily or as directed by a health professional.

Cautions: Do not use by mouth, in nostrils, on wounds, or on damaged skin. Do not use on children under 2 years of age. Ask a doctor before use if you have a cough that occurs with too much phlegm (mucus).

DEODORANTS

Most deodorants today are loaded with toxic chemicals ranging from aluminum to antifreeze. As the chemicals leach through the skin into the blood and tissues, they can create a toxic buildup in the body that can lead to cancer, liver damage, and neurological diseases.

Young Living deodorants are clinically proven to inhibit the growth of odor-causing bacteria and maintain the balance of skin microbiome. They are pH balanced and formulated without aluminum, parabens, phthalates, talc, alcohol, mineral oil, synthetic perfumes, dyes, artificial colors, fragrances, preservatives, or gluten-containing ingredients. They are clinically proven to inhibit the growth of odor-causing bacteria and maintain the balance of the skin microbiome and are made with the natural fragrances of therapeutic-grade essential oils.

Perils of Aluminum

Glen Scott, MD, of Cincinnati, and Patricia Saunders, a government microbiologist, warned of aluminum neurotoxicity, causing the FDA to require aluminum-bearing antiperspirants to carry a renal dysfunction warning (June 9, 2003).

According to the Antiperspirant Products Final Monograph, the FDA is "concerned that people with renal dysfunction may not be aware that the daily use of antiperspirant products containing aluminum may put them at higher risk because of exposure to aluminum in the product." Young children are "at higher risk resulting from exposure to aluminum." Parents and others "must keep these products away from children and seek professional assistance if accidental ingestion occurs."[1]

Sources of Aluminum Exposure and Contamination

Many over-the-counter deodorants, antiperspirants, baby wipes, skin creams, suntan lotions, toothpastes, and buffered aspirin contain aluminum. Additionally, aluminum is found in some medical vaccinations, intravenous solutions, wound and antacid irrigations, ulcer treatments, blood oxygenation treatments, bone or joint replacement treatments, and burn treatments. Foods containing aluminum include baking powder, cake mixes, frozen dough, pancake mixes, self-rising flour, grains, and processed cheese. Aluminum cans, aluminum foil, disposable turkey roasting pans, and other containers are also sources of aluminum contamination.

Studies of Aluminum Toxicity

"Regardless of the host, the route of administration, or the speciation, aluminum is a potent neurotoxicant."

—MJ Strong, Department of Clinical Neurological Sciences, University of Western Ontario, Canada [2]

"Aluminum is acutely toxic to fish in acid waters. The gill is the principal target organ and death is due to a combination of ionoregulatory, osmoregulatory, and respiratory dysfunction. The mechanism of epithelial cell death is proposed as a general mechanism of aluminum-induced accelerated cell death."

—C Exley, University of Stirling, Scotland [3]

"Experimental evidence is summarized to support the hypothesis that chronic exposure to low levels of aluminum may lead to neurological disorders."

—JG Joshi, Department of Biochemistry, University of Tennessee [4]

"This data defines a new model in which aluminum kills liver cells by mechanisms distinct from previously recognized pathways of lethal cell injury. It is hypothesized that aluminum binds to cytoskeletal proteins intimately associated with the plasma membrane. This interaction eventually disrupts the permeability barrier function of the cell membrane, an event that heralds the death of the hepatocyte."

—JW Snyder, et al. Department of Pathology, Thomas Jefferson University, Philadelphia, Pennsylvania [5]

> "Epidemiological studies from Norway and England suggest a relation between the frequency of Alzheimer's disease and the concentration of aluminum in the drinking water. Estimates, made in this study, show that the role of aluminum from toothpastes may be even more important than that from the drinking water. For that reason we determined in samples of toothpastes taken from the Benelux market which brands contained aluminum. This appeared to be the case for about 22% of the brands which according to the manufacturers cover about 60% of the market."
>
> —RM Verbeeck, Laboratory for Analytical Chemistry, State University, Ghent, Belgium [6]

> "Attention was first drawn to the potential role of aluminum as a toxic metal over 50 years ago. . . . The accumulation of aluminum is associated with the development of toxic phenomena; dialysis encephalopathy, osteomalacic dialysis, osteodystrophy, and an anemia. Aluminum has also been implicated as a toxic agent in the etiology of Alzheimer's disease, Guamiam amyotrophic lateral sclerosis, and parkinsonism-dementia."
>
> — CD Hewitt, et al., University of Virginia [7]

CinnaFresh™ Deodorant

CinnaFresh Deodorant is clinically shown to help maintain your skin's delicate microbiome, giving you the protection and confidence you deserve. This all-natural deodorant has essential oils and other powerful natural ingredients strong enough to help inhibit the growth of odor-causing bacteria but gentle enough to not disturb the skin's microbiome.

Ingredients: Caprylic/capric triglyceride, Beeswax, Arrowroot root powder, Tapioca starch, Cocoa seed butter, Mango seed butter, Triethyl citrate, Safflower seed oil, Grapefruit extract, Sodium bicarbonate, Black Cumin seed oil, Zinc oxide, Vitamin E, Clove bud oil, Sodium Caproyl/Lauroyl Lactylate, Kaolin, Lemon peel oil, Cinnamon Bark oil, Eucalyptus Radiata, Rosemary leaf oil, Sage oil

Essential Oils: Clove, Lemon, Cinnamon Bark, Eucalyptus Radiata, Rosemary, Sage

Directions: Apply 3-4 light strokes to underarms daily. Turn dial to raise product.

Cautions:

Allergen Warning: Contains coconut and bee product.

CinnaGuard™ Deodorant

CinnaGuard Deodorant is clinically shown to help maintain the balance of the skin's natural microbiome, which means that your skin is shielded from unwanted external and environmental influences, while offering dynamic protection from odor-causing bacteria.

Ingredients: Caprylic/capric triglyceride, Beeswax, Arrowroot root powder, Tapioca starch, Cocoa seed butter, Mango seed butter, Triethyl citrate, Safflower seed oil, Grapefruit seed extract, Sodium bicarbonate, Black cumin seed oil, Zinc oxide, Tocopherol, Sodium caproyl/Lauroyl lactylate, Lemon peel oil, Kaolin, Thyme leaf oil, Geranium flower oil, Tea Tree leaf oil, Lavender oil, Rosemary leaf oil, Sage oil

Essential Oils: Lemon, Thyme, Geranium, Tea Tree, Lavender, Rosemary, Sage

Directions: Apply 3-4 light strokes to underarms daily. Turn dial to raise product.

Cautions:

Allergen Warning: Contains coconut and bee product.

Valor® Deodorant

Start your day with boldness. Valor Deodorant helps you feel courageous and provides the protection you need against odor without using aluminum or harsh chemical additives. It combines the odor-absorbing properties of arrowroot powder with pure essential oils and has a motivating scent that powers you throughout your day while protecting you from emitting offensive odors.

Ingredients: Caprylic/capric triglyceride, Beeswax, Arrowroot root powder, Tapioca starch, Cocoa seed butter, Mango seed butter, Triethyl citrate, Safflower seed oil, Sodium bicarbonate, Glycerin, Black cumin seed oil, Zinc oxide, Tocopherol, Sodium caproyl/lauroyl lactylate, Kaolin, Grapefruit extract, Black Spruce leaf oil, Camphor wood oil, Blue Tansy flower oil, Frankincense oil, Geranium flower oil, Sage oil

Essential Oils: Black Spruce, Camphor, Blue Tansy, Frankincense, Geranium, Sage

Directions: Apply 3-4 light strokes to underarms daily. Turn dial to raise product.

Cautions:

Allergen Warning: Contains coconut and bee product.

HAIR CARE

Many personal care products on the market today, including shampoos and conditioners, contain harmful chemicals. Unfortunately, too much of the public is unaware of the dangers and continue using these harmful products on themselves and their families, simply because they are uninformed and bombarded with so much advertising touting the beauty and benefits of synthetic products. Besides that, too many believe natural products do not work as effectively as their synthetic counterparts.

Recognizing that what you put on your body is as important as what you put in your body, the Young Living signature hair care line contains unique formulations of pure, therapeutic-grade essential oils and other plant-based ingredients to ensure not only a safe and toxin-free experience but also an effective one.

Benefits of the Young Living hair care products include sustainable plant-based products that are derived from actual botanicals, not synthesized in a lab; contain safe ingredients that have been shown by modern research to have no health risks; use recyclable packaging; and are not tested on animals. Our products are equally as good for the environment as they are for you.

Copaiba Vanilla Moisturizing Conditioner

Plant-based, safe, and environmentally responsible, Copaiba Vanilla Moisturizing Conditioner is a rich, hydrating conditioner for dry or damaged hair.

Formulated with botanical extracts, vitamins, silk proteins, and the benefits of pure copaiba and vanilla essential oils, this gentle conditioner protects without over-drying for a soothing aromatherapy experience.

Ingredients: Water, Cetearyl alcohol, Behenamidopropyl dimethylamine, Glyceryl stearate, Glycerin, Levulinic acid, p-Anisic Acid, Lactic acid, Inulin, Hydrolyzed algin, Chlorella vulgaris, Orbignya speciosa kernel oil, Astrocaryum murumuru seed butter, Potassium sorbate, Silk protein, Panthenol, Soybean seed extract, Palm fruit extract, Rice extract, Undaria pinnatifida extract, Phytic acid, Wolfberry fruit extract, Rosemary leaf extract, Equisetum arvense extract, Yucca schidigera root extract, Lavender oil, Copaiba resin oil, Geranium flower oil, Vanilla absolute, Lime oil

Essential Oils: Lavender, Copaiba, Geranium, Lime

Directions: Use daily to hydrate dry or damaged hair.

Cautions:

Allergen Warnings: Contains corn, soy, and coconut/palm ingredients

Copaiba Vanilla Moisturizing Shampoo

Copaiba Vanilla Moisturizing Shampoo calms and moisturizes dry, irritated scalps and is a natural sealant that can help tame flyaways and lock in moisture. Plant-based, safe, and environmentally responsible, this shampoo is a rich, hydrating cleanser for dry or damaged hair.

Ingredients: Water, Decyl glucoside, Coco-betaine, Lauryl glucoside, Coco-glucoside, Glyceryl oleate, Sorbitan sesquicaprylate, Glycerin, Levulinic acid, p-Anisic acid, Behenamidopropyl dimethylamine, Lactic acid, Inulin, Xanthan gum, Sodium phytate, Wolfberry fruit extract, Potassium sorbate, Panthenol, Silk protein, Rosemary leaf extract, Equisetum arvense extract, Yucca schidigera root extract, Hydrolyzed algin, Chlorella vulgaris, Soybean seed extract, Palm fruit extract, Rice extract, Undaria pinnatifida extract, Lavender oil, Copaiba resin oil, Geranium flower oil, Vanilla absolute, Lime oil

Essential Oils: Lavender, Copaiba, Geranium, Lime

Directions: Use daily to hydrate dry or damaged hair.

Cautions:

Allergen Warnings: Contains corn, soy, and coconut/palm ingredients

Lavender Mint Daily Conditioner

Plant-based, safe, and environmentally responsible, Lavender Mint Daily Conditioner is an invigorating moisturizing conditioner suitable for noncolor-treated hair. Containing botanical extracts, vitamins, silk protein, and the benefits of pure Lavender and mint essential oils, this conditioner provides an invigorating aromatherapy experience suitable for all hair types.

Ingredients: Water, Cetearyl alcohol, Glycerin, Behenamidopropyl dimethylamine, Glyceryl stearate, Lactic acid, Inulin, Peppermint oil, Sodium levulinate, Orbignya speciosa kernel oil, Astrocaryum murumuru seed butter, Lavender oil, Potassium sorbate, Hydrolyzed silk, Sodium anisate, Panthenol, Spearmint leaf extract, Undaria Pinnatifida extract, Phytic acid, Soybean seed extract, Hydrolyzed algin, Palm fruit extract, Rice extract, Wolfberry fruit extract, Rosemary leaf extract, Equisetum arvense extract, Yucca schidigera root extract, Chlorella vulgaris extract

Essential Oils: Lavender, Peppermint

Directions: After shampooing, apply liberally to wet hair. Leave on for several seconds for light conditioning or for at least one minute for deeper nourishment.

Cautions:

Allergen Warnings: Contains corn, soy, and coconut/palm ingredients

Lavender Mint Daily Shampoo

Lavender Mint Daily Shampoo contains Lavender essential oil to soothe the scalp and calm unmanageable hair and Peppermint essential oil to stimulate the blood flow to the hair follicle—allowing hair to better absorb nutrients.

Plant-based, safe, and environmentally responsible, this shampoo is an invigorating cleansing blend suitable for noncolor-treated hair.

Ingredients: Water, Decyl glucoside, Coco betaine, Lauryl glucoside, Sorbitan sesquicaprylate, Behenamidopropyl dimethylamine, Lactic acid, Glycerin, Inulin, Coco-glucoside, Glyceryl oleate, Peppermint oil, Xanthan gum, Lavender oil, Sodium levulinate, Sodium anisate, Spearmint leaf extract, Sodium phytate, Panthenol, Hydrolyzed silk, Rosemary leaf extract, Equisetum arvense extract, Yucca schidigera root extract, Undaria pinnatifida extract, Wolfberry extract, Soybean seed extract, Palm fruit extract, Rice extract, Potassium sorbate, Hydrolyzed algin, Chlorella vulgaris extract

Essential Oils: Lavender, Peppermint

Directions: Massage gently into wet hair and scalp, then rinse thoroughly. Repeat if desired.

Cautions:

Allergen Warnings: : Contains corn, soy, and coconut/palm ingredients

Lavender Conditioner

Lavender Conditioner moisturizes and conditions without weighing down the hair. It enriches the hair with MSM, amino acids, a multivitamin complex, and pure, therapeutic-grade essential oils.

Ingredients: Natural vegetable fatty acid base, Dimethyl sulfone (MSM), Milk protein, Phospholipids, Chenopo-dium quinoa extract, Hydrolyzed soy protein, Retinyl palmitate, Ascorbic acid, Rosemary leaf extract, Amino acids, Glycoprotein, Sage leaf extract, Horsetail extract, Lavender oil, Coltsfoot flower extract, Hydrolyzed wheat protein, Grape seed extract, Tocopheryl acetate, Panthenol, Cetyl triethylmonium dimethicone PEG-8 Phthalate, PEG-8 Dimethicone, Acetamide MEA, Dimethiconol panthenol, Keratin, Linoleic acid, Hyaluronic acid, Sorbitol, Wheat germ oil, Dimethiconol cysteine, Jojoba oil, Tocopherol sulfur, Guar gum, Clary oil, Lemon peel oil, Jasmine oil

Essential Oils: Lavender, Clary Sage, Lemon, Jasmine

Cautions:

Allergen Warning: Contains wheat, milk, and soy product.

Lavender Shampoo

Lavender Shampoo contains all-natural ingredients for gently cleansing and moisturizing hair. It is fortified with a vitamin complex, including panthenol and vitamins A, C, and E. It also contains MSM, which provides sulfur to help build and strengthen hair, essential oils for healthy hair and scalp, and a beautiful fragrance.

Ingredients: Coconut oil, Olive fruit oil, Decyl glucoside, Dimethyl sulfone (MSM), Water, PEG-8 Dimethi-cone, Soybean protein, Wheat protein, Oat kernel protein, Lemon peel extract, Sugar maple extract, Orange fruit extract, Aloe vera leaf gel, Retinyl palmitate, Lavender oil, Ascorbic acid, Sweet almond oil, Tocopheryl ac-etate, Panthenol, Dimethyl lauramine oleate, Grape seed extract, Acetamide MEA, Dimethiconol panthenol, Keratin, Linoleic acid, Linolenic acid, Hyaluronic acid, Sorbitol, Wheat germ oil, Dimethiconol cysteine, Jojoba seed oil, Tocopherol sulfur, Guar gum, Orbignya oleifera seed oil, Saponaria officinalis leaf/root extract, PG-Hydroxyethylcellulose cocodimonium chloride, Inositol, Cetyl Triethylmonium Dimethicone PEG-8 Phthalate, Niacin, Clary oil, Lemon peel oil, Jasmine oil

Essential Oils: Lavender, Clary Sage, Lemon, Jasmine

Directions: Use daily to cleanse and strengthen hair.

Cautions:

Allergen Warning: Contains coconut, soy, and wheat products.

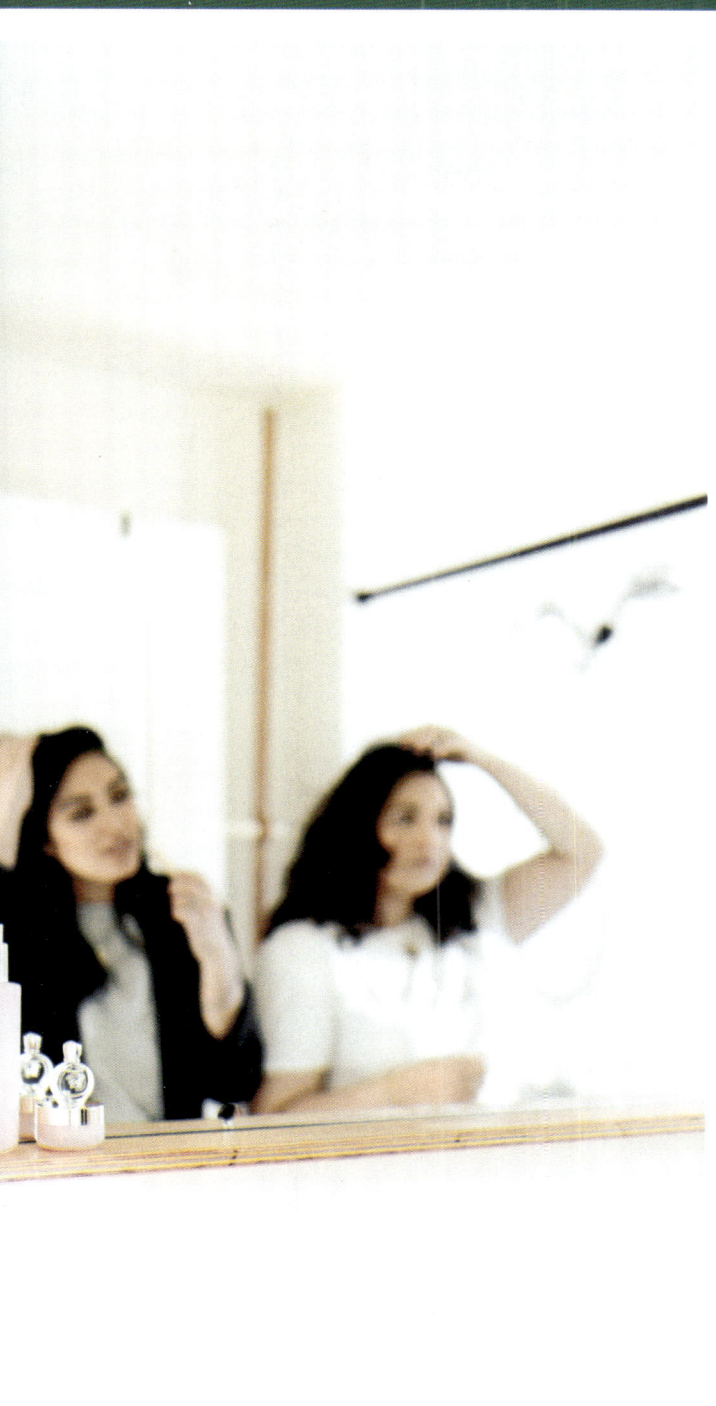

Mirah Lustrous Hair Oil™

Mirah Lustrous Hair Oil does double-duty as a hair treatment or styling aid. It adds body and shine while taming flyaway hair. This exotic hair oil is 100 percent plant-based and fragrant from a special blend of essential oils.

Ingredients: Caprylic/capric triglyceride, Grape seed oil, Isoamyl laurate, Crambe abyssinica seed oil phytosterol esters, Camellia seed oil, Argan kernel oil, Passionfruit seed oil, Marula seed oil, Monoi flower extract, Black Spruce leaf oil, Geranium flower oil, Tocopherol, Orange peel oil, Lavender oil, Sage oil, Ylang Ylang flower oil, Rose flower oil

Essential Oils: Black Spruce, Geranium, Orange, Lavender, Sage, Ylang Ylang, Rose

Directions: Apply a small amount to damp hair from mid-length to ends before blow-drying or air-drying, or smooth through dry hair to eliminate frizz and create a shiny finish.

Caution:

Shutran® Beard Oil

While grooming unruly facial hair, Shutran Beard Oil softens and conditions with its 100 percent natural formula. Men will enjoy the light, masculine scent from the Shutran essential oil blend.

Ingredients: Caprylic/capric triglyceride, Sunflower seed oil, Apricot kernel oil, Wolfberry seed oil, Tocopherol, Idaho Blue Spruce branch/leaf/wood oil, Ylang Ylang flower oil, Ocotea leaf oil, Hinoki oil, Davana flower oil, Cedarwood bark oil, Lavender oil, Coriander seed oil, Lemon peel oil, Northern Lights Black Spruce oil

Essential Oils: Idaho Blue Spruce, Ylang Ylang, Ocotea, Hinoki, Davana, Cedarwood, Lavender, Coriander, Lemon, Northern Lights Black Spruce

Directions: Use the dropper to dispense a dime-sized amount of oil into the palm of your hand. Gently work the oil into your facial hair, then groom and style it as normal. Rinse excess oil from your hands with warm, soapy water.

Cautions:

Allergen Warning: Contains coconut ingredients.

HAND SANITIZER

Thieves® Hand Sanitizer

This all-natural hand cleaner is designed to sanitize and refresh the hands. Thieves Hand Sanitizer conveniently promotes good hygiene whenever water or washing facilities are not available.

It contains Thieves blend essential oil, known for the powerful, antibacterial properties that penetrate the skin as the ethanol in this hand sanitizer evaporates. It also contains active skin-moisturizing ingredients to prevent dry skin.

Ingredients: Active: Ethyl alcohol. Inactive: Water, Aloe vera leaf powder, Glycerin, Hydroxylpropylcellulose, Peppermint oil, Clove bud oil, Lemon peel oil, Eucalyptus Radiata leaf oil, Rosemary leaf oil, Cinnamon Bark oil

Essential Oils: Peppermint, Thieves Blend: [Clove, Lemon, Cinnamon Bark, Eucalyptus Radiata, Rosemary]

Directions: Apply a small amount to the palm of the hand and rub in until completely absorbed. Use as often as necessary.

Cautions: Do not use on or near the face. If contact occurs with eyes, flush thoroughly with clean, cool water for several minutes. Avoid contact with broken skin. If symptoms persist, contact your physician. For children under 6, use adult supervision. Not recommended for infants.

Hormone Balancing
Prenolone® Plus Body Cream

Prenolone Plus Body Cream contains pregnenolone, DHEA, blue and black cohosh, and Ylang Ylang, Clary Sage, and other essential oils to nourish the skin and help maintain healthy estrogen levels.

Ingredients: Water, Dimethyl sulfone (MSM), Caprylic/capric triglyceride, Sorbitol, Lecithin, Pregnenolone acetate, Shea butter, Wolfberry seed oil, Glyceryl stearate, Aloe vera leaf juice, Sodium PCA, Stearic acid, English marigold flower extract, Roman Chamomile flower oil, Rosebud flower extract, Green tea leaf extract, St. John's wort extract, Gingko biloba leaf extract, Grape seed extract, Algae extract, Prasterone (DHEA), Tocopheryl acetate, Hydrolyzed wheat protein, Locust bean gum, Sea salt, Flax seed oil, Wheat germ oil, Ylang Ylang flower oil, Allantoin, Wild yam root extract, Eleuthero root extract, Clary oil, Kelp extract, Retinyl palmitate, Tocopheryl linoleate, Black cohosh root, Blue cohosh root, Geranium flower oil, Bergamot peel oil, Fennel oil, Sage oil, Blue Yarrow oil, Ascorbic acid

Essential Oils: Roman Chamomile, Ylang Ylang, Clary Sage, Geranium, Bergamot, Fennel, Sage, Blue Yarrow

Directions: Begin using one day after menstrual cycle ends or as desired. Apply $\frac{1}{4}$–$\frac{1}{2}$ teaspoon 2 times a day for 21 consecutive days. Discontinue for 7 days, then repeat. Massage thoroughly into soft tissue areas of the body until absorbed. Individual needs may vary.

Cautions:

Allergen Warning: Contains wheat products.

Progessence™ Plus

As women age, progesterone levels drop, and staying hormonally balanced becomes increasingly challenging, causing everything from sleep and mood disorders to more serious health concerns. Progesterone deficiency is something that affects all women.

Progessence Plus increases hormonal balance the way nature intended. It is a balancing blend designed to enhance the natural effects of progesterone. Pure USP-grade, super-micronized progesterone from wild yam is purified into a pure, therapeutic-grade essential oil-infused serum.

The first-ever, pure progesterone serum on the market, Progessence Plus has a pleasant aroma, is easily portable, is easily absorbed into the skin, and does not require cycling the application sites like other progesterone supplements.

Progessence Plus contains Sacred Frankincense, Bergamot, and Peppermint essential oils, plus vitamin E for increased skin benefits.

Ingredients: Balsam Copaiba resin oil, Sacred Frankincense oil, Cedarwood bark oil, Caprylic/capric triglyceride, Tocopherols, Bergamot peel oil (Furocoumarin-free), Peppermint oil, USP-grade progesterone (from wild yam extract), Clove bud oil

Essential Oils: Copaiba, Sacred Frankincense, Cedarwood, Bergamot (Furocoumarin-free), Peppermint, Clove

Directions: Apply 2-4 drops to the stomach, feet, or inner thighs each day, rotating application sites to avoid applying to the same area 2 days in a row. For added effect, 1-2 extra drops may be applied. Do not exceed 2 applications per day.

Cautions: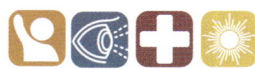

Allergen Warning: This product contains an ingredient known to the state of California to cause cancer.

Regenolone™ Moisturizing Cream

Regenolone is a natural moisturizer formulated to support proper estrogen levels in women. It contains wild yam, black and blue cohosh, Peppermint, and Wintergreen to invigorate the skin and enhance absorption.

Ingredients: Water, Dimethyl sulfone (MSM), Caprylic/capric triglyceride, Sorbitol, Lecithin, Pregnenolone acetate, Wintergreen leaf oil, Shea butter, Wolfberry seed oil, Glyceryl stearate, Aloe vera leaf juice, Roman Chamomile flower extract, Calendula flower extract, Green tea leaf extract, Ginkgo biloba leaf extract, St. John's wort flower/leaf/stem extract, Rosa canina flower extract, Sodium PCA, Stearic acid, Grape seed extract, Peppermint oil, Algae extract, Balsam Canada needle oil, Oregano leaf oil, Hydrolyzed wheat protein, Tocoph-erol acetate, Carob gum, Trace minerals, Linseed seed oil, Wheat germ oil, Wild yam root extract, Eleuthero root extract, Kelp extract, Retinyl palmitate, Tocopheryl linoleate, Blue cohosh rhizome/root, Black cohosh root, Ascorbic acid

Essential Oils: Wintergreen, Peppermint, Balsam Canada (Grand Fir), Oregano

Directions: Apply a dime-sized amount directly on dry skin as needed, not to exceed five applications per day.

Cautions:

Allergen Warning: Contains coconut and wheat products.

Shutran®

Shutran is an empowering essential oil blend that is specifically designed for men to boost feelings of masculinity and confidence.

Ingredients: Idaho Blue Spruce branch/leaf/wood oil, Ylang Ylang flower oil, Ocotea leaf oil, Hinoki, Da-vana flower oil, Cedarwood bark oil, Lavender oil, Coriander seed oil, Lemon peel oil, Northern Lights Black Spruce oil

Essential Oils: Idaho Blue Spruce, Ylang Ylang, Ocotea, Hinoki, Davana, Cedarwood, Lavender, Coriander, Lemon, Northern Lights Black Spruce

Directions: Apply to desired area. In case of sensitivity, dilute 15 drops in 10 ml of V-6 or other pure carrier oil.

Caution:

LIP BALMS

Cinnamint™ Lip Balm

Moisturize and protect your lips with an all-natural lip balm. Featuring pure Cinnamon Bark and Peppermint essential oils, Cinnamint Lip Balm helps prevent skin dehydration for soft, smooth lips.

Ingredients: Coconut oil, Beeswax, Jojoba seed oil, Sweet almond oil, Wolfberry seed oil, Rose hip seed oil, Tocopherol, Peppermint oil, Orange peel oil, Spearmint leaf extract, Cinnamon Bark oil

Essential Oils: Peppermint, Orange, Spearmint, Cinnamon Bark

Directions: Apply to lips as needed.

Caution:

Allergen Warning: Contains bee product, nut, soy, and coconut/palm ingredients

Grapefruit Lip Balm

This balm is infused with grapefruit essential oil, Wolfberry seed oil, and antioxidants that seal in moisture to prevent dehydration for smooth, supple lips.

Ingredients: Coconut oil, Beeswax, Jojoba seed oil, Sweet almond oil, Grapefruit peel oil, Wolfberry seed oil, Rose hip seed oil, Tocopherol

Essential Oils: Grapefruit

Directions: Apply to lips as needed.

Caution: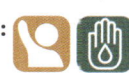

Allergen Warning: Contains bee product, nut, soy, and coconut/palm ingredients

Lavender Lip Balm

This balm soothes dry, chapped lips with gentle, protective Lavender essential oil and the moisturizing benefits of jojoba oil and vitamin E.

Ingredients: Coconut oil, Beeswax, Jojoba seed oil, Sweet almond oil, Wolfberry seed oil, Rose hip seed oil, Tocopherol, Lavender oil

Essential Oils: Lavender

Directions: Apply to lips as needed.

Caution:

Allergen Warning: Contains bee product, nut, soy, and coconut/palm ingredients

MAKEUP
Savvy Minerals by Young Living®

You care about what goes on your skin, so your makeup must be non-comedogenic (i.e., will not clog your pores and cause blackheads). The ingredients must be responsibly sourced, natural, plant based, toxin-free, cruelty-free and essential oil-infused.

You want only the best, natural ingredients. No toxins allowed! This includes parabens, phthalates, petrochemicals, talc, bismuth, synthetic fragrances or colorants, and cheap, synthetic fillers.

Savvy Minerals are naturally derived cosmetic products with ingredients that are Seed to Seal® verified and not tested on animals. With Savvy Minerals, your look will be radiant and natural.

To learn more about Savvy Minerals products and to choose the makeup tones and shades most suited to you, check the Savvy Minerals by Young Living booklet, SavvyMinerals.com, or Young Living.com.

Savvy Minerals Products

Blush shades: Awestruck, Captivate, Charisma, I Do Believe You're Blushin', Serene, Smashing

Bronzer shades: Crowned All Over, Summer Loved

Concealer: Light 1, Light 2, Medium 1, Medium 2, Dark 1, Dark 2

Eyeshadow shades: Best Kept Secret [Matte], Envy, Freedom, Inspired, Overboard, Residual, Wanderlust

Eyeshadow Palette: Natural Quartz

Eyeshadow Palette: Sahara Sunset

Eyeliner shade: Jetsetter

Foundation Powder shades: Cool No. 1, Cool No. 2, Cool No. 3, Dark No. 1, Warm No. 1, Warm No. 2, Warm No. 3

Hydrating Primer

Lip Gloss shades: Abundant, Anchors Aweigh, Embrace, Headliner, Maven, and Rockin'

Lip Luxe

Lip Scrub, Poppy Seed

Lipstick shade: Mic Drop

Lipstick Cinnamint-infused shades: Icon, Posh, Siren, Untamed

Lipstick Tangerine-infused shade: Bedazzled

Liquid Foundation: Buff, Caramel, Cocoa, Fresh Beige, Hazelnut, Honey, Ivory, Natural Beige, Pecan, Porcelain, Sand Beige, Tan, Truffle

Mascara, Lengthening: Black

Mascara, Volumizing: Black

Mattifying Primer

Misting Spray

Multitasker shades: Dark, Light

Veil shade: Diamond Dust

The tools for your best look, the Savvy Minerals Accessories, are made of the highest-quality, vegan-friendly materials. The Essential Brush Set contains Foundation Brush, Blush Brush, Blending Brush, Eye Shadow Brush, and Veil Brush. Other brush offerings that are available include Concealer Brush, Contour Brush, Bronzer Brush, Eyeliner Brush, and Eyebrow Brush.

Introduced at the 2018 Young Living Convention, the Savvy Minerals by Young Living® Kabuki Brush's densely packed bristles give you flawless makeup application and coverage. The high-quality bristles will feel heavenly against your skin.

Note: Prior preparation with Young Living's ART® Gentle Cleanser, ART Light Moisturizer, ART Refreshing Toner, ART Intensive Moisturizer, ART Renewal Serum, ART Sheerlumé Brightening Cream, Boswellia Wrinkle Cream, or Sandalwood Moisturizing Cream will enhance the Savvy Minerals collection. The time-tested, reformulated Satin Facial Scrub, Mint; Orange Blossom Facial Wash; Orange Blossom Facial Moisturizer; and other Young Living personal care products are also wonderful additions to your skin care routine.

MASSAGE OILS

Massage and therapeutic touch have long been part of both physical and emotional healing. Massage improves circulation and lymphatic drainage and aids in the elimination of tissue wastes. Massage also opens and increases the flow of energy, balancing the entire nervous system and helping to release physical and emotional disharmony.

When essential oils are combined with massage, the benefits are numerous. The oils bring peace and tranquility as well as keen mental awareness.

The unrefined carrier vegetable oils are rich in fat-soluble nutrients and essential fatty acids.

Cel-Lite Magic™ Massage Oil

Cel-Lite Magic Massage Oil enhances circulation and provides nutrients that help reduce the appearance of fat and cellulite. This massage oil is formulated with pure vegetable oils, vitamin E, Grapefruit essential oil to improve skin texture, and Juniper essential oil to detoxify and cleanse.

Ingredients: Caprylic/capric triglyceride, Grape seed oil, Grapefruit peel oil, Cypress leaf/nut/stem oil, Cedarwood bark oil, Juniper aerial parts oil, Wheat germ oil, Clary [Sage] oil, Sweet almond oil, Olive fruit oil

Essential Oils: Grapefruit, Cypress, Cedarwood, Juniper, Clary Sage

Directions: Massage on locations where firming and toning are desired. Shake well before using.

Caution: Avoid contact with sensitive tissues. If contact occurs, flush area with V-6 or pure vegetable oil (olive, etc.) and consult a health care practitioner immediately.

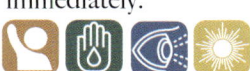

Allergen Warning: Contains coconut, nut, and wheat products.

Dragon Time™ Massage Oil

Dragon Time Massage Oil combines specially blended vegetable oils with pure Lavender, Ylang Ylang, and other essential oils that deliver natural phytoestrogens to balance and stabilize the body. Containing a blend of essential oils that have been researched in Europe for their balancing effects on hormones, this massage oil is recommended for both young and mature women.

Ingredients: Caprylic/capric triglyceride, Grape seed oil, Lavender oil, Fennel oil, Clary [Sage] oil, Sage oil, Ylang Ylang flower oil, Wheat germ oil, Blue Yarrow oil, Sweet almond oil, Olive fruit oil, Jasmine oil

Essential Oils: Lavender, Fennel, Clary Sage, Sage, Ylang Ylang, Blue Yarrow, Jasmine

Directions: Shake well before using. Gently massage onto lower abdomen and lower back or add approximately ½ ounce to bath water.

Caution: If contact occurs with eyes, flush area with warm water and consult a health care professional immediately.

Allergen Warning: Contains coconut, nut, and wheat products.

Ortho Ease® Massage Oil

Ortho Ease Massage Oil is a calming blend of vegetable oils and therapeutic-grade essential oils. This unique blend is anti-inflammatory and painkilling, ideal for strained, swollen, or torn muscles and ligaments. It also combats insect bites, dermatitis, and itching.

Ingredients: Fractionated coconut oil, Wintergreen leaf oil, Grape seed oil, Peppermint oil, Juniper oil, Eucalyptus Globulus leaf oil, Lemongrass oil, Marjoram leaf oil, Thyme oil, Eucalyptus Radiata leaf oil, Vetiver root oil, Wheat germ oil, Sweet almond oil, Olive fruit oil

Essential Oils: Wintergreen, Peppermint, Juniper, Eucalyptus Globulus, Lemongrass, Marjoram, Thyme, Eucalyptus Radiata, Vetiver

Directions: Shake well before using. Gently massage into areas of body experiencing stress.

Caution: If contact with eyes or mucous membranes occurs, flush area with warm water and consult a health care professional immediately. Not for use on children under 2 years of age.

Allergen Warning: Contains coconut, nut, and wheat products.

Ortho Sport® Massage Oil

Ortho Sport Massage Oil is an anti-inflammatory and painkilling complex of vegetable and essential oils. Ideal for strained, swollen, or torn muscles and ligaments. It has a higher phenol content than Ortho Ease and produces a greater warming sensation.

Ingredients: Caprylic/capric triglyceride, Grape seed oil, Wintergreen leaf oil, Peppermint oil, Oregano oil, Eucalyptus Globulus leaf oil, Elemi gum oil, Vetiver root oil, Lemongrass oil, Thyme oil, Wheat germ oil, Sweet almond oil, Olive fruit oil

Essential Oils: Wintergreen, Peppermint, Oregano, Eucalyptus Globulus, Elemi, Vetiver, Lemongrass, Thyme

Directions: Shake well before using. Thoroughly massage into areas of the body feeling stress following exercise.

Caution: Not for use on children under 2 years of age.

Allergen Warning: Contains coconut, nut, and wheat products.

Relaxation™ Massage Oil

Relaxation Massage Oil promotes tranquility in the body, mind, and spirit and eases tension to restore vitality. This formula blends specially selected vegetable oils with soothing essential oils for maximum stress relief and relaxation.

Ingredients: Caprylic/capric triglyceride, Grape seed oil, Tangerine peel oil, Lavender oil, Spearmint leaf extract, Ylang Ylang flower oil, Peppermint oil, Coriander seed oil, Bergamot peel oil (Furocoumarin-free), Wheat germ oil, Sweet almond oil, Olive fruit oil, Geranium flower oil

Essential Oils: Tangerine, Lavender, Spearmint, Ylang Ylang, Peppermint, Coriander, Bergamot (Furocoumarin-free), Geranium

Directions: Shake well before using. Gently massage onto skin as needed.

Caution: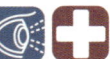

Allergen Warning: Contains coconut, nut, and wheat products.

Sensation™ Massage Oil

Sensation Massage Oil inspires the senses and encourages feelings of passion, romance, and youthfulness. This special blend of vegetable oils and essential oils leaves skin feeling silky, smooth, and soft.

Ingredients: Caprylic/capric triglyceride, Grape seed oil, Ylang Ylang flower oil, Coriander seed oil, Bergamot peel oil (Furocoumarin-free), Wheat germ oil, Jasmine oil, Sweet almond oil, Olive fruit oil, Geranium flower oil

Essential Oils: Ylang Ylang, Coriander, Bergamot (Furocoumarin-free), Jasmine, Geranium

Directions: Shake well before using. Massage liberally onto skin as desired.

Caution: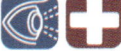

Allergen Warning: Contains coconut, nut, and wheat products.

V-6™ Vegetable Oil Complex

V-6 Vegetable Oil Complex is comprised of nourishing, antioxidant vegetable oils that are colorless and odorless. It is used to create custom massage oils or to dilute essential oils for sensitive skin. V-6 has a long shelf life, does not clog pores, and will not stain clothes.

Ingredients: Caprylic/capric triglyceride, Sesame seed oil, Grape seed oil, Sweet almond oil, Wheat germ oil, Sunflower seed oil, Olive fruit oil

Directions: Mix 1 drop of chosen essential oil in 1-8 teaspoons (5-40 ml) of V-6 Vegetable Oil Complex and apply. May also be used to create your own massage oil blend for topical applications by adding 15-30 drops of essential oil to $^1/_8$-$^1/_4$ cup (30-60 ml) of V-6. V-6 may be applied to skin prior to the application of essential oils. Stronger oils (e.g., Cinnamon Bark, Clove, Peppermint, Thyme, and Oregano) require more dilution than gentler oils (e.g., Spruce, Fennel, Sage). Shake well before using.

Cautions: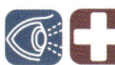

Allergen Warning: Contains coconut, nut, and wheat products.

ORAL HEALTH CARE

The Dirtiest Place on the Body

It is common medical knowledge that the dirtiest part of the body is not the colon or bowels—but the mouth. The back of the tongue is literally teeming with pathogenic microorganisms.

According to Dr. John Richter, founder of the Richter Center for the Diagnosis and Treatment of Breath Disorders, "more bacteria per square inch live on the back of the tongue than on any other part of the body."[8]

The problem is that few people use a toothbrush to remove these bacteria, and even if the tongue were to receive a thorough scrubbing, many would remain and quickly repopulate the mouth.

U.S. Surgeon General

Few people realize how important good oral hygiene is to wellness and reducing the risk of serious chronic diseases such as heart disease and cancer. According to the U.S. Surgeon General, "The terms oral health and general health should not be interpreted as separate entities. Oral health is integral to general health."[9]

Effectiveness of Chemical Constituents Against Strains of Bacteria

Bacteria	Cinnamaldehyde from Cassia/Cinnamon essential oil	Thymol from Thyme essential oil	Carvacrol from Oregano essential oil	Eugenol from Clove essential oil
Streptococcus mutans	250	250	250	500
Streptococcus sanguis	250	125	125	250
Streptococcus milleri	31	125	125	125
Streptococcus mitis	125	125	125	250
Peptostreptococcus anaerobius	500	500	500	1000
Prevotella buccae	125	250	250	500
Prevotella oris	63	250	250	500
Prevotella intermedia	125	125	125	250

MIC µg/ml (PPM or parts per million)

Didry N, Dubreuil L, Pinkas M. Activity of thymol, carvacrol, cinnamaldehyde and eugenol on oral bacteria. Pharm Acta Helv. 1994 July; 69(1):25-8.

The Heart Disease Link

"Periodontal disease increases the body's burden of inflammation," says periodontist Dr. Hatice Hasturk of the Harvard-affiliated Forsyth Institute, a not-for-profit research organization focused on oral health. Long-term (chronic) inflammation is a key contributor to many health problems, especially atherosclerosis."[10]

The same oral pathogen Porphyromonas gingivalis that causes gum disease also contributes to the inflammation along arteries and arterial damage that leads to heart and vascular disease.

The Cancer Link

Studies show a clear link between poor dental hygiene (i.e., gingivitis, cavities) and cancer.

A fascinating longitudinal study published in the British Medical Journal followed 1,390 Swedish patients over the course of 25 years. Those with the most dental plaque (bacteria) were twice as likely to die of cancer as those who had low-to-normal levels.

"Poor oral hygiene, as reflected in the amount of dental plaque, was associated with increased cancer mortality," concluded researchers from the prestigious Karolinska Research Institute in Sweden."[11]

Oil Pulling

One of the oldest and most powerful ways of improving oral health is the ancient Ayurvedic practice of "oil pulling." Traditionally using sesame seed oil, this technique involves swishing vegetable oil in the mouth for 5 to 15 minutes. It is important to push the oil under the tongue and between the teeth where most of the pathogenic microorganisms reside. The swishing action with the oil literally "pulls" or "extracts" inflammation-causing bacteria and fungi from the crevices in the mouth, which will then be spit out (not swallowed or gargled). A modern version of this practice replaces sesame seed oil with coconut oil. The coconut oil version has been reported to not only improve oral health but also sinus function as well.

A new advancement in the practice of oil pulling is to combine coconut oil with an antiseptic essential oil such as Clove. This can magnify the effectiveness of oil pulling to a huge degree, especially because the germ-killing Clove oil will penetrate the nooks and crannies of the mouth along with the coconut oil to provide far-reaching dis-infecting benefits far exceeding that of the vegetable oil alone (which only mechanically removes microbes without actually killing them).

Oral Hygiene: The Next Level

Combining oil pulling with a water-soluble antiseptic such as xylitol further improves oral hygiene. A five-carbon sugar derived from birch tree sap, xylitol is found in dental products such as chewing gum and reduces plaque and dental decay.

Because xylitol is water-soluble, it acts on a completely different level than oil-based solutions. Using a two-pronged approach in which both oil-soluble and water-soluble oral disinfectants are combined, xylitol takes oral health to an entirely new level and creates an unmatched oral treatment-care system that is revolutionizing the way people approach general health.

Brushing Teeth: Cosmetic Only

Most toothpastes work to prevent cavities by merely hardening the tooth enamel with fluoride or using abrasive salts to mechanically scrub away microorganisms from teeth and gums.

The problem is that brushing is not enough to reduce the persistent inflammation and disease-causing bacteria, fungi, and viruses in the mouth. Such microorganisms typically hide between teeth and under the tongue. While brushing mechanically removes some of the plaque and pathogens, it still leaves countless microorganisms behind to later reinfest the mouth. Oral hygiene could be vastly improved by adding proven and potent antiseptics to the toothpaste matrix, rather than relying on either fluoride or scrubbing.

Antibacterial and Antiseptic

Essential oils are ideal for use in oral care products because they are both antiseptic and nontoxic, a rare combination. Jean Valnet, MD, who used essential oils for decades in his clinical practice, emphasized this: "Essential oils are especially valuable as antiseptics because their aggression toward microbial germs is matched by their total harmlessness toward tissue." [12]

Thieves AromaBright, Thieves Whitening, and KidScents toothpastes and Thieves Fresh Essence Plus Mouth-wash all use pure, therapeutic-grade essential oils at the heart of their formulas. These oils include Peppermint, Wintergreen, Eucalyptus Globulus, Thyme, and a proprietary blend of pure, therapeutic-grade essential oils called Thieves, which includes Clove, Lemon, Cinnamon Bark, Eucalyptus Radiata, and Rosemary.

Thieves blend was tested at Weber State University in Ogden, Utah, and found to dramatically inhibit the growth of many types of bacteria (both gram-negative and gram-positive), including Micrococcus luteus and Staphylococcus aureus.

Even more remarkably, this blend exhibited a 99.96 percent kill rate against tough gram-negative bacteria like Pseudomonas aeruginosa. These bacteria, because of their thicker cell walls, tend to be far more resistant to antiseptics.

The Strength of Thyme Essential Oil

A comprehensive 2002 survey of medical literature has shown that Thyme essential oil is one of the strongest natural antiseptics known.

Researchers found that Thyme essential oil kills over 60 different strains of bacteria (both gram-negative and gram-positive) and 16 different strains of fungi.

A 1994 study by Nicole Didry at the College of Pharmaceutical and Biological Sciences in Lille, France, found that Thyme essential oil, even in very small concentrations (500 parts per million or less), killed the pathogenic organisms responsible for tooth decay, gingivitis, and bad breath—Streptococcus mutans, Streptococcus sanguis, Streptococcus milleri, Streptococcus mitis, Peptostreptococcus anaerobius, Prevotella buccae, Prevotella oris, and Prevotella intermedia. [13]

Clinical Research on Essential Oils in Dental Hygiene

Over 100 studies have documented how essential oils kill the microbes that cause tooth decay and gingivitis. According to Christine Charles and colleagues in a study published by the Journal of the American Dental Association, "The efficacy of an essential-oil-containing antiseptic mouth rinse has been demonstrated in numerous double-blind clinical studies." [14]

Researchers at the University of Maryland have also stated in the Journal of Clinical Periodontology that "Antiseptic mouth rinses are well known for their antibacterial effectiveness and are widely used for the prevention and treatment of periodontitis and to prevent the formation of supragingival plaque." [15]

Removing Plaque Naturally

Most toothpastes use questionable chemicals such as pentasodium triphosphate and tetrasodium pyrophosphate to control plaque, the scale that builds up on teeth and irritates gums, leading to gingivitis, tooth loss, and periodontal disease. Plaque is a bacterial community called a biofilm that is extremely difficult to eradicate.

However, studies published in the American Journal of Dentistry have documented the significant plaque-reducing effects of zinc citrate. Among these clinical studies was a randomized, double-blind, six-month trial that showed that zinc citrate-containing toothpaste could reduce plaque by 26 percent. [16]

Essential Oils as Effective Antiseptic Mouth Rinses

Essential oils have proven to be even more effective as antiseptic mouth rinses than even FDA-recognized, plaque-control, antiseptic drugs, such as stannous fluoride.

A 2015 study published in the journal PLoS found that an essential oil mouth rinse containing essential oil constituents thymol, menthol, methyl salicylate, and eucalyptol was as effective as a 0.2 percent solution of chlorhexidine against plaque biofilm without the gastrointestinal and tooth-staining effects of chlorhexidine. [17]

Excess Abrasion Destroys Tooth Enamel

The problem with many common brand toothpastes is that they contain very large-sized abrasive particles that can quickly wear away tooth enamel.

Because tooth enamel is not regenerated by the body, its loss is permanent. It is never replaced. As tooth enamel is lost, the softer dentin material underneath is exposed, thereby greatly enhancing the risk of dental decay and tooth loss.

To preserve dental enamel, toothpaste (dentifrice) should have extremely fine particles, which should be fine enough to not damage or wear away irreplaceable enamel but yet be sufficiently strong to remove the biofilm of dental plaque (caused by Streptococcus mutans bacteria) that can cause tooth decay, gingivitis, and dental disease.

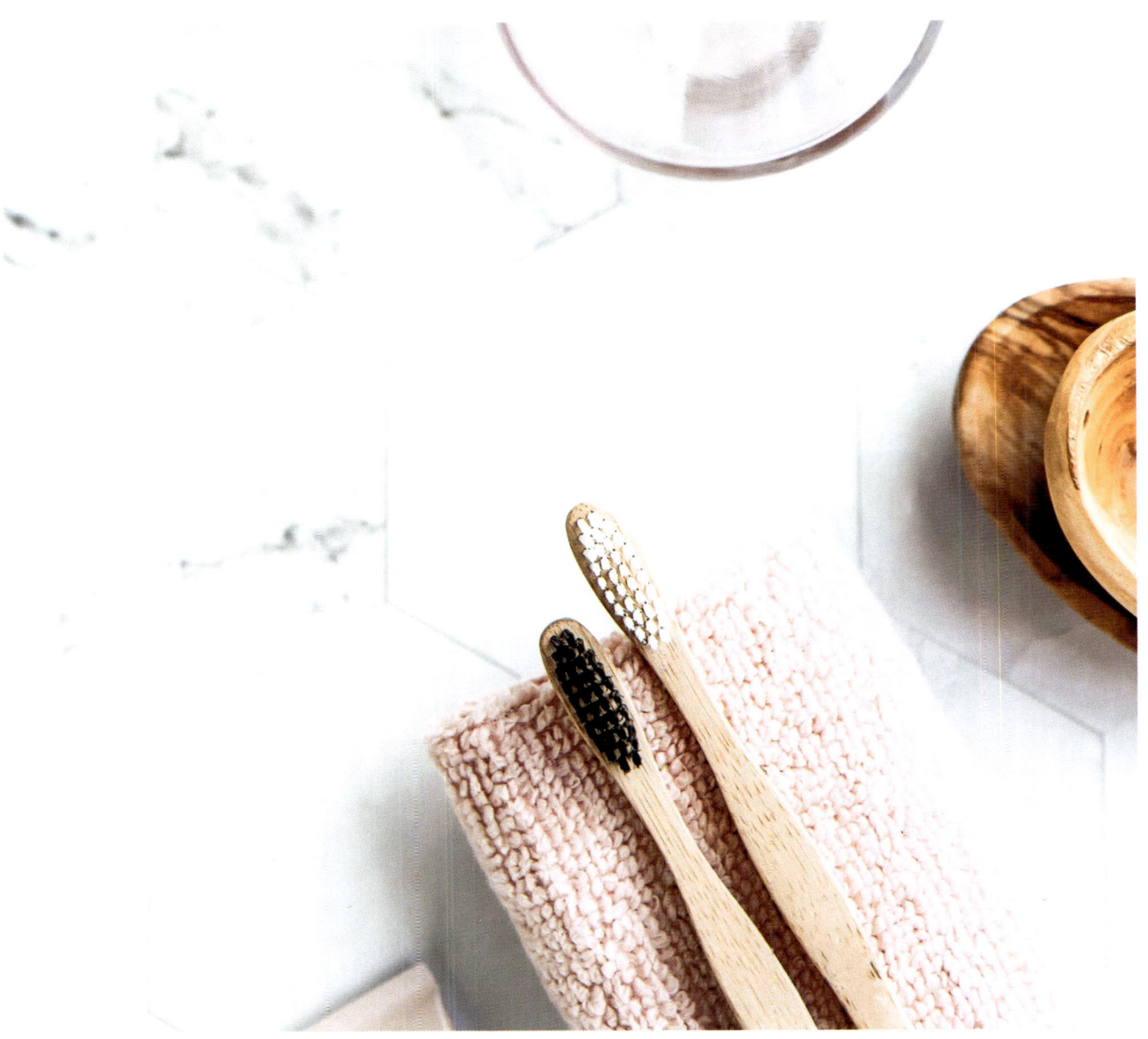

Key Differences Between Thieves Toothpastes

Oral Health Care Ingredient	AromaBright	Dentarome Ultra	Dentarome Plus
Calcium carbonate	✓	✓	
Sodium bicarbonate	✓		✓
Virgin Coconut Oil	✓		
Xylitol	✓	✓	
Thieves Essential Oil Blend	✓	✓	✓
Ocotea Essential Oil	✓		
Peppermint Essential Oil	✓		✓
Spearmint Essential Oil	✓		
Wintergreen Essential Oil		✓	✓
Lecithin	✓	✓	

"The essential oils of thyme, clove, and cinnamon possess significant inhibitory effects against 23 different genera of bacteria."

— International Journal of Food Microbiology

Chlorhexidine in Mouthwashes Increases Blood Pressure

On March 18, 2019, Reader's Digest[18] reported on a hidden danger of using commercial mouthwashes. A study published in Frontiers in Cellular and Infection Microbiology found that a balanced oral microbiome can be disturbed by mouthwashes containing the antiseptic compound chlorhexidine.[19]

Beneficial oral bacteria convert the dietary nitrate found in vegetables into nitric oxide. Nitric oxide is key in maintaining healthy blood pressure. In the study, people using mouthwash with chlorhexidine had a "significant" increase in systolic blood pressure. Study author Nathan Bryan said their findings could explain why two out of three people with high blood pressure cannot manage it with medication.

Not all mouthwashes have this problem. Essential oils with antibiotic properties do not harm beneficial bacteria. Kurt Schnaubelt, PhD, stated that "So-called good bacteria such as acidophilus and bifidus are able to metabolize the phenylpropanoids of essential oils. Pathogenic bacteria such as klebsiella or E. coli are destroyed by them."[20]

A 2009 study tested eight essential oils against the 12 major species of intestinal bacteria. Four of the essential oils tested "displayed the greatest degree of selectivity, inhibiting the growth of potential pathogens at concentrations that had no effect on the beneficial bacterial examined."[21] [Emphasis added.]

Toothpaste Solutions (see chart)

The Thieves line of toothpastes represent a comprehensive, powerful, natural, and novel approach to dental health.

Thieves AromaBright contains the key components of sodium bicarbonate and calcium carbonate. This combination is far more effective than each alone in promoting oral health and beauty. Sodium bicarbonate greatly enhances the antiseptic action of the essential oils, while calcium carbonate is essential for brightening teeth. In fact, these two carbonate salts are superior to enzymes in promoting tooth whiteness.

Thieves AromaBright also includes the powerful anti-inflammatory essential oil Ocotea, essential for reducing oral inflammation, gingivitis, and periodontitis. Ocotea is rich in alpha humulene and beta caryophyllene, which are some of the best-studied essential oil compounds to combat inflammation.

KidScents® Toothpaste

KidScents Toothpaste is a safe, natural alternative to commercial brands of toothpaste. It's the perfect choice for parents who want a safe, all-natural toothpaste for their kids.

Formulated with Slique Essence essential oil blend, this toothpaste gently cleans teeth and tastes great without synthetic dyes or flavors.

Thieves essential oil blend is used as a gum health agent with antibacterial properties.

KidScents Slique Toothpaste is perfect for children of all ages, and it makes a great training toothpaste for children during the crucial first years while they develop their primary teeth. Calcium carbonate, baking soda, and xylitol are used as tooth and gum health agents.

Ingredients: Water, Calcium carbonate, Coconut oil, Sodium bicarbonate, Glycerin, Xylitol, Xanthan gum, Grapefruit peel oil, Stevia rebaudiana leaf extract, Tangerine peel oil, Lecithin, Spearmint leaf extract, Lemon peel oil, Ocotea leaf oil, Clove bud oil, Cinnamon Bark oil, Eucalyptus Radiata leaf oil, Rosemary leaf oil

Contains NO fluoride, sodium lauryl sulfate, sugar, synthetic chemicals, or colors

Essential Oils: Grapefruit, Tangerine, Spearmint, Lemon, Ocotea, Clove, Cinnamon Bark, Eucalyptus Radiata, Rosemary

Safe, Natural Products | Chapter 6

Oral Health Care Ingredient	Thieves AromaBright	Common Brand
Primary Active Ingredient	Thieves Essential Oil Blend*	Stannous Fluoride, Sodium Fluoride
Germ-killing Ingredients	Essential Oils of Clove, Cinnamon Bark, and Eucalyptus Radiata	None
Antimicrobial Enhancer	Lemon Essential Oil**	None
Treats Tooth Sensitivity Agent	Clove Essential Oil	Potassium Nitrate
Foaming Agent	None	Poloxamer 407, PEG-12, Sodium Lauryl Sulfate***
Plaque Control	Sodium Bicarbonate	None
Tooth and Gum Health Agents	Virgin Coconut Oil, Peppermint Essential Oil, Ocotea Essential Oil	Tetrasodium Pyrophosphate
Moisturizer	Vegetable Glycerin	Propylene Glycol, PEG-6, Glycerin
Sweetener	Xylitol, Pure Stevia Extract	Sorbitol, Sodium Saccharin
Coloring	None	Titanium Dioxide, FD&C Blue #1, Yellow #5
Cleansing Agent	Nano-sized Calcium Carbonate	Abrasive Hydrated Silica, Mica, Sodium Hexametaphosphate
Flavoring	Spearmint Essential Oil	"Flavor" (Artificial and/or Natural Chemicals)
Warnings on Usage	None	Warning: When using this product, do not use for sensitivity for longer than four weeks, unless recommended by a dentist.
Warnings on Ingestion	None	Warning: Keep out of reach of children. If more than used for brushing is accidentally swallowed, get medical attention or contact a poison control center right away.

Directions: Apply a small amount of toothpaste on a brush, brush teeth, and rinse thoroughly after each meal or as directed by a dentist or doctor. Supervise children until good brushing and rinsing habits are established. Do not swallow. Intended for children 2 years of age and older. For children under 2 years of age, consult a dentist or doctor before use.

Caution:

Allergen Warning: Contains coconut product.

Thieves® AromaBright® Toothpaste

Thieves AromaBright Toothpaste gently removes stains while polishing and brightening the appearance of teeth for a sparkling smile. Significant attributes include:

- Anti-stain whitening enzymes
- Time-released essential oil mouthwash
- Therapeutic-grade essential oil blend of Thieves
- A low-abrasion formula
- Special plaque-control agents
- All food-grade, edible ingredients

Ingredients: Water, Calcium carbonate, Coconut oil, Sodium bicarbonate, vegetable Glycerin, Xylitol, Xanthan gum, Peppermint leaf oil, Spearmint leaf

Comparing Mouthwashes

	Thieves Fresh Essence Mouthwash	Common Brand
Active Ingredients	Thieves*, Thyme oil, Eucalyptus oil, Wintergreen oil, Peppermint oil, Thymol, 1,8-cineole, Methyl Salicylate, Menthol	None
Base	Water	Alcohol, SD Alcohol
Sweetener	Stevioside, Sorbitol	Sodium Saccharin
Coloring	None	D&C Yellow #10, FD&C Green #3, FD&C Blue #1, FD&C Yellow #5
Flavoring	Peppermint	Artificial Sources
Preservatives	None	Benzoic Acid, Polysorbate 80
Dispersant	Natural Lecithin	Poloxamer 403, Sodium Hydroxide (Lye), Synthetic Glycerine

* A proprietary blend of Clove, Lemon, Cinnamon, Eucalyptus Radiata, Rosemary

extract, Stevia rebaudiana leaf extract, Lecithin, Clove bud oil, Ocotea leaf oil, Cinnamon Bark oil, Lemon peel oil, Eucalyptus Radiata leaf oil, Rosemary leaf oil

Essential Oils: Peppermint, Spearmint, Clove, Ocotea, Cinnamon Bark, Lemon, Eucalyptus Radiata, Rosemary

Contains NO fluoride, sodium lauryl sulfate, sugar, synthetic chemicals, or colors.

Directions: Apply toothpaste to brush, brush teeth, and rinse thoroughly after each meal or as directed by a dentist or doctor. Do not swallow. For children under 2 years of age, consult a dentist or doctor before use.

Caution:

Allergen Warning: Contains coconut product.

Thieves® Dental Floss

Flossing is an essential part of the tooth-cleaning process because it removes plaque from between teeth and at the gum line, where periodontal disease often begins.

Thieves Dental Floss is made with strong fibers that resist fraying and easily glide between teeth for those hard-to-reach places. This floss combines the traditional benefits of regular dental floss with the antibacterial benefits of Thieves essential oil blend. The floss is infused with essential oils that help fight infection and cavities.

Ingredients: Thieves: [Clove bud oil, Lemon peel oil, Cinnamon Bark oil, Eucalyptus Radiata leaf/twig oil, Rosemary leaf oil], Peppermint leaf oil

Essential Oils: Thieves: [Clove, Lemon, Cinnamon Bark, Eucalyptus Radiata, Rosemary], Peppermint

Thieves® Whitening Toothpaste

Thieves Whitening Toothpaste is great for the entire family. It combines safe, pure ingredients to whiten teeth, fight plaque, support healthy gums, and remove stains, yet doesn't damage enamel. This exclusive formula is free of fluoride and other harsh ingredients and delivers a superior clean.

Ingredients: Glycerin, Water, Silica, Xylitol, Calcium hydroxyapatite, Sodium myristoyl glutamite, Calcium car-bonate, Perlite, Sodium bicarbonate, Zinc citrate trihydrate, Menthol, Orange peel oil, Spearmint leaf ex-tract, Xanthan gum, Stevia, Clove bud oil, Peppermint oil, Cocos nucifera (Coconut) oil, Lemon peel oil, Cinnamon Bark oil, Eucalyptus leaf oil, Rosemary leaf oil.

Essential Oils: Orange, Spearmint, Clove, Peppermint, Lemon, Cinnamon Bark, Eucalyptus Radiata, Rosemary

Directions: Brush after each meal or as directed by a dentist or doctor. Apply toothpaste to a soft-bristled tooth-brush. Brush with gentle, circular stokes for at least 2 minutes, and rinse thoroughly after use. Do not swallow. For children under 2, consult a dentist or doctor before use.

Cautions: For external use only. Contains xylitol for effectively reducing the risk of tooth decay. While xylitol is nontoxic to humans, it can cause adverse reactions in our fury family members and should not be used to clean pets' teeth.

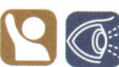

Allergen Warning: Contains coconut product.

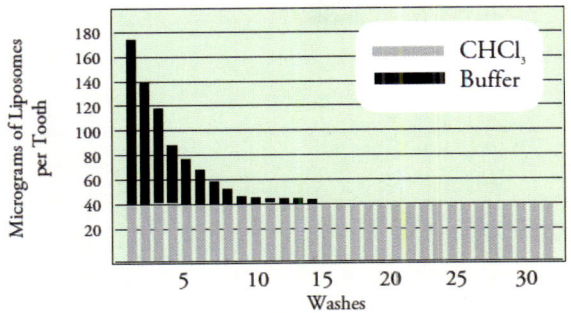

Figure 1. A saliva-coated human tooth was dipped in a solution of dental liposomes and rinsed repeatedly with 1.0 ml of water.

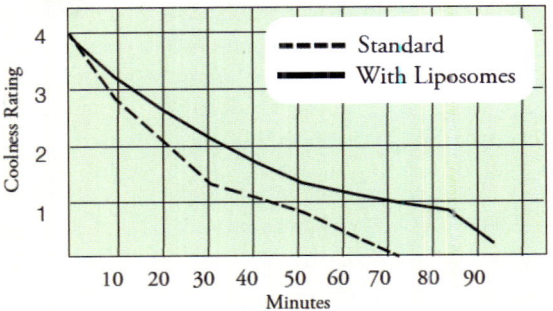

Figure 2. Lozenges made with mucin-binding system to release menthol flavor slowly are compared to control menthol lozenges. Timing began when the lozenge was completely dissolved in the mouth.

Critical Kill Time Against Representative Oral Pathogens

	TYPES of MOUTH RINSES		
	Essential Oil	Stannous Fl	Sterile Water Control
Fusobacterium nucleatum	<0.5 min	<0.5 min	>5 min
Streptococcus mutans	<0.5 min	<1 min	>5 min
Prevotella intermedia	<0.5 min	<2 min	>5 min
Lactobacillus casei	<0.5 min	>2 min	>5 min
Candida albicans ATCC 28366	<0.5 min	>5 min	>5 min
Candida albicans ATCC 18804	<0.5 min	>5 min	>5 min

Pan, et al., 1999

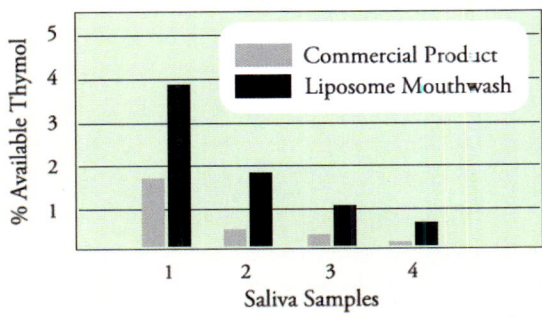

Figure 3. The retention of thymol was measured over a period of five minutes in various saliva samples. The level of thymol remaining in the saliva dropped off rapidly following usage of the commercial product. However, following usage of the liposome-based mouthwash, there was a significantly higher level of thymol in each saliva sample analyzed.

Slique® Gum

This unique chewing gum promotes a healthy mouth and helps with appetite control. It is infused with Frereana Frankincense resin, famous for its tooth and gum benefits. Natural sweeteners and the act of chewing alleviate snack cravings, making this gum a helpful tool in weight management. Peppermint and Spearmint essential oils freshen the breath.

Ingredients: Isomalt, Frereana Frankincense resin, Gum base, Sorbitol, Natural flavors, Calcium stearate, Natural green color (Red cabbage juice, Turmeric, Soy protein isolates), Stevia leaf extract, Monk fruit extract, Peppermint oil, Spearmint leaf oil, Xylitol

Essential Oils: Peppermint, Spearmint

Directions: Chew 1 gum tablet before or after meals as desired.

Cautions: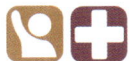

Allergen Warning: Contains soy product.

Slow-Release Systems for Oral Soft Tissues

Liposomal systems that adhere to mucous membranes are designed to slowly release beneficial chemical compounds in the mucous membranes of the mouth and nose. This is useful in the slow release of flavors.

For example, a breath lozenge containing menthol that is contained in a mucin-binding system can provide extended oral freshness longer than a standard menthol lozenge (Figure 1).

In another study, two thymol-based mouthwashes were compared side by side. The first was a standard commercial product with no liposome-based delivery; the second used a liposomal delivery system. The results of the experiment are illustrated in Figure 2.

The level of thymol measured in saliva over a period of five minutes was measured. With the commercial product, thymol levels dropped off quickly, whereas with the liposome-based mouthwash, a significantly higher level of thymol was found in each saliva sample.

Thieves® Cough Drops

Thieves Cough Drops are an over-the-counter product that soothes sore throats, relieves coughs, and cools nasal passages. They are free from sugar, dyes, preservatives, and artificial flavors. With the Thieves blend and Lemon and Peppermint essential oils, these sweet, spicy drops taste great and provide effective relief in combination with natural menthol.

Ingredients: Menthol, Cinnamon Bark oil, Clove bud oil, Eucalyptus Radiata leaf oil, Isomalt, Lemon peel oil, Pectin, Peppermint aerial parts oil, Rosemary leaf oil, Stevia leaf extract, Water

Essential Oils: Thieves: [Cinnamon Bark, Clove, Eucalyptus Radiata, Lemon, Rosemary], Peppermint

Directions: Adults and children 5 years and over: dissolve 1 drop slowly in mouth and repeat every 2 hours as needed. Children under 5 years of age: ask a doctor.

Caution: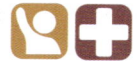

Thieves® Hard Lozenges

Thieves Hard Lozenges deliver the cleansing power of Thieves essential oil blend with the sweet flavor of Peppermint, Lemon, and other natural ingredients for long-lasting relief. Both adults and children have found it to ease the pain of a sore throat and help with dryness. A convenient and portable way to enjoy this favorite dietary supplement.

Thieves is university tested for its ability to kill 99.6 percent of bacteria tested.

Ingredients: Lemon peel oil, Peppermint oil, Clove flower bud oil, Cinnamon Bark oil, Eucalyptus Radiata leaf oil, Rosemary leaf oil, Isomalt, Water, Stevia leaf extract, Pectin

Essential Oils: Lemon, Thieves: [Clove, Lemon, Cinnamon Bark, Eucalyptus Radiata, Rosemary], Peppermint

Directions: Dissolve 1 lozenge in mouth as needed.

Cautions: Swallowing lozenges whole may cause choking.

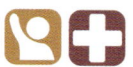

Thieves® Mints

Infused with the power of Thieves and Peppermint essential oils, Thieves Mints dissolve easily in the mouth and provide a healthy, sugar-free alternative to freshen your breath.

Thieves is university-tested for its ability to kill 99.6 percent of bacteria tested.

Ingredients: Sorbitol, Calcium stearate, Clove bud oil, Lemon peel oil, Cinnamon Bark oil, Eucalyptus Radiata leaf oil, Rosemary leaf oil, Peppermint oil, Stevia leaf extract

Essential Oils: Thieves blend: [Clove, Lemon, Cinnamon Bark, Eucalyptus Radiata, Rosemary], Peppermint

Directions: Dissolve 1 mint in mouth, as desired.

Cautions: Swallowing mints whole may cause choking.

Thieves® Fresh Essence Plus™ Mouthwash

Essential Oil Mouth Rinses Reduce Plaque and Fight Tooth Decay

A number of clinical studies over the past 20 years have documented the ability of essential oil mouth rinses to control plaque and fight gingivitis.

Typical of these is a 1999 study at Humboldt University in Berlin, Germany. Researchers using an observer-blind, randomized, cross-over design found that median plaque reductions generated by twice-daily essential oil mouth rinses were 23 percent greater than a placebo. The essential oils used were thyme, peppermint, wintergreen, and eucalyptus.[22]

"A meta-analysis of 16 six-month studies involving 4,016 patients showed that 'in patients with gingivitis, EO-containing mouthwashes are more efficacious for the reduction of plaque and gingival inflammation than mechanical plaque control either alone (placebo) or in combination with mouthwashes with cetylpyridinium chloride (CPC).'"[23]

Benefits of Liposomes in Thieves Fresh Essence Plus Mouthwash

Controlled-release liposomes are a key ingredient in Thieves Fresh Essence Plus Mouthwash. These liposomes adhere to either tooth enamel or mucous membranes in the mouth. The two primary benefits of using liposome technology are:

1. **Controlled release of active ingredients**

2. **Ingredient protection**

The controlled-release aspect of liposome technology is enhanced through the use of a patented "liposome anchoring" system. Liposomes that adhere to dental enamel can be used to improve dental health because they contain active materials to prevent plaque formation, treat periodontal disease, and prevent dental caries. These active materials can be released slowly, enhancing their benefits.

The ability of dental liposomes to slowly release their therapeutic cargo is demonstrated in Figure 3.

A saliva-coated tooth is dipped into a solution containing dental liposomes. The liposomes contain a test material. The tooth is sequentially washed with 1.0 ml of buffer 30 times. The test material is removed slowly with the washes. Even after 30 washes, some active material is retained on the tooth. Thieves Fresh Essence Plus Mouthwash combines Thieves essential oil blend and Peppermint, Spearmint, and Vetiver essential oils for an extra clean mouth and fresh breath. It contains only natural ingredients and uses a patented, time-release technology for lasting freshness.

Ingredients: Water, Colloidal silver, Peppermint oil, Lecithin, Quillaja saponaria wood extract, Potassium sorbate, Stevia rebaudiana leaf extract, Clove bud oil, Spearmint leaf extract, Lemon peel oil, Cinnamon Bark oil, Vetiver root oil, Eucalyptus Radiata leaf oil, Rosemary leaf oil, Tocopheryl, Citric acid

Essential Oils: Peppermint, Thieves: [Clove, Lemon, Cinnamon Bark, Eucalyptus Radiata, Rosemary], Spearmint, Vetiver

Directions: Rinse mouth with 1 tablespoon or capful for 30-60 seconds or as needed. May be used to ease a painful sore throat or upset stomach. For children under 2 years of age, consult a dentist or doctor before use.

Caution:

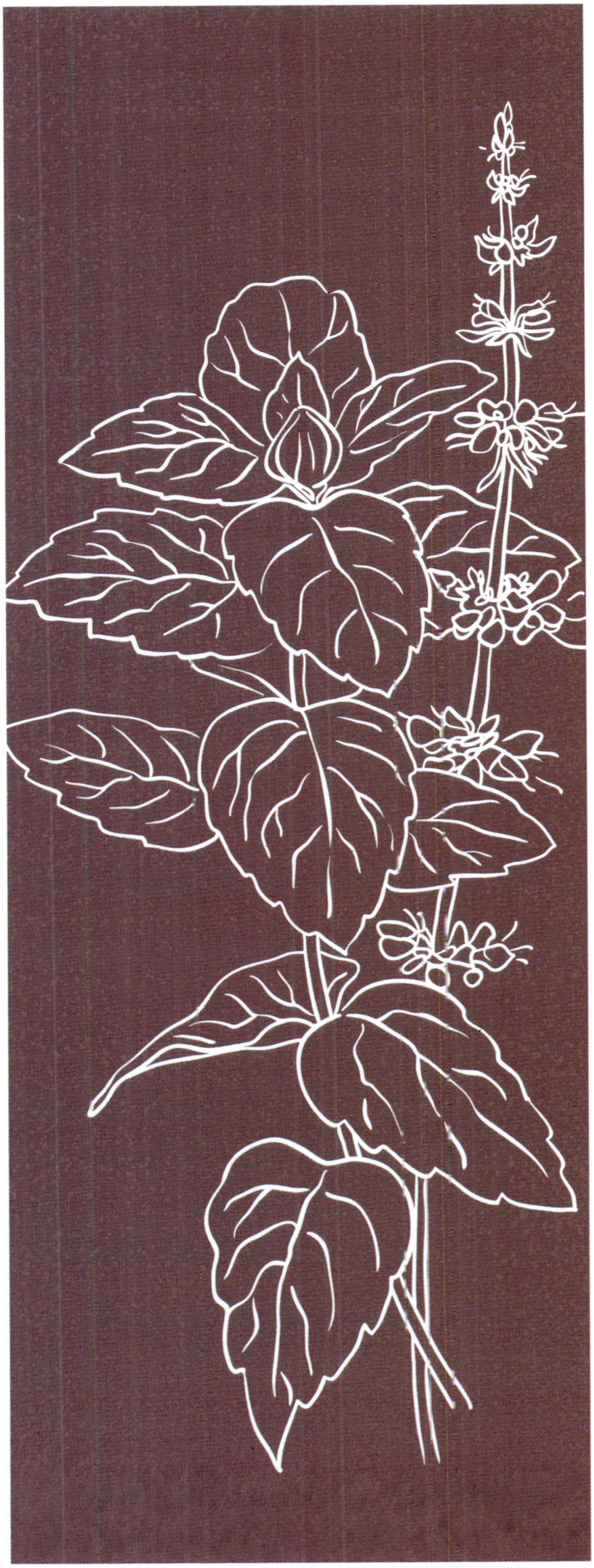

PAIN RELIEF

CBD Muscle Rub (See also BLENDS, CBD Oil Blends, Nature's Ultra and Young Living)

CBD, or cannabidiol, is a plant-based compound found in hemp. It is pure and has 0.0 percent THC, which is the mind-altering chemical found in marijuana. Nature's Ultra CBD is tested and verified through third-party testing to ensure that you're getting a high-quality product free from solvents, heavy metals, gluten, and pesticides.

CBD Muscle Rub from Nature's Ultra takes the hot-and-cold sensation of menthol and gives it a boost by infusing it with an array of all-natural Young Living essential oils that work hard together to soothe your hard-working body.

Certified by a third-party lab: Contains 0% THC and 99%+ CBD; 100% pure, therapeutic-grade essential oils

Ingredients: Camellia leaf oil, Beeswax, Shea butter, Safflower, Menthol, Squalane, Jojoba seed oil, Camphor, Tea Tree, Lemon, Peppermint, Clove, Vitamin E, Arnica flower, CBD, Wormwood oil, Wintergreen, Helichrysum

Essential Oils: Camphor, Tea Tree, Lemon, Peppermint, Clove, Wintergreen, Helichrysum

Directions: Apply to clean skin and massage well. Do not apply to the face or broken or sensitive skin. Do not refrigerate. Keep at room temperature to preserve freshness. Store away from humidity, heat, and light.

Cautions:

Cool Azul® Pain Relief Cream

Young Living's Cool Azul Pain Relief Cream provides penetrating and cooling relief from minor muscle and joint aches, simple backache, arthritis, strains, bruises, and sprains. This plant-based formula combines the power of Wintergreen essential oil and Cool Azul essential oil blend, while remaining free of synthetic ingredients. Get lasting comfort you can feel.

Ingredients: Active: Methyl salicylate, Menthol. Inactive: Aloe vera leaf, Safflower oil, Glyceryl monostearate, Cetyl alcohol, Stearyl alcohol, Glycerin, Squalane, Rosa moschata oil, Mangifera indica seed butter, Benzyl alcohol, Camphor white oil, Sodium anisate, Water, Peppermint oil, Sage oil, Alcohol, Chamomile, Camellia oleifera leaf, Balsam Copaiba resin oil, Oregano leaf oil, Melaleuca Quinquenervia (Niaouli) oil, Ecuadorian (Plectranthus) Oregano, Sodium levulinate, Lavender oil, White Cypress Pine oil, Elemi leaf oil, Vetiver oil, Caraway oil, Dorado Azul seed oil, German Chamomile flower oil

Essential Oils: Peppermint, Sage, Copaiba, Oregano, Melaleuca Quinquenervia (Niaouli), Ecuadorian (Plectranthus) Oregano, Lavender, White Cypress Pine, Elemi, Vetiver, Caraway, Dorado Azul, German Chamomile (Matricaria)

Directions: Adults and children 12 years of age and older: Apply to affected area not more than 3-4 times daily. Children under 12 years of age: Ask a doctor.

Cautions: Use only as directed. Do not bandage tightly or use with a heating pad. Do not apply to wounds or damaged, broken, or irritated skin. If severe burning sensation occurs, discontinue use immediately. Do not expose the area treated with product to heat or direct sunlight. If swallowed, get medical help or contact a Poison Control Center right away.

Allergy Alert: If prone to allergic reaction from aspirin or salicylates, consult a doctor before use.

Cool Azul® Sports Gel

With 10-percent essential oils, Cool Azul Sports Gel is great to use before or after physical activity.

Ingredients: Aloe leaf extract, Olive fruit oil, Glycerin, Wintergreen leaf oil, Peppermint oil, Menthol, Sage oil, Arnica flower extract, Balsam Copaiba resin, Camphor, Sodium hyaluronate, Sunflower Lecithin, Xanthan gum, Oregano oil, Niaouli leaf oil, Ecuadorian (Plectranthus) Oregano oil, Lavender oil, Water, Matricaria flower extract, Blue Cypress wood oil, Elemi leaf extract, Willow bark extract, Vetiver root oil, Levulinic acid, Caraway seed oil, Dorado Azul seed oil, German Chamomile flower oil, p-Anisic acid

Essential Oils: Wintergreen, Peppermint, Sage, Copaiba, Oregano, Melaleuca Quinquenervia (Niaouli), Ecuadorian (Plectranthus) Oregano, Lavender, Blue Cypress, Elemi, Vetiver, Caraway, Dorado Azul, German Chamomile (Matricaria)

Directions: Shake well before use. Rub and massage generously into skin.

Caution: Proceed with caution when applying to sensitive skin.

SHAVING

Mirah® Shave Oil

Mirah Shave Oil is formulated with a rich blend of essential oils, emollients, and botanical ingredients for a luxuriously close shave. Exotic baobab, meadowfoam, and avocado oils work together with our exclusive Mirah essential oil blend to reduce razor drag, bumps, and nicks.

Ingredients: Caprylic/capric triglyceride, Avocado fruit oil, Meadowfoam seed oil, Camellia seed oil, Baobab seed oil, Ylang Ylang flower oil, Idaho Blue Spruce branch/leaf/wood oil, Ocotea leaf oil, Coriander seed oil, Davana flower oil, Cedarwood bark oil, Lemon peel oil, Jasmine oil, Royal Hawaiian Sandalwood oil, Lavender oil, Rose flower oil

Essential Oils: Ylang Ylang, Idaho Blue Spruce, Ocotea, Coriander, Davana, Cedarwood, Lemon, Jasmine, Royal Hawaiian Sandalwood, Lavender, Rose

Directions: Pump shave oil into hands and rub a thin layer over skin. Shave.

Caution:

Shutran® Aftershave Lotion

This aftershave lotion is light and soothing and moisturizes the skin with pure essential oils like Ylang Ylang, Lavender, and Northern Lights Black Spruce, as well as with other natural botanicals, including aloe and argan oil.

Ingredients: Water, Glycerin, Caprylic/capric triglyceride, Jojoba seed oil, Coconut oil, Polyglyceryl-10 pentastearate, Sunflower seed wax, Witch hazel leaf extract, Argan kernel oil, Lauryl laurate, Sunflower seed oil, Benzyl alcohol, Aloe leaf juice powder, Sodium levulinate, Behenyl alcohol, Sodium stearoyl lactylate, Xanthan gum, Sodium anisate, Citric acid, Menthol, Sodium hyaluronate, Dandelion root extract, Agar, Idaho Blue Spruce branch/leaf/wood oil, Ylang Ylang flower oil, Ocotea leaf oil, Hinoki oil, Davana flower oil, Cedarwood bark oil, Lemon peel oil, Coriander seed oil, Lavender oil, Northern Lights Black Spruce oil

Essential Oils: Idaho Blue Spruce, Ylang Ylang, Ocotea, Hinoki, Davana, Cedarwood, Lemon, Coriander, Lavender, Northern Lights Black Spruce

Directions: Apply a small amount to face after shaving. Can also be applied in between shaves to keep skin moisturized.

Caution:

Allergen Warning: Contains coconut product.

Shutran® Shave Cream

Made with pure essential oils and moisturizing botanicals, Shutran Shave Cream delivers an incredibly close, smooth shave. Combining hydrating palm, grape seed, and olive oils; naturally derived vitamin E complex; and mango and cocoa butter, this luxurious shave cream provides a frictionless glide to reduce razor burn and nicks.

Ingredients: Aloe vera leaf juice, Caprylic/capric triglyceride, Zinc oxide, Palm oil, Grape seed oil, Olive fruit oil, Mango seed butter, Glyceryl stearate, Palm butter, Cocoa seed butter, Cera alba, Xanthan gum, Glycerin, Cetearyl alcohol, Menthol (natural source), Tea Tree leaf oil, Sugarcane extract, Tocopherol, Honey, Sodium PCA, Sodium stearoyl lactylate, Water, Idaho Blue Spruce branch/leaf/wood oil, Bamboo extract, Camellia oleifera leaf extract, Levulinic acid, Ocotea leaf oil, Ylang Ylang flower oil, Hinoki oil, p-Anisic acid, Cedarwood bark oil, Coriander seed oil, Davana flower oil, Lavender oil, Lemon peel oil, Northern Lights Black Spruce oil

Essential Oils: Tea Tree, Idaho Blue Spruce, Ocotea, Ylang Ylang, Hinoki, Cedarwood, Coriander, Davana, Lavender, Lemon, Northern Lights Black Spruce

Directions: Wet area with warm water. Apply a thin, even layer. Shave; rinse razor after each stroke. Rinse area with water.

Caution:

Allergen Warning: Contains coconut/palm products.

SKIN CARE

Human skin is like a large sponge and absorbs trace amounts of almost everything with which it comes in contact—both harmful and beneficial. The skin is especially vulnerable to solvents and petroleum-based chemicals. When some of these chemicals come in contact with the skin, they can be absorbed in far higher volumes than other types of substances.

Chinese Secret to Youthful Skin

For centuries, the Chinese living in Inner Mongolia have been using a very unusual vegetable oil with exceptional benefits for the skin: wolfberry seed oil. This rare and expensive oil is painstakingly extracted from the seeds of the Ningxia variety of the Lycium berry. Not only is the oil rich in vitamin E, linoleic, and linolenic acids, but it also has an unusual chemistry that makes it ideal for nourishing and hydrating the skin. "The wolfberry seed oil is one of the best oils for the skin," according to researcher Sue Chao. "It is sought after throughout Asia and has some very unusual regenerative properties, such as protecting aging skin and adding luster to skin."

This means that many questionable petrochemicals commonly found in personal care products, such as sodium lauryl sulphate (SLS), triethanolamine (TEA), polyethylene glycol (PEG), and quaterniums (ammonium salt), can be absorbed into the skin. Over time, some of these chemicals may accumulate in the organs and tissues and result in mounting brain, nerve, and liver damage.

A Troubling Trend

The most troubling indication that showed that the synthetic chemicals in cosmetics and shampoos may be leaching into our bodies was provided by the government-funded Human Adipose Tissue Survey. According to this study, almost every person tested showed measurable levels of petroleum-based, carcinogenic chemicals, such as toluene, benzene, and styrene, in their fatty tissues.[24]

This is why increasing numbers of health professionals are recommending personal care formulas that are completely natural and free of synthetic or petroleum-based ingredients.

"To stay healthy, people have to do more than just exercise and eat healthy," states former Denver physician Terry Friedmann, MD. "Consumers should also avoid personal care products that contain toxic synthetic ingredients that can penetrate the skin and accumulate in their tissues. In some cases, these products can have a greater impact on health than either diet or exercise."

Many of the skin care products found here contain wolfberry seed oil, a costly, unusual ingredient that makes important contributions to healthy skin. Along with wolfberry seed oil, these unique products contain MSM, an essential nutrient that has an unsurpassed ability to strengthen the skin.

"MSM is absolutely dynamite for the skin," said international fashion model Teri Williams Secrest, who was a cover model for Vogue Magazine. She continued: "In my experience, it is the single most important nutrient to support healthy skin and hair."

Ronald Lawrence, MD, PhD, agrees, "The importance of MSM for healthy skin and hair cannot be overemphasized. In my clinical practice, I have seen the difference that MSM makes. It is outstanding whether applied topically or taken as a dietary supplement."

In addition to wolfberry seed oil and MSM, these skin products also contain therapeutic-grade essential oils that have a long history of use in skin care. Pure Myrrh, Sandalwood, Geranium, Lavender, Ylang Ylang, Frankincense, and Roman Chamomile essential oils have been used to preserve the health of the skin throughout recorded history.

Also included in these personal care products is a proprietary blend of antioxidant herbal extracts such as ginkgo biloba, orange blossom, witch hazel, cucumber, horse chestnut, and aloe vera gel, as well as special blends of pure vegetable oils such as almond, jojoba, avocado, and rose hip seed oils.

"They feel fabulous on my skin," raved Kay Cansler, a former Director of Educational Diagnostics, in an interview. "Without question, these are products for the new millennium. I have been using them for six months, and I can feel and see a huge difference. I am very, very impressed."

Acne Treatment, Maximum Strength

This maximum-strength formula takes on acne and blemishes like pimples and blackheads. With maximum-strength salicylic acid naturally derived from Wintergreen essential oil, Tea Tree oil adds cleansing power, while Manuka oil fights blemishes. Extracts of chamomile make sure this formula also moisturizes, leaving your skin soft and smooth.

Ingredients: Active: Salicylic acid. Inactive: Water, Glycerin, Cetostearyl alcohol, Lactobacillus reuteri, Cetyl al-cohol, Coco-caprylate, Coconut alkanes, Cetearyl olivate, Aloe vera leaf, Starch-potato, Sorbitan olivate, Citric ac-id monohydrate, Sodium hydroxide, Xanthan gum, Coco-caprylate/caprate, Alpha-tocopherol acetate, Sunflow-er oil, Phytate sodium, Manuka oil, Frankincense oil, Rosemary leaf oil, Tea Tree oil, Geranium flower oil, Lavender oil, Chamomile, Salix alba bark, Tocopherol

Essential Oils: Manuka, Frankincense, Rosemary, Tea Tree, Geranium, Lavender

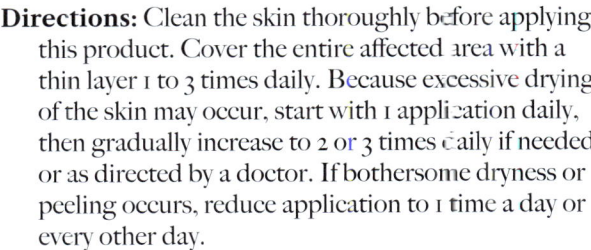

Directions: Clean the skin thoroughly before applying this product. Cover the entire affected area with a thin layer 1 to 3 times daily. Because excessive drying of the skin may occur, start with 1 application daily, then gradually increase to 2 or 3 times daily if needed or as directed by a doctor. If bothersome dryness or peeling occurs, reduce application to 1 time a day or every other day.

Caution: When using this product, skin irritation and dryness is more likely to occur if you use another topical acne medication at the same time. If irritation occurs, use only one topical acne medication at a time. If eye contact occurs, rinse thoroughly with water. If swallowed, get medical help or contact Poison Control right away.

Allergen Warning: Contains coconut/palm ingredients

ART® Beauty Masque

The ART Beauty Masque features a concentrated formula designed to soothe skin and leave it feeling healthier and looking more radiant. This exotic blend of orchid petals and essential oils helps nourish stressed areas and promotes a more youthful appearance. It is suitable for all skin types.

Ingredients: Water, Glycerin, Trehalose, Lactobacillus ferment, Sea water, Astragalus membranaceus root extract, Speranskia tuberculata whole plant extract, Morus alba leaf extract, Sodium hyaluronate, Orchid flower extract, Torenia concolor whole plant extract, Angelica polymorpha sinensis root extract, Boswellia carterii (Frankincense) resin extract, Safflower flower extract, Dipotassium glycyrrhizate, Kelp extract, Copaiba oil, Lime oil, Cedarwood wood oil, Vanilla fruit extract, Ocotea leaf oil, Lavender oil

Essential Oils: Stress Away blend: [Copaiba, Lime, Cedarwood, Ocotea, Lavender]

Directions: Wash and dry face. Remove masque from pouch and unfold with the plastic lining facing out. Place over entire face and remove the lining. Use hands to gently smooth masque for even coverage. Leave masque on for 20 minutes, then gently remove and discard. Use a damp cloth to remove any residue. For best results, use 3-4 times weekly in combination with ART Renewal Serum.

Cautions: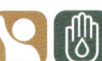

ART® Chocolate Masque

Available at Beauty School, the ART Chocolate Masque combines pure essential oils with exclusive Ecuadorian cacao to help nourish, soothe, and hydrate your skin.

Ingredients: Theobroma cocoa extract, Sacred Sandalwood oil, Frankincense oil, Geranium flower oil, Ylang Ylang flower oil

Essential Oils: Sacred Sandalwood, Frankincense, Geranium, Ylang Ylang

Directions: Place 1 piece of the ART Chocolate Masque in a double boiler pot. Allow chocolate to melt at a low temperature, not to exceed 113°F (about 45°C). Before applying, test the masque to ensure that it is not too hot. Apply using a facial brush, small spatula, or fingertips. Spread liberally over face and neck, avoiding the eyes and mouth. Leave masque on for 25-30 minutes and gently remove with lukewarm water. May also be used on hands.

Cautions: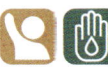

ART® Creme Masque

The ART Creme Masque is a blend of pure essential oils and spa-quality botanicals that help restore the look of youthfulness to the skin. We use hyaluronic acid and an exclusive blend of essential oils to moisturize and nourish skin, leaving it visibly more radiant. Other natural ingredients like cucumber extract, aloe vera, vitamin C, and green tea are added to soothe, protect, and tighten skin.

Ingredients: Water, Caprylic/capric triglycerides, Dicaprylyl carbonate, Hydroxypropyl starch phosphate, Sorbitol, Squalane, Cetearyl olivate, Sorbitan olivate, Aloe vera leaf juice, Oat kernel extract, Maltodextrin, Panthenol, Sodium hyaluronate, ART Creme Masque Essential Oil Blend: [Vetiver oil, Davana flower oil, Roman Chamomile flower oil, Ylang Ylang flower oil, Geranium flower oil, Vanilla oil 16x, Ocotea leaf oil, Jasmine oil], Coconut alkanes, Coco-caprylate/caprate, Camellia oleifera leaf extract, Pectin, Glycerin, Cetyl palmitate, Sorbitan palmitate, Tocopheryl acetate, Cucumber fruit extract, Xanthan gum, Caprylyl glycol, Phenoxyethanol, Sodium ascorbyl phosphate, Sodium gluconate, Soy lecithin, Hexylene glycol,

Essential Oils: Vetiver, Davana, Roman Chamomile, Ylang Ylang, Geranium, Vanilla, Ocotea, Jasmine,

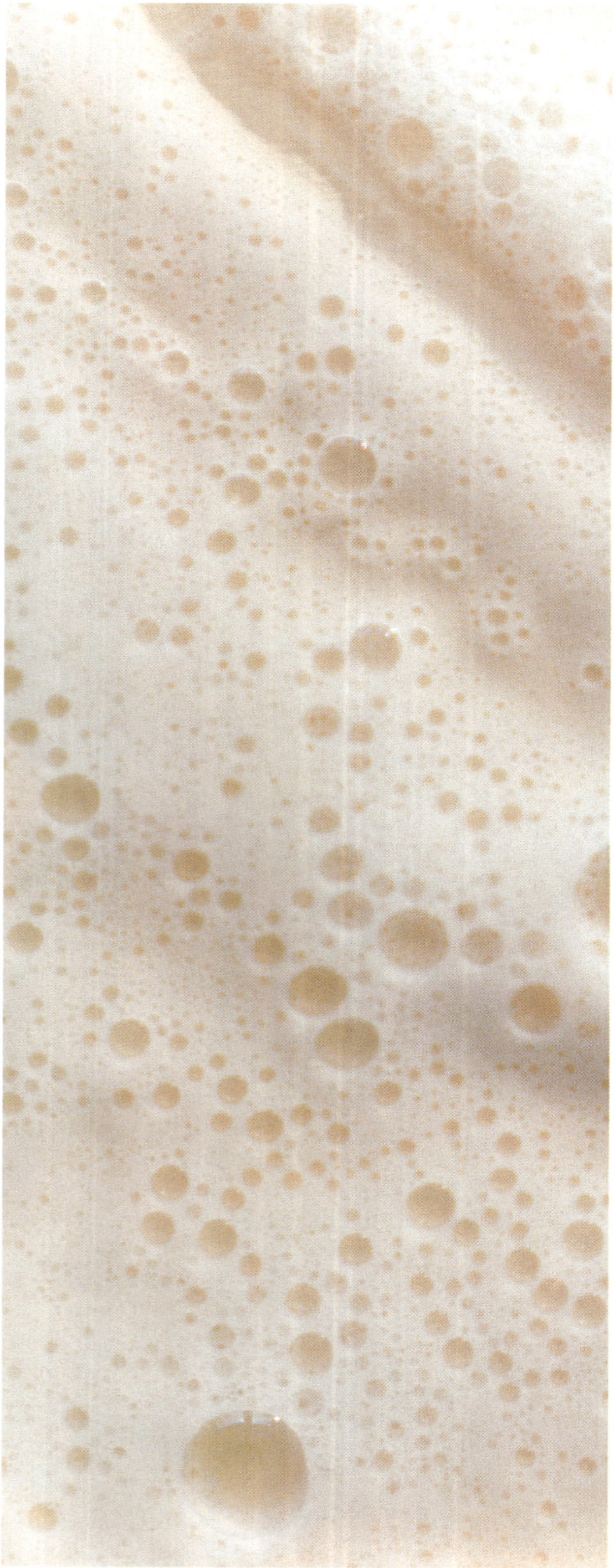

Directions: Wash and dry face. Apply evenly to face, avoiding eyes, and leave on for 20 minutes. Remove residue with moist towel. You may also use the masque overnight to help deepen the moisturizing effect. Use 2-3 times per week.

Cautions: Patch test on small area of face before use. Do not use if irritation or redness occurs.

Allergen Warning: Contains coconut/palm and soy products

ART® Gentle Cleanser

This unique foaming cleanser was designed to cleanse the skin by gently removing oil, dirt, and makeup.

ART Gentle Cleanser is formulated from naturally occurring sugars and contains ingredients that penetrate the epidermis to remove unwanted oils and impurities. One quarter of this cleanser is composed of pure, therapeutic-grade essential oils that were specifically selected for their skin-enhancing benefits.

Ingredients: Water, Disodium cocoyl glutamate, Coco-glucoside, Glycerin, Decyl glucoside, Polyglyceryl-4 caprate, Sodium cocoyl threoninate, Sodium cocoyl glutamate, Benzyl alcohol (natural), Glyceryl oleate, Sodium levulinate, Sodium anisate, Sodium phytate, Frankincense oil, Royal Hawaiian Sandalwood wood oil, Orchis mascula flower extract, Melissa leaf oil, Lemon peel oil, Lavender oil

Essential Oils: Frankincense, Royal Hawaiian Sandalwood, Melissa, Lemon, Lavender

Directions: Apply to wet hands and massage gently over face and neck with a circular motion. Rinse with warm water. Use 2 times daily for a refreshing cleanse in the morning and a thorough cleanse at night. It is suitable for all skin types.

Cautions:

Allergen Warning: Contains coconut/palm ingredients

ART® Intensive Moisturizer

ART Intensive Moisturizer is infused with exotic botanicals and essential oils, providing lasting hydration that produces the qualities of young-looking skin.

Ingredients: Water, Glycerin, Coco-caprylate, Cetearyl alcohol, Glyceryl stearate, Olive fruit unsaponifiables, Apple fruit extract, Astrocaryum murumuru seed butter, Diheptyl succinate, Capryloyl glycerin/sebacic acid co-polymer, Pentaclethra macroloba seed oil, Benzyl alcohol, Sodium stearoyl glutamate, Physalis angulata extract, Caprylic/capric triglyceride, Hinoki oil, Sodium levulinate, Royal Hawaiian Sandalwood wood oil, Cedarwood bark oil, Ylang Ylang flower oil, Frankincense oil, Alcohol denatured, Sodium anisate, Guar gum, Hibiscus syriacus callus extract, Terminalia ferdinandiana fruit extract, Xanthan gum, Sodium phytate, Sodium hyaluronate, Tocopherol, Sunflower seed oil

Essential Oils: Hinoki, Royal Hawaiian Sandalwood, Cedarwood, Ylang Ylang, Frankincense

Directions: Apply on clean, dry face and neck with an upward, outward motion. Use morning, night, and throughout the day.

Caution: Patch test on small area of face before use.

Allergen Warning: Contains coconut/palm ingredients

ART® Light Moisturizer

ART Light Moisturizer helps your skin retain proper hydration. With Young Living's essential oils and naturally derived ingredients, your face will feel soft and supple.

Ingredients: Water, Glycerin, Coco-caprylate, Coconut alkanes, Polyglyceryl-6 distearate, Cetearyl alcohol, Microcrystalline cellulose, Olive fruit unsaponifiables, Cupuacu seed butter, Benzyl alcohol (natural), Jojoba esters, Squalane, Sodium levulinate, Coco-caprylate/caprate, Cellulose gum, Cetyl alcohol, Polyglyceryl-3 beeswax, Royal Hawaiian Sandalwood wood oil, Xanthan gum, Sodium anisate, Senna alexandrina seed polysaccharide, Dipotassium glycyrrhizate, Prickly pear leaf cell extract, Frankincense oil, Summer snowflake bulb extract, Sodium phytate, Asteriscus graveolens flower/fruit/leaf/stem extract, Purple orchid flower extract, Aloe vera leaf juice, Tocopherol, Sunflower seed oil

Essential Oils: Royal Hawaiian Sandalwood, Frankincense

Directions: After cleansing and toning skin, apply moisturizer over dry face and neck. For best results, apply both morning and night and as needed throughout the day.

Cautions: Discontinue use if irritation occurs.

Allergen Warning: Contains coconut/palm and bee products

ART® Refreshing Toner

A necessary step in any comprehensive skin care regimen, ART Purifying Toner helps support cleansing by removing unwanted oil, dirt, and impurities that can accumulate on the skin.

Designed to work in synergy with the other products in the ART Skin Care System, the Purifying Toner contains the essential oils of Frankincense and Sandalwood for their ability to replenish and revitalize skin, Lemon and Peppermint to cleanse and energize, and Melissa and Lavender to soothe and balance.

This mild formula absorbs quickly and leaves skin feeling clean, smooth, and soft. It minimizes oily shine and reduces the appearance of pores.

Ingredients: Water, Alcohol, Heptyl glucoside, Witch hazel water, Glycerin, Betaine, Peppermint oil, Royal Hawaiian Sandalwood wood oil, Frankincense oil, Orchis mascula flower extract, Aloe vera leaf juice, Green tea leaf extract, Lavender oil, Lemon peel oil, Melissa leaf oil

Essential Oils: Peppermint, Royal Hawaiian Sandalwood, Frankincense, Lavender, Lemon, Melissa

Directions: Shake well. After cleansing, gently sweep over face and neck with a cotton ball. Use in the morning and evening as needed.

Cautions: Discontinue use if irritation occurs.

ART® Renewal Serum

ART Renewal Serum is an intricate blend of exotic botanicals chosen for their unique ability to soothe and protect the most delicate areas of the face. These premium ingredients work in harmony to deeply nourish, hydrate, and help restore youthfulness to skin.

Ingredients: Water, Glycerin, Selaginella lepidophylla extract, Lactobacillus ferment, Snow lotus whole plant extract, Vanilla extract, Niacinamide,

Astragalus membranaceus root extract, Glycine tomentella root extract, Morus alba leaf extract, Phalaenopsis orchid flower extract, Torenia concolor extract, Sodium hyaluronate, Ascorbyl glucoside, Matricaria (German Chamomile) flower oil, Myrrh resin oil, Frankincense oil, Spatholobus suberectus extract, Angelica polymorpha sinensis root extract, Liquidambar formosana fruit extract, Crocus sativus flower extract, Sensation Oil Blend: [Coriander seed oil, Ylang Ylang flower oil, Bergamot peel oil (Furocoumarin-free), Jasmine oil, Geranium flower oil]

Essential Oils: Sensation Blend: [Coriander, Ylang Ylang, Bergamot (Furocoumarin-free), Jasmine, Geranium]

Directions: Apply 2-3 pumps on clean skin before your moisturizer, morning and evening. Wash face. Apply to delicate areas of face 2 times daily and allow to absorb. For added moisture benefits, use ART Beauty Masque or ART Creme masque 2-3 times a week or as needed.

Cautions: Discontinue use if irritation occurs.

ART® Sheerlumé™ Brightening Cream (See also BLOOM Brightening Cream)

This advanced formula combines a perfect blend of essential oils with skin-nourishing ingredients to visibly brighten and balance skin tone, unveiling a more radiant, youthful-looking glow.

Ingredients: Water, Glycerin, Coconut alkanes, Caprylic/capric triglycerides, Glyceryl stearate SE, Cetearyl alcohol, Licorice root extract, Sodium stearoyl lactylate, Hydrocotyl extract, Theobroma grandiflorum seed butter, Physalis angulata extract, Batyl alcohol, Alcohol denat., Coco-caprylate/caprate, Plumeria acutifolia flower extract, Sodium PCA, Meadowfoam seed oil, Terminalia ferdinandia fruit extract, Lilium candidum leaf cell extract, Sodium citrate, Honeysuckle flower extract, Citric acid, Mallow extract, Peppermint leaf extract, Primula veris extract, Alchemilla vulgaris extract, Veronica officinalis extract, Melissa officinalis extract, Achillea millefolium extract, Honeysuckle flower extract, Sodium phytate, Tocopherol, Vetiver root oil, Blue Cypress wood oil, Davana flower oil, Royal Hawaiian Sandalwood wood oil, Clove bud oil, Jasmine flower extract, Carrot Seed oil, Spearmint leaf extract, Geranium flower oil, Sacred Frankincense oil

Essential Oils: Vetiver, Blue Cypress, Davana, Royal Hawaiian Sandalwood, Clove, Jasmine, Carrot Seed, Spearmint, Geranium, Sacred Frankincense

Directions: First, cleanse and tone skin, then apply a thin layer to face and neck, morning and night. For added moisture benefits, layer with your favorite Young Living moisturizer. May be used on the hands.

Cautions: Discontinue use if irritation occurs.

Allergen Warning: Contains corn, soy, and coconut/palm ingredients

BLOOM by Young Living Brightening Cleanser

BLOOM by Young Living Brightening Cleanser is a nourishing facial wash that reveals radiant skin while leaving your face feeling fresh and smooth.

Ingredients: Water, Disodium cocoyl glutamate, Decyl glucoside, Glycerin, Sodium laurylglucosides hydroxy-propylsulfonate, Glyceryl oleate citrate, Glyceryl Caprylate/Caprate, Sucrose cocoate, Plumeria acutifolia flower ex-tract, Sorbitan sesquicaprylate, Sodium lauroyl lactylate, Cetyl alcohol, Citric acid, Pentaclethra macroloba seed oil, Benzyl alcohol, Glyceryl caprylate, Caprylic/Capric triglyceride, Xanthan gum, Sodium levulinate, Licorice root extract, Cetearyl alcohol, Sodium PCA, Sodium chloride, Sodium nisate, Mica, Glyceryl undecylenate, Sodium hyaluronate, Sodium phytate, Titanium dioxide, Vetiver root oil, Blue Cypress wood oil, Davana flower oil, Royal Hawaiian Sandalwood wood oil, Clove bud oil, Jasmine oil, Carrot Seed oil, Spearmint leaf extract, Geranium flower oil, Frankincense oil, Alcohol, Tocopherol

Essential Oils: Vetiver, Blue Cypress, Davana, Royal Hawaiian Sandalwood, Clove, Jasmine, Carrot Seed, Spearmint, Geranium, Frankincense

Directions: Wet skin with lukewarm water and gently massage a small amount of cleanser into skin. Rinse thoroughly and pat dry, repeating both morning and night.

Cautions: Discontinue use if irritation occurs.

Allergen Warning: Contains coconut/palm ingredients

BLOOM by Young Living Brightening Essence

BLOOM by Young Living Brightening Essence helps brighten and improve your skin's complexion. This luminous, gel-textured essence infuses moisture into skin, boosting the absorption of your moisturizer.

Ingredients: Water, Glycerin, Apple fruit extract, Sea water, Levulinic acid, Xanthan gum, Benzoic acid, Licorice root extract, Sodium hyaluronate, Sodium levulinate, Sodium phytate, Caprylyl/capryl glucoside, Lepidium meyenii root extract, Maltodextrin, Lilium canadidum leaf cell extract, Mica, Sodium cocoyl glutamate, Phenethyl alcohol, Titanium dioxide, Glyceryl caprylate, Saccharide isomerate, Citric acid, Chlorella vulgaris extract, Polyglyceryl-6 oleate, Vetiver root oil, Blue Cypress wood oil, Davana flower oil, Lactic acid, Sodium surfactin, Royal Hawaiian Sandalwood wood oil, Clove bud oil, Jasmine oil, Carrot Seed oil, Spearmint leaf extract, Geranium flower oil, Frankincense oil

Essential Oils: Vetiver, Blue Cypress, Davana, Royal Hawaiian Sandalwood, Clove, Jasmine, Carrot Seed, Spearmint, Geranium, Frankincense

Directions: Gently shake before use. Pour a generous amount onto the palm of your hand. Rub hands together and lightly press palms into your skin from the center of face outward, including your neck and décolletage. Repeat morning and night.

Cautions: Discontinue use if irritation occurs.

Allergen Warning: Contains coconut/palm ingredients

BLOOM by Young Living Brightening Lotion

(See also ART Sheerlumé Brightening Cream)
BLOOM by Young Living Brightening Lotion, featuring the Sheerlumé™ Brightening Complex, is infused with the most advanced natural ingredients, brightening the skin's appearance while boosting natural radiance. Its lightweight hydration helps fortify the skin's moisture barrier and antioxidants help minimize the appearance of future damage.

Ingredients: Water, Glycerin, Caprylic/capric triglyceride, Glyceryl stearates, Sodium stearoyl lactylate, Plumeria acutifolia flower extract, Canarium indicum seed oil, Benzyl alcohol, Coconut alkanes, Sea water, Theobroma grandiflorum seed butter, Licorice root extract, Maltodextrin, Sodium levulinate, Sodium PCA, Lilium candidum leaf cell extract, Jojoba esters, Xanthum gum, Palmaria palmate extract, Alcohol, Centella asiatica extract, Sodium anisate, Sodium hyaluronate, Lecithin, Achillea millefolium extract, Alchemilla vulgaris extract, Mallow extract, Melissa officinalis leaf extract, Peppermint leaf extract, Primula veris extract, Veronica officinalis extract, Coco-caprylate/caprate, Sodium phytate, Alpinia officinarum root extract, Citric acid, Phenethyl alcohol, Vetiver root oil, Blue Cypress wood oil, Davana flower oil, Sodium carrageenan, Royal Hawaiian Sandalwood, Clove bud oil, Jasmine oil, Carrot Seed oil, Spearmint leaf extract, Geranium flower oil, Frankincense oil, Xylitol, Caprylic acid, Sea salt, Tocopherol

Essential Oils: Vetiver, Blue Cypress, Davana, Royal Hawaiian Sandalwood, Clove, Jasmine, Carrot Seed, Spear-mint, Geranium, Frankincense

Directions: Gently press and pat a small amount of cream evenly over face, neck and décolletage. Repeat morning and night.

Cautions: Discontinue use if irritation occurs.

Allergen Warning: Contains coconut/palm ingredients

Boswellia Wrinkle Cream™

Boswellia Wrinkle Cream contains the pure essential oils of Frankincense, Sandalwood, Myrrh, Ylang Ylang, and Geranium that moisturize while minimizing shine, relaxing facial tension, and reducing the effects of sun damage. It tones, refines, and brightens the appearance of maturing skin.

This wrinkle cream may help build collagen and when used daily may help minimize and prevent wrinkles.

Ingredients: Water, Cetearyl alcohol, Caprylic/capric triglyceride, Sweet almond seed extract, Glycerin, Glyceryl stearate, Olive fruit oil, Stearic acid, Barley extract, Sodium stearoyl lactylate, Geranium flower oil, Ylang Ylang flower oil, Sodium levulinate, Sorbic acid, Sandalwood wood extract, Phellodendron amurense bark extract, Shea Butter, Myrrh oil, Frankincense oil, Royal Hawaiian Sandalwood wood oil, Sodium anisate, Sodium hyaluronate, Allantoin, Xanthan gum, Panthenol, Sodium PCA, Wolfberry seed oil, Grape seed oil, Calendula officinalis flower extract, Roman Chamomile flower oil, Rose flower oil, Orange flower extract, St. John's wort flower/leaf/stem extract, Kelp extract, Ginkgo biloba leaf extract, Sodium phytate, Tocopheryl acetate, Retinyl palmitate, Aloe vera leaf juice, Sodium hydroxide, Citric acid

Essential Oils: Geranium, Ylang Ylang, Myrrh, Frankincense, Royal Hawaiian Sandalwood, Roman Chamomile, Rose

Directions: After cleansing skin, use upward strokes to apply a small amount to face and neck.

Cautions: Discontinue use if irritation occurs.

Allergen Warning: Contains coconut/palm and nut products

CBD Beauty Boost

The soothing ingredients of Nature's Ultra CBD Beauty Boost work to maintain an even skin tone and reduce the appearance of fine lines and wrinkles. Just one daily dropper of this Smart Spectrum blend will moisturize your skin and promote a youthful glow. It is ideal for all skin types, so it's the perfect way to pamper yourself every day.

Rose essential oil is produced by steam distilling Damask rose petals. Each dropper contains the oils from one full Damask rose.

This hemp-based product has been verified by an accredited third-party lab and contains 0.0 percent THC.

One full dropper contains 20 mg of naturally derived cannabidiol (CBD) from the USA. There are 30 full droppers per bottle.

Ingredients: Grape seed oil, Tamanu seed oil, Cannabidiol (CBD), Tocopherol, Rose flower oil, Sunflower seed oil

Essential Oils: Rose

Directions: For best results, shake well before use. Add ¼-1 dropper (according to preference) in the palm of your hand and mix with your favorite Young Living beauty products. Apply evenly to face, neck, chest, or anywhere you could use a moisturizing boost.

Cautions: Not intended for children or women who are pregnant or breastfeeding.

ClaraDerm™

ClaraDerm spray soothes dry, chapped, or itchy skin. Its gentle blend is particularly helpful in relieving skin irritations, burning, and itching in sensitive female areas.

Its formula can assist in controlling rashes, candida, etc. It is especially suited for the vaginal area before and after childbirth. ClaraDerm is expertly formulated with a blend of Lavender, Frankincense, and other essential oils.

Ingredients: Caprylic/capric triglyceride, Myrrh oil, Tea Tree leaf oil, Lavender oil, Frankincense oil, Helichrysum flower oil, Roman Chamomile flower oil

Essential Oils: Myrrh, Tea Tree, Lavender, Frankincense, Helichrysum, Roman Chamomile

Directions: Spray topically as needed. ClaraDerm may be used before and after childbirth.

Cautions: Possible skin/surface area sensitivity.

Allergen Warning: Contains coconut/palm ingredients

Insect Repellent

At last, protection from insects without synthetic chemicals like DEET and phthalates! Young Living's Insect Repellent is made of naturally derived, plant-based ingredients.

Ingredients: Sesame oil, Citronella oil, Lemongrass oil, Rosemary oil, Geranium oil, Spearmint oil, Thyme oil, Clove oil, Vitamin E

Essential Oils: Citronella, Lemongrass, Rosemary, Geranium, Spearmint, Thyme, Clove

Directions: Dispense into hand and apply evenly over exposed skin. Reapply as needed. Animals: Suitable for use on animals. When applying to animals, wipe on desired area on animal. Avoid contact with animal's eyes, nose, mouth, and open wounds.

Cautions: Causes eye irritation. Adult supervision required when applying to children. Do not apply to children's hands. Prolonged or frequently repeated skin contact may cause allergic reactions in some individuals. Avoid contact with clothing, as product can stain fabrics.

LavaDerm™ After-Sun Spray

Menthol from mint, with cooling and skin-supporting Lavender and Helichrysum essential oils, will ease itchy, irritated skin from sunburn or insect bites. LavaDerm After-Sun Spray will return the joy to your outdoor time. It is formulated without alcohol, parabens, phthalates, petrochemicals, animal-derived ingredients, synthetic preservatives, and synthetic fragrances.

Ingredients: Active: Menthol. Inactive: Water, Olive oil, Glycerin, Safflower oil, Sunflower oil, Jojoba oil, Polyglyceryl-10 pentastearate, Glyceryl monocaprylate, Helianthus annuus seed wax, European elderberry, Xanthan gum, Docosanol, Sodium stearoyl lactylate, Lavender oil, aloe vera leaf, Glyceryl monoundecylenate, Phytate sodium, Northern Lights Black Spruce oil, Helichrysum flower oil, Citric acid

Essential Oils: Lavender, Northern Lights Black Spruce, Helichrysum

Directions: Shake well. Adults and children 2 years of age and older: Apply to affected area not more than 3 to 4 times daily. Children under 2 years of age, ask a doctor.

Cautions: Stop use and ask a doctor if condition worsens or if symptoms last more than 7 days or clear up and occur again within a few days. If swallowed, get medical help or contact Poison Control right away.

LavaDerm Cooling Mist™

Lavender essential oil has been highly regarded as a burn treatment since cosmetic chemist René Gattefossé used the oil to heal a severe burn he suffered in a laboratory explosion. Lavender oil has both antiseptic properties and an ability to reduce the formation of scar tissue.

LavaDerm Cooling Mist assists in the healing of most topical burns, ranging from sunburn to second-degree thermal burns. It also contains a highly purified concentrate of aloe vera gel, freshly processed from the leaves of Aloe barbadensis.

Ingredients: Water, Aloe vera leaf extract, Glycerin, Potassium sorbate, Sodium levulinate, Lavender oil, Sodium anisate, Trace mineral complex, Northern Lights Black Spruce oil, Helichrysum flower oil, Citric acid

Essential Oils: Lavender, Northern Lights Black Spruce, Helichrysum

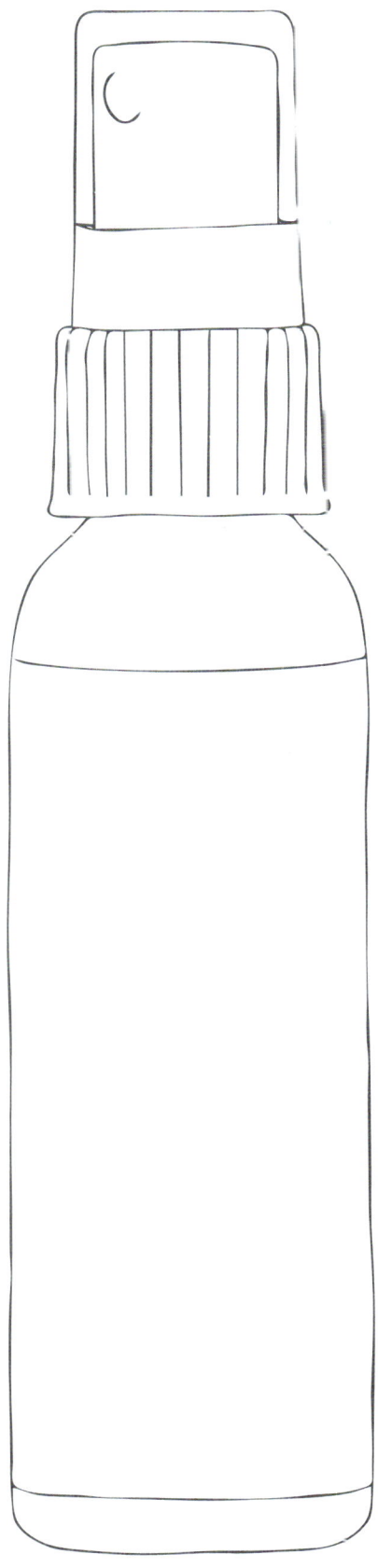

Directions: Shake well before use. Spray evenly over desired area. Repeat every 10-15 minutes as needed to keep the skin cool and promote tissue regeneration.

Cautions: Discontinue use if irritation occurs.

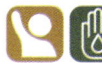

Mineral Sunscreen Lotion – SPF 50

Now you can have sun protection without harsh chemicals! Young Living's Mineral Sunscreen Lotion – SPF 50 protects with plant- and mineral-based ingredients. The non-greasy lotion is fast-absorbing and provides powerful, high-sun protection against UVA and UVB rays without synthetic UV-blocking ingredients. This leaves no white residue and is dermatologist tested.

Ingredients: Active: Zinc oxide. Inactive: Medium-chain triglycerides, Yellow wax, Castor oil, Coco-caprylate/caprate, Coconut oil, Tocopherol, Polyglyceryl-3 ricinoleate, Sunflower oil, Isostearic acid, Helichrysum flower oil, Lavender oil, Myrrh oil, Labdanum (Cistus) oil, Ylang Ylang flower oil, Carrot seed oil, Frankincense oil

Essential Oils: Helichrysum, Lavender, Myrrh, Labdanum (Cistus), Ylang Ylang, Carrot Seed, Frankincense

Directions: Apply liberally 15 minutes before sun exposure. Reapply after 80 minutes of swimming or sweating, immediately after towel drying, and at least every 2 hours. For children under 6 months, ask a doctor.

Cautions: Rinse with water to remove. Do not use on damaged or broken skin.

Allergen Warning: Contains coconut/palm ingredients

Mirah™ Luminous Cleansing Oil

With soothing essential oils of Sacred Sandalwood and Rose, Mirah Luminous Cleansing Oil leaves your complexion clean and well-hydrated.

Ingredients: Sunflower seed oil, Grape seed oil, Caprylic/capric triglyceride, Jojoba seed oil, Isoamyl laurate, Meadowfoam seed oil, Polyglyceryl-2 sesquioleate, Kukui seed oil, Babassu kernel oil, Polyglyceryl-2 caprate, Argan kernel oil, Rice bran extract, Watermelon seed oil, Marula seed oil, Sacred Sandalwood oil, Rosemary leaf oil, Bergamot peel oil, Ylang Ylang flower oil, Geranium flower oil, Lemon peel oil, Sunflower extract, Tocopherol, Coriander seed oil, Tangerine peel oil, Jasmine oil, Roman Chamomile flower oil, Palmarosa oil, Rose flower oil

Essential Oils: Sacred Sandalwood, Rosemary, Bergamot, Ylang Ylang, Geranium, Lemon, Coriander, Tangerine, Jasmine, Roman Chamomile, Palmarosa, Rose

Directions: Apply 3-4 pumps to dry hands and massage onto face to cleanse and remove makeup. Rinse with warm water.

Cautions:

Allergen Warning: Contains coconut/palm ingredients

Orange Blossom Facial Wash

This gentle, soap-free facial wash cleanses the skin without stripping natural oils. It contains MSM for softening, kelp to improve elasticity, and Lavender to soothe acne-prone skin and other problem areas.

Ingredients: Water, Decyl glucoside, Glycerin, Aloe vera leaf juice, Coco-glucoside, Glyceryl oleate, Glyceryl caprylate, Citric acid, Xanthan gum, Sunflower seed oil, Balsam copaiba resin, Lavender oil, Levulinic acid, Glyceryl undecylenate, Carapa guaianensis seed oil, Euterpe oleracea fruit oil, Sodium levulinate, Patchouli oil, Rosemary leaf oil, Lemon peel oil, Calendula officinalis flower extract, Camellia sinensis leaf extract, Matricaria flower extract, Chlorella vulgaris extract, Orange flower extract, Orange peel extract, Lemon peel extract, Hypericum perforatum flower/leaf/stem extract, Kelp extract, Apple fruit extract, Rosa centifolia flower extract, Sugarcane extract

Essential Oils: Lavender, Patchouli, Rosemary, Lemon

Directions: Wet your face with warm water. Put a small amount of wash into the palm of your hand. Gently lather over face and neck with warm water. Rinse and pat dry.

Cautions: Discontinue use if irritation occurs.

Allergen Warning: Contains wheat product and coconut/palm ingredients

Orange Blossom Moisturizer

Apply this refreshing moisturizer after cleansing face and neck. The rich botanicals will leave your skin soft and enriched.

Ingredients: Water, Caprylic/capric triglyceride, Glycerin, Glyceryl stearate, Coco-caprylate, Cetearyl alcohol, Leuconostoc/radish root ferment filtrate, Olive fruit oil, Cocoa seed butter, Microcrystalline cellulose, Grape seed oil, Rose hips fruit oil, Andiroba seed oil, Coconut oil, Xanthan gum, Cellulose gum, Sunflower seed oil, Tocopherol acetate, Lavender oil, Ruttnera lamellosa oil, Citric acid, Licorice root extract, Sodium phytate, Patchouli oil, Rosemary leaf oil, Lemon peel oil, Tocopherol, Camellia sinensis leaf extract, Orange peel extract, Lemon peel extract, Lecithin, Apple fruit extract, Sugarcane extract, Calendula officinalis flower extract, Matricaria flower extract, Chlorella vulgaris extract, Orange flower extract, Hypericum perforatum flower/leaf/stem extract, Kelp extract, Rosa centifolia flower extract

Essential Oils: Lavender, Patchouli, Rosemary, Lemon

Directions: Cleanse face and neck with Orange Blossom Facial Wash or preferred cleanser. After patting face dry, apply Orange Blossom Moisturizer morning and night, or as needed. Non-comedogenic; does not clog pores.

Cautions:

Rose Ointment™

Rose Ointment is a deeply soothing and nourishing blend for dry skin. Rose essential oil and vitamin A improve skin texture, while Tea Tree and Rose work to rejuvenate rough, irritated skin.

Use Rose Ointment over essential oils to lock in their benefits. Though not recommended for burns initially, this ointment can be very beneficial in maintaining, protecting, and keeping the scab soft.

Ingredients: Sunflower seed wax, Astrocaryum murumuru seed butter, Caprylic/capric triglyceride, Sunflower seed oil, Raspberry seed oil, Castor seed oil, Jojoba seed oil, Marula seed oil, Avocado oil, Argan kernel oil, Rhus verniciflua peel wax, Passionfruit seed oil, Tocopherol, Rose hip seed extract, Pomegranate seed oil, Glycerin, Sea Buckthorn fruit oil, Palmarosa oil, Patchouli oil, Coriander seed oil, Myrrh oil, Grape seed extract, Bergamot peel oil (Furocoumarin-free), Carrot Seed oil, Tea Tree leaf oil, Ascorbyl palmitate, Ylang Ylang flower oil, Geranium flower oil, Rose flower oil

Essential Oils: Palmarosa, Patchouli, Coriander, Myrrh, Bergamot (Furocoumarin-free), Carrot Seed, Tea Tree, Ylang Ylang, Geranium, Rose

Directions: Apply to desired areas several times a day. Can be used with or without essential oils. If essential oils are used, apply oils to skin first. Do not use on heat-stressed skin.

Cautions:

Allergen Warning: Contains wheat, coconut/palm, and bee products.

Sandalwood Moisture Cream™

Sandalwood Moisture Cream is an ultra-hydrating moisturizer infused with pure essential oils. MSM—a naturally occurring, plant-based chemical—softens skin and promotes elasticity. When used daily after cleansing and toning, this moisture cream promotes younger, healthier skin.

Ingredients: Water, Glycerin, Cetearyl alcohol, Glyceryl stearate, Caprylic/capric triglycerides, Olive fruit oil, Stearic acid, Pichia anomala extract, Barley extract, Sodium stearoyl lactylate, Shea butter, Sandalwood extract, Phellodendron amurense bark extract, Sodium levulinate, Sorbic acid, Coriander seed oil, Royal Hawaiian Sandalwood, Lavender oil, Sodium anisate, Allantoin, Xanthan gum, Ascorbic acid, Sodium PCA, Bergamot peel oil (Furocoumarin-free), Myrrh oil, Hydrolyzed wheat protein, Rose hips seed oil, Wolfberry seed oil, Calendula officinalis flower extract, Chamomile flower extract, Ginkgo biloba leaf extract, Grape seed oil, Kelp extract, Orange flower extract, Rosebud flower extract, St. John's wort extract, Rosemary leaf oil, Sodium phytate, Tocopheryl acetate, Retinyl palmitate, Hydrolyzed wheat starch, Ylang Ylang flower oil, Aloe vera leaf juice, Geranium flower oil, Sodium hyaluronate, Sodium hydroxide, Citric acid

Essential Oils: Coriander, Royal Hawaiian Sandalwood, Lavender, Bergamot (Furocoumarin-free), Myrrh, Rosemary, Ylang Ylang, Geranium

Directions: Massage a generous amount gently onto face, neck, and other desired areas using gentle, upward strokes. Use daily after cleansing and toning your skin.

Cautions: Discontinue use if irritation occurs.

Allergen Warning: Contains wheat and coconut/palm products.

Satin Facial Scrub, Mint™

Satin Facial Scrub, Mint is a gentle, exfoliating scrub designed for normal skin. It contains jojoba oil, mango butter, MSM, aloe, and Peppermint essential oil to minimize the appearance of pores and rejuvenate dull skin.

This revolutionary formula gently eliminates layers of dead skin cells and can be used as a drying face mask to draw impurities from the skin.

Ingredients: Water, Decyl glucoside, Glycerin, Caprylic/capric triglyceride, Xanthan gum, Sunflower seed oil, Apricot seed powder, Glyceryl caprylate, Pectin, Mango seed butter, Stearic acid, Cetearyl alcohol, Coconut oil, Peppermint oil, Coco-glucoside, Glyceryl oleate, Levulinic acid, Glyceryl undecylenate, Stearyl alcohol, Cetearyl glucoside, Sodium levulinate, Tocopheryl acetate, Citric acid, Raspberry fruit extract, Tocopherol, Cetyl alcohol, Arachidyl alcohol

Essential Oils: Peppermint

Directions: Apply directly to moistened skin in a circular motion. Rinse thoroughly; pat dry.

Cautions: Discontinue use if irritation occurs.

Allergen Warning: Contains wheat, coconut, and soy products.

Shutran® 3-in-1 Men's Wash

This triple-combination body wash cleanses face, hair, and skin. Rich in essential and vegetable oils, Shutran 3-in-1 Men's Wash is hypoallergenic and will nourish skin and banish dryness.

Ingredients: Water, Decyl glucoside, Glycerin, Sodium laurylglucosides hydroxypropylsulfonate, PCA glyceryl oleate, Xanthan gum, Glyceryl caprylate, Sodium caproyl/lauroyl lactylate, Pumpkin seed extract, Sodium chloride, Sodium levulinate, Virola sebifera nut oil, Glyceryl undecylenate, Idaho Blue Spruce branch/leaf/wood oil, Sodium phytate, Aloe vera leaf juice powder, Nigella sativa seed extract, Ylang Ylang flower oil, Ocotea leaf oil, Hinoki oil, Davana flower oil, Cedarwood bark oil, Lavender oil, Coriander seed oil, Lemon peel oil, Northern Lights Black Spruce leaf oil, Citric acid

Essential Oils: Idaho Blue Spruce, Ylang Ylang, Ocotea, Hinoki, Davana, Cedarwood, Lavender, Coriander, Lemon, Northern Lights Black Spruce

Directions: Lather over hair, body, and face. Rinse.

Cautions:

Wolfberry Eye Cream™

Wolfberry Eye Cream is a natural, water-based moisturizer. Containing the antiaging properties of wolfberry seed oil, this cream soothes tired eyes and minimizes the appearance of bags, circles, and fine lines.

Ingredients: Water, Sorbitol, Glycerin, Cetearyl alcohol, Glyceryl stearate, Sodium stearoyl lactylate, Oat kernel extract, Stearic acid, Caprylic/capric triglycerides, Alfalfa seed extract, Hydrolyzed lupine protein, levulinic acid, p-Anisic acid, Sandalwood extract, Phellodendron amurense bark extract, Barley extract, Olive fruit oil, Lavender oil, Coriander seed oil, Roman Chamomile flower oil, Frankincense oil, Geranium flower oil, Bergamot peel oil (Furocoumarin-free), Ylang Ylang flower oil, Wolfberry seed oil, Avocado oil, Kukui seed oil, Rose hips seed oil, Sweet almond oil, Jojoba seed oil, Mango seed butter, Sorbic acid, Witch hazel extract, Allantoin, Xanthan gum, Shea butter, Retinyl palmitate, Sodium PCA, Ascorbyl palmitate, cucumber fruit extract, Hydrolyzed soy protein, Hydrolyzed wheat protein, Hydrolyzed wheat starch, Horse chestnut seed extract, Centella asiatica extract, Sodium phytate, Sodium hyaluronate, Green tea leaf extract, Ascorbic acid, Sodium hydroxide, Citric acid

Essential Oils: Lavender, Coriander, Roman Chamomile, Frankincense, Geranium, Bergamot (Furocoumarin-free), Ylang Ylang

Directions: After cleansing and toning, massage gently onto soft skin under eyes. Use in the evening.

Cautions: Discontinue use if irritation occurs.

Allergen Warning: Contains corn, gluten, nut, soy, and coconut/palm ingredients.

SOAPS, ALL NATURAL

The Body's Largest Organ: The Skin

With skin covering approximately 22 square feet on the outside surface of the human body, it is the largest human organ and the first line of defense against harmful substances, infection, and dehydration. In adults, the skin is between 15 and 20 percent of total body weight.

Because of its large surface area, the skin can soak in many types of toxins and petrochemicals. This can result in cancer-causing compounds leaching into the body and accumulating in fat.

Many people complain that commercial soaps make their skin feel dry and itchy, or worse. Trapped "free alkali" is the most common irritant in soap, which is made from oils (acids) mixed with water and alkali (a base).

Acids and bases neutralize each other to form a salt—in this case, soap—with glycerin as a byproduct.

Oils that do not combine with the alkali are "free," which creates a "superfatted" soap. These mild soaps are exceptionally good for the skin, even though they have a reduced lather and shelf life. Alkali that is not neutralized by essential oils is "free alkali," which makes soap harsh and drying.

The handcrafting process for natural soap removes the excess alkali that is left in commercial soaps.

Benefits of Handmade, Natural Soaps

Handcrafted in small batches, natural bar soaps are not only pure, natural, and nontoxic, but they are also good for the skin.

Handmade soaps have a "hand-lotion-in-the-soap" effect, created by the natural vegetable oils and waxes in the soap, as well as an emulsion of water and glycerin that is formed when the soap was made. While the "hand-lotion-in-the-soap" effect may reduce lathering, this is what makes handmade soap extraordinarily mild and moisturizing for dry and sensitive skin.

Secret to Creating the Best Handmade Soap

The best handmade soaps are made exclusively with natural ingredients that are blended in small batches and poured into wooden block molds.

The soap is then wire cut into bars, dried on oak frames, and aged for over four weeks in a humidity- and temperature-controlled curing room. The extended curing process is usually time consuming and expensive, but it effectively eliminates most of the free alkali from the bar soap, a major cause of dryness and irritation.

Handmade, natural soap can be made from a number of vegetable ingredients, such as the saponified oils of palm, coconut, and olive and may include pure,

Safe, Natural Products (Do-It-Yourself)

First-aid Spray
Ingredients
- 2 drops Lavender
- 3 drops Tea Tree
- 2 drops Cypress
- 3 droppers (for dropping each oil into spray bottle)
- 8 oz. distilled water
- 1 spray bottle
- 1 sterile gauze pad

Directions

This first-aid spray is for minor cuts and abrasions. If you have a serious cut or wound, consult your physician.

Pour distilled water into spray bottle. Add the drops of essential oils, and shake to mix. Clean all cuts and abrasions thoroughly and then spray the area with the first-aid spray.

You may want to cover the area with the sterile gauze to which you have applied 3 drops of Lavender.

This application should be repeated 2 times daily as necessary. After 3 days, you should allow the cut or abrasion to be exposed to the air, if possible.

Spa Foot Scrub
Ingredients
- $\frac{1}{4}$ cup sea salt or Epsom salts
- Almond, coconut, avocado, or grape seed oil
- 10 to 15 drops of Lavender

Directions

Treat your feet to a luxurious spa experience to exfoliate and pamper your feet. Mix ingredients and massage your feet with this mixture, which will soothe and soften your feet. Be sure to rinse and dry your feet when finished.

therapeutic-grade essential oils. In addition, rosemary extract can be used as a natural preservative.

The result is a soap that does more than just cleanse the skin. It can also act as a therapeutic skin treatment with powerful antioxidant and skin-protecting properties that may be used to treat eczema, psoriasis, dermatitis, pigmentation, inflammation, and more.

"Natural" Can be Unnatural

Unfortunately, the term "natural" can be used in very deceptive ways. If an ingredient is a five-generation derivative of coconut meat, some will claim it to be natural, even if you can't pronounce the name of the ingredient.

The main ingredients in many mass-produced bar soaps are substances known as "sodium tallowate" and "potassium tallowate." These are the fatty remains of slaughtered cows, sheep, and horses.

Brains, fatty tissues, and other unwanted parts of dead and sometimes diseased animals are collected into large vats and used to create "tallow." This tallow is shipped to commercial soap makers, where it is processed into bar soaps.

Unfortunately, the U.S. Food and Drug Administration does not regulate the ingredients in soap.

Some ingredients in mass-marketed soap, including isopropyl alcohol, fragrances, DEA, FD&C colors, propylene glycol, and triclosan, have been proven harmful to human health.

Isopropyl alcohol's drying effects can remove the skin's protective oils and cause irritation.

DEA (diethanolamine) is a hormone-disrupting chemical known to form cancer-causing nitrates and nitrosa-mines. Dr. Samuel Epstein of the University of Illinois has found that repeated skin applications of DEA-based detergents resulted in a major increase in the incidence of liver and kidney cancers.

Regarding coal tar-derived FD&C colors, A Consumer's Dictionary of Cosmetic Ingredients states that "many pigments cause skin sensitivity and irritation . . ., and absorption (of certain colors) can cause depletion of oxygen in the body and death."[25]

Instead of synthetic colors, German Chamomile may be used. Rich in chamazulene, an intense blue pigment, German Chamomile actually has anti-inflammatory properties that accelerate skin healing.

Moreover, other compounds in German Chamomile and other essential oils combine therapeutic action with delightful aromas.

Peppermint oil imparts a delightfully fresh fragrance to soap, while containing compounds such as menthol that act as pain relievers and anti-inflammatory agents.

Sadly, many of the compounds in the commercial fragrances used in bath and body products are carcinogenic or otherwise toxic.

The word "fragrance" on a soap label refers to over 4,000 ingredients, most of which are synthetic.

Not only are fragrances potentially carcinogenic, but according to Home Safe Home author Debra Lynn Dadd, "Clinical observation by medical doctors has shown that exposure to synthetic fragrances can affect the central nervous system, causing depression, hyperactivity, irritability, inability to cope and other behavioral changes."[26]

A surprising number of people experience a dry-skin reaction from many common synthetic fragrances.

BAR SOAPS

Moisturizing, all-natural bar soaps are created through a proprietary soap-making process derived from a 16th century Spanish recipe that was combined with modern technology and a proprietary blend of ultra-pure ingredients.

Hand poured and cured for almost a month, these bar soaps are unlike any other soaps on earth. Mild and long-lasting, the soaps are made with pure, therapeutic-grade essential oils that are redefining natural skin therapy.

Benefits

- Contain less than 1 percent free alkali; the proprietary soap-making process minimizes the presence of irritating, skin-drying, alkali salts
- Use a moisturizing, vegetable base that contains over 50 percent moisturizers
- Include pure, therapeutic-grade essential oils, many of which have been studied for their antiseptic, anti-inflammatory, and antifungal properties and are added at the optimum moment of the soap-making process to preserve their beneficial compounds
- Contain only the finest organic ingredients, including:
- Saponified oils of palm, coconut, jojoba, and olive
- Organic oatmeal
- Pure, therapeutic-grade essential oils

- Ningxia wolfberry seed oil
- Liquid aloe vera extract
- Rosemary extract (as an antioxidant)
- Glycerin

Charcoal Bar Soap

Natural charcoal's gentle exfoliating power will help cleanse the pores of impurities and deodorize the skin, while Young Living's Orange Blossom essential oil blend helps the skin stay hydrated and moisturized.

Ingredients: Sodium palmate, Sodium palm kernelate, Water, Glycerin, Olive fruit oil, Lavender oil, Charcoal powder, Sodium gluconate, Patchouli oil, Rosemary leaf oil, Lemon peel oil, Wolfberry seed oil, Jojoba seed oil, Sunflower seed oil, Oat bran, Aloe vera leaf extract, Orange flower extract

Essential Oils: Lavender, Patchouli, Rosemary, Lemon

Directions: Work soap into a lather with water. Apply generously to face and body. Rinse thoroughly.

Cautions: If contact occurs, flush eyes liberally with clean, cool water for several minutes. If redness or irritation occurs, discontinue use. If symptoms persist, contact your physician.

Allergen Warning: Contains coconut/palm products.

Lavender-Oatmeal Bar Soap

Lavender-Oatmeal Bar Soap is a gentle formula that creates a creamy lather with a relaxing and calming scent. It naturally cleanses and is suitable for all skin types, making a soap that the whole family can enjoy. It is formulated with 100 percent vegetable base and naturally derived ingredients, which includes oats that gently exfoliate and remove flaky, dull skin and excess oil. Infused with five therapeutic-grade essential oils, it moisturizes and soothes skin for a more radiant appearance and a soft, supple feeling.

Ingredients: Sodium palmate, Sodium palm kernelate, Water, Glycerin, Oat kernel flour, Olive fruit oil, Laven-der oil, Sodium gluconate, Caprylic/capric triglyceride, Coriander seed oil, Oat bran, Bergamot peel oil (Furocoumarin-free), Jojoba seed oil, Wolfberry seed oil, Oat kernel meal, Aloe vera leaf extract, Rosemary leaf extract, Ylang Ylang flower oil, Geranium flower oil

Essential Oils: Lavender, Coriander, Bergamot (Furocoumarin-free), Ylang Ylang, Geranium

Directions: Work soap into a lather with water. Apply generously to face and body. Rinse thoroughly.

Cautions: If contact occurs, flush eyes liberally with clean, cool water for several minutes. If redness or irritation occurs, discontinue use. If symptoms persist, contact your physician.

Allergen Warning: Contains coconut/palm products.

Lemon-Sandalwood Cleansing Soap

Lemon-Sandalwood Cleansing Soap is cleansing and purifying to the skin. Lemon oil is highly antifungal, so this soap can be effective at combating ringworm, athlete's foot, and other fungal infections. Sandalwood has been shown to protect the skin against viruses such as the human papilloma virus, which is related to herpes.

Ingredients: Sodium palmate, Sodium palm kernelate, Water, Glycerin, Lemon peel oil, Olive fruit oil, Sodium gluconate, Royal Hawaiian Sandalwood wood oil, Jojoba seed oil, Wolfberry seed oil, Oat bran, Aloe vera leaf extract, Rosemary leaf extract,

Essential Oils: Lemon, Royal Hawaiian Sandalwood

Directions: Work soap into a lather with water. Apply generously to face and body. Rinse thoroughly.

Cautions: If contact occurs, flush eyes liberally with clean, cool water for several minutes. If redness or irritation occurs, discontinue use. If symptoms persist, contact your physician.

Morning Start® Moisturizing Soap

Morning Start Moisturizing Soap contains Lemongrass, Peppermint, Rosemary, and Juniper oils that revitalize the mind and awaken the skin each morning. Lemongrass has been documented as a powerful antifungal agent in clinical studies, ideal for combating ringworm, athlete's foot, and other fungal skin conditions.

Ingredients: Sodium palmate, Sodium palm kernelate, Water, Glycerin, Olive fruit oil, Lemongrass oil, Rosemary leaf oil, Juniper oil, Peppermint oil, Jojoba seed oil, Wolfberry seed oil, Oat bran, Aloe vera leaf extract, Rosemary leaf extract

Essential Oils: Lemongrass, Rosemary, Juniper, Peppermint

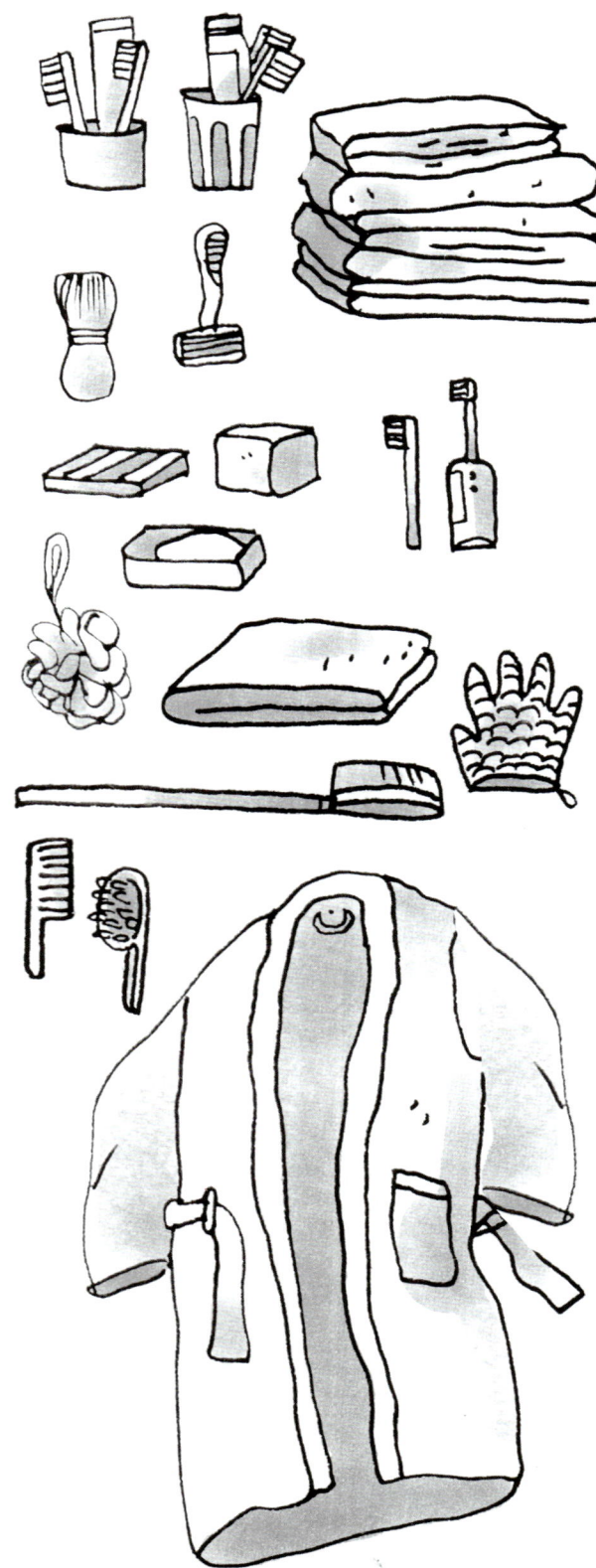

Directions: Work soap into a lather with water. Apply generously to face and body. Rinse thoroughly.

Cautions: If contact occurs, flush eyes liberally with clean, cool water for several minutes. If redness or irritation occurs, discontinue use. If symptoms persist, contact your physician.

Peppermint-Cedarwood Moisturizing Soap

Peppermint-Cedarwood Moisturizing Soap offers ultra-cleansing benefits to cleanse and invigorate the skin. It also contains a blend of essential oils designed to combat pain and itching. Analgesic and pain-relieving, Peppermint-Cedarwood Moisturizing Soap eases tendon, ligament, bone, and muscle pain.

Ingredients: Sodium palmate, Sodium palm Kernelate, Water, Glycerin, Peppermint oil, Olive fruit oil, Sodium gluconate, Cedarwood wood oil, Jojoba seed oil, Wolfberry seed oil, Oat bran, Aloe vera leaf extract, Rosemary leaf extract

Essential Oils: Peppermint, Cedarwood

Directions: Work soap into a lather with water. Apply generously to face and body. Rinse thoroughly.

Cautions: If contact occurs, flush eyes liberally with clean, cool water for several minutes. If redness or irritation occurs, discontinue use. If symptoms persist, contact your physician.

Sacred Mountain™ Moisturizing Soap

Sacred Mountain Moisturizing Soap soothes dehydrated skin, and the essential oil blend of Sacred Mountain promotes feelings of protection and empowerment. Designed for oily skin, this soap dissolves away excess sebum and gently exfoliates.

Ingredients: Sodium palmate, Sodium palm kernelate, Water, Glycerin, Olive fruit oil, Black Spruce leaf oil, Ylang Ylang flower oil, Sodium gluconate, Idaho Grand Fir needle oil, Jojoba seed oil, Wolfberry seed oil, Cedarwood wood oil, Oat bran, Aloe vera leaf extract, Rosemary leaf extract

Essential Oils: Black Spruce, Ylang Ylang, Idaho Grand Fir, Cedarwood

Directions: Work soap into a lather with water. Apply generously to face and body. Rinse thoroughly.

Cautions: If contact occurs, flush eyes liberally with clean, cool water for several minutes. If redness or irritation occurs, discontinue use. If symptoms persist, contact your physician.

Shutran® Bar Soap

Enriched with aloe, wolfberry seed oil, and Shutran essential oil blend, this vegan-friendly bar soap's creamy lather leaves skin feeling smooth, clean, and refreshed.

Ingredients: Sodium palmate, Sodium palm kernelate, Water, Glycerin, Olive fruit oil, Shea butter, Idaho Blue Spruce branch/leaf/wood oil, Sodium gluconate, Ylang Ylang flower oil, Ocotea leaf oil, Hinoki oil, Wolfberry seed oil, Jojoba seed oil, Davana flower oil, Cedarwood bark oil, Lavender oil, Coriander seed oil, Lemon peel oil, Carbon, Northern Lights Black Spruce oil, Aloe leaf extract, Rosemary leaf oil

Essential Oils: Idaho Blue Spruce, Ylang Ylang, Ocotea, Hinoki, Davana, Cedarwood, Lavender, Coriander, Lemon, Northern Lights Black Spruce, Rosemary

Directions: Work soap into a lather with water. Apply generously to face and body. Rinse thoroughly.

Cautions: If contact occurs, flush eyes liberally with clean, cool water for several minutes. If redness or irritation occurs, discontinue use. If symptoms persist, contact your physician.

Thieves® Cleansing Soap

Thieves Cleansing Soap is enriched with the powerful Thieves essential oil blend, moisturizing plant oils, and botanical extracts to help cleanse, purify, and promote soft, healthy skin. Thieves is known for its antibacterial and antiseptic properties, making this soap ideal for purifying the skin.

Ingredients: Sodium palmate, Sodium palm kernelate, Water, Glycerin, Olive fruit oil, Clove bud oil, Sodium gluconate, Lemon peel oil, Cinnamon Bark oil, Eucalyptus Radiata leaf oil, Rosemary leaf oil, Jojoba seed oil, Wolfberry seed oil, Oat bran, Aloe vera leaf extract, Rosemary leaf extract

Essential Oils: Thieves Blend: [Clove, Lemon, Cinnamon, Eucalyptus Radiata, Rosemary]

Directions: Work soap into a lather with water. Apply generously to face and body. Rinse thoroughly.

Cautions: If contact occurs, flush eyes liberally with clean, cool water for several minutes. If redness or irritation occurs, discontinue use. If symptoms persist, contact your physician.

Valor® Moisturizing Soap

Valor Moisturizing Soap is made with the empowering scent of Valor essential oil blend. Its all-natural ingredients help moisturize, cleanse, and rejuvenate the skin.

Ingredients: Sodium palmate, Sodium palm kernelate, Water, Glycerin, Olive fruit oil, Caprylic/capric triglyceride, Sodium gluconate, Northern Lights Black Spruce oil, Camphor wood oil, Jojoba seed oil, Wolfberry seed oil, Oat bran, Blue Tansy flower oil, Frankincense oil, Geranium oil, Aloe vera leaf extract, Rosemary leaf extract

Essential Oils: Northern Lights Black Spruce, Camphor (Ho Wood), Blue Tansy, Frankincense, Geranium

Directions: Work soap into a lather with water. Apply generously to face and body. Rinse thoroughly.

Cautions: If contact occurs, flush eyes liberally with clean, cool water for several minutes. If redness or irritation occurs, discontinue use. If symptoms persist, contact your physician.

Allergen Warnings: Contains coconut/palm ingredients

FOAMING HAND SOAPS

Christmas Spirit® Foaming Hand Soap

Ring in the holiday season with this fresh, festive blend of Orange, Cinnamon Bark, and Black Spruce! This foaming hand soap that incorporates the holiday blend favorite of Christmas Spirit is a gentle yet effective way to stay clean, refresh your skin, and enjoy festive finger foods with clean hands that are free of harsh, drying chemicals. The joyous blend of this holiday aroma will evoke the spirits of Christmases past, present, and yet to come!

Ingredients: Water, Alcohol denatured, Decyl glucoside, Cocamidopropyl hydroxysultaine, Orange peel oil, Cetyl hydroxyethylcellulose, Cinnamon Bark oil, Black Spruce leaf oil,

Cinnamomum cassia oil, Glycerin, Sodium hydroxide, Camellia sinensis leaf extract, Ginkgo biloba leaf extract, Aloe vera leaf juice powder, Tocopheryl acetate, Citric acid.

Essential Oils: Orange, Cinnamon Bark, Black Spruce

Directions: Pump foam onto hands, lather, and rinse thoroughly.

Cautions: If contact occurs, flush eyes liberally with clean, cool water for several minutes. If redness or irritation occurs, discontinue use. If symptoms persist, contact your physician.

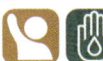

Lavender Foaming Hand Soap

Lavender Foaming Hand Soap cleanses and conditions your hands without leaving them dry or irritated. Infused with Lavender essential oil, vitamin E, and aloe, this soap is effective yet gentle enough for the most sensitive skin.

Ingredients: Water, Decyl glucoside, Cocomidopropyl hydroxysultaine, Lavender oil, Myrrh resin oil, Green tea leaf extract, Retinyl palmitate (Vitamin A), Aloe vera leaf juice, Lemon oil, p-Anisic acid, Tocopheryl acetate (Vitamin E), Ginkgo biloba leaf extract, Glycerin, Citric acid, Levulinic acid, Phytic acid, Cetyl hydroxyethylcellulose, Sodium hydroxide, Potassium sorbate

Essential Oils: Lavender, Myrrh, Lemon

Directions: Pump foam onto hands, lather, and rinse thoroughly.

Cautions: If contact occurs, flush eyes liberally with clean, cool water for several minutes. If redness or irritation occurs, discontinue use. If symptoms persist, contact your physician.

Lushious Lemon Foaming Hand Soap

This bright, citrusy aroma invigorates the spirit while the gentle, plant-based formula gently gets rid of grime and leaves skin soft and refreshed. This is a gentle, effective alternative to commercial soaps and is family friendly.

Ingredients: Water, Decyl glucoside, Alcohol denat., Cetyl Hydroxyethylcellulose Ylang Ylang flower oil, Eucalyptus Globulus leaf oil, Lemon Myrtle leaf oil, Lemon peel oil, Spearmint leaf extract, Cinnamomum cassia oil, Glycerin, Sodium hydroxide, Ginkgo biloba leaf extract, Camellia sinensis leaf extract, Aloe barbadensis leaf juice powder, Tocopherol, Sunflower seed oil, Citric acid

Essential Oils: Ylang Ylang, Eucalyptus Globulus, Lemon Myrtle, Lemon, Spearmint

Directions: Pump foam onto hands, lather, and rinse thoroughly.

Cautions: If contact occurs, flush eyes liberally with clean, cool water for several minutes. If redness or irritation occurs, discontinue use. If symptoms persist, contact your physician.

Thieves® Foaming Hand Soap

Thieves Foaming Hand Soap is a natural hand-cleansing formula that contains Thieves essential oil blend, known for its powerful antibacterial properties. Thieves essential oil blend penetrates beneath the skin's surface, providing a long-lasting barrier of protection. This gentle, foaming soap also contains ingredients such as vitamin E, aloe vera, and ginkgo biloba to moisturize and soften the skin and provide a balanced pH to support the skin's natural moisture complex.

Ingredients: Water, Decyl glucoside, Cocamidopropyl hydroxysultaine, Alcohol denatured, Clove bud oil, Cetyl hydroxyethylcellulose, Orange oil, Lemon peel oil, Cinnamon Bark oil, Eucalyptus Radiata leaf oil, Rosemary leaf oil, Ginkgo biloba leaf extract, Camellia sinensis leaf extract, Sodium hydroxide, Tocopherol acetate, Retinyl palmitate, Aloe vera leaf juice, Citric acid

Essential Oils: Thieves: [Clove, Lemon, Cinnamon Bark, Eucalyptus Radiata, Rosemary], Orange

Directions: Pump foam onto hands, lather, and rinse thoroughly.

Cautions: If contact occurs, flush eyes liberally with clean, cool water for several minutes. If redness or irritation occurs, discontinue use. If symptoms persist, contact your physician.

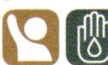

ENDNOTES

1. Shuren J. Antiperspirant drug products for over-the-counter human use; final monograph. Rockville (MD): Food and Drug Administration (US); 2003 Jun. 21 p. RIN 0910–AA01.

2. Strong MJ, Garruto RM, Joshi JG, Mundy WR, Shafer TJ. Can the mechanisms of aluminum neurotoxicity be integrated into a unified scheme? J Toxicol Environ Health. 1996 Aug 30;48(6):599-613.

3. Exley C, Chappell JS, Birchall JD. A mechanism for acute aluminium toxicity in fish. J Theor Biol. 1991 Aug 7;151(3):417-28.

4. Joshi JG. Aluminum, a neurotoxin which affects diverse metabolic reactions. Biofactors. 1990 Jul;2(3):163-9.

5. Snyder JW, Serroni A, Savory J, Farber JL. The absence of extracellular calcium potentiates the killing of cultured hepatocytes by aluminum maltolate. Arch Biochem Biophys. 1995 Jan 10;316(1):434-42.

6. Verbeeck RM, Driessens FC, Rotgans J. Aluminum in toothpastes and Alzheimer's disease. Acta Stomatol Belg. 1990 Jun;87(2):141-4.

7. Hewitt CD, Savory J, Wills MR. Aspects of aluminum toxicity. Clin Lab Med. 1990 Jun;10(2):403-22.

8. ProFresh.com [Internet]. Philadelphia (PA): ProFresh International Corporation; c2018. A message from Dr. Richter; [cited 2018 Oct 12]. Available from: https://www.profresh.com/about/dr-richter-message/.

9. Oral health in America: a report of the surgeon general (executive summary) [Internet]. Bethesda (MD): National Institute of Dental and Craniofacial Research (US); [updated 2018 Jul; cited 2018 Oct 12]. Available from: https://www.nidcr.nih.gov/research/data-statistics/surgeon-general.

10. The Forsyth Institute [Internet]. Cambridge: Harvard School of Dental Medicine Affiliate; c2014. The connection between mouth bacteria and inflammation in heart disease; 2015 Apr 17 [cited 2019 Apr 11]. Available from: https://forsyth.org/news-press-room/connection-between-mouth-bacteria-and-inflammation-heart-disease#.XK-L-uhKiUk.

11. Söder B, Yakob M, Meurman JH, Andersson LC, Söder PÖ. The association of dental plaque with cancer mortality in Sweden. A longitudinal study. BMJ Open. 2012 Jun 11;2(3). pii: e001083.

12. Valnet. Jean. The practice of aromatherapy. New York (NY): Random House UK; c1982. 280 p.

13. Didry N, Dubreuil L, Pinkas M. Activity of thymol, carvacrol, cinnamaldehyde and eugenol on oral bacteria. Pharm Acta Helv. 1994 Jul;69(1):25-8.

14. Marcelo WBA, Charles CA, Weinstein RB, McGuire JA, Parikh-Das AM, Du Q, Zhang J, Berlin JA, Gunsolley JC. Meta-analysis of the effect of an essential oil–containing mouth-rinse on gingivitis and plaque. Journal of the American Dental Association. 2015 Aug;146(8):610-622.

15. Fine DH, Markowitz K, Furgang D, Goldsmith D, Charles CH, Lisante TA, Lynch MC. Effect of an essential oil-containing antimicrobial mouth rinse on specific plaque bacteria in vivo. J Clin Periodontal 2007 Aug;34(8):652-7. Epub 2007 May 29.

16. Santos SL, Conforti N, Mankodi S, Kohut BE, Yu D, Wu MM, Parikh R. Anticalculus effect of two zinc citrate/essential oil-containing dentifrices. Am J Dent. 2000 Sep;13(Spec No):11C-13C.

17. Quintas V, Prada-López I, Donos N, Suárez-Quintanilla D, Tomás I. Antiplaque effect of essential oils and 0.2% chlorhexidine on an in situ model of oral biofilm growth: a randomised clinical trial. PLoS One. 2015 Feb 17;10(2):e0117177. eCollection 2015.

18. The Hidden Danger of Using Mouthwash, Jen McCaffrey, Reader's Digest, 3-19-2019.

19. Tribble GD, Angelov N, Weltman R, Wang B-Y, Eswaran SV, Gay IC, Parthasarathy K, Dao D-H V, Richardson KN, Ismail NM, Sharina IG, Hyde ER, Ajami NJ, Petrosino JF, Bryan NS. Frequency of Tongue Cleaning Impacts the Human Tongue Microbiome Composition and Enterosalivary Circulation of Nitrate. Front Cell Infect Microbiol. 2019 Mar 1;9:39.

20. Schnaubelt, K. Medical Aromatherapy. Frog. Ltd. North Atlantic Books, 1999, 235.

21. Hawrelak JA, Cattley T, Myers SP. Essential oils in treatment of intestinal dysbiosis; A preliminary in vitro study. Altern Med Rev. 2009 Dec;14(4):380-4.

22. Riep BG, Bernimoulin JP, Barnett ML. Comparative antiplaque effectiveness of an essential oil and an amine fluoride/stannous fluoride mouthrinse. J Clin Periodontal. 1999 Mar;26(3):164-8.

23. Richards D. Effects of essential oil mouthwashes on plaque and gingivitis. Evid Based Dent. 2017 Jun 23;18(2):39-40.

24. National Human Adipose Tissue Survey 1990. Washington: Environmental Protection Agency; 1990. 8 p.

25. Winter, Ruth. A consumer's dictionary of cosmetic ingredients. 7th ed. New York (NY): Three Rivers Press; c2009. 576 p.

26. Dadd, Debra Lynn. Home Safe Home: Protecting Yourself and Your Family from Everyday Toxics and Harmful Household Products. New York (NY): Penguin Putnam; c1997. 464 p.

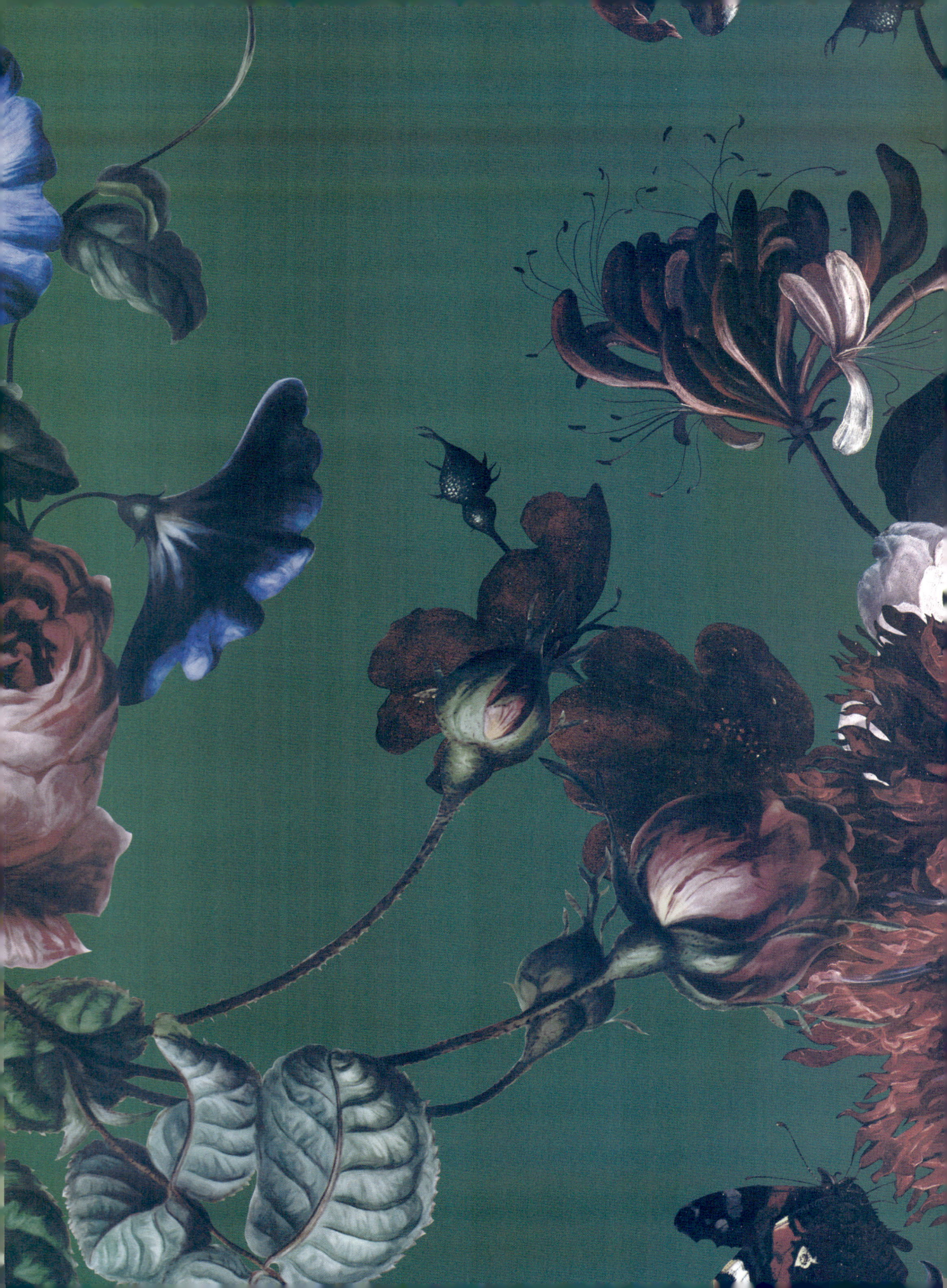

Healthy Choices for Children

Being conscious of what you put in your body is very important. However, since your skin is your largest organ, being careful what you put on it is equally important.

Our KidScents proprietary blends and other products are safe alternatives to products for children commonly found in the market today. You'll love our kid-focused essential oil blends and other products.

You will find our KidScents products free from chemicals, sulfates, toxins, synthetic colorants, dyes, artificial flavors, and preservatives.

You can feel safe using these high quality, essential oil-infused products for your children.

KIDSCENTS® PERSONAL CARE FOR CHILDREN

KidScents® Bath Gel

KidScents Bath Gel is a safe, gentle formula with a neutral pH balance perfect for young skin. This hypoallergenic gel is enriched with nourishing botanicals for a natural clean that is gentle on sensitive skin. Babassu oil acts as a light, non-greasy moisturizer that absorbs quickly, while aloe vera soothes and cools the skin. It contains no mineral oils, synthetic perfumes, artificial colorings, or toxic ingredients.

Ingredients: Water, Decyl glucoside, Glycerin, Sodium laurylglucosides hydroxypropylsulfonate, Xylityl sesquicaprylate, Xanthan gum, Citric acid, Benzyl alcohol, Sodium chloride, Tangerine peel oil, Sodium gluconate, Anhydroxylitol, Aloe barbadensis leaf juice, Lemon peel oil, Orbignya oleifera seed oil, Agar, Kiwi fruit extract, Cucumber fruit extract

Essential Oils: Tangerine, Lemon

Directions: Apply a small amount of KidScents Bath Gel to washcloth or directly to the skin. Rub gently, then rinse. Use as you would a liquid soap.

Cautions: Keep out of children's eyes and mouth. Do not expose to excessive heat or direct sunlight. Avoid contact with severely damaged skin.

Allergen Warnings: Contains corn, gluten, wheat, soy, and coconut/palm ingredients

CAUTIONS

Note which cautions are applicable to which oil under each oil's listing. Not all cautions apply to all oils.

 Keep out of reach of children.

 For external use only.

 Avoid contact with eyes and mucous membranes.

 If you are pregnant, nursing, taking medication, or have a medical condition, consult a health professional prior to use.

 Flammable. Keep away from fire, heat, or sparks. Do not store above room temperature.

 PH = Photosensitizing. Avoid direct sunlight or UV rays (e.g., sunlamps, tanning beds, etc.) for up to 12 hours after applying oil. Sunlight should be avoided for 24 hours after applying some oils, shown as (24).

 May stain some surfaces, skin, or clothing.

 Some oils might cause a stinging, burning sensation, rash, redness, pain, blisters, inflammation, swelling, itching, or darkening of the skin. Test for sensitivity on a small area of skin on the underside of your arm and apply as needed.

These statements have not been evaluated by the Food and Drug Administration. These products are not intended to diagnose, treat, cure, or prevent any disease. Consult individual product labels for safety information.

Bolded ingredients are essential oils.

All Young Living Vitality™ essential oils are Non-GMO Project Verified! To receive this certification, all Vitality oils passed through third-party verification, auditing, and testing.

KidScents® Lotion

KidScents Lotion is safe, gentle, and pH neutral, ideal for young skin. It restores moisture to children's skin with its gentle and nourishing ingredients. Mango seed butter and aloe also soften skin and allow it to quickly absorb the naturally derived botanical ingredients. It contains no mineral oils, synthetic perfumes, artificial colorings, or toxic ingredients.

Ingredients: Water, Aloe barbadensis leaf juice, Glycerin, Meadowfoam seed oil, Apple fruit extract, Isoamyl laurate, Ethylhexyl olivate, Glyceryl stearate, Glyceryl stearate citrate, Cetearyl alcohol, Babassu seed oil, Cetyl alcohol, Mango seed butter, Raspberry seed oil, Sodium levulinate, Watermelon seed oil, Benzyl alcohol, Oat bran extract, Rice bran extract, Tangerine peel oil, Glyceryl caprylate, Sodium anisate, Xanthan gum, Lemon peel oil, Squalane, Orange peel extract, Rosemary leaf extract, Sodium phytate, Sunflower extract, Tocopherol, Alcohol, Citric acid, Sodium hydroxide

Essential Oils: Tangerine, Lemon

Directions: Apply liberally to skin as needed.

Cautions: Avoid contact with severely damaged skin.

KidScents® Shampoo

KidScents Shampoo contains the finest natural ingredients for gently cleansing children's delicate hair. Strengthened with botanicals and plant extracts, this hypoallergenic, non-irritating shampoo helps your little one's hair feel smooth and hydrated without over-drying tender skin. A mild formula designed to provide the perfect pH balance for children's hair, it contains no mineral oils, synthetic perfumes, artificial colorings, or toxic ingredients.

Ingredients: Water, Glycerin, Decyl glucoside, Cetyl betaine, Lauryl glucoside, Sorbitan oleate, decylglucoside crosspolymer, Tangerine peel oil, Xanthan gum, Sodium levulinate, Lemon peel oil, Sodium anisate, PCA glyceryl oleate, Citric acid, Hydrolyzed jojoba esters, Acetic acid/vinegar [derived from apple sources]

Essential Oils: Tangerine, Lemon

Directions: Apply a small amount to hair. Lather, then rinse.

Cautions: Avoid contact with severely damaged skin.

KidScents® Toothpaste

KidScents Toothpaste is a safe, natural alternative to commercial brands of toothpaste. Formulated with Slique Essence® and Thieves® essential oil blends, this toothpaste gently cleans teeth and tastes great without synthetic dyes or flavors. Slique Essence is antibacterial, antifungal, a lipid regulator, and a glucose regulator. Thieves is antiseptic, antimicrobial, and combats plaque-causing micro-organisms.

KidScents Toothpaste is perfect for children, and it makes a great training toothpaste for children during the crucial first years while they develop their primary teeth. Calcium carbonate, baking soda, and xylitol are used as tooth and gum health agents. It includes an amazing blend of highly antiviral, antiseptic, antibacterial, and anti-infectious essential oils.

Ingredients: Water, Calcium carbonate, Coconut oil, Sodium bicarbonate, Glycerin, Xylitol, Xanthan gum, Grapefruit peel oil, Stevia leaf extract, Tangerine peel oil, Lecithin, Spearmint leaf extract, Lemon peel oil, Ocotea leaf oil, Clove bud oil, Cinnamon Bark oil, Eucalyptus Radiata leaf oil, Rosemary leaf oil

Essential Oils: Grapefruit, Tangerine, Spearmint, Lemon, Ocotea, Clove, Cinnamon Bark, Eucalyptus Radiata, Rosemary

Directions: Brush teeth thoroughly after meals or at least 2 times daily. Do not swallow. Intended for children 2 years and older. Children under 2 years of age: Consult a dentist or doctor before use.

Cautions: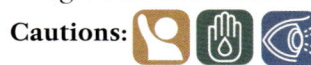

Allergen Warnings: Contains coconut product.

KidScents® Tender Tush™

KidScents Tender Tush is a gentle ointment designed to protect and nourish young skin and promote healing. This ointment soothes dry, chapped skin and offers protection for delicate skin. It is also great for expectant mothers who are concerned about having stretch marks.

Ingredients: Coconut oil, Cocoa seed butter, Olive fruit oil, Sweet almond oil, Beeswax, Wheat germ oil, Sacred Sandalwood oil, Coriander seed oil, Roman Chamomile flower oil, Lavender oil, Frankincense oil, Bergamot peel oil (Furocoumarin-free), Cistus oil, Ylang Ylang flower oil, Geranium flower oil

Essential Oils: Sacred Sandalwood, Coriander, Roman Chamomile, Lavender, Frankincense, Bergamot (Furocoumarin-free), Cistus, Ylang Ylang, Geranium

Directions: Apply liberally to diaper area as often as needed to help soothe diaper rash, redness, or irritation.

Cautions: Avoid contact with severely damaged skin.

Allergen Warnings: Contains coconut, bee, and wheat products.

KIDSCENTS® NUTRITIONAL SUPPORT FOR CHILDREN

KidScents® MightyPro™

Support is here for children's digestive and immune health with a delicious wolfberry punch flavor. This KidScents supplement delivers the synergistic power of pre- and probiotics with over 8 billion active, live cultures of the friendly bacteria needed for optimal health.

Ingredients: Fructooligosaccharides, Lactobacillus paracasei Lpc-37, Lactobacillus acidophilus LA-14, Ningxia wolfberry fruit powder, Lactobacillus plantarum LP-115, Lactobacillus rhamnosus GG AF, Streptococcus thermophilus, Lactobacillus rhamnosus 6594, Bifidobacterium infantis BI-26, Xylitol, Erythritol, Natural fruit punch flavor, Citric acid

Directions: For children 2 years and above, empty entire content of 1 packet into mouth and allow it to dissolve. Take 1 packet daily with food to provide optimal conditions for healthy gut bacteria. Can be combined with cold food or drinks. Do not add to warm or hot food or beverage.

Cautions: Do not exceed recommended dosage. Adults may also take this supplement. Not intended for animals.

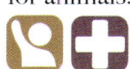

KidScents® MightyVites™

KidScents MightyVites is a whole-food multinutrient that contains super fruits, plants, and vegetables that deliver the full spectrum of vitamins, minerals, antioxidants, and phytonutrients, specifically designed for children's developing bodies. Following in the footsteps of the Master Formula™ reformulation, MightyVites benefit from Orgen-kids®, a nutrient-dense, food-based superfruit, plant, and vegetable complex.

Orgen-kids® is formulated with Orgen-FA®, which is the best source for natural folate available. Orgen-FA® is 100 percent USDA Certified Organic and does not contain synthetic folic acid or additives. It is extracted using hot water and is no different than the folic acid that is produced when boiling broccoli.

Children's diets often need a bridge between what they are eating and what they should be eating. To fuel growth and normal activity levels, a child's diet must provide plenty of vitamins and minerals as well as support the storing of nutrients in preparation for the accelerated growth spurts of the teenage years.

The Ningxia wolfberry fruit is the highest antioxidant food known, making it an excellent whole food with 18 amino acids; 21 trace minerals; vitamins A, B1, B2, B6, B12, C, D, and E; polyphenols; carotenoids; magnesium; and potassium.

This super-enriched, chewable vitamin is perfect for children to energize, build their bodies, and protect their entire system the way Mother Nature intended.

Ingredients: Vitamin A (as beta carotene from organic food blend), Vitamin C (from organic food blend), Vitamin D (as cholecalciferol), Vitamin E (from organic food blend), Thiamin (from organic food blend), Riboflavin (from organic food blend), Niacin (from organic food blend), Vitamin B6 (from organic food blend), Folate (from organic food blend), Vitamin B12 (from organic food blend), Biotin (from organic food blend), Pantothenic acid (from organic food blend), Magnesium (from organic food blend), Zinc (from organic food blend), Selenium (from organic food blend), Natural sweetener (Erythritol, Oligosaccharide), Malic acid, Stevia, Silica, Magnesium stearate

MightyVites Wild Berry Blend: Orgen-Kid [Curry leaf extract, Guava fruit extract, Lemon peel extract, Sesbania leaf extract, Amala fruit extract, Holy Basil aerial parts extract, Annatto seed extract], Beet root juice powder, Orange fruit juice powder, Strawberry fruit juice powder, Wolfberry fruit powder, Citrus flavonoids, Barley grass leaf powder, Broccoli sprout powder

Directions: Children 4-12 years old, take 4 chewable tablets daily. Can be taken separately or in 1 daily dose.

Cautions: Do not exceed recommended dosage.

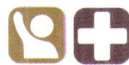

KidScents® MightyZyme™

KidScents MightyZyme is an all-natural, vegetarian, chewable tablet designed to give children added enzyme nutrition to prevent enzyme depletion, which is a precursor to body dysfunction that can impede growth and brain development. Children today face a world of fast foods and nutritionally depleted foods that are practically devoid of enzymes critical for the proper function of everything from breathing, thinking, circulation, and digestion.

MightyZyme combines nine different digestive enzymes with several other nutrients to support healthy digestion and relieve occasional symptoms—such as stomach pressure, bloating, gas, pain, and minor cramping—that may occur after eating.

MightyZyme chewable tablets address each of the digestive needs of growing bodies and assist with normal digestion of all foods, including proteins, carbohydrates, and fats. They energize, build, and protect your child's whole system, the way Mother Nature intended.

Ingredients: Calcium (from calcium carbonate), MightyZyme Blend: [Lipase, Alfalfa leaf powder, Amylase, Protease 4.5, Bromelain, Carrot root powder, Peptidase, Phytase, Protease 6.0, Protease 3.0, Peppermint aerial parts oil, Cellulase], Sorbitol, Dextrates, Natural mixed berry flavor, Microcrystalline cellulose, Magnesium stearate, Steric acid, Silica, Apple juice powder, Stevia leaf extract

Essential Oil: Peppermint

Directions: For children age 6 or older: chew 1 tablet 3 times daily prior to or with meals. For children ages 2-6 years of age: chew ½ to 1 tablet (crushed if needed and mixed with yogurt or applesauce).

Cautions: Do not exceed recommended dosage. Do not expose to excessive heat.

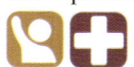

KidScents® Unwind™

With Young Living's Unwind, you can offer your children an all-natural way to help them find their calm state as they settle down for bed and helps ease occasional irritability. Unwind also provides terrific next-day benefits like improved focus and mental clarity both at home and in the classroom. One stick pack helps promote a calm, restful, and relaxed state, giving children the focus they need to succeed.

Ingredients: Xylitol (contains Sodium carboxyl methyl cellulose), Magnesium (from Magnesium citrate,

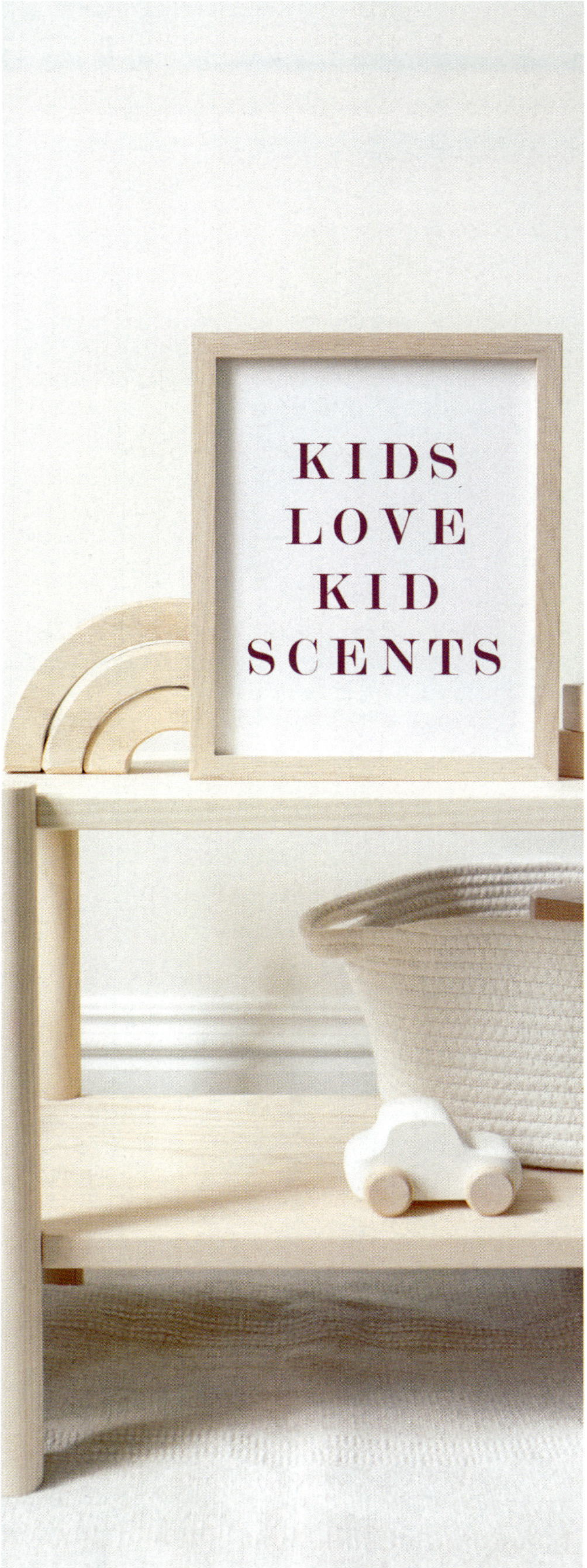

Oxide, Hydroxide), L-theanine, 5-HTP (Griffonia simplicfolia seed extract), Natural watermelon flavor, Stevia leaf extract, Lavender flower essential oil, Roman Chamomile flower essential oil

Essential Oils: Lavender, Roman Chamomile

Directions: Consume 1 stick pack before bedtime.

Cautions: For human consumption only; not intended for animal use.

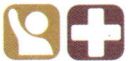

KIDSCENTS® OIL COLLECTION & KIDSCENTS® ROLL-ON COLLECTION

The KidScents Oil Collection includes six oil blends formulated especially for kids to help them through the common ups and downs of childhood.

The KidScents Roll-On Collection includes the same six oil blends and gives children an easy-to-apply way of using the oils themselves.

KidScents® GeneYus™ & KidScents® GeneYus™ Roll-On

Diffuse KidScents GeneYus or use the roll-on to help young minds focus and concentrate on projects.

Ingredients: Caprylic/capric triglyceride, Sacred Frankincense, Blue Cypress, Cedarwood Bark, Idaho Blue Spruce, Melissa, Palo Santo, Northern Lights Black Spruce, Sweet almond oil, Vetiver, Bergamot, Myrrh, Geranium, Sacred Sandalwood, Ylang Ylang, Coriander, Black Spruce, Hyssop, Rose

Directions: Aromatic: 6o. Topical: Neat. Apply 2-4 drops directly to desired area. Recommended application is for children ages 2-12. Dilution not required, except for the most sensitive skin. Use as needed.

Cautions: To be applied only by a trusted adult or under adult supervision.

Allergen Warnings: Contains coconut product.

KidScents® KidPower & KidScents® KidPower Roll-On

KidPower is a unique, everyday blend formulated to help inspire feelings of confidence, courage, and positivity at home, at school, or at play. Apply KidPower on your children's wrists or back of their necks to inspire, motivate, and empower them for their best day every day or diffuse daily to promote feelings of courage and inspire positivity to help them find their power within.

Medical Properties and Uses: Promotes peaceful feelings, prompts spiritual feelings, balances the senses, energizes, relaxes, promotes a comforting environment, uplifting

Ingredients: Fractionated coconut oil, Orange, Vanilla, Black Spruce, Ho Wood, Blue Tansy, Frankincense, Geranium

Directions: Aromatic: 6o. Topical: Neat. Recommended application is for children ages 2-12. To be applied only by a trusted adult or under adult supervision.

Cautions:

Allergen Warnings: Contains coconut product.

KidScents® Owie™ & KidScents® Owie™ Roll-On

Apply Owie topically to improve the appearance of your child's skin and help heal wounds. This relaxing blend provides a calming aroma along with oils that support the appearance of healthy skin.

Ingredients: Caprylic/capric triglyceride, Idaho Grand Fir, Tea Tree, Helichrysum, Elemi, Cistus, Clove

Directions: Aromatic: 6o. Topical: Neat. Apply 2-4 drops directly to desired area. Recommended application is for children ages 2-12. Dilution not required, except for the most sensitive skin. Use as needed.

Cautions: To be applied only by a trusted adult or under adult supervision.

Allergen Warnings: Contains coconut product.

KidScents® SleepyIze™ & KidScents® SleepyIze™ Roll-On

SleepyIze calms and relaxes the mind and body prior to bedtime for kids. It's an excellent way to help your child naturally relax at the end of the day.

Ingredients: Caprylic/capric glycerides, Lavender, Geranium, Roman Chamomile, Bergamot, Tangerine, Sacred Frankincense, Valerian, Rue

Directions: Aromatic: 6o. Topical: Neat. Apply 2-4 drops directly to desired area. Recommended application is for children ages 2-12. Dilution not required, except for the most sensitive skin. Use as needed.

Cautions: To be applied only by a trusted adult or under adult supervision.

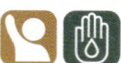

Allergen Warnings: Contains coconut product.

KidScents® SniffleEase™ & KidScents® SniffleEase™ Roll-On

SniffleEase is a refreshing, rejuvenating blend formulated just for kids for when they have congestion. The aroma promotes feelings of health and wellness while also assisting in releasing feelings of discomfort. The natural, relaxing, soothing vapors help promote wellness when inhaled and inspire calm breathing.

Ingredients: Caprylic/capric triglyceride, Eucalyptus Blue, Palo Santo, Lavender, Dorado Azul, Camphor (Ravintsara), Eucalyptus Globulus, Myrtle, Pine, Marjoram, Eucalyptus Radiata, Eucalyptus Citriodora, Cypress, Black Spruce, Peppermint

Directions: Aromatic: 6o. Topical: Neat. Apply 2-4 drops directly to desired area. Recommended application is for children ages 2-12. Dilution not required, except for the most sensitive skin. Use as needed.

Cautions: To be applied only by a trusted adult or under adult supervision.

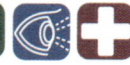

Allergen Warnings: Contains coconut product.

KidScents® TummyGize™ & KidScents® TummyGize™ Roll-On

TummyGize is a quieting, relaxing blend that can be applied to little tummies that are upset. It also supports proper digestion. This comforting, peaceful blend can be diffused or gently massaged directly onto the tummy for a sense of balance and grounding.

Ingredients: Caprylic/capric triglyceride, Spearmint, Peppermint, Tangerine, Anise, Fennel, Cardamom, Ginger

Directions: Aromatic: 6o. Topical: Neat. Apply 2-4 drops directly to desired area. Recommended application is for children ages 2-12. Dilution not required, except for the most sensitive skin. Use as needed.

Cautions: To be applied only by a trusted adult or under adult supervision.

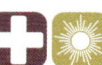

Allergen Warnings: Contains coconut product.

SEEDLINGS® BABY PRODUCTS

Your baby's health is safeguarded with all-natural, plant-derived formulas in the Seedlings product line. Gentle essential oils add a calming effect that enriches your baby's bathing experience.

Seedlings® Baby Lotion

Keep your baby's skin soft and hydrated with this baby lotion made from plant-based, naturally derived ingredients. You will also love the calming influence of its lavender-infused essential oil blend.

Ingredients: Water, Caprylic/capric triglyceride, Glycerin, Glyceryl stearate, Coco-caprylate, Cetearyl alcohol, Sodium stearoyl glutamate, Glyceryl caprylate, Xanthan gum, Cellulose gum, Apple fruit extract, Sodium levulinate, Lavender oil, Glyceryl undecylenate, Sodium anisate, Murumuru seed butter, Mango seed butter, Cocoa seed butter, Safflower seed oil, Coriander seed oil, Sodium chloride, Bergamot peel oil (Furocoumarin-free), Marigold flower extract, Sodium hydroxide, Achiote seed extract, Ylang Ylang flower oil, Geranium flower oil, Tocopheryl acetate

Essential Oils: Lavender, Coriander, Bergamot (Furocoumarin-free), Ylang Ylang, Geranium

Directions: Apply a small amount to your hands. Rub hands together to warm the lotion and gently massage into baby's skin.

Caution: To be applied only by a trusted adult. Discontinue use if skin irritation occurs.

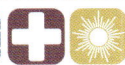

Allergen Warnings: Contains coconut product.

Seedlings® Baby Oil

Your baby's delicate skin will thrive with this naturally derived, plant-based formula. With no mineral oil or dangerous phthalates, Seedlings Baby Oil nourishes your baby's skin while providing the calming scent of appropriately diluted, pure essential oils. It absorbs smoothly; provides a light, calm aroma; and promotes a relaxing environment. It is vegan friendly and suitable for everyday use.

Ingredients: Caprylic/capric triglyceride, Apricot kernel oil, Safflower seed oil, Prickly pear seed oil, Mixed tocopherols, Lavender oil, Coriander seed oil, Bergamot peel oil (Furocoumarin-free), Ylang Ylang flower oil, Geranium flower oil

Essential Oils: Lavender, Coriander, Bergamot (Furocoumarin-free), Ylang Ylang, Geranium

Directions: Apply a small amount to your hands. Rub hands together to warm the oil and gently massage into baby's skin.

Caution: To be applied only by a trusted adult. Discontinue use if skin irritation occurs.

Allergen Warnings: Contains coconut product.

Seedlings® Baby Wash & Shampoo

Gentle and mild, Young Living's Baby Wash & Shampoo is 100 percent plant based. Your baby's tender skin will be cleansed without overdrying. The calming essential oil blend adds a light and calming scent to enrich baby's bathing experience. It leaves skin and hair clean and soft and makes tangles easy to comb out. This product is sulfate-free, vegan friendly, and perfect for everyday use.

Ingredients: Water, Sodium lauryl glucosides hydroxypropylsulfonate, Glycerin, Decyl glucoside, Glyceryl caprylate, Xanthan gum, Sodium chloride, Sodium levulinate, Glyceryl undecylenate, Lavender oil, Marigold flower extract, Caprylic/capric triglyceride, Coriander seed oil, Eyebright extract, Bergamot peel oil (Furocoumarin-free), Citric acid, Ylang Ylang flower oil, Geranium flower oil

Essential Oils: Lavender, Coriander, Bergamot (Furocoumarin-free), Ylang Ylang, Geranium

Directions: Wet hair and skin with warm water. Apply a small amount to a moistened washcloth or hand and gently lather over entire body and scalp.

Caution: To be applied only by a trusted adult. Discontinue use if skin irritation occurs.

Allergen Warnings: Contains coconut product.

Seedlings® Baby Wipes

These soft, thick wipes do double-duty for diaper changes and feeding clean-ups. Formulated with cleansing botanicals and without harsh chemicals, this baby-safe essential oil blend leaves a delicate, calming scent. Dermatologist tested and hypoallergenic for worry-free care.

Ingredients: Water, Aloe vera leaf juice, Soapberry fruit extract, Glycerin, Phenethyl alcohol, Apple fruit extract, Marigold flower extract, Glyceryl caprylate, Lavender oil, Witch hazel leaf extract, Caprylic/capric triglyceride, Coriander seed oil, Bergamot peel oil (Furocoumarin-free), Ylang Ylang flower oil, Geranium flower oil

Essential Oils: Lavender, Coriander, Bergamot (Furocoumarin-free), Ylang Ylang, Geranium

Directions: Close lid firmly after each use to keep moist. Do not flush.

Cautions: To be applied only by a trusted adult.

Allergen Warnings: Contains coconut product.

Seedlings® Calm

This soothing, gentle blend is formulated for children, with its soft, relaxing, floral notes. A great way to spread the scent of your favorite Seedlings products around your child's room or the whole house.

Ingredients: Lavender oil, Caprylic/capric triglyceride, Coriander seed oil, Bergamot peel oil, Ylang Ylang flower oil, Geranium flower oil

Directions: Aromatic only: 30.

Cautions: To be handled only by a trusted adult or under adult supervision. For aromatic use only. Clean the diffuser thoroughly after each use.

Allergen Warnings: Contains coconut product.

Seedlings® Diaper Rash Cream

With 100 percent naturally derived ingredients, Seedlings Diaper Rash Cream provides extra-gentle protection when used at the first sign of diaper rash. It soothes irritation, protecting baby's tender skin. This soothing cream is vegan friendly and formulated without lanolin, parabens, phthalates, petrochemicals, animal-derived ingredients, synthetic preservatives, synthetic fragrances, or synthetic dyes and colorants.

Ingredients: Active: Zinc oxide. Inactive: Coconut oil, Beeswax, Castor oil, Mango butter, Sunflower oil, Safflower oil, Cocoa butter, Arrowroot, Avocado oil, Astrocaryum murumuru seed butter, Glyceryl rosinate, Kaolin, Lavender oil, Tocopherol, Tamanu oil, Grape seed oil, Sea buckthorn seed oil, Glyceryl oleate, Olive oil unsaponifiables, Black Spruce leaf oil, Helichrysum flower oil, Marigold flower, Chamomile, Lavender flower extract, Broadleaf plantain, Chickweed

Essential Oils: Lavender, Black Spruce, Helichrysum

Directions: Change wet and soiled diapers promptly. Cleanse the diaper area and allow to dry. Apply cream liberally with each diaper change, especially at bedtime or anytime when exposure to wet diapers may be prolonged.

Caution: Stop use and ask a doctor if condition worsens, symptoms last more than seven days, or symptoms clear up and occur again within a few days. If swallowed, get medical help or contact a Poison Control Center right away.

Allergen Warnings: Contains coconut and bee products.

Seedlings® Linen Spray

Capture the clean-air freshness of clothes drying in the sun with this alcohol-free spray, made with 100 percent naturally derived ingredients. Crib sheets, blankets, even car seats can be freshened with the calming aroma of the essential oils in this formula. With a naturally derived, vegan formula, this calming spray is gentle enough for babies and parents alike.

Ingredients: Water, Glyceryl caprylate, Glycerin, Caprylyl/capryl glucoside, Sodium levulinate, Glyceryl undecylenate, Sodium anisate, Lavender oil, Sodium cocoyl glutamate, Polyglyceryl-5 oleate, Caprylic/capric triglyceride, Coriander seed oil, Citric acid, Bergamot (Furocoumarin-free) peel oil, Ylang Ylang flower oil, Geranium flower oil

Essential Oils: Lavender, Coriander, Bergamot (Furocoumarin-free), Ylang Ylang, Geranium

Directions: Shake well before each use. Spray on linens as needed. Do not spray directly on skin or face.

Caution: To be applied only by a trusted adult. Discontinue use if skin irritation occurs.

Allergen Warnings: Contains coconut products

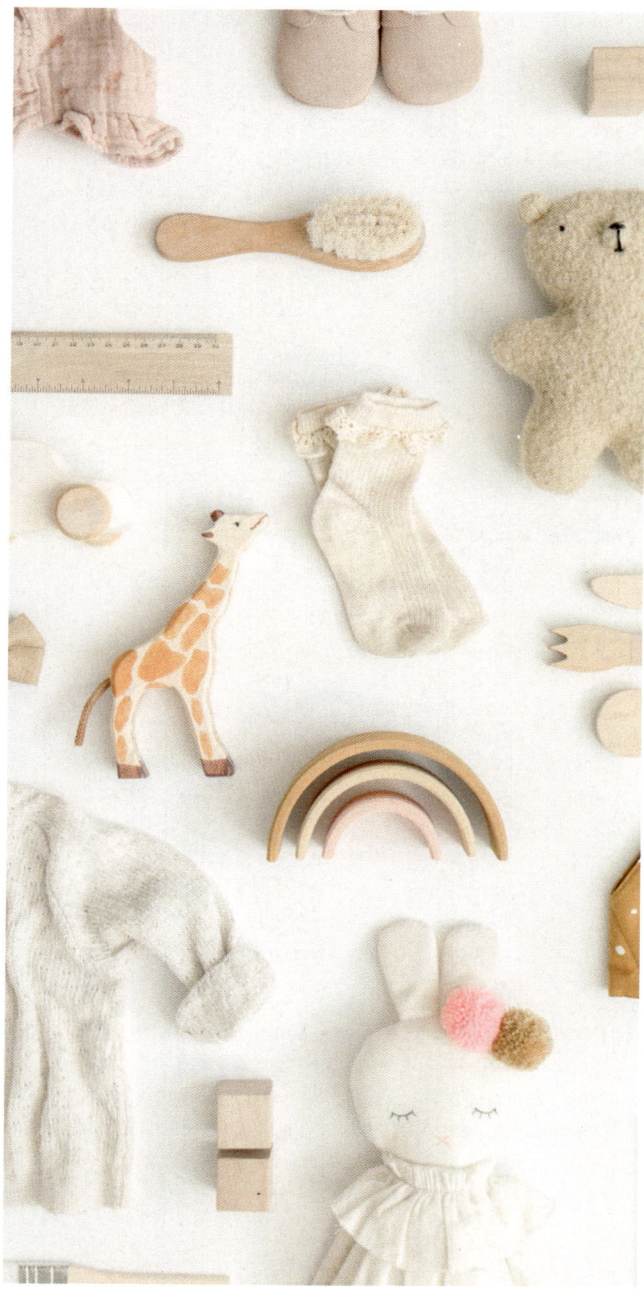

Protecting Your Home

Essential oils have been used since the beginning of time for a vast array of applications. They were most noticeably used for religious ceremonies, healing, perfumery, cosmetics, and beautifying the body, etc.

Over the last three or four decades, the perfume and food-flavoring industries have used the majority of the essential oil production in the world for commercial purposes. However, in the last few years, since essential oils have made their re-entrance into our modern world on a more dramatic scale, they are being used for many things.

If you start reading labels, you will be astounded at how many products contain essential oils. It is easy to understand why they would be used in toothpastes, mouthwashes, deodorants, perfumes, sprays, sauces, preservatives, liquors, air fresheners, and pharmaceuticals. But could you imagine that they would be used in glues, tapes, cements, paints, paint removers, upholstery materials, finishing materials, carbon papers, crayons, inks, ribbons, writing papers, labels, wrappers, polishes, cleaners, solvent lubricating oils and waxes, greases, rubber toys, waterproofing compounds, and plastics?

What you will read in this chapter are but a few of the many ways you can use essential oils to deodorize and protect your home. It is for you to make those discoveries and share them with your family and friends.

THIEVES® PRODUCTS

Protect yourself from harmful bacteria and viruses naturally. Thieves products provide a natural, safe, and highly effective defense against germs that can make us sick. Every day we touch door handles, tabletops, and other surfaces covered with bacteria. Chemical-filled antibacterial soaps and hand sanitizers may or may not be effective but are filled with synthetic ingredients that can be highly toxic.

All-natural Thieves household products contain the proven antibacterial and antiviral properties of the Thieves essential oil blend, other complementary essential oils, and plant-based ingredients. With their eco-friendly packaging and effective results, Thieves natural household products should be in every home.

A September 2018 Canadian study found a connection between exposure to household cleaning disinfectants in infants of 3-4 months and higher body mass index (BMI) in children three years of age, possibly caused

CAUTIONS

Note which cautions are applicable to which oil under each oil's listing. Not all cautions apply to all oils.

 Keep out of reach of children.

 For external use only.

 Avoid contact with eyes and mucous membranes.

 If you are pregnant, nursing, taking medication, or have a medical condition, consult a health professional prior to use.

 Flammable. Keep away from fire, heat, or sparks. Do not store above room temperature.

 PH = Photosensitizing. Avoid direct sunlight or UV rays (e.g., sunlamps, tanning beds, etc.) for up to 12 hours after applying oil. Sunlight should be avoided for 24 hours after applying some oils, shown as (24).

 May stain some surfaces, skin, or clothing.

 Some oils might cause a stinging, burning sensation, rash, redness, pain, blisters, inflammation, swelling, itching, or darkening of the skin. Test for sensitivity on a small area of skin on the underside of your arm and apply as needed.

These statements have not been evaluated by the Food and Drug Administration. These products are not intended to diagnose, treat, cure, or prevent any disease. Consult individual product labels for safety information.

Bolded ingredients are essential oils.

All Young Living Vitality™ essential oils are Non-GMO Project Verified! To receive this certification, all Vitality oils passed through third-party verification, auditing, and testing.

by alteration of the children's gut microbiota. However, the use of eco-friendly products was associated with decreased odds of overweight or obesity.1

Thieves essential oil blend or Thieves household cleaning products will not cause this change in children's gut microbiota.

Essential oil expert Kurt Schnaubelt has written that essential oils do not kill beneficial bacteria. He explains that phenylpropanoids such as cinnamic aldehyde, eugenol, and carvacrol are antimicrobial. However, they are also unique in the way that beneficial probiotic bacteria can harmlessly metabolize them.2

Thieves blend consists of Clove, Lemon, Cinnamon Bark, Rosemary, and Eucalyptus Radiata essential oils.

Thieves® Automatic Dishwasher Powder

This gentle yet effective formula uses Thieves, Lemongrass, and Orange essential oils combined with other naturally derived ingredients to safely tackle even stuck-on food, and it dries without hard water spots for sparkling dishes.

Ingredients: Sodium carbonate, Sodium citrate dihydrate, Sodium percarbonate, Sodium silicate, Soapberry fruit extract, Tapioca maltodextrin, Silica, Protease, Sunflower seed oil, Amylase, Orange peel oil, Lemongrass oil, Clove bud oil, Lemon peel oil, Cinnamon Bark oil, Rosemary leaf oil, Eucalyptus Radiata leaf oil

Essential Oils: Orange, Lemongrass, Thieves blend: [Clove, Lemon, Cinnamon Bark, Rosemary, Eucalyptus Radiata]

Directions: Place 1 scoop in the dishwasher dispenser. Use 2 scoops for heavy loads or with hard water.

Cautions: In case of eye contact, immediately flush thoroughly with water. If swallowed or inhaled, drink plenty of water and seek medical help. Flush immediately if product comes in contact with skin.

Thieves® Dish Soap

Thieves Dish Soap naturally and effectively cleans your dishes without chemicals, dyes, or synthetics. Featuring Thieves, Jade Lemon, Bergamot, and other plant-based ingredients, this dish soap leaves dishes sparkling clean.

Ingredients: Water, Decyl glucoside, Sodium lauroyl lactylate, Sodium oleate, Lauryl glucoside, Sodium carbonate, Caprylyl glucoside, Lemon peel oil, Bergamot peel oil (Furocoumarin-free), Jade Lemon peel oil, Clove bud oil, Cinnamon Bark oil, Eucalyptus Radiata leaf oil, Rosemary leaf oil

Essential Oils: Bergamot (Furocoumarin-free), Jade Lemon, Thieves blend: [Clove, Lemon, Cinnamon Bark, Eucalyptus Radiata, Rosemary]

Directions: Dispense a small amount of soap with warm running water. Add additional soap as needed.

Cautions: In case of eye contact, flush thoroughly with water. If swallowed, drink plenty of water to dilute.

Thieves® Foaming Hand Soap

A natural alternative to chemical soaps, Thieves Foaming Hand Soap contains the essential oil blend Thieves, known for its powerful cleansing and antibacterial properties. Thieves essential oil blend penetrates beneath the skin's surface, providing a long-lasting barrier of protection. This gentle, foaming soap also contains ingredients such as vitamin E, aloe vera, and ginkgo biloba to moisturize and soften the skin and provide a balanced pH to support the skin's natural moisture complex.

Ingredients: Water, Decyl glucoside, Cocamidopropyl hydroxysultaine, Alcohol denat., Clove bud oil, Cetyl hydroxyethylcellulose, Orange peel oil, Lemon peel oil, Cinnamon Bark oil, Eucalyptus Radiata leaf oil, Rosemary leaf oil, Ginkgo biloba leaf extract, Camellia sinensis leaf extract, Sodium hydroxide, Tocopheryl acetate, Retinyl palmitate, Aloe vera leaf juice, Citric acid

Essential Oils: Orange, Thieves blend: [Clove, Lemon, Cinnamon Bark, Eucalyptus Radiata, Rosemary]

Directions: Pump foam onto hands, lather, and then rinse thoroughly.

Cautions: If contact occurs, flush eyes liberally with clean, cool water for several minutes. If redness or irritation occurs, discontinue use. If symptoms persist, contact your physician.

Thieves® Fruit & Veggie Soak

Formulated with DiGize®, Purification®, and Thieves essential oil blends, the Thieves Fruit & Veggie Soak safely and efficiently cleans large amounts of produce at one time.

Ingredients: Water, Decyl glucoside, Glycerin, Citric acid, Sodium citrate, Tarragon oil, Ginger root oil, Peppermint oil, Juniper oil, Fennel oil, Lemongrass oil, Clove bud oil, Rosemary leaf oil, Citronella oil, Anise seed oil, Lemon peel oil, Patchouli oil, Cinnamon Bark oil, Tea Tree leaf oil, Lavandin oil, Eucalyptus Radiata oil, Tunisian Myrtle oil, Moroccan Myrtle oil

Essential Oils: Tarragon, Ginger, Peppermint, Juniper, Fennel, Lemongrass, Thieves blend: [Clove, Lemon, Cinnamon Bark, Eucalyptus Radiata, Rosemary], Citronella, Anise, Patchouli, Tea Tree, Lavandin, Tunisian Myrtle, Moroccan Myrtle

Directions: Pour 1 fl. oz. (2 tablespoons) for every gallon of water. Make enough solution to completely cover produce. Soak produce in solution for 1-2 minutes. Rinse under running water.

Cautions: Do not expose to direct sunlight.

Thieves® Fruit & Veggie Spray

Powered by six essential oils, the Thieves Fruit & Veggie Spray is formulated to quickly and naturally clean fruits and vegetables.

Ingredients: Water, Citric acid, Decyl glucoside, Glycerin, Sodium citrate, Lime rind oil, Clove bud oil, Lemon peel oil, Cinnamon Bark oil, Eucalyptus Radiata leaf oil, Rosemary leaf oil

Essential Oils: Lime, Thieves blend: [Clove, Lemon, Cinnamon Bark, Eucalyptus Radiata, Rosemary]

Directions: Spray to cover produce. Rub for 30 seconds. Rinse under running water.

Cautions: Do not expose to direct sunlight.

Thieves® Household Cleaner

Thieves Household Cleaner offers a nontoxic, biodegradable, all-purpose cleaning solution using therapeutic-grade essential oils as emulsifiers and germ and fungus killers. Containing Thieves essential oil blend, proven in a 1997 Weber State University (Ogden, Utah) study to kill over 99.96 percent of bacteria like Pseudomonas aeroginosa, this cleaner is fully biodegradable and complies with EPA standards.

Ingredients: Water, Alkyl polyglucoside, Sodium methyl 2-sulfolaurate, Clove bud oil, Lemon peel oil, Tetrasodium glutamate diacetate, Cinnamon Bark oil, Rosemary leaf oil, Eucalyptus Radiata leaf oil, Disodium 2-sulfolaurate

Essential Oils: Thieves blend: [Clove, Lemon, Cinnamon Bark, Eucalyptus Radiata, Rosemary]

Directions: Use for household cleaning purposes as needed. Dilute or use straight for extra strength. Dilution ratios are listed on the label. Before using this product to clean wood or other finished surfaces, plastics, and fabrics, perform a spot test in an inconspicuous area.

Cautions: In case of eye contact, flush thoroughly with water. If swallowed, drink plenty of water and consult a physician.

Thieves® Laundry Soap

With a plant-based formula, Thieves Laundry Soap gently and naturally washes clothes without using chemicals or synthetics. Natural enzymes and powerful essential oils enhance the formula's strength and give a pleasant, light citrus scent.

Ingredients: Water, Decyl glucoside, Glycerin, Sodium oleate, Lauryl glucoside, Caprylyl glucoside, Sodium carbonate, Alpha amylase, Lipase, Protease, Sodium gluconate, Carboxymethyl cellulose, alpha-amylase, protease, lipase, Lemon peel oil, Bergamot peel oil (Furocoumarin-free), Jade Lemon peel oil, Clove bud oil, Cinnamon Bark oil, Rosemary leaf oil, Eucalyptus Radiata leaf oil

Essential Oils: Jade Lemon, Bergamot (Furocoumarin-free), Thieves blend: [Clove, Lemon, Cinnamon Bark, Eucalyptus Radiata, Rosemary]

Directions: Follow garment-care label instructions. Add clothes. Start machine and add the proper amount of soap for load size. Standard: ½ cap for conventional washers; ¼ cap for High Efficiency (HE) washers. Adjust for smaller, larger or heavily soiled loads. To pretreat, pour onto stained fabric, gently rub, and soak. This natural formula is safe to add directly to clothes.

Cautions: In case of eye contact, flush thoroughly with water. If swallowed, drink plenty of water and consult a physician.

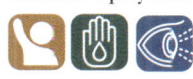

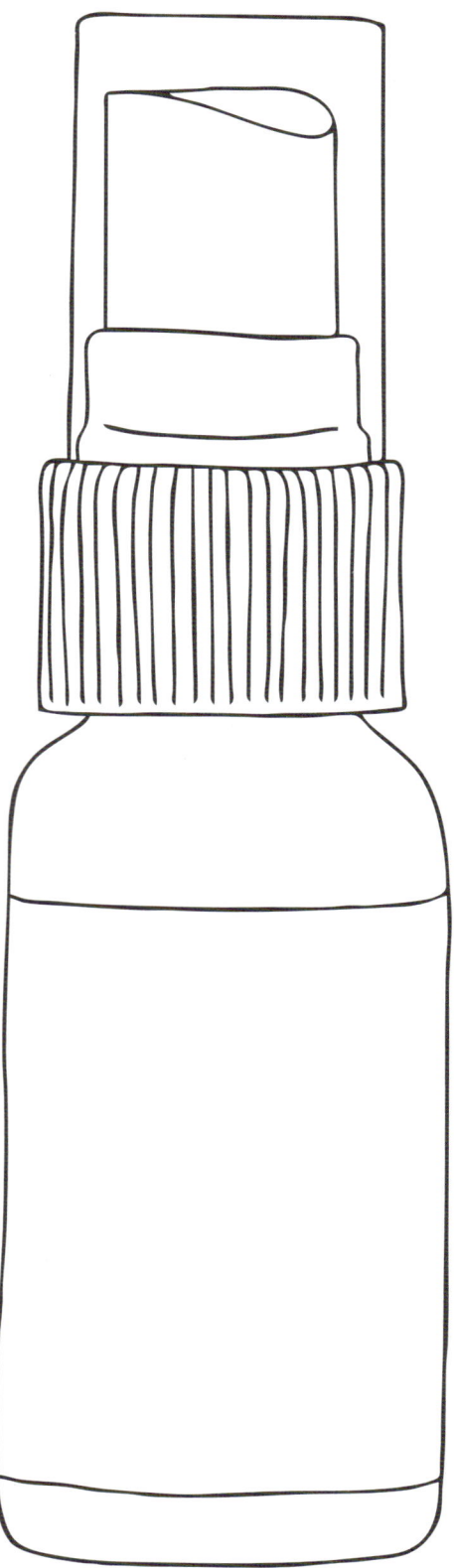

Thieves® Spray

Thieves Spray is an all-natural, petrochemical-free antiseptic spray ideal for purifying small surfaces like doorknobs, handles, toilet seats, and more. Containing Thieves essential oil blend, proven in a 1997 Weber State University (Ogden, Utah) study to kill bacteria like Pseudomonas aeroginosa, this antiseptic spray may be used to spray any surface that needs cleaning and protection from dust, mold, fungi, and other undesirable microorganisms.

Ingredients: Alcohol denat., Water, Caprylic/capric triglyceride, Clove bud oil, Lemon peel oil, Cinnamon Bark oil, Eucalyptus Radiata leaf oil, Rosemary leaf oil, Lecithin, Quillaja saponaria wood extract

Essential Oils: Thieves blend: [Clove, Lemon, Cinnamon Bark, Eucalyptus Radiata, Rosemary]

Directions: Spray on surfaces such as kitchen and bathroom counters, public seats, and anywhere germs may be present. Clean as needed.

Cautions: Not for use on infants or on sensitive areas of the body.

Thieves® Waterless Hand Sanitizer

An all-natural hand cleaner, Thieves Waterless Hand Sanitizer conveniently promotes good hygiene whenever water or washing facilities are not available. This sanitizer contains the essential oil blend of Thieves, known for its powerful antibacterial properties that penetrate the skin as the ethanol evaporates. It is effective at eliminating 99.99 percent of many common harmful germs and bacteria. It also contains active moisturizing ingredients to prevent dry skin.

Ingredients: Active: Ethyl Alcohol. Inactive. Alcohol, Water, Aloe vera leaf, Glycerin, Hydroxypropyl cellulose, Peppermint oil, Clove bud oil, Lemon peel oil, Eucalyptus Radiata leaf oil, Rosemary leaf oil, Cinnamon Bark oil

Essential Oils: Thieves blend: [Clove, Lemon, Cinnamon Bark, Eucalyptus Radiata, and Rosemary]

Directions: Dispense directly on hands and rub in thoroughly. Use daily as often as necessary to sanitize hands. Use adult supervision for children under 6.

Cautions: Do not use on or near the face. If contact occurs, flush eyes liberally with clean, cool water for several minutes. If symptoms persist, contact your physician.

Thieves® Wipes

Thieves Wipes are antiseptic cleaners infused with Thieves essential oil blend, proven in a 1997 Weber State University (Ogden, Utah) study to kill bacteria like Pseudomonas aeroginosa and are ideal for use on door handles, toilet seats, and any surface in need of cleaning and protection from dust, mold, and undesirable microorganisms.

Ingredients: Alcohol, Water, Clove bud oil, Lemon peel oil, Cinnamon Bark oil, Eucalyptus Radiata leaf oil, Rosemary leaf oil, Sunflower lecithin, Quillaja saponaria extract

Essential Oils: Thieves blend: [Clove, Lemon, Cinnamon Bark, Eucalyptus Radiata, Rosemary]

Directions: Wipe surfaces to clean as needed. Ideal for use on door handles, toilet seats, and anywhere undesirable organisms may be present.

Cautions: Not recommended for use on infants or sensitive areas of the body.

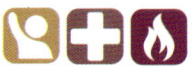

PERSONAL USES FOR ESSENTIAL OILS

There are far too many uses of essential oils to list here; nevertheless, they have really taken their place in our world. You will have many fun and amazing experiences as you use them in your daily household activities. How nice to open the dryer door and take a breath of the fresh smell of Lemon as you take out your clothes.

Laundry Freshener
Ingredients
- 2 drops Lavender (or Lemon)
- 2 drops Tea Tree

Directions
There is nothing new about the idea of scented laundry. Our ancestors used to dry their clothes on rosemary or lavender bushes to scent them. It was also popular to lay sprigs of lavender between the clean linens in cupboards to keep them smelling fresh.

Today you may add Lavender, known for its fresh scent; Tea Tree, known for its disinfecting power; or any other oil of your choice to a washcloth and put this into your washer with the rest of your laundry. You may also add a washcloth with Lavender, Lemon, or other essential oil to your dryer for fresh-smelling linens and towels.

Kitchen Deodorizing Spray

Thieves Household Cleaner and Thieves Spray are wonderful for deodorizing and cleaning the air, countertops, and appliances. Here's another spray you can have fun with as well.

Ingredients
- 4 drops Lemon
- 4 drops Lavender
- 2 drops Rosemary
- 2 drops Eucalyptus Globulus
- 1 quart distilled water

Directions
The kitchen and bathroom are often sources of odors and bacteria. This spray deodorizes and cleans the air instead of merely covering up odors.

Fill a 1-quart spray bottle with the distilled water, add the essential oils, and mix by shaking. You may use this to deodorize and freshen the air after cooking or to wipe work areas, cupboards, sinks, tiles, or woodwork. It will deodorize and help keep the areas disinfected.

Use as directed. Kitchen deodorizing spray is safe for your family and the environment.

Essential Oils for Cooking

Many essential oils and some essential oil blends may be used as ingredients for cooking and baking, in addition to their uses as supplements. Please see the Vitality essential oils and blends and their usage directions in Chapter 6 (Single Oils) and Chapter 7 (Essential Oil Blends).

Directions
When using essential oils for cooking and baking, keep in mind that they are very concentrated. You will need only 1 or 2 drops per recipe that serves at least 4 people if the oils are added after cooking and baking. However, you may find that you will need more drops of oil if they are added before cooking and baking.

Examples
Here are some examples of uses. Be creative; see what your family likes. You may find that you can include the oils in many of your own favorite recipes. The essential oils are better added at the end of cooking or boiling to keep the flavor strong.

- Season salad dressings with Lemon Vitality, Rosemary Vitality, Clove Vitality, Orange Vitality, Cinnamon Bark Vitality, Tangerine Vitality, Peppermint Vitality, or any other oil or blend of your choice.

- Season cakes, frostings, puddings, fruit pies, and salads with Lemon Vitality, Orange Vitality, Cinnamon Bark Vitality, Lavender Vitality, Clove Vitality, Spearmint Vitality, Nutmeg Vitality, Peppermint Vitality, or any other oil or blend of your choice.

- Flavor homemade ice cream with Lavender Vitality, Lemon Vitality, Orange Vitality, Peppermint Vitality, Slique Essence, or any other oil or blend of your choice.

- Season meat with Oregano Vitality, Basil Vitality, Clove Vitality, Rosemary Vitality, Nutmeg Vitality, Thyme Vitality, or any other oil or blend of your choice.

- Add Lavender Vitality, Lemon Vitality, Orange Vitality, Tangerine Vitality, Clove Vitality, Spearmint Vitality, Cinnamon Bark Vitality, Peppermint Vitality, Slique Essence, or any other oil or blend of your choice to your favorite herbal tea after brewing.

- For a cold drink that even children will love, add Lemon Vitality, Orange Vitality, Spearmint Vitality, Peppermint Vitality, Citrus Fresh Vitality, Slique Essence, or any other oil or blend of your choice to a pitcher of iced, distilled water as an alternative to sweetened sodas.

- Flavor honey by stirring in an essential oil or blend of your choice. If the honey is too solid to stir, warm it on low heat until it becomes liquid and then stir in the essential oil.

Have fun cooking and baking with the essential oils and blends of your choice.

ENDNOTES

1. Tun MH, Mahoney JJ, Konya TB, Guttman DS, Becker AB, Mandhane PJ, Turvey SE, Subbarao P, Sears MR, Brook JR, Lou W, Takarao TK, Scott JA, Kozyrskyj AL. Postnatal exposure to household disinfectants, infant gut microbiota and subsequent risk of overweight in children. Canadian Medical Association Journal. 2018 Sep 17;190(37): 1097-107.
2. Schnaubelt, Kurt. Medical aromatherapy: healing with essential oils. Berkeley (CA): Frog; c1999. 235 p.

Veterinary Medicine

Essential oils have been used very successfully on many kinds of animals, and veterinarians have now witnessed the use of essential oils with almost every form of the animal kingdom. The amazing realization that every animal in nature could be exposed to nature's powerful medicine has propelled the use of essential oils to include all species, from honeybees to elephants. In general, animals respond to essential oils in much the same way as humans.

How Much Should I Use?

That being said, most animals are more sensitive to the effects of essential oils than humans. Their keen sense of smell can be more than 10,000 times more sensitive than humans'. That alone can be enough to oversensitize them. They often seem to have a natural affinity to the healing influence of the oils.

Hair follicles may enhance the absorption of essential oils. Since animals clearly have more hair follicles than humans, we can see the potential for animals to effectively absorb essential oils, even from exposure to basic diffusion.

The sensitivity to essential oils, which was once thought to be purely an animal trait, may have a great deal to do with the density, or number, of hair follicles on a particular animal. The more follicles per square inch of skin, the more enhanced the absorption of essential oils. Therefore, cats can absorb more essential oils through their skin more efficiently than a horse or a dog with a coarser hair coat. When we consider which animal species seem most sensitive to exposure to essential oils, it often has a strong correlation with density of hair follicles.

While adjusting a dosage proportionately based on the animal's body weight is a sound first start, one must consider this enhanced ability for absorption as well. It would seem logical that if the protocol for a human being weighing 160 pounds calls for 3-5 drops, then a horse at 1,600 pounds or more could use as much as 10 times that amount, and a dog weighing 16 pounds would need as little as one tenth of that amount. Although this increase for the horse is likely accurate for oral use, topical applications may actually require less, considering hair follicle density per square inch of skin.

In animals smaller than humans, protocols are often adjusted based on body weight. If one drop of an essential oil can aid a headache in a 160-pound human, a bird weighing less than 1 pound may receive therapeutic levels from the minute amount of oils associated with water-based diffusion. Wide ranges of safety within the animal kingdom have been documented when therapeutic-grade oils are used.

Start with protocols that are known to be used for your particular species of animal, using small amounts initially and then gradually increasing in concentration and frequency. It is easy to reapply essential oils in an hour or more if additional oil is needed, but it's impossible to take back what has already been applied.

Applying oils to the feet has long been considered the safest location for humans. However, evidence suggests that animals come into contact with more toxins through their "feet." Applying essential oils (especially neat) to the pads and feet of dogs and cats may create discomfort due to interaction with everyday exposure to toxic residue that may have built up on the "feet." This phenomenon—known as bio-accumulation—results from exposure to fabric softeners, floor cleaners, lawn and ice-melting chemicals, outdoor pollutants, chemical-laden human skin care and beauty products, topical medications, hand sanitizers, air fresheners, odor eliminators, etc. Large animals such as horses and cows generally tolerate well the application of essential oils along the hooves and along the frog or coronet band regions. Proper oil selection and application with personal safety in mind should be considered.

With small dogs, cats, and exotic pets, essential oils should generally be diluted prior to application. Animals are more sensitive to essential oils than humans for many reasons, so to achieve the best results with them, understanding each species' unique needs, appropriate dilution, and applications of the oils is important.

Some species are more sensitive to the chemical constituents of the oils. For example, cats are notoriously deficient in the Cytochrome P450 liver pathway, which is responsible for the metabolism and excretion of many chemicals from their bodies.

This requires that a different approach be considered when using essential oils on cats. When choosing oils high in phenols and eugenols, such as Oregano, Thyme, Clove, and Cinnamon, do so with veterinary supervision, increased dilutions, and decreased frequency of application. For more information, please see the Essential Oils Animal Desk Reference.

Essential Oils Complete Home Reference | First Edition

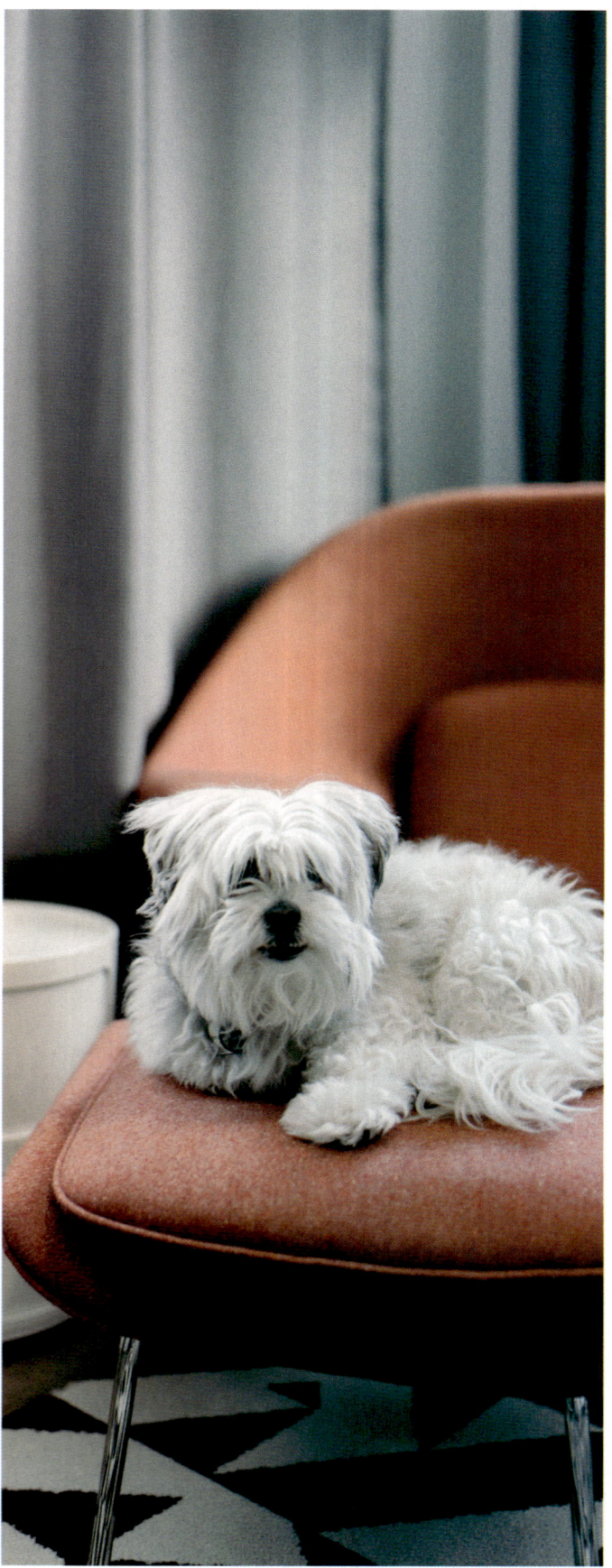

Percentages

A clear understanding about how to dilute essential oils is critical for proper use, especially for animals, but understanding the percentages of dilution can be difficult. Confusion can be created when someone is uncertain if the oil should be used at 90 percent "strong" or 90 percent "diluted." In most situations, describing the dilution of essential oils in terms of how many drops of essential oils are added to the number of drops of carrier oil is easier to understand.

A solution referred to as 90 percent is 1 drop of essential oil in 9 drops of carrier oil. An 80 percent solution is 2 drops of essential oil in 8 drops of carrier oil. Below is a quick reference for the percent of dilution in terms of drops of essential oil per carrier oil.

90%	=	1 drop essential oil	+ 9 drops carrier oil
80%	=	2 drops essential oil	+ 8 drops carrier oil
70%	=	3 drops essential oil	+ 7 drops carrier oil
60%	=	4 drops essential oil	+ 6 drops carrier oil
50%	=	5 drops essential oil	+ 5 drops carrier oil

(also called 50:50 = 1 drop essential oil + 1 drop carrier oil)

40%	=	6 drops essential oil	+ 4 drops carrier oil
30%	=	7 drops essential oil	+ 3 drops carrier oil
20%	=	8 drops essential oil	+ 2 drops carrier oil
10%	=	9 drops essential oil	+ 1 drop carrier oil

General Guidelines

- For small animals (cats, small dogs, and exotics): Apply 3-5 drops of diluted (80-90 percent) oil mixture per application.
- For larger animals (large dogs, goats, and pigs): Apply 3-5 drops neat (dilute if using oils high in phenol) per application.
- For large animals (cattle, horses, and elephants): Apply 10-15 drops neat (dilute if using oils high in phenol) per application.

Aversions to Essential Oils

For those new to essential oils, start with very light, "species-specific" applications. When animals appear to "dislike" essential oils, they may have been exposed to an inappropriate amount or use of the essential oil.

Aversion to a negative event is strongly ingrained in an animal's memory, according to a lecture presented by Dr. Temple Grandin, PhD and professor of animal science at Colorado State University. If an animal experiences a negative event along with a particular scent, future use of that scent may "remind" an animal of that past occurrence.

An animal in close proximity to an essential oil may exhibit behavior that is interpreted as an aversion to that oil. In reality, the olfactory receptors may have been overwhelmed. Animals don't need to have close contact with the oil to experience its benefits. To quote Stanley Coren and Sarah Hodgson: "In humans, the area containing odor analyzers in the brain is the size of a postage stamp. The same area in a dog may be just under 8.5" x 11"."

We do not need to avoid using essential oils around our animals, but we do need to understand and respect that some animals can smell the essential oil from across the room (or across the football field) with the bottle still closed.

Before Using Essential Oils

When using essential oils to address specific health concerns, consult with a veterinarian and have blood and urine evaluations performed prior to using essential oils. Work with your veterinarian to determine the frequency of follow-up examinations and laboratory testing. It is important to address the underlying root cause of the condition, rather than just using essential oils to address the symptoms.

The vast majority of essential oils available today are nontherapeutic oils. Adulterated, synthetic, and contaminated oils should not be used and may be toxic to both you and your animal. Using these types of oils may result in adverse reactions, including, but not limited to, skin issues, vomiting, and diarrhea. When you use therapeutic-grade oils on top of areas that have poor-quality oils or other toxins stored within them, you run the risk of having skin irritations and outbreaks.

TECHNIQUES FOR DIFFERENT ANIMAL SPECIES

The use of essential oils has been documented in almost every species; however, each species has a slightly different set of techniques and methods used to safely and easily expose them to essential oils.

Fish

Fish are exposed to plant matter decomposing in their water environment. Peppermint and Lemon essential oils and Purification essential oil blend have been used frequently and with great results for a multitude of concerns from fungal infections to parasites and bacterial concerns.

Start by introducing very small amounts of oil into a glass aquarium or pond by dipping a toothpick into the oil and then putting the toothpick into the water. After several days, amounts can be increased according to the volume of water in the enclosure. Often, when drops of essential oil are placed on the water's surface, fish will orally ingest the oil droplets. This is truly an amazing sight to see.

Insects

Likewise, insects can be affected by essential oils. For example, honeybees are suffering from mysterious conditions. Dripping essential oils like Frankincense onto cotton balls and placing them in or around the beehive is currently being used to boost honeybee health.

Essential oils are also used as pest control to repel insects.

Birds

Birds (especially parrots) are a more recent addition to the world of veterinary aromatherapy. Pet birds are extremely sensitive to household toxins, and even the spraying of an air freshener or the burning of a candle can be dangerous to a bird. Since many household fragrances are created with poor-grade, adulterated, or synthetic essential oils, it was commonly thought that all essential oils were toxic to birds. This has been found to be untrue. While birds have a distinct way in which they should be exposed to essential oils, they not only benefit from but also thrive with the addition of essential oils into their lives.

A favorite technique that is being used currently with thousands of birds is the Feather Spray Recipe. This amazing spray was created by Leigh Foster and carries benefits for everything from bacterial, viral, and fungal conditions to cancer prevention and immune system support.

Feather Spray Recipe

Place 20 drops of Lavender, 20 drops of Lemon, and 20 drops of Orange essential oils into a 4-ounce glass spray bottle. Add distilled water to fill the bottle. Shake well before each application and then mist the bird directly with the spray up to 2 times a day. Birds love this spray, including those who routinely dislike a shower from a traditional spray bottle.

Diffusing

Diffusing from one of the water-based diffusers is recommended for use with birds. Air diffusers may be used; however, they require being farther away from the bird or used in a much larger room (such as a barn or large aviary). Almost all essential oil singles and blends have been diffused around birds from water-based diffusers such as the Aria Ultrasonic Diffuser.

In general, start with 3 drops of oil added to the water in the diffuser. Monitor the bird(s) closely for the first 5-10 minutes of diffusing and gradually increase the length of time and frequency. Often, you can diffuse on an almost continual basis—bringing amazing benefits and health to your birds.

Exotic Pets

You can use essential oils for ferrets in the same way as for cats. For other exotic animals, start with water-based diffusing, as outlined for birds. For animals that may soak in water, such as turtles or lizards, the recommendations made for fish can easily be used. Many exotic pets enjoy small amounts of Citrus Fresh or other citrus oils added to their drinking water. Use approximately 1 drop per liter of water. Make sure that the animal drinks adequately and that plastic dishes are not used to hold the water. Glass, ceramic, and stainless-steel water containers are recommended for use with essential oils.

Cats

Cats present their own unique controversies and requirements for essential oil use. Most cat owners would agree that cats have distinct opinions of the world, and this certainly holds true for aromatherapy. Diffusing is usually a method that is well tolerated by all cats, especially from water-based ultrasonic diffusers.

Many misconceptions have been made about what cats like or don't like. Apparently, these generalizations may have been made based on individual reports and not from cats as a species. For example, one cat may dislike citrus oils, but then another cat is found to be attracted to them. Allowing cats to show you their individual preferences is a good idea. If a cat leaves or enters the room when you diffuse a certain essential oil, you will quickly find out its preferences every time that particular oil is diffused.

The wisest choice is to use oils that are used often or have been used with many cats and to use them with techniques that cats enjoy. The best choice is to first select an oil that is known to be very safe and well-tolerated by cats.

Presented here are the application methods most commonly used on cats. Start with techniques that are widely used and shown to be safe. Animals are individuals so there could be a specific cat that will not respond well to an application method or that may prove to be more sensitive than another cat. Common sense and a tailored approach for each cat are important. A good policy is to consult with a veterinarian and have blood and urine evaluations done prior to starting the use of essential oils.

Diffusing

Diffusing by a water-based ultrasonic diffuser is the most tolerated by cats. Start by adding 3-5 drops of essential oil to the diffuser. If cats tolerate and like particular essential oils, concentrations and times may be increased.

Kitty Raindrop Technique (KRDT)

This technique was created by Leigh Foster and used on many of her own rescued cats prior to its now mainstream use. Although this technique includes oils that are typically contraindicated for cats, veterinarians and cat owners alike have witnessed amazing health benefits with this technique. The formula and technique were designed specifically for cats, and it is remarkable to watch them enjoy this application.

Kitty Raindrop Solution

Add 4 drops each of Oregano (or Plectranthus Oregano), Thyme, Basil, Cypress, Wintergreen, Marjoram, and Peppermint to a 30-ml (1-ounce) glass essential oil bottle. Add V-6 Vegetable Oil Complex to fill the remainder of the bottle, creating a Kitty Raindrop Massage Oil Blend.

Mix by rocking the bottle; then apply approximately 6 drops of the solution up the spine of the cat, from tail to head. Next, gently stroke or feather the Kitty Raindrop Massage Oil Blend up the back of the cat, similar to the methods used with the human Raindrop Technique. Amazingly, cats often enjoy this backward stroke! If you encounter one that does not, just pet the cat "normally" from head to tail or omit the strokes all together.

Balancing the cat with Valor (neat or diluted) can be performed prior to the KRDT. Place Valor in the palms of your hands, and then rub your hands together, allowing the Valor to almost completely absorb into your palms. Place your hands over the shoulder and rump area, and the balancing procedure is completed much like that described for humans. In some situations, this step is omitted, mainly in cats who are unable to be handled easily.

Petting the Cat

This method is well-tolerated by cats and seems to be far superior to dripping oils directly onto their skin. Since hair follicles may enhance absorption, spreading the essential oils over a larger area of the cat may indeed prove more effective. This method involves placing a neat or diluted oil into your hand. Circling your hands together, the essential oils can absorb in varying degrees into your skin. Once you have the amount of oil on your hands that you desire—which can vary from completely absorbed to a thin coating—you simply pet your cat.

Even with oils completely absorbed into your hand, if you smell your cat after petting, you will find that it smells like essential oils. Since cats groom themselves, oral ingestion of the essential oil is also likely to occur.

Kitty Litter

Kitty litter is possibly one of the easiest methods by which to expose cats to the health benefits of essential oils. It not only replaces the toxic fragrances found in commercial kitty litter, but it also offers a way to provide preventive and continued health benefits from essential oils on a regular basis.

Initially, stay with your same brand of kitty litter, making sure it's unscented. Add 1-3 drops of your chosen essential oil to 1 cup of baking soda. Store this mixture in a glass jar and allow it to "marinate" for several hours, shaking the mixture several times. Later, you may find you can add more essential oil drops to this recipe.

Sprinkle a small amount of the baking soda mixture onto your kitty litter. Mix well. Provide a separate litter box that does not contain essential oils to make sure that your cat does not have an aversion to the essential oil that was selected. Once you are sure your cat is using the litter box with your oil selection and concentration, you can then omit the use of the plain litter box.

Selecting and rotating various oils can bring big benefits to your cat. Copaiba can aid with arthritis pains, DiGize or DiGize Vitality can aid in intestinal upset, and Frankincense or Frankincense Vitality may bring anticancer benefits. The choices are endless and can provide powerful preventive measures to your feline friends.

Dogs

Dogs come in various sizes, so techniques will often need to be modified accordingly. Dogs the size of cats and smaller may initially do best when exposed to essential oils with the recommendations made for cats. Larger concentrations of oils may then be used as needed. On average, dogs can use oils more freely and easily than cats and smaller-sized animals, much like we would use oils for young children.

Raindrop Technique

Raindrop Technique has become a very common and regular treatment course for animals. This powerful technique is indicated for almost any concern; however, streamlining this application into approximately 15-20 minutes is mandatory to be able to provide the procedure to every patient who is in need. When possible, a full Raindrop Technique, similar to that described and used for humans, is recommended.

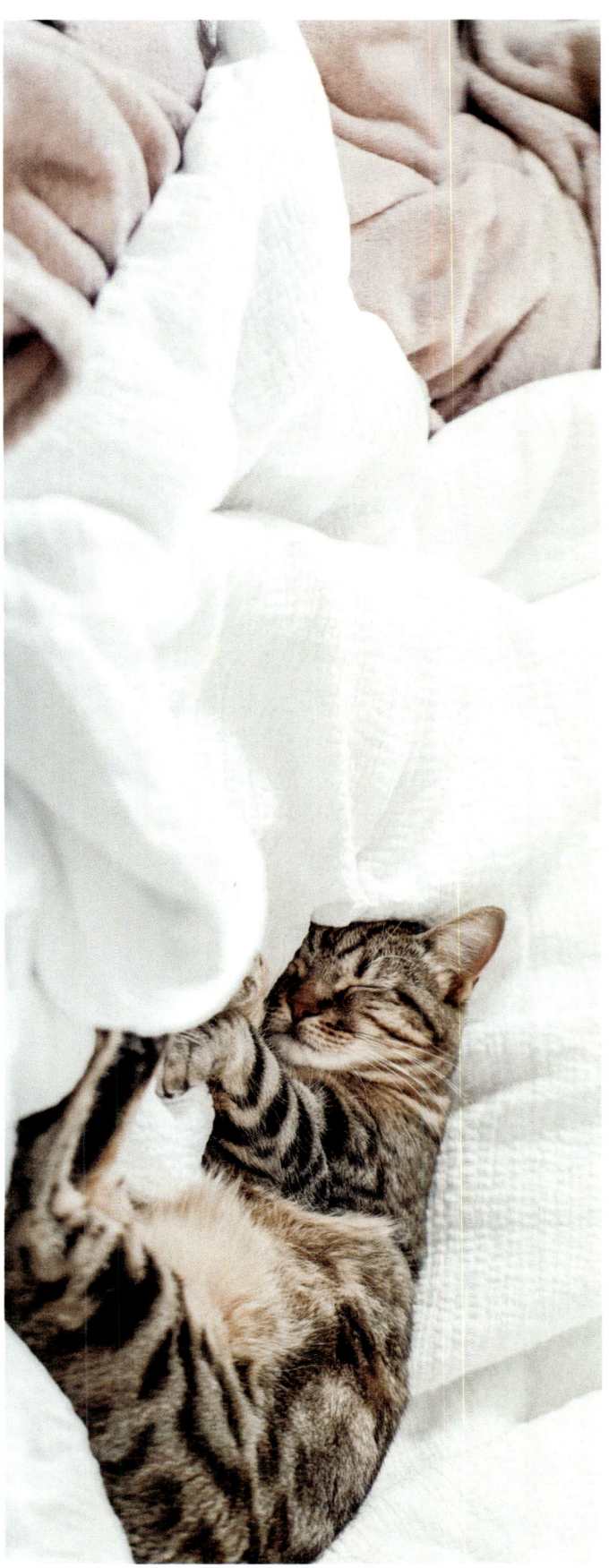

However, when multiple animals in a hospital, farm, or household would benefit from a Raindrop Technique, the oils are far more important than the actual procedure. Learning the very simple and basic procedure allows for a level of comfort to be established, and future skills may be incorporated when the facilitator is ready.

Balancing with Valor can occur as an optional step for dogs as well. Several drops are placed into the palms of your hand, generally neat, and are usually left "wet" in the palm. The hands are placed over the shoulder and rump, and balancing is performed, much as it is described for humans.

Next, the Raindrop Technique oils are applied one at a time up the spine, dripping from approximately 6 inches above the dog. The oils are not mixed together for dogs as they are for cats. Some dogs may require oils to be diluted prior to application, and in that case, we generally dilute each oil individually.

Very small or sensitive dogs can benefit from the Kitty Raindrop Technique as well. For very small dogs, generally under 20 pounds (9 kg), approximately 3 drops of each oil should be applied. For dogs 20-50 pounds (9-23 kg), approximately 3-6 drops of each oil are applied. Dogs over 50 pounds (23 kg) can generally receive approximately 6-9 drops of each Raindrop oil.

The sequence of oil application is generally:
- Oregano (or Plectranthus Oregano)
- Thyme
- V-6 Vegetable Oil Complex
- Basil
- Cypress
- Wintergreen
- Marjoram
- Peppermint

After each oil is dripped up the spine, the oils are stroked up the back from tail to head. For this abbreviated version of the Raindrop Technique, don't be concerned with the length of the strokes or how many times you perform them. Stimulating the spinal area over which the oils are dripped is the main goal, and even normal petting can accomplish this when needed.

So, if Oregano and Thyme are applied and stroked in, a fairly generous strip of V-6 should also be applied along the spine. Fur does not need to be parted for any part of the application, except with extremely long-haired dogs whose hair naturally parts.

The V-6 is massaged in, and then the rest of the essential oils are dripped on in sequence and stroked in, right on top of the V-6. It has a much better handling quality and does not leave as much of a greasy residue behind (for fur or furniture).

After all the essential oils are applied and stroked in, Vita Flex may also be performed up the spine in a final closing procedure.

If irritation to the skin or animal occurs at any stage of the Raindrop Technique, it is suggested that you stop the procedure and not apply any more oils. Apply more V-6 to the area of detoxification and irritation and allow approximately 10-15 minutes for full calming effects to be seen. Generally, do not try to "fix" any skin irritation by applying another calming or skin-soothing essential oil to the site.

Kitty Raindrop for Dogs

Many dogs have been exposed to toxic chemicals, repeat vaccinations, or chronic medications and are in great need of detoxification. Since essential oils are so powerful in evoking this detoxification, sometimes more is not better. For dogs that do have a larger need for detoxification, using diluted or milder oils will gradually detoxify them in a more comfortable manner. After a time, their body will grow healthier, and they will be able to enjoy a full-fledged Raindrop Technique.

For dogs less than 20 pounds, use the Kitty Raindrop Massage Oil Blend and use the same technique as for cats. For larger dogs between 20 and 45 pounds, increase the drops of each oil in the blend to 10 drops each.

Petting the Dog

Just as described for cats, petting dogs is a wonderful application method. You can usually have much more essential oil on the palms of your hands prior to petting dogs, and dilution is not commonly needed.

Diffusing

Dogs benefit greatly from regular daily diffusion and tolerate well both air-style and water-based diffusing. The previous directions regarding diffusing may be followed for dogs as well.

Small Ruminants, Pigs

These animals can often be exposed to oils in similar ways as dogs. Raindrop Technique is often used. Diffusing for these animals is best with a direct oil diffuser such as the AromaLux™ Atomizing Diffuser or a large-volume, water-based diffuser, as they are often in barns or larger areas. Oral essential oils are commonly used and are easily added to feed.

Horses

Favorite methods of oil use for horses include Raindrop Technique, oral oils, oils in feed, topical applications (neat or diluted), massage, and petting. Oils can be added to the water trough, as long as there is also non-oiled water available.

Cattle and Livestock

Oils are used similarly to horses for these animals. Regular use of oils in feeds, water, udder washes, and post-milking teat dips are wonderful ways to provide health benefits on a routine basis.

How to Administer Essential Oils Internally

For ingestion, the essential oils can be put into a capsule or mixed with the animal's food. A few drops can be added to soft, moist foods or to gravy on food when giving to dogs or cats. Mixing an essential oil with NingXia Red juice and giving it orally by syringe or mixing with food are common practices. Some animals will also ingest essential oils added to their drinking water. Have a second water source without oils available.

For large animals, the animal's bottom lip can be pulled out, and, as in the case of horses, 5 to 15 drops of oil dropped in. The animal will feel the effect quickly because capillaries in the lip will carry the oil into the bloodstream immediately. For a large dog, 1 to 3 drops are sufficient. Oral dosing in cats is often met with profuse salivation. This response can be seen with medications and supplements as well as essential oils.

When treating animals with essential oils internally, it is critical to make certain the oils used are pure and free of chemicals, solvents, and adulterants.

Applying Essential Oils to a Jittery, Resistant Animal

If you have a high-spirited, jittery animal that will not be still to receive the application, apply Peace & Calming, Stress Away, and/or Valor on yourself first. As you approach the animal, it should react more calmly as it smells the aroma.

Kneel or squat beside the animal and remain still for several minutes so that it can become accustomed to the smell. As the animal breathes in the fragrances, it will become calmer and easier to manage.

Other Helpful Tips

- When treating large animals for viral or bacterial infection, arthritis, or bone injury, generally use the same oils and protocols recommended for humans.

- When applying to large, open wounds or hard-to-reach areas, it helps to put the oils in a spray bottle. Dilute the oils with V-6 Vegetable Oil Complex, other vegetable oils, or olive oil, and spray the mixture directly on the location.

- After applying oil to an open wound, cover the wound with Animal Scents Ointment to seal and protect it from further infection. The ointment will also prevent the essential oils from evaporating. Use the Seedlings Diaper Rash Cream to cover and dry an area where you do not want more moisture, such as a hot spot.

- There is no right or wrong way to apply essential oils. Every animal is a little different. Use common sense and good judgment as you experiment with different methods. Observe carefully how the animal responds to the treatment.

- Take special care not to get essential oils in the animal's eyes. Make sure you have a carrier oil available to flush the eye if required.

- Make sure the animal is drinking pure water. Chlorinated water will suppress thyroid and immune function in animals even quicker than in humans. When that happens, you will suppress the healing process of that animal, whether it is a dog, horse, or cat.

- Quality protein is vitally important to promote healing, which makes the use of organic or non-GMO feed essential. The addition of enzymes and probiotics maximize digestion and protein assimilation.

ANIMAL SCENTS® PRODUCTS

Nutritional supplementation is a great blessing for our animals, but the value is determined by quality, quantity, and frequency.

CAUTIONS

Note which cautions are applicable to which oil under each oil's listing. Not all cautions apply to all oils.

 Keep out of reach of children.

 For external use only.

Bolded ingredients are essential oils.

Animal Scents Cat Treats

These treats for your favorite kitty have naturally derived, grain-free ingredients. They are flavored with Ginger oil, creating a delicious treat for your furry friends. These treats are made without wheat, soy, or corn fillers for the good health of your pet.

Ingredients: Chicken meal, Pea protein, Tapioca starch, Pea powder, Chicken fat, Chicken, Natural flavor palatability enhancer for dry cat food, Brewer's dried yeast, Potassium chloride, Calcium carbonate, Glucono-delta-lactone, Citric acid (preservative), Mixed tocopherols (preservative), Rosemary extract, **Ginger**

Directions: 5-10 lbs. (6-9 treats), 10-15 lbs. (10-14 treats), 15 lbs. and over (up to 15 treats). Feeding guidelines are based on the recommendation that cats receive no more than 10 percent of their daily calories from treats. Intended for intermittent or supplemental feeding only.

Cautions: Choking hazard. Not for human consumption. Always offer sufficient water when giving your pets treats or food. Make sure your pet chews the treat completely, as gulping any item can be harmful to your pet. This product is not recommended for pets with a history of gulping, choking, or poor chewing capability. Always consult with your veterinarian about the proper nutrition for your pets.

Animal Scents Dental Pet Chews

Animal Scents Dental Pet Chews are a fast and easy way to clean your pet's teeth without having to use a toothbrush. Their naturally derived ingredients help to freshen your pet's breath; your pet will love it and so will you.

Ingredients: Potato starch, Pork gelatin, Dried plain beet pulp, Rice syrup, Pea fiber, Coconut oil, Calcium carbonate, Salt, Natural poultry flavor, Sunflower lecithin, Glycerin, Dried kelp, Dill, Parsley, Mixed tocopherols (preservative), Green tea extract, Rosemary extract (flavor), **Spearmint**

Directions: For 20+ lb. pets: give 2 chews per week. For 5-19 lb. pets: give ½ a chew 2 times a week. This product is intended for intermittent or supplemental feeding only. Adjust diet as needed to accommodate this chew. Consult a veterinarian for pets that are pregnant or under 5 lbs. before use.

Cautions: Always offer sufficient water when giving your pet treats or food. Make sure your pet chews the treat completely, as gulping any item can be harmful. This product is not recommended for pets with a history of gulping, choking, or poor chewing capability. Always consult with your veterinarian about the proper nutrition for your pet. Choking hazard. Not for human consumption.

Animal Scents Ointment

Animal Scents Ointment is blended with Tea Tree and Myrrh, two of nature's most powerful essential oils. It is a protective and soothing salve formulated for external use on animals. Tested in the field for many years, this ointment is typically used for minor skin irritations, cuts, and abrasions. It is designed to cover infected wounds and seal in the essential oils.

Animal Scents Ointment offers an effective yet gentle and safe approach to soothing your pets without using harmful chemicals or synthetic products.

Ingredients: Apricot kernel oil, Sunflower seed oil, Sunflower seed wax, Caprylic/capric triglyceride, Mango seed butter, Castor seed oil, Avocado oil, Tocopherol, Glycerin, Tamanu seed oil, Jojoba oil, **Palmarosa, Carrot Seed, Geranium, Patchouli, Coriander,** Grape seed extract, **Idaho Grand Fir, Myrrh, Tea Tree, Bergamot** (Furocoumarin-free), Ascorbyl palmitate, Rose hip seed oil, **Ylang Ylang**

Directions: Clean area and apply as needed. If using Young Living essential oils, apply oil(s) prior to application of Animal Scents Ointment.

Cautions: Specially formulated for veterinary use.

Animal Scents Shampoo

Animal Scents Shampoo is formulated to clean all types of animal fur and hair. It has insect-repelling and killing properties and is designed to rid hair of lice, ticks, and other insects. This all-natural shampoo contains five powerful essential oils that are blended to gently cleanse, increase luster, and enhance grooming without the harmful ingredients often found in pet care products.

Ingredients: Water, Decyl glucoside, Coco betaine, Lauryl glucoside, Coco-glucoside, Glycerin, Glyceryl oleate, Citric acid, Xanthan gum, Inulin, Sodium levulinate, Sodium anisate, Lavandin, Lemon, Geranium, Citronella (Cymbopogon nardus), Citronella (Cymbopogon winterianus), Sodium phytate, Northern Lights Black Spruce, Vetiver

Directions: Pour a small amount of shampoo into your palms and rub gently between your hands. Massage thoroughly into your pet's wet coat. Lather. Rinse thoroughly. Repeat if necessary.

Cautions: Specially formulated for veterinary use.

ANIMAL SCENTS ESSENTIAL OIL BLENDS

Animal Scents Infect Away™

Infect Away utilizes six essential oils for a gentle cleansing effect on your animal. For best results, use as the second part to a three-part system, with PuriClean being used first, then Infect Away, followed by Mendwell. It supports a healthy skin barrier.

Ingredients: Caprylic/capric glycerides, Myrrh, Patchouli, Dorado Azul, Palo Santo, Ecuadorian (Plectranthus) Oregano, Ocotea

Directions: Carefully apply according to the size and species of the animal. Additional dilution is recommended for smaller species.

Cautions: Specially formulated for veterinary use. Take extra care when using essential oils around cats, especially those with citric ingredients.

Animal Scents Mendwell™

Mendwell is a blend of oils that supports healthy skin repair and is specifically formulated for animals. For best results, use as the last step in a three-part system, with PuriClean and Infect Away being used first.

Ingredients: Caprylic/capric glycerides, Geranium, Lavender, Hyssop, Myrrh, Frankincense

Directions: Carefully apply according to the size and species of the animal. Additional dilution is recommended for smaller species.

Cautions: Specially formulated for veterinary use. Take extra care when using essential oils around cats, especially those with citric ingredients.

Animal Scents ParaGize™

Created with animals in mind, ParaGize is a proprietary blend of essential oils that promotes healthy digestion and helps expel worms and parasites.

Ingredients: Caprylic/capric glycerides, Ginger, Anise, Peppermint, Cumin, Spearmint leaf extract, Rosemary, Tarragon, Juniper, Fennel, Lemongrass, Patchouli

Directions: Carefully apply according to the size and species of the animal. Additional dilution is recommended for smaller species.

Cautions: Specially formulated for veterinary use. Take extra care when using essential oils around cats, especially those with citric ingredients.

Animal Scents PuriClean™

PuriClean is a unique blend of eleven essential oils that is specifically formulated for animals that cleanses and refreshes the skin. For best results, use as the first step in a three-part application, with Infect Away and Mendwell being used after PuriClean.

Ingredients: Caprylic/capric glycerides, Patchouli, Lavender, Mountain Savory, Palo Santo, Cistus, Lemongrass, Citronella, Rosemary, Tea Tree, Lavandin, Myrtle

Directions: Carefully apply according to the size and species of the animal. Additional dilution is recommended for smaller species.

Cautions: Specially formulated for veterinary use. Take extra care when using essential oils around cats, especially those with citric ingredients.

Products for First Aid for Animals

Animal Scents Ointment to seal and disinfect open wounds.

Copaiba for bruising and soreness on small animals; used as a replacement for traditional Non-Steroidal Anti-Inflammatory Drugs (NSAIDs).

Exodus II for infection and inflammation and to promote tissue regeneration.

Helichrysum as a topical anesthetic and for neurologic conditions.

Palo Santo, one of the most versatile essential oils for animals, is purifying, cleansing, tissue-regenerating, anti-inflammatory, and anesthetic. It is used for bruised bones and ligaments, cuts, and wounds. It also repels flies.

Lavender for tissue regeneration, infection, and calming. Effective against ringworm.

Melrose for disinfecting and cleaning wounds; accelerates healing of wounds.

Mountain Savory for reducing inflammation and infection.

Myrrh for infection, inflammation, and promoting tissue regeneration

Ocotea for bruising and soreness on large animals; oil of choice for diabetes.

Ortho Ease Massage Oil and Ortho Sport Massage Oil to dilute essential oils and act as a pain reliever and anti-inflammatory; also has insect-repelling actions.

PanAway as a pain killer if the pain originates from a broken bone rather than an open wound. Make sure there is no visible, open, raw tissue because it will sting and traumatize the animal. Instead, use Helichrysum and Idaho Balsam Fir to reduce bleeding and pain.

Purification for washing and cleansing wounds is more effective than using iodine or hydrogen peroxide. It also repels ticks and mites.

Roman Chamomile for tissue regeneration and calming.

Thieves for inflammation, infection, bacteria, proud flesh (a condition where new tissue continues to rebuild itself, causing excessive granulation), and promoting tissue regeneration.

Valerian for controlling internal or external pain.

Vetiver for controlling internal or external pain.

Animal Scents T-Away™

T-Away is formulated with a powerful combination of essential oils to promote new levels of emotional freedom and joyful feelings.

Ingredients: Caprylic/capric glycerides, Tangerine, Lavender, German Chamomile, Frankincense, Valerian, Royal Hawaiian Sandalwood™, Ylang Ylang, Orange, Black Spruce, Geranium, Davana, Angelica, Rue, Helichrysum, Hyssop, Spanish Sage, Citrus Hystrix leaf extract, Patchouli, Coriander, Blue Tansy, Bergamot (Furocoumarin-free), Rose, Lemon, Jasmine, Roman Chamomile, Palmarosa

Directions: Carefully apply according to the size and species of the animal. Additional dilution is recommended for smaller species.

Cautions: Specially formulated for veterinary use. Take extra care when using essential oils around cats, especially those with citric ingredients.

ANIMAL TREATMENT

Arthritis (common in older animals and purebreds)

Ortho Ease Massage Oil, Ortho Sport Massage Oil, or PanAway: Massage Ortho Ease, Ortho Sport, or PanAway on location or put several drops of PanAway in animal feed.

Use Raindrop-like application of PanAway, Wintergreen, Pine, or Spruce and massage the location. For larger animals, use at least two times more oil than a normal Raindrop Technique would call for on humans.

Copaiba can be given orally as a replacement for traditional NSAIDs.

For prevention: AminoWise, Pure Protein Complete, BLM Caps, AgilEase, and/or Sulfurzyme in feed or fodder. Small animals need 1/8 to 1/4 serving per day. Large animals need 2 to 4 servings per day.

Birthing
Gentle Baby

Bleeding
Geranium, Helichrysum, and Cistus: For internal hemorrhage, the use of Cistus orally is recommended.

Bones (pain and spurs on all animals)
R.C., PanAway, Wintergreen, Copaiba, Frankincense, Idaho Grand Fir, any variety of Spruce is recommended. All conifers are very powerful in the action for bones and in promoting bone health. AgilEase, BLM caps, SuperCal Plus, and Sulfurzyme are excellent supplements for building animal bones.

Bones (fractured or broken)
In conjunction with veterinary care, mix PanAway with 15-25 drops of Wintergreen and Spruce. Cover the area. After 15 minutes, rub in 10-15 more drops of Wintergreen and Spruce and cover with Ortho Sport Massage Oil.

Calming
Peace & Calming, T-Away, Trauma Life, Stress Away, Tranquil, Grounding, and Lavender; domestic animals respond very quickly to smell.

Colds and Flu
For small animals, put 1-3 drops of Exodus II, ImmuPower, DiGize, or DiGize Vitality in feed or fodder. For large animals, use 10-20 drops. Use Raven, R.C., or Breathe Again for respiratory effects.

Colic
For large animals like cows, put 10-20 drops of DiGize or DiGize Vitality in feed or fodder or apply topically to abdomen. For small animals, use 1-3 drops.

Horse Colic Protocol: In addition to veterinary care, administer 5-20 drops of Peppermint or Peppermint Vitality and 5-20 drops of DiGize or DiGize Vitality orally and apply to the umbilical area of the abdomen. Repeat every 20 minutes, as needed.

Dull Coat
Animal Scents Shampoo, PuriClean, Rosemary, Sandalwood, Sulfurzyme, OmegaGize3, Cedarwood

Fleas and Other Parasites
Singles: Lemongrass, Tea Tree, Eucalyptus (all types), Peppermint

Blends: Purification, Citronella, Palo Santo, Cedarwood, ParaGize, DiGize; also add 1-2 drops of above oils to Animal Scents Shampoo.

Oils repel fleas and other external parasites. Wash blankets with Thieves Laundry Soap, with oils added to the wash during the rinse cycle. Also, place 1-2 drops of Purification on the collar to help eliminate fleas.

For internal parasites, rub ParaGize and/or DiGize on the abdomen daily or use ParaFree.

Inflammation
Apply Copaiba, Ortho Ease Massage Oil, Ortho Sport Massage Oil, PanAway, Pine, Wintergreen, Deep Relief Roll-On. or Spruce on location. Put Sulfurzyme and/or AgilEase in feed. Mineral Essence may also be helpful.

Insect Repellent
Use Purification. Put 10 drops each of Palo Santo, Kunzea, Eucalyptus Globulus, and Peppermint in an 8-ounce spray bottle with water.

Alternate formula: Put 2 drops Cedarwood, 2 drops Eucalyptus Globulus, and 5-10 drops Purification in a spray bottle of water. Shake vigorously and spray over area.

Ligaments/Tendons (torn or sprained)
Apply Lemongrass and Palo Santo (equal parts) on location. For small animals or birds, dilute essential oils with V-6 Vegetable Oil Complex (2 parts carrier oil to 1 part essential oil). Palo Santo is an excellent oil for use on smaller animals and is generally milder than Lemongrass.

Mineral Deficiencies
Mineral Essence. In one case, an animal stopped chewing on furniture once his mineral deficiency was met. Mineral deficiency is also an important aspect of anxiety in animals, so supplementing with Mineral Essence can show beneficial calming effects.

Mites (ear mites)
Apply Purification and/or Melrose to a cotton swab and swab just the inside of the ear flap and the base of the ear, avoiding putting oils directly in the ear canal.

Nervous Anxiety
Valor, T-Away, Trauma Life, Roman Chamomile, Geranium, Lavender, Valerian, Stress Away, Peace & Calming, Inner Child, Tranquil

Pain

Helichrysum, PanAway, Relieve It, Cool Azul Pain Relief Cream, Deep Relief Roll-On, Cool Azul, Cool Azul Sports Gel, Clove, or Peppermint diluted 50/50 with V-6 Vegetable Oil Complex

Sinus Problems

Diffuse Raven, R.C., Pine, Myrtle, Dorado Azul, and/or Eucalyptus Radiata in the animal's sleeping quarters or sprinkle on the bedding. Thieves, Super C, Exodus II, Allerzyme, and ImmuPro have been reported as being extremely beneficial for sinus and lung congestion.

Skin Cancer

Frankincense, Lavender, Clove, Myrrh, Ledum, Sacred Frankincense, Sacred Sandalwood; apply neat, then dilute if required.

Ticks

To remove ticks, apply 1 drop of Thieves or Peppermint on a cotton swab and apply directly to the tick. Then wait for it to release its head before removing from the animal's skin.

Trauma

T-Away, Trauma Life, Valor, Peace & Calming, Melissa, Gentle Baby, Lavender, Valerian, Roman Chamomile, SARA, Release, Stress Away

Tumors or Cancers

Mix Frankincense with Ledum, Lavender, Citrus oil of choice, or Clove and apply on the area of the tumor.

Upset

Peace & Calming, T-Away, Trauma Life, and Lavender. Domestic animals respond very quickly to the smell.

Worms and Parasites

ParaGize, ParaFree, DiGize, Fennel, Patchouli, Thieves

Wounds (open or abrasions)

PuriClean, Infect Away, Mendwell, Melrose, Helichrysum, Animal Scents Ointment, ClaraDerm, LavaDerm

SPECIFIC CARE FOR HORSES

Bruised Ankle (e.g., from hobble injury)

Copaiba, PanAway, Idaho Grand Fir, Melrose, Cool Azul, Cool Azul Pain Relief Cream, Ortho Sport Massage Oil, Ortho Ease Massage Oil, Relieve It, Wintergreen, Idaho Blue Spruce, Cool Azul Sports Gel, and Deep Relief Roll-On to reduce tenderness, bruising, and inflammation

Cancer

Sacred Frankincense or Frankincense. Alternate with Clove oil every four days. Keep saturated with Sacred Frankincense or Frankincense. If the area is open, put a saturated or cotton gauze plug in the opening to hold the oil in the tumor cavity. Continue for up to six months.

Colic (the leading cause of death in horses)

Symptoms

- Pawing the ground with head down
- Stretching out as if to urinate
- Lying down and looking bloated
- Excessive or no churning or rumbling in the stomach
- Biting or looking toward the stomach area

Causes

- Eating off the ground and a mineral imbalance (getting too much dirt or sand in the gut; accumulated dirt can cause the gut to twist, abscess, and spasm)
- Parasites
- Eating too much alfalfa and not enough feed; alfalfa can stress the kidneys and livers of horses. In general, grass hay is best for horses of all kinds.
- Abrupt feed changes
- Getting too hot
- Drinking too much cold water immediately after exercise

Treatment Protocol

Encourage the horse to stand or continue walking to prevent it from lying down and rolling. Keep the horse's head tied up to prevent him from rolling.

1st hour, after calling the vet:

Internal Use

- Mix 8 to 10 opened Detoxzyme capsules with 15 drops of DiGize Vitality in a NingXia Red base, then syringe down the throat.

Animal Care | Chapter 9

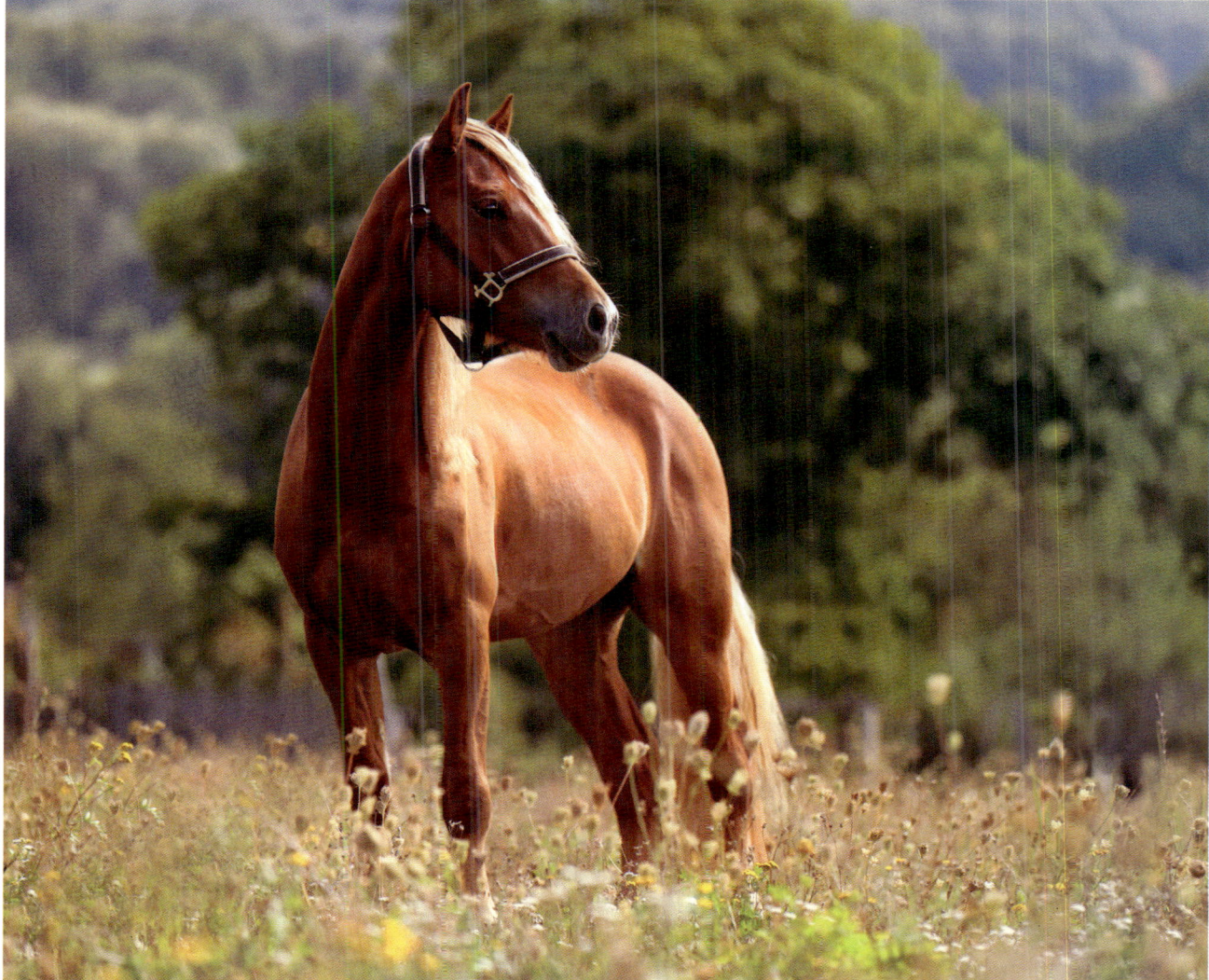

- Place 10-30 drops Peppermint and/or Peppermint Vitality inside the horse's lip.
- Do not feed the horse until it starts defecating or as directed by the attending veterinarian.

Massage
- Rub 10 drops DiGize or Peppermint up each flank and massage out toward umbilical area.
- Rub 10 drops DiGize and/or Peppermint around the coronet band.
- Rub DiGize on auricular points of ears.

Enema
- Mix 30 drops of DiGize in 6 oz. V-6 Vegetable Oil Complex or olive oil and insert in the horse's rectum as an enema. Do not use castor oil, as it dehydrates the colon.
- Walk the horse at least 15 minutes every hour.

2nd hour
- Put 10-20 drops DiGize Vitality in the mouth and on the flanks and coronet band.

4th hour
- Repeat 1st-hour protocol except for enema.

6th hour
- Repeat 1st-hour protocol. Call your vet and prepare to trailer the horse to a clinic or referral facility.

8th hour
- If the horse is improving, repeat 1st-hour protocol, except for enema, every two hours until the horse's bowels are moving well.

Emphysema, Heaves, COPD, or Asthma
Daily Regimen

- Mix 30 drops each of R.C. and Raven in 4 ounces of V-6 Vegetable Oil Complex and insert into the rectum.
- Put 15 drops each of R.C. and Raven in the bottom lip. Use R.C. or Raven in an equine nebulizer in a sterile saline base.
- Massage oils on the chest between the front legs and on auricular points of the ears.
- Apply Raindrop Technique down the spine and neck hair.
- Administer 4 Inner Defense.

Fractures/Bone Chips
Apply mixture of:
- 5 drops Wintergreen
- 5 drops Idaho Grand Fir
- 2 drops Oregano (or Plectranthus Oregano)

Add 2 tablespoons Sulfurzyme to feed.

Continue the above regimen daily for 3 months.

Case History

In 1997 a horse's back hock was fractured when two 50-cent-sized pieces splintered off. The animal was diagnosed with stage five lameness, and the vet urged the owners to have the animal euthanized.

After Wintergreen essential oil was applied for several months, the bone regenerated, and the break healed. The horse returned to the jousting arena stronger and more powerful than ever and spent several more years entertaining the crowds.

Note: Other oils that may be effective for this condition include Helichrysum, Northern Lights Black Spruce, and Idaho Grand Fir. Sulfurzyme may be used internally.

Hide Injuries
Case History

A four-month-old colt had the hide on one side of its body stripped off. The wound was sprayed with Melrose to disinfect and Helichrysum to control the pain. The wound was then sealed with the formula now known as Animal Scents Ointment. Within several months, the hair and skin had completely grown in, and the animal had made a full recovery.

Hoof Infections
Case History

In 2000 a show horse received some kind of severe bite on the pastern. Although the vet diagnosed a rattlesnake bite, it may have been caused by something else.

Two weeks later, the entire pastern and coronet band were inflamed (the size of a cantaloupe), and the rotting, decaying flesh revealed a large hole where the bone was visible and had separated from the hoof.

The vet suggested amputating the foot. Instead, the following protocol was initiated:

- **Day 1:** The wound was cleaned and disinfected with Thieves and Helichrysum, and the foot was bandaged. This treatment decreased pain enough to allow the mare to put weight on the foot.
- **Day 2:** The swelling had dropped by 50 percent. The wound was again cleaned with Thieves and Helichrysum and then packed with Animal Scents Ointment.
- **Days 3 to 14:** The wound was washed morning and night with Thieves, Melrose, and Helichrysum and packed with Animal Scents Ointment.
- **Result:** Today the animal walks with no discomfort. A brand-new hoof has appeared with only a small scar on the wound site. Although there was minor swelling in the pastern for a while, it had faded eight months later.

Imprinting on New Foals
Recommended Essential Oils and Blends: Valor, Highest Potential, Frankincense, Sacred Frankincense, The Gift, 3 Wise Men, Northern Lights Black Spruce, Idaho Grand Fir, Palo Santo, Idaho Blue Spruce, Sacred Mountain, Joy, Surrender, Acceptance

After the mare and foal have bonded, pick up the foal and hold it in your arms. Massage 5-6 drops of oil along the spine and massage the oil residue from your hands on each ear. Then rub oils all over the colt's body a few drops at a time. Lay the colt in your lap and position it with its head back, stroke its neck, and pass all the way over its nose (avoid putting any oils on the nose as it is very sensitive). Repeat every day for 21 days.

Jitteriness
To calm a horse, apply a few drops of oil on your hands and put one hand on the base of the tail and the other on the withers. The animal should relax. Relaxation is the first step to healing.

Put several drops of T-Away, Vetiver, Trauma Life, Stress Away, Grounding, Surrender, Peace & Calming, or Peace & Calming II in your hand and briefly hold it up to the animal's muzzle or nostrils. If the horse pulls away and returns several times, perhaps out of curiosity or thinking that food may appear, feed it some grain as a reward and then put your hand with oil on its muzzle and gently rub it in.

As the horse relaxes, work your hand around the side of its jaw and up along the neckline to the ears. Then rub its ears and the top of its head and crop. As the horse relaxes further, you can add more oil to the palm of your hand (Peace & Calming, Peace & Calming II, or Valerian) and continue rubbing its ears, head, and crop.

Kidney Failure
- Administer 1-3 droppers full of K&B tincture morning and night.
- Using a Raindrop application on the spine, apply 5 drops each of Cypress and Juniper daily for 10 days.
- Use Geranium and Lemongrass on BL23 acupressure point.
- Use Celery Seed Vitality on the back coronary bands (Ting points).

Laxative for Foals
Put 4 drops of DiGize Vitality in bottom lip daily until bowels are moving. Rub 4-10 drops of Release on the belly and under the tail.

Open Wounds
Case History
A large thoroughbred gelding was attacked by a cougar that clawed a chunk of flesh half the size of a soccer ball out of the horse's buttocks. The horse bled terribly, blood squirting from ruptured blood vessels.

The vet said the prognosis was grim because there was too much torn, damaged, and removed tissue. Even if the horse didn't die, the wound would leave a sizeable scar and indentation.

Treatment Protocol
Day 1
To reduce the pain and stop the bleeding, a 5-cc hypodermic syringe was filled with Helichrysum and sprayed into the wound. The horse became less jittery, and the bleeding stopped. Several minutes later, a larger 10-cc syringe of Purification was sprayed into the open wound. It took over 15 ml of Purification to spray down and cover the entire wound.

After several hours, the wound was sprayed with Melrose to disinfect it and was packed with Animal Scents Ointment. To keep hair out of the wound and reduce the possibility of infection, the tail was wrapped and tied up. Because there was no way to cover or close the wound, the horse was kept in the stable to prevent him from moving around. The horse was closely monitored to reduce the possibility of infection caused by the animal lying down, rolling around, or scratching the wound.

Days 2-7
The horse's grain was supplemented with crushed up Essentialzyme, the yellow capsule in Essentialzymes-4, and four scoops of Pure Protein Complete, which is dense in the nutrients required for healing and tissue rebuilding.

Three times a day, the open wound was irrigated with Purification and Helichrysum. The vet came regularly to monitor the horse's progress. He remarked that he had never seen muscle tissue regenerate to such a degree.

Weeks 2-4
Two times a day, the open wound was irrigated with Purification and Helichrysum.

Weeks 5-8
Once a week, the wound was irrigated with Purification and Helichrysum until it was closed.

Results
Today, no indentation or concavity is visible, only a small, circular 2-inch scar.

Puncture Wounds
Mix 1cc of Thieves in 12cc's of carrier oil and flush thoroughly. Follow with Helichrysum and Copaiba and seal with Animal Scents Ointment. Encourage drainage by hot packing or hydrotherapy. Repeat 1-2 times per day, until healing is complete from the inside out. If drainage is purulent (contains pus), contact your veterinarian.

Saddle Sores and Raw Spots
(i.e., where packs rub against flesh)

Use PuriClean, Infect Away, and Mendwell as a three-part system. You may also use Melrose and Animal Scents Ointment for at least 3 days.

Scours (diarrhea caused by bacteria)
- Put 5 drops ParaGize in a foal's lower lip and rub on its flank. For a full-size horse, use Thieves or DiGize Vitality and Copaiba in the horse's lower lip and rub 5-8 drops in the flank.
- Place ICP in water and pour it down the throat. Continue for four days. Administer Life 9 or an equine probiotic.

Screw Worm

There is a round worm called a bore or screw worm that bores into the spine of horses (especially wild horses). It will cause a huge boil-like abscess on the spine. When lanced, a larva worm will come out of that abscess. Sometimes the abscess will actually break open and ooze.

Pour Thieves into the hole to flush out the larva worm and then fill the hole with a mixture of 12 drops of Melrose and 5 drops of Exodus II. Dilution may be required.

Strangles (Streptococcus equi infection)

- Perform the Raindrop Technique with Thieves.
- Apply 4-10 drops of Thieves Vitality on the inside of the bottom lip (for a large horse, 8-15 drops).
- After 6-12 hours, repeat Raindrop Technique with Ravintsara and Lemongrass. Put 2 drops of Oregano Vitality and 2 drops of Thyme Vitality on the inside of the bottom lip (for a large horse, 4-10 drops each).
- Repeat the oral steps every 4-6 hours until the horse begins to improve. As the horse continues to improve, alternate treatments.
- Cover abscesses with Ravintsara and Thieves and then poultice.
- Use Seedlings Diaper Rash Cream or Thieves Dentarome Ultra Toothpaste to draw out infection.

Swollen Sheath

Geldings and stallions occasionally suffer from swollen sheath with or without an abscess and infection. It can be caused by:

- Eating hay too rich in protein. Ideal levels of protein should be 12 to 15 percent, and alfalfa hay can have protein as high as 26 percent.
- High sugar levels
- Lack of routine cleaning and urethral obstruction from accumulated smegma (bean)
- Injury (breeding, getting kicked)
- Cancer
- Not extending the penis and letting it clean off

Treatment

- Put on rubber gloves.
- Lightly coat the shaft with Animal Scents Ointment to soften any debris.
- Clean inside the sheath and remove debris with Thieves dish soap and water or a cap of Thieves Household Cleaner diluted in a half gallon of water. If infected, clean twice a day until infection and swelling subside.

Maintenance

- The sheath should be cleaned out every 4-6 months. Make sure the horse is fed adequate water and grass hay and gets sufficient exercise to increase circulation.
- Apply Copaiba and Cypress to any outside swollen tissues.
- Perform a Raindrop Technique every 3 to 6 months.

Umbilical Cords of Newborn Foals

Instead of iodine, put Myrrh oil on the umbilical cord of newborn foals and a circle of Melrose around the base of the navel. Myrrh will dry the umbilical cord and facilitate a good separation. Exodus II can also be used to treat infections in a foal's umbilical cord prior to veterinary examination.

RAINDROP TECHNIQUE® FOR HORSES

Although many veterinarians have developed their own variations of this technique, the simplicity of this procedure is what makes it effective.

Raindrop Technique for horses is similar to that for humans, except that the majority of the oils are also used on the eliminative energetic acupressure meridians (Kidney, Liver, Spleen, Lung, and Large Intestine) on the inside of the legs to prime the body for release and to acquaint the body with the energy of the oils.

Starting Point

Apply 6 drops of Valor to the tailbone (the base of the tail where it connects with the spine). Next, place one hand on the withers and the other on the tailbone and hold for 5 minutes. There is no difference energetically whether you use your right or left hand in these spots. Once the horse relaxes (i.e., drops its head and droops its eyelids), the procedure can start.

Don'ts

- Do not spend too much time stroking the horse's spine. Usually, three repetitions are sufficient.
- Do not work or ride a horse or put him in the sun for 12-24 hours after a Raindrop.

How to Apply Oils

- Perform Raindrop 2-4 days prior to shows or other stressful events.

- As much as possible, maintain contact with the horse while doing a Raindrop.
- Some horses are very reactive to the hotter oils and require a large strip of V-6 down the back prior to putting oils on the back for the first time or two a Raindrop is done. Today's horses are exposed to more toxins—both internally and externally—than in years past. Putting a layer of V-6 down first minimizes potential uncomfortable reactions of the horse. This also mitigates erroneous interpretation of any topical changes the owner may observe.
- Hold the oil 6 inches above the spine as you drop it in.
- For coarse-haired animals, stroke in the oils using small, circular motions, working from the base of the tail to the shoulders of the spine
- For fine-haired animals, stroke in the oils using regular Raindrop Technique straight strokes.
- Spend enough time massaging to get the oils down into the skin and not sitting on top of the hair.
- Remember to have lots of carrier oil handy.
- When dripping the oils on the spine, use 12 drops on a draft horse, 6 drops on a saddle horse, or 3-4 drops on a miniature horse, Shetland, or Welch pony.

Additional Tips
- Carefully use your fingertips and thumb tips to perform Vita Flex along the auricular points of the ear. Be gentle. If you inflict even a little discomfort, the horse will distrust you and pull away.
- Stretching the spine is problematic in horses, so instead, place one hand over the tail, the other hand on the withers, and focus moving the energy along the spine.
- Rubbing oils around the coronet band will allow the oils to reach the bloodstream and travel through the nerves in the legs to the spine.
- Drip Marjoram and Aroma Siez into the hair of the outside muscles away from the spine and rub in with a larger circular motion massage. Palo Santo, Cypress, Copaiba, or Melrose—which are anti-inflammatory, anesthetic, insect-repelling, relaxing, and healing—can also be used. This is important because horses used for packing, riding, or working have extra stress placed on the spine and muscles in the back.
- Use a stool (mounting block) to reach both sides of the spine without having to break contact, potentially creating tension in the animal. Above all, stay in a safe position.
- Some people mistakenly believe that if they don't have all the oils in the Raindrop Kit, they can't do a Raindrop. You do not need to apply every oil to have an effective treatment. You can perform an excellent, beneficial Raindrop Technique with one oil, if that's all you have. Using just Oregano (or Plectranthus Oregano) and Thyme, or Palo Santo can produce excellent results. Similarly, Melrose, Tea Tree, Australian Kuranya, or Mountain Savory can also be used.
- It is okay to stroke oils down off the hips and down the legs.
- It is okay to put a hot towel on the spine. In fact, it is recommended as long as there are no neurological issues.
- Following a Raindrop Technique, you can apply a saddle blanket and then a horse blanket and leave the animal standing in the stall. Usually after about 10 minutes, it will lie down and go to sleep.
- The carrier oils in the Raindrop will flatten the coat muscles that keep a horse's back warm. Keep a blanket on the horse to help maintain warmth in a frigid climate until all oils are absorbed.

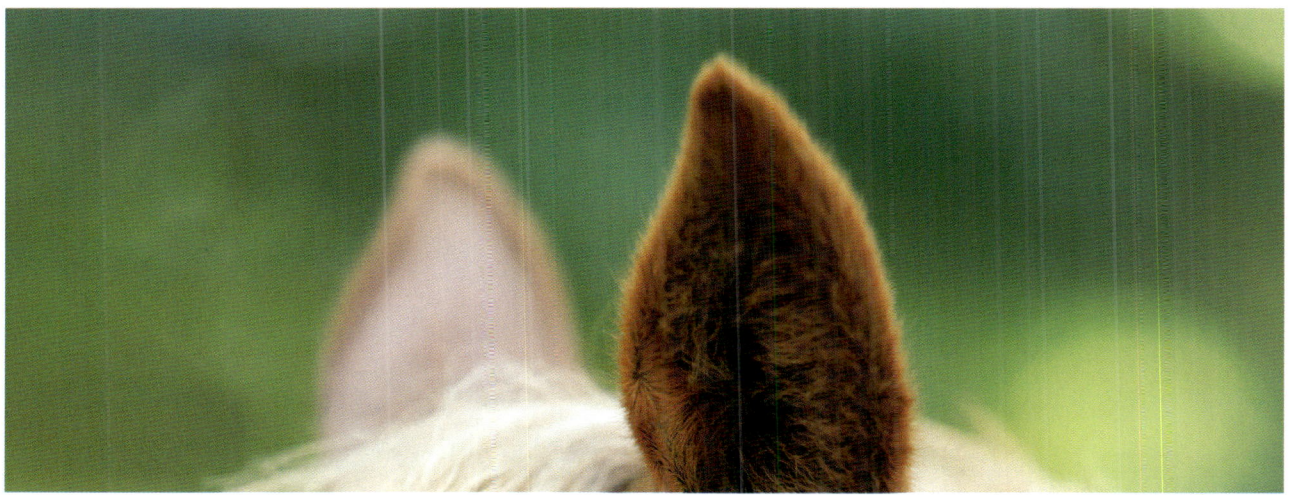

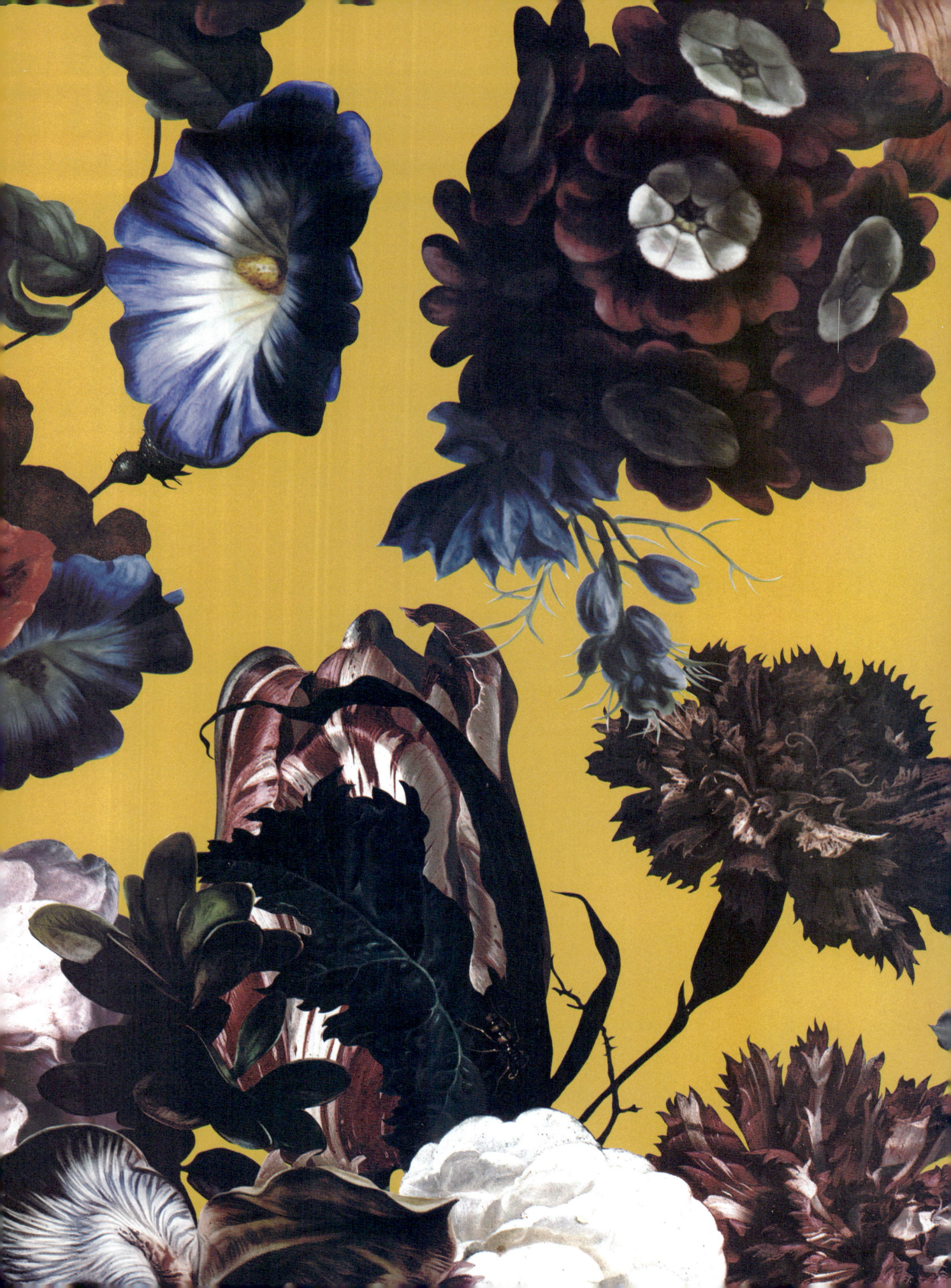

Techniques for Essential Oil Application

THE USE OF DIFFERENT TECHNIQUES

People use essential oils in many creative ways for healing and supporting the human body that open a world of great discovery and untapped potential. It does not seem to matter how the essential oils are used, as long as their energy penetrates the body through direct application, inhalation, or ingestion.

The possibilities become very exciting as the essential oils are used by new and/or inexperienced individuals, and they begin to discover unexpected and fascinating benefits. However, as with any natural substance, essential oils should be used carefully, intelligently, and most importantly, with common sense. Keeping this in mind, common sense will enable you to enjoy the benefits and immense pleasure in using the essential oils as you learn to apply them through these techniques. They have brought Peace & Calming, Joy, Harmony, and Abundance to thousands of people throughout the world.

The five specific techniques explained in this chapter have been studied and used in research as the development of their application has been refined and documented. Numerous doctors and health professionals are now acknowledging the benefits of these natural techniques, and thousands of individuals throughout the world have had tremendous benefits.

This knowledge is available to those who are interested in learning about essential oils, God's gifts that Mother Nature eagerly provides, and ways to use these brilliant but simple techniques to help themselves, their families and friends, and those in their world of influence.

VITASSAGE™ ESSENTIAL OIL DISPENSING MASSAGER

The Vitassage is a one-of-a-kind creation by D. Gary Young that incorporates Young Living essential oils into the massage experience.* Three stainless-steel roller balls simultaneously disperse up to three different oils onto the skin, while the powerful vibration technology allows the oils to penetrate deep into stressed tissue.

The Vitassage offers the power of Young Living's pure, therapeutic-grade essential oils and massage to both professionals and casual users alike.

- The ultimate aromatherapeutic massage experience
- Profound vitality using YL patent-pending* aroma vibration
- Sliding mechanism for independent oil dispersion
- Unique 2-ml bottle replacement system that allows for customizable oil combinations

*Pat. No. 9205020

NEURO AURICULAR TECHNIQUE

D. Gary Young developed the Neuro Auricular Technique (NAT), which integrates the use of pure, therapeutic-grade essential oils with acupressure by using a small, pen-shaped instrument with a rounded end to apply the oils to the acupressure meridians or Vita Flex points on the ears.

He discovered that using essential oils in conjunction with acupressure was extremely beneficial. Interestingly, he found that acupressure stimulation on specific neurological points with the essential oils evoked a quicker response to specific conditions. The combination of acupressure with essential oils seemed to substantially increase benefits in targeted areas.

The Neuro Auricular Technique has shown remarkable benefits in both the emotional and physical realm. When working on a physical need, an emotional release is often experienced that can bring about a positive attitude of hope and renewed vitality.

The Neuro Auricular Technique has been extremely beneficial in delivering the oils to the exact location of neurological damage related to spinal cord injury.

It is a program that Gary researched, developed, and taught worldwide to doctors and other health practitioners. It has proven to have tremendous results and has the potential to be a well-known modality in the future.

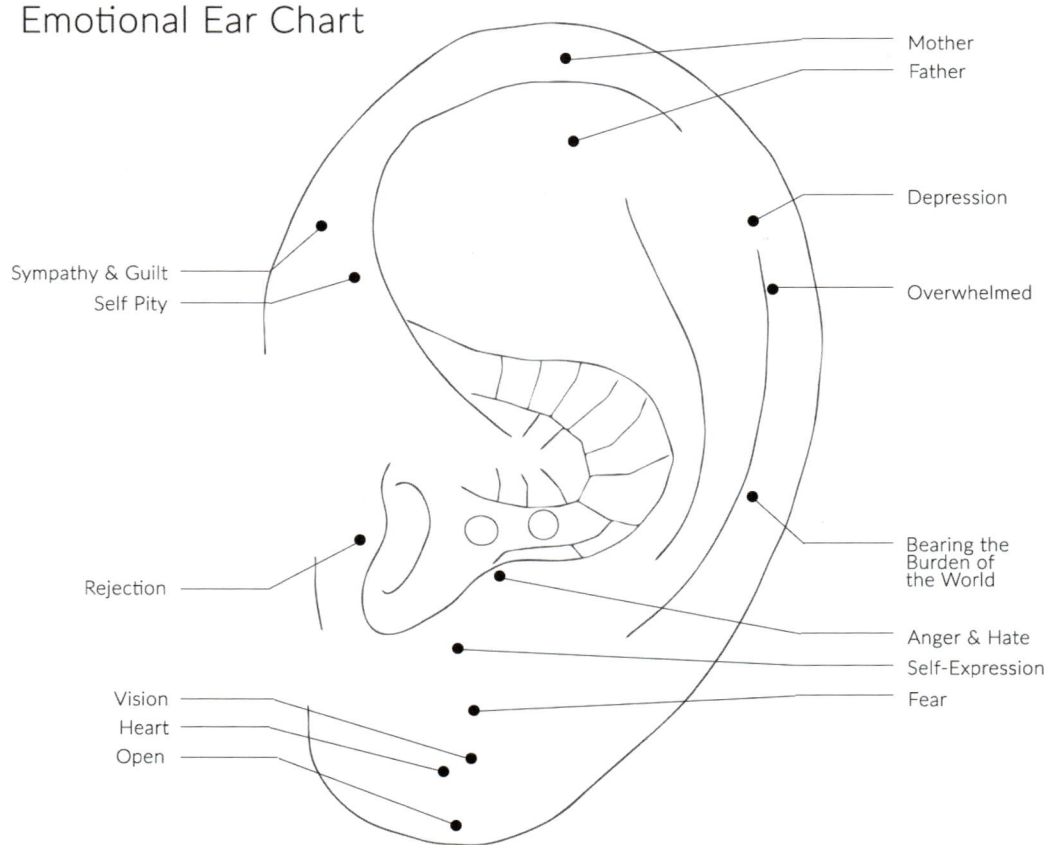

LYMPHATIC PUMP

Maintaining lymph circulation is one of the keys to keeping the immune system adequately functioning. This technique is designed to promote lymph circulation. It is an excellent tool for those who are sedentary or bedridden.

1. With the recipient lying on his or her back, hold one leg with one hand just above the ankle with your palm on the underside of the leg (covering the Achilles tendon).
2. Place the other hand on the bottom of the recipient's foot with your palm over the ball of the foot and your fingers curled around the toes.
3. Push the top of the foot away from you (See Figure A).
4. Then pull the foot toward you by the toes until the ball of the foot is as close to the table as possible (See Figure B).
5. Check with the recipient during the pump to verify that the muscles in the foot are not being overextended. This should be an active process, but not a painful one.
6. Pull and push the foot using this "pumping motion" at least 10 times on each leg for maximum benefit. Note that the recipient's entire body should move during each step of the Lymphatic Pump.

VITA FLEX TECHNIQUE

Vita Flex means "vitality through the reflexes" and is an easy way to apply essential oils through the bottoms of the feet. It is a very important technique that can facilitate the relief of pain and suffering quickly, as well as improve physical and emotional well-being.

It helps identify different structural and health needs of the body and, together with the Raindrop Technique, increases the opportunity for healing and rejuvenation. Vita Flex is a specialized form of hand and foot massage

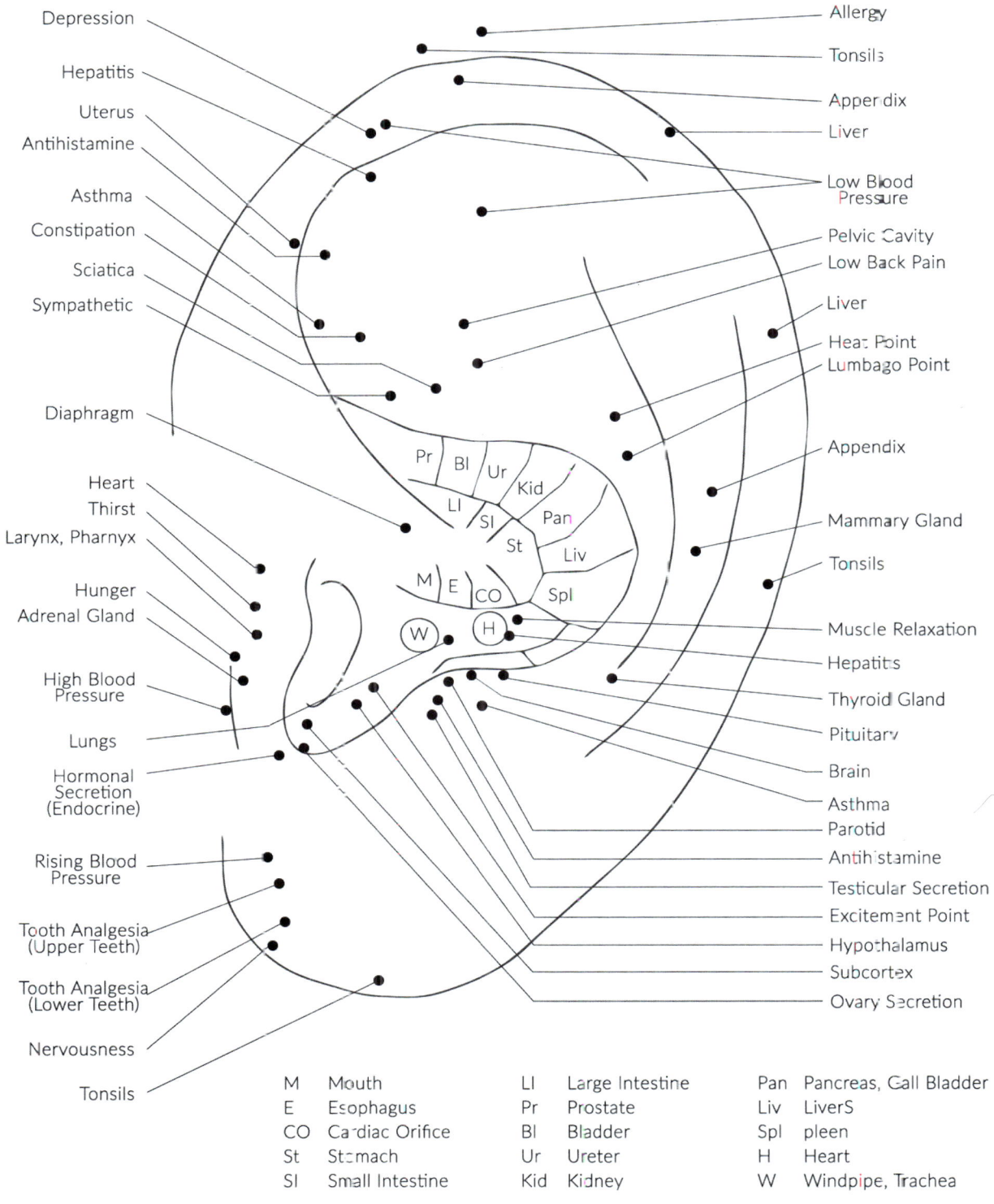

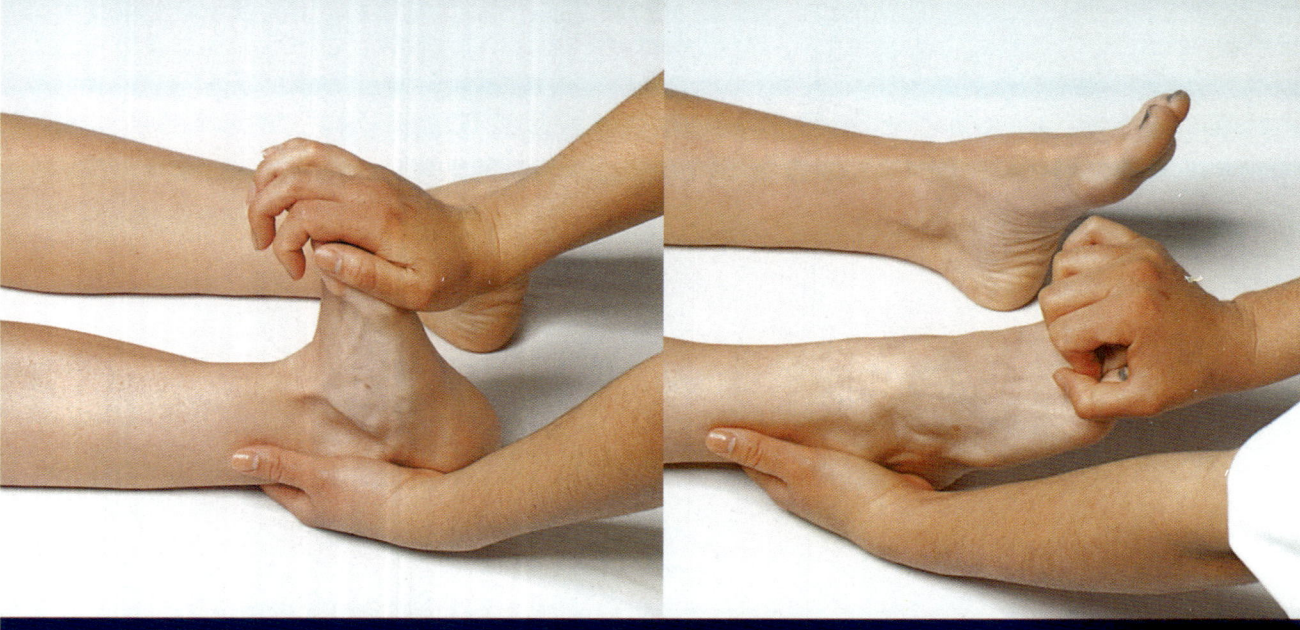

Figure A — Pushing the foot

Figure B — Pulling the foot

that is exceptionally effective in delivering the benefits of essential oils throughout the body. It is said to have originated in Tibet thousands of years ago and was perfected in the 1960s by Stanley Burroughs long before acupuncture was popular in Western medicine.

Vita Flex is based on a complete network of reflex points that stimulate all the internal body systems. When the fingertips connect to specific reflex points with essential oils using the special Vita Flex application, an electrical charge is released that sends energy through the neuroelectric pathways.

This electrical charge follows the pathways of the nervous system to the point of breakage in the electrical circuit, usually related to an energy block caused by toxins, damaged tissues, or loss of oxygen.

More than 1,500 Vita Flex points are located throughout the body in comparison to only 365 acupuncture points used in reflexology. Vita Flex is similar to but different from reflexology. As it is used today, reflexology has a tendency to ground out the electrical charge from constant compression and rotation pressure, which causes cell separation and loss of oxygen to subdermal tissues, causing further injury.

In contrast to the steady stimulation of reflexology, Vita Flex uses a rolling and releasing motion that involves placing the fingers flat on the skin, rolling up onto the fingertips, and continuing over onto the fingernails, using medium pressure, and then sliding the hand forward about $\frac{1}{2}$ inch, continually repeating this rolling and releasing technique until the specific Vita Flex area is covered. This rolling motion is repeated over the area three times.

Vita Flex corrects weakened or injured areas through the electrical reflex points, preventing further injury and stress and allowing for quicker, more efficient healing. Combining the electrical frequency of the oils and that of the person receiving the application creates rapid and phenomenal results.

This ancient technique has brought healing of a greater dimension to our modern world with its complete, scientific, workable system of controls that releases the unlimited healing power within the human body.

The diagram of the nervous system shows the points on the spine and their electrical connection to specific areas throughout the entire body.

Vita Flex on the Hands

The hands also have specific reflex points that correspond to different organs and systems of the body. Although the hands are smaller and perhaps not as comfortable to work on, if you are in a hurry or are unable to get to the feet, there are still definite benefits in using the Vita Flex technique on the hands.

Vita Flex Foot Chart

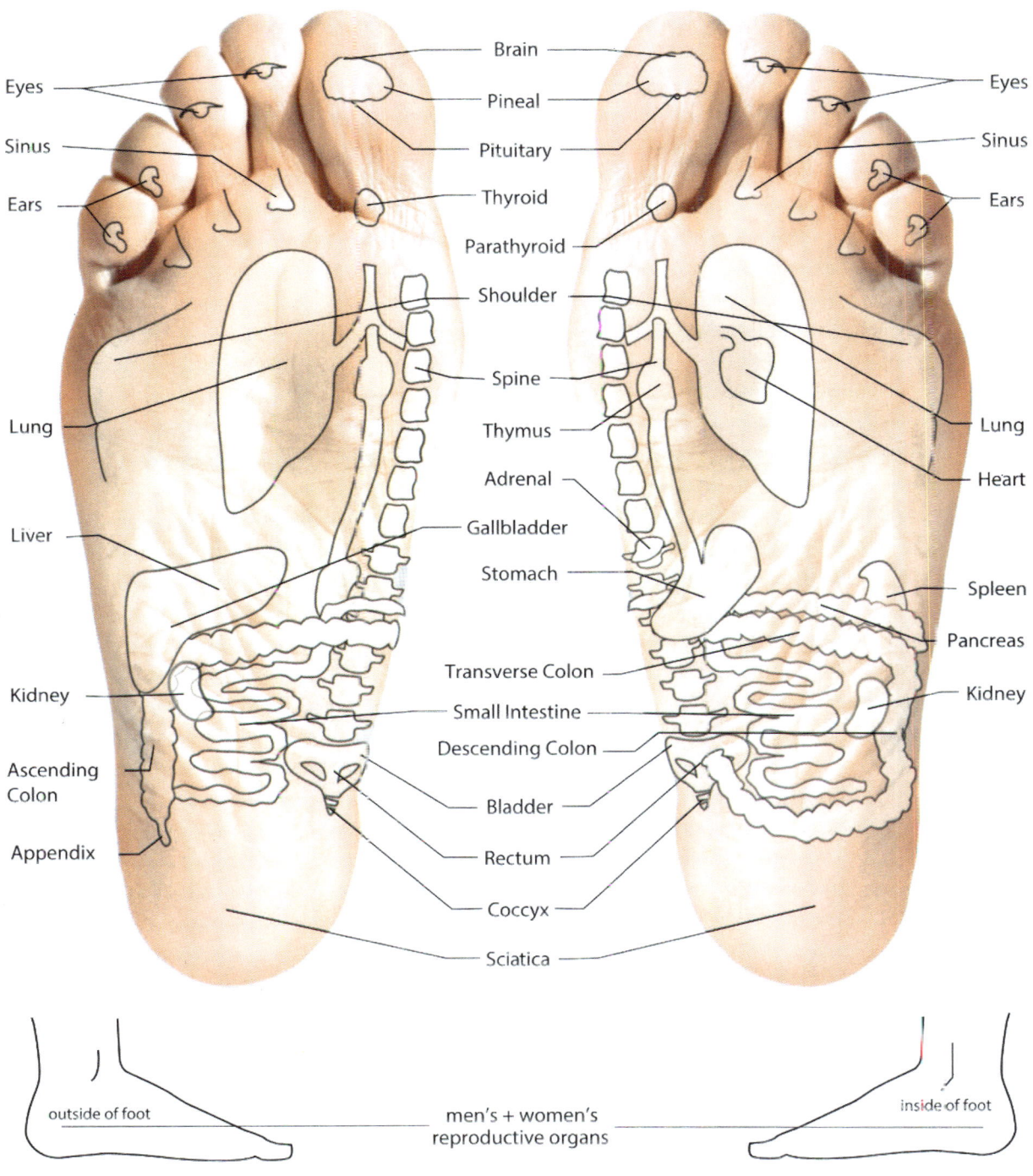

Nervous System Connection Points

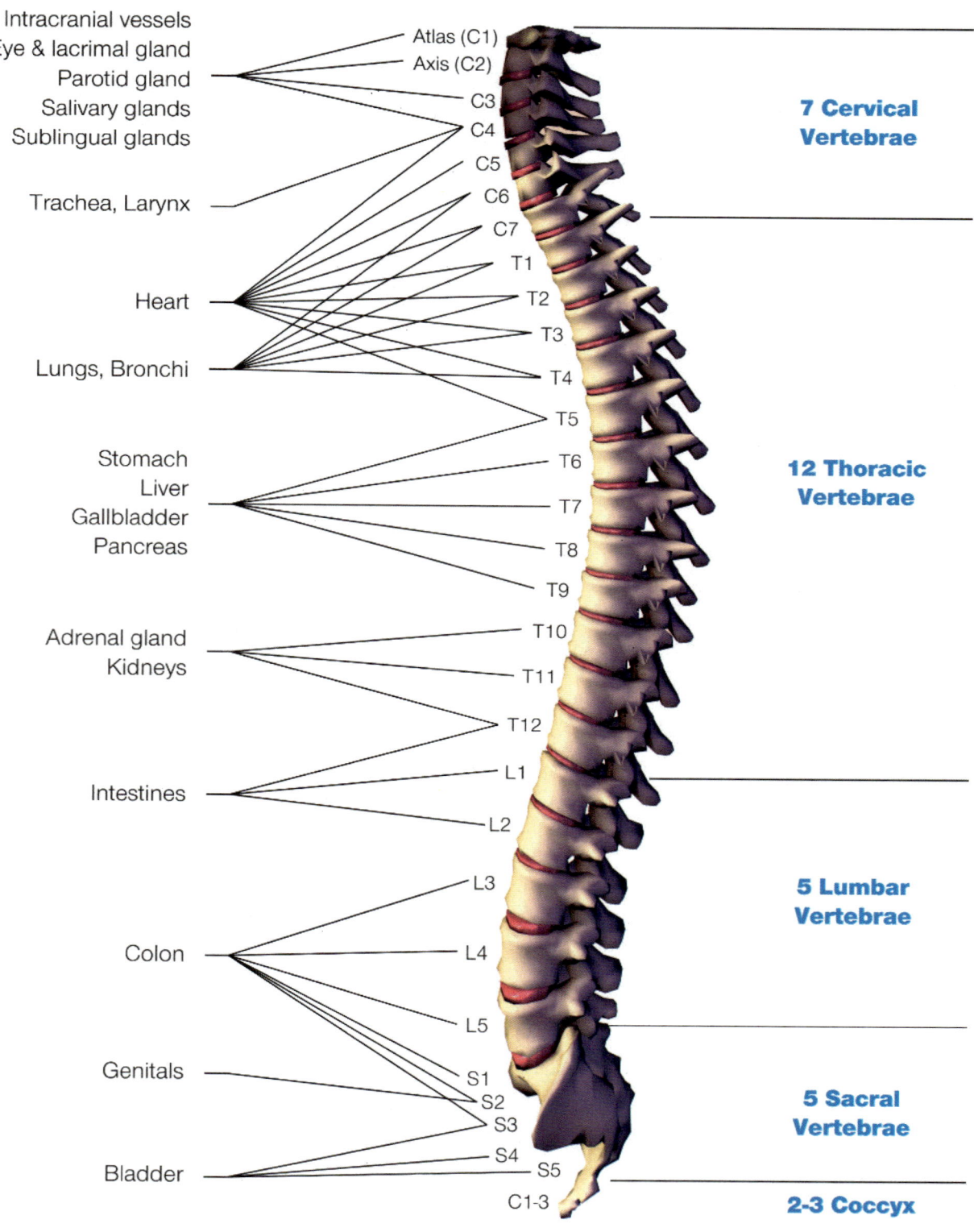

Palm of Left Hand

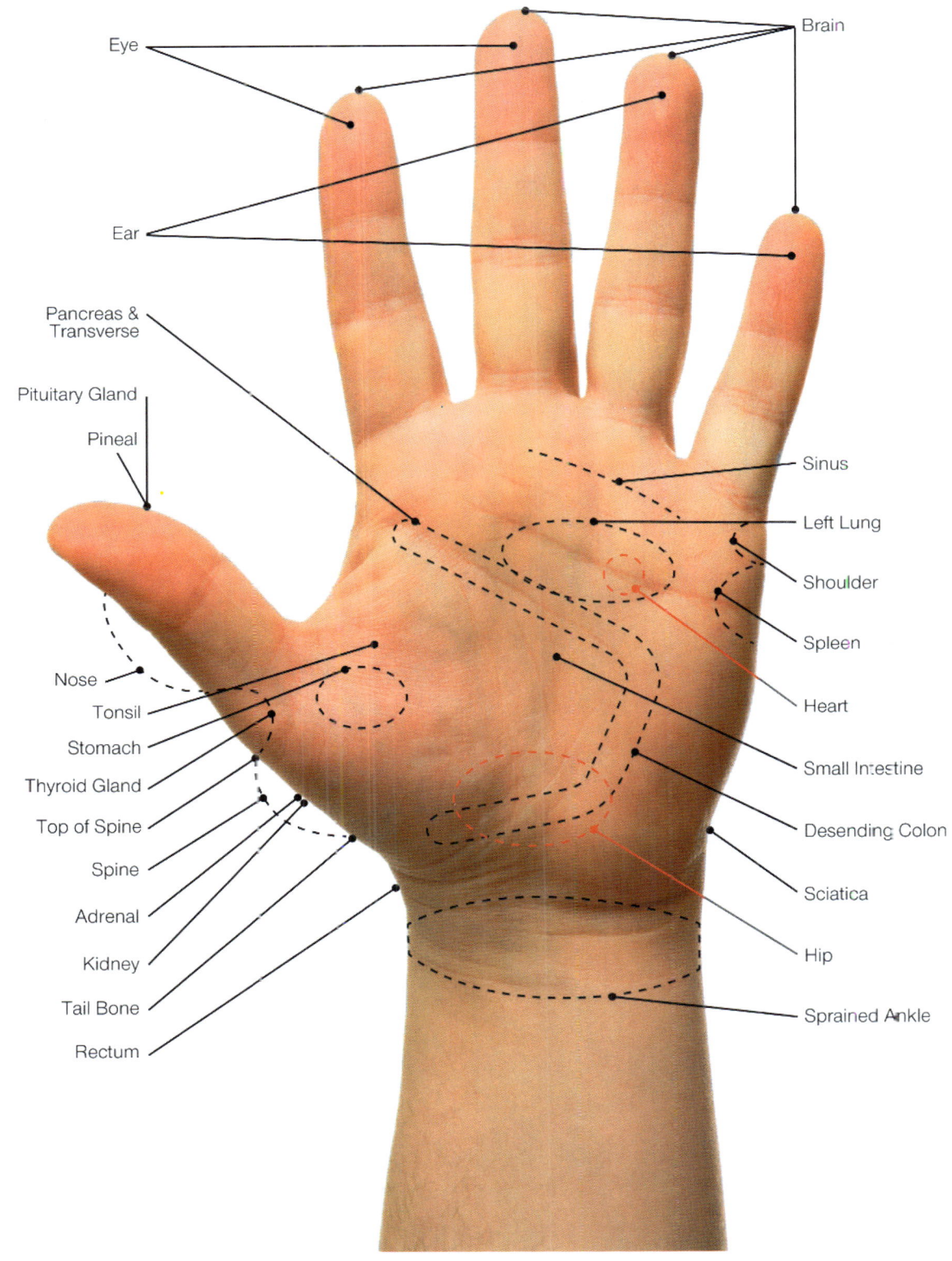

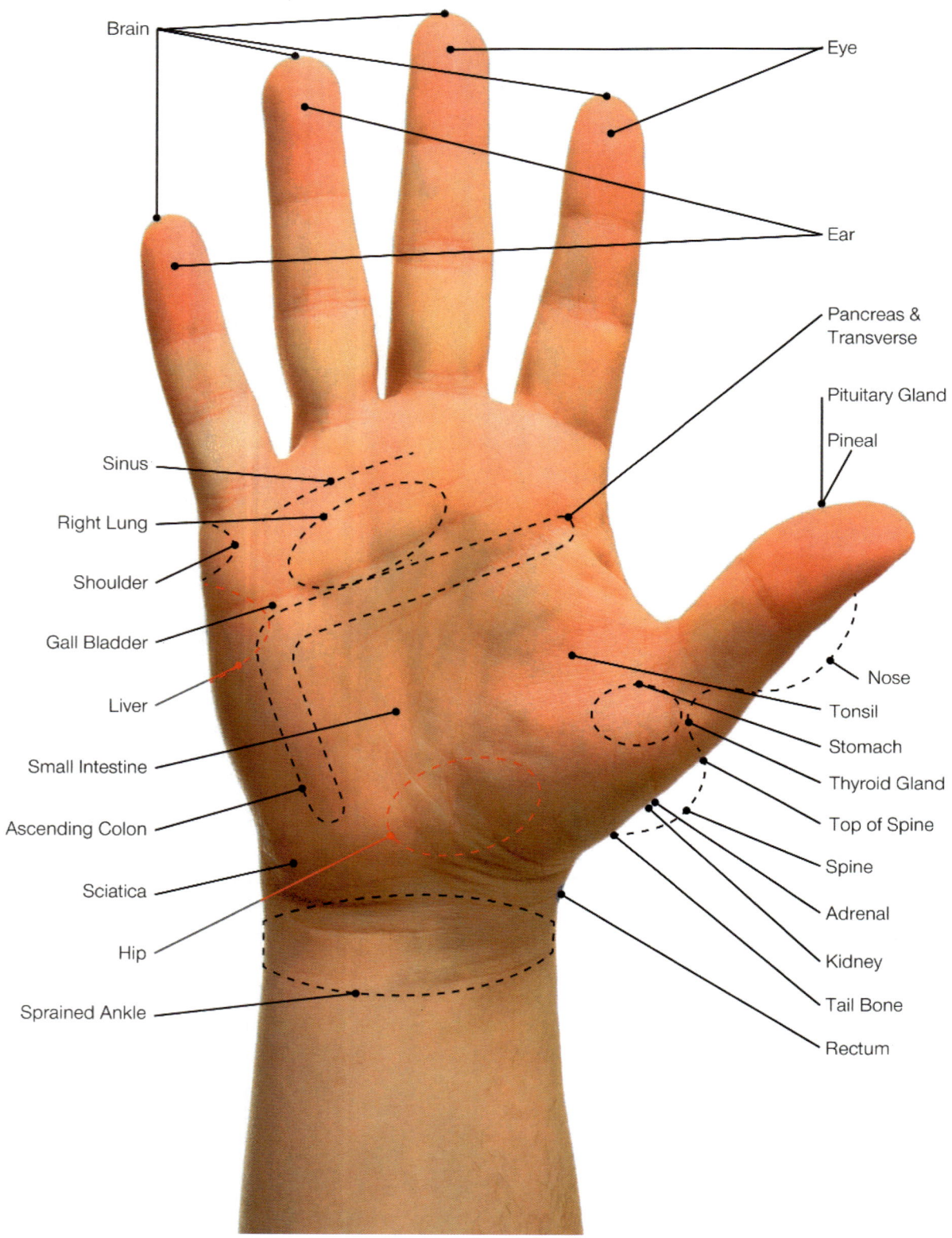

RAINDROP TECHNIQUE®

Most people would agree that massage is soothing, relaxing, and pleasurable. But Raindrop Technique is unquestionably far superior as it combines essential oils with special massage techniques to add greater therapeutic benefits to a pleasurable massage.

Anyone who has experienced Raindrop Technique is very quick to get on the massage table again to enjoy and discover new benefits of this most remarkable application of essential oils.

Raindrop Technique is one of the safest, most noninvasive regimens available for spinal health. It is also an invaluable method to promote healing from within using topically applied essential oils.

The Development of the Raindrop Technique

D. Gary Young developed the Raindrop Technique based on his research of essential oils and their antimicrobial properties, his knowledge of the Vita Flex technique and its reflex points on the feet, and fascinating information on the light stroking called effleurage and its effect on the muscular and nervous systems.

Lakota Indians

While visiting with the Lakota people, Gary learned that for several generations before the U.S./Canadian border was established, the Lakota Indians migrated across it into the northern regions of Saskatchewan and Manitoba. There, they often witnessed the Northern Lights, or Aurora Borealis. Those who were ill or had complicated health problems would stand facing the Aurora Borealis, hold their hands toward the lights, and inhale deeply.

The Lakota believed that when the Aurora Borealis was visible, the air was charged with healing energy. They would mentally "inhale" this energy, allowing it to pass through their spine and on to other afflicted areas of the body through neurological pathways. Many experienced dramatic healing effects through this practice.

Eventually, after the border divided the U.S. from Canada, making migrations to the north impossible, the Lakota began practicing this energy process mentally, coupled with light stroking to facilitate the spreading of energy through the body.

Effleurage

It is believed that the Lakota people continued their practice of mentally processing energy, coupled with effleurage, to distribute healing energy throughout the body. Gary said that he did not know if this is where the effleurage he taught (feathered finger-stroking) first originated, but it has become associated with this healing technique.

Gary found that when this practice of effleurage was coupled with the therapeutic power of essential oils and the stimulation of Vita Flex, its effects were greatly heightened. Since this therapeutic practice was adopted in 1989, Raindrop Technique has been embraced by massage therapists, chiropractors, and other medical professionals around the world for its help with relaxation, correction of spinal misalignments, and antiviral effects.

Statistical Validation

In 2001 David Stewart, PhD, circulated a questionnaire to over 2,000 health practitioners, massage therapists, aromatherapists, and their clients to gain insight on the results that were accruing from Raindrop Technique. He received 422 responses summarizing the experiences of some 14,000 Raindrop sessions. His findings are summarized in his booklet A Statistical Validation of Raindrop Technique (available through Life & Science Publishing; order online at mylsp.com or by calling toll-free 1.800.336.6308).

Overall, the respondents who had received a Raindrop Technique rated it positive (97 percent), pleasant (98 percent), resulted in improved health (89 percent), resulted in an improved emotional state (86 percent), and would choose to receive Raindrop Technique again (99.9 percent).

Consistent with the French Model

The use of undiluted essential oils in Raindrop Technique is consistent with the French model for aromatherapy—which is the most extensively practiced and studied model in the world. Having used essential oils clinically since the 1920s, the French have consistently recommended neat (undiluted) use of essential oils.

An illustrious roster of 20th century French physicians provides convincing evidence that undiluted essential oils have a valuable place in the therapeutic arsenal of clinical professionals. René Gattefossé, PhD; Jean Valnet, MD; Jean-Claude Lapraz, MD; Daniel Pénoël, MD; and many others have long attested to the safe and effective use of undiluted essential oils and the dramatic and powerful benefits they can impart.

Skin Warming or Reddening

In the case of Raindrop Technique, the use of certain undiluted essential oils typically causes minor reddening and "heat" in the tissues. Normally, this is perfectly safe and not something to be overly concerned about. Individuals who have fair skin such as blondes and redheads or those persons whose systems are toxic are more susceptible to this temporary reddening.

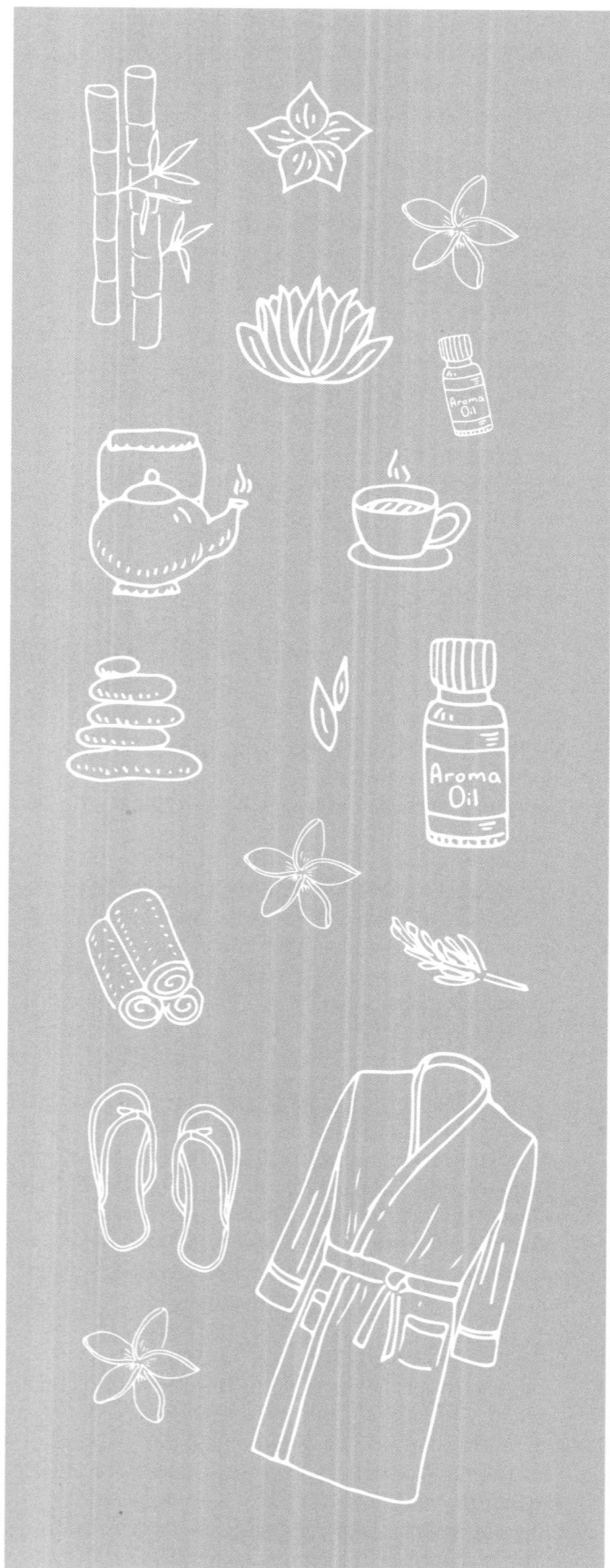

If the reddening or heat becomes excessive, it can be remedied within a minute or two by immediately applying several drops of V-6™ Vegetable Oil Complex or a pure, high-quality vegetable oil like jojoba, almond, avocado, olive, or coconut oil on the affected area. This effectively dilutes the oils and the warming effect.

Temporary, mild warming is normal for Raindrop Technique. Typically, it is even milder than that of many capsicum creams or sports ointments. Indeed, rather than being a cause for concern, this warming indicates that positive benefits are being received.

In cases where the warmth or heat exceeds the comfort zone of the recipient, as mentioned before, the facilitator can apply any pure vegetable oil to the area until the comfort level is regained, and reddening dissipates (usually within two to five minutes).

Note: If a rash should appear, it is an indication of a chemical reaction between the oils and synthetic compounds in the skin cells and the interstitial fluid of the body (usually from conventional personal care products). Some misconstrue this as an allergic reaction, when, in fact, the problem is not caused by an allergy but rather by foreign chemicals already imbedded in the tissues. Essential oils are known to digest toxic waste, chemicals, and other unwanted toxins in the body, and sometimes that process starts to work very quickly.

Medical Professionals

A number of medical professionals throughout the United States have adopted Raindrop Technique in their clinical practice and have found it to be an outstanding method to relieve the problems associated with sciatica, scoliosis, kyphosis, and chronic back pain.

Ken Krieger, DC, stated, "As a chiropractor, I believe that the dramatic results of Raindrop Technique are enough for me to rewrite the books on scoliosis."

Similarly, Terry Friedmann, MD, stated that "...these essential oils truly represent a new frontier of medicine; they have resolved cases that many professionals had regarded as hopeless."

Microorganisms May Cause Scoliosis and Sciatica

A growing amount of scientific research shows that certain microorganisms lodge near the spinal cord and contribute to deformities. These pathogens create inflammation, which, in turn, contorts and disfigures the spinal column.

Raindrop Technique uses a sequence of highly antimicrobial essential oils dropped on the back as a noninvasive therapy for fighting against pathogens lying dormant against the spine, which alleviates symptoms of scoliosis, ky-phosis, and other back ailments, while strengthening the immune system.

Studies at Western General Hospital in Edinburgh, Scotland, linked virus-like particles to idiopathic scoliosis.[1,2]

Researchers at the University of Bonn have also found that the varicella zoster virus can lodge in the spinal ganglia throughout life.[3]

Research in 2001 further corroborated the existence of infectious microorganisms as a cause of spinal pain and inflammation. Alistair Stirling and his colleagues at the Royal Orthopedic Hospital in Birmingham, England, found that 53 percent of patients with severe sciatica tested positive for chronic, low-grade infection by gram-negative bacteria (particularly Propionibacterium acnes), which triggered inflammation near the spine. Stirling suggested that the reason these bacteria had not been identified earlier was because of the extended time required to incubate disc material (seven days).[4]

The tuberculosis mycobacterium has also been shown to contribute to spinal disease and possible deformations. Research at the Pasteur Institute in France, published in The New England Journal of Medicine, documented increasing numbers of patients showing evidence of spinal disease (Pott's disease) caused by tuberculosis.[5,6,7,8]

In addition, vaccines made from live viruses have been linked to spinal problems. A 1982 study by Pincott and Taff found a connection between oral poliomyelitis vaccines and scoliosis.[9]

Raindrop Technique is a powerful, noninvasive technique utilizing the antiviral, antibacterial, and anti-inflammatory action of several key essential oils to assist the body in maintaining or retraining the spinal column's natural curvature.

During the past 18 years, this technique has helped alleviate or resolve many cases of scoliosis, kyphosis, and chronic back pain and has eliminated the need for back surgery for hundreds of people.

Powerful Antibacterial Agents

Essential oils are some of the most powerful inhibitors of microbes known and, as such, are an important new weapon in combating many types of tissue infections. A 2015 study tested a number of essential oils against several gram-positive and gram-negative bacteria like Klebsiella pneumoniae, Pseudomonas aeruginosa, Staphylococcus aureus, and E. coli. The study authors concluded that the "components of essential oil of thyme and pine are highly active against foodborne pathogens, generating the largest zones of inhibition."[10]

Similarly, basil essential oil also demonstrated strong bactericidal action against microorganisms Aeromonas hydrophila and Pseudomonas fluorescens.[11]

A study at the Central Food Technological Research Institute in Mysuru, India, found that a large number of essential oil components had tremendous germ-killing effects, inhibiting the growth of Staphylococcus, Micrococcus, Bacillus, and Enterobacter strains of bacteria. These germ-killing compounds included menthol (found in Peppermint), eucalyptol (found in Rosemary, Eucalyptus Radiata, and Peppermint), linalool (found in Marjoram), and citral (found in Lemongrass).[12]

A 2001 study conducted by D. Gary Young, Diane Horne, Sue Chao, and colleagues at Weber State University in Ogden, Utah, found that Oregano, Thyme, Peppermint, and Basil exhibited very strong antimicrobial effects against pathogens such as Streptococcus pneumoniae, a major cause of illness in young children and death in elderly and immune-weakened patients.[13] Many other studies confirm these findings.[14]

The ability of essential oils to penetrate the skin quickly and pass into body tissues to produce therapeutic effects has also been studied. Hoshi University researchers in Japan found that cyclic monoterpenes (including menthol, which is found in Peppermint) are so effective in penetrating the skin that they can actually enhance the absorption of water-soluble drugs.[15] North Dakota State University researchers have similarly found that cyclic monoterpenes such as limonene and other terpenoids such as menthone and eugenol easily pass through the dermis, magnifying the penetration of pharmaceutical drugs such as tamoxifen.[16]

Ingesting Essential Oils

It is interesting to note that many essential oils used in Raindrop Technique—in addition to being highly antimicrobial—are also among those classified as GRAS (Generally Regarded As Safe) for internal use by the U.S. Food and Drug Administration. These include Basil, Marjoram, Peppermint, Oregano, and Thyme. These and many other essential oils on the GRAS list have had a long history for decades as foods or flavorings, with virtually no adverse reactions. It is interesting how the people of the world were ingesting essential oils long before the FDA determined they were safe.

In sum, Raindrop Technique is a safe, noninvasive way to achieve spinal health. It is an invaluable method to promote healing from within using topically applied essential oils.

Physical Relief and Emotional Release

With the development of Raindrop Technique in 1991, nine Naturally Therapeutic oils were chosen that would synergistically combine to kill viral and bacterial pathogens, reduce inflammation, support the immune system, ease respiratory discomfort, relax stressed muscles, and relieve the body of bone and joint discomfort.

The intent was that this combination of oils would also balance the energy, lift the spirit by reducing stress, and calm a troubled and confused mind. This began a new realm of healing that emerged from within the confines of emotional bondage.

In the cerebral cortex is a structure called the amygdala that is affected only by scent. It is here that the emotions and memories of life are stored. Since some essential oils have the ability to cross the blood-brain barrier and stimulate the amygdala, buried feelings of past trauma, emotional upset, and unhappy memories are often released to the cognizant mind, bringing those feelings and consequences to the surface of awareness.

Many physical and emotional problems become dim or completely disappear as the foundation of the emotion is discovered and released. Raindrop Technique has vast benefits only to be realized by the individual receiving the application. It is unique for each individual and is very personal and specific to each person's needs.

Children tend to respond even faster than adults because they do not have any preconceived ideas about what they want to have happen or experience. They just love it and often fall asleep, while the essential oils and the touch of massage fill them with peace and contentment as body systems harmonize together.

Raindrop Technique is an experience for everyone at any age for whatever the need or desire may be, and perhaps it is just a time of quiet relaxation and enjoyment.

Raindrop Technique and Essential Oils

Raindrop Technique is one of the safest, most noninvasive regimens available for spinal health. It is also an invaluable method for promoting healing from within using topically applied essential oils.

Single Oils
- **Oregano:** Awakens receptors, kills pathogens, and helps digest toxic substances on the receptor sites
- **Thyme:** Kills pathogens and digests waste and toxic substances on the receptor sites
- **Basil:** Releases muscle tension
- **Cypress:** Improves circulation and nourishes the pituitary gland
- **Wintergreen:** Reduces pain
- **Marjoram:** Strengthens muscles
- **Peppermint:** Promotes greater oil penetration

Essential Oil Blends
- **Valor:** Structural balancing and alignment
- **Aroma Siez:** Muscle relaxation and pain reduction
- **White Angelica:** Protection for adversarial energies

Simple Explanation

The oils are dispensed like drops of rain from a height of about 6 inches above the back. Starting from the low back, the oils are feathered with the back of the fingers up along the vertebrae, out over the back muscles, and over the shoulders to the neck. Although the entire technique takes from 30-45 minutes to complete, the oils continue to work for several days as the healing and realignment processes take place.

Many recipients feel the benefits of the oils for several days afterward, as they recognize that the pain has decreased or is completely gone, there is no fever, they have more mobility, and they have an overall feeling of peace and a renewed zest for life.

Experiencing the wonderful results of a first-time Raindrop application does not mean that all the desired benefits will be realized. One Raindrop session might be just a time to balance and relax the body. Some individuals may feel they want to have Raindrop once a week, once a month, or every three or four months. Other individuals working on structural realignment or needing emotional support may choose to have Raindrop done on a weekly basis to continue with their progress.

It is important to recognize that a healthy body is not attained by doing just one thing. It is a result of a well-rounded program of exercise, proper diet, and sufficient sleep. Health is everything we do, say, see, eat, and think, along with drinking plenty of water and getting enough sleep.

Preparation

to properly perform the Raindrop Technique, the following items are necessary and the guidelines should be followed:

1. A massage table or comfortable, flat surface.

The surface should be high enough that the facilitator can perform the technique without back strain. Use sheets or towels as a barrier, being sensitive to the fact that essential oils may damage or stain vinyl and other fabrics.

2. Respect the receiver's modesty at all times.

The use of a blanket or sheet provides the best protection. Make sure the environment and your actions promote a sense of security and protection for the receiver.

3. Raindrop Technique Kit®:

- Valor
- Thyme
- Cypress
- Marjoram
- Peppermint
- V-6 Vegetable Oil Complex
- Ortho Ease Massage Oil
- Oregano
- Basil
- Wintergreen
- Aroma Siez
- White Angelica*

* White Angelica is needed but is not included in the kit.

Be sure to remember the following:

1. The Raindrop Technique should be performed only if the facilitator is feeling balanced and focused. Time should be spent developing clarity and energy for transfer to the receiver during the technique.

2. Both facilitator and receiver should be relaxed and comfortable. Appropriate clothing should be worn.

3. An environment should be created that is warm, quiet, relaxing, and comfortable. Soft music and lighting generally prove to be beneficial to the receiver.

4. Both the facilitator and the receiver should remove all jewelry. This includes watches, pendants, chains, rings, bracelets, belts, earrings, etc. These items produce an electrical energy that may interfere with the technique. Metal eyeglasses are acceptable.

5. Facilitators should make sure their fingernails are clipped and filed to prevent scratching the receiver's skin, particularly when performing Vita Flex. Nails should also be free of polish, since essential oils can remove polishes and lacquers.

6. Inquire as to whether the receiver has been exposed to chemicals or has worked in a toxic environment.

7. Ask the receiver if he or she needs to use the restroom prior to beginning.

8. Request permission to begin the Raindrop Technique.

9. It is necessary to access the receiver's back for application of the oils. The use of clothing that fully exposes the spine works best. If modesty can be preserved, remove all clothing from the waist up for easier application.

10. To begin, the receiver should lie as straight as possible on his or her back, face up, on the massage table. Arms should rest alongside the body with the palms touching the sides of the thighs. This will help direct the flow of energy and keep it connected to the receiver.

11. Once contact is made with the receiver, the facilitator should maintain a constant physical connection. This promotes feelings of calmness and security while developing a sense of trust with the facilitator.

12. While applying the Raindrop Technique, use caution when working near the spine or applying direct pressure.

13. Offer assistance to the receiver when dismounting the table.

14. Have plenty of water available for the receiver after the Raindrop Technique is complete.

15. Provide detailed instructions to the receiver for post-Raindrop Technique care.

Caution: Some of the oils may feel hot to the receiver. You may apply V-6 at any time. This will create a cooling effect on the area of discomfort.

Overview of the Application:

Step 1: Balance energy. Apply Valor on the soles of the feet. If a second person is assisting, then that person can put the oils on the shoulders.

Step 2: Vita Flex Technique. Work the same Raindrop Technique oils into the spinal reflex areas of the feet.

Vita Flex facilitates quick absorption of the oils through the bottoms of the feet and prepares the body for Raindrop on the back. It is also highly relaxing.

Step 3: The 5-step Feathering Technique. Use with each of the oils as they are applied on the back, starting at the base of the spine and working upward to stimulate the cell receptors and activate energy centers along the spine, as well as to distribute the oil drops over the back for rapid penetration.

Step 4: Feather 3-5 drops of Oregano from the spine outward.

Step 5: Feather 3-5 drops of Thyme from the spine outward.

Step 6: Stretch and release. Feather 4-6 drops of Basil along both sides of the spine and feather out and upward. Then take hold of the feet and gently pull to stretch the spine, releasing tension from the vertebra, back muscles, and tissue.

Step 7: Finger Straddle Massage. Apply 5-8 drops of Cypress on the spine and feather, then perform the Spinal Finger Straddle.

Step 8: Vita Flex Thumb Roll. Apply 5-8 drops of Wintergreen on the spine and feather, then perform the Vita Flex Thumb Roll.

Step 9: Circular Hand Massage. Apply 8-10 drops of Marjoram on the back and feather, then perform the Circular Hand Massage.

Step 10: Palm Slide. Apply 8-10 drops of Aroma Siez over the entire back and feather, then perform the Palm Slide.

Step 11: Feather 3-5 drops of Peppermint on the spine.

Step 12: Feather 8-10 drops of Valor over the back.

Explanation of Terms:

Facilitator: The person conducting the Raindrop Technique. If there are two facilitators, one will work at the feet, and the other will work at the shoulders.

Receiver: The person receiving the Raindrop Technique

Malleolus: Hammer-shaped protuberance at each side of the ankle joint

Sacrum: Base of the spine

Atlas: Hairline or top of the neck

Lumbar: Part of the back between the lowest ribs and the pelvis

Cervical: Upper part of the spine/neck

Thoraces: Middle of the spine

Feather: Alternating the use of the hands to brush the backs of your fingertips along the spine from sacrum to atlas

Spinal Tissue Pull: Using circular, clockwise motions with fingertips to gently pull the muscle tissue away from the spine

Finger Straddle: Straddling the spine with the index and middle fingers and using the bottom edge of the right hand to create a sawing motion over the straddled fingers, while at the same time slowly pulling hands toward the atlas

Thumb Roll: Rolling thumbs along either side of the spine, moving toward the atlas

Circular Hand Massage: Rotating hands, palms down, along the spine in a clockwise motion

Palm Slide: Sliding palms in opposite directions along the spine

Fan: Using long strokes with the hands to fan up the spine and to the sides

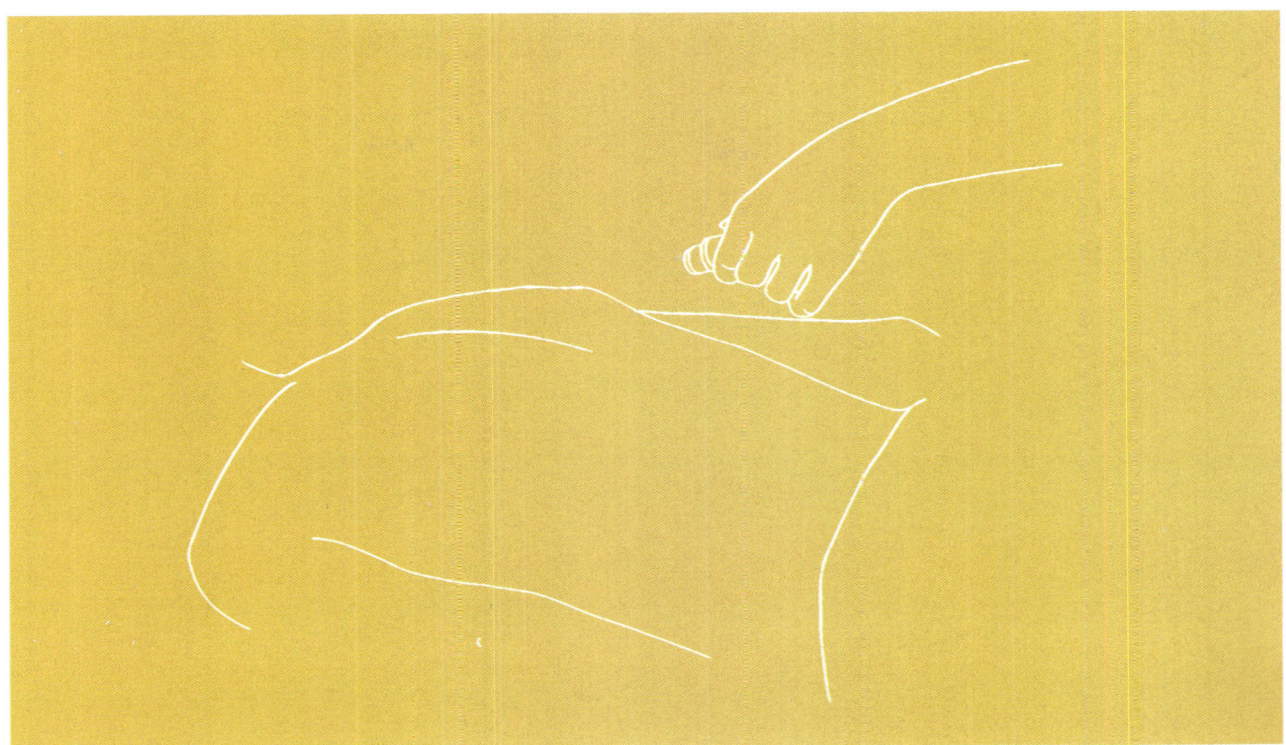

1. BALANCING BODY ENERGY

Application of Valor

Valor serves as the foundation for all work performed during the Raindrop Technique. This essential oil blend helps regulate the electromagnetic energy that flows through the body and balances the receiver's emotional, spiritual, and physical energy. By balancing these energies, the receiver's connections are dramatically improved.

Only one facilitator is needed to perform this process by using the foot application. If two facilitators are present, work in unison: one at the shoulders and one at the feet. Both will apply Valor and remain in contact until the energy is balanced.

Shoulder Application

1. The facilitator applies White Angelica essential oil blend to the shoulders, back of the neck, and thymus area before starting the Raindrop Technique.
2. The facilitator places 3 drops of Valor in each hand.
3. With both palms up, cup under the receiver's right shoulder with the right hand and under the left shoulder with the left hand.
4. Hold this position until the facilitator at the feet completes the same technique.
5. Continue to the foot application as described.

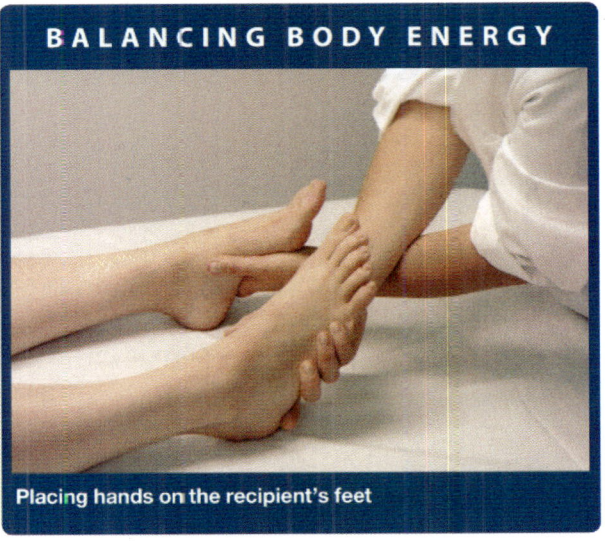

Placing hands on the recipient's feet

Foot Application

1. Facing the receiver, place 6 drops of Valor in each hand.
2. Make contact with the receiver's feet, with the palm of the right hand to the right foot and the palm of the left hand to the left foot. The feet should be held snug with the palms of the hands against the soles of the feet. The facilitator should have firm, but comfortable, contact with the receiver.

VITA FLEX ON THE SOLES OF THE FEET

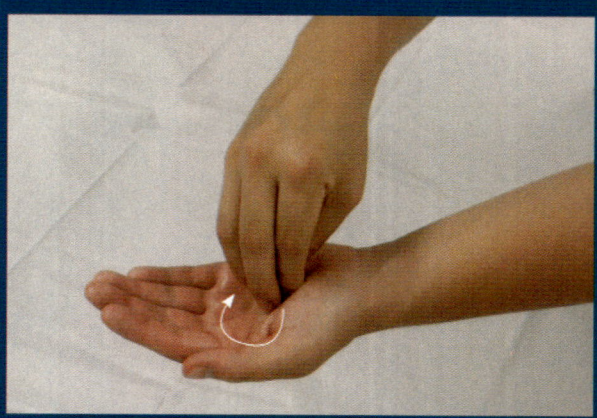
Dipping fingertips into essential oil

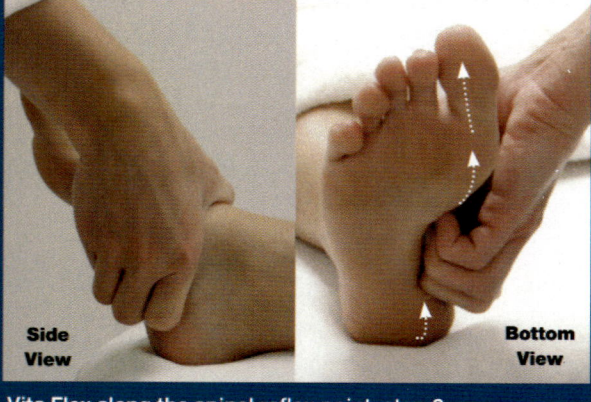
Vita Flex along the spinal reflex point, step 2

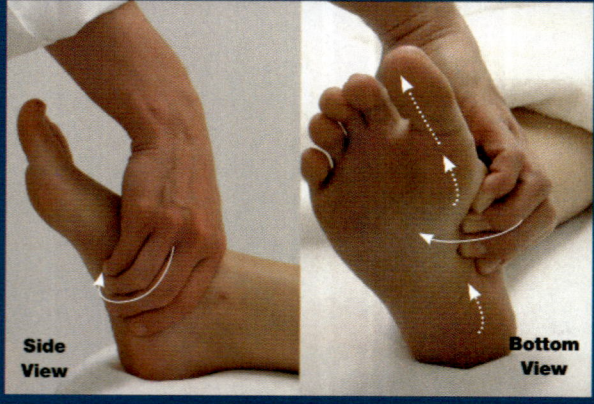
Vita Flex along the spinal reflex point, step 1

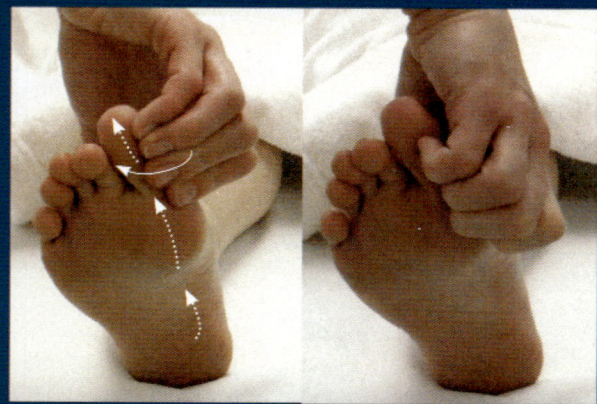
Vita Flex at the big toe, step 1   Vita Flex at the big toe, step 2

2. VITAFLEX

To use this technique, nine essential oils are applied to the spinal Vita Flex area on the soles of the feet. These nine oils and blends, in application sequence, are:

1. Oregano
2. Thyme
3. Basil
4. Cypress
5. Wintergreen
6. Marjoram
7. Peppermint
8. Aroma Siez
9. White Angelica

Things to Remember

1. Always begin with the right foot for consistency purposes.
2. Use firm, but not painful, pressure; roll and press to the first knuckle.
3. Move slowly and evenly, one finger width at a time.
4. Repeat everything in threes.

Procedure

The following procedure is to be repeated for each of the seven oils, using the appropriate sequence (see the 10 Steps for Vita Flex worksheet for more detailed instructions).

1. Place 2-3 drops of essential oil (1-2 drops for smaller feet) in the palm of the left hand. Dip the fingertips of the right hand in the oil and stir clockwise three times to energize the oil. Apply along the spine Vita Flex points (bottom inside edge of the foot from heel to the tip of the big toe).
2. Cup the hand so that the fingertips rest on the Vita Flex points at the heel while the thumb rests on the top of the foot.
3. Rock the hand forward so the nail ends up flat against the bottom of the foot (about half a finger length). Then rock backward to the original position.
4. Continue this technique all the way up the foot to the tip of the big toe. End with several Vita Flexes on the neck and center pad of the big toe.

Repeat two times before moving to the other foot.
5. Continue this process with the remaining oils.

Remember: Right hand to right foot and left hand to left foot. Do both right and left feet before moving to the next oil in the sequence.

3. SPINAL APPLICATION OF ESSENTIAL OILS

After Vita Flex is complete, have the receiver turn over and lie on their stomach. Be sure that the receiver is comfortable, and modesty is respected. The receiver should place their arms comfortably along the sides of the body. The entire back needs to be exposed for application of the Raindrop oils. The oils will be applied from the sacrum to the atlas.

Feather strokes are used in addition to stretching, Vita Flex, and rubbing techniques. For both Vita Flex and other procedures within the Raindrop, specific steps are performed three complete times.

The oils used here mirror those that were used in the Vita Flex application and should be used in the same sequential order.

A. OREGANO
1. Hold the bottle 6 inches above the skin and evenly place 2-4 drops of Oregano along the spine, extending from the sacrum to the atlas.

Feather
2. Use 6-inch brush strokes to "feather" up the spine. To feather, gently brush the back of the fingertips up the spine while alternating hands.
3. Use 12-inch brush strokes to feather up the length of the spine.
4. Feather the entire length of the spine using three long brush strokes.
5. Repeat this process two or three more times.

Fan
6. Use 6-inch fanning strokes to fan up the spine and to the sides of the receiver. To fan, gently brush the back of the fingertips up and away from the spine.
7. Fan the entire length of the spine using three long fanning strokes.

Note: Do not repeat this process.

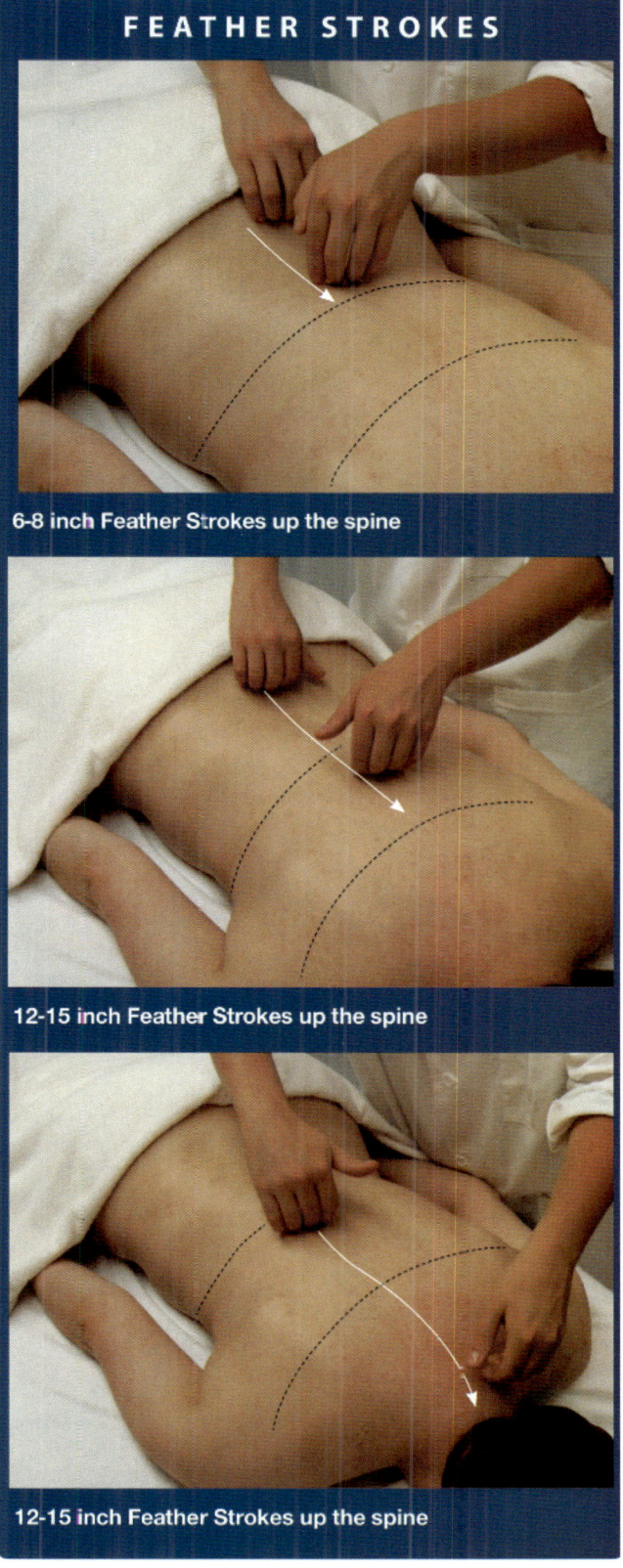

FEATHER STROKES

6-8 inch Feather Strokes up the spine

12-15 inch Feather Strokes up the spine

12-15 inch Feather Strokes up the spine

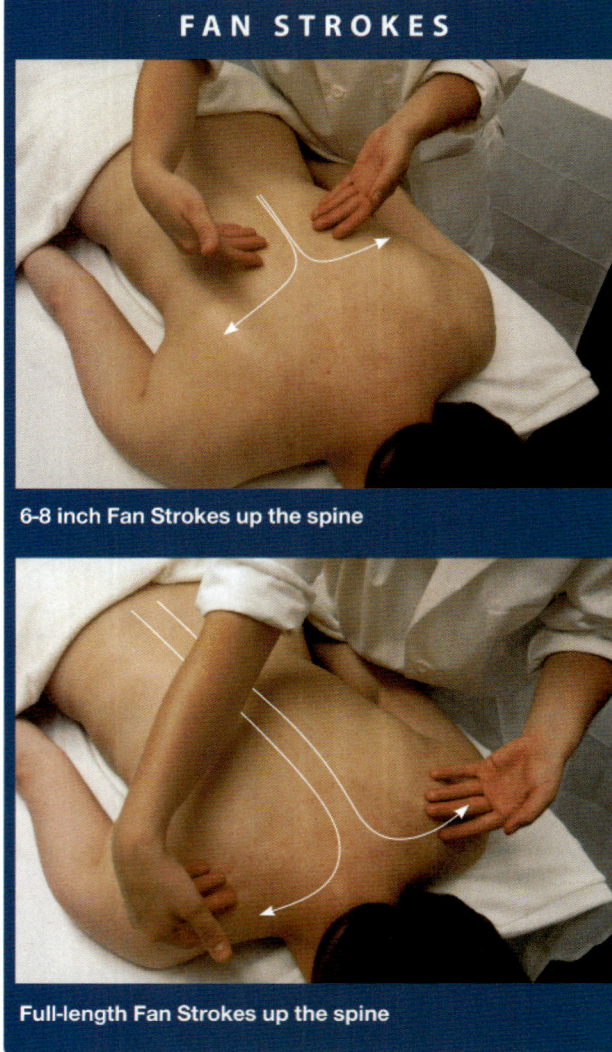

6-8 inch Fan Strokes up the spine

Full-length Fan Strokes up the spine

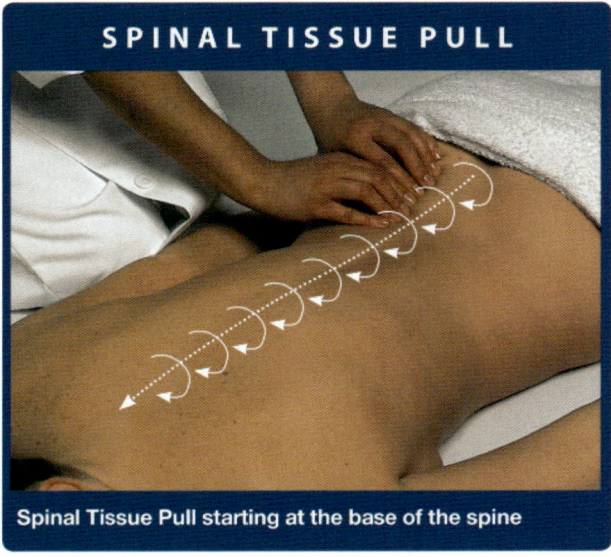

Spinal Tissue Pull starting at the base of the spine

B. THYME
1. Hold the bottle 6 inches above the skin and evenly place 2-4 drops of Thyme along the spine, extending from the sacrum to the atlas.
2. Immediately feather up the spine according to the technique previously described.

C. BASIL
1. Apply 3-4 drops of Basil evenly along both sides of the spine.
2. Immediately feather up the spine according to the technique previously described.

Spinal Tissue Pull

3. Alongside the spine, place hands side by side with fingers curved and the heels of the hands resting on the back. Complete three rotations using the pads of the fingertips to create small, circular, clockwise motions that gently pull the muscle tissue away from the spine.
4. After finishing one side of the spine, move to the other side of the receiver and repeat the procedure on the opposite side. Do not apply direct pressure to the spinal vertebrae.
5. Repeat this step two more times.

D. CYPRESS
1. Hold the bottle 6 inches above the skin and evenly place 4-6 drops of Cypress along both sides of the spine, extending from the sacrum to the atlas.
2. Immediately feather up the spine according to the technique previously described.

Finger Straddle

3. Stand on the receiver's left side, near the shoulder area, facing the receiver's feet.
4. With the index and middle fingers of the left hand, straddle the spine at the sacrum. Place the bottom edge of the right hand ulna or pinky-side down, just below the middle joints of the two straddling fingers.
5. Apply moderate, downward pressure with the straddling fingers while pulling them slowly to the atlas of the spine. At the same time, saw with the right hand using short, rapid, back-and-forth motions.
6. Once at the atlas, use the straddled fingers to gently pull toward the head three times.
7. Repeat this process two more times.

E. WINTERGREEN
1. Hold the bottle 6 inches above the skin and evenly space 6-10 drops of Wintergreen along both sides of the spine, extending from the sacrum to the atlas.
2. Immediately feather up the spine according to the technique previously described.

Techniques for Essential Oil Application | Chapter 10

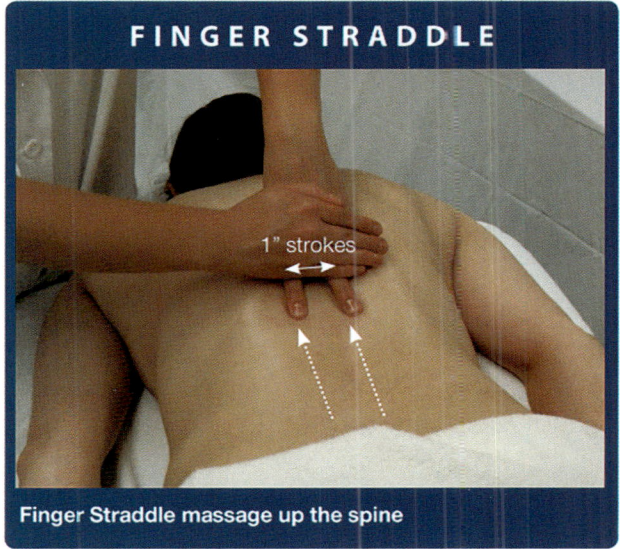

Finger Straddle massage up the spine

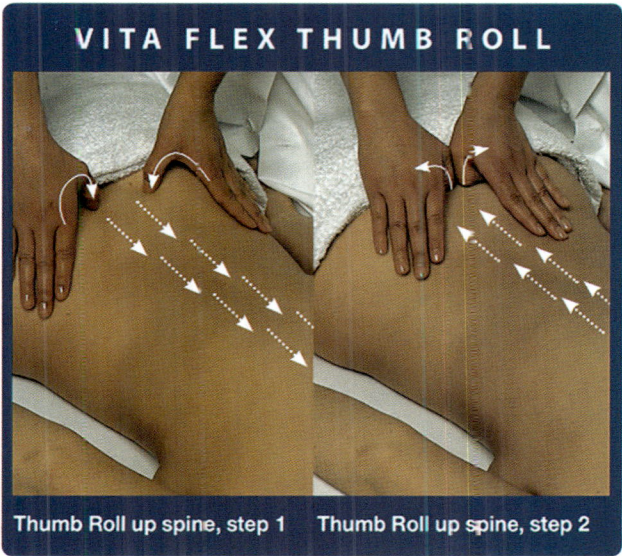

Thumb Roll up spine, step 1   Thumb Roll up spine, step 2

Vita Flex Thumb Roll
3. At the sacrum, place both thumbs 1 inch apart on either side of the spine with the tip of the thumbs down, one slightly higher on the back than the other.
4. Begin rolling thumbs from the tip to the nail, back and forth, working up the spine in small increments from the sacrum to the atlas, applying mild pressure the entire time.
5. Continue to roll your thumbs lightly over onto the knuckles and then back to their stand-up position. When doing this process, the knuckles should make contact with the spine. Work up the spine 1 inch at a time.
6. Repeat this step two more times.

Note: For clients who have neurological conditions, it is important to work down from the atlas to the sacrum instead of working up the spine.

F. MARJORAM
1. Hold the bottle 6 inches above the skin and evenly space 10-15 drops of Marjoram over the entire back, extending from the sacrum to the atlas.
2. Immediately feather as needed to evenly distribute the oil.

Circular Hand Massage
3. Place your hands palms down on the lower right side of the back. Rotate hands in a firm, clockwise motion up the right side of the spine.
4. Walk to the left side of the receiver and place your hands palms down on the lower left side of the back. Rotate hands in a firm, clockwise motion up the left side of the spine. Walk back to the right side of the receiver.
5. Repeat steps 3 and 4 two more times.

G. AROMA SIEZ
1. Hold the bottle 6 inches above the skin and evenly place 10 drops of Aroma Siez all over the back, extending from the sacrum to the atlas.
2. Immediately feather as needed to evenly distribute the oil.

Palm Slide
3. Place both hands palms down on the receiver's back on each side of the spine near the sacrum. One hand should be slightly higher than the other.
4. Slide palms, with mild downward pressure, in opposite directions, working slowly up the spine using a back-and-forth motion up to the nape of the neck.
5. Slide back to the base using the same movements.
6. Repeat this process two more times.

H. PEPPERMINT
1. Hold the bottle 6 inches above the skin and evenly space 3-5 drops of Peppermint along the spine, extending from the sacrum to the atlas.
2. Immediately feather up the spine according to the technique previously described.

I. VALOR
1. Hold the bottle 6 inches above the skin and evenly space 10-12 drops of Valor along the spine, extending from the sacrum to the atlas
2. Immediately feather up the spine according to the technique previously described.

First Edition | Essential Oils Complete Home Reference | 665

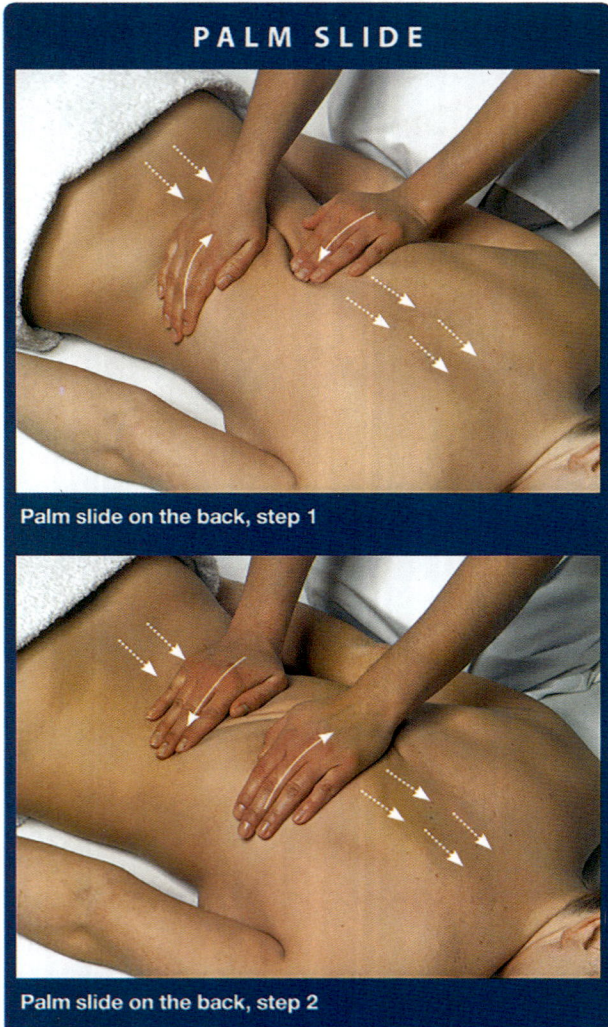

PALM SLIDE

Palm slide on the back, step 1

Palm slide on the back, step 2

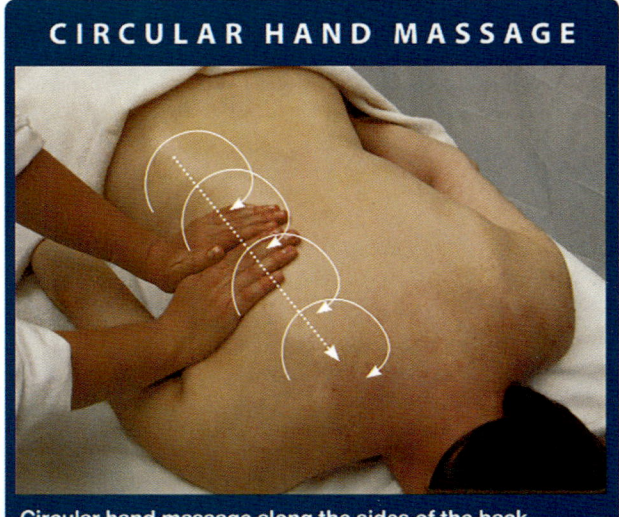

CIRCULAR HAND MASSAGE

Circular hand massage along the sides of the back

4. LYMPHATIC PUMP (BRAIN STEM PUMP TECHNIQUE)

1. Have the receiver lie facing up.
2. Place both hands under the back of the head with fingertips resting at the base of the skull.
3. Gently pull the head toward you in a soft, rocking motion, so the entire body moves. Sustain motion for one minute, then rest for one minute.
4. Repeat this process one more time. This movement provides an excellent lymphatic pump effect.

5. STRETCH AND RELAX PULL

1. Sit so that your shoulders are parallel to the receiver's shoulders.
2. Hold the receiver's head, using the cranial hold, with your less dominant hand under the base of the receiver's head and the dominant hand cradling the chin.
3. Next, place together your pointer finger and your middle finger and place them under the receiver's chin, just above the Adam's apple, keeping your ring and pinky fingers from touching the receiver's throat.
4. Pull straight back, gently toward you, with the hand under the base of the skull and gently pull with the fingers on the chin. Hold for three to five seconds and gently release.
5. Repeat this movement two more times.

Note: If another facilitator is available to assist with this process, they should stand at the feet of the receiver and hold the ankles. When the gentle pull is being done at the head, the facilitator at the feet holds the ankles and gently pulls and then releases at the same time as the facilitator at the head.

FINAL NOTES

- Finish by having the receiver place White Angelica on their shoulders, back of the neck, and thymus.
- It is possible that the receiver may have some emotions surface during the application of the Raindrop Technique. Be sure to have the emotional oils ready to assist them through the process of releasing those emotions.
- It is important that BOTH the receiver and facilitator drink plenty of water when giving and receiving the Raindrop Technique.

Customizing Raindrop Technique

Raindrop Technique may be customized to address different health issues that are not directly related to back problems. Lung infections, digestive complaints, hormonal problems, liver insufficiencies, and other

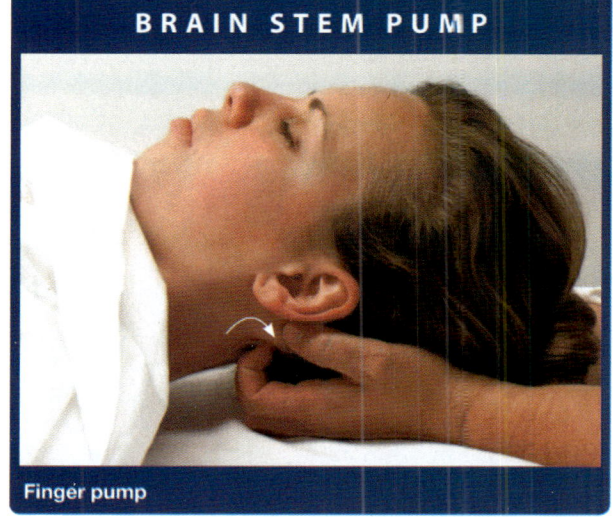

BRAIN STEM PUMP

Finger pump

problems can all be dealt with by substituting standard Raindrop Technique essential oils with other oils that are specifically targeted for those body systems.

As a rule, when customizing, start with Valor, Oregano, and Thyme. For extra antiviral effect, add Mountain Savory. The other essential oils such as Basil, Wintergreen, Marjoram, Thyme, or Cypress can be omitted or replaced by essential oils specific for the condition being targeted.

For example, if targeting a lung infection, replace Basil and Wintergreen with Ravintsara. Cypress is replaced with Eucalyptus Radiata, and Marjoram is replaced with R.C.

Use Chapter 15, "*The Personal Usage Guide*," to see other essential oils that would be applicable for what the individual needs are.

The basic Raindrop Technique has several variations, but these variations are not easy to explain and require class instruction and demonstration. It would be informative to attend a Raindrop Technique Training with a Young Living trainer and learn the Raindrop Technique from someone who has the knowledge of essential oils and their application.

Raindrop Technique has assisted both professionals and lay people to achieve true balance in the body. Out of the thousands of Raindrop Technique sessions that have been performed, hundreds of instances have been reported where the results were amazingly profound and immediate. Here are just a few examples:

A young man from Denver, Colorado, who suffered from chronic scoliosis, was able—for the first time in eight years—to fully bend over after the application of Raindrop Technique. With an overhead camera televising an image of his spine as he bent over, an audience of over 400 watched the vertebrae in his spine literally move into place. When he stood up, he was measured and had gained an inch in height.

Another instance involved a professional model in her early 40s who had developed early adult-onset scoliosis. She had to alter clothing so that it would fit properly for modeling sessions. She was not able to sit still for any length of time. After a Raindrop session, her spine straightened to such a degree that she, too, had gained an inch in height. She followed up with more sessions, and in the next few months reported that all discomfort was gone. She now dances and rides horses, pain free.

It is quite common for individuals with scoliosis who receive Raindrop Technique to gain $\frac{1}{2}$ inch or more in stature from a single application.

Many others have reported pain relief, congestion relief, and cold and flu relief as a result of Raindrop Technique, which is why it has captured so much interest among those involved in the healing arts.

ENDNOTES

1. Green RJ, Webb JN, Maxwell MH. The nature of virus-like particles in the paraxial muscles of idiopathic scoliosis. J Pathol. 1979 Sep;129(1):9-12.
2. Webb JN, Gillespie WJ. Virus-like particles in paraspinal muscle in scoliosis. Br Med J. 1976 Oct 16;2(6041):912-3.
3. Wolff MH, Buchel F, Gullotta F, Helpap B, Schneweiss KE. Investigations to demonstrate latent viral infection of varicella-Zoster virus in human spine ganglia. Verh Dtsch Ges Pathol. 1981;65:203-7.
4. Stirling A, Worthington T, Rafiq M, Lambert PA, Elliott TS. Association between sciatica and Propionibacterium acnes. Lancet 2001 Jun 23;357.9273):2024-5.
5. Nagrath SP, Hazra DK, Pant PC, Seth HC. Tuberculosis spine—a diagnostic conundrum. Case report. J Assoc Physicians India. 1974 May;22(5):405-7.
6. Jenks FJ, Stewart B. Images in clinical medicine. Vertebra tuberculosis. N Engl J Med. 1998 June 4;338(23):1677.
7. Monaghan D, Gupta A, Barrington NA. Case report: tuberculosis of the spine—an unusual presentation. Clin Radiol. 1991 May;43(5):360-2.
8. Petersen CK, Craw M. Radiological differentiation of tuberculosis and pyogenic osteomyelitis: a case report. J Manipulative Physiol Ther. 1986 Mar;9(1):39-42.
9. Pinott IR, Taffs LF. Experimental scoliosis in primates: a neurological cause. J Bone Joint Surg Br. 1982;64(4):503-7.
10. Ozogul Y, Kuley E, Ucar Y, Ozogul F. Antimicrobial impacts of essential oils on food-borne pathogens. Recent Pat Food Nutr Agric. 2015;7(1):53-61.
11. Wan J, Wilcock A, Coventry MJ. The effect of essential oils of basil on the growth of Aeromonas fluorescens. Journal of Applied Microbiology. 1998;84:152-158.
12. Moleya V, Narasimhan. Antibacterial activity of essential oil components. Int J Food Microbiol. 1992 Aug;16(4):337-42.
13. Horne D, Holm M, Oberg C, Chao S, Young DG. Antimicrobial effects of essential oils on Streptococcus pneumoniae. Journal of Essential Oil Research. 2001 Sep/Oct;13:387-392.
14. Moleyar V, Narasimham P. Antibacterial activity of essential oil components. International Journal of Food Microbiology 1992;16:337-32.
15. Obata Y, Takayama K, Maitani Y, Machida Y, Nagai T. Effect of pretreatment of skin with cyclic monoterpenes on permeation of diclofenac in hairless rat. Biol Pharm Bull. 1993 Mar;16(3) 312-4.
16. Zhao K, Singh J. Mechanisms of percutaneous absorption of tamoxifen by terpenes: Eugenol, d-limonene and menthone. Control Release. 1998 Nov 13;55(2-3):253-60.

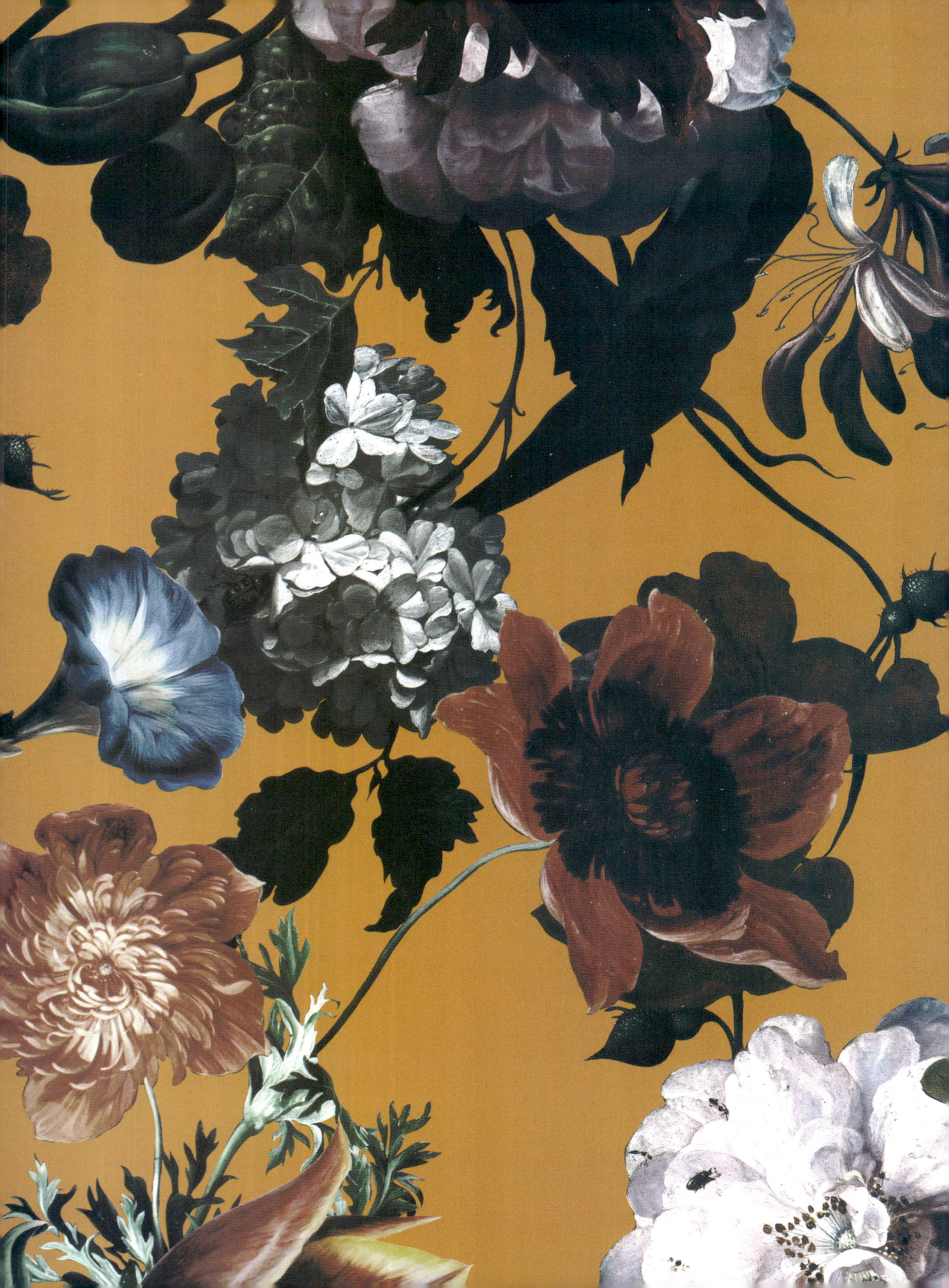

Spiritual, Mental & Emotional Support | Chapter 11

Support With Essential Oils

For literally thousands of years, the sacred smoke of frankincense rose in fragrant columns from temples across the ancient world. Why was it given so much importance in worship and as an offering to the gods? Why do some churches even today still burn frankincense for an incense as a major rite of their worship services?

The Appeal of Frankincense

The appeal of frankincense has not lessened as ancient days have rolled into the 21st century. As essential oils have gained prominence in our world, people are drawn to the rich aromas of frankincense and myrrh. Fittingly, it is only in our time that scientists have discovered that our bodies are apparently "hardwired" to have feelings of peace, awe, and reverence when using frankincense.

A young Israeli researcher named Arieh Moussaieff joined others from the Hebrew University in studying the Jerusalem Balsam, an herbal remedy that was formulated in 1719 in the Saint Savior monastery pharmacy in the old city of Jerusalem. Of the five different formula variations, the researchers chose to focus on one found in manuscript form in the monastery's archives. It contained four plants: olibanum (Boswellia [frankincense] species), myrrh (Commiphora species), aloe (Aloe species), and mastic (Pistacia lentiscus L.). The study that was published in 2005 showed the formula to have anti-inflammatory, antioxidative, and antiseptic properties.[1]

In further frankincense studies, Dr. Moussaieff discovered that a component in frankincense resin provides protection for the nervous system. He was also the lead researcher on a study that made news around the world. He noticed:

. . . the resin's antidepression and antianxiety properties and, investigating further, found that they act on a previously unknown pathway in the brain that regulates emotion. These findings not only help explain the ubiquity of frankincense in religion, they also hint that the active compounds may be used in the future to treat any number of neurological diseases, from Parkinson's to depression.[2]

Dr. Moussaieff's study was published in 2008 and documented for the first time that an ion channel in the brain (TRPV3) that was previously known only to be implicated in the perception of warmth in the skin had the much more important effect of causing antidepression and antianxiety behavioral changes when triggered by a component of frankincense, incensole acetate. Dr. Moussaieff's study concluded that, "TRPV3 channels in the brain may provide a biological basis for deeply rooted cultural and religious traditions."

Truly, can one come to any other conclusion than we are hardwired to experience calming and mood-enhancing effects when inhaling the scent of Boswellia carterii or Boswellia sacra, the two frankincense species known and loved for thousands of years?[3]

You may wonder if being uplifted in mood and having your anxiety quelled by Sacred Frankincense or Frankincense is really a requisite for worship or meditation. The ancient Egyptians apparently thought so, even though they had no idea how frankincense actually accomplished this. The late Professor Gonzague Ryckmans wrote that the Egyptian word for frankincense is SNTR, and it can be translated as "scent of the deity" or "what qualifies man to communicate with the deity."[4]

Religion scholar Scott Hahn, PhD, wrote a chapter on incense in his book, Signs of Life: 40 Catholic Customs and Their Biblical Roots. He wrote: "Incense became the most emblematic form of worship. Grains of incense, once dropped into a thurible with hot coals, rise heavenward as fragrant smoke. It's meant to be an outward sign of the inner mystery that is true prayer."[5]

Hahn mentioned that from Psalm 141:2 in the Old Testament ("Let my prayer be counted as incense before you,") to Philippians 4:18 in the New Testament ("an odour of a sweet smell, a sacrifice acceptable, wellpleasing to God"), incense permeates the Bible. The last book of the New Testament, Revelation, also connects incense with prayer: ". . . and there was given unto him much incense, that he should offer it with the prayers of all saints upon the golden altar which was before the throne. And the smoke of the incense which came with the prayers of the saints, ascended up before God out of the angel's hand" (Rev. 8:3-4).

Hahn also observed that some biblical people used incense and prayer merely as a rote ritual or offered it to strange gods, causing Isaiah to declare these words of the Lord: "Bring no more vain offerings; incense is an abomination to me" (Isaiah 1:13).

True worship is always within a sincere heart. Hahn notes that, "In fact, through the prophet Malachi, he [God] foretold a day when 'from the rising of the sun to its setting . . . in every place incense shall be offered unto my name, and a pure offering' (Malachi 1:11)."[6]

First Edition | Essential Oils Complete Home Reference | 669

How to Enhance Worship and Meditation with Essential Oils

When you want to be "centered" and to quiet your busy mind during meditation so that you can focus on worshipful prayer, Frankincense brings peace and a sense of calming to your heart. You need not burn the precious resin to achieve this calmness. Simply breathe in deeply the aroma of Sacred Frankincense or Frankincense.

You may wish to apply a few drops of these precious oils on your crown chakra and over your heart. Imagine being away from the busyness of life and perhaps resting on a solitary hill in Oman that overlooks the blue waters of the Arabian Sea, looking in the other direction and feeling the quietness of the immense desert with mystifying sand dunes that seem to shimmer in the sun, or taking refuge under a large frankincense tree that offers a little shade and a place of rest.

Prayer and meditation are ways of preparing that many energy workers and healers use before they begin their day.

The negative energy that also inhabits this world can have no influence while you become quiet and communicate with God. Simply apply a few drops of Angelica on your shoulders to wrap yourself in its energetic protection. A drop of rose oil over your heart or on the crown chakra can also help you rise up to a meditative state above the worries of the world.

It is a scientific fact that meditating is healthful, and prayer is calming to the soul. You may find singing a quiet hymn a joyful experience. Poet Paul Gerhardt (1607-1676) wrote that hymns can be offerings to God: "Hymns of praise are incense and rams."

Mental and Emotional Support

Today we live in a society of emotional turmoil. More and more the evidence is accumulating that our emotional health can have a profound effect on our physical health. More than ever before, researchers are probing the impact that emotional states have on the physical condition of the body.

Many doctors are recognizing the possibility that many diseases are caused by emotional problems that link back to infancy and childhood—and perhaps even to the womb. These emotional problems can compromise body systems and even genetic structuring through a process that creates the equivalent of a molecular "memory" in key organs and structures of the body.

The idea that memories and traumas can be embedded in the brain is not new, but scientists are now saying that these brain imprints may extend throughout the body.

Well-known author and Georgetown University research professor Candace Pert states, "Repressed traumas caused by overwhelming emotion can be stored in a body part, thereafter affecting our ability to feel that part or even move it."[7]

"To some degree, all of the organ systems in the human body have 'memory,'" agrees Bruce D. Perry, MD, PhD. "All nerve cells 'store' information in a fashion that is contingent upon previous patterns of activity," he noted. Dr. Perry is with the Child Trauma Program sponsored jointly by Baylor College of Medicine and Texas Children's Hospital. Perry says further that the ability to "carry elements of previous experience forward in time is the basis of the immune, the neuromuscular, and the neuroendocrine systems."[8]

Sense of Smell Links Emotion and Memory

As scientists have studied to understand the neural basis of emotion, they have discovered that the limbic system of the brain plays a vital role in interpreting and channeling intense experiences, particularly memories of fear or trauma. Interestingly, the two parts of the limbic system that play a major role in emotional processing—the amygdala and the hippocampus—are located within less than an inch of the olfactory nerve (see diagram).

Olfaction, or smell, is the sense that is physically the closest to the limbic system structures of the amygdala, which is involved in experiencing emotion and emotional memory, and the hippocampus, which encompasses both the working memory and short-term memory. This gives you an idea of how closely linked the sense of smell is to emotion and memory.

In 1989 researchers agreed that the amygdala—one of several structures in the cerebral cortex—plays a major role in storing and releasing emotional trauma and that aromas have a profound effect in triggering those responses.

Joseph Ledoux, MD, of the New York Medical University, was one of the first to suggest that the use of aroma could be a major breakthrough in helping to release hidden and suppressed feelings and memories of emotional bondage.

Fear and trauma can produce conditioned emotional responses that—unless released—will not only hamper our ability to live and enjoy life fully but can also limit the ability of some body systems to function properly, particularly the immune system. This can result in unexplained pain and illness as well as depression and other psychological issues.

Energy Centers (Chakras) and Associated Glands

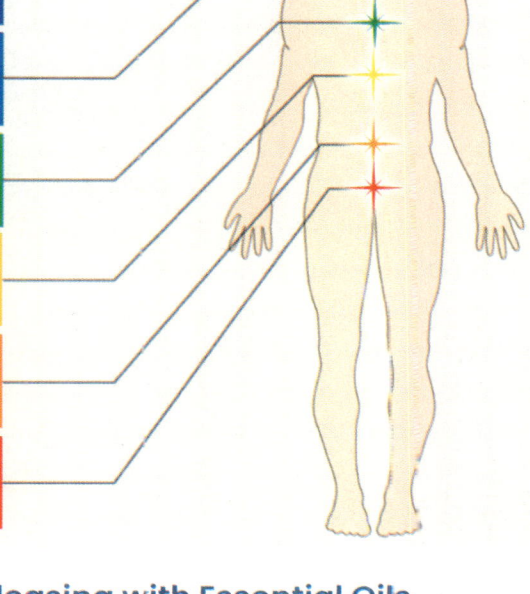

CROWN—Thought—Violet
Pineal: Controls cerebrum, right-brain hemisphere, central nervous system, and right eye

THIRD EYE—Light—Indigo
Pituitary: Controls endocrine system, left-brain hemisphere, left eye, nose, ears, sinuses, and parts of nervous system

THROAT—Ether/Sound—Blue
Thyroid: Controls jaw, neck, throat, voice, airways, upper lungs, nape of neck, and arms

HEART—Air/Touch—Green
Thymus: Controls heart, blood circulation, immune system, lower lungs, rib cage, skin, upper back, and hands

SOLAR PLEXUS—Fire/Sight—Yellow
Pancreas: Controls liver, digestive system, stomach, spleen, gall bladder, muscles, autonomic nervous system, and lower back

SACRAL—Water/Taste—Orange
Adrenal: Controls all solid parts—spinal column, bones, teeth, nails; also controls blood and building of cells, kidneys, and bladder

BASE/ROOT—Earth/Smell—Red
Reproductive: Controls pelvic area, sex organs, potency, and fluid functions

Many of the constituents in essential oils—particularly sesquiterpenes—can increase blood oxygen levels in the brain. The stimulation of both aroma and oxygenation seems to affect the amygdala in ways that facilitate the release of stored emotional blocks, both in the subconscious and in various body systems.

Combining the aroma of essential oils and oxygenation regularly over time—accompanied by mental focus and intent—has proven to be effective in many cases for resolving unexplained physical problems that were rooted in past emotional trauma.

Relaxing with Essential Oils

Another way in which essential oils can assist in helping people to move beyond emotional blocks is through their relaxing effect. The aldehydes and esters of certain essential oils such as Lavender, Rue, Frankincense, etc., are very calming and sedating to the nervous system (including both the sympathetic and parasympathetic systems). These substances allow us to relax instead of getting caught in an anxiety spiral.

Anxiety creates an acidic condition that activates the transcript enzyme, which then transcribes that anxiety on the RNA template and stores it in the DNA. That emotion then becomes a predominant factor in our lives from that moment on.

Releasing with Essential Oils

The process of emotional release using essential oils should not be dramatic, but gentle, occurring step-by-step over a period of time. Application of the oils accompanied by mental focus and relaxation should occur multiple times per day. Some emotional blocks will require only a day or two to begin releasing, while others may require weeks.

Many essential oil blends have been created precisely for the purpose of helping to release emotional patterns. The protocol outlined below is one that can be used very flexibly. One can use just the first step or two, a selection of steps, or all of the steps, depending on inclination and need. Each succeeding step involves another essential oil, which may further stimulate the release process.

It is important to remember that this process should not be uncomfortable. As you reach a step during which you begin to feel uncomfortable, there is no need to go further. It is better to wait for a future application when you feel confident before going to the next step. The applications should be accompanied by mental effort focusing on replacing negative emotions with positive emotions and images.

Note: Some people may find the idea that essential oil scents can be healing and therapeutic just a bit strange or somewhat "woo-woo." Perhaps a testimonial will be instructive.

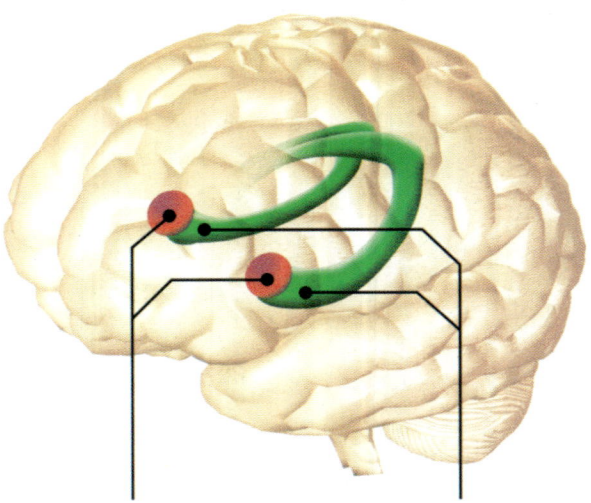

Amygdala
Influences behaviors and activities. It is also concerned with emotions such as anger and jealousy, as well as drives such as hunger, thirst, and sexual desire.

Hippocampus
Involved with recognizing new experiences, learning, and memory—especially short-term memory.

A lady in her early forties tells of her experience. She had the opportunity to smell several essential oil blends and was drawn to the blend of Release. Her friend gave it to her so that she could experiment to see if she noticed anything. Day after day she opened the bottle, inhaled deeply, and put it on her wrists so that she could smell it throughout the day.

A few months later she had a marvelous dream that went back to a long-repressed memory. A new experience occurred in the dream that gave balance and perspective to the traumatic memory. She was able to heal her feelings as though they just "wafted away in a gentle breeze."

It was many months later that she realized that it was the power of the oil blend Release that allowed this healing to take place. You would have a difficult time telling this lady that oils cannot possibly be healing!

"LETTING GO" WITH ESSENTIAL OILS

There is a very simple guideline for "letting go" of some old emotional baggage, releasing, allowing the uplifting feeling of peace and emotional freedom to take root.

Emotional health is a precious gift to our physical health and well-being.

It is important to be in a quiet place and setting with no cell phone, no TV, and no noisy environment.

STEP 1. Valor should be the first blend used when preparing for an emotional release. It helps balance the energies within the body and gives courage, confidence, and self-esteem. Apply 3-6 drops on each foot and top of shoulders, then cup hands and breathe in the beautiful strength-giving aroma as it balances the body.

STEP 2. Harmony is an exquisite blend of 12 essential oils and promotes physical and emotional healing through harmonic balance of the energy centers of the body, enabling energy to flow more efficiently. It helps reduce stress and creates an overall sense of well-being. Apply a drop on each of the chakra points.

STEP 3. Sacred Frankincense helps to regulate emotions, reduces the feelings of stress, and is very calming. It eases the depression around the traumatic experiences of life, whether in times of bereavement, divorce, or other emotional losses. It promotes confidence and purpose as the feelings of negativity disappear and stimulates the body's immune system.

When used during yoga, meditation, or prayer, the fullness and capacity of this oil brings support physically, emotionally, and spiritually, offering healing to those who use it. Placing this oil on the temples, back of neck, top of head, and over the heart allows the opportunity for deeper spiritual connection.

STEP 4. The 3 Wise Men blend was formulated to open the subconscious mind through pineal stimulation to release deep-seated trauma encoded in the DNA. This blend opens the crown chakra and stimulates the limbic system, bringing a sense of grounding and uplifting through positive memory recall. Place 2-3 drops on the crown of the head.

STEP 5. Release helps a person let go of the energy that comes from anger and hate held within the cells of the liver in order to create emotional peace and well-being. Freedom comes from being at peace rather than from harboring negative emotions. Rub 1-2 drops over the front and back of the liver area in a clockwise circular motion.

STEP 6. Idaho Grand Fir is a wonderful aroma that is very grounding and relaxing to the body. It helps with the effects of seasonal affective disorder, lifting depression. This strengthening oil stimulates the immune system, creating an increase of energy and sense of well-being. Rub a drop on the brain stem and under the nose. Breathe in the fortifying and balancing fragrance, bringing in the feeling of security.

STEP 7. Inner Child is a blend that may stimulate childhood memory. When children experience abuse or trauma, they can become "disconnected" from their inner child or identity. This disconnection may not be apparent until many years later, manifesting itself as a "midlife crisis." The Inner Child fragrance may stimulate memory response, helping one reconnect with his or her fundamental identity. This is an essential step or condition to achieving emotional balance. Apply 1 drop under the nose and 1 drop around the navel.

STEP 8. Forgiveness has high electrical frequencies that can help release negative memories to facilitate forgiveness, letting go, and moving on. Apply 1-2 drops around the navel and massage in a clockwise motion.

STEP 9. Grounding may be helpful in situations where one is overexcited about new ideas or wants to escape into a protective fantasy. In this kind of mental state, it is easy to make choices that lead to bad relationships, bad business decisions, and other unfortunate circumstances. We seek for an escape because we have no anchor to know how to deal with negative emotions.

The aroma of Grounding helps restore confidence and peace, enabling us to deal logically and peacefully with life's decisions. Apply 1-2 drops to the back of the neck and on the sternum.

STEP 10. Hope is formulated to reconnect with a feeling of strength and optimism for the future. Hope must be in place in order to move forward in life. Hopelessness can cause a loss of vision of goals and dreams, making it impossible to release emotional blocks. This aroma may also help in overcoming tendencies toward depression. Massage 1 drop on the outer edge of each ear.

STEP 11. Joy is an exotic blend of Ylang Ylang, Bergamot, and pure Bulgarian Rose oil and produces a magnetic energy to attract love and enhance self-love, bringing joy to the heart. Apply 1-2 drops over the heart area and massage in a clockwise motion.

STEP 12. Present Time has an empowering fragrance that gives a feeling of being "in the moment." One can only progress through emotional release when in the present time. Apply 1-2 drops on the thymus (top of the sternum) in a clockwise circular motion.

STEP 13. SARA is an essential oil blend formulated specifically for opening the limbic system to release the memories of serious trauma connected with Sexual And/or Ritual Abuse. Apply 1 drop over the energy centers (chakras), navel, and chest.

STEP 14. White Angelica is an amazing blend of 18 different oils, some of which were used during ancient times to increase the aura around the body, bringing a delicate sense of strength and protection. Its frequency protects against negative energies and helps to create a feeling of wholeness and oneness with the Creator. Apply 1-2 drops on the crown and on the shoulders.

STEP 15. Take time while still in the quiet, meditative space and select an oil or oil blend of your choice to enhance this process, reflect on your goals, your dreams, and on the positive things in your life, along with the things that you are choosing to change in your life.

Place a couple of drops of your oil or blend of choice over your heart, back of neck, and then, cupping your hands together, breathe in the life-giving, minute, fragrant molecules.

This can be a fortifying process, so take time to write some notes about your experience.

You can choose many oils and blends for this quiet time such as Rose, Ylang Ylang, Sacred Frankincense, Frankincense, Northern Lights Black Spruce, Highest Potential, Gathering, The Gift, Envision, Motivation, Into the Future, Magnify Your Purpose, Joy, Gratitude, Believe, Build Your Dream, Light the Fire, Live Your Passion, Transformation, Freedom, etc. They are all wonderful oils and oil blends to anchor emotional balance and stability.

When you are finished with your quiet time or meditation, do not distract your focus by immediately watching TV or going out to a social event. Remember that the oils may continue to work on an emotional level for several days.

Several oils you can carry with you that are easily available are the roll-on oils of Valor, Tranquil, RutaVaLa, and Stress Away, for those times when you need some emotional support immediately. Use them on a regular basis, especially at nighttime before you go to sleep. Roll the oils on behind your neck and along the rims of your ears; rub some on your hands until dry and then rub inside the pillow cover; or rub some on the pillow for a wonderful, aromatic, wafting fragrance to lull you off to sleep.

For a much more thorough explanation of emotional release and for specific emotional issues, consult the two books by Karol K. Truman entitled Feelings Buried Alive Never Die (1999/2017, Olympus Distributing) and Healing Feelings from Your Heart (2000, self-published) and the book by Dr. Carolyn L. Mein entitled Releasing Emotional Patterns with Essential Oils (2014, CreateSpace). These books are available through Life Science Publishing.

OILS FOR SPECIFIC EMOTIONAL CHALLENGES

Abuse
Singles: Geranium, White Angelica, Ylang Ylang, Palo Santo, Ocotea, Frankincense, Sacred Frankincense, Angelica

Blends: SARA, Hope, Gary's Light, Freedom, Joy, Peace & Calming, Inner Child, SleepyIze, Grounding, Trauma Life, Release, Valor, Valor Roll-On, Forgiveness, One Heart

Agitation
Singles: Idaho Blue Spruce, Bergamot, Cedarwood, Idaho Grand Fir, Jade Lemon, Clary Sage, Frankincense, Sacred Frankincense, Geranium, Juniper, Davana, Kunzea, Lavender, Myrrh, Marjoram, Rose, Ylang Ylang, Laurus Nobilis, Cistus, Hinoki

Blends: Peace & Calming, Peace & Calming II, Gary's Light, Freedom, Joy, Valor, Valor Roll-On, AromaEase, KidScents KidPower, KidScents KidPower Roll-On, Tranquil Roll-On, Harmony, Forgiveness, One Heart, Seedlings Calm, RutaVaLa, RutaVaLa Roll-On, Abundance, Australian Blue

Anger
Singles: Idaho Blue Spruce, Bergamot, Cedarwood, Frankincense, Sacred Frankincense, Lavender, Myrrh, Orange, Rose, Roman Chamomile, Ylang Ylang, Laurus Nobilis, Jade Lemon, Pine, Angelica

Blends: Release, Gary's Light, Valor, Valor Roll-On, Sacred Mountain, AromaEase, KidScents KidPower, KidScents KidPower Roll-On, Harmony, Hope, Forgiveness, Freedom, SleepyIze, Transformation, Seedlings Calm, Present Time, Trauma Life, Joy, Tranquil Roll-On, Surrender, Christmas Spirit, One Heart, White Angelica

Antagonism
Singles: Idaho Blue Spruce, Cedarwood, Palo Santo, Idaho Grand Fir, Roman Chamomile, Frankincense, Sacred Frankincense, Jade Lemon, Jasmine, Orange, Ylang Ylang, Cistus, Palmarosa, Pine

Blends: Peace & Calming, Peace & Calming II, Gary's Light, Freedom, Egyptian Gold, Joy, Harmony, Hope, Valor, Valor Roll-On, SleepyIze, Acceptance, AromaEase, KidScents KidPower, KidScents KidPower Roll-On, Humility, Surrender, One Heart, Release, RutaVaLa, RutaVaLa Roll-On

Anxiety
Singles: Idaho Blue Spruce, Orange, Roman Chamomile, Ylang Ylang, Lavender, Sacred Frankincense, Frankincense, Davana, Clary Sage, Jade Lemon, Angelica, Laurus Nobilis, Hinoki, Cistus, Palmarosa, Pine

Blends: Freedom, Valor, Valor Roll-On, Gary's Light, SleepyIze, Hope, Peace & Calming, KidScents KidPower, KidScents KidPower Roll-On, AromaEase, Tranquil Roll-On, Joy, Present Time, The Gift, Seedlings Calm, Reconnect, Abundance, Surrender, Believe, Shutran, White Angelica, One Heart, Australian Blue

Apathy
Singles: Frankincense, Sacred Frankincense, Geranium, Marjoram, Jasmine, Orange, Peppermint, Rose, Sacred Sandalwood, Royal Hawaiian Sandalwood, Jade Lemon, Angelica, Thyme, Ylang Ylang, Lime

Blends: Joy, Harmony, Valor, Valor Roll-On, Gary's Light, 3 Wise Men, Hope, Believe, White Angelica, KidScents KidPower, KidScents KidPower Roll-On, Motivation, Live with Passion, Live Your Passion, Highest Potential, Build Your Dream, One Heart, Shutran, KidScents GeneYus

Boredom
Singles: Cedarwood, Northern Lights Black Spruce, Black Pepper, Roman Chamomile, Sacred Frankincense, Frankincense, Juniper, Lavender, Rosemary, Jade Lemon, Thyme, Ylang Ylang

Blends: Build Your Dream, Dream Catcher, Light the Fire, Journey On, Gary's Light, Citrus Fresh, Motivation, Transformation, Inner Child, KidScents KidPower, KidScents KidPower Roll-On, Valor, Valor Roll-On, KidScents GeneYus, Awaken, Live with Passion, Live Your Passion, Gathering, En-R-Gee

Concentration
Singles: Cedarwood, Cypress, Juniper, Lavender, Lemon, Jade Lemon, Lemon Myrtle, Basil, Helichrysum, Myrrh, Orange, Peppermint, Rosemary, Sacred Sandalwood, Royal Hawaiian Sandalwood, Ylang Ylang

Blends: Brain Power, Clarity, Reconnect, KidScents GeneYus, Highest Potential, Common Sense, Awaken, Gathering, Fulfill Your Destiny, Dream Catcher, Build Your Dream, Light the Fire, Gary's Light, KidScents KidPower, KidScents KidPower Roll-On, Citrus Fresh, Magnify Your Purpose, Brain Power, Freedom

Spiritual, Mental & Emotional Support | Chapter 11

Confusion

Singles: Cedarwood, Northern Lights Black Spruce, Peppermint, Sacred Frankincense, Frankincense, Jade Lemon, Ginger, Juniper, Copaiba, Lemon Myrtle, Rosemary, Basil, Thyme, Ylang Ylang

Blends: Clarity, Light the Fire, Gary's Light, Reconnect, One Heart, KidScents GeneYus, Citrus Fresh, Common Sense, Harmony, Valor, Valor Roll-On, AromaEase, KidScents KidPower, KidScents KidPower Roll-On, Freedom, Journey On, Present Time, Awaken, Brain Power, Gathering, Grounding, Abundance, SleepyIze, Shutran, Build Your Dream

Daydreaming

Singles: Ginger, Cedarwood, Ocotea, Northern Lights Black Spruce, Lemon, Peppermint, Rose, Rosemary, Tangerine, Jade Lemon, Lemon Myrtle, Spearmint

Blends: Reconnect, KidScents GeneYus, Sacred Mountain, Gathering, Common Sense, Harmony, Present Time, Dream Catcher, Build Your Dream, 3 Wise Men, Magnify Your Purpose, Journey On, Envision, Light the Fire, Live with Passion, Live Your Passion, One Heart, KidScents KidPower, KidScents KidPower Roll-On, Brain Power, Highest Potential

Depression

Singles: Sacred Frankincense, Idaho Blue Spruce, Frankincense, Copaiba, Palo Santo, Jade Lemon, Lemon, Sacred Sandalwood, Royal Hawaiian Sandalwood, Geranium, Lavender, Angelica, Orange, Grapefruit, Cistus, Ylang Ylang, Hinoki, Melissa, Lime, Palmarosa, Pine, Tsuga, Mastrante

Blends: Valor, Valor Roll-On, Gary's Light, AromaEase, Freedom, Motivation, Live with Passion, Live Your Passion, Hope, Believe, Christmas Spirit, Reconnect, Shutran, Citrus Fresh, Journey On, Brain Power, Present Time, Envision, KidScents KidPower, KidScents KidPower Roll-On, Sacred Mountain, Harmony, Highest Potential, Build Your Dream, Light the Fire, Joy, Australian Blue, Dragon Time, En-R-Gee, Gentle Baby, SARA, One Heart, White Angelica

Despair

Singles: Cedarwood, Northern Lights Black Spruce, Sacred Frankincense, Idaho Blue Spruce, Frankincense, Lavender, Geranium, Jade Lemon, Lemon, Orange, Peppermint, Rosemary, Thyme, Cistus, Ylang Ylang, Hinoki, Melissa, Lime, Palmarosa, Pine, Tangerine, Tsuga, Mastrante

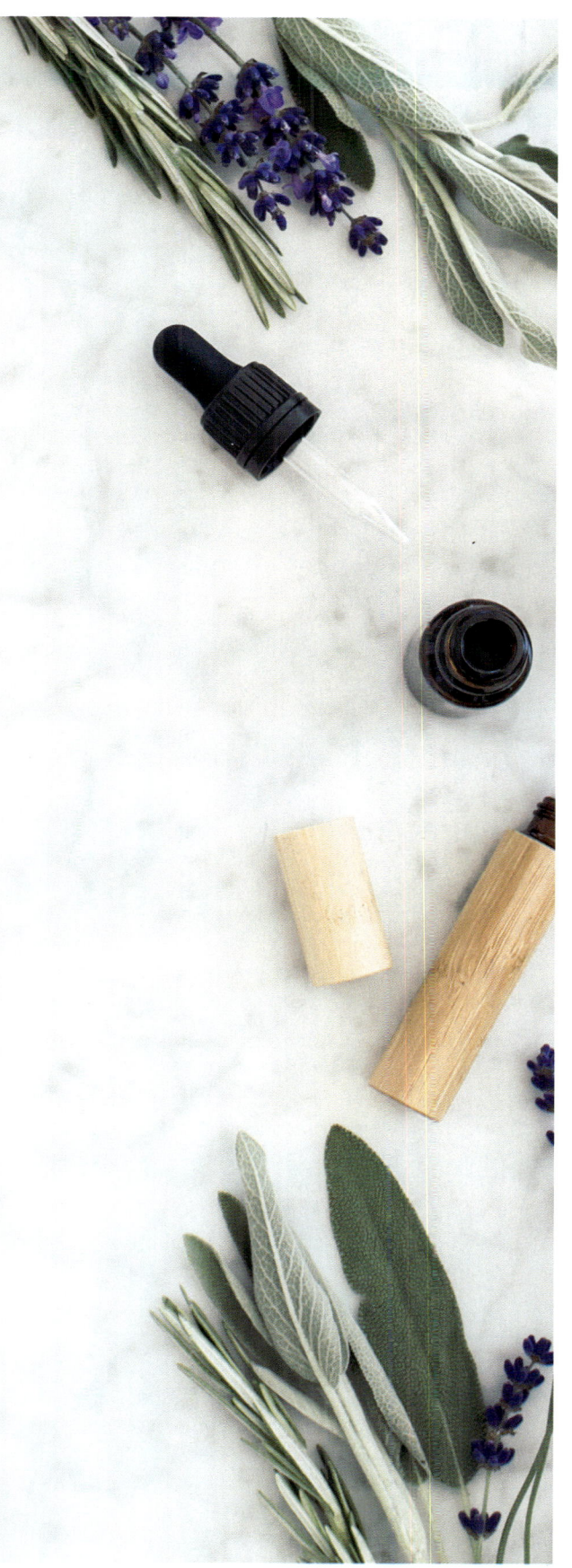

First Edition | Essential Oils Complete Home Reference | 675

Blends: Joy, Believe, Gary's Light, Christmas Spirit, Freedom, Reconnect, InTouch, AromaEase, Valor, Valor Roll-On, SleepyIze, Harmony, Seedlings Calm, Gathering, Grounding, Inner Child, Forgiveness, One Heart, Motivation, Hope, KidScents KidPower, KidScents KidPower Roll-On, Journey On, RutaVaLa, RutaVaLa Roll-On, Citrus Fresh, Abundance, Australian Blue, En-R-Gee, Gentle Baby, SARA, Build Your Dream, Light the Fire

Despondency
Singles: Idaho Blue Spruce, Geranium, Sacred Frankincense, Frankincense, Jade Lemon, Ginger, Orange, Rose, Ylang Ylang, Idaho Grand Fir, Hinoki, Melissa, Lime, Cistus, Nutmeg, Palmarosa, Pine, Tangerine, Tsuga, Mastrante

Blends: Inspiration, Reconnect, Gary's Light, Common Sense, Shutran, Harmony, Christmas Spirit, Valor, Valor Roll-On, Hope, Freedom, Joy, Build Your Dream, KidScents KidPower, KidScents KidPower Roll-On, Light the Fire, Present Time, Gathering, One Heart, Inner Child, Trauma Life, Australian Blue, AromaEase, Envision, SleepyIze, Citrus Fresh, En-R-Gee, Gentle Baby

Disappointment
Singles: Copaiba, Sacred Frankincense, Frankincense, Palo Santo, Geranium, Ginger, Juniper, Lavender, Jade Lemon, Northern Lights Black Spruce, Orange, Thyme, Ylang Ylang, Hinoki, Laurus Nobilis, Melissa, Cistus, Tangerine, Tsuga, Mastrante

Blends: Hope, Joy, Gary's Light, Christmas Spirit, Valor, Valor Roll-On, Reconnect, SleepyIze, Present Time, Harmony, Build Your Dream, Dream Catcher, KidScents KidPower, KidScents KidPower Roll-On, Light the Fire, Abundance, Release, Freedom, Gathering, Magnify Your Purpose, Live with Passion, Live Your Passion, Believe, Journey On, One Heart, Shutran, AromaEase, Motivation, Australian Blue

Discouragement
Singles: Idaho Blue Spruce, Bergamot, Idaho Grand Fir, Cedarwood, Sacred Frankincense, Frankincense, Geranium, Juniper, Lavender, Jade Lemon, Lemon, Orange, Northern Lights Black Spruce, Hinoki, Melissa, Cistus, Davana, Laurus Nobilis, Lime, Cardamom, Nutmeg, Palmarosa, Pine, Tangerine, Tsuga, Mastrante

Blends: Valor, Valor Roll-On, Shutran, SleepyIze, Light the Fire, Gary's Light, The Gift, Sacred Mountain, Freedom, Common Sense, Hope, Joy, KidScents KidPower, KidScents KidPower Roll-On, Build Your Dream, Dream Catcher, Release, Reconnect, One Heart, Abundance, Into the Future, Magnify Your Purpose, Envision, Believe, AromaEase, Gathering, Christmas Spirit, Australian Blue, Citrus Fresh, En-R-Gee

Failure
Singles: Copaiba, Sacred Frankincense, Frankincense, Palo Santo, Geranium, Ginger, Juniper, Lavender, Jade Lemon, Northern Lights Black Spruce, Orange, Thyme, Ylang Ylang, Hinoki, Laurus Nobilis, Melissa, Cistus, Tangerine, Tsuga, Mastrante

Blends: Hope, Joy, Christmas Spirit, Valor, Valor Roll-On, Reconnect, SleepyIze, Present Time, Harmony, Build Your Dream, Dream Catcher, Light the Fire, Gary's Light, KidScents KidPower, KidScents KidPower Roll-On, Abundance, Release, Freedom, Gathering, Magnify Your Purpose, Live with Passion, Live Your Passion, Believe, Journey On, One Heart, Shutran, AromaEase, Motivation, Australian Blue

Fear
Singles: Idaho Blue Spruce, Palo Santo, Cypress, Roman Chamomile, Geranium, Juniper, Myrrh, Northern Lights Black Spruce, Orange, Sacred Frankincense, Angelica, Hinoki, Jade Lemon, Cistus, Pine, Tangerine, Tsuga

Blends: Freedom, Valor, Valor Roll-On, AromaEase, SleepyIze, Freedom, Present Time, The Gift, Tranquil Roll-On, Release, Hope, White Angelica, KidScents KidPower, KidScents KidPower Roll-On, Trauma Life, Seedlings Calm, Gratitude, Gathering, Abundance, Highest Potential, Gary's Light, Shutran, Australian Blue, Light the Fire, Christmas Spirit

Forgetfulness
Singles: Cedarwood, Roman Chamomile, Sacred Frankincense, Frankincense, Rosemary, Copaiba, Idaho Grand Fir, Peppermint, Thyme, Jade Lemon, Lemon Myrtle, Ylang Ylang

Blends: Reconnect, KidScents GeneYus, Clarity, Valor, Valor Roll-On, Present Time, Gathering, 3 Wise Men, Dream Catcher, KidScents KidPower, KidScents KidPower Roll-On, Citrus Fresh, Acceptance, Brain Power, Highest Potential, Egyptian Gold, Gathering

Forlorn
Singles: Idaho Blue Spruce, Bergamot, Idaho Grand Fir, Cedarwood, Sacred Frankincense, Frankincense, Geranium, Juniper, Lavender, Jade Lemon, Lemon, Orange, Northern Lights Black Spruce, Hinoki, Melissa, Cistus, Davana, Laurus Nobilis, Lime, Cardamom, Nutmeg, Palmarosa, Pine, Tangerine, Tsuga, Mastrante

Blends: Valor, Valor Roll-On, Gary's Light, Shutran, SleepyIze, Light the Fire, The Gift, Sacred Mountain, Freedom, Common Sense, Hope, Joy, KidScents KidPower, KidScents KidPower Roll-On, Build Your Dream, Dream Catcher, Release, Reconnect, One Heart, Abundance, Into the Future, Magnify Your Purpose, Envision, Believe, AromaEase, Gathering, Christmas Spirit, Australian Blue, Citrus Fresh, En-R-Gee

Frustration
Singles: Idaho Blue Spruce, Roman Chamomile, Palo Santo, Ocotea, Ginger, Juniper, Lavender, Jade Lemon, Lemon, Orange, Peppermint, Thyme, Ylang Ylang, Northern Lights Black Spruce, Hinoki, Melissa, Cistus, Angelica, Davana, Palmarosa, Tangerine

Blends: Valor, Valor Roll-On, Light the Fire, Hope, AromaEase, Present Time, Sacred Mountain, 3 Wise Men, Humility, Peace & Calming, Peace & Calming II, White Angelica, Gary's Light, SleepyIze, Hope, Freedom, Reconnect, KidScents GeneYus, KidScents KidPower, KidScents KidPower Roll-On, Tranquil Roll-On, Seedlings Calm, Release, Surrender, One Heart, Gratitude, Gathering, Abundance, Shutran, Australian Blue

Grief
Singles: Bergamot, Palo Santo, Roman Chamomile, Clary Sage, Eucalyptus Globulus, Juniper, Lavender, Hinoki, Laurus Nobilis, Melissa, Cistus, Tsuga, Davana, Jade Lemon, Mastrante

Blends: Valor, Valor Roll-On, SARA, Gary's Light, Journey On, AromaEase, Seedlings Calm, KidScents KidPower, KidScents KidPower Roll-On, SleepyIze, Release, Freedom, Inspiration, Inner Child, Gathering, Harmony, Present Time, Magnify Your Purpose, Abundance, Australian Blue, Christmas Spirit, Egyptian Gold, One Heart

Guilt
Singles: Roman Chamomile, Cypress, Juniper, Geranium, Sacred Frankincense, Frankincense, Northern Lights Black Spruce, Rose, Jade Lemon, Thyme

Blends: Valor, Valor Roll-On, SARA, Gary's Light, AromaEase, Release, One Heart, Freedom, SleepyIze, Inspiration, Common Sense, Inner Child, KidScents KidPower, KidScents KidPower Roll-On, Gathering, Harmony, Present Time, Magnify Your Purpose, Gratitude, Egyptian Gold

Horror
Singles: Gary's Light, White Angelica, Idaho Blue Spruce, Palo Santo, Cypress, Roman Chamomile, Geranium, Juniper, Myrrh, Northern Lights Black Spruce, Orange, Sacred Frankincense, Angelica, Hinoki, Jade Lemon, Cistus, Pine, Tangerine, Tsuga

Blends: Freedom, Valor, Valor Roll-On, One Heart, AromaEase, SleepyIze, Freedom, Present Time, The Gift, Tranquil Roll-On, Release, Hope, Trauma Life, Seedlings Calm, KidScents KidPower, KidScents KidPower Roll-On, Gratitude, Gathering, Abundance, Highest Potential, Shutran, Australian Blue, Light the Fire, Christmas Spirit

Irritability
Singles: Idaho Blue Spruce, Idaho Grand Fir, Lavender, Ocotea, Melissa, Palo Santo, Copaiba, Dorado Azul, Valerian, Ylang Ylang, Angelica, Jade Lemon, Davana, Tangerine, Cistus, Tsuga, Palmarosa

Blends: Valor, Valor Roll-On, Freedom, Hope, AromaEase, Peace & Calming, Peace & Calming II, KidScents KidPower, KidScents KidPower Roll-On, SleepyIze, Release, Surrender, Seedlings Calm, Transformation, Forgiveness, Gary's Light, Harmony, Present Time, Inspiration, White Angelica, One Heart, Abundance, Dragon Time, Lady Sclareol

Jealousy
Singles: Ocotea, Palo Santo, Idaho Grand Fir, Dorado Azul, Sacred Frankincense, Frankincense, Lemon, Orange, Rose, Angelica, Rosemary, Thyme

Blends: The Gift, Sacred Mountain, Valor, Valor Roll-On, White Angelica, Joy, KidScents KidPower, KidScents KidPower Roll-On, Harmony, Gary's Light, SleepyIze, Humility, Forgiveness, Surrender, Release, One Heart, Gratitude

Mood Swings

Singles: Idaho Blue Spruce, Idaho Grand Fir, Clary Sage, Sage, Geranium, Juniper, Fennel, Lavender, Peppermint, Rose, Jasmine, Rosemary, Jade Lemon, Lemon, Northern Lights Black Spruce, Angelica, Yarrow, Hinoki, Laurus Nobilis, Melissa, Cistus, Lime, Ylang Ylang, Davana, Nutmeg, Vetiver

Blends: Peace & Calming, Peace & Calming II, Reconnect, KidScents GeneYus, AromaEase, RutaVaLa, RutaVaLa Roll-On, Gathering, Valor, Valor Roll-On, SleepyIze, Dragon Time, Mister, Harmony, Joy, KidScents KidPower, KidScents KidPower Roll-On, One Heart, Seedlings Calm, Present Time, Freedom, Envision, Magnify Your Purpose, Abundance, White Angelica, Brain Power, Australian Blue, Christmas Spirit, Tranquil Roll-On, Egyptian Gold, En-R-Gee, Shutran, Lady Sclareol

Obsessiveness

Singles: Clary Sage, Ocotea, Palo Santo, Cypress, Geranium, Lavender, Ylang Ylang, Jade Lemon, Patchouli

Blends: Sacred Mountain, The Gift, Valor, Valor Roll-On, Forgiveness, Acceptance, Humility, Inner Child, Present Time, Awaken, Motivation, Surrender, Transformation, AromaEase, KidScents KidPower, KidScents KidPower Roll-On, Release, Common Sense, Joy, One Heart, Gratitude

Panic

Singles: Idaho Blue Spruce, Bergamot, Idaho Grand Fir, Roman Chamomile, Myrrh, Sacred Frankincense, Frankincense, Lavender, Marjoram, Rosemary, Jade Lemon, Thyme, Ylang Ylang, Northern Lights Black Spruce, Angelica, Davana, Cistus, Palmarosa, Pine

Blends: Gary's Light, White Angelica, Harmony, Valor, Valor Roll-On, AromaEase, SleepyIze, Freedom, RutaVaLa, RutaVaLa Roll-On, The Gift, Gathering, Peace & Calming, Peace & Calming II, Seedlings Calm, Trauma Life, Tranquil Roll-On, Awaken, Grounding, KidScents KidPower, KidScents KidPower Roll-On, Abundance, Believe, Reconnect, One Heart, Shutran, Australian Blue

Resentment

Singles: Jasmine, Rose, Ocotea, Jade Lemon, Palo Santo, Angelica

Blends: Forgiveness, RutaVaLa, RutaVaLa Roll-On, Harmony, Believe, Common Sense, Humility, White Angelica, One Heart, KidScents KidPower, KidScents KidPower Roll-On, Surrender, Joy, Release, AromaEase, SleepyIze

Restlessness

Singles: Idaho Blue Spruce, Bergamot, Ocotea, Idaho Grand Fir, Dorado Azul, Sacred Frankincense, Frankincense, Geranium, Lavender, Jade Lemon, Orange, Ylang Ylang, Sacred Sandalwood, Northern Lights Black Spruce, Angelica, Valerian, Cistus, Davana, Cardamom, Palmarosa

Blends: Reconnect, KidScents GeneYus, RutaVaLa, RutaVaLa Roll-On, Gary's Light, AromaEase, Common Sense, Peace & Calming, Peace & Calming II, Freedom, Journey On, Tranquil Roll-On, Build Your Dream, The Gift, Sacred Mountain, Gathering, Valor, Valor Roll-On, Seedlings Calm, Inspiration, Acceptance, Surrender, Light the Fire, Live with Passion, Live Your Passion, White Angelica, KidScents KidPower, KidScents KidPower Roll-On, One Heart, Shutran, SleepyIze, Abundance

Sadness

Singles: Bergamot, Palo Santo, Roman Chamomile, Clary Sage, Eucalyptus Globulus, Juniper, Lavender, Hinoki, Laurus Nobilis, Melissa, Cistus, Tsuga, Davana, Jade Lemon, Mastrante

Blends: Valor, Valor Roll-On, SARA, Journey On, AromaEase, Seedlings Calm, SleepyIze, Release, Freedom, Inspiration, Inner Child, KidScents KidPower, KidScents KidPower Roll-On, Gathering, Harmony, One Heart, Gary's Light, Present Time, Magnify Your Purpose, Abundance, Australian Blue, Christmas Spirit, Egyptian Gold

Shock

Singles: Idaho Blue Spruce, Helichrysum, Basil, Dorado Azul, Copaiba, Roman Chamomile, Ylang Ylang, Rosemary, Cardamom

Blends: Gary's Light, White Angelica, Clarity, Common Sense, Reconnect, AromaEase, KidScents KidPower, KidScents KidPower Roll-On, Valor, Valor Roll-On, Inspiration, Joy, SleepyIze, Tranquil Roll-On, Grounding, Trauma Life, Freedom, One Heart, Brain Power, Australian Blue, Abundance

Sorrow

Singles: Bergamot, Palo Santo, Roman Chamomile, Clary Sage, Eucalyptus Globulus, Juniper, Lavender, Hinoki, Laurus Nobilis, Melissa, Cistus, Tsuga, Davana, Jade Lemon, Mastrante

Blends: Valor, Valor Roll-On, SARA, Gary's Light, Journey On, AromaEase, Seedlings Calm, KidScents KidPower, KidScents KidPower Roll-On, SleepyIze, Release, Freedom, Inspiration, Inner Child, Gathering, Harmony, One Heart, Present Time, Magnify Your Purpose, Abundance, Australian Blue, Christmas Spirit, Egyptian Gold

Stress

Singles: Idaho Blue Spruce, Roman Chamomile, Ylang Ylang, Angelica, Frankincense, Sacred Frankincense, Davana, Cistus, Cardamom, Cedarwood, Hinoki, Laurus Nobilis, Melissa, Lime, Jade Lemon, Clove, Dill, Palmarosa

Blends: Stress Away, Stress Away Roll-On, Shutran, White Angelica, Gary's Light, One Heart, Seedlings Calm, AromaEase, SleepyIze, Freedom, Reconnect, KidScents GeneYus, KidScents KidPower, KidScents KidPower Roll-On, Tranquil Roll-On, Release, Hope, Journey On, Magnify Your Purpose, Christmas Spirit, Live with Passion, Live Your Passion, Light the Fire, Citrus Fresh, En-R-Gee, Into the Future, Highest Potential, Gathering, Mister, RutaVaLa, RutaVaLa Roll-On, Transformation, InTouch

Terror

Singles: Idaho Blue Spruce, Palo Santo, Cypress, Roman Chamomile, Geranium, Juniper, Myrrh, Northern Lights Black Spruce, Orange, Sacred Frankincense, Angelica, Hinoki, Jade Lemon, Cistus, Pine, Tangerine, Tsuga

Blends: White Angelica, Gary's Light, Freedom, Valor, Valor Roll-On, AromaEase, SleepyIze, Freedom, Present Time, The Gift, Tranquil Roll-On, Release, Hope, One Heart, Trauma Life, Seedlings Calm, KidScents KidPower, KidScents KidPower Roll-On, Gratitude, Gathering, Abundance, Highest Potential, Shutran, Australian Blue, Light the Fire, Christmas Spirit.

ENDNOTES

1. Moussaieff A, Fride E, Amar Z, Lev E, Steinberg D, Gallily R, Mechoulam R. The Jerusalem balsam: from the Franciscan monastery in the Old City of Jerusalem to Martindale 33. Journal of Ethnopharmacology. 2005;101(1-3):16-26.

2. Moussaief A, Rimmerman N, Bregman T, Straiker A, Felder CC, Shoham S, Kashman Y, Huang SM, Hyosang L, Shohami E, Mackie K, Caterina MJ, Walker JM, Fride E, Mechoulam R. Incensole acetate, an incense component, elicits psychoactivity by activating TRPV3 channels in the brain. The FASEB Journal. 2008;22(8):3024-34.

3. Ibid.

4. Ryckmans, G. Der Weihrauch: Geschichte, Bedeutung, Vervendung, Regensburg, 1977:17.

5. Hahn S. Signs of life: 40 Catholic customs and their Biblical roots. New York: Doubleday; 2009. p 159.

6. Ibid:158.

7. Pert, C. Molecules of emotion: the science behind mind-body medicine. New York: Touchstone; 1997. p. 141.

8. Perry B. Splintered reflections: images of the body in trauma. ed. Jean Goodwin, Reina Attias. New York: Basic Books; 1999. Memories of fear: How the brain stores and retrieves physiologic states, feelings, behaviors and thoughts from traumatic events.

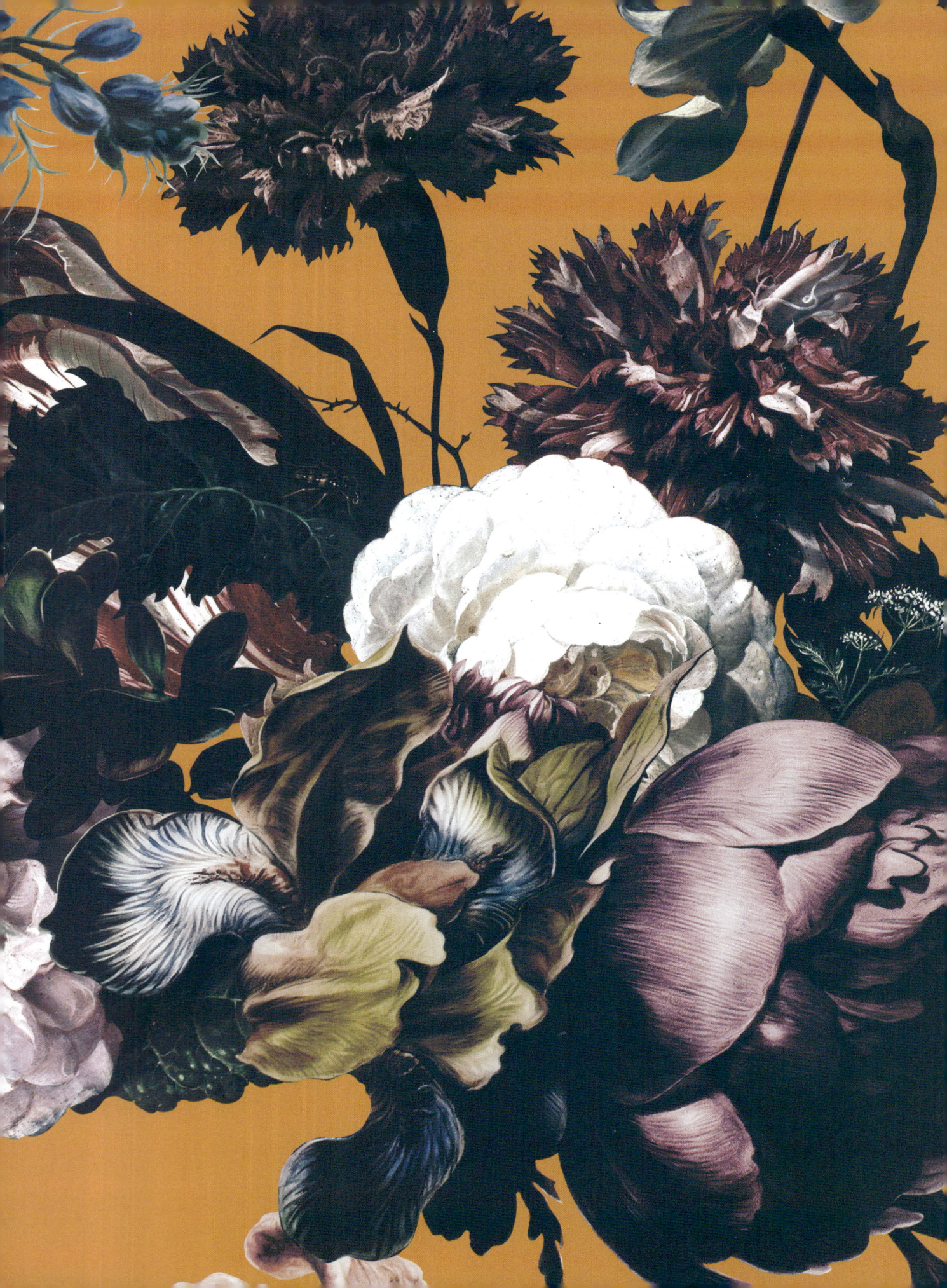

The Importance of Cleansing

As the human body ages, there is a greater buildup of chemical contamination in our tissues. As toxins accumulate, the body is more likely to suffer the energy-robbing effects of poor health and degenerative diseases.

This is why cleansing the body is so important. When the body is purging itself of heavy metal contamination, undigested foods, and internal pollution, it relieves enormous stress on the organs and tissues, enhances immune function, and reduces stress on the liver.

Cleansing helps with weight reduction and brings back the creative energy, motivation, and vitality that are especially healing when suffering from degenerative diseases.

Everyone Needs Cleansing

Babies, who are at the beginning of their lives, and the elderly, who have lived long lives, all need cleansing.

All of us are stressed, to a lesser or greater degree, by an ever-mounting buildup of toxins, chemicals, bacteria, parasites, industrial wastes, herbicides, pesticides, additives, and heavy metals we unknowingly absorb from our food, cosmetics, air, water, and even from the mercury fillings in our teeth.

Moreover, humans are subjected to concentrated doses of potentially harmful chemicals, hormones, and antibiotics from the meats and dairy products consumed.

According to a 1990 survey taken by the Environmental Protection Agency (EPA), every single person tested showed some evidence of petrochemical pollution in their body tissues and fat. Some of the chemicals found included styrene (used in plastics), xylene (a solvent in paint and gasoline), benzene (a chemical found in gasoline), and toluene (another carcinogenic solvent).

If that survey were taken today, how many more chemicals and pollutants would be found? How much radiation contamination is our world experiencing from just the atomic energy disaster in Japan? It all adds up to a world of disease and suffering.

Inflammation is one of the main factors contributing to disease in the human body today, heart disease being a prime example. Many people do not understand how someone relatively healthy, with low cholesterol levels, normal arterial function, and healthy arterial walls, can unexpectedly suffer a heart attack, yet it happens all too often. The explanation is inflammation.

What causes this inflammation and how does it occur in the body? Inflammation has various causes: bacterial infection (such as Chlamydia pneumoniae), poor diet, chemicals, hormonal imbalance, or physical injury.

Inflammation can come just from an organ or a body system not functioning properly—a system plugged with a vast number of toxins and waste debris, unable to absorb all the necessary life-giving nutrients.

A protein called "C-reactive" is released by the liver when inflammation is present. The level of this protein indicates the degree of inflammation in places like the linings of the arteries of the heart.

Accumulation of C-reactive protein and an excess of blood protein plasma can change pH in the blood and cellular function, hasten the onset of tumors, and cause a predisposition for heart disease. In fact, C-reactive protein testing may help doctors predict heart attack or stroke risk.

Cleansing gives the body the strength to fight off the disease and not be encumbered or overloaded with the accumulation of toxins, mucous, and parasites that have built up over the years.

LIVER HEALTH

The Importance of Liver Health

"The liver is one of the most important organs in the body, playing a major role in detoxifying the body. When the liver is damaged due to excess alcohol consumption, viral hepatitis, or poor diet, an excess of toxins can build up in the blood and tissues that can result in degenerative disease and health."

— D. Gary Young, ND
Essential Oils Integrative Medical Guide

The quality of virtually every bodily function depends on the liver. Essential for life, the liver is responsible for removing and neutralizing toxins and germs from the blood, promoting digestion, maintaining hormone balance, regulating blood sugar levels, and making proteins that regulate blood clotting.

Cumulative liver stress caused by toxins, poor diet, or disease inevitably leads to irreversible liver damage and death. The first stage is a condition known as fatty liver in which fat deposits accumulate and poison the liver. It has been estimated that five percent of the general population and 25 percent of patients with obesity and diabetes suffer from fatty liver.

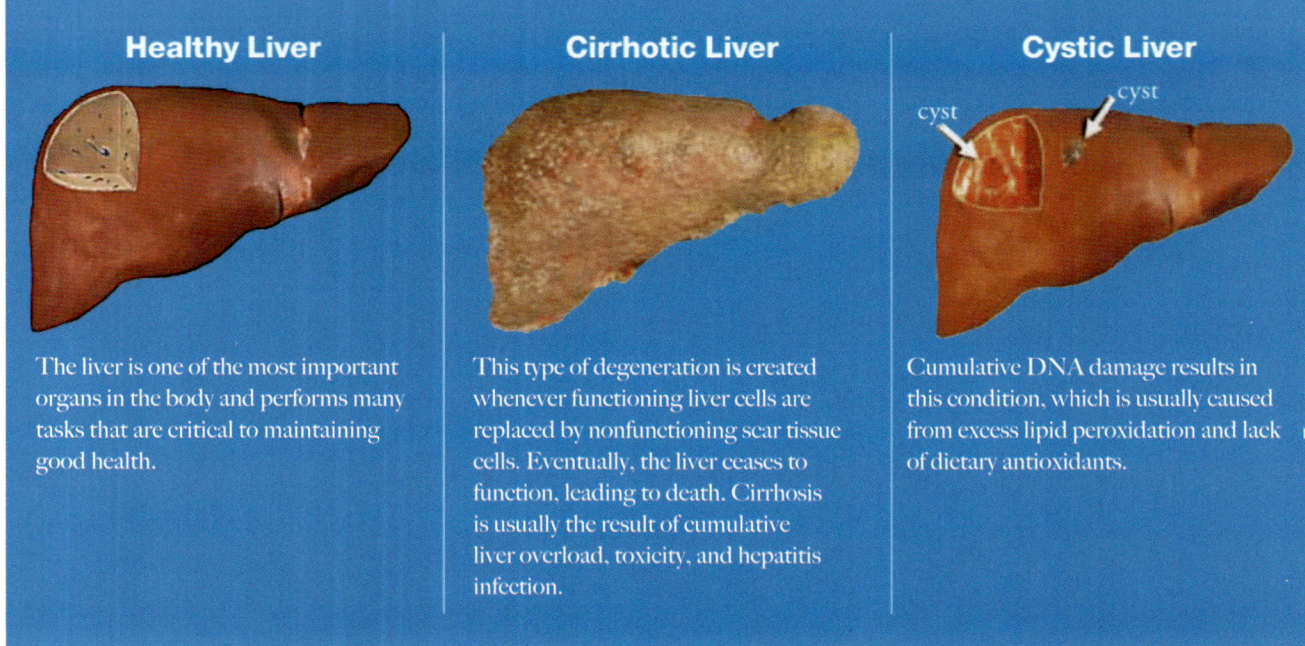

Healthy Liver
The liver is one of the most important organs in the body and performs many tasks that are critical to maintaining good health.

Cirrhotic Liver
This type of degeneration is created whenever functioning liver cells are replaced by nonfunctioning scar tissue cells. Eventually, the liver ceases to function, leading to death. Cirrhosis is usually the result of cumulative liver overload, toxicity, and hepatitis infection.

Cystic Liver
Cumulative DNA damage results in this condition, which is usually caused from excess lipid peroxidation and lack of dietary antioxidants.

With time, fatty liver eventually progresses to cirrhosis, a condition in which nonfunctioning scar tissue replaces working tissue; it is the eighth leading cause of death by disease, killing over 41,000 people in 2017 in the U.S.

The liver is one of the most important organs in the body. It is pivotal for purifying the blood and plays a key role in converting carbohydrates to energy, as well as storing energy in the form of glycogen and fats. It is also responsible for these vital functions:

- Filtering and processing all food, nutrients, alcohol, drugs, and other materials that enter the bloodstream and letting them pass, breaking them down, or storing them
- Manufacturing bile needed to emulsify fats for digestion
- Making and breaking down many hormones, including cholesterol, testosterone, and estrogen
- Regulating blood sugar levels

Virtually every function of the human body depends on the liver. Beyond the physiological importance of the liver, it is the anchor of many emotions, meaning that many of the negative emotions we experience are stored in the liver.

With the health challenges we all face in our modern world, it has never been more important to maintain a fully functioning, healthy liver. An overburdened liver can negatively affect our energy, digestion, skin, and blood. That is why cleansing and detoxifying the liver is so fundamental for good health.

Facts About the Liver
- About one fourth of your total blood volume passes through your liver every minute.
- It is the largest organ in the body, essential for life.
- It produces bile to help absorb fats and fat-soluble vitamins.
- It removes or neutralizes poisons from the blood.
- It removes germs and bacteria from the blood.
- It makes proteins that regulate blood clotting.

Things that Stress the Liver
- **Blocked bile ducts**—When the ducts that carry bile out of the liver are blocked, bile backs up and damages liver tissue (biliary cirrhosis).
- **Chronic hepatitis B and C**—The hepatitis virus is a major cause of chronic liver disease and cirrhosis in the United States. Hepatitis viral infections cause inflammations and low-grade damage to the liver, which eventually lead to cirrhosis and death.
- **Diabetes, protein malnutrition, obesity, and corticosteroid use**—Any of these can cause nonalcoholic steatohepatitis (NASH). NASH results in deadly fat buildup and eventual cirrhosis in the liver.
- **Exposure to chemicals and parasites**—Toxins, pharmaceutical drugs, and parasites contribute to liver problems. Many pesticides, petrochemicals, and environmental toxins are potent liver stressors. Parasitic infection (schistosomiasis) can also contribute to cirrhosis.

| **Extreme Fatty Liver** | **Fatty Liver** | **Haemo-type Liver** |

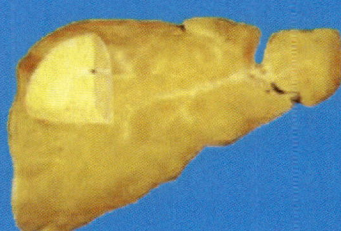 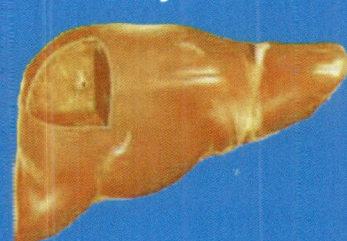 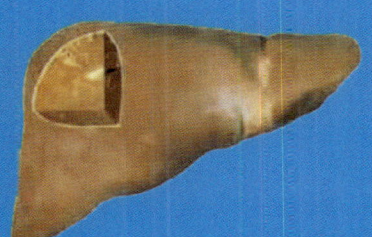

This becomes more common later in life or because of severe liver stress. A liver that displays this level of fatty degeneration will eventually become scarred and contribute to cirrhosis. Overcooked and refined foods can also contribute to the progression of severe fatty liver.

This disease is found in 5 percent of the general population and over 25 percent of patients with obesity and type II diabetes. The condition usually comes from cumulative liver stress caused by excess sugars in the diet, deficiency in choline, chemical stress and toxicity, lipid peroxidation (fats becoming rancid in the liver), and/or alcohol.

Hemochromatosis is excess iron absorption from the diet, which can lead to cumulative liver damage, cirrhosis, diabetes, and heart disease.

Acetaminophen can also stress the liver, as can reactions to prescription drugs. Acetaminophen is found in both over-the-counter and prescription drugs; and accidental overdoses each year result in more than 56,000 emergency room visits, 1,600 cases of acute liver failure, and 458 deaths, according to a 2002 study.

On January 13, 2011, the FDA announced that products containing acetaminophen cannot contain more than 325 milligrams of acetaminophen, and the labels must warn of the potential risk of severe liver injury.

- **Inherited diseases**—Alpha-1 antitrypsin deficiency, Wilson's disease, galactosemia, and glycogen storage diseases are inherited disorders that result in faulty production, processing, and storage of enzymes, proteins, and metals by the liver.
- **Iron overload**—Excess iron in the diet can stress the liver, especially in individuals who are genetically unable to dispose of or sequester dietary iron (hemochromatosis).
- **Nonalcoholic steatohepatitis (NASH)**—This condition causes fat buildup and eventual cirrhosis of the liver. This type of hepatitis appears to be associated with diabetes, protein malnutrition, obesity, coronary artery disease, and corticosteroid treatment.
- **Poor diet**—Excess intake of refined carbohydrates and sugars can cause fatty liver or liver degeneration over time. Diabetes, protein malnutrition, obesity, and corticosteroid treatment can also cause fatty liver.

- **Coffee and colas**—Because the liver is the cleansing organ of the body, it has to cleanse and filter the toxins and waste out of the blood. If the liver is too overloaded and cannot function optimally, then other systems begin to break down, and the liver starts to deteriorate.

  Coffee is a drink loved by millions of people all over the world, but that does not change the fact that it has damaging effects on the liver and other organs of the body.

  - Coffee promotes aging because of high amounts of cadmium.
  - Cadmium, a toxic heavy metal, interferes with immune function, nerve conduction, and hundreds of other physiological systems.
  - High quantities of cadmium in the diet have been correlated with shortened life span.
  - Cadmium stays locked in the body for decades. Researchers estimate that its biologic half-life is up to 38 years, according to the Agency for Toxic Substances & Disease Registry.
  - Coffee blocks the absorption of zinc, which is one of the few minerals that can counteract and neutralize cadmium.
  - The caffeine in coffee and colas acts as both a stimulant and a diuretic and is related to lower calcium and trace mineral levels in the body.

Signs of an Overloaded and/or Toxic Liver

Here are some clues that could mean your liver is in trouble:

- Abdominal bloating and/or pain after eating
- Allergies
- Bad breath
- Bruising and bleeding easily—This is caused when the liver is unable to produce sufficient clotting proteins.
- Chemical intolerance
- Coated tongue when going without food for a half or full day
- Decreased sensitivity to medication—Because of the liver's inability to remove drugs from the blood at the usual rate, drugs take longer than expected to be effective.
- Diarrhea
- Disorientation or confusion
- Edema and ascites—Excessive fluid in the abdomen between the lining and the abdominal organs is caused when the liver stops making the protein albumin, holding water in the leg (edema) and abdomen (ascites), often referred to as fluid retention.
- Excessive alcohol intake
- Excessive body heat
- Excessive gas
- Fatty liver
- Fever
- Forgetfulness, poor concentration, or disturbed sleep
- Frequent headaches or migraines
- Frequent or continued fatigue
- Gallbladder problems
- Gallstones
- Headaches
- High blood pressure
- High cholesterol
- Hormonal imbalance
- Inability to lose weight
- Irritable bowel syndrome (IBS)
- Itching—Intense itching may be a result of bile waste residue deposited in the skin.
- Jaundice—The liver's inability to cleanse the blood may result in yellowing of the skin and eyes.
- Loss of appetite
- Lowered immunity—A liver not able to work at the optimum level will result in immune system dysfunction, which leads to infection and many other problems.
- Mood or behavior swings
- Nausea
- Oily skin
- Over-burdened immune system
- Overweight
- Poor and inadequate digestion
- Portal hypertension—When the flow of blood through the portal vein is slowed, pressure increases inside.
- Rashes
- Recurring colds, fevers, and mucus
- Skin blemishes
- Sleepiness
- Sluggish metabolism
- Sugar cravings
- Swollen abdomen
- Unpleasant moods
- Varices (distended veins)—When blood from the intestines and spleen backs up into blood vessels in the stomach and esophagus, the varices swell and are more likely to burst.
- Vomiting
- Weakness
- Weight loss

- Caffeine increases the stress hormone cortisol in the body, which, if produced in excess, can result in high blood pressure, adrenal exhaustion, and diabetes.

  Colas containing phosphoric acid can leach magnesium from the body. Magnesium deficiency is directly linked to degenerative diseases like heart disease and diabetes.

- **Viruses**—The hepatitis B and C viruses are major causes of chronic liver disease and cirrhosis in the United States. Hepatitis viral infections cause inflammation and low-grade damage to the liver that eventually leads to cirrhosis and death.

A 2003 case study conducted by Roger Lewis, MD, at the Young Life Research Clinic in Springville, Utah, evaluated the efficacy of Helichrysum, Ledum, and Celery Seed, essential oils in the JuvaCleanse blend, in treating cases of advanced hepatitis C.

In one case, a male, age 20, was diagnosed with a hepatitis C viral count of 13,200. After taking two capsules (approximately 750 mg each) of JuvaCleanse per day for a month with no other intervention, the patient's viral count dropped to 2,580, an over 80 percent reduction.

Nonalcoholic Fatty Liver Disease

Nonalcoholic fatty liver disease is caused not by alcohol but by excess fat accumulation in the liver that affects up to 40 percent of the people in the United States, according to the American Liver Foundation. It has been reported that this condition is even appearing in children. Medscape reported that choline deficiency has been suggested as a possible cause of NAFLD, although further evaluation is needed.

ALKALINITY

The Importance of Alkalinity to Health

The pH of the blood is very tightly controlled by the body. When serum pH becomes too acidic, then calcium is robbed from the bones, and biochemical changes begin to slowly tax and stress liver tissues.

As the liver's ability to filter becomes impaired, the blood becomes increasingly acidic. Unfriendly bacteria and fungi that populate our intestinal tracts thrive in an acidic environment and are responsible for secreting mycotoxins, which are the root cause of many debilitating human conditions.

In fact, many researchers believe that most diseases can be linked to blood and intestinal acidity, which contributes to an acid-based yeast and fungus dominance.

Maintaining healthy pH levels is essential to keeping your skin happy, especially on your face.

The symptoms of excess internal acidity include:
- Fatigue/low energy
- Unexplained aches and pains
- Overweight conditions/obesity
- Low resistance to illness
- Unbalanced blood sugar
- Allergies
- Headaches
- Irritability/mood swings
- Indigestion
- Colitis/ulcers
- Diarrhea/constipation
- Urinary tract infections
- Flaking skin
- Rectal itch/vaginal itch

The pH scale is between 0 and 14. The lower the number, the more acidic; the higher the number, the more alkaline. Neutral pH is 7.0, which is also the pH of water. A healthy range for PH is between 6.0 and 7.5. However, pH levels vary throughout the body. Low pH, acidic, is best for digestion in the stomach, while higher pH, alkaline, is best for the blood.

The ideal pH for human blood is between 7.4 and 7.6. Preserving this alkalinity (pH balance) is the bedrock on which sound health and strong bodies are built. When the blood loses its alkalinity and starts to become more acidic, the foundation of health is undermined. This creates an environment where we become vulnerable to disease, runaway yeast, and fungus overgrowth.

When yeast and fungus decline in the body, so do their production of mycotoxins, the poisonous waste products and byproducts of their life cycles.

There are numerous varieties of these mycotoxins, many of which are harmful to the body and must be neutralized by our immune systems. When our bodies are overwhelmed by large quantities of these toxins, our health becomes impaired, and we become susceptible to disease and illness.

Many cancers have been linked to mycotoxins. For example, the fungus Aspergillus flavus, which infests stored peanuts, not only generates cancer in laboratory animals but has been documented as the prime culprit in many liver cancers in humans.

By balancing the body's pH and creating a more alkaline environment, you can rein in the microbial overgrowth and choke off the production of disease-producing mycotoxins. With pH balance restored, the body can regain vigor and health.

How to Restore Alkalinity

Some of the most common varieties of pathogenic bacteria, yeast, and fungi that live in the intestines are inactive. However, when the body is weakened by illness, stress, and excess acidity caused by stress or high acidic foods, these bacteria become harmful and active, changing into an invasive mycolic form. Here are six suggestions to help you achieve and maintain an alkaline pH blood environment.

1. **Carefully monitor your diet.** Avoiding yeast- and fungus-promoting foods is a crucial factor in combating excess acidity and fungus overgrowth. Meats, sugars, dairy products, pickled foods, and malted products can be especially acidic. On the other hand, garlic is excellent for controlling fungi and yeast. Other high-alkaline, fungus-inhibiting foods include green and yellow vegetables, watermelon, cucumbers, strawberries, apples, asparagus, lemons, broccoli, avocados, cabbage, celery, spinach, chia seeds, cold-pressed coconut oil, extra virgin olive oil, beans, and whole nuts.

   The natural ratio between alkaline and acidic foods in the diet should be 4:1—four parts alkaline foods to one part acidic. JuvaPower is a mixture of extremely alkaline and high-antioxidant foods that nourish the liver and combat toxic acidity.

   The pH of a raw food does not always determine its acidity or alkalinity in the digestive system.

Some foods, like lemons, might be acidic in their natural state but when consumed and digested are converted into alkaline residues.

Thus, the true determinant of a food's pH is whether it is an alkaline-ash or acidic-ash food. In this case, lemons are an alkaline-ash food.

2. **Avoid the use of antibiotics.** The overuse of antibiotics for incidental, minor, or cosmetic conditions not only increases the resistance of pathogenic microorganisms, but it kills the beneficial bacteria in your body, leaving the mycotoxin-generating yeast and fungi intact. This is why many women suffer outbreaks of yeast infections after antibiotic use.

3. **Use essential oils.** Many essential oils possess important antimicrobial, antibacterial, and antifungal properties. Clove and Thyme essential oils have been documented to kill over 15 different strains of fungi.

   Essential oils work best when blood and tissues are alkaline. When our systems become acidic—due to poor diet, illness, or emotional stress—essential oils lose some of their effectiveness. So the best way to enhance the action of essential oils is to alkalize your body.

4. **Increase alkaline minerals.** Increasing the intake of calcium can dramatically boost blood and intestinal alkalinity.

   - Calcium and magnesium-rich supplements such as MegaCal and SuperCal Plus can help alkalinize both blood and body tissues.
   - AlkaLime is an outstanding source of alkaline salts that can help reduce internal acidity.
   - Mineral Essence supplies the body with more than 60 of the most efficiently absorbed ionic minerals available.
   - JuvaPower is also rich in minerals and yeast-fighting phytonutrients.

5. **Lower stress.** Emotional and psychological tension can be especially damaging to body systems and act as a prime promoter of acid formation in the body. To properly appreciate how acidic stress can be, just think back to the last time you were seriously stressed out and had to reach for an antacid tablet to soothe your heartburn or stomach discomfort.

   Blends of essential oils high in sesquiterpenes such as Myrrh, Sandalwood, and Cedarwood can produce profound balancing and calming effects on emotions. They work by affecting the limbic system of our brain, the seat of our emotions.

6. **Boost friendly flora.** From 3 to 4 pounds of beneficial bacteria permanently reside in the intestines of the average adult. Not only are they the first line of defense against foreign invaders, but they are also absolutely essential for health, energy, and optimum digestive efficiency. These intestinal houseguests not only control mucus and debris, but they also produce B vitamins and vitamin K and maintain the all-important pH balance of the body.

   These friendly floras are also important in counteracting and opposing yeast and fungus overgrowth.

   Using an acidophilus and bifidus supplement (such as Life 9 and KidScents MightyPro) may be especially valuable in boosting levels of naturally occurring beneficial bacteria in the body and preventing fungal and yeast overgrowth. They also help the body maintain proper pH balance for nutrient digestion and absorption.

   Ideally, the lactobacillus acidophilus and bifidobacterium cultures must be combined with plantain to pro-mote implantation on the intestinal wall. Life 9 capsules are most beneficial at night while the body is busy cleansing and repairing while you sleep.

   Research indicates a significant proportion of bacteria from many acidophilus supplements do not reach the lower intestine alive, or they arrive in such a weakened state that they are not of much benefit. Combining the acidophilus and bifidus cultures is stronger in helping these cultures adhere to the intestinal walls.

   An even more effective means of fortifying the friendly flora in our intestines is by consuming fructooligosaccharides (also known as FOS).

   FOS is one of the most powerful natural agents for feeding our friendly flora and is made up of medium-chain sugars that cannot be used by pathogenic yeast and fungi. The end result is that FOS starves fungi while feeding the acidophilus and bifidus cultures that are our main defense against disease.

   But FOS is far more than just an outstanding means of rebuilding and protecting the beneficial bacteria inside the body. Over a dozen clinical studies have documented the ability of fructooligosaccharides to prevent constipation, lower blood sugar, reduce cholesterol levels, and even prevent cancer.

Testing Your pH

You can easily test your pH at home by purchasing small litmus-paper strips at your drug store or pharmacy. To get the most accurate reading, expose the strip to a sample of your saliva immediately after awakening in the morning and before eating breakfast. Color changes on the litmus paper will determine pH; check the instructions in your kit for specific details on how to read the litmus paper.

CLEANSING PROGRAMS

Cleansing and the commitment you make to it is a personal choice. You have to decide what program you want to follow and then discipline yourself to accomplish what you desire. Even drinking enough water takes discipline.

However, the reward is worth the denial of food and the pleasure of eating. You cannot put a price on health, because the price of not having good health is too high. You simply have to plan your protocol, get started, and stay with it. Those are the only requirements.

The Ideal Program

The ideal cleansing program requires a high consumption of water, and that means distilled or purified water, never chlorinated tap water. You should work up to drinking a gallon of water each day. Then with strong digestive enzymes, minerals, high-potency herbs, and therapeutic-grade essential oils, the body is ready to go to work.

Essential oils have a special, lipid-soluble makeup, which gives them a remarkable ability to penetrate cell membranes, break up undigested food, and digest toxins. Essential oils deliver oxygen that inhibits the growth of many types of microbes. In fact, many essential oils have been studied and documented for their unique antimicrobial, antifungal, and antiparasitic properties. Some oils, like Rosemary, have demonstrated significant antiseptic activity, with documented research appearing in many scientific journals.

Cleanse Often

Cleansing should be done two to three times a year, but eating healthy, cleansing foods and supplements should be a daily part of your life throughout the year. It is important to have this kind of awareness at a young age to be able to enjoy the "older" years without health problems. Just because an individual is 40 years old does not mean that the body has to start breaking down and taking on disease.

Naturally, with age comes a greater buildup of debris in our bodies caused by the food we eat and the pollutants in our environment, as well as less production of stomach acids and enzymes. Without proper enzyme production, the body is not able to properly break down undigested proteins and other fermenting debris that obstruct our digestive system and impede the assimilation of nutrients.

Cleanse Completely

It is difficult to control internal pollution with a simple one-time fix or a single magic bullet. Complete

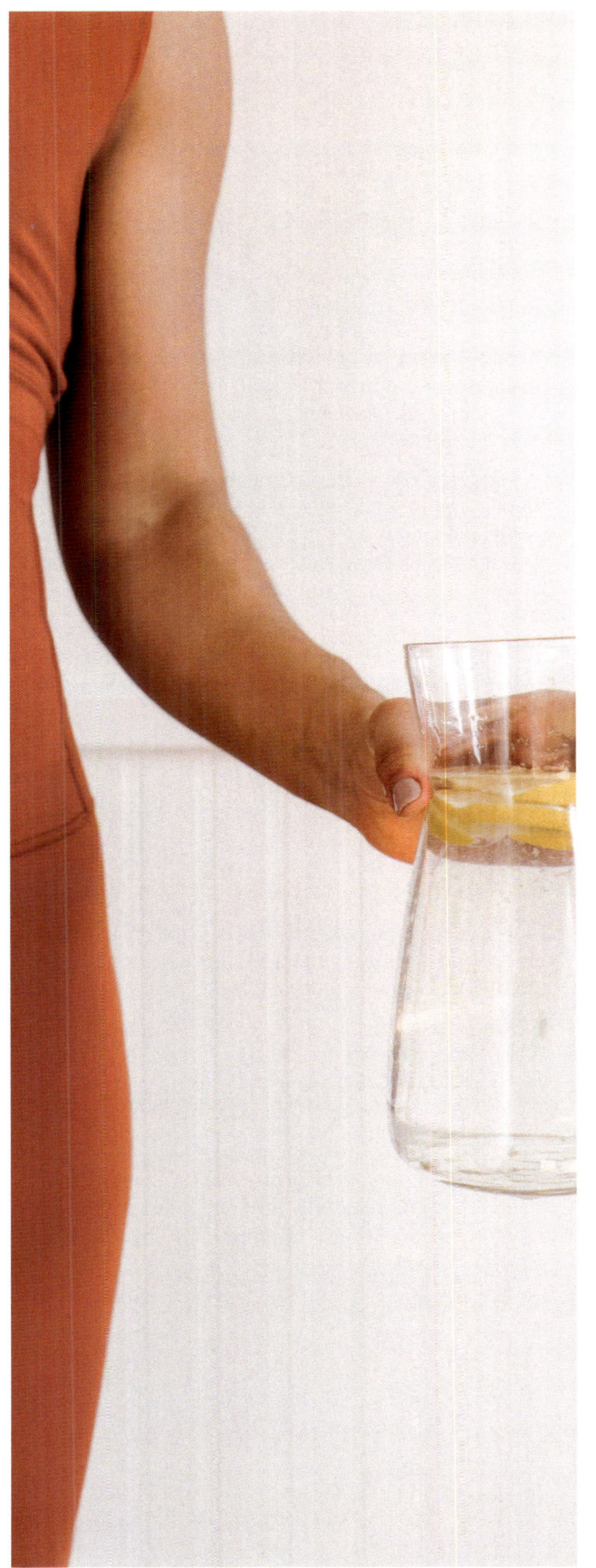

> ### Consult Your Physician
>
> Anyone cleansing or fasting for more than three days should do so under the supervision of a health care professional.
>
> Never begin a shut-down fast unless you have been fasting regularly for at least two years. This type of fast should always be done under supervision.

cleansing requires many different solutions targeted at specific systems of the body. Cleansing the liver requires a different combination of herbs, oils, and minerals than those required for the colon, for example.

A complete cleansing requires a broad array of products that are effective against a wide variety of contaminants and microorganisms, not just one or two. Contaminants, like heavy metals, need a different set of tools to deactivate and purge them from the body than parasites do.

Essential oils are an important part of a complete cleansing program. Essential oils are highly antibacterial, antifungal, antiviral, and anti-inflammatory. They digest and chelate toxic chemicals and poisons in the body. Essential oils promote the body's production of enzymes, which improve colon peristalsis, the key to waste elimination.

Fasting

Fasting is the avoidance of solid food, with liquid intake varying from no liquids (one to two days) to just water or water and fresh juices. A fast can last 24 hours or several weeks.

Fasting has long been a tradition in Judaism, Christianity, and the Eastern religions. Religious fasting can in-volve purification, penitence, or preparation for approaching God. It has been called "nature's single-greatest healing therapy."

An increasing number of doctors are recognizing that fasting can be physically healing while allowing us to focus our energy inward, bringing clarity and change.

Fasting is generally safe, but those with medical conditions should check with their health care professional.

An extremely important benefit of fasting is the elimination of toxins. By minimizing the work our digestive system must do, we allow it to repair itself and expel stored toxins.

In the beginning of a fast, the liver will convert stored glycogen to energy. As the fast continues, some proteins will break down unless calories are provided through juices and sweeteners such as maple syrup or Yacon Syrup.

The first two to four days of the fast are often the most difficult, since you will be overcoming the powerful psychological need to eat. As the body begins to cleanse itself of parasites and putrefying toxins, a person may experience a sudden surge in energy and well-being.

Tapeworms, pinworms, roundworms, etc., may be seen in the stools after four to six days. As the cleansing progresses, the mind will become sharper, the memory will improve, and the spirit will become more buoyant.

Pregnant or lactating women should not fast.

Cleansing Through Fasting

This is the most disciplined, comprehensive way to cleanse the body. It is a time when the body can work on revitalizing cells and stopping degeneration that has already started. It enables the body to cleanse and rebuild an overworked liver. This is when longevity is put in motion.

A true fast consists of only water, but very few people are able to sustain this type of fast. There are other options, though.

The Master Cleanse—
Stanley Burroughs (Lemonade Diet)

The Master Cleanse, as it is called, was developed by Stanley Burroughs and has been used successfully by thousands of people. It takes time, but although it is still a liquid diet, it provides certain nutrients to sustain the body and help with cleansing. Stay focused and determined and you will have success too.

The Master Cleanse is a mixture of lemon juice, Grade B maple syrup, and cayenne pepper that is consumed throughout the day and is the source of calories, vitamins, and minerals for the body. The Master Cleanse is for almost anyone, except young children, diabetics, and those who are very weak and cannot stay with their own commitment of cleansing or who need supervised help.

Most people can safely cleanse for at least seven to ten days. As with any program of caloric restriction, however, it is strongly recommended that you consult with your health care professional before undertaking any extended fast or cleanse.

The Master Cleanse Protocol

- Squeeze the juice from $\frac{1}{2}$ fresh organic lemon.
- Mix juice into 8 ounces distilled water.
- Add 1-2 tablespoons Grade B maple syrup or Yacon Syrup.
- Add up to 1/10 teaspoon cayenne (red) pepper (capsicum).

Start with a pinch or two of cayenne pepper and gradually increase to 1/10 teaspoon. Do not put it in capsules and swallow separately. The cayenne pepper is specific to the formula, and the action of the formula changes with it. If sent directly to the stomach, it can cause inflammation and excessive mucus that may lead to sinusitis or too much bowel mucus and can even contribute to inflammatory bowel syndrome.

Drink 6 to 12 10-ounce glasses of lemonade daily. Every time you begin to feel hunger, have another glass of lemonade. Remember, it is extremely important to also drink water to help flush out toxins.

Grade B maple syrup contains minerals and nutrients that support the body nutritionally during the cleansing period. Diabetics should substitute molasses for maple syrup. Available at most health food stores, about ¼ to ½ tablespoon is usually sufficient for sweetening.

Contrary to popular belief, lemon is not acidic in the body. As the lemon juice mixes with the saliva, it gradually starts to change its pH, and then in the stomach it turns completely alkaline as it mixes with the hydrochloric acid.

If an acid-like reaction is observed when using lemon with water, it is because of the minerals in the water. Distilled water will not react in this manner.

Cayenne pepper is a blood vessel dilator, thermal warmer, and provider of vitamin A. People who have Type O blood tend to have poor circulation and will need to drink the lemonade every ½ hour to maintain proper blood sugar levels, or else the body temperature may drop during the cleanse.

Cayenne is a thermogenic herb known for its ability to warm and improve circulation. When used in a dietary program, it can promote greater fat burning. Moderate exercise enhances the cleansing action of the program.

During the middle and later phases of the Master Cleanse, typically between day three and day seven, the body chemistry changes, and energy levels usually begin to rise. You may experience minor discomfort such as headaches, upset stomach, or low energy, while toxins and parasites are released from the body.

If your energy decreases, then drink another glass of the juice. Sometimes when on this type of cleanse, if you are not watching the clock to make sure you are drinking the juice on a regular schedule, you may feel weak and develop a headache.

A Blood Type O person will need to drink it more often than a Blood Type A person. Remember—drinking plenty of water is also very important.

These symptoms should pass. If not, ask your health care professional to monitor the situation, gently come off the lemon cleanse, or begin to add foods that are cleansing such as salads, fruits, etc. Grapefruit makes a good cleansing juice. Follow the recipe and sweeten to taste.

You can also experiment with adding different essential oils like Lemon, Orange, or Grapefruit, which will provide additional benefit. Add only 1 drop of oil per glass as the oils are very concentrated.

Wanting to Eat

If you feel that you need or want to eat, add only foods that are compatible with your cleansing program. Salads, vegetables, fruit, Pure Protein Complete, ICP, and JuvaPower are immensely supportive to the elimination process.

Take different enzymes at varied times for their particular benefits: Allerzyme, Detoxzyme, Essentialzyme, Essentialzymes-4, and MightyZyme increase the enzymatic action for better detoxification.

See the recipes at the end of this section for healthy eating choices with or without your cleansing program. Use them as examples and modify them for your taste.

A Positive Mental Attitude Is Important

Having a positive attitude during cleansing or fasting is important. If you are learning how to fast, start by fasting one day a week. Start on a Sunday or a day that is more restful and not filled with normal, everyday stress. The biggest obstacle to successful cleansing is fear of failure and not knowing what to expect.

When fasting for 24 hours, it is easiest to begin at noon and finish at noon on the following day or fast from one dinner to the next.

Again, drink plenty of water, as water is the catalyst to all cleansing. At the beginning of the fast, you might experience some unpleasant side effects such as headache, nausea, bloating, or irritability. These symptoms are part of the cleansing response and are often a result of toxins and waste matter being purged from the body, which usually begins to take place within 12 to 36 hours.

If you experience these symptoms, simply cut back on fluid intake and drink vegetable juices such as carrot and celery. Try mixing carrot, celery, spinach, and broccoli together and see how your body feels.

Carrot juice with a little apple juice or apple and lemon juice promotes continuous cleansing. A mixture of 6 ounces of carrot juice, 1 ounce of apple juice, and ½ ounce of lemon juice will help keep the pH balanced, slow down any diarrhea, and keep the cleansing action going.

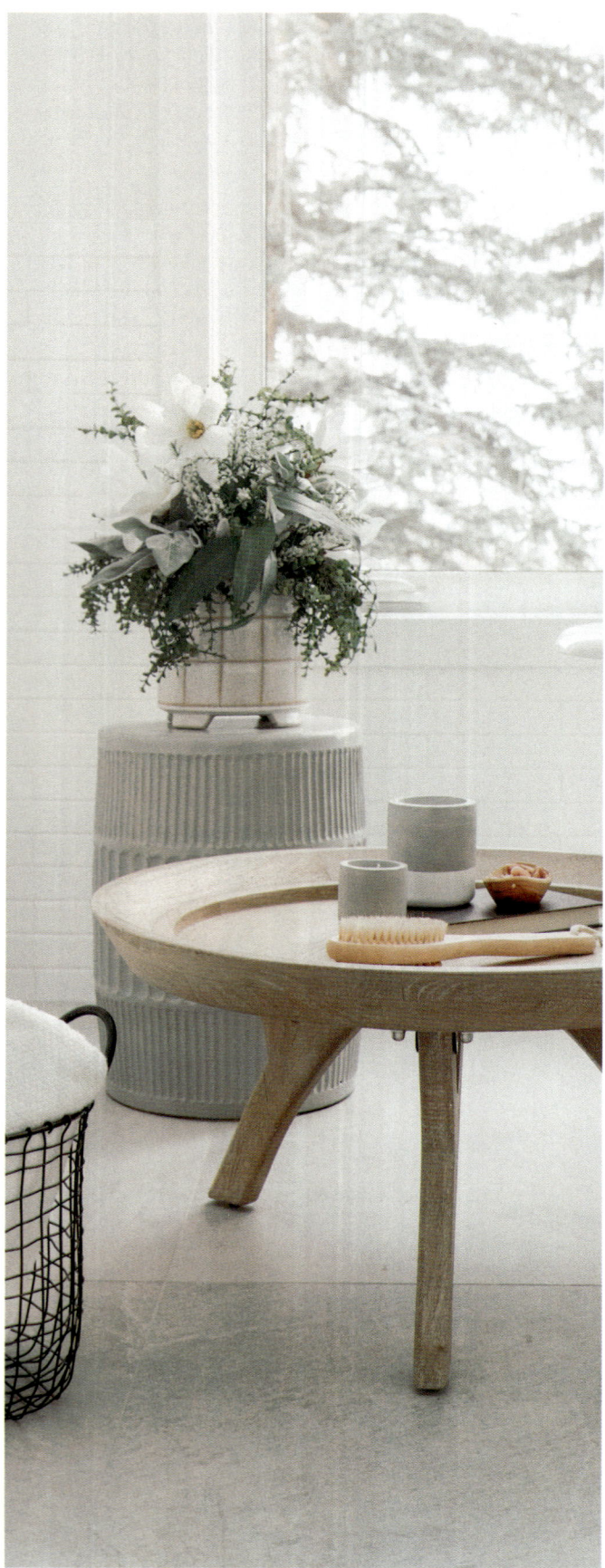

Nausea and bloating are an indication that the poisons are being released at a very rapid rate and may be backing up into the liver. Keeping the liver cleansed and flushed is extremely important.

The essential oil of Ledum works well as a diuretic and dilates the bile duct between the liver and kidneys. One or two capsules morning or night is probably sufficient. Other essential oil blends such as GLF, JuvaCleanse, and JuvaFlex all aid in the cleansing process.

Peristalsis is the wave-like motion of the intestines as they move waste matter out of the body. A spastic or prolapsed colon from loss of peristalsis or restrictions from kinks, loops, or twists in the colon make proper elimination difficult and often painful.

Colon Hydrotherapy Cleanse

Colon hydrotherapy is a powerful treatment for cleansing the colon and helps restore peristalsis. Make an appointment with a colon hydrotherapist to have a colonic treatment or buy a colema board to give yourself a colonic at home. Portable colon hydrotherapy units are also available for home use. The Colonet JR-4 is an advanced, free-gravity-flow, in-home enema unit that is lightweight, portable, and specifically designed for easy use in a private bathroom.

Colon Cleanse Recipe #1
- 5 drops Rosemary
- 5 drops ParaFree
- 5 drops Basil
- 4 drops Fennel

Colon Cleanse Recipe #2
- 15–20 drops of ParaFree

Add to colonic water and mix well.

During cleansing, you might have an unexpected emotional clearing. Various essential oils have a direct effect on the emotional centers of the brain. They can help control, calm, release, and facilitate the emotional response.

Essential oil blends such as Release, Inner Child, Valor, Gary's Light, SARA, Grounding, Peace & Calming, and Peace & Calming II offer good emotional support during such times. Roll-on blends such as Stress Away Roll-On, Tranquil Roll-On, Breathe Again Roll-On, Valor Roll-On, and RutaVaLa Roll-On are easy to carry in your pocket and can offer immediate relief.

The essential oils of Valerian, Roman Chamomile, Idaho Grand Fir, and Lavender are very calming and relaxing. In addition, Peace & Calming, Peace &

Calming II, Release, Seedlings Calm, and JuvaFlex oil blends, used topically or diffused, promote a calming environment. Most citrus oils contain aldehydes that are very calming as well. Vitamin B12 (Super B) and folic acid are also important for emotional stability.

Liquid Cleansing Recipes

There are many other liquid recipes and protocols for easier and simpler cleansing. Some of the recipes are used as daily maintenance with or without food, and some are used for one or two weeks with or without food. Some are specific for a particular need, some are used once a year, some are used once a month, and some are used just for the experience. Whatever the reason, your body will benefit with improved health and vitality.

Vital Life Juice Recipe

D. Gary Young first created this recipe over 35 years ago for detoxification of patients with degenerative disease. Since that time, it has been very successful in providing the needed benefits to those with greater health challenges. It has become a very popular juice for many who just want the concentrated nutrients and a simple cleansing.

Use a juicer (not a blender):

- 3 ounces beet juice
- 1 ounce celery juice
- 1 ounce carrot juice
- 1/3 ounce white radish juice
- 1/3 ounce red potato juice (optional)
- 1/8 ounce ginger (Whole ginger may be juiced while juicing other vegetables.)

Directions:

- Drink $\frac{1}{4}-\frac{1}{2}$ cup every 2-3 hours.
- The potato is optional except when fighting liver cancer.
- The Vital Life Juice is good to drink while on the Master Cleanse.

Grapefruit Juice Recipe

This fruit has a history of cleansing and promoting fat burning. It is simple to make and enjoyable to drink throughout the day.

- About $\frac{1}{2}$ cup freshly pressed grapefruit juice
- 1 quart distilled or purified water
- 3 drops Spearmint
- 3 drops Tangerine
- Maple syrup or Yacon Syrup to taste

The more frequent the elimination, the better. There may be some discomfort or bloating if the body is not eliminating several times a day. There should be at least 2-3 or more bowel movements every day to constantly be moving the waste out of the body that is being loosened from the various organs and intestines.

If there is some discomfort and elimination is slow, add ComforTone, one of the first herbal supplements formulated with essential oils to help relieve constipation, enhance colon and digestive functions, and dispel parasites and toxins. Increase the number of enzyme capsules as well.

Cleansing with Supplements
Blood Cleanse

The tincture Rehemogen contains herbs that were traditionally used by Native Americans for cleansing and purifying the blood. It builds red blood cells and is recommended for any blood disorder.

- Put 2-3 droppers of Rehemogen (50-75 drops) in distilled water and drink every 2-3 hours.
- Rehemogen and JuvaTone together work well to assist in cleansing the blood and the liver.

Enzymes and Daily Maintenance

- Take 2-3 enzyme capsules of your choice 3 times daily before meals.
- Always carry enzymes with you when eating out or remember to take them when you return home. If you have eaten a heavy meal at night, be sure to take your enzymes before going to bed to keep the food digesting and prevent fermenting.
- A, B, and AB blood types: 2-4 capsules
- O blood types: 3-6 or more capsules, if necessary

Enzyme Cleanse

Enzymes break down foods and proteins that might otherwise ferment and putrefy in the gastrointestinal tract. Undigested foods tax our bodies, sap our energy, and spur the overgrowth of yeast, fungi, parasites, bacteria, and microorganisms that contribute to viral conditions, gastritis, Crohn's disease, diverticulitis, and other inflammatory conditions.

Inadequate digestive enzyme activity has also been linked to chronic inflammation elsewhere in the body such as fibromyalgia, inability to gain or lose weight, bad breath, body odor, skin rashes, and migraines.

Enzymes like pancreatin, pancrelipase, chymotrypsin, and trypsin are very efficient in breaking down proteins.

However, if the body is acidic, chymotrypsin, trypsin, and other enzymes will not effectively activate in the body.

Vegetable enzymes from the unripe papaya and pineapple (papain and bromelain) provide enzyme support.

Digestive enzymes promote complete digestion and help those who have difficulty digesting and assimilating food. As we age, we need more enzymes for complete digestion. Enzymes are essential in unlocking and metabolizing the vitamins, minerals, and amino acids in food.

Detoxzyme, Allerzyme, Essentialzyme, Essentialzymes-4, and MightyZyme all help digest cooked and processed foods that lack the natural enzymes of fresh foods.

Enzyme Ramping Protocol

Essentialzyme was formulated in 1984 with this protocol for someone suffering from a degenerative disease such as cancer.

Most people would not need to follow this protocol, but it will help you to understand the commitment it takes to fight disease.

Phase 1: Take 3 caplets 3 times daily. Increase by 1 caplet every day until you become nauseated. Then discontinue Essentialzyme for 24 to 36 hours.

Phase 2: Take 4 caplets 3 times daily. Increase daily by 1 caplet until you become nauseated. Rest (discontinue) again for 24–36 hours.

Phase 3: Take 5 caplets 3 times daily. Increase daily by 1 caplet until you become nauseated. Rest again for 24–36 hours.

Phase 4: Start again with the amount that you were taking before the nausea occurred the third time. For example: If you were taking 18 caplets, you would have been taking 6 caplets 3 times a day when you became nauseated. Therefore, start Phase 4 again with 6 caplets 3 times daily and continue with this amount for 6 weeks.

Phase 5: In the 7th week, start the enzyme-ramping program all over again. This means to begin Phase 1 again and increase the amount by 1 each day until nausea or vomiting starts again. Repeat and continue for 6 weeks as previously described.

If your doctor determines that you are in remission, you can maintain with 5-10 caplets daily for one year, 6 days a week.

Maintenance: Take 5-10 Essentialzyme caplets 3 times daily.

Caution: This is a very rigorous program, so you should consult with your doctor or health care professional before starting and have your doctor monitor your progress during the program.

Heavy Metals Cleanse

Heavy metals are some of the most toxic poisons on earth and can slowly accumulate in human tissues and cause neurological diseases, cardiovascular problems, and some types of cancers.

The problem is that heavy metals such as mercury and lead form insoluble metallic salts that become trapped in the fat and kidneys and cannot be easily excreted from the liver. Because the liver plays a major role in trapping and stabilizing mercury, liver cleansing using essential oils can be an outstanding treatment in purging the body of heavy metal contamination that contributes to many chronic neurological diseases.

Mercury is present in harmful amounts in almost every person in the United States, due to the consumption of seafood (methyl mercury levels in canned tuna are especially problematic) and amalgam dental fillings (which are about 50 percent mercury).

According to the Mercury Policy Project, dental amalgam is the largest source of mercury pollution to reach wastewater treatment plants.

Mercury discharges [in wastewater] from dental offices far exceeded all other commercial and residential sources. EPA cited an estimate in 2007 that 36 percent of the mercury reaching municipal sewage treatment plants is released by dental offices. Other investigations have put the figure closer to 50 percent.

According to Mercola.com, a 44-pound child consuming 6 ounces of tuna a week would be exposed to 4 times the EPA reference dose for mercury, and a 120-pound woman consuming the same amount would be exposed to $1\frac{1}{2}$ times the EPA reference dose.

Women of childbearing age in the United States suffer from tissue levels of mercury that can be dangerous to a developing fetus.

Clinical Studies with Heavy Metals

Clinical studies show that the essential oil blends of JuvaCleanse, JuvaFlex, and GLF, which contain the essential oils of Helichrysum, Ledum, and Celery Seed, dramatically amplified the elimination of heavy metals from the body, especially mercury, one of the most toxic of all nonradioactive metals.

Mercury is particularly damaging to the brain and nervous system because it passes through the blood-brain barrier, accumulates indefinitely in motor neurons, and destroys healthy growth of the dendrites.

JuvaCleanse may be applied over the liver and also taken as a dietary supplement. Put 10-20 drops into one 00 capsule and take it in the morning and evening.

The Importance of Cleansing | Chapter 12

Food "Ash" pH

pH measures below +7.0 are considered acidic; those above +7.0 are considered alkaline. The determination of whether a food is acid or alkaline is not gauged by its pH but by the pH of its residues (ash) or metabolites.

Alfalfa Grass .... +29.3	Buttermilk .... +1.3	Cumin .... +1.1
Almond .... +3.6	Cabbage, Green	Currant .... -8.2
Apricot .... -9.5	December Harvest .... +4.0	Currant, Black .... -6.1
Artichokes .... +1.3	Cabbage, Green	Currant, Red .... -2.4
Asparagus .... +1.1	March Harvest .... +2.0	Dandelion .... +22.7
Avocado (Protein) .... +15.6	Cabbage, Red .... +6.3	Date .... -4.7
Banana, Ripe .... -10.1	Cabbage, Savoy .... +4.5	Dog Grass .... +22.6
Banana, Unripe .... +4.8	Cabbage, White .... +3.3	Eggs .... -18.0 to -22.0
Barley Grass .... +28.7	Cantaloupe .... -2.5	Endive, Fresh .... +14.5
Barley Malt Syrup .... -9.3	Caraway .... +2.3	Fennel .... +1.3
Beans, French Cut .... +11.2	Carrot .... +9.5	Fig Juice Powder .... -2.4
Beans, Lima .... +12.0	Cashews .... -9.3	Filbert .... -2.0
Beans, White .... +12.1	Cauliflower .... +3.1	Fish, Fresh Water .... -11.8
Beef .... -34.5	Cayenne Pepper .... +18.8	Fish, Ocean .... -20.0
Beer .... -26.8	Celery .... +13.3	Flax Seed Oil .... -1.3
Beet, Fresh Red .... +11.3	Cheese, Hard .... -18.1	Flax Seed .... +3.5
Beet Sugar .... -15.1	Cherry, Sour .... +3.5	Fructose .... -9.5
Biscuit, White .... -6.5	Cherry, Sweet .... -3.6	Garlic .... +13.2
Blueberry .... -5.3	Chia, Sprouted .... +28.5	Gooseberry, Ripe .... -7.7
Borage .... +3.2	Chicken .... -18.0 to -22.0	Grapefruit .... -1.7
Brazil Nuts .... -0.5	Chives .... +8.3	Grapes, Ripe .... -7.6
Bread, Rye .... -2.5	Coconut, Fresh .... +0.5	Hazelnut .... -2.0
Bread, White .... -10.0	Coffee .... -25.1	Honey .... -7.6
Bread, Whole-grain .... -4.5	Comfrey .... +1.5	Horseradish .... +6.8
Bread, Whole-meal .... -6.5	Corn oil .... -6.5	Juice, Natural Fruit .... -8.7
Brussels Sprouts .... -1.5	Cranberry .... -7.0	Juice, White Sugar
Buckwheat Groats .... +0.5	Cream .... -3.9	Sweetened Fruit .... -33.4
Butter .... -3.9	Cucumber, Fresh .... +31.5	Kamut Grass .... +27.6

One of the most difficult aspects of cleansing is refraining from food or reducing food intake. Additionally, most of the food we eat is not very complimentary to our cleansing. If you eat in a healthy manner that will not compromise your cleansing program, you will not defeat your purpose. Too many people feel confused and do not know what foods are basically supporting to the cleansing process.

ComforTone—Herbal Colon Cleanse

ComforTone is formulated with cascara sagrada, diatomaceous earth, apple pectin, bentonite, licorice root, psyllium, cayenne pepper, and garlic. These herbs are particularly effective in purging the colon of toxins and impurities, which is just as important as cleansing the small intestine.

Waste products and gases held in the colon have a much higher concentration of toxic byproducts than those in the small intestine. When these leach into the organs and tissues, they can wreak havoc in our bodies.

The essential oil blends of DiGize and JuvaFlex, formulated with the single oils of Peppermint, Rosemary, Tarragon, Ginger, Anise, and Fennel, promote peristalsis and increase digestive secretions for better digestion.

ComforTone Protocol

- Taking 2 capsules every morning and night for two days should increase bowel movements to three to four daily.
- If elimination does not improve, then increase capsules to 3 each night and morning.
- Do not exceed 10 capsules per day without advice from a health care practitioner.
- If you start to have cramps, you may be dehydrated and may have a spastic or prolapsed colon, causing loss of peristalsis. This is when colon hydrotherapy may be helpful.

Food "Ash" pH (cont.)

Food	pH	Food	pH	Food	pH
Ketchup	-12.4	Papaya	-9.4	Soybeans, (Cooked, then Ground)	+12.8
Kohlrabi	+5.1	Peach	-9.7	Soybeans, Fresh	+12.0
Lecithin, Pure (Soy)	+38.0	Peanuts	-12.8	Spelt	+0.5
Leeks (Bulbs)	+7.2	Pear	-9.9	Spinach (other than March)	+13.1
Lemon, Fresh	+9.9	Peas, Fresh	+5.1	Spinach, March Harvest	+8.0
Lentils	+0.6	Peas, Ripe	+0.5	Straw Grass	+21.4
Lettuce	+2.2	Pineapple	-12.6	Strawberry	-5.4
Lettuce, Fresh Cabbage	+14.1	Pistachios	-16.6	Sugar Cane Juice Dried (Sucanat)	-9.6
Lettuce, Lamb's	+4.8	Plum, Italian	-4.9	Sugar Cane, Refined (White)	-17.6
Limes	+8.2	Plum, Yellow	-4.9	Sunflower Oil	-6.7
Liquor	-28.6 to -38.7	Pork	-38.0	Sunflower Seeds	-5.4
Liver	-3.0	Potatoes, Stored	+2.0	Sweeteners, Artificial	-26.5
Macadamia Nuts	-11.7	Primrose	+4.1	Tangerine	-8.5
Mandarin Orange	-11.5	Pumpkin	-5.6	Tea (Black)	-27.1
Mango	-8.7	Quark	-17.3	Tofu	+3.2
Margarine	-7.5	Radish, Sprouted	+28.4	Tomato	+13.6
Marine Lipids	+4.7	Radish, Black (Summer)	+39.4	Turbinado	-9.5
Mayonnaise	-12.5	Radish, Red	+16.7	Turnip	+8.0
Meats, Organ	-3.0	Radish, White (Spring)	+3.1	Veal	-35.0
Milk Sugar	-9.4	Raspberry	-5.1	Walnuts	-8.0
Milk, Homogenized	-1.0	Rhubarb Stalks	+6.3	Watercress	+7.7
Millet	+0.5	Rice, Brown	-12.5	Watermelon	-1.0
Molasses	-14.6	Rice Syrup, Brown	-8.7	Wheat Germ	-11.4
Mustard	-19.2	Rose Hips	-15.5	Wheat Grass	+33.8
Nut, Soy (Soaked, then Air Dried)	+26.5	Rutabaga	+3.1	Wheat	-10.1
Olive Oil	+1.0	Sesame Seeds	+.5	Wine	-16.4
Onion	+3.0	Shave Grass	+21.7	Zucchini	+5.7
Orange	-9.2	Sorrel	+11.5		
Oysters	-5.0	Soy Flour	+2.5		
		Soy Sprouts	+29.5		

- Aloe vera juice and/or prune juice work as natural laxatives. Drink 8 ounces a day and take 5-6 capsules of ComforTone and 1-2 tablespoons of JuvaPower in water morning and night.

- Drink half your body weight of water in fluid ounces daily, and, when cleansing, drink 20 percent more water. It softens clay-like, hard waste matter trapped in tissue pockets in the intestinal tract, caused from not drinking enough fluids.

- When bowel movements increase up to three to four times per day, you know ComforTone is working. If when you stop taking ComforTone your bowel movements slow down or become sluggish, then begin again until ComforTone is again working.

- If diarrhea occurs for more than one or two days, stop the ComforTone, rest for one to two days, and then start again with a smaller amount. ComforTone is safe and can be very helpful during an entire pregnancy, if necessary. A little diarrhea is easier to take care of than the misery of being constipated. The object is to eliminate easily and often.

- ComforTone and JuvaPower work very well together for synergistic cleansing through the digestive system.

ICP—Intestinal Fiber Cleanse

Coarsely ground grains rich in soluble and semi-soluble fiber are some of the best intestinal cleansers known. ICP's psyllium powder and husks, rice bran, oat bran, flax seed, and fennel seed help loosen and expel undigested and fermenting materials from the intestines that block nutrient absorption and cause poison to be reabsorbed into the body.

Fibers act as a biochemical sponge for the body, absorbing impurities, gases, and toxins and increasing the flow of waste matter through the intestines, helping to minimize the exposure to harmful substances. The slower the "transit time" of waste matter through the intestinal tract, the higher the incidence of disease.

Fiber satisfies the appetite by giving people a feeling of fullness without adding excessive calories. Fiber may also help balance blood sugar levels. It also helps maintain regularity as we age, preventing and overcoming constipation, diarrhea, and gas.

The essential oil blend DiGize and the supplement Digest & Cleanse are formulated with the single oils of Fennel, Tarragon, Ginger, Lemongrass, Rosemary, Basil, Bergamot, and Melissa that not only help dissolve and chelate toxins but also combat pathological microorganisms that reside in the intestines.

ICP Protocol
When the bowels are moving regularly:
- Take 1 tablespoon ICP mixed in a glass of water morning and night for 2-3 days.
- After 2-3 days, increase dosage to 2 tablespoons morning and night while you cleanse. Drink plenty of water.
- Maintenance dosage: Take 2 tablespoons 3-4 times per week.
- Beta-carotene, found in carrot juice and beet juice, also helps with elimination.
- Carrot Seed oil detoxifies the liver and in combination with the essential oils of Geranium and Lemongrass may help in eliminating gallstones, cleansing the bowel, and relieving flatulence.
- Lemon, Frankincense, and Idaho Grand Fir help dissolve, eliminate, and decrease the pain of kidney stones.
- Ledum, Juniper, and Geranium also work well together for an intestinal cleanse.
- DiGize, Fennel, Tarragon, and Peppermint help relieve flatulence.

To maintain a healthy colon, it is best to stay away from processed and pasteurized dairy products, including all cheeses except goat cheese. Avoid refined white sugar, white flour, processed salt, starchy processed foods, and fried foods. These are deadly to the intestinal tract.

Breads made from hybrid wheat and other grains are also damaging to the digestive tract. Both whole wheat and white bread are converted into sugar by the body, and the sugar turns to fat.

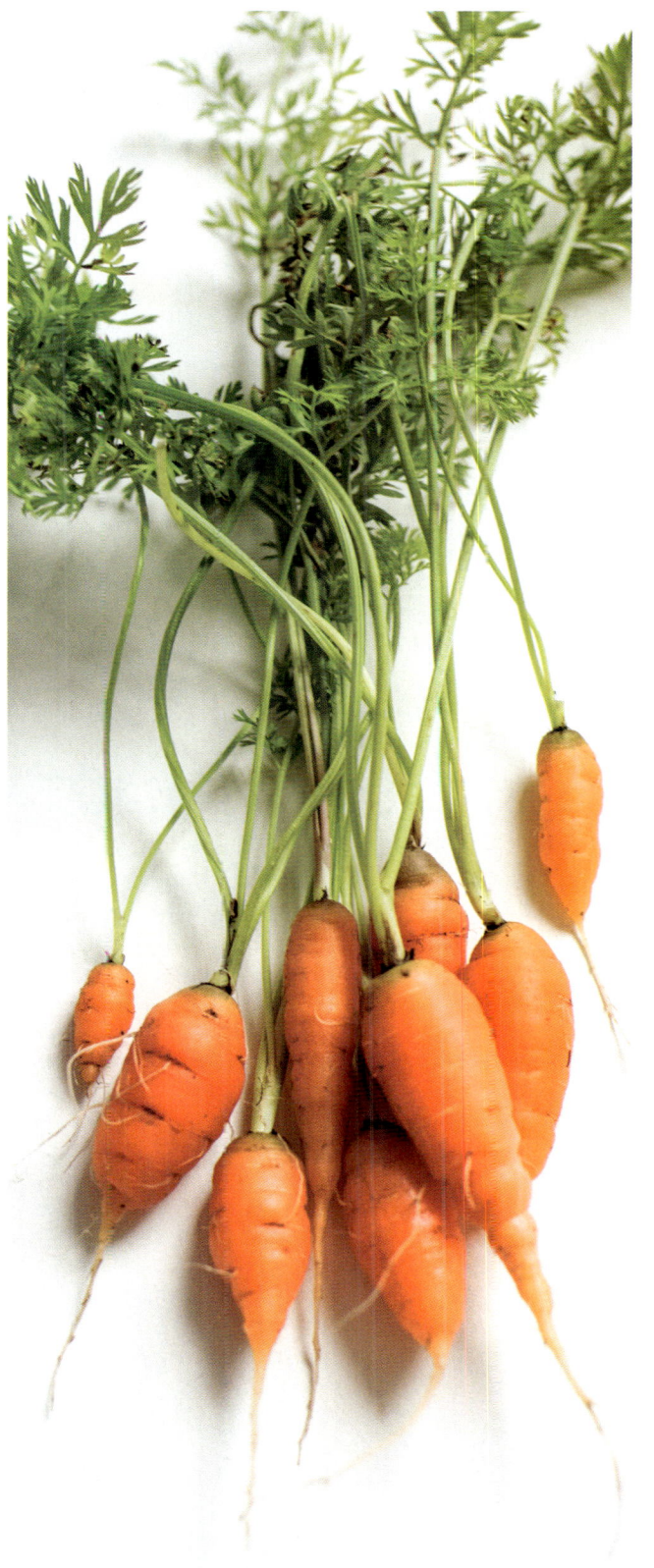

If you have heartburn while taking ComforTone or ICP, your digestive system is obviously not working properly. If the cleansing process reduces the intestinal flora, begin adding the following to the program:

- Essentialzyme: Take 1-3 caplets per meal and up to 6 with heavy meat meals late in the day or at night. Oils that can accelerate digestion are Tarragon, Fennel, and the essential oil blend of DiGize. Take 3 or 4 drops of each essential oil mentioned above in a double oo capsule before or after a meal to enhance digestion.

- Take 5 capsules of Life 9 at nighttime to help build up the intestinal flora. Consume organic yogurt or kefir without sugar or artificial sweeteners ½ hour before meals on an empty stomach.

These supplements provide the stomach with the friendly bacteria and enzymes necessary for good digestion, conversion, and assimilation. Master Formula, MultiGreens, and Mineral Essence provide trace minerals that the body requires to produce enzymes.

When taken together, ComforTone and Essentialzyme have synergistic effects, so less of each is required to achieve similar benefits.

Liver Cleansing Supplements

The Juva products will bring restoration and support for optimal liver function.

- **JuvaCleanse**
  This oil blend was formulated with Celery Seed, Helichrysum, and Ledum essential oils to help detoxify while enhancing liver function. It offers both hepatoprotective activity and antioxidant protection. Antioxidants neutralize the effects of free radicals, the oxidizing agents that cause aging and degenerative conditions.

- **JuvaFlex**
  With the essential oils of Fennel, Rosemary, Blue Tansy, Geranium, Roman Chamomile, and Helichrysum, this blend provides liver and digestive system support.

- **JuvaPower**
  This dietary supplement is delicious and a convenient addition to a healthy diet with advanced phytonutrient fibers to cleanse the liver and intestines simultaneously. It contains the highest acid-binding foods for superior results.

- **JuvaTone**
  This dietary supplement provides choline, a nutrient that is known for supporting optimal liver health, along with healing herbs and essential oils, including Lemon, German Chamomile, Geranium, and Blue Tansy.

Liver Cleanse Recipes

This liver cleanse, designed by D. Gary Young, will help detoxify the liver and maximize normal liver function in a natural, effective way.

This program combines the Master Cleanse, Vital Life Juice (recipe below), salads, and the nutritional supplements for a minimum of five days.

Immediately after you awaken (6 a.m.):

Drink a 10-ounce glass of Master Cleanse:
- 10 ounces purified water
- ½ lemon (squeezed)
- Pinch of cayenne pepper
- 2 teaspoons maple syrup or Yacon Syrup

Then take the following supplements:

- 2 JuvaTone
- 2 Detoxzyme
- 1 Essentialzymes-4 (white capsule)
- 20 drops JuvaCleanse in one oo capsule

Wait for 30-60 minutes and then drink ¼ cup Vital Life Juice.

Vital Life Juice Recipe:

Mix in a juicer (not a blender):
- 3 ounces beet juice
- 1 ounce carrot juice
- 1 ounce celery juice
- 1/3 ounce white radish juice
- 1/8 ounce ginger (Whole ginger may be juiced while juicing other vegetables.)
- 1/3 ounce red potato juice (optional)

7 a.m.: Drink 10 ounces of the Master Cleanse drink.

8 a.m.: Eat quinoa and oatmeal with coconut or other alternative milk.

9 a.m.–10 a.m.: Drink Vital Life Juice followed by 1 package of Slique Shake and 1 tablespoon JuvaPower in liquid of choice.

11 a.m.: Drink 10 ounces of the Master Cleanse drink.

12 noon–Lunch: Lunch may include any of the salad recipes that follow. Eat lunch along with drinking the Master Cleanse drink. One tablespoon of JuvaPower may be added to the salad.

1 p.m.: Drink 10 ounces of the Master Cleanse drink.

2 p.m.: Drink Vital Life Juice.

3 p.m.: Drink Slique Shake and NingXia Red.

4 p.m.: Drink Vital Life Juice.

6 p.m.: Eat a salad of your choice, white basmati rice with coconut or other alternative milk, or one of the dinner recipes listed below. If you have not used JuvaPower before, take 1 tablespoon of JuvaPower at dinnertime along with 2 Allerzyme capsules.

7 p.m.: Drink Master Cleanse drink.

8 p.m.: Drink Vital Life Juice.

9 p.m.: Take 2 JuvaTone, 2 Detoxzyme, 1 Essentialzymes-4 (white capsule), and 1 Essentialzymes-4 (yellow capsule), followed by 1 capsule of JuvaCleanse and the Master Cleanse drink.

Drink 2-4 ounces of NingXia Red during the day as desired.

If there are any problems with bowel function or movement, incorporate ComforTone and ICP into one of your drinks. This will enhance the cleansing action of the liver.

You may want to check with your health care professional before beginning any dietary change, especially if serious degenerative disease is a condition.

ParaFree and Parasites

Almost everyone has parasites in one form or another. For the most part, they go entirely unnoticed until the person begins to feel "achy" and fatigued.

Pure essential oils have some of the strongest antiparasitic properties known, including Thyme, Clove, Anise, Nutmeg, Fennel, Vetiver, Cumin, Tea Tree, Ledum, Melissa, and Bergamot. ParaFree, DiGize, Digest & Cleanse, and Inner Defense are supplements that aid the body in killing and ridding itself of parasites.

ParaFree Protocol

- Take 3-6 ParaFree softgels 2-3 times daily for 1 week. Rest for 1 week to allow the parasite eggs to hatch.
- Start again and continue for 3 weeks and then rest for 3 weeks. Repeat this cycle three times.

ESTABLISHING AND MAINTAINING GOOD HEALTH

Babies and Children

Babies and children respond very well to essential oils and nutritional supplements. The only difference is the amount. KidScents MightyZyme, MightyVites, and MightyPro are products specific to children. The Super C Chewables and NingXia Red are good companions.

Children have an innate sense about essential oils. Most children are very drawn to the aromas. They love to have them massaged on their feet and backs as much as they love to feel them in their own hands and massage them on someone else. They just want to put them on without questions and concerns.

- **Babies:** Put 1-2 drops of oil in your hand and rub your hands together until they are practically dry. Then hold them over any area of the baby. This works very well without direct application.
- **Direct application:** Mix 1-2 drops of an essential oil in V-6 Vegetable Oil Complex and apply to the bottoms of feet.
- **Children:** Put 1-2 drops on bottoms of feet or anywhere else on the body as long as the oil is diluted in V-6 Vegetable Oil Complex or in any vegetable oil. Although dilution is recommended, it is not always necessary. The essential oil roll-ons are perfect for babies and children of all ages as well as for adults.

Balancing Body Frequency

When the body is overloaded with toxins and is not able to cleanse properly, the endocrine system is not able to maintain good electrical balance throughout the physical body. The first solution is to begin a cleanse, as has been written about in this chapter.

- If the imbalance is due to allergies in the sinuses, throat, or pituitary, apply 1-3 drops of The Gift, Valor, Sacred Mountain, etc., to the crown of the head, the forehead, and the thymus.
- The essential oil blends Release, Freedom, Harmony, Reconnect, etc., stimulate harmony and balance by releasing memory trauma from liver cells, where many of the emotions of anger, hate, and frustration are stored. Apply neat or diluted with V-6 or other massage oil over liver, apply compress over liver, or massage Vita Flex points on feet and hands.
- Sandalwood (both Sacred Sandalwood and Royal Hawaiian Sandalwood) oxygenates the pineal/pituitary gland, thus improving attitude and body balance. Rose has a frequency of 320 MHz, the highest of all oils. Its beautiful fragrance is aphrodisiac-like and almost intoxicating. The frequency of every cell is enhanced, bringing balance and harmony to the body. Rose is stimulating and elevating to the mind, creating a sense of well-being.
- A blend of 5 drops each of Frankincense, Myrrh, and Idaho Grand Fir with 1 drop of Rose oil is very helpful for depression. Put a drop of the blend on the thumb and press the thumb against the roof of the mouth. This opens the cranial

sutures and is a powerful way to amplify the benefits and change the feelings of depression, sadness, despair, etc.

- Idaho Grand Fir rubbed under the nose and even up the nostrils is very uplifting and mood enhancing. There is usually an immediate, noticeable change of emotion.

- Lavender, Aroma Ease, Harmony, Peace and Calming, Peace & Calming II, Gary's Light, One Heart, etc., are excellent for calming a troubled mind and creating a peaceful environment.

- Harmony will probably work in most situations because it brings harmonic balance to the energy centers of the body.

- Inner Child, Reconnect, SARA, Release, InTouch, etc., stimulate memory response, enabling a person to get in touch with the feelings connected to trauma and negative memories and to let them go, thus allowing the person to create positive attitudes and intentions for the future.

- For overall body electrical imbalance, put 1–2 drops of Sacred Frankincense, 3 Wise Men, Reconnect, Gathering, Inspiration, etc., in each palm. Rub the hands together and then hold the right palm over the navel and the left palm over the thymus and take three slow, deep breaths.

Next, place the dominant hand over the navel, the other hand over the thymus, and rub clockwise three times. This works through the body's electrical field by pulling the frequency in through the umbilicus, the thymus, the olfactory, and then to the limbic system in the brain to create electrical balance.

The same procedure may be repeated with any of the different oils. Grounding is good for balancing frequencies when disrupted by disease.

- Harmony on the energy centers (or chakras) helps to balance the body, thus improving the healing process and facilitating the release of stored emotions.

- Massage 3–4 drops of Thieves on the bottoms of the feet.

The energy points corresponding to the endocrine glands are:

- The crown (top) of the head (pineal)
- Forehead (pituitary)
- Neck (thyroid)
- Thymus
- Solar plexus (adrenal)
- Navel (pancreas)
- Groin (ovaries/gonads)

Other oils and oil blends that can be used to balance frequency are Frankincense, Sacred Frankincense, The Gift, Gary's Light, Common Sense, Idaho Grand Fir, Valor, 3 Wise Men, Gathering, Northern Lights Black Spruce, Highest Potential, Transformation, Joy, White Angelica, and many others.

Any of the roll-ons really work well in applying oils to the energy points of the body: RutaVaLa, Tranquil, Stress Away, Valor, Thieves, and Breathe Again. You can also transform your favorite Young Living oils and blends into easy-to-use roll-on bottles by inserting an AromaGlide™ advanced roller fitment into any 5-ml or 15-ml bottle with an "Sb" marking on the bottom.

Fortifying the Immune System

The immune system must be strong and responsive in order to combat all types of disease brought on by pollution and undigested toxins that can lower the immune system response. Dietary supplements containing essential oils can boost and strengthen the immune system.

ImmuPro—combines complex polysaccharides, beta glucans, minerals, essential oils, and melatonin, one of the most powerful immune stimulants known.
- Take 1 or more chewable tablets at night before retiring. If you take them during the day, you will probably feel like you would like to take a nap.

Exodus II and Thieves—are essential oil blends that contain immune-stimulating and antimicrobial-compounds. Because essential oils have such complex chemistry, viruses and bacteria have difficulty living in an essential oil solution.
- **Massage:** 3–6 drops on thymus, throat, bottoms of feet, or wherever desired
- **Maintenance:** 2–4 capsules daily
- **Health challenges:** 6–10 capsules 3 times daily for 10 days and then reduce

Sulfurzyme—contains MSM and Ningxia wolfberry for powerful nutritional support.
- **Maintenance:** 1–2 teaspoons daily in water or juice or as needed
- **Additional health support:** Begin with 1–2 teaspoons daily and work up to 3–4 tablespoons daily or more if desired

ImmuPower—is an essential oil blend used to strengthen, build, and protect the body.
- **Maintenance:** 1 capsule 3-4 times weekly
- **Pneumonia, flu, or colds:** 4 capsules daily for 10 days, rest 4 days, and then 1 capsule daily for another 10 days

Inner Defense—Take 2-4 capsules daily

OmegaGize3—Take 1-2 capsules daily

Super B—Take 1 tablet daily after eating

Thyromin—is a very unique blend of glandular extracts, herbs, amino acids, minerals, and essential oils to support the thyroid. This gland regulates body metabolism and temperature and is important for immune function.
- **Maintenance:** Take 1 capsule immediately before going to bed.
- **Additional health support:** Take 3 capsules immediately before going to bed and 2 in the morning.

Mineral Essence—is a precisely balanced complex of essential oils and more than 60 trace minerals that are essential to a healthy immune system. It includes well-known antioxidants and immune supporters such as zinc, selenium, and magnesium.
- **Maintenance:** Take 1-2 droppers 1-3 times daily in water or NingXia Red.
- **Additional health support:** Take 2-5 droppers 2 times daily.

Singles: Sacred Frankincense, Palo Santo, Eucalyptus Blue, Ocotea, Ravintsara, Thyme, Oregano, Ecuadorian Oregano, Rosemary, Mountain Savory, Melissa, Lemon, Cinnamon, Lemon Verbena, Clove, Cistus, Tea Tree, Myrrh, Myrtle

Blends: The Gift, Gary's Light, Thieves, Melrose, Purification, ImmuPower, Exodus II, DiGize, GLF, JuvaCleanse, JuvaFlex, Longevity Softgels

Supplements: Super Vitamin B, Super Vitamin D, Master Formula, MultiGreens, Slique Shake, Pure Protein Complete, Rehemogen, AlkaLime, Life 9, NingXia Red, JuvaTone, Super C, and Inner Defense

NingXia Red juice is the highest-ranked antioxidant liquid dietary supplement that combines the wolfberry fruit (Lycium barbarum), pomegranates, blueberries, raspberries, and other fruit juices with essential oils. It is delicious and provides a great many nutrients that promote strength, vitality, and longevity.

DAILY MAINTENANCE
Strength-building Protocol

Nutritional supplements enhanced with essential oils can help support and balance body systems. The following products will nourish, strengthen, and build your body.

Slique Shake—Vegan protein drink with Chinese wolfberries
- Mix 1 package in water or milk of choice and drink 2-3 times daily. It can be mixed in orange or apple juice, but this may make it too sweet and lower the pH. It also may be mixed with cereal, fruits, desserts, or other foods.
- Combine equal parts Slique Shake and Pure Protein Complete for a high-powered protein blend.
- Drink as needed or as a meal replacement.

Essentialzyme—Enzyme-rich ingredients for better digestion and nutrient absorption for improved mental clarity and physical activity
- O Blood Type: 3-5 caplets daily (depending on type of food eaten and time of day)
- B Blood Type: 4-6 caplets daily
- A Blood Type: 5-7 caplets daily (A types tend to have more digestive needs.)

Note: When eating heavy protein foods after 3 p.m., take Essentialzymes-4 (yellow capsule), which will help with evening and nighttime digestion.

MultiGreens—Protein-rich chlorophyll to facilitate balanced pH
- O Blood Type: 8-10 capsules daily
- B Blood Type: 6-8 capsules daily
- A Blood Type: 4-6 capsules daily

Super Vitamin C—Properly balanced with rutin, biotin, bioflavonoids, and trace minerals, Super Vitamin C works synergistically in balancing the electrolytes and increasing the absorption rate of vitamin C.

Without bioflavonoids, vitamin C has a hard time getting inside cells, and without proper electrolyte balance and trace minerals, it will not stay there long.

Super Vitamin C Chewable—This is the only chewable vitamin C in the world that combines citrus

A Simple Guide for Daily Maintenance	
Longevity Vitality (oil blend)	Children over age 8: 6 drops per capsule 2 times daily or in yogurt; Adults: 20 drops per capsule, 1-2 capsules, 2 times daily or in yogurt
Longevity Softgels	1 softgel 1 time daily with food
Melrose	Children over age 8: 6 drops per capsule 2 times daily or in yogurt; Adults: 20 drops per capsule, 1-2 capsules, 2 times daily or in yogurt
Super C	1-4 tablets daily or as needed
Super C Chewable	1 chewable 3 times daily or as needed
Thyromin	1-2 capsules daily
Citrus Fresh	Put 2 drops in a capsule and take up to 3 times daily or take in yogurt.
EndoFlex	Dilute 1 drop with 1 drop of V-6 or other pure carrier oil. Put in a capsule and take up to 3 times daily.
Allerzyme	1 capsule 3 times daily just prior to meals or as needed
Detoxzyme	1-2 capsules 3 times daily between meals or as needed
DiGize	Dilute 1 drop with 4 drops of V-6 or other pure carrier oil. Put in a capsule and take 1 daily.
Essentialzyme	Take 1 caplet 1 hour before meals.
ICP	Mix 2 rounded teaspoons with at least 8 ounces of warm water or juice 1 time daily.
JuvaPower	Sprinkle 1 tablespoon on food or stir 4-8 ounces into purified drinking water or rice or almond milk and drink. Take 3 times daily.

essential oils, citrus bioflavonoids, and whole-food, natural vitamin C in one tablet.

It is a powerful antioxidant vitamin with minerals, bioflavonoids, and trace minerals to balance electrolytes and assist in the absorption of vitamin C.

Pure essential oils of Orange, Grapefruit, Tangerine, Lemon, and Lemongrass help increase digestion and nutrient absorption and are enjoyed by both adults and children.

Super Vitamin Cal Plus or Mega Vitamin Cal—
Contain minerals, calcium, magnesium, potassium, and zinc combined with essential oils to maintain proper health. Take 2-6 capsules or 1-2 scoops daily or as needed.

Sulfurzyme—A natural form of dietary sulfur to support normal metabolic functions, circulation, and help strengthen the body's natural defense system. It builds strong hair and nails.

- Start: 1-2 teaspoons daily for 1-2 days
- Increase: 1-2 tablespoons 2 times daily for maximum results

Maintenance Protocol

Our lifestyles should incorporate cleansing at all times. The intensity of cleansing depends on the individual. ComforTone, Essentialzyme, Detoxzyme, JuvaPower, and ICP taken at the same time provide a powerful, synergistic cleansing force.

- **ComforTone:** 3-5 capsules morning and night
- **Essentialzyme:** 3 caplets 3 times daily to digest toxic waste from everyday metabolism
- **Detoxzyme**: 2 capsules morning and noon, 4 capsules at night
- **ICP:** 1 teaspoon of powder in water, carrot juice, or apple juice morning and night
- **JuvaPower:** 1-2 tablespoons of powder in water 2 times daily

Good Eating Habits

Breakfast is the most important meal of the day. Some people work for an hour or two or more prior to having breakfast to promote appetite and prime the digestive system.

Before you begin to eat, be sure to drink a large glass of water to help move the nutrients through the body. Protein and complex carbohydrate foods are best for energy conversion in the morning. Strawberries or raspberries are the only fruits recommended to eat with cereal.

Plain yogurt or kefir without sweeteners are good sources of acidophilus and bifida bacteria cultures essential for proper intestinal flora. Sugar, synthetic sweeteners, and other foods high on the glycemic index should be avoided.

Sometimes people who have health challenges or digestive systems that do not function properly feel better eating fruit like papaya, mango, pineapple, and watermelon, which are easier to digest.

Cereals can include Einkorn, Einkorn Flakes, oatmeal, millet, barley, quinoa, or a mixture of these, with your choice of milk.

However, it is best not to tax the body with too many grains, which make digestion more difficult.

Bread is better toasted to change it from a wet food

ENVIRONMENTAL PROTECTION

(see also Chapter 19)

Daily radiation bombardment from our highly technical, electrical world does not make the body healthier. If you know you have been exposed to radiation, feel fatigued from it, or have been flying on commercial airlines (which have greater exposure to radiation due to the high altitude), an increased daily number of antioxidant supplements is needed.

An important supplement to take when flying is Thyromin, which supports the thyroid. Increase the number of antioxidant supplements you take 10 days before flying and increase the number for 10 days after traveling.

Suggestions: Inner Defense, Super C (tablets or Chewable), Detoxzyme, Essentialzyme, Essentialzymes-4, NingXia Red, and many others.

Although the Environmental Protection Kits, QuadShield and EndoShield, are no longer sold as kits, the products may be purchased separately and are convenient, easy ways to help you maintain your protection against the dangers of daily radiation bombardment and, in the case of a more serious threat, radioactive poisoning. Refer to the chart titled Environmental Protection Kits for products and details about how these products can protect you, your family, your friends, and those around you from the dangers of environmental pollution and potential daily radiation exposure.

Restoring Proper Bowel Flora

Antibiotics, chemotherapy, or radiation destroy the good bacteria in the body. A good probiotic that contains acidophilus and bifidus, such as Life 9 probiotic and KidScents MightyPro, will help restore proper flora in the digestive system.

Take 5 capsules at night daily for one week after finishing with antibiotics or other medicines. Plain, unflavored yogurt or kefir taken before lighter meals also helps provide friendly bacteria.

For patients undergoing radiation, saturate the site 10 days prior to treatment with Tea Tree and Melaleuca Quinquenervia oils. Take 4 double oo capsules per day before, during, and for 30 to 60 days following radiation treatment.

Environmental Protection Kits

The QuadShield and EndoShield kits each combine four powerful products to help people protect themselves against daily radiation bombardment of cell phones, computers, electrical appliances, and other potential dangers.

The QuadShield kit contains Longevity Softgels, the essential oil blend Melrose, and the nutritional supplements Super C (Tablets or Chewable), and Thyromin.

The EndoShield kit contains Longevity Softgels and the essential oil blends Melrose, EndoFlex, and Citrus Fresh.

To create the kits, purchase products separately.

The Japanese earthquake of March 11, 2011, taught the world that nuclear power plants are vulnerable to natural disasters, and years of use have caused deterioration and weakness.

Of the 104 nuclear power plants in the United States, six are identical to the damaged Fukushima plant, 17 others are very similar, and several are close to major earthquake faults.

The "giant" that has been sleeping since the days of the Three Mile Island and Chernobyl disasters has awakened.

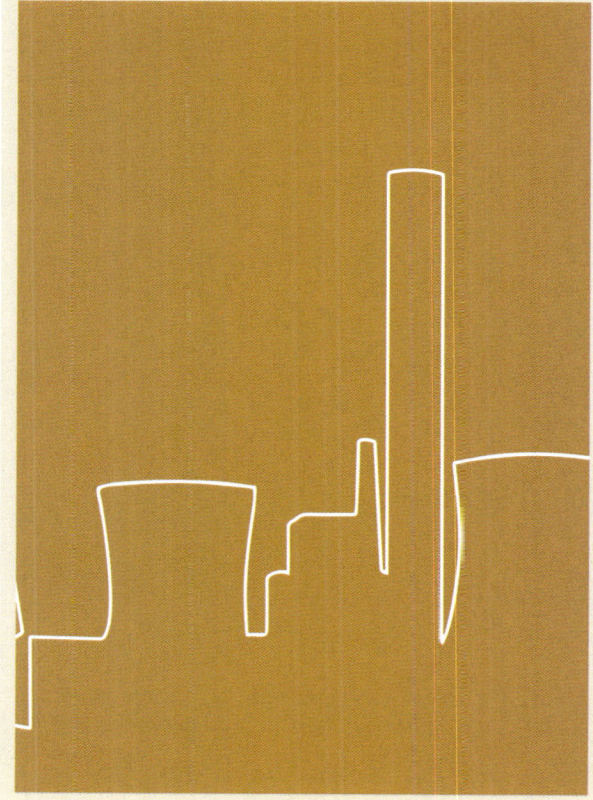

Environmental Protection Kits

QuadShield™

Longevity Softgel—The essential oils in Longevity Softgels increase the oxygen and ATP (adenosine triphosphate) cellular fuel for increasing cell life and immunity for stronger resistance against damage from environmental pollution.
- **Children and teens ages 10–18:** 1-2 capsules daily
- **Adults:** 2–4 capsules daily

Melrose—This blend is formulated with two species of Melaleuca oil: M. alternifolia, also known as Tea Tree, and M. quinquenervia, also known as Niaouli, which were found through research by Daniel Pénoël, MD, and Pierre Franchomme, PhD, to prevent cellular damage from environmental pollution and potential daily radiation exposure.
- **Children ages 1–3:** 1 drop in yogurt or other liquid
- **Children ages 4–7:** 2 drops in yogurt or other liquid
- **Children 8 and older:** 6 drops per capsule 1-3 times daily or in yogurt or other liquid
- **Adults:** 20 drops per capsule, 1-2 capsules, 1-3 times daily or in yogurt or other liquid

Super C (Tablet or Chewable)—Super C provides the body with 2,166 percent of the recommended dietary intake of the powerful antioxidant vitamin C and is enhanced with minerals, bioflavonoids, and pure Orange, Lemon, and other essential oils. It is a natural antioxidant and free-radical scavenger that supports the immune system and protects healthy cells from becoming damaged by the effects of environmental pollution.
- **Children ages 1–3:** 1-2 MightyVites daily
- **Children ages 4–7:** 2-3 MightyVites or Super C Chewables daily
- **Children 8 and older:** 3-4 MightyVites or Super C Chewables daily
- **Adults:** 4-6 tablets daily

Thyromin—Thyromin contains ingredients that give support and nutrition to both the thyroid and adrenal glands for a healthier glandular system.
- **Children:** continue to use MightyVites 2-4 daily
- **Adults:** only 1 capsule, 3 times daily

NingXia Red—Drink 4-6 oz. of NingXia Red for a delicious and healthy addition to your diet.

EndoShield™

Longevity Softgel—The essential oils in Longevity Softgels increase the oxygen and ATP (adenosine triphosphate) cellular fuel for increasing cell life and immunity for stronger resistance against damage from environmental pollution.
- **Children and teens ages 10–18:** 1-2 capsules daily
- **Adults:** 2-4 capsules daily

Melrose—This blend is formulated with two species of Melaleuca oil: M. alternifolia, also known as Tea Tree, and M. quinquenervia, also known as Niaouli, which were found through research by Daniel Pénoël, MD, and Pierre Franchomme, PhD, to prevent cellular damage from environmental pollution and potential daily radiation exposure.
- **Children ages 1–3:** 1 drop in yogurt or other liquid
- **Children ages 4–7:** 2 drops in yogurt or other liquid
- **Children 8 and older:** 6 drops per capsule 1-3 times daily or in yogurt or other liquid
- **Adults:** 20 drops per capsule, 1-2 capsules, 1-3 times daily or in yogurt or other liquid

EndoFlex—This blend contains oils very specific to the thyroid while at the same time addressing the entire endocrine system. Myrtle oil stimulates and promotes good thyroid health when combined with Spearmint, encouraging better circulation, stronger metabolism, and production of digestive enzymes. Geranium contains esters that protect the thyroid, which may explain why it is so heralded in French publications as a general tonic for the body. It supports the thyroid in being able to uptake iodine from food.
- **Children ages 1–3:** 1 drop in yogurt or other liquid
- **Children ages 4–7:** 2 drops in yogurt or other liquid
- **Children 8 and older:** 6 drops per capsule 2 times daily or in yogurt or other liquid
- **Adults:** 20 drops per capsule, 1-2 capsules, 1-3 times daily or in yogurt or other liquid

Citrus Fresh—This blend combines six citrus oils that are naturally antioxidant, antibacterial, and increase the uptake of vitamin C.
- **Children ages 1–3:** 1 drop in yogurt or other liquid
- **Children ages 4–7:** 2 drops in yogurt or other liquid
- **Children 8 and older:** 6 drops per capsule 2 times daily or in yogurt or other liquid
- **Adults:** 20 drops per capsule, 1-2 capsules, 1-3 times daily or in yogurt or other liquid

NingXia Red—Drink 4-6 oz. of NingXia Red for a delicious and healthy addition to your diet.

to a dry food, making it more digestible. However, bread made with today's modern hybrid wheat is not healthy for the body. A and B blood types gain weight more easily than O types because of the difference in digestive systems.

Breakfast is the best time to eat proteins such as beans, rice, eggs, fish, etc., providing more energy and stamina throughout the day. Be sure to take 1-3 Essentialzymes-4 (yellow capsule) with high-protein meals.

Lunch should consist of carbohydrates such as mixed vegetables or salads (particularly greens) along with free-range chicken or turkey or fresh-caught fish (not farm raised). Drink plenty of water with every meal.

A simple meal of organic, white basmati rice with cinnamon, maple syrup, or Yacon Syrup with your choice of milk is a perfect acid-binding food for an evening meal. White basmati rice is an alkaline food that is easier for the body to digest at night. A Slique Shake drink is also a simple replacement meal in the evening.

Dinner should be eaten in the late afternoon or early evening, if possible. It is much better to eat a bigger meal midday and a lighter meal in the evening. Both fruit and solid vegetables are suitable for evening meals. If an individual must eat a large, heavy meal late in the day or evening, Essentialzyme or Essentialzymes-4 (yellow capsule) is needed to promote proper digestion, reduce gas, and prevent putrefaction and fungal growth in the intestines.

RECIPES—DELICIOUS AND NUTRITIOUS

These recipes for salads and smoothies are very tasty and give great ideas for nutritious eating while you are on a cleansing program. Everyone loves smoothies as a treat anytime, especially children.

Smoothie and Popsicle Recipes
Created by Vallorie Judd

Protein Power
(A nutritional protein drink for all ages!)
- 1-2 scoops Balance Complete
- $\frac{1}{2}$ cup carrot juice
- $\frac{1}{2}$ cup fresh coconut milk
- 1 drop Orange essential oil
- $\frac{1}{4}$-$\frac{1}{2}$ cup water or an equivalent amount of ice

Directions
- Blend and enjoy nutrition at its best! It tastes like a "Creamsicle" but even better.
- This can be enjoyed fresh or frozen in little containers for a frozen "Proteinsicle."
- The carrot juice provides enzymes, and the coconut milk is full of essential omegas.
- It also makes a great replacement meal and is very satisfying to children who want to eat all the time.

Variations
- Use 1 scoop Pure Protein Complete and 1 scoop Balance Complete.
- Mangos are another wonderful fruit to blend into the protein drinks.
- Another healthful drink can be made using kefir (probiotics) and pineapple (bromelain).

Pina Colada Delight
- 1 cup kefir milk
- 1 cup coconut milk
- 1-2 scoops Balance Complete or Pure Protein Complete
- $\frac{1}{2}$ cup fresh, chopped pineapple
- 1 frozen banana (or fresh banana with ice cubes)
- $\frac{1}{2}$ cup ice cubes or water

Directions
- Blend and enjoy as a nutritious drink or freeze for a frozen treat.
- If you do not have kefir, then use coconut milk in its place.

Frozen NingXia Popsicles
- 1 cup NingXia Red
- $\frac{1}{4}$-$\frac{1}{2}$ cup water
- $\frac{1}{2}$ cup blueberries
- $\frac{1}{2}$ cup strawberries
- 1 drop Orange or Lemon oil (optional)

Directions

Blend and pour into Popsicle trays and freeze. Also, the next recipe is very delicious!

NingXia Red Watermelon Juice or Popsicles
- $\frac{1}{4}$-$\frac{1}{2}$ cup NingXia Red
- 1 cup watermelon juice

Directions
- Mix together.
- Drink fresh or freeze for Popsicles.

Recipes for Healthful Eating
Created by D. Gary Young

The following recipes, created by D. Gary Young, are compatible meals with any cleansing program and are examples of healthful eating anytime.

Note: Basmati white rice is acid binding; brown rice is acid forming.

Beet Salad with Apples and Carrots
- 3 medium cooked beets, diced
- 1 large apple, diced (Golden Delicious or Gala)
- 3 carrots, diced
- 2 fresh limes
- 2 tablespoons coconut, avocado, or olive oil
- 1 dash of JuvaPower
- 1 dash of cayenne pepper
- 2 teaspoons maple syrup or Yacon Syrup
- 1 head romaine lettuce
- 1 head red leaf lettuce

Directions
- Grate or dice the carrots and apples.
- Steam the beets for 1 minute and then run under icy water for 3 minutes to prevent overcooking.
- Slice, dice, and mix together. Squeeze limes for juice.

Spinach Delight
- 2 bunches spinach leaves, torn
- 4 tablespoons sesame seeds
- 2 cups coconut, avocado, or olive oil
- 2 squeezed lemons
- 1 tablespoon JuvaPower
- 1 dash Tabasco sauce
- 1 can diced water chestnuts
- 6 button mushrooms
- 2 beets, steamed, chilled, and diced
- 4 figs, diced

Directions
- Mix together and add a dressing of your choice.

Mandarin Avocado Salad
- 4 heads romaine lettuce, chilled and torn
- 1 avocado, peeled and chopped
- 3 fresh mangos, chilled and diced
- 1 small red pepper, finely chopped
- 1 small green pepper, finely chopped
- 8 green onions, finely chopped
- 1 tablespoon fresh chives, finely chopped

Directions
- Mix together, then add dressing.

Tuna Mandarin Salad
- Use the same recipe as Mandarin Avocado Salad but add fresh albacore tuna.

Essential Rice Salad
- 3 cups cooked basmati rice, chilled
- 1 cup cooked corn kernels
- 1 cup chopped celery
- 1 cup chopped almonds
- 1 cup grated carrots
- 3 green onions, finely sliced
- 2 tablespoons sesame seeds, toasted
- 4 cups raisins

Directions
- After cooking rice, place it in the refrigerator.
- When rice is chilled, toss all ingredients in a salad bowl along with the dressing of your choice.

Bean Salad
- 1 cup chickpeas (garbanzo beans)
- 1 cup kidney beans
- 2 cups butter beans
- 1 cup black eyed beans
- 1 cup pinto beans
- 2 cups diced green beans

Directions
- Soak all beans for 12 hours, except the green beans.
- Next, boil for approximately 30 minutes and let simmer for 40 minutes or until beans are tender.
- Rinse, dry, and chill in the refrigerator.
- Add a dressing of your choice and serve.

Garden Salad
- 2 heads romaine lettuce, torn
- 1 head red leaf lettuce, torn
- 1 bunch spinach leaves, torn
- 2 cups snow pea sprouts or pea sprouts
- 3 cups alfalfa, chopped
- 1 cup watercress, chopped
- 4 cups fresh dill, finely chopped
- 8 basil sprigs, chopped
- 4 fennel sprigs, chopped

Directions
- Mix together and add the dressing of your choice.

Potato/Vegetable Salad
- 1 dozen small red potatoes
- 4 teaspoons paprika
- 2 tablespoons organic coconut, avocado, or olive oil
- 2 cups broccoli
- 6 cups romaine lettuce, torn
- 2 cups green beans or spinach, chopped
- 2 cups alfalfa sprouts
- 2 cups bean sprouts
- 1 cup finely sliced red cabbage

Directions
- Boil the potatoes in water for 20 minutes, with or without skins.
- Mix the potatoes, paprika, and oil.
- Preheat oven to 400°F and place potato mixture in a glass casserole dish; bake for 5-10 minutes on the top rack of the oven.
- Steam the broccoli, then wait for 5 minutes and remove from heat.
- Run under cold water for 30 seconds, then drain well.
- Mix lettuce and spinach/greens.
- Cut the broccoli lengthwise and dice. Add the greens, cabbage, and dressing of your choice.
- Use JuvaPower with an additional pinch of cayenne pepper for extra flavor.

Minestrone Soup
- 1 cup basmati rice, cooked
- 2 cups navy beans, cooked
- 2 cups green beans, diced
- 2 teaspoons oregano, chopped
- 2 teaspoons basil, chopped
- 2 drops coconut oil
- 2 large potatoes, diced
- 3 average-size zucchinis, chopped
- 2 large, whole leeks
- 4 celery stalks, diced
- 2 large carrots, diced
- 10 cups vegetable or chicken stock
- 2 garlic cloves, minced
- 1 large onion, chopped
- 2 cups mushrooms, sliced
- 4 large tomatoes, diced
- 1 tablespoon JuvaPower

Directions
- Cook beans and rice separately. It will take approximately 45 minutes to cook the beans and 20-30 minutes to cook the rice.
- Mix all the rest of the ingredients and let simmer in the chicken stock for 15 minutes.
- When beans appear to be tender (but not mushy) and the rice is done, add beans and rice to the vegetable mixture.
- Add 1 tablespoon of JuvaPower and let simmer for 15 minutes.

Pumpkin Pinch
- 3 butternut squash, diced
- 2 cups winter squash, diced
- 1 cup acorn squash, diced
- 2 onions, diced
- 1 garlic clove, minced
- 6 cups vegetable stock
- 4 bunches of fresh basil, chopped
- Coriander, to taste
- 2 tablespoons soy sauce
- 1 dash cayenne pepper
- 1 tablespoon JuvaPower
- 4 bunches flat-leaf parsley, chopped and minced
- 2 bay leaves (remove after cooking)
- 1 cup milk of choice

Directions
- Place all vegetables, onion, garlic, and vegetable stock in a large pot and simmer slowly (approximately 45 minutes to 1 hour).
- Add herbs, spices, soy sauce, pepper, JuvaPower about halfway through.
- Blend soup in a food processor until smooth, then add milk.
- Tastes great over basmati rice.

Dinner Delight
- 1 large winter squash or butternut squash
- 2 tablespoons organic coconut or avocado oil
- 1 tablespoon sesame seeds
- 1 cup basmati rice
- 1 onion, chopped
- 1 stalk celery, chopped
- 1 carrot, chopped
- Ginger root, minced
- Garlic clove, minced
- 1 bunch brussels sprouts, chopped
- 1 medium-size zucchini, chopped or sliced
- Shrimp and red snapper

Directions
- Cover squash with coconut or avocado oil and sesame seeds and bake at 350°F for 45-60 minutes until completely done.

- Cook basmati rice.
- Cook all the vegetables and spices together in a frying pan for about 20 minutes or until they start to become soft. Then add shrimp or fish and cook together on low heat for 15 to 20 minutes or until done.
- Take squash out of the oven and serve with vegetables, shrimp, or fish.

Stir Fry
- 1 lb. brussels sprouts
- 1-2 teaspoons coconut or avocado oil
- 10 scallions, minced
- 2 garlic cloves, minced
- 2 tablespoons ginger
- 2 red chili peppers, minced
- 1 teaspoon sesame oil
- 1 tablespoon mild chili powder

Directions
- Cook brussels sprouts in water for 10 min., let cool, and dice.
- Then mix the brussels sprouts with the rest of the ingredients.
- Stir in hot frying pan or wok until tender.
- Eat with rice or potatoes.

Chicken with Onion Pineapple Sauce
- 2 cloves of garlic, minced
- 1 onion, chopped
- 6 chicken breasts
- 1 red pepper, chopped
- 1 pineapple, cubed
- $\frac{1}{2}$ cup water
- JuvaPower
- Mixed herbs/seasonings for chicken
- Basmati white rice (optional)

Directions
- Sauté garlic and onions in a small amount of coconut or avocado oil; you also can use a small amount of water in a frying pan until lightly cooked.
- Add chicken and red pepper; brown with the onion and garlic.
- Add spices, water, and $\frac{1}{2}$ of the cubed pineapple.
- Put a lid on the pan and let cook for about $\frac{1}{2}$ hour until the chicken is cooked.
- Take the other half of the pineapple and process in a blender; pour over chicken and stir.
- Sprinkle a liberal amount of JuvaPower into the sauce. Let simmer for about 5 minutes.
- This becomes like gravy. You can add a mixture of flour, guar gum, or natural thickener for a more gravy-like texture.
- This is great served over basmati white rice and served with baked sweet potatoes and salad.

Gary's Chocomolie
- 1 cup avocado
- 4 tablespoons carob
- 16 dates
- 2 teaspoons vanilla extract
- 2 tablespoons maple syrup or Yacon Syrup
- 34 ounces water

Directions
- Blend until thick and creamy.
- Chill in the fridge or freezer for $\frac{1}{2}$ hour.
- This is wonderful on organic, einkorn pancakes or waffles with yogurt or over rice milk ice cream with sliced bananas.
- This can also be used as the filling to a precooked einkorn pie crust and then topped with yogurt and sliced bananas.
- This pudding may also be flavored with a drop of Peppermint oil, Orange oil, or a combination of both.
- This is really a delicious recipe!

Acorn Squash Apple Crisp
Created by Vallorie Judd
- 1 acorn squash washed and cut in half with seeds and pulp removed
- 1 Jonagold apple or other good baking apple, peeled and cored
- $\frac{1}{4}$ cup Yacon Syrup
- 1 teaspoon cinnamon
- $\frac{1}{4}$ cup Organic Dried NingXia Wolfberries

Directions
- Take acorn squash and cut a small piece off the bottom of it to help it sit level.
- Slice half an apple into $\frac{1}{2}$ of the acorn squash; do the same for the other half.
- Mix Yacon Syrup, wolfberries, and cinnamon in a bowl, then pour half of it into each halved acorn squash.
- Divide topping and cover the top of each half of the acorn squash with the apple inside of it.

- Sprinkle extra cinnamon over the top of the oatmeal topping (see below).
- Bake for about 30 minutes or until the squash and apple are soft from baking.
- Top with rice milk ice cream or goat yogurt.

Topping
- ¼–½ cup butter, coconut butter, or half-and-half
- ¾–1 cup oatmeal
- ¼ cup einkorn, oat, or other flour
- ½ cup Yacon Syrup
- Put cinnamon oil on toothpick and stir into Yacon Syrup

Quinoa Oatmeal Breakfast
- 2 cups organic, old-fashioned rolled oatmeal
- 4 cups water
- ½ cup quinoa

Directions
- Rinse quinoa and add to water.
- Boil for about 5 to 10 minutes.
- Add oatmeal and cook slowly for 10 minutes until thick.

About Quinoa

Thousands of years ago, quinoa (keen-wah) was a key source of nourishment for the Incas, who grew it high in the arid Andes Mountains.

Today, it is known as a "super grain" because it's so good for you. It is rich in essential amino acids, protein, calcium, iron, potassium, and B vitamins such as riboflavin, not to mention magnesium, zinc, copper, manganese, and folate, a water-soluble B vitamin that occurs naturally in food.

The seed of a spinach-like plant, quinoa is most often creamy in color, but it also comes in pink, red, yellow, orange, or black. When cooked, it expands and releases its germ, a delicate, white fibrous ring that is pleasantly crunchy.

Look for quinoa in the health-foods or bulk-foods section of your supermarket or health food store. If the price looks a little high to you, keep in mind that quinoa triples in volume when cooked.

To make a quick, nutritious, and tasty side dish for dinner, combine ½ cup rinsed quinoa with 1 cup water in a covered saucepan and bring to a boil. Reduce to a simmer for 15 minutes, checking to be sure it does not dry out. When seeds have tripled in size and spiral-shaped white germs are prominent, toss with butter, olive or avocado oil, chopped garlic, and/or fresh herbs.

For additional recipes using essential oils and nutritious ingredients, see The Young Living Cookbook, From Our Fields to Your Table. The recipes were submitted by Young Living members and employees and can be ordered through Young Living (YoungLiving.com).

Delicious and fun products can also be made with einkorn wheat. Baking & Cooking with Einkorn by Heidi Ellis contains lots of hints, tricks, and recipes for baking and cooking with einkorn and is available through Life Science Publishing (DiscoverLSP.com). Young Living also carries a selection of einkorn products.

For more information on liver cleansing and a detailed daily protocol, consult Re-JUVA-nate Your Health, a book on liver cleansing by D. Gary Young, also published by Life Science Publishing (DiscoverLSP.com).

Cooking with Essential Oils

Essential oil-enhanced cooking can be a lot of fun. A healthier lifestyle way of eating starts with your food preparation. When you have finished cooking your meats, add 2–3 drops of Fennel, Basil, Rosemary, or Thyme and let the meat cool in the covered pot, so the oils can penetrate and soak into the meat.

After steaming vegetables, add 1–2 drops of Lemongrass, Melissa, Ocotea, Peppermint, Spearmint, or Lemon to enhance the enzymatic action of the food and increase the natural enzyme secretion in your gastrointestinal (GI) tract.

When making apple pie, pumpkin pie, carrot cake, etc., add 3–4 drops of Cinnamon, Ocotea, Nutmeg, or other oils you desire according to taste. Essential oils kill unfriendly and unwanted microbes that can survive cooking.

Healthy Snacks

Everyone loves to snack, so why not snack in a healthy way? Slique Shake, Gary's True Grit Wolfberry Crisp Bars (Chocolate Coated), Protein Power Bites, Slique Bars, Slique Bars (Chocolate-Coated), and Ecuadorian Dark Chocolessence bars are always a treat. They add protein, good fiber, and are packed with nutrients and essential oils that support and strengthen the body. Organic Dried Ningxia Wolfberries and Gary's True Grit Einkorn Granola, and Gary's True Grit Wolfberry Flakes Cereal are also great snacks.

ENDNOTES

1. National Vital Statistics Report (US). Deaths: final data for 2015. Atlanta (GA): Centers for Disease Control (US); November 27, 2017. https://www.cdc.gov/nchs/data/nvsr/nvsr66/nvsr66_06.pdf.

2. Lee WM. Acetaminophen and the U.S. acute liver failure study group: lowering the risks of hepatic failure. Hepatology. 2004;40(1):6-9.

3. FDA drug safety communication: prescription acetaminophen products to be limited to 325 mg per dosage unit; boxed warning will highlight potential for severe liver failure [Internet]. U.S. Food & Drug Administration. January 13, 2011. Available from: https://www.fda.gov/Drugs/DrugSafety/ucm239821.htm.

Building Blocks of Health

ENZYMES: THE KEY TO DIGESTION

Enzymes are biological catalysts that speed up the chemical reactions in all living things. Without enzymes nothing would work. Our food would sit for weeks in our stomachs, and we would eventually die. Enzymes are absolutely vital to human health and are the foundation on which life is perpetuated. The purpose of enzymes is to break molecules apart or put them together, which they do very quickly and efficiently. There are specific enzymes for each chemical reaction needed to make each individual cell work properly.

Enzymes are like other proteins, consisting of long chains of amino acids that are held together by peptide bonds. Amino acids are organic compounds made of carbon, hydrogen, oxygen, nitrogen, and sometimes sulfur that are bonded in various formations. There are strings of 50 or more amino acids known as proteins that are large molecules that promote growth, repair damaged tissue, strengthen the immune system, and make enzymes. Enzymes facilitate chemical reactions but are not affected by the reactions.

Many body processes that normally require high temperatures, such as processing starch, would have to come to the boiling point outside our stomachs. But with the catalytic enzyme action, starches are easily converted naturally to usable energy in the body.

Over 3,000 known enzymes in the body perform every type of chemical conversion imaginable. They control the body's vital metabolic processes and are present in every biological system. Enzyme conversion creates energy and builds new cells. All living cells require nutrients and enzymes to divide, grow, and perform their normal activities. Enzymes turn the food we eat into energy and facilitate the use of this energy. There are two major enzyme systems in the human body: metabolic and digestive.

Metabolic enzymes help run all the body systems. They speed up the chemical conversion within the cells for detoxification and the production of energy and are produced in the organs of the body, such as the liver, pancreas, and gallbladder. Enzymes enable us to move, think, see, hear, and feel, which, in reality, comprise the complete control mechanism of the body. One researcher found over 98 enzymes carrying out metabolic functions in the arteries alone.

Digestive enzymes break down the food we eat to release the nutrients for absorption. They are perhaps the most talked-about enzymes, because food is the fuel for life. These enzymes are secreted along the digestive tract, where food is broken down and essential nutrients, vitamins, and minerals that sustain life are released to be absorbed into the blood stream and carried throughout the body.

The waste continues through the digestive tract and is discarded. However, if the waste does not move, causing constipation, then the waste begins to break down into putrefaction that the body will reabsorb as poison, creating all types of body dysfunction. Digestive enzymes include ptyalin, pepsin, trypsin, lipase, protease, and amylase. Another enzyme, cellulase, needed for the digestion of fiber, is not manufactured by the body, so it must come from the food we eat and the supplements we take.

Heat is an enemy to enzymes, and when temperatures exceed 118 degrees, the enzymes begin to break down; at 120 degrees, the enzymes are totally destroyed, whether through pasteurization, sterilization, or commercial food preparation, etc., and the food becomes difficult to digest. It follows, then, that cooking is an enemy to enzymes. The body secretes its own digestive enzymes for breaking down food, but when the naturally occurring enzymes in the food have been destroyed, the body is greatly taxed in its digestive function.

Amylase, found in the saliva of adults, breaks down carbohydrates and simple sugars found in vegetables and fruits. However, it is not produced in the bodies of infants when they are born. Their digestive systems are able to produce protease, cellulase, maltase, lipase, lactase, and sucrase; but they do not produce the enzyme amylase, which comes in a very high level from the mother's milk and supplies the baby adequately through nursing. If the infant's body produced amylase and the baby was receiving amylase through the mother's milk, it would simply be too much and would overload the infant's system.

All animal milk contains amylase for the same purpose of nourishing their offspring. Many people choose to give their babies goat milk because it is closest to the chemical structure of human milk and is easy to digest; but, of course, the best source of amylase comes from the mother of the infant.

A vegetable source of amylase is made, but it is never as effective as true amylase. Primary sources of amylase are raw fruits and vegetables, sprouted seeds, raw nuts, whole grains, and legumes.

Enzyme Quick Reference Guide

Please copy this page for a quick, daily reference. Keep it in the kitchen or carry it with you when traveling.

Open Capsules:

All capsules may be opened and enzymes sprinkled on any food or mixed in any liquid.

Combinations:

If more than one enzyme is recommended, you may take just one or a combination and see how your body responds. Basically, any combination is acceptable.

Key:

Essentialzyme (caplet)

Essentialzymes-4 (two capsules):

E-4 yellow capsule: for proteins, carbohydrates, sugars, and starches

E-4 white capsule: for fats

Example:

If for your evening meal you eat chicken, salad, vegetable, bread, juice, and apple pie, you will need more enzymes to digest during the night: 2 E-4 yellow, 2 Essentialzyme, 1 Allerzyme, and 6 Detoxzyme. If it seems like too many, just reduce the number. For children: 3 MightyZyme, 1 E-4 yellow, 1 Detoxzyme

Standard Dosages:

For each meal:
Adults: 2–4
Children: 1–2
Babies: ¼ to ½

Check with your health care professional regarding children younger than 2 years of age.

Choices:

The first enzyme listed is usually the first choice in combination with any others as desired.

Start the Morning: **Essentialzyme** (Adults: 2–4; Children: 1–2 or MightyZyme 1–3; Babies: ¼ to ½) Essentialzyme is an overall enzyme that supports the pancreas, which regulates glucose the body needs throughout the day for energy.

General Food Categories:

Carbohydrates, fruits, vegetables	**E-4 yellow**, Detoxzyme, Allerzyme, MightyZyme
Fats	**E-4 white, E-4 yellow**, Essentialzyme, MightyZyme
Protein of any kind	**E-4 yellow**, Detoxzyme, MightyZyme
Sugars, starches	**E-4 yellow**, Allerzyme, Essentialzyme, MightyZyme

Specific Foods:

Eggs, meat, fish	**E-4 yellow**, Essentialzyme, Detoxzyme, MightyZyme
Grains, oatmeal, wheat toast	**E-4 yellow**, Allerzyme, Detoxzyme, MightyZyme
Meat with pasta, salad, cheese	**E-4 yellow**, Essentialzyme, Allerzyme
Meat with salad, bread, dessert	**E-4 yellow**, Detoxzyme
Milk, yogurt, kefir	**E-4 white**, Allerzyme, MightyZyme
Pasta, cheese, bread	**Essentialzyme**, E-4 yellow, Detoxzyme
Rice, vegetables, fruit	**Allerzyme**, E-4 yellow, MightyZyme
Salad *(no meat)*, vegetables	**E-4 yellow**, Allerzyme, Detoxzyme, MightyZyme
Sweets *(ice cream, frozen Rice Dream, cookies, cake, candy bars, granola bars, apple pie)*	**E-4 yellow**, Allerzyme, Detoxzyme

Carbohydrate Categories:

Carbohydrates *(simple: refined sugars, fruits)*	**Allerzyme**, Detoxzyme, E-4 yellow, MightyZyme
Carbohydrates *(complex: vegetables, fruits, grains, beans, rice, bread, some milk products)*	**E-4 yellow**, Allerzyme, Essentialzyme, E-4 white

Bedtime: **Detoxzyme:** 5–15 as desired; MightyZyme: 3–4

Children are often given a milk formula that usually comes as a powder to be mixed with water. There are many different kinds of formula powders, and perhaps some are better than others. But the formulas are all still processed and "chemicalized" with ingredients that cause various problems that parents don't link to the synthetic milk. Unfortunately, much of the public is still very uneducated in the field of health and nutrition.

Many parents unknowingly mix their powdered formula with chlorinated tap water—**poison!** Then they heat the bottle in the microwave—**deadly!**

Heating the bottle or food in the microwave not only kills the nutrients but also poses a danger to the child. Anything heated in a microwave oven becomes hot on the inside first and yet feels cool on the outside. So if the bottle temperature feels nice and warm, it is probably extremely hot inside. It's a horrible experience for the unsuspecting child to get lips, mouth, and throat burned from the scalding milk.

Another threat is that the bottle could become so hot that it explodes, burning the person who opens the door and touches the bottle. Microwave cooking? Don't do it! Besides, who wants to eat the plastic chemicals that have leached into the food?

How many babies on formula seem to cry a lot and keep their parents walking the floor all night? The baby can't tell you his stomach hurts and that his body does not want "that milk." How many babies have skin rashes, are not developing normally, or do not seem very happy? There can be any number of causes, but chemicals and processed foods are not healthy for anyone, and for an infant or growing baby, the negative effects can be more dramatic.

Unfortunately, too many children are not being nursed. Perhaps the mother is physically not able to nurse, she has to get back to work, or she is just too busy. The reason does not matter; the results are the same—an amylase deficiency, which usually starts an allergic condition where the children begin to develop allergies to starches, usually proteins, and certainly sugars.

Unknowingly, parents, trying to help the child, rush to the doctor or the hospital, where more chemicals are put into this little, growing body, only to have more problems created that can become lifelong. If we just did things Mother Nature's way to begin with, we would not have to even be talking or writing about all this negative "stuff."

In the last couple of decades, science and technology have made it possible for us to supplement our diet with all kinds of nutritional supplements. With enzyme supplementation, children and adults alike do not have to suffer because of digestive problems and insufficient nutrient absorption.

Protease and amylase are the two most important enzymes that children need. You can take a protease enzyme first because protein takes a little longer to break down than starches, carbohydrates, and even lipids. Amylase breaks down the simple sugars that have to be in the bloodstream in order for the body to utilize protein. By taking protease and amylase together, the body is able to digest the sugar and facilitate the assimilation of protein.

It is extremely important that children who were not nursed, or drank some kind of formula, have enzyme supplementation as well. In order for children to be healthy and free of allergies, they must have amylase.

MightyZyme, a chewable multienzyme for children, is easy for children to ingest. Children who were not nursed and therefore did not get the needed amylase should take 1-2 tablets a day until about the age of ten. At about this age, it is good to have the child start taking the adult enzymes, which have a broader nutritional profile and are a little stronger.

Many children prefer the adult enzymes and begin taking them as early as seven or eight years old. However, many children have difficulty swallowing capsules, so they can be opened and emptied into yogurt, kefir, oatmeal, NingXia Red, or anything that will help them "get it down."

Below is a list of a few digestive enzymes, their actions, and the supplements in which they can be found. This will give you an idea of their critical importance in digestion, without which there will be minor and major dysfunction in the body. If any enzymes are missing or are insufficient in quantity, the body cannot perform optimally.

- **Alpha-Galactosidase** digests complex carbohydrate sugars found in vegetables, grains, nuts, seeds, and beans and prevents gas, bloating, cramping, and flatulence produced from fermented sugars (Allerzyme, Detoxzyme).

- **Amylase,** found in saliva, breaks down carbohydrates and simple sugars found in vegetables and fruits (Allerzyme, Essentialzymes-4 [yellow capsule], Detoxzyme, KidScents MightyZyme).

- **Bromelain** is the enzyme found in pineapple that promotes digestion in systems lacking sufficient digestive enzymes. It helps break down protein and the digestion of trypsin or pepsin. It can ease heartburn, nausea, and diarrhea (Allerzyme, Detoxzyme, Essentialzyme, Essentialzymes-4 [yellow capsule], KidScents MightyZyme).

- **Cellulase** is an enzyme not found in humans. It digests cellulose fiber and lessens malabsorption (Allerzyme, Detoxzyme, KidScents MightyZyme).
- **Invertase** hydrolyzes (liquefies) sucrase to glucose and fructose, promotes longer shelf life, and has broad activity range over pH 3.5 – 5.5 (Allerzyme, Detoxzyme).
- **Lactase** digests lactose, the sugar found in milk and dairy products (Allerzyme, Detoxzyme).
- **Lipase** breaks down fats in most dairy products, vegetables, nuts, oils, and meats (Allerzyme, Detoxzyme, Essentialzymes-4 [yellow and white capsules], KidScents MightyZyme).
- **Malt Diastase** (Maltase) breaks down disaccharide maltose into glucose or malt sugars (Allerzyme).
- **Pancreatin** is an enzyme composition that combines amylase, lipase, and protease to help break down starches and fats, metabolizes complex proteins, and removes dead and dying tissue (Essentialzymes-4 [white capsule], Essentialzyme).
- **Peptidase** promotes the hydrolysis of peptides into amino acids, which are the break-down product of protein absorbed in the gut (Allerzyme, Essentialzymes-4 [yellow capsule], KidScents MightyZyme).
- **Phytase** breaks down indigestible forms of phosphorus found in grains and oil seeds, releasing digestible phosphorus, calcium, and other nutrients (Detoxzyme, Essentialzymes-4 [yellow capsule], KidScents MightyZyme).
- **Protease** breaks down proteins in meats, nuts, eggs, and cheese (Allerzyme, Detoxzyme, Essentialzymes-4 [yellow capsule], KidScents MightyZyme).
- **Trypsin** is a pancreatic enzyme that hydrolyzes protein, operates at a pH of 7-12, and is used in baby food to predigest protein. It also breaks down the protein membrane surrounding cancer cells to digest and eliminate as toxic waste from the body (Essentialzyme).

Betaine HCL (hydrochloric acid) helps to break down fats and proteins and is found in Essentialzyme. It is important to have adequate levels of stomach acid for the absorption of protein, calcium, vitamin B12, and iron. Healthy stomach acid kills disease-causing microbes and parasites that are in the food we eat. Stomach acid decreases with age, which leaves us vulnerable to the attack of unwanted microbial invaders that bring disease and create unhealthy conditions in the body.

Food enzymes naturally come from the raw food we eat. However, the enzymes in a particular food are only for that specific food and have little effect on other foods. Some digestive enzymes are present in the food we eat; some are produced by the body itself.

Enzymes are very sensitive to heat, pH, and metal ions and are easily destroyed or rendered inactive. Commercially grown foods that are sprayed with chemicals are also devoid of enzymatic activity.

Enzymes are completely destroyed when cooked, boiled, heated, grilled, or baked, which means that enzymes are also destroyed in all processed food.

This means that we should avoid processed foods whenever possible, as they are devoid of the necessary enzymes for digestion and usually contain enzyme inhibitors to increase shelf life. Inhibitors block the enzymatic process, which stresses the body into an out-of-balance condition.

A lack of digestive enzymes in the food we eat forces the body to overproduce its own digestive enzymes and limits its ability to produce metabolic enzymes, which are also crucial for health and normal metabolism.

This limitation occurs because both digestive enzymes and metabolic enzymes are created from the same enzyme precursors (PST) that are produced in the liver.

The production of these precursors is limited in the human body, so when the digestive system must overproduce digestive enzymes due to an enzyme-less diet, it causes a harmful underproduction of metabolic enzymes, which are involved in every process of the human body.

The immune system, circulatory system, liver, kidneys, spleen, pancreas, and even our ability to see, breathe, and think depend upon these metabolic enzymes.

When the diet is supplemented with digestive enzymes that are naturally present in whole, raw, or uncooked foods, two powerful benefits are created:

1. The body is able to extract the maximum nutritional value from the food.
2. The body can reduce its internal production of digestive enzymes, which allows for higher production of metabolic enzymes, crucial for daily metabolism, health, and detoxification.

When we put food into our mouth, amylase in the saliva begins to break down complex carbohydrates into simple sugars. While the food is still in our mouth, our stomach begins to produce pepsin, which, like protease, helps digest protein.

When the food enters the small intestine, the pancreas secretes pancreatic juice, which contains three enzymes that break down carbohydrates, fats, and proteins that pass into the small intestine.

The enzymes from the food mix with the nutrients and travel in the blood plasma, which is the watery liquid in which the red blood cells are suspended. This is how the body absorbs and uses the enzymes for the vast number of catalytic activities that aid the body in everything from growth to fighting infection.

Ancient cultures prized the natural enzymes in foods—especially meats. They probably did not know how the enzymes worked or what worked, but they knew that something happened when food was allowed to cure because it gave them more strength, endurance, and vitality.

That is why we read about the tradition of curing and why many ancient cultures aged or cured meats, which allowed the natural enzymes present in the flesh to predigest it, thereby easing the burden on their own digestive system and conserving their own limited pool of enzymes.

When meat is predigested, it places less stress on the body's own enzyme bank. Predigestion also enhances the breakdown of peptide chains and proteins into free-form amino acids, the building blocks of every major body function, from immunity to growth.

Every protein that enters the human body via digestion has to be broken down into amino acids before it can be fully utilized. Meats that are not completely digested contain large protein fragments that cannot benefit the body.

In fact, these protein fragments can cause allergic reactions if the body's antibodies mistake them for foreign microorganisms.

Even worse, these protein fragments can become trapped in the intestines, where they will ferment and promote parasite proliferation and disease.

Cathepsin, a natural enzyme present in all animal flesh, starts the aging or "curing" process to slowly digest the meat. This is not unlike the process that ripens bananas. A green banana starts out high in starch. As it ages or ripens, the natural amylase in the banana converts the starches into sugar. In effect, the amylase is digesting the banana, eventually turning it brown.

As soon as an animal is dead, cathepsin begins to predigest the meat. It begins splitting large peptide protein chains into smaller, more digestible ones. When the meat is eaten after it has been hung for two to three weeks, the digestive system now has a far easier job completing its breakdown and liberating the vital

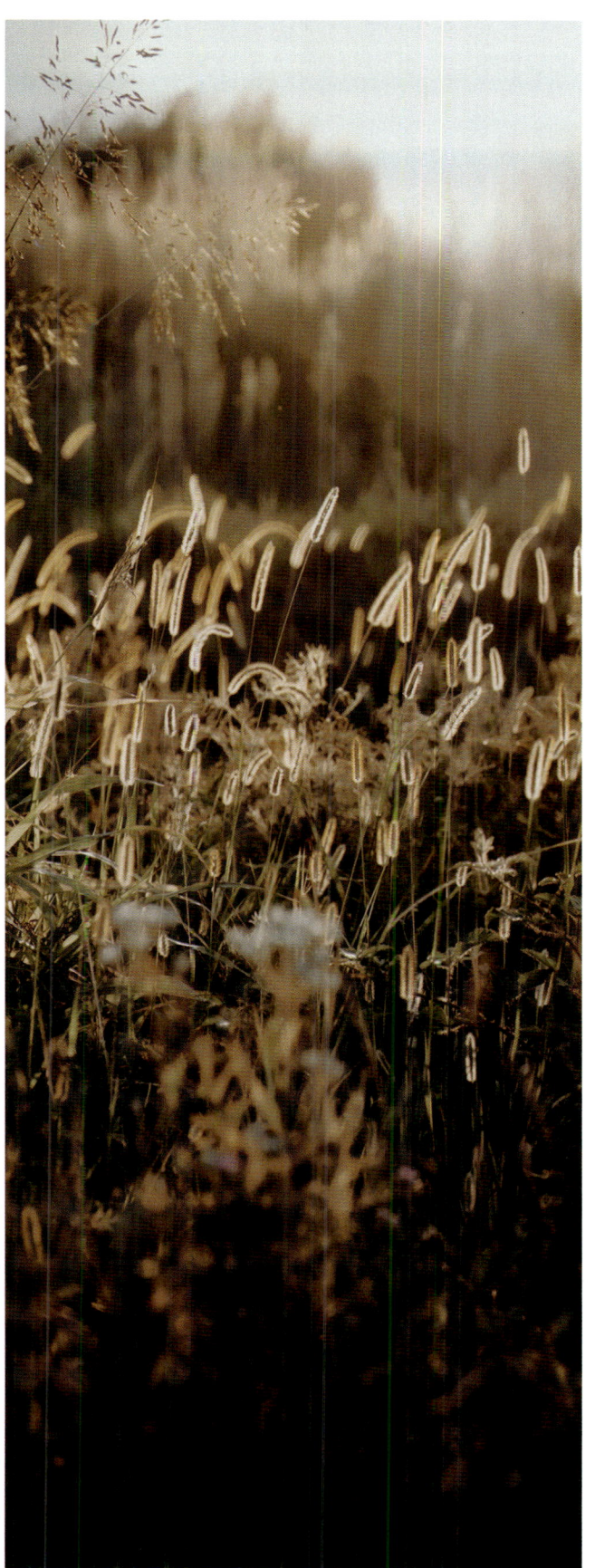

free-form amino acids, the building blocks of all bodily processes.

This explains why when an animal such as a dog or a cow is killed and left to rot, the vultures can be seen sitting on the fence for days, just waiting until the enzymes have done their job. Then the birds have a feast and eat the dead animal to the bones.

The history of enzymes is rather interesting. Long before chemists determined that there was some kind of chemical reaction taking place in organic substances, common people were making soaps, fermenting wine to make vinegar, and baking breads and pastries and many other things through these enzymatic reactions. Early in the 19th century, scientists began to investigate this unusual change in substances.

The well-known French chemist Louis Pasteur (1822-1895) called these catalysts ferments. A few years later, the German biochemist Eduard Buchner (1860-1917) isolated these catalysts and determined that they were chemicals, which were later named "enzymes."

This began the most revealing scientific journey into the world of enzymatic activity and the discovery of their purpose in all living organisms. It is fascinating to think about how this phenomenon has been observed and used from the beginning of time and was never understood or explained until modern science had the technology to give us that information.

The remarkable physical strength and endurance exhibited by the pioneers and Native Americans may have been due to their consumption of enzyme-rich raw and unprocessed foods, despite the sometimes-meager rations of less than 4 ounces of food a day. We have been taught that you must eat to have strength. But there is more to it than that. You must be able to digest what you eat and assimilate the nutrients in order to sustain health and strength.

On the average, only 8 percent of the food we consume is metabolized to sustain normal bodily functions. The remainder passes through undigested. Even worse, only 1 to 2 percent of the nutrient value of the food that we consume reaches our cells.

Many people today suffer with wheat and grain allergies, perhaps caused by the fact that when the grains are cut during the harvest, they are not bundled and left standing in the fields for a few days before threshing, as was the practice many years ago.

The purpose of leaving the bundled grains standing in the field was so that the dew at night or the rain would soften the shell. Then the next day the sun would evaporate the moisture, stimulating the enzymatic process within the kernels. This began the germination to prepare the grains for digestion.

Without the germination process, the enzymes in the kernels remain inactive and, therefore, do not have the ability to digest the grain, which makes it even worse for people who have low sulfur levels and phenolic sensitivity.

Most often, the PST pathway becomes blocked and cannot digest the gluten in the grains. PST (phenol-sulfotransferase) is a Phase II enzyme that detoxifies leftover hormones and a wide variety of toxic molecules—such as phenols—that are produced in the body and even in the gut by bacteria, yeast, and other fungi as well as food dyes and chemicals.

A four-year study (2000-2004) conducted by the Young Life Research Clinic in Springville, Utah, found that people with gluten intolerance and even celiac disease had no allergic reaction after eating grains grown from nonhybrid seed with no chemical sprays, harvested with horses, and then left to stand in the field for seven to eight days before threshing.

Egyptian hieroglyphics depict the ancient process of grain harvesting. The grain was cut with a scythe, tied into sheaves, and left to stand in the field for several days. It was then loaded into ox carts, hauled to the threshing site, and thrown into a big stone grinder operated by an ox team. The stone rolled around on the grain, cracking the hulls. With the sifting of the wind, the chaff was blown off, and the grain was picked up by slaves and carried in baskets to the storehouse.

Stone-ground, whole wheat bread that is rich in enzymes, vitamin E, and other nutrients is, sadly, a thing of the past. Today, modern technology brings grain to us via a machine called a combine. The combine cuts the grain, almost instantly separates the kernel from the husk, and delivers the grain ready for market on the same day it was cut. It is then further processed to strip out the vitamin E and other oils. Most of it is then bleached, leaving only a tiny fraction of the grain's initial enzymes.

To maximize the enzymes in a food, the fruit of the plant needs to mature on the stalk or stem to the point of "ripening" or readiness to sprout. This is when the enzyme content of the food is the highest. Unfortunately, many fruits, vegetables, and grains are harvested when they are immature and assumed to ripen "in transit," resulting in a food that has a far lower enzyme content.

In order for grains to fully digest in the human body, they must contain a full complement of their natural enzymes. Every food has its own specific enzymes. In order for a grain to have viable enzymes, it must have time to germinate. Once it germinates, its enzymes are released from the bondage of enzyme inhibitors. This is why sprouted grains are so health-giving—the enzyme inhibitors have been deactivated and can no longer counteract the natural enzymes present in the food.

Early signs of enzyme deficiency can manifest with many complaints. Heartburn, gas, bloating, fatigue, headaches, stomachaches, diarrhea, constipation, chronic fatigue, yeast infections, nutritional deficiencies, pain, joint stiffness, skin eruptions, psoriasis, eczema, and colon, liver, pancreas, and intestinal problems are just a few.

Many enzymes are not only deficient but are also inactive. At the Young Life Research Clinic in Springville, Utah, D. Gary Young tested over 21 different enzyme products from 21 different manufacturers and did not find a single one that was effective in a clinical environment. The patients were closely monitored, their food intake measured, and their blood and digestive systems regularly tested and analyzed. The clinic staff found that patients were simply not obtaining value from their food because their enzymes were inactive.

How are enzymes destroyed or rendered inactive?

1. Planting, growing, and cultivating food grown with chemical fertilizers, herbicides, and pesticides will produce a crop basically devoid of enzymes.
2. Heat begins to break down the enzymes at 118°F and totally destroys them at 120°F.
3. Pasteurization, sterilization, microwaving, chemical processing for freezing, and any other modern processes kill the enzymes or render them inactive.

Dr. Francis M. Pottenger, Jr., conducted an amazing study with over 900 cats. He fed one group of cats raw milk and meat. They lived healthy and disease-free. They produced healthy litters generation after generation. He fed another group of cats pasteurized milk and cooked food. After the first generation, this group became lethargic and began to suffer from allergies, infections, and other diseases, including heart, kidney, and lung diseases. Each succeeding generation of cats that ate cooked food suffered more diseases. By the third generation, the cats were unable to reproduce.[1]

Another study showed that after eating cooked food, the human body reacted just as if suffering from an acute illness. Within 30 minutes of eating cooked food, white blood cell counts increased dramatically, as though the body were fighting an infectious disease.

In a very interesting experiment, one group of pigs was fed enzyme-rich raw potatoes, and another group was fed enzyme-deficient cooked potatoes. The pigs eating cooked potatoes gained weight rapidly. The pigs that were eating raw potatoes did not get fat.

Obesity is an area of deep concern. Dr. David Galton at the Tufts University School of Medicine tested people weighing 230-240 pounds. He found that almost all of them were lacking lipase enzymes in their fatty tissues. Lipase, found abundantly in raw foods, is a fat-splitting enzyme that aids the body in digestion. Lipase activity breaks down and dissolves fat throughout the body. Without lipase, fats are kept and stored in tissues. We see this manifest around the waistline, hips, and thighs.

It is astounding to see the obesity levels of children and adults not only in America but around the world, which have reached epidemic proportions. Childhood obesity has more than tripled in the past 30 years. About 35 percent of children and teens between the ages of 2 and 19 are overweight, and almost 17 percent are obese.

According to the latest data from The State of Obesity, a report issued by the Robert Wood Johnson Foundation released in September 2018, almost 40 percent of adults aged 20 and over in the United States were overweight, and two thirds of U.S. adults were overweight or obese (68.6 percent).[2] According to the latest data from the World Health Organization, over 50 percent of men and women in the European Region were overweight, and roughly half of the women and men who were overweight were obese.[3]

These statistics are frightening when you look at the rapid increase in numbers. No wonder physical and mental problems as well as diseases are becoming more prominent in children and young adults. Clinics and hospitals are full of people suffering from problems due to being overweight. It is certainly possible that this overweight problem is due partly to chronic enzyme and nutrient deficiencies.

Our food is processed and devoid of nutrients and enzymes, so seeing such deterioration of our health is not surprising. Even our fresh fruits and vegetables are grown in polluted water and air and sprayed with a myriad of pesticidal and herbicidal chemicals.

There are even chemicals to induce plant growth and produce a perceived beautiful quality. It is hard to know the difference between and impossible to see the contamination and food devoid of nutrients when we walk through a well-organized grocery store and see such beautiful produce and products on the shelves.

We have a better chance of buying nutritious food when we buy organic food rather than nonorganic food, but even then, we don't know all the conditions under which the food is grown. The food may not be directly sprayed, but that does not change the quality of air and water. Government regulations for the organic food industry are allowing "less dangerous" chemicals to be used in organic farming, but we want to avoid all chemicals whenever possible.

Besides that, we do not know what is done to the

Carbohydrates, Proteins and Sugars

This partial list of complex and simple carbohydrates, proteins, and sugars might help you determine which supplement you want to take for different foods.

Carbohydrates (Complex)
Essentialzyme™ and Essentialzymes-4™ (yellow capsule):

Vegetables: spinach, lettuce, zucchini, asparagus, artichokes, cabbage, sweet potatoes, carrots, cucumbers, potatoes, radishes, broccoli, cauliflower, onions, peas, celery, sprouts, dill pickles, eggplant

Fruits: grapefruit, apples, prunes, pears, plums, strawberries, oranges

Grains: barley, einkorn, spelt, buckwheat, whole wheat, oat bran, wild rice, brown rice, multigrain breads, lentils, granola

Beans: pinto, soy, garbanzo, kidney, navy

Milk products: skim milk, soy or almond milk, low-fat yogurt

Carbohydrates (Simple)
Essentialzyme™ and Essentialzymes-4™ (white capsule):

Table sugar, corn syrup, fruit juice, cake, honey, milk, yogurt, jam, chocolate, white-flour pasta, white-flour bread, most packaged cereals

Proteins
Essentialzyme™ and Essentialzymes-4™ (yellow capsule):

Meat such as beef, chicken, turkey, bison, elk, venison, fish, nuts, nut butters (almonds, peanuts, etc.)

---

harvest after it leaves the farm. Preserving freshness is critical to the brokers and retailers, and how long is the food kept in storage before it goes on the shelf for the buyer? These are all things to consider.

Can we live without enzymes? The evidence is voluminous. Our bodies would cease to function without them. It would be ideal if we could consciously eat raw, unprocessed foods rich in enzymes in order to maintain an ample reserve in the body to maintain optimal health and effectively prevent and fight disease.

Unfortunately, most of our food supply does not contain the quantity of enzymes needed for proper digestion and conversion. That is why enzymes are added to so many commercial products. When you read product labels, you will be amazed to see such phrases as "enzyme enriched," "enzymes added," or "enzymes for better digestion," etc. We eat too much processed and devitalized food. So what do we do? How do we solve this problem?

Enzyme supplementation is the modern-day solution. Science has come a long way in its ability to manufacture high-quality enzymes that are absorbable and usable. Medical research shows that enzyme supplements can help fight illness, reduce or block the development of life-threatening diseases, and slow the effects of aging. There are enzymes specific to a particular need, and there are enzymes that provide overall enzymatic needs.

The best time to ingest protein is in the early morning or by mid-afternoon. You must have glucose in the blood to absorb protein. Because your body operates on glucose and protein primarily, it is better to put that in your body in the morning than at night when there is little or no activity. Protein at night is more difficult for the body to digest because it just sits in the stomach while the body is working to detoxify and cleanse.

Water is the activator of your enzymes. To activate your vegetable enzymes, you must have minerals and water. Water activates and creates enzyme saturation to the food that you have ingested. Water carries up to 18 percent oxygen, providing greater enzymatic action, so by drinking water with your meal, your food will digest better, giving you better nutrient availability, much more so than if you do not drink water with your meal.

To begin your day with breakfast, take 2 Essentialzymes-4 (yellow capsules) and 1 Essentialzyme, which help to supply both metabolic and digestive enzymes and at the same time target the carbohydrates and proteins that you've ingested for your morning meal.

There is an old belief system that says, "never drink with a meal." This is both correct and incorrect at the same time. All of the Young Living enzyme supplements contain raw, plant-extracted enzymes that require two things to activate them—minerals and water.

However, if you drink milk with your meal, thus saturating your food with lactose, you will need a high-lactose enzyme for digestion that can create fermentation along with the other foods that you have eaten, so you will want to take 1-2 Essentialzymes-4 (white capsules). If you drink apple juice, orange juice, or other juices high in sugar with your meal, you will need a high-sucrase enzyme to digest the simple carbohydrates (sugars) and proteins in the juices, so you will want to take 1-2 Essentialzymes-4 (yellow capsules).

Essential oils are an ingenious addition to enzyme supplementation. They support enzyme conversion with many added benefits specific to each oil. Many oils—such as Tarragon, Ginger, Peppermint, Juniper, Rosemary, Lemongrass, Anise Seed, Fennel, and Patchouli—are natural enzyme promoters in the body. They help increase the oxygen for the uptake of ATP, adenosine triphosphate, one of the most important (if not the most important) molecules that exists in the body.

ATP provides the chemical energy of fuel within the cells for all processes of human metabolism. Each enzyme supplement contains various oils for the promotion of natural enzyme activity. Enzymes and essential oils work in a synergistic way to promote a healthier digestive system.

Enzymes can be taken in many different quantities for many different needs. Different enzyme supplements may be combined or added for specific digestive functions. Most people are enzyme deficient, which is very detrimental to the healthy state of the body. Optimal digestion and metabolism are dependent on the presence and activation of enzymes.

It is not likely that you will do something wrong by taking too many or combining too many enzymes if you are just using common sense. The body will tell you by how you feel and by the increase in energy that you might experience.

Pay attention to an increase in clarity of thought, awareness, ability to respond faster, more energy to get things done, and not feeling tired or feeling less tired at the end of the day. These are all indicators that things are working better in the body. Minerals, vitamins, enzymes, and water must all be present and work together for a balanced process of nutrient conversion, absorption, and utilization.

Allerzyme is a complex blend of enzymes used to help the body utilize nutrients, combat allergies, expel waste, and prevent gas and bloating. As children reach the age of ten, it is a good time for them to begin taking adult enzymes, which are more complete. Allerzyme (1-2 capsules daily) is a good companion for children because it specifically contains amylase and protease, along with a full complex of enzymes, such as bromelain, to help prevent or alleviate symptoms of allergies, aiding in better digestive function.

Detoxzyme contains amylase and bee pollen rich in amino acids, which are important for healthy body function in the promotion of enzyme development and performance. Detoxzyme is a vegetarian-based enzyme used to help digest milk products, meats, and nuts and to eliminate toxic chemicals and waste.

Detoxzyme can be taken more heavily for a detoxification program, anywhere from 4-6 capsules morning and midday and 6-10 in the evening. Your body can utilize a lot of Detoxzyme. You will know when it is enough if you start to have diarrhea.

The essential oil of Cumin has been recognized as a very powerful detoxifying agent. Combined with Anise Seed and Fennel, it creates nice stimulation of the hydrochloric acid and pepsin that are naturally occurring in the gastrointestinal tract for more effective digestion and cleansing.

Before going to bed, take anywhere from 2 to 10 Detoxzyme, because during the night your body is going through metabolic processes of digestion and assimilation. The liver is detoxifying and "dumping" the waste into the colon to be released in the morning.

Essentialzyme is a multienzyme complex originally formulated to combat degenerative disease. It digests the protein shell around cancer cells so that it can digest and remove the dead cells. It is also used to promote balanced digestion and nutrient assimilation.

It takes a combination of enzymes, minerals, proteins, lipase, and fat for building hormones. Carrot powder is very nourishing, as carrots are one of the highest-enzyme foods that you can eat.

Periodically, a carrot juice fast can be very beneficial for one to two days to build a ready supply of natural enzymes, giving the body an extra boost in detoxifying and cleansing. Alfalfa sprout powder contains 21 minerals, which are critical for the activation of enzymes.

Start your morning with Essentialzyme. Adults: 3-4 before eating and 3-4 after eating. More caplets can be taken if needed. Children: 1 before eating and 1 after eating or both together. It is best to drink water or herbal tea. Drinking smoothies or juices complicates and compromises the ability to digest efficiently.

Essentialzymes-4 (yellow capsule) is a powerful plant enzyme complex and is very specific for the digestion of proteins in meats, eggs, cheese, and other foods high in proteins. It also assists the body in the digestion of sugars and starches found in vegetables and fruits. The essential oils of Anise Seed, Peppermint, and Rosemary are specific for stimulating the production of natural protease in the body.

When eating meals with meat such as beef, chicken, turkey, elk, venison, bison, etc., taking 1 Essentialzymes-4 (yellow capsule) before dinner and 1-2 Allerzyme after dinner works well in aiding digestion to prevent bloating and in helping to alleviate that heavy, lethargic feeling after eating so much.

When overcoming allergies, Essentialzymes-4 (yellow capsule) gives added benefit in breaking down carbohydrates. Take 1-2 Allerzyme for greater support in fighting allergies. If you are still eating proteins at lunchtime but adding carbohydrates like a salad combined with bread and dessert, take 1-2 Essentialzymes-4 (yellow capsules).

If you have a food allergy, a metabolic problem from gastrointestinal surgery, disease in the gastrointestinal tract, or are amylase deficient, take 1-2 Essentialzymes-4 (yellow capsules) with 3-4 Essentialzyme to meet digestive needs.

Essentialzymes-4 (white capsule) contains powerful, fat-digesting enzymes for dairy products, meats, and vegetables and promotes greater nutrient absorption. It is specific for digesting the lipids or fats in foods like avocados, olives, vegetable oils, and meats. Undigested lipids can contribute to gallstones by plugging the pathway out of the gallbladder for the bile and by also causing congestion and plugging the liver, causing increased fat deposits.

Essentialzymes-4 is an important supplement in fat reduction for overweight conditions. Take 1-2 capsules 2 or 3 times a day or as desired. It also contains barley grass, a complex green that is high in minerals needed for enzyme activation.

MightyZyme is formulated especially for children, providing a full spectrum of nutrients and enzymes combined with Ningxia wolfberry. Because MightyZymes are chewable and crunchy, children often think that they are a treat and are happy to eat them. They are a great snack to put in school lunches. Interestingly, many adults prefer MightyZyme over other supplements and eat several daily.

Although enzyme supplementation is a blessing to our modern society, not many people really know the importance of enzymes in our diet. Their function is not well understood and is oftentimes confusing. However, more is being written about enzymes, and more people are beginning to add enzyme supplements to their diet. Many people have different ideas about how they should be used or taken, so perhaps the following suggestions will be helpful.

1. Some people open the capsules and sprinkle the enzymes onto their food, but not very hot food, to get the digestive process started.

2. Because it takes a while for a caplet or capsule to dissolve in your stomach, it is a good idea to take your enzyme caplets and capsules about 30 minutes before eating.

3. Drink plenty of water with your meal because enzymes need water for activation.

4. Chew your food well so that the digestive enzyme cellulase can be released from the fiber; otherwise, you could experience a stomachache with gas and bloating.

5. Eat fresh fruits and vegetables to increase your enzyme intake.

6. Be careful not to eat too many foods that contain enzyme inhibitors, which neutralize some of the enzymes that your body produces. Be moderate in eating such foods as raw seeds, nuts, beans, grains, and especially peanuts and raw wheat germ. Enzyme inhibitors are found in potatoes, concentrated in the potato eyes. Lesser amounts of inhibitors are present in peas, beans, lentils, and egg whites.

7. Traditionally, seeds, nuts, beans, and grains were soaked or partially sprouted before they were eaten. These foods contain many enzyme inhibitors such as phytic acid that can tax the digestive system if eaten excessively.

   Phytic acid is important because it prevents premature germination and stores nutrients for plant growth. However, it combines with minerals such as iron, copper, calcium, magnesium, and zinc in the intestinal tract and interferes with nutrient absorption.

   Soaking these types of foods in an acid medium such as lemon juice or whey or even in water neutralizes the enzyme inhibitors and can make the vitamin and mineral content more available.

8. You can also destroy the inhibitors by cooking, but then that destroys the enzymes. The better way is by soaking, rinsing, germinating, and sprouting. This destroys the inhibitors while increasing enzyme production.

9. Another way to neutralize these inhibitors is to take extra enzymes when eating ungerminated or unsprouted seeds and nuts.

10. Fermentation also neutralizes damaging chemicals found in grains and beans. Fermentation adds many beneficial micro-

organisms to foods, making them more digestible, which increases the flora in the intestinal tract.

A diet in unfermented whole grains can lead to mineral deficiencies and bone loss. The easiest way to cause fermentation is to put the beans, seeds, and grains in water, add whey or yogurt, and let them stand for seven or eight hours. A local health food store should carry whey or yogurt powder. Beans are even better if left in water for 12 hours.

11. Kefir is a special culture used in milk that promotes fermentation and a fermented milk drink that produces many enzymes during its creation.

12. Small amounts of salt can also work as an enzyme inhibitor, so be careful. Besides the fact that salt is not the best choice to use in your diet because of the numerous health problems it can cause, it would be best to just eliminate it from your diet. Salt certainly has a place in the balance of diet, but today, white table salt is overused and becomes an enemy to the body.

The choice is yours. When you come to understand the critical importance of enzymes and the life-giving role they perform in our bodies, you have certainly discovered many possible explanations for health problems that you or those around you may have.

You can also see how you might prevent future health problems from arising. Knowledge gives hope, especially when products are available that can increase your potential for vibrant health and longevity.

For those who are already on a path of a healthier lifestyle, it is critical to spread this information to others who are searching for answers and to help those who do not know what questions to ask. We need to educate, strengthen, uplift people everywhere, and protect our children and the babies yet to be born.

MINERALS: WE CAN'T LIVE WITHOUT THEM

A mineral is a solid chemical substance that is naturally formed through geological processes. All minerals come from the ground and make their way into our bodies through the foods we eat that grow in the ground and the foods we eat that come from the animals that live off the land. Fruits, vegetables, meats, nuts, grains, poultry, and dairy products provide a rich source of minerals that our bodies need to live and function properly in conjunction with vitamins and other nutrients such as enzymes.

The difference between vitamins and minerals is that vitamins contain carbon, classifying them as organic substances. Minerals do not contain carbon and are therefore classified as inorganic.

There are two categories of minerals: major, or large minerals, and trace minerals. The difference between them is determined by how much the body needs. The body needs a daily minimum of 100 milligrams of major minerals and less than 100 milligrams daily of trace minerals.

Minerals are a major part of every cell in all forms of life. Enzymes need minerals to build strong, healthy organisms, whether they are human, animal, or plant. All foods have minerals, but some have more than others. Plants take the minerals from the ground; we eat the plants and take the minerals from them, use the ones we need, and eliminate the ones we don't need.

We really don't give any thought to it until something starts to go wrong in our bodies. Then we start looking and asking for answers. Becoming educated about how our body works and what it needs is a key to staying healthy. But too often we wait until we have problems before we start to educate ourselves.

Unfortunately, our soil is devitalized of many nutrients and contaminated with chemicals from the pollution in the air and water and from man-made products that are sprayed to supposedly protect our crops and help them grow. Perhaps in days gone by, we could get the minerals and vitamins we needed from rich topsoil, but foods grown commercially today don't produce the quality crops that can provide the nutrients we need.

We would all do well to grow our own organic gardens, but few can do so, and often those who have the ground available are too busy. "It's just too much work." So what do we do? With a little education and awareness, we can start to improve our diet with fresh, organic fruits and vegetables and buy foods that specifically say they are grown and produced in a natural environment. This is especially true of eggs and meat products.

Commercial food companies have been promoting the vitamin and mineral content of their products for quite some time. We see "fortified with vitamins and minerals" on many labels. Perhaps this list below will give you an idea of the importance of having good mineral balance in your body.

Major Minerals

Calcium builds strong bones and teeth and is needed for muscle growth. It helps to normalize blood clotting and may help to prevent bone loss and osteoporosis. It is most effective in combination with vitamins A, C, D, iron, magnesium, manganese, and phosphorus. **Food**

sources: milk products such as yogurt and cheese, whole grains, unrefined cereals, green vegetables, sardines, salmon, soybeans, and peanuts.

Phosphorus maintains healthy bones and teeth and is found in every cell to help make energy. **Food sources:** fish, poultry, beef, eggs, milk products, almonds, lentils, peanuts, pumpkin seeds, and whole wheat.

Magnesium helps muscles and nerves, keeps the heart rhythm smooth, and keeps bones strong. **Food sources:** green vegetables, legumes, nuts, seeds, whole wheat, and milk products.

Sodium ions regulate blood and body fluids. Sodium also maintains proper acid-base balance in the transmission of nerve impulses, smooth heart function, and good blood pressure (See Chloride below). **Food sources:** barley, beets and beet greens, carrot juice, celery, kelp, some cheeses, milk from goats and cows, and buttermilk.

Potassium supports the muscular and nervous systems and maintains electrolyte balance between blood and body tissues (See Chloride below). **Food sources:** prunes, prune juice, bamboo shoots, chard, sweet potato (must be cooked with whole skin), beet greens, orange juice, white beans, dates, yogurt, raisins, clams, tomato puree, blackstrap molasses, halibut, yellow tuna, Pacific rockfish, Pacific cod, winter squash, soybeans, kidney beans, lentils, plantains, apricots, prunes, and bananas.

Sulfur is found in all cells and especially in cartilage and keratin. It is important for healthy hair, skin, and nails and helps to maintain oxygen balance for healthy brain function. **Food sources:** garlic, onions, cabbage, cau-liflower, asparagus, dried beans, nuts, chives, fish, and eggs.

Chloride is an electrolyte—along with potassium and sodium—that keeps the body fluids in balance. The cells need potassium on the inside and sodium on the outside. Sodium and potassium have a positive electrical charge and constantly move into the cells and then out of the cells to maintain balance. Chloride has a negative charge, which balances with the sodium and potassium. This constant movement allows these minerals to carry nutrients into the cells and waste out of the cells.

Chloride helps alleviate fluid retention and keeps sodium balanced to maintain good blood pH and healthy kidney function. Chloride also helps with digestion in the production of hydrochloric acid. **Food sources**: seaweed, sea salt, rye, tomatoes, lettuce, celery, and olives.

Trace Minerals

Chromium improves the efficiency of insulin in metabolizing carbohydrates and helps maintain normal blood pressure. **Food sources:** lean meats, whole grains, liver, cheese, eggs, and brewer's yeast.

Copper strengthens the metabolic processes in the body in combination with amino acids and vitamins. It fortifies enzymatic reactions in the utilization of iron and benefits connective tissue, hair, eyes, aging, and energy production. It supports the thyroid, smooths the heart rhythm, promotes wound healing, and prevents the buildup of cholesterol. **Food sources:** meat, liver, seafood, beans, whole grains, soy flour, wheat bran, almonds, avocados, barley, garlic, nuts, oats, molasses, beets, and lentils.

Iodine makes two thyroid hormones: triiodothyronine and thyroxine, which control and regulate basal metabolic rate, which determines how fast and efficiently the body burns calories. It is very important for proper cell metabolism. Thyroid hormones help control the mental development of children and their overall growth. Iodine is an effective antiseptic for cleaning wounds and healing the skin. **Food sources:** kelp (sea vegetable), vegetables grown in iodine-rich soil, yogurt, cow's milk, eggs (whole: cooked or boiled), strawberries, mozzarella cheese, and often fish and shellfish.

Iron is necessary for the production of hemoglobin, the primary component of red blood cells that carries oxygen to every cell of the body and removes carbon dioxide. Iron cannot function properly without calcium and copper and is necessary for the metabolism of B vitamins. **Food sources:** liver, beef, baked beans, white beans, soy beans, lima beans, black-eyed peas, fish, chicken, oatmeal, rye bread, whole wheat bread, prune juice, prunes, dried apricots, raisins, plums, spinach, peas, asparagus, Brewer's yeast, kelp, squash, molasses, wheat bran, pumpkin seeds, squash seeds, and sunflower seeds.

Manganese, although needed only in small amounts, is an antioxidant that fights free radicals. Manganese-activated enzymes help metabolize cholesterol, carbohydrates, and amino acids. It also helps to heal wounds and helps bones and cartilage to form properly. Manganese aids the body in the use of vitamin B_1, biotin, and vitamin C. **Food sources:** leafy vegetables, whole grains, pecans, almonds, peanuts, brown rice, whole wheat bread, pinto beans, lima beans, navy beans, spinach, sweet potatoes, avocados, eggs, and pineapple.

Molybdenum is found in most plants and animal tissue. It is essential to the enzymatic action of protein synthesis and the use of iron in the body. Food sources:

meats, whole grains, buckwheat, barley, wheat germ, legumes, lima beans, sunflower seeds, and dark green leafy vegetables.

Selenium is an important antioxidant that protects against the formation of free radical cells and works well with vitamin E. It is needed by the white blood cells to fight microorganisms and is important to the T-cells of the immune system to produce cytokines, which work as messengers between the cells. It appears that low selenium causes a risk of viral infections. It may be no coincidence that flu viruses and viruses like Bird Flu originate in a large area of China with selenium-deficient soil. Research has shown that selenium prevents and fights against cancer. **Food sources:** bran, broccoli, onions, tomatoes, tuna, and wheat germ.

Zinc is one of the most important minerals used by the body; it helps in the production of over 100 enzymes your body needs. It supports growth, builds immunity, maintains your senses of smell and taste, helps to heal wounds, and is critical for DNA synthesis. **Food sources:** beef, lamb, crabmeat, turkey, chicken, lobster, clams, salmon, milk, cheese, yeast, beans, whole grain cereals, brown rice, whole wheat bread, potatoes, yogurt, and pumpkin seeds.

Minerals are extremely important, but few people know why. The body needs iron to make the hemoglobin found in red blood cells. Calcium is necessary for kidney, muscle, and nerve function. The thyroid cannot work without iodine. The thyroid controls many functions in the body, and one of them is to produce energy. How often do we hear, "If you don't have enough energy, your thyroid must be low"? Manganese, selenium, and zinc work as antioxidants and help in the healing of wounds, the growth of the skeletal system, and the protection of cell membranes. Chromium helps keep the arteries clear.

The information about minerals is voluminous, and to really understand their purpose and how they work takes a lot of time, study, and research. But there is no doubt about their importance in maintaining a well-functioning body. Because the nutrients in so much of our food are depleted, how do our bodies get the nutrients that are needed to achieve and maintain optimal health? In the past, doctors and scientists have said that supplementation was not necessary because we could get all the nutrients we needed if we ate properly.

Today, the story is different. Even the Food and Drug Administration (FDA) is regulating the food industry and requiring that certain vitamins and minerals be added to commercial foods. More and more, people are turning to supplementation.

Most liquid minerals don't taste very good. It's

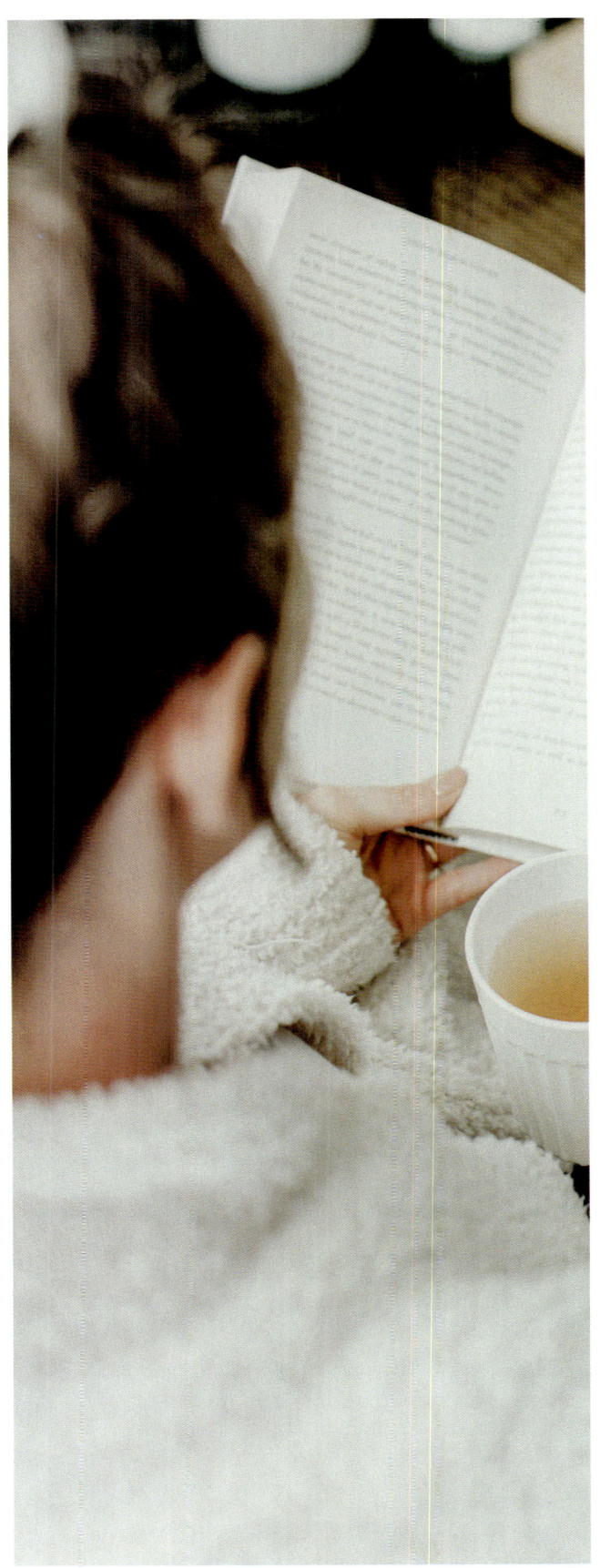

easy to swallow capsules or tablets, but liquid minerals are different. Some taste so awful that no one wants to consume them. However, there is one that isn't bad tasting at all—Mineral Essence. As a liquid, it is much easier and quicker for the body to assimilate and is more efficient.

Mineral Essence is an organic, liquid ionic mineral complex with more than 60 very fine ionic minerals that assimilate much easier than other mineral compounds that are taken from dirt, rocks, or other sources. Mineral Essence is uniquely formulated with essential oils to enhance its bioavailability, supplying the body with the most efficient and best-balanced mineral formula that we have found at the present time.

Minerals are essential for activating certain enzymes for digestion and metabolic function, and the minerals found in Mineral Essence are very specific for the promotion of a healthy digestive tract, reducing the risk of candida and food allergens.

Some people like to drink it in cold juice such as NingXia Red wolfberry juice or some other combination that they have discovered that helps with the taste. However, the benefits far outweigh any resistance to the taste. When one thinks of sustaining life without dysfunction or disease, Mineral Essence is certainly worth putting to the test.

WATER: THE PURITY OF LIFE

Nothing is more refreshing when you are hot and thirsty than a drink of clear, cold, spring water. However, water is not only refreshing, but it is absolutely essential to life. Most of us probably don't think of water as one of the body's building blocks, but water is the second most critical substance we need for maintaining life. Without water, life ceases to exist. Water is the activator of all body functions and facilitates growth, development, strength, and vitality. The only substance more important to the body than water is oxygen.

The human body on average is over 70 percent water. Certain vital organs and systems have an even higher concentration: the brain is over 75 percent, the blood is over 80 percent, and the liver is amazingly made up of 96 percent water. To a large degree, we are what we drink.

Water is crucial for our body's self-cleansing system. We are certainly aware of the body's normal elimination processes, but the body also eliminates waste through exhalation and perspiration, both of which require water. Our kidneys cannot cleanse efficiently if our system does not have enough water to carry the waste away.

Water (H_2O) plays a role in nearly every chemical reaction in the body. Aside from aiding in digestion and absorption of food, water regulates body temperature and blood circulation, carries nutrients to cells, and removes toxins and other wastes. Water also protects joints, tissues, and organs, including the spinal cord, from shock and damage.

The ideal amount of water to consume is half your body weight in ounces per day. That means if you weigh 160 pounds, you should drink 80 ounces of water or about ten 8-ounce glasses per day. Lack of water or a state of dehydration will cause many maladies such as hypertension, asthma, allergies, migraine headaches, dizziness, and many more.

The amount of water we drink greatly affects our energy level. Over 80 percent of our population suffers from low energy because they don't drink enough water. Science has proven that if the average person drops as little as 5 percent in body fluids, he or she will suffer a 25 to 30 percent loss of energy. A 15 percent drop in body fluids will cause death.

The liver needs water to metabolize fat into useable energy. Therefore, drinking pure water will help metabolize and shed stored fat, resulting in more energy and less fat.

All day long we lose water from our bodies. When we breathe, we lose moisture to the air every time we exhale—as much as 2 cups a day. We also lose water through evaporation from the surface of our skin, even without rigorous exercise; and, of course, we also pass water in our urine. A healthy adult can lose 8 to 10 cups of water a day. With exercise, the amount greatly increases. Many drinks like soda, coffee, and tea contain caffeine, which has a diuretic effect, leading to increased loss of fluids through frequent urination.

The function of every cell in our body is controlled by electrical signals sent through our nervous system from the brain. Our nerves, in reality, are an elaborate system of tiny waterways. If the fluid inside our nerves thickens due to dehydration or is contaminated with synthetic chemicals or toxic heavy metals like lead, the vital signals can get distorted.

Many experts now believe that the distortion of these signals may be the root cause of many degenerative diseases and neurological illnesses, including Attention Deficit Disorder, Chronic Fatigue Syndrome, anxiety, depression, and even Alzheimer's disease.

Because water is such a major factor in brain and nervous system functions, its purity is probably the most basic component for longevity. Proper digestion and nutrient absorption depend on a healthy intake of water. We must drink plenty of pure water for our bodies to convert and assimilate the nutrients from our food and the supplements we take.

The amount of pure water we drink determines how efficiently our body can detoxify by excreting the body's waste. Water is the body's primary means of flushing out toxins, the key to disease prevention. Every day we are exposed to hundreds of harmful substances. Our air, food, and everything we touch contains traces of harmful chemicals. Unfortunately, we can't keep toxins from getting into our body, but we can help our body get rid of them by drinking plenty of pure water. The more pure water we drink, the more we allow our body to detoxify and purify itself.

Because water is so crucial to life, it is crucial that we drink pure water. Constantly drinking water that is contaminated will eventually lead to a miserable state of health and early death.

Finding pure drinking water is becoming a challenge. Our increasingly polluted world has made it necessary for the Environmental Protection Agency to set water standards. The EPA screens for the presence of suspended solids, oil, grease, fecal coliform bacteria, chemicals, and heavy metals. Unfortunately, 65 percent of the major source of pollution does not come from industrial sites, which can be regulated, but from stormwater runoff.

Rainfall encountering pollutants from agricultural and industrial operations absorbs these chemicals and transports them into lakes and rivers. Today, about 35 percent of water pollution comes from actual industrial sites.

Excessive and uncontrolled use of chemical fertilizers and pesticides promotes contaminated agricultural runoff. This not only pollutes the surface drains, but the water trickling down to lower layers of soil also causes a severe contamination of the natural aquifer.

The World Health Organization (WHO) reports that 25-30 percent of all hospital admissions are connected to water-borne bacterial and parasitic conditions, and 60 percent of infant deaths are caused by water infections.

The long-term effects on human health of pesticides and other pollutants include colon and bladder cancer, miscarriages, birth defects, deformation of bones, and sterility.

Contamination of fresh water with radionuclides, which can result from mining, testing, disposing, and manufacturing of radioactive material and transportation accidents, has led to increased incidences of cancer, developmental abnormalities, and death.

Cesspools of stagnant, dirty water, both in rural and urban areas, account for a large number of deaths caused by potentially fatal diseases like cholera, malaria, dysentery, and typhoid.

Nitrate concentration in water above 45 mg/l makes it unfit for drinking by infants. The nitrates are reduced in the body to nitrites and cause a serious blood condition called "Blue Baby Syndrome." Higher concentrations of nitrates cause gastric cancer. Untreated and highly toxic industrial sewage is also used for irrigation near major cities, which contaminates crops and consequently affects consumers.

According to EPA reports, 40 million Americans are exposed to levels of lead in water that exceed the EPA-proposed maximum contaminant allowances. Even at low levels, lead in water causes reduced birth weight, premature births, delayed mental development, and impaired mental abilities. In 2014 between 6,000 and 12,000 children in Flint, Michigan, were exposed to high levels of lead in their drinking water.

Using information gathered from the EPA, the National Resources Defense Council (NRDC) reports that more than 25 million Americans drink tap water polluted with fecal matter, pesticides, toxic chemicals, radiation, and lead.

The tap water in some cities has parasites in it, so it is not good drinking water. Tap water contains chlorine, which kills bacteria but is very bad for you to drink. In the book Natural Cures,[4] Kevin Trudeau says, "All tap water is poisonous. All tap water is loaded with chlorine and chlorine byproducts. Chlorine sears your arteries and, along with hydrogenated oil and homogenized dairy products, causes heart disease. Most tap water also has fluoride, which is one of the most poisonous and disease-causing agents [that] you can put in your body. Do not drink or use tap water except for washing your floor." Tap water is not pure drinking water.

The purpose of water is not nutrition. The purpose of water is to transport things. It brings the nutrition in and takes the waste out.

Paul Bragg, ND, PhD, says in The Shocking Truth About Water,[5] "The greatest damage done by inorganic minerals—plus waxy cholesterol and salt—is to the small arteries and other blood vessels of the brain. Hardening of the arteries and calcification of the blood vessels starts on the day you start taking inorganic chemicals and minerals from tap water into our bodies."

Municipal or city water should be avoided if possible, and that includes public swimming pools as well. Most municipal waters have a high concentration of aluminum due to the use of aluminum hydroxide for water treatment. Moreover, the addition of chlorine results in the creation of cancer-causing chemicals when dissolved; organic solids are chemically altered by chlorination. While there is a trend toward replacing chlorination with peroxide treatment of water, it will be decades before peroxide is adopted as a standard.

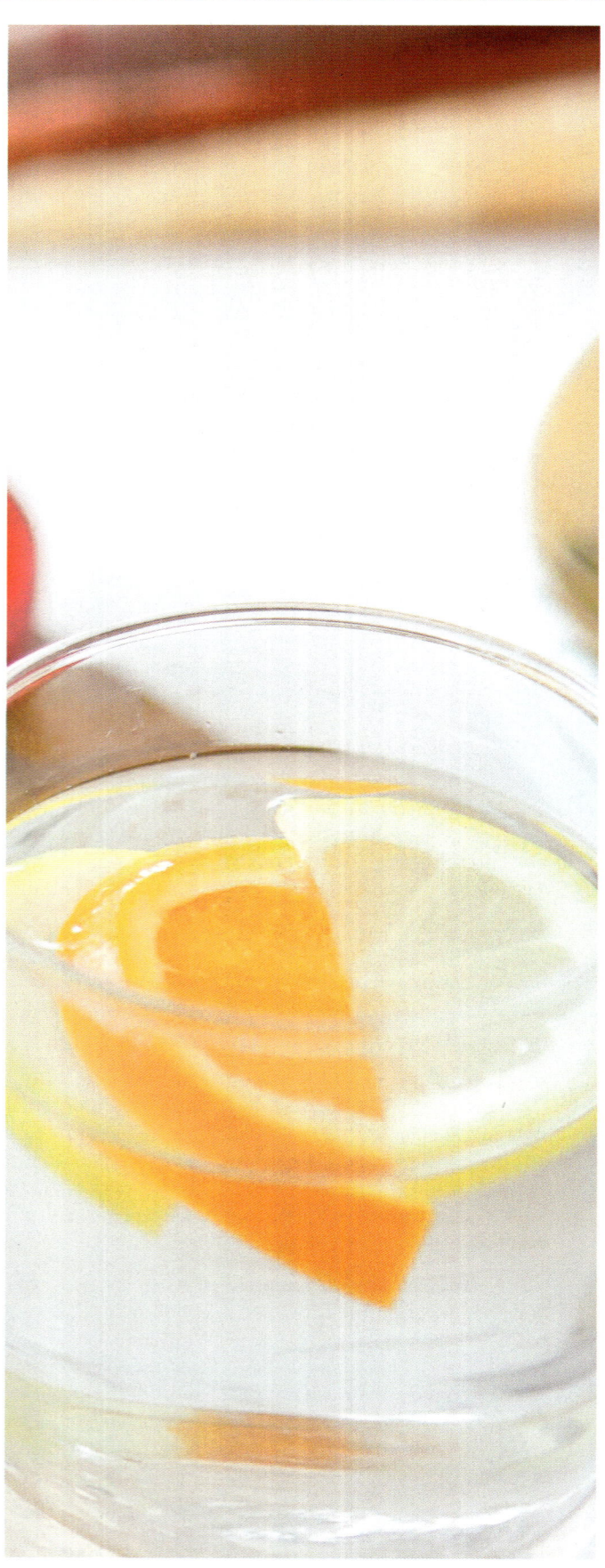

Chlorine

Have you noticed when you walk near an enclosed swimming pool area of a hotel that you have to hold your breath to block the horrible smell of chlorine? Chlorine is one of the most reactive and toxic elements known to man. It is very damaging to the thyroid, which is a major, regulating organ in the body. When it malfunctions, major health issues arise. When put in the public water supply as a disinfectant, chlorine creates disinfection byproducts (DBP) that can cause cancer, birth defects, and spontaneous abortions. This information makes "chlorinated sugar" (i.e., Splenda®) not quite so desirable.

Besides being used in the water supply, chlorine is also chemically bonded in the manufacture of numerous industrial chemicals. Many toxic herbicides, fungicides, and insecticides are created by attaching one or more chlorine molecules to a carbon skeleton. Once ingested or inhaled, chlorinated chemicals penetrate the fat cells and become trapped.

Some of the most common and toxic of these chemicals include a quartet of chlorinated carcinogenic chemicals known as trihalomethanes (THMs): chloroform, bromoform, bromodichloromethane, and chlorobromomethane. These trihalomethanes are created when chlorine reacts with naturally occurring organic matter in raw water.

THMs are very volatile and can mix with both air and water. From the air they can be inhaled during bathing as well as consumed with potable water. Showering, washing dishes, and flushing a toilet can also contaminate the air with trihalomethanes.

Once inhaled or ingested, THMs accumulate in the fat cells—the same way dioxins do. Once trapped inside the body, they chemically bind with and damage DNA.

A California Department of Health study surveyed 5,144 pregnant women to determine the effects of THM in the drinking water.[6] They measured levels of THM from water tests obtained from public utility records and matched these against the study group.

They found that pregnant women who consumed more than five glasses of water a day containing more than 75 ppb (parts per billion) had double the risk of spontaneous abortion. Women who drank less water or who drank water with lower levels of THM had substantially lower risk of miscarriage. Women who drank filtered water also had significantly lower risk of miscarriage.

Researchers at the University of North Carolina at Chapel Hill also examined the link between THM and miscarriages in populations living throughout central North Carolina.[7] They found that women who suffered the highest exposure to THM in their drinking water tripled the risk of miscarriage.

Another study conducted by the U.S. Department of Health and Human Services examined the effect of THM in the water supply of 75 towns throughout the state of New Jersey.[8] When scientists compared levels of THMs to the frequency of birth defects, they found that women who consumed water exceeding 80 ppb THMs had triple the risk of giving birth to infants with neural tube defects. The authors suggested that one of the reasons for this may be the fact that vitamin B12 may be disrupted in the body due to chloroform, a common THM.

Another statewide study in New Jersey also linked THMs in drinking water to a doubled risk of neural tube defects.[9]

An even larger epidemiological study by the National Institute of Public Health in Norway surveyed the effects of chlorinated water on 141,077 infants born in Norway between 1993 and 1995.[10] Researchers found that the higher the chlorine content of the water and the higher the organic matter in the water, the higher the risk for birth defects, including cardiac defects, respiratory tract defects, and urinary tract defects.

Murray S. Malcolm, MD, a public health physician in New Zealand, spearheaded a countrywide study that examined the role of THMs in triggering birth defects and cancer. He concluded, "A quarter of all bladder, colon, rectal cancers, and birth defects may be preventable by reducing disinfection byproducts (i.e., THMs) exposure."[11]

A Solution

There are many ways of avoiding chlorine and the many other toxic chemicals found in water, but it isn't necessarily simple. It is most important that we avoid these chemicals in any way possible. The cost of the physical problems that contaminated water can bring can be astronomical.

Bottled water is probably one of the easiest ways to avoid contamination, but can you be certain that this water is free of chemicals and safe to drink? Regardless of cost, the bottled water you buy may simply be tap water put through a filtration process. Naturally, there are many reliable water bottling companies, but regulation in this industry is vague, and so we must be aware all the time of the water we choose to drink.

Buying drinking water does not protect consumers from inhaling vapors. Reports from the EPA indicate that entities such as mining companies and electrical power plants release 7.8 billion pounds of toxic substances per year onto the land, into the water, and into the air,

and the amount is increasing. The NRDC reports that over 940,000 Americans are sickened by contaminated tap water annually. In addition, the council reports that contaminated tap water kills 900 people each year.

Many people today are investing in water purifiers for home and business alike. There are many and varied types of purifiers. Some attach under the sink to filter the water as it comes through the tap. Other filtration systems work for the entire house and filter the water as it comes into the house from the outside. You need to weigh the cost with the perceived benefit and make the best decision you can.

Many choose to drink distilled water to be sure of getting pure water, although there has always been controversy over drinking purified versus distilled water, which almost becomes a personal preference. You can distill the water or let it stand unsealed, which allows the chlorine to evaporate over time.

Naturally, adding an essential oil will always be of great benefit to help maintain the purification of the water. Essential oils like Lemon, Clove, Orange, Cinnamon, Peppermint, etc., purify your water and taste great as well. Distilled water washes out the system. With the help of essential oils in distilled water, the body can excrete petroleum residues, metals, inorganic minerals, and other toxins.

One drop per glass is generally enough. Put the oil in a glass or container first and then fill the container with water. Since oil does not mix with water, putting the oil in first will help disperse it through the water.

Several drops of oil can be put in the end of the carbon filter of a water purification system so that when the water leaves the filter, it carries oil molecules with it as it goes into the water system of your house. This can drop nitrate levels by up to 3,000 ppm.

The inhalation of trihalomethanes in a vapor form that occurs with hot water while showering is more toxic than drinking chlorinated water. A good showerhead filter is important to be able to shower and bathe in chlorine-free water.

While carbon filters are good for removing chlorine from water, the best water purifiers have preflash or preboiling chambers to flash off volatile gases such as chlorine and petroleum products. The steam should rise at least 15 inches to balance the pH and fall 15 inches to oxygenate again.

One very popular water purification system is the ion exchange used with "hard" water, or water with dissolved minerals. Water is passed through a filter, exchanging charged particles (ions) in the water for charged particles in the filter. Most units use salt, with sodium and chloride ions exchanging for the contaminated ions in the water. Since the minerals are replaced with salt, at least one cold water tap needs to be left out of the system so that drinking water is not loaded with sodium.

Types of Water Filtration Cartridges for Home Systems

Many types of filters may be purchased for home use, but only three of them are discussed below.

A dual-gradient filter has one layer wrapped around the other to provide finer filtration than is found in most other filters. In the second layer, the water flows through a high-powered carbon briquette filter system, not available through retail channels. The dual-gradient cartridge has three times the dirt-holding capacity of similarly sized cartridges. It removes sediment such as dirt, sand, grit, rust, etc., from the water to extend the life of the charcoal filters. In addition, the inner layers reduce the levels of fine particles.

The carbon briquette filter system contains a superior carbon-briquette cartridge of bonded powdered charcoal. The powdered consistency of the briquette allows for increased surface contact that results in maximum absorption of chlorine. The 0.5-micron post filter greatly reduces bacteria, including giardia and cryptosporidium. This carbon filter removes trihalomethanes, which might otherwise be consumed, absorbed through the skin, or inhaled during a shower. It also reduces lead and removes pesticides, odors, and objectionable tastes.

A UV filtration unit is sold separately. It kills all types of viruses, bacteria, and fungi and is often combined with other types of carbon filters to add to the purification of the water and your protection.

Water is life itself, and pure water is critical, no matter what the cost. With anything less than pure water, the body cannot perform its metabolic functions in an efficient, healthy way. We need to study and become knowledgeable about the overwhelming damage that comes from drinking contaminated water and the undeniable benefits and health that come from drinking pure water. Think of your family, your friends, and all the children who are not aware of this crucial aspect in our lives. Make them aware so that the best choices are made to attain a vibrant life.

ENDNOTES

1. Pottenger FM. Pottenger's cats: a study in nutrition. 2nd ed. Lemon Grove (CA): Price-Pottenger Nutrition Foundation; 1983. 126 p.
2. Warren M, Beck S, Rayburn J. State of obesity issue report. Princeton (NJ): Robert Wood Johnson Foundation; 2018 Sept; 68 p.
3. Global health observatory (GHO) data: obesity situation and trends [Internet]. World Health Organization. Geneva, Switzerland.
4. Trudeau, Kevin. Natural cures "they" don't want you to know about. Elk Grove Village (IL): Alliance Publishing Group Inc; 2004. 572 p.
5. Bragg PC, Bragg P. The shocking truth about water. Santa Barbara (CA): Bragg Live Foods; c1985. 121 p.
6. Windham GC, Wallker K, Anderson M, Fenster L, Mendola P, Swan S. Chlorination by-products in drinking water and menstrual cycle function. Environmental Medicine. 2003 June;111(7):935-941.
7. Savitz DA, Andrews KW, Pastore LM. Drinking water and pregnancy outcome in central North Carolina: source, amount, and trihalomethane levels. Environ Health Perspect. 1995 June;103(6):592-6.
8. Bove FJ, Fulcomer MC, Klotz JB, Esmart J, Dufficy EM, Savrin JE. Public drinking water contamination and birth outcomes. Am J Epidemiol. 1995 May 1;141(9):850-62.
9. Klotz JB, Pyrch LA. Neural tube defects and drinking water disinfection by-products. Epidemiology. 1999 Jul;10(4):383-390.
10. Magnus P, Jaakkola JJ, Skrondal A, Alexander J, Becher G, Krogh T, Dybing E. Water chlorination and birth defects. Epidemiology. 1999 Sept;10(5):513-517.
11. Malcolm MS, Weinstein P, Woodward AJ. Something in the water? A health impact assessment of disinfection by-products in New Zealand. N Z Med J. 1999 Oct 22;112(1098):404-407.

Longevity & Vitality – Special Features

LIVING LONGER WITH ESSENTIAL OILS

Essential oils and aromatics were some of the most highly prized natural remedies of the ancient world. References to cassia, clove, frankincense, myrrh, cinnamon, and rosemary appear in many historical manuscripts, including the Old and New Testaments, the writings of Hippocrates, Avicenna, Egyptian hieroglyphics, and other ancient writings, pictographs, and legends.

Intriguing new research offers a fascinating glimpse into the far-reaching potential of essential oils, like thyme, to reverse or slow the aging process by acting as powerful antioxidants that protect tissues and organs from damaging stress and deterioration.

Other essential oils such as clove and lemon have been shown to not only act as powerful antioxidants but also to protect cellular DNA from damage and to act as potent antiseptics with broad-spectrum, germ-killing properties.

Frankincense, myrrh, and balsam have been used since the beginning of mankind and even anciently were known for their spiritual and physical healing properties.

Essential oils have their own specific chemical constituents that target particular body functions for maintaining good health and emotional well-being. Hundreds of essential studies document the value of these oils in fighting physical and mental dysfunction as well as chronic and life-threatening diseases.

AGING: THE POWER OF ESSENTIAL OILS

There is much controversy and many theories over the causes of aging and premature death. Some researchers believe that declining levels of hormones from the pituitary and hypothalamus are the culprits. Still others blame the buildup of lipofuscin, a brownish pigment that accumulates inside the cells, particularly nerve and heart muscle cells.[1]

However, the oxidative, stress-free theory of aging is the most persuasive and substantiated. One scientific thought is that aging is caused by cumulative, oxidative stress to the cell walls, receptors, and DNA. Rogue electrons that are generated from normal metabolic and immune functions attack proteins and disrupt DNA, eventually overloading the natural repair abilities of the body, which sometimes leads to disease and death.[2,3,4]

Many researchers have focused on damage to the DNA as the cause of aging. DNA is a nucleic acid that contains the blueprint for genetic instructions or cellular activity used in the growth and function of all living organisms. Few scientists have understood how devastating free radical damage can be to fats—especially the unstable polyunsaturated fatty acids (PUFAs) that form the phospholipid membranes of almost every cell in the body. When these fatty membranes are attacked by free radicals, ion transport and hormone receptors are disrupted.[5] As cell membranes become less fluid, they lose their ability to function normally. This can hasten the onset of tissue and organ damage and lead to premature death.

One of the most easy-to-understand examples of the detrimental effects of cell membrane deterioration occurs in the blood vessel walls. As the blood vessels lose their flexibility, the risk of hypertension (high blood pressure) increases, as does the incidence of arteriosclerosis.

Free radical damage seems to escalate with age because antioxidant protection declines as we grow older. Free radical scavengers, such as superoxide dismutase (SOD) and glutathione peroxidase, show a steady decline along with other antioxidants. This means that the older we become, the less efficient the body is in neutralizing free radicals and combating the oxidative damage that gradually weakens and eventually destroys key organs.

Levels of polyunsaturated fats such as DHA (docosahexaenoic acid) are also crucial for healthy brain and eye function. DHA occurs in unusually high concentrations in the cerebral cortex—the most advanced part of the brain structure, where logic and reasoning take place. When DHA becomes oxidized and loses its double bonds because of free radical attacks, brain and cognitive function can deteriorate. This can lead to memory loss, dementia, and even death. By protecting fats like DHA from free radical attack, hydrolysis, or oxidation, brain health can be significantly improved.[6,7,8,9]

Essential Oils vs. Fatty Oils

Fatty oils are very different from essential oils. Cottonseed, almond, olive, corn, sunflower, and canola oil are all fatty oils that are usually pressed from a seed or fruit. They are greasy in texture and have little odor, being simple mixtures of several different fatty acids (i.e., capric, stearic, and oleic).

In contrast, essential oils are usually steam distilled from leaves, flowers, roots, and bark. They have strong odors and are not greasy. Because many are lighter than water, they float and tend to evaporate very easily. Essential oils are complex mosaics of hundreds of aromatic molecules (i.e., terpenes, sesquiterpenes, and phenols) that usually have a ring-like structure.

CAPRIC FATTY ACID (from coconut oil)

THYMOL (from thyme ess. oil)

The root of the problem is that DHA and other long-chain PUFAs are very unstable and vulnerable to chemical alteration and oxidation. This means that the antioxidant function of the body must work overtime to protect the PUFAs in order to sustain health. An even greater problem is that with age, the liver slows down the production of PUFAs and thus becomes less and less able to replace the dwindling supply of PUFAs needed to sustain the brain, tissues, and other organs.[10]

Therefore, the longevity of the organism is strongly linked to preserving the integrity of the polyunsaturated fats that comprise cells, nerves, and other tissues. Preventing the degradation of these fats from free radical damage can forestall the signs of accelerated aging.

Research: Antioxidative Properties of Essential Oils

In the late 1980s, Dr. Radwan Farag of the biochemistry department of the University of Cairo was among the first to show in vitro how selected essential oils were able to significantly slow the rancidity or oxidation of fatty oils such as cottonseed oil. He dosed samples of cottonseed oil with 200 ppm of thyme oil (55.7 percent thymol and 36 percent p-cymene) and 400 ppm of clove oil (85.3 percent eugenol). After comparing the essential oil-treated samples with untreated control samples, he found that both thyme and clove oils showed significant protection against rancidity to the cottonseed oil. Thyme oil reduced rancidity by 20 percent, while clove oil reduced the rancidity by almost 30 percent.[11] A second study by Dr. Farag and his colleagues showed that essential oils such as thyme (Thymus vulgaris), clove (Syzygium aromaticum), rosemary (Rosmarinus officinalis), and sage (Salvia officinalis) arrested the oxidation of linoleic acid, a polyunsaturated omega-6 fatty acid.[12]

In addition, Dr. Farag demonstrated the safety of these essential oils in vivo. When he added thyme and clove oils to rat feed rations at up to six times the minimum concentration needed to stall fat oxidation, none of the rats studied suffered any negative side effects. Essential oil-fed rats exhibited no difference in protein, cholesterol, and liver enzyme levels (SGPT, SGOT) when compared with a control group.[13]

Protecting Fats and Phospholipids in Animals

Almost a decade after Farag's groundbreaking research, another series of more intensive in vivo studies was begun at the Scottish Agricultural College in the United Kingdom and the Semmelweis University of Medicine in Hungary. In these clinical trials, researchers found that daily lifelong feeding of thyme and clove oils to laboratory animals preserved key antioxidant levels in the liver, kidneys, heart, and brain. Even more importantly, essential oils arrested the oxidation and destruction of long-chain PUFAs throughout the organism.

One of the first studies to document these remarkable antioxidant effects was conducted at the Semmelweis University of Medicine in 1993. Researchers fed different groups of mice with daily doses of 0.72 mg of essential oils, including thyme, clove, nutmeg, and black pepper. Groups of younger mice, 6 months old, were treated for 5 weeks, while groups of 22-month-old mice were treated for 21 weeks. Following treatment, the livers of the animals were examined for levels of C_{20} and C_{22} polyunsaturated fatty acids, which usually decline substantially during the animal's lifetime.

The results were phenomenal. According to the researchers, ". . . dietary administration of the volatile oils to the aging mice had a marked effect on fatty acid distribution by virtually restoring the proportions of the polyunsaturated fatty acids within the phospholipids to the levels observed in young mice."[14]

Another randomized, controlled animal study at Semmelweis University in 1987 showed that these same essential oils—thyme, clove, nutmeg, and pepper—restored DHA in the eyes to much younger levels. As a long-chain polyunsaturated fatty acid (PUFA) that is very fragile and easily oxidized, DHA is absolutely crucial for normal eye health. Declining levels of DHA have been directly linked to heightened risk of age-related macular degeneration, the leading cause of blindness in old age.[15]

In this case, dietary supplementation of just 3.9 mg per day of essential oils to laboratory animals over a 17-month period was sufficient to markedly slow DHA loss in their eyes.

BRAIN FUNCTION: ESSENTIAL OILS TO THE RESCUE

The brain is another organ where DHA is essential to health. Karesh Youdim and his colleagues at the Scottish Agricultural College tested the ability of essential oils to preserve DHA levels in the brains of 100 animal subjects. Feeding them a daily dose (42.5 mg/K of body weight) of thyme oil (48 percent thymol) over the course of their lifetimes (about 28 months), the researchers achieved stunning results: thyme oil dramatically slowed age-related DHA and PUFA degeneration in the brain. In other words, the essential oil of thyme was able to partially prevent brain aging through protection of essential fatty acids. An analysis of the data showed that the DHA levels in 28-month-old animals' brains were almost the same as that of 7-month-olds. In human terms, this was equivalent to an 80-year-old having the brain chemistry of a 20-year-old.[16]

Thyme oil supplements also slowed the decline of total brain antioxidant levels that occurs with age. Lifelong supplementation with thyme oil in laboratory rats resulted in antioxidant levels dropping by only 29 percent, compared with a 45 percent fall for untreated animals.

Even more startling is the fact that thyme essential oil also preserved levels of PUFAs in the animals' hearts, livers, and kidneys, while at the same time raising total antioxidant levels—including key antioxidants such as glutathione peroxidase and superoxide dismutase. This was accomplished by feeding laboratory rats thyme oil supplements (42.5 mg/K of body weight) daily throughout their lives.[17]

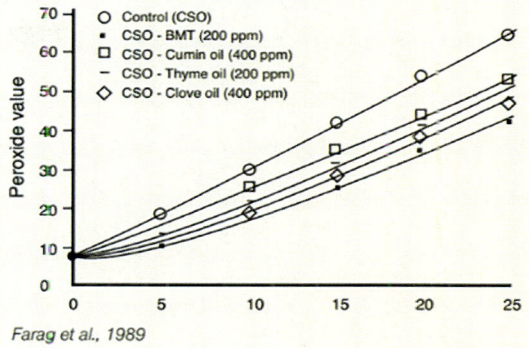

Thyme and Clove Essential Oils Slow the Oxidation of Cottonseed Oil

Farag et al., 1989

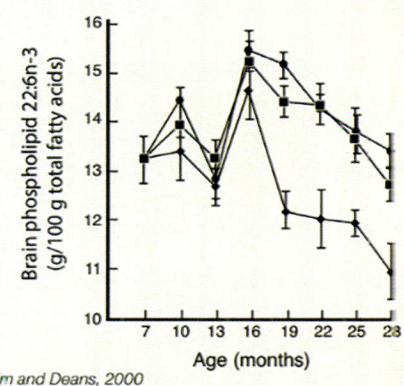

Thyme Oil Arrests the Breakdown of Phospholipids in the Brain of Test Animals

Youdim and Deans, 2000

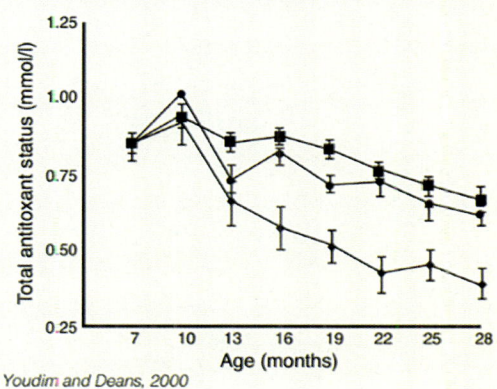

Thyme Oil Increases Total Antioxidant Activity in the Brain of Test Animals

Youdim and Deans, 2000

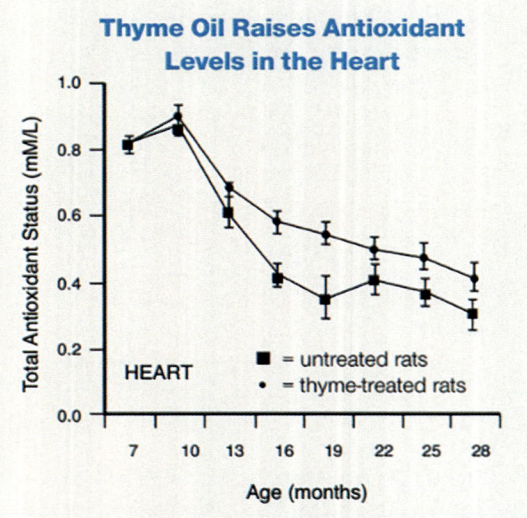

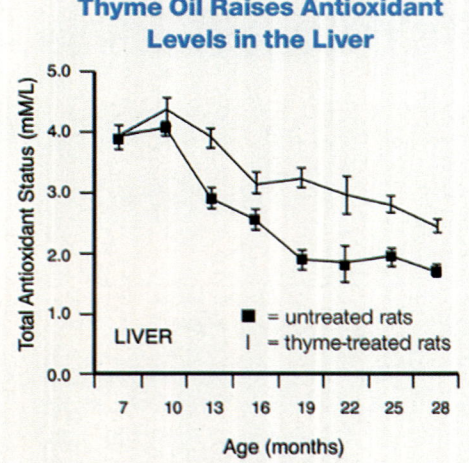

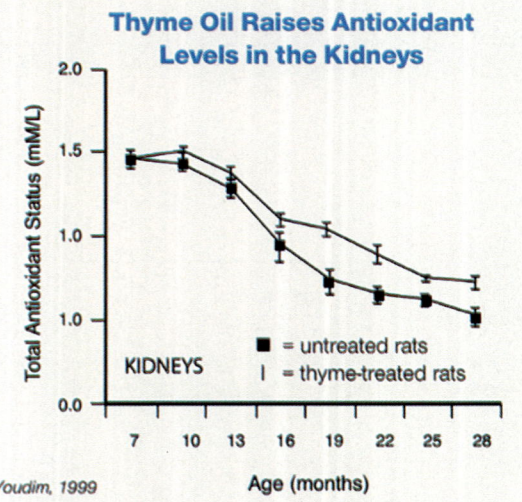

Youdim, 1999

CLOVE OIL: A POWERFUL ANTIOXIDANT

Clove oil also has potent antioxidant-boosting properties. Animal studies conducted at LKT Laboratories in Minneapolis, Minnesota, found that five compounds within clove oil significantly increased levels of GST (glutathione S-transferase), one of the most important detoxifying enzymes in the human body, critical for neutralizing potential cancer-causing chemicals.

Just 60 mg of each of the five compounds of b-caryophyllene, b-caryophyllene oxide (sesquiterpenes), a-humulene and a-humulene epoxide I (terpenes), and eugenol fed to rats over the course of six days (3 doses of 20 mg each) resulted in a doubling of GST activity in the liver and a quadrupling of GST level in the small bowel mucosa. The authors concluded that ". . . these sesquiterpenes show promise as potential anti-carcinogenic agents."[18] Other research has shown that clove essential oil exhibits pronounced antitumoral and DNA-protectant effects.[19,20]

Essential oils may do more than just raise antioxidant levels and block damage to PUFAs. They may also protect cellular DNA from damage that can eventually lead to mutations and subsequent tumor growth. In a 1986 study, Yokota, et al., found that a diet including 5 percent eugenol, the main chemical constituent in clove oil, helped protect test animals against the mutagenic and cancer-causing effects of the chemical benzoapyrene.[21] Yokota and Iwano, et al., completed five more eugenol and rat liver studies, finding in 2013 that dietary eugenol increased xenobiotic-metabolizing enzymes that are known to protect against cancer.[22]

How Five Constituents in Clove Oil Raise Glutathione Levels

Compound	Liver Levels of GST	Small Bowel Levels of GST
Control	0.74	0.25
Compound 1	1.92	0.75
Compound 2	2.13	1.20
Compound 3	1.47	0.63
Compound 4	1.54	0.81
Compound 5	1.26	0.59

Zheng et al., 1992.

FLUORIDE: CLASSIFIED AS A NEUROTOXIN

Fluoride is a cumulative toxin found in drinking water and in dental products like toothpaste and mouthwash. Overuse leads to enamel-damaging fluorosis and a host of more serious health problems.

The global leader in clinical neurology, The Lancet Neurology journal, reported in the March 2014 journal that fluoride has been added to the list of known neurotoxins, such as arsenic, lead, and mercury.

Drop in IQ with Increased Fluoride Exposure

Two internationally known researchers, Philippe Grandjean, MD, PhD, Department of Environmental Health at Harvard, and Philip J. Landrigan, MD, MSc, of the Department of Environmental Medicine at the University of Southern Denmark, warned of "a pandemic of developmental neurotoxicity" in their 2014 study. The authors stated, "All but one of the 27 studies documented an IQ deficit associated with increased fluoride exposure."[23]

Now the Journal of the American Medical Society (JAMA) Pediatrics reported in August 2019 a study of 601 Canadian mother and child pairs. The women drank fluoridated water during pregnancy at the recommended level of 0.7 mg fluoride per liter of drinking water. Urine samples were taken throughout the pregnancies. At follow-up of the women's three- and four-year-old children, a 4.9-point drop in IQ was found in males. Study author Christine Till, said, "that translates to millions of IQ levels lost" [https://www.ncbi.nlm.nih.gov/pubmed/31424532]. Boys are known to have a higher prevalence of autism and attention-deficit disorder, the common neurodevelopmental disorders.

An August 21, 2019, CNN article stated the reaction to this study by Dr. Pamela Den Besten, professor at the University of California San Francisco's School of Dentistry. She said she preferred fluoride strategies not requiring ingestion, and women could drink bottled water with lower-fluoride content during pregnancy.

Danger: Is Anyone Listening?

When the evidence that fluoride is more harmful than helpful is so overwhelming, we have to ask—why is it still being added to the drinking water of 170 million Americans?

A British newspaper—The London Observer—stated one possible answer succinctly: "If health scares about fluoride were to be recognised in the courts, the litigation, especially in the U.S., could be expected to run for decades. Consequently, scientists have been inhibited from publicizing any adverse findings."[24]

Below is a prime example of how research showing fluoride dangers is first ignored, then falsely refuted, and finally, suppressed.

Fluoride and Increased Risk of Bone Cancer for Boys

Evidence that fluoride in tap water can cause bone cancer (osteosarcoma) was first reported in 1990. Osteosarcoma is a deadly form of cancer that is usually fatal within three years. An animal study by the National Toxicology Program showed strong evidence of a link between fluoridated water and bone cancer in male rats. Several human studies followed this that also showed a link between fluoride and osteosarcoma.[25, 26]

Harvard dental professor Dr. Chester Douglass stepped up with a small study (too small to be conclusive) that did not find a link between fluoridation and osteosarcoma. In 1992 Douglass submitted a proposal to the National Institutes of Health (NIH) for a more comprehensive study of this issue. He received $1.3 million for his study. During this time Douglass continually voiced concern that worry over osteosarcoma could have consequences for fluoridation health policies. No concern was expressed for cancer risks for young boys because of fluoridation.

Although Douglass' research did find a statistical link between fluoride and osteosarcoma in boys (not in girls), he continually summarized his work as showing a lower risk for cancer in fluoridated areas.

One of his doctoral students, Elise Bassin, studied the relationship between fluoridation, growth spurts, and osteosarcoma. Her thesis, completed in 2001 but not published until 2006, stated: "Among males, exposure to fluoride at or above the target level was associated with an increased risk of developing osteosarcoma. The association was most apparent between ages five to ten, with a peak at six to eight years of age."[27]

WebMD wrote about Bassin's research and thought it ironic that Douglass, who led her PhD dissertation committee, warned that her results were based on a subset of exposed people. Bassin specifically looked at the subgroup of people most likely to be affected by fluoridation: children. Her analysis was limited to those who got bone cancer by the age of 20.

WebMD Health writer Daniel J. DeNoon explained why Dr. Bassin looked at this subset:

[It's] because most cases of osteosarcoma occur either during the teen years or after middle age. Fluoride collects in the bones, and it's particularly likely to accumulate in the bones during periods of rapid bone growth. So Bassin looked at fluoride exposures during childhood for 103 under-20 osteosarcoma patients and compared them with 215 matched people without bone cancer. Her study took into account how much fluoride was in the water in the communities where children actually lived and the history of municipal, well water, or bottled water use.[28]

It is of interest that if one goes by Douglass' warning to factor in all age groups (including adults), the overall risk for osteosarcoma will likely be diminished statistically. However, the fact remains that fluoride is a risk factor for bone cancer in young boys.

While Douglass approved Bassin's thesis and quoted from it, he did not mention that her findings were exactly opposite of his conclusion. The Fluoride Action Network [FAN] wrote that in March 2004, "In his final report to the NIH, Douglass again summarized the results of his first study as showing no significant association between fluoridation and osteosarcoma. As with his report to the NRC [National Research Council], Douglass referenced Bassin's thesis without mentioning the fact that her findings contradicted his summary."[29]

The Environmental Working Group brought an ethics charge against Douglass in 2005. After a 13-month study, The Harvard Medical School and School of Dental Medicine circled the wagons and concluded, "Douglass did not intentionally omit, misrepresent, or suppress research findings. . . ."[30]

In the face of such outright erroneous reports of his findings, we have to wonder if Douglass has conflicts of interest. The FAN article on the Harvard investigation notes:

. . . in addition to being a professor of Dentistry at Harvard . . . Douglass serves as Editor of COLGATE's 'Oral Care Report.' Colgate is one of the world's largest manufacturers of fluoride toothpaste. If fluoride were found to cause osteosarcoma in children, the potential for legal litigation against Colgate would exist not only in the U.S. but also in many other countries as well.

Colgate, however, is not Douglass' only possible conflict of interest. Douglass, who has been a long-time proponent of fluoridation, is the Chairman of the Board of Trustees for the Delta Dental Foundation of Massachusetts, an organization that—along with its other state affiliates—actively promotes and funds water fluoridation programs in recent years.

The question raised by FAN is a fair one: is it reasonable to believe that these associations with pro-fluoride organizations make it more difficult for Douglass to report a linkage between fluoridation and childhood bone cancer? The late Dr. John Colquhoun posed the question: "How many cavities would have to be saved to justify the death of one young man from osteosarcoma?"[31]

Fluoride Fluorosis Warning

In November 2010 the CDC (Centers for Disease Control and Prevention) released a data brief reporting that 41 percent of adolescents ages 12 to 15 had dental fluorosis from ingesting too much fluoride.[32] Fluorosis leaves white markings or spots on tooth enamel. The spots may be prominent enough to be disfiguring. The more severe forms of fluorosis actually damage tooth enamel. Besides being in drinking water, fluoride is found in dental products like toothpaste and mouth rinses, prescription fluoride supplements, and fluoride applied by dental professionals.

HHS and the EPA (Environmental Protection Agency) announced in 2015 that HHS' proposed recommendation of 0.7 milligrams of fluoride per liter of water replace the current recommended range of 0.7 to 1.2 milligrams.[33]

Bill Osmunson, DDS and president of Washington Action for Safe Water, said, "Fluorosis is the first clinical sign of fluoride poisoning. Excess fluoride does not affect only teeth. It also harms bones, kidneys, thyroid, brains, and other organs. Fluoride is not a nutrient and the body has no need for any of it."[34]

Fluoride and Endocrine Function

The U.S. National Research Council (NRC) reported that "several lines of information indicate an effect of fluoride exposure on thyroid function."[35]

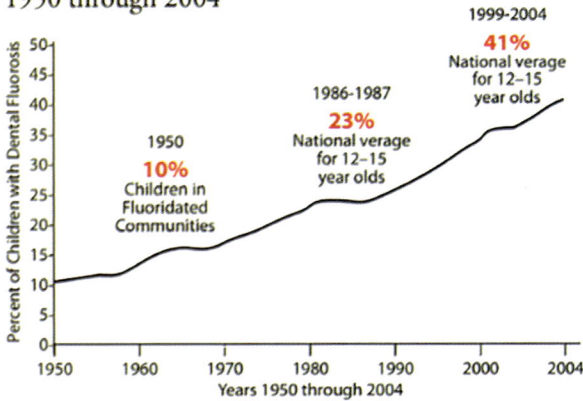

Beltran ED, et al. (2010) Prevalence and Severity of Dental Fluorosis in the United States, 199–2004. NCHS Data Brief No. 53. Figure 3.

National Research Council. (1993). Health Eddects of Ingested Fluoride. National Academy Press, Washington DC. p. 4-5.

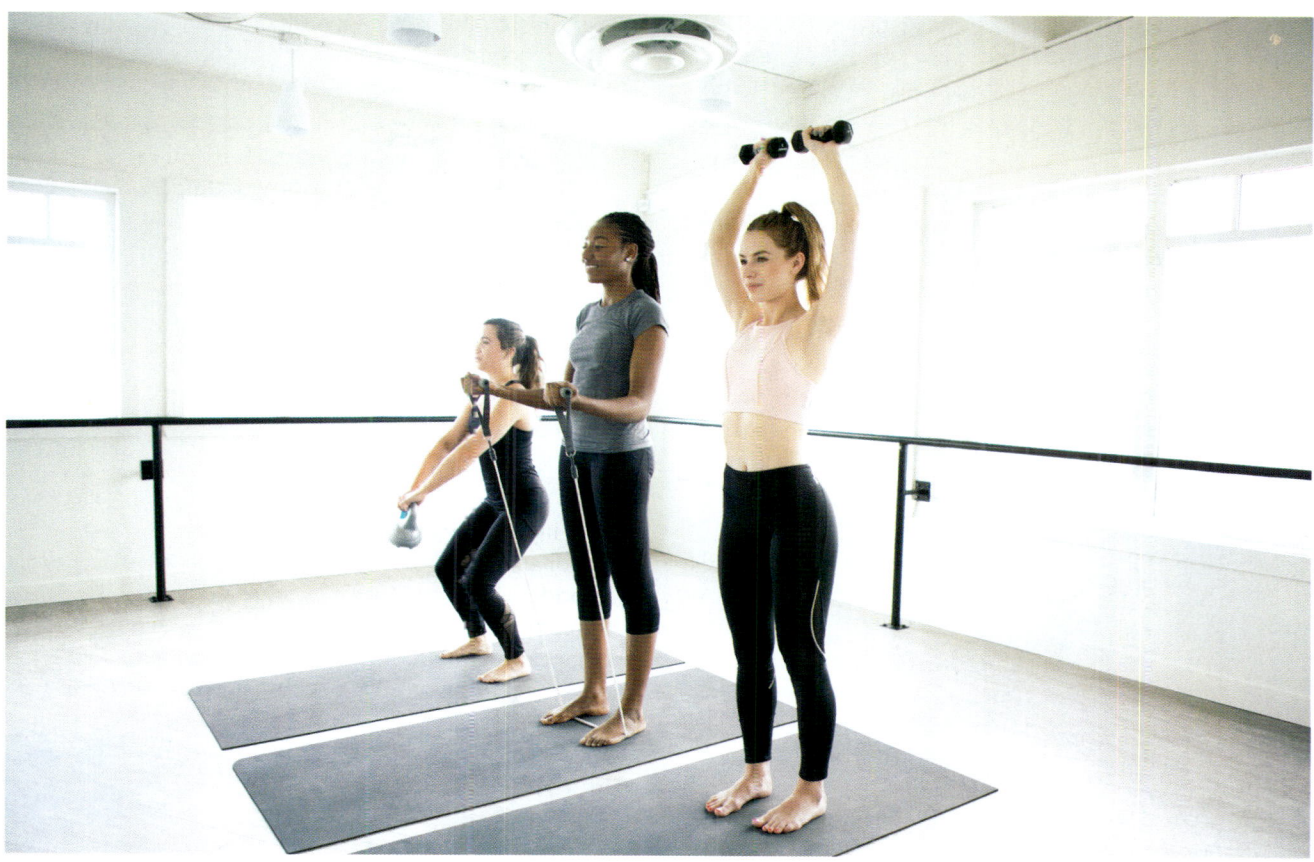

How many people know that until the 1970s, European doctors prescribed fluoride to suppress thyroid function in patients with hyperthyroidism (overactive thyroid)? It was an effective medication in reducing thyroid activity at as low a dose as 2 mg a day. People with fluoridated water may be ingesting doses (up to 6.6 mg a day) that were once used by doctors to reduce thyroid activity. Could this have anything to do with an increase of hypothyroidism (underactive thyroid) in the U.S.?

The NRC concluded its review of fluoride in drinking water with this statement:

". . . evidence of several types indicates that fluoride affects normal endocrine function or response; the effects of the fluoride-induced changes vary in degree and kind in different individuals. Fluoride is therefore an endocrine disrupter in the broad sense of altering normal endocrine function or response." The report cited possible mechanisms such as inhibition of hormone secretion "by effects on things such as calcium balance and inhibition of peripheral enzymes that are necessary for activation of the normal hormone."[36]

A 2010 Chinese study on the effects of fluoride on human hypothalamus-hypophysis-testis axis hormones showed that fluoride can cause reproductive endocrine-disturbing effects, more severe in males than in females.[37]

Fluoride and Bone Fractures

Fluoride is an equal-opportunity hydrofluoric-acid salt. It can be counted on to increase hip fractures in the elderly[38] and bone fractures in children with fluorosis.[39]

Remember that 41 percent of 12-15-year-olds and 36 percent of 16-19-year-olds have fluorosis. That means one out of every three American teenagers has not only mottled teeth but is at increased risk for bone fractures.

But the dental fluorosis now affecting American youth has more dangers than a marred smile and increased risk for bone fractures. A 2011 study of fluorosis served up several vital pieces of information. First, chronic fluoride poisoning is called fluorosis. Second, researchers in Ankara, Turkey, investigated the effects of fluorosis on the cardiovascular system in children.

The conclusion is so technical that clarification from a health professional is added in brackets:

Endemic fluorosis is a risk factor for decrease in calcium and FT4 levels [FT4 is free thyroxine, the major form of thyroid hormone in the blood] increase in sodium levels and QT prolongation [prolonged QT Syndrome is a cause of sudden death that occurs due to a cardiac arrhythmia]. These findings might be related with some cardiovascular system dysfunctions such as arrhythmias [irregular heartbeat] or syncope [temporary loss of consciousness described as fainting or passing out]. Subjects with fluorosis should be monitored in terms of long QT and QTc intervals.[40] [Emphasis added]

When an EKG is given, five peaks are tracked on a graph: P Q R S T. Electrical activity between the Q peak and the T peak is called the QT interval. A "long QT" is a genetic disorder that can lead to early death.

In a study in Circulation, the journal of the American Heart Association, the authors investigated 328 families with this disorder and found that by age 12 years, 50 percent of the young family members with long QT syndrome, "had experienced at least one syncopal [fainting] episode or death."[41] Fluorosis is a risk factor for triggering either arrhythmia or sudden death in those (69 percent of whom are female) with this genetic disorder.

Recently, the EPA rejected a petition to change the source of fluoride in U.S. drinking water. William Hirzy, a chemistry researcher at American University in Washington, D.C., who worked at the EPA for 27 years, and colleagues presented research showing that fluorosilicic acid is often contaminated with arsenic. Fluorosilicic acid is a by-product of phosphate fertilizer manufacturing and is the fluoride form added to drinking water. Hirzy, et al., found that pharmaceutical-grade sodium fluoride contains about 100 times less arsenic than fluorosilicic acid and thus carries a 100-fold lower risk of cancer. The EPA upheld Dr. Hirzy's findings on arsenic in August of 2013 but said the cost of switching to the purer form of fluoride is prohibitive.

Dr. Hirzy stated: "If this stuff (hydrofluorosilicic acid) gets out into the air, it's a pollutant; if it gets into the river, it's a pollutant; if it gets into the lake, it's a pollutant; but if it goes right straight into your drinking water system, it's not a pollutant. That's amazing."[42]

Perhaps it's time to ask the FDA why Americans are forced to drink such a harmful chemical and to ask dentists why they continue to promote fluoride toothpastes.

FRANKINCENSE: A GIFT TO THE WORLD

Research has shown that certain specifies of frankincense have an important impact on longevity and vitality.

Four Questions to Ask About Frankincense

Be sure to ask the following four questions before you buy frankincense essential oil from any manufacturer:

1. Have company owners and officials actually traveled to the Middle East to meet the people and find verifiable frankincense sources?
2. Does the company own the sophisticated, technical instruments needed to test for purity? Does it employ scientists with the credentials (a PhD in chemistry) and training to use this technology correctly?
3. Does the company invest in a library of innovative, peer-reviewed research?
4. Does the company meet and work with leading botanists and cutting-edge scientists in the field of frankincense research?

Only one essential oil company can answer "yes" to every single question: Young Living Essential Oils, the World Leader in Essential Oils.

Three Different Frankincense Species

ThePlantList.org[43] identifies 44 different varieties of frankincense (Boswellia species). These three are the most well-known species: Boswellia carterii from East Africa (Somalia and Yemen), Boswellia sacra from Oman, and Boswellia frereana from Somalia.

Boswellia carterii: Frankincense

"The oleogum resin known as frankincense or olibanum has been obtained since ancient times from several species of Boswellia in the family Burseraceae," according to Hepper.[44]

A 2009 study discusses where the four most important frankincense species are found:

There are numerous species and varieties of frankincense trees, including Boswellia serrata in India, Boswellia carterii in East Africa [Somalia and Yemen], and China [Frankincense is believed to have been cultivated at one time in China, although the current status is unsure.], Boswellia frereana in Somalia, and Boswellia sacra in Arabia, each producing a slightly different type of resin.[45]

Boswellia carterii is among the most studied frankincense species. The 2009 study mentioned above—which had significant scientific impact—is titled "Frankincense oil derived from Boswellia carteri induces tumor cell specific cytotoxicity." [In the scientific literature, Boswellia carterii is also listed as Boswellia carteri]. One of the study's authors, H. K. Lin, PhD, of the University of Oklahoma, has spoken at many Young Living International Grand Conventions.

Dr. Lin's groundbreaking study notes: "Frankincense oil containing 1,200 mg/ml frankincense gum resin was obtained from Young Living Essential Oils (Lehi, UT)."

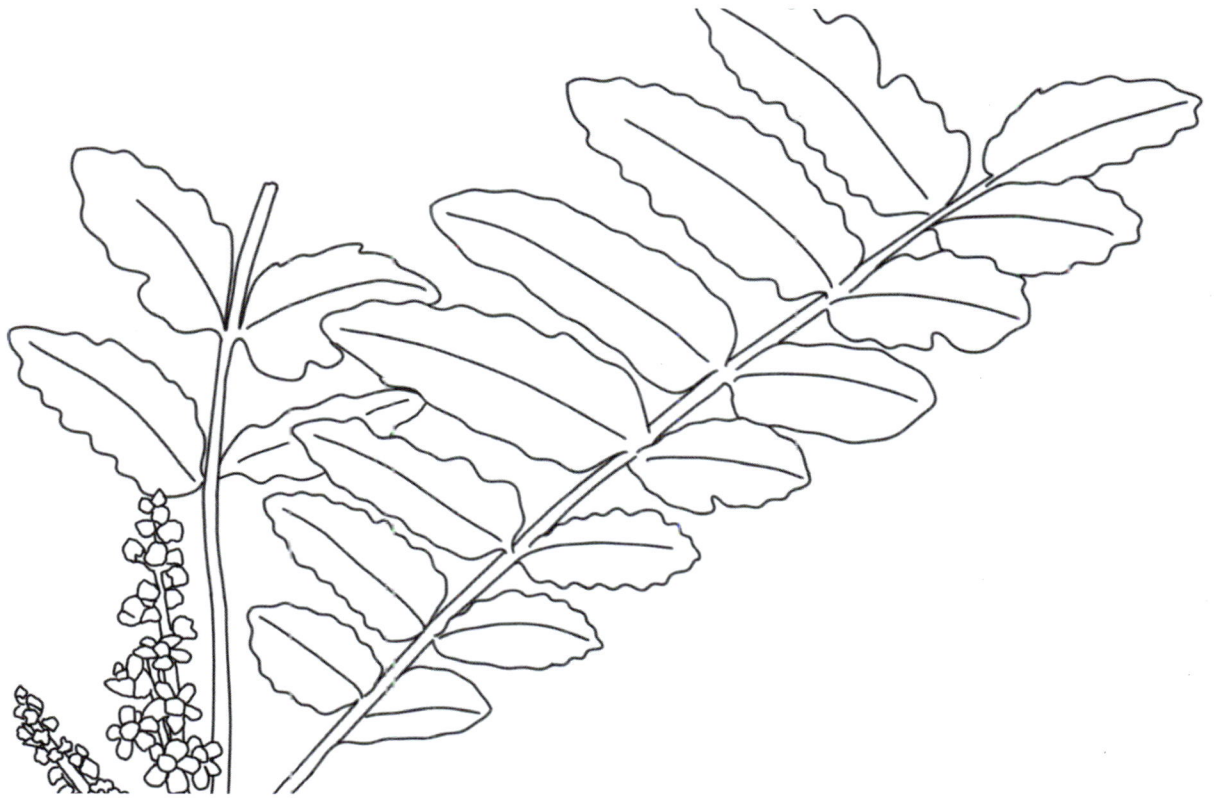

Other essential oil companies falsely make this claim, but the study clearly states that the frankincense oil was obtained from Young Living.

The study states: "This is the first report demonstrating that frankincense oil can discriminate between bladder cancer cells and normal urothelial cells in a cell culture system and utilizing microarray technology to identify potential biological pathways activated by frankincense oil." [46]

Researchers in Tokyo, Japan, discovered that the extract of Boswellia carterii contains 15 triterpene acids, including 7 beta-boswellic acids, as well as the physiologically active diterpene incensole and its acetate, and that this extract "exhibited potent cytotoxic activities against three human neuroblastoma cells." [47]

Researchers from the University of Maryland explained how a purified mixture of boswellic acids from B. carterii resin exhibits not only anti-inflammatory properties but also immunomodulatory activity. [48]

Boswellia sacra: Sacred Frankincense

In Juliet Highet's book on frankincense, she writes: "The international aromatic trade has a grading system for frankincense depending upon size, colour, degree of transparency, and of course fragrance, but it is generally acknowledged that the premium resin comes from Boswellia sacra." [49]

Ahmed Al-Harrasi and Salim Al-Saidi are scientists at the Department of Chemistry, College of Science, Sultan Qaboos University in Oman. Dr. Harrasi's study, "Phytochemical Analysis of the Essential Oil from Botanically Certified Oleogum Resin of Boswellia sacra (Omani Luban)," explains that: "Boswellia sacra is a tree indigenous to the Dhofar region of the Sultanate of Oman." [50]

Mahmoud Suhail, MD, Young Living's partner in the Omani frankincense venture and a noted researcher, said, "Boswellia sacra is the only frankincense species native to Arabia." This is documented by the U.S. National Plant Germplasm System. [51] Dr. Suhail also cited a book commissioned by His Majesty Sultan Qaboos Bin Said, Sultan of Oman, called Plants of Dhofar: The Southern Region of Oman, Traditional, Economic and Medicinal Uses, which states:

Several species of Boswellia including B. sacra, B. papyrifera (from tropical NE Africa), B. frereana (from Somalia) and B. serrata (from India) produce an oleogum-resin, which is exploited as the frankincense or olibanum of commerce—the different species each producing a distinct type and quality of the resin. Only one species, B. sacra, is found in Arabia. [52]

Omani frankincense, Boswellia sacra, is regarded the world over as the rarest, most sought-after aromatic in existence. After careful negotiations with Omani officials, Gary Young was granted permission to build a Young Living distillery in Oman. Until this partnership, no Omani frankincense had been officially exported except that purchased by Saudi royals.

Boswellia sacra has been the focus of research conducted by Young Living Essential Oils' scientists and their colleagues documenting that sacra and carterii are separate species,[53] analyzing a case report showing that B. sacra may provide a non-surgical treatment for basal cell carcinoma,[54] and studies showing that B. sacra induces human pancreatic cancer cell death in cultures[55] and induces cancer cell death in human breast cancer cells.[56]

Imagine the joy it brought Gary Young to be the one to reintroduce Omani frankincense to the world. Young Living is distilling Boswellia sacra essential oil in partnership with Mahmoud Suhail, MD, in Muscat, Oman.

The Science Behind Spirituality

During one of his overseas trips in 2009, former Young Living researcher Marc Schreuder made a vital connection with an Israeli scientist named Arieh Moussaieff, who created headlines around the world when he and an international team of researchers discovered unique capabilities of a diterpene of certain Boswellia species.

Incensole acetate may be the reason frankincense has been part of religious and cultural ceremonies dating back to ancient times. Moussaieff's team discovered that this diterpene triggered an ion channel in the brain with hitherto unknown effects. The areas of the brain affected are known to be involved in emotions. The diterpene, incensole acetate, had antianxiety and antidepressant effects.

One of the media headlines was quite instructive: "Incense is psychoactive: Scientists identify the biology behind the ceremony." If you inhale frankincense with this diterpene, you will be calmed down if you are anxious, and if you are depressed, you will feel happier. What better steps to take to commune with Deity? Incensole acetate is found in B. carterii and B. sacra.

Dr. Moussaieff's studies have shown indeed that incensole acetate is responsible for the remarkable spiritual effects of frankincense.[57] But he also discovered a neuroprotective activity of incensole acetate.[58] An article about Dr. Moussaieff's work stated:

In his doctoral work at the Hebrew University of Jerusalem, Moussaieff isolated the active compounds in the [frankincense] resin. When tested on mouse models of human head injury, he found that some of these substances provide protection for the nervous system. He later noted the resin's anti-depression and anti-anxiety properties and, investigating further, found that they act on a previously unknown pathway in the brain that regulates emotion.[59]

Young Living's Frankincense (Boswellia carterii) and Sacred Frankincense (Boswellia sacra) both contain incensole acetate.

Boswellia frereana: Frereana Frankincense

Boswellia frereana is a rather unusual frankincense species. It is not found in Oman but grows only in Somalia, a country with a troubled history. Independent testing has questioned whether some frereana currently being sold by other essential oil companies is truly a pure, quality essential oil. Gary Young traveled to Somalia in November 2013 to investigate sourcing. He made contact with harvesters who wanted to sell their best frereana resins to Young Living.

While in great demand as incense, frereana does not have the same chemical configuration as other frankincense species. It does not contain boswellic acids, nor does it contain incensole acetate. It does, however, contain unique constituents that have definite anti-inflammatory activities different than other frankincense species.

Unfortunately, Boswellia frereana has not been the focus of many research studies. As of 2019, seven frereana studies found on PubMed, an online database of biomedical literature, only three discuss its benefits. Two of these studies show efficacy against inflammatory conditions. The first, a 2006 study by Frank and Unger in the Journal of Chromatography A, reported that "frankincense from B. frereana also potently inhibited the activity of CYP enzymes [involved in inflammation] but did not contain any of the characteristic boswellic acids."[60]

The second study was published in 2010 in the journal Phytotherapy Research. The researchers noted that "This is the first report detailing the anti-inflammatory efficacy of B. frereana in auricular cartilage."[61]

Without question, Young Living Essential Oils is the world leader in frankincense. D. Gary Young made more than 15 trips to the Middle East to study the Boswellia species so that he could find the best varieties possible to bring to market. Through his company, he invested in trained personnel, instruments, and scientific research to back up his own personal studies. No other essential oil company invests in scientific research like Young Living does.

FREQUENCY: OUR ELECTRICAL ENERGY

"Because science has long taught us to rely on what we can see and touch, we often don't notice that our spirit, thoughts, emotions, and body are all made of energy.

"Everything is vibrating. In fact, each of us has a personal vibration that communicates who we are to the world and helps shape our reality," said Penny Pierce, author of Frequency: The Power of Personal Vibration.[62]

When studying the topics of vibration, frequency, and energy, it is a wise man or woman who realizes he or she does not know everything. Who is to argue with the German biophysicist Fritz-Albert Popp (author of 150 scientific studies), who proposed that all living things emit light energy, and that includes humans. Dr. Popp has written:

We know today that man, essentially, is a being of light. And the modern science of photobiology . . . is presently proving this. In terms of healing the implications are immense. We are still on the threshold of fully understanding the complex relationship between light and life, but we can now say emphatically, that the function of our entire metabolism is dependent on light.[63]

Certainly, more than one gifted energy worker has been able to "see" light and energy shooting up from certain essential oils like Young Living's Frankincense.

The original publication of the *Essential Oils Desk Reference* (1999) (EODR) included information on bio-frequency and disease. Many people copied and disseminated the information, most often without acknowledging this as Bruce Tainio's work. Unfortunately, he did not continue with his studies, and so no further research has been conducted.

The theory of bio-frequency continues to be investigated by researchers, and much of the information from the 1999 EODR deserves to be reviewed in light of recent scientific advances.

A groundbreaking study reported on research that has been conducted with energetic measurements of essential oils using Raman spectroscopy, which is based on the incidence of a monochromatic light source, which, upon reaching the oil in question, undergoes scattering of light, allowing researchers to obtain information about the chemical compound indicating that the components show energy bands [Emphasis added].[64]

Science is proving long-held theories.

Bio-frequency and Disease

Frequency is defined as a measurable rate of electrical energy that is constant between any two points. When there is frequency, there is electromagnetic potential. We are being influenced by the magnetic action (or attraction) of the frequencies that surround us each day, and these frequencies influence our state of well-being. Everything has an electrical frequency measured in megahertz.

Robert O. Becker, MD, documents the electrical frequency of the human body in his book The Body Electric.[65]

A "frequency generator" was developed in the early 1920s by Royal Raymond Rife, MD. He found that by using certain frequencies, he could destroy a cancer cell or virus. He found that these frequencies could prevent the development of disease, and others would destroy disease.

Nikola Tesla said that if you could eliminate certain outside frequencies that interfered with our own electrical frequencies, we would have greater disease resistance.

Björn Nordenström, a radiologist from Stockholm, Sweden, wrote the book Biologically Closed Circuits. He discovered in the 1980s that by putting an electrode inside a tumor and running a milliamp DC (Direct Current) through the electrode, he could dissolve the cancer tumor and stop its growth. He found electropositive and electronegative energy fields in the human body.[66]

Bruce Tainio of Tainio Technology in Cheney, Washington, developed new equipment to measure the bio-frequency of humans and foods. He used this bio-frequency monitor to determine the relationship between frequency and disease.

Measuring in megahertz, he found that:

- Processed/canned food had a zero MHz frequency.
- Fresh foods had 20-27 MHz.
- Dry herbs had 15-22 MHz.
- Fresh herbs had 20-27 MHz.
- Essential oils started at 52 MHz and went as high as 320 MHz (which is the frequency of rose oil).

Fresh foods and herbs can be higher in frequency if grown organically and eaten freshly picked. It is believed that a healthy body typically has a frequency ranging from 62 to 78 MHz, while disease may begin at 58 MHz. According to Dr. Rife's theories, every disease has a frequency, and a substance with a higher frequency will alter the disease that is at a lower frequency.

Clinical research shows that essential oils have the highest frequency of any natural substance known to man and can create an environment in which microbes cannot live. That would certainly indicate that the oil frequencies are several times greater than frequencies of herbs and foods.

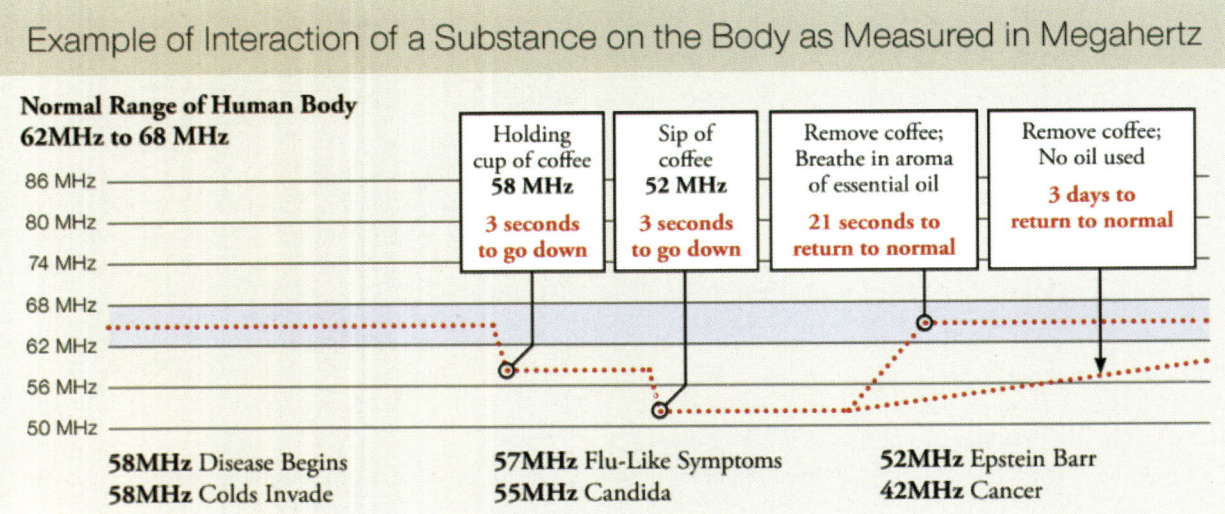

Truly, the chemistry and frequencies of essential oils have the ability to help man maintain an optimal health frequency.

For years, research has been conducted on the use of electrical energy to reverse disease. Scientists in the field of natural healing have believed there has to be a more natural way to increase the body's electrical frequency. This led to the research and subsequent discovery of electrical frequencies in essential oils.

Patients felt better emotionally when oils were diffused in their homes. It seemed that, within seconds, these patients were calmer and less anxious with a little exposure and inhalation. Certain oils acted within one to three minutes; others acted within seconds. It is fascinating to think that an oil applied to the bottoms of the feet can travel to the brain and take effect within one minute. The more results that have been seen, the more research that has been initiated.

Unhealthy Substances Cause Frequency Changes

In one test, the frequencies of two individuals—the first, a 26-year-old male and the second, a 24-year-old male—were measured at 66 MHz each.

The first individual held a cup of coffee (without drinking any), and his frequency dropped to 58 MHz in three seconds. He put the coffee down and inhaled an aroma of essential oils. Within 21 seconds, his frequency had returned to 66 MHz.

The second individual took a sip of coffee, and his frequency dropped to 52 MHz in the same three seconds. However, no essential oils were used during the recovery time, and it took three days for his frequency to return to its normal 66 MHz.

One surprising aspect of this study measured the influence that thoughts have on the body's electrical frequency. Negative thoughts lowered the measured frequency by 12 MHz, and positive thoughts raised the measured frequency by 10 MHz. It was also found that prayer and meditation increased the measured frequency levels by 15 MHz.

Raising Your Frequency

It has been demonstrated that we can change lower, depressed feelings and negative attitudes with the application of essential oils that carry frequencies in the higher range, resulting in a positive change of attitude and mood, thereby uplifting our spirits.

Essential oils and oil blends with higher frequency ranges work in the emotional and spiritual regions. Essential oils and blends that have a lower frequency have a more profound effect on making structural/physical changes. Oils with a frequency of 78 and below are believed to work specifically with harmonizing and balancing the physical body. Single oils may be added to a blend to increase effect.

Inhaling essential oils is particularly beneficial because the sense of smell is the only one of our senses that directly affects the amygdala, part of the limbic system of the brain, where emotions and memory are stored and released. This is why essential oils can have immediate and profound physiological and psychological effects.

This testing of the oils created a lot of interest and perhaps a better understanding of the functionality of the oils in relationship to their frequency. The frequencies should not be considered absolute, because any outside interference can minutely alter the number. However, these are as accurate as was possible at that time, and they are certainly within range and accurate to their point of usage and frequency potential.

Frequencies of Essential Oils Singles and Blends

SINGLE ESSENTIAL OILS
Angelica .... 85 MHz
Basil .... 52 MHz
Frankincense .... 147 MHz
Galbanum .... 56 MHz
German Chamomile .... 105 MHz
Helichrysum .... 181 MHz
Juniper .... 98 MHz
Lavender .... 118 MHz
Melissa (Lemon Balm) .... 102 MHz
Myrrh .... 105 MHz
Peppermint .... 78 MHz
Ravintsara .... 134 MHz
Rose .... 320 MHz
Sandalwood .... 96 MHz

ESSENTIAL OIL BLENDS
3 Wise Men .... 72 MHz
Abundance .... 78 MHz
Acceptance .... 102 MHz
Aroma Life .... 84 MHz
Aroma Siez .... 64 MHz
Awaken .... 89 MHz

Brain Power .... 78 MHz
Christmas Spirit .... 104 MHz
Citrus Fresh .... 90 MHz
Clarity .... 101 MHz
Dragon Time .... 72 MHz
Dream Catcher .... 98 MHz
EndoFlex .... 138 MHz
En-R-Gee .... 106 MHz
Envision .... 90 MHz
Exodus II .... 180 MHz
Forgiveness .... 192 MHz
Gathering .... 99 MHz
Gentle Baby .... 152 MHz
Grounding .... 140 MHz
Harmony .... 101 MHz
Hope .... 98 MHz
Humility .... 88 MHz
ImmuPower .... 89 MHz
Inner Child .... 98 MHz
Inspiration .... 141 MHz
Into the Future .... 88 MHz
Joy .... 188 MHz
JuvaFlex .... 82 MHz

Live with Passion .... 89 MHz
Magnify Your Purpose .... 99 MHz
Melrose .... 48 MHz
Mister .... 147 MHz
Motivation .... 103 MHz
M-Grain .... 72 MHz
PanAway .... 112 MHz
Peace & Calming .... 105 MHz
Present Time .... 98 MHz
Purification .... 46 MHz
Raven .... 70 MHz
R.C. .... 75 MHz
Release .... 102 MHz
Relieve It .... 56 MHz
Sacred Mountain .... 176 MHz
SARA .... 102 MHz
Sensation .... 88 MHz
Surrender .... 98 MHz
Thieves .... 150 MHz
Trauma Life .... 92 MHz
Valor .... 47 MHz
White Angelica .... 89 MHz

FREQUENCY OF THE HUMAN BODY

The following frequency charts will stimulate your curiosity and intellectual mind. To some people, they will make absolute sense, and to others, no sense. We do not often hear it taught that sickness, disease, depression, negative thoughts, and emotions are of a low frequency, and it is perhaps a new thought for many people.

Few people relate to the idea that devitalized and processed food; consumer products made with chemicals, drugs, alcohol, tobacco; and polluted air and water envelope us in an environment of low frequencies.

It has been said that the lower the frequency, the closer we come to sickness, disease, and eventually death. The higher the frequency, the closer we come to God and a life of happiness, health, and prosperity.

Frequency is a fascinating subject, and these charts are great food for thought, whether it be in your realm of belief or mere supposition. Open your mind to greater awareness and the vast possibilities of how you might increase the frequency to which the vibration of your body and soul harmonically resonate.

Normal Human Frequency
The normal body frequency ranges between 62 and 68 MHz and appears to drop somewhat during sleep, but it is still maintained within those markers.

Daily activity and emotions will always cause frequency to vary. However, with proper diet, exercise, pure water, enough rest, a positive attitude, and an environment of peace and harmony, whether at work or at home, the body should be able to stay consistently within the proper and balanced range of frequency.

Frequency Fluctuation Causes Cellular Breakdown
As the body picks up more negative energy particles, the frequency fluctuation begins to cause cellular breakdown. When the frequency exceeds the normal energy cycle on the negative side, a greater electrical charge is produced, causing negative attitudes, depression, and unhappy experiences. Frequencies too far from normal will cause a cellular breakdown that leads to disease.

Alternating Static and Incoherent Frequencies
Static and incoherent frequencies fracture the human, animal, and plant electrical fields, resulting in cellular degeneration, disease, and death.

Research was conducted with exposure of plants to classical, harmonic, beautiful music versus hard rock, noisy, nonharmonic music. With the beautiful music, the plants thrived; and with the other music, they died. It is the same with the human body.

A noisy room with a lot of talking, laughing, and loud music tends to be a very unproductive environment, creating tension and agitation. Road rage has become an evil that has developed because of vast numbers of cars stuck on roadways, with thousands of car engines racing, horns blaring, and people staring at tall buildings and billboards, feeling trapped, angry, and wanting to fight—a very destructive, incoherent frequency.

Why is it that people want to flee to the mountains, away from tall buildings, computers, cell phones, and other people? Has society become so immune and unaware that people just continue to live in oblivion, wondering why they are tired, unmotivated, and sick?

There is so much peace and harmony in the environment of God's creations, away from man's cement and asphalt, electrical wiring, gadgets of all kinds, and millions of people scurrying thousands of different directions, all at the same time.

We live in an environment of incoherent frequency. No wonder there is so much more disease, depression, frustration, and irritation than there ever was even 50 years ago.

Negative Magnetic Field

The shaded areas in the following chart indicate the negative electromagnetic field that accumulates negatively charged magnetic particles. Daily radiation from cell phones, computers, electrical appliances and gadgets, cars, and x-ray equipment used at the dentists' and doctors' offices all contribute to this toxic build up.

These magnetic particles travel in the airways and spread dramatically throughout the environment. Too much magnetic accumulation in the body without daily cleansing and protection results in untold cellular damage that leads to body malfunction, deterioration, disease, and death.

Spiritual Frequencies

As spiritual frequency increases, the negative curve decreases. Man must maintain a connection with the earth in order to remain grounded and to keep the physical body on the earth plane.

Frequency most likely elevates during times of

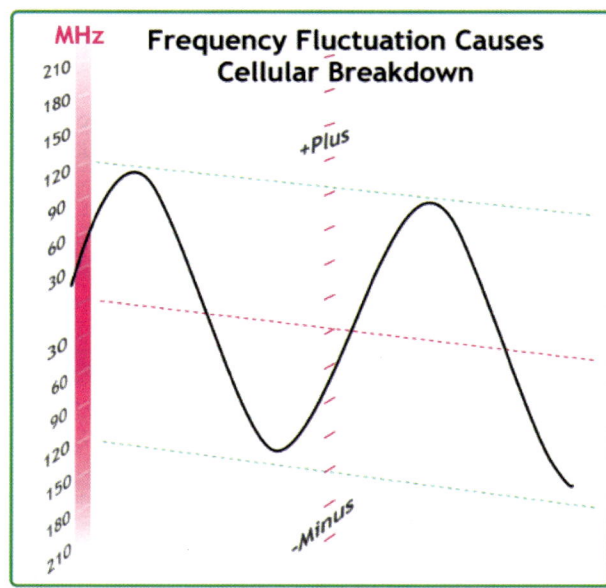

heightened spiritual or intuitive awareness. Visions, out-of-body experiences, going beyond life for a short time (as when someone dies and then is revived a short time later) will carry higher frequencies when the spirit is in

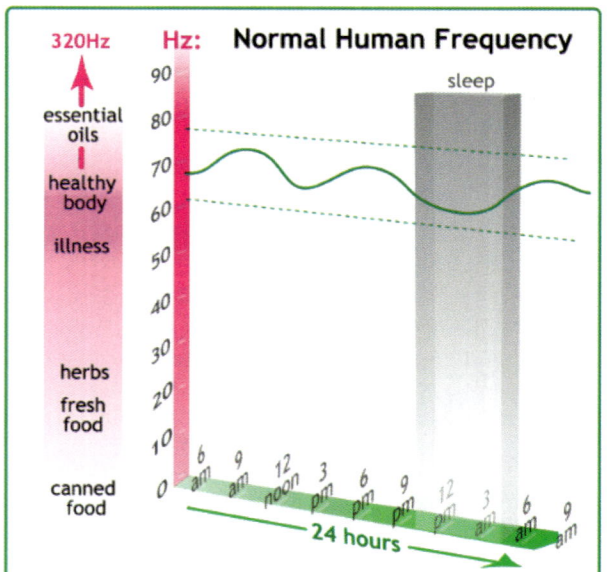

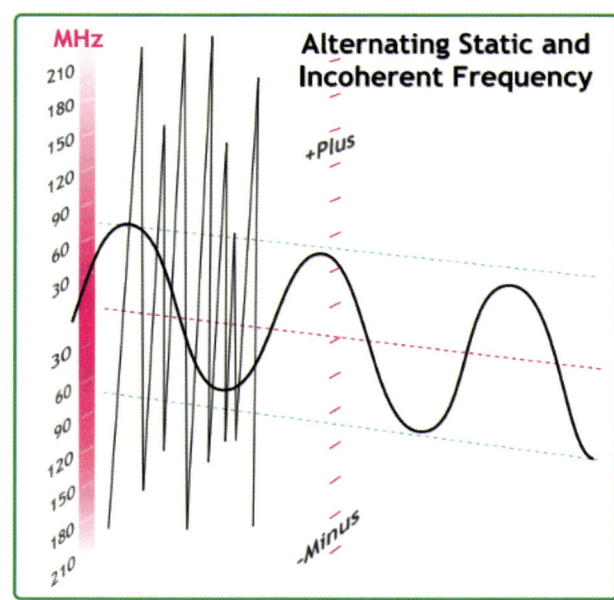

tune with spiritual dimensions. The exact copy on the minus side is the pseudo effect called spiritualism, where deception is so strong.

MICROBES: HOW ESSENTIAL OILS FIGHT THEM

Another method by which aromatics and essential oils may exert a life-lengthening effect is through their ability to inhibit the growth of bacteria, fungi, and viruses. Some bacteria, such as Chlamydia pneumoniae, have been implicated as one of the true causes of heart disease. Viruses such as HIV and hepatitis have resulted in liver failure and premature death. Fungi, like Candida albicans, have been implicated in cancer due to their secretion of mycotoxins.

One of the most comprehensive studies to probe the powerful antimicrobial effects of essential oils was the research directed by D. Gary Young and conducted with Sue Chao at Weber State University in Ogden, Utah. Using disc diffusion assays, they tested the killing power of 67 different Young Living essential oils against a variety of yeast, molds, gram-negative bacteria, and gram-positive bacteria. Cinnamon Bark, Clove, Thyme, Peppermint, Oregano, and Mountain Savory exerted the strongest antimicrobial properties.[67]

In further tests the following year, the researchers successfully proved the ability of Thyme, Oregano, and Clove essential oils to destroy colonies of Streptococcus pneumoniae, the bacteria responsible for many types of throat, sinus, and lung infections.[68]

The spread of dangerous methicillin-resistant Staphylococcus aureus (MRSA) spurred further research by D. Gary Young, Sue Chao, and her colleagues at the Department of Microbiology at Weber State University. Their study, "Inhibition of methicillin-resistant Staphylococcus aureus (MRSA) by essential oils" was published in Flavour and Fragrance Journal in 2008. This study showed that of Young Living's 64 blends, 52 exhibited inhibitory action against MRSA, with R.C. showing the strongest action. Of 91 single essential oils, 78 showed inhibition, with Lemongrass having the strongest action.[69]

MICROWAVE COOKING: SCIENTIFIC FACTS AND SOLUTIONS

Microwave ovens can be found in almost every home and restaurant because they are extremely convenient for thawing, cooking, and heating food. Yet what is the price for this convenience?

Fact: Decreased Nutritional Value

In a study conducted by Dr. Radwan Farag, dean of the Biochemistry Department at Cairo University, he discovered that just two seconds of microwave energy destroys all the enzymes in food, thus increasing our

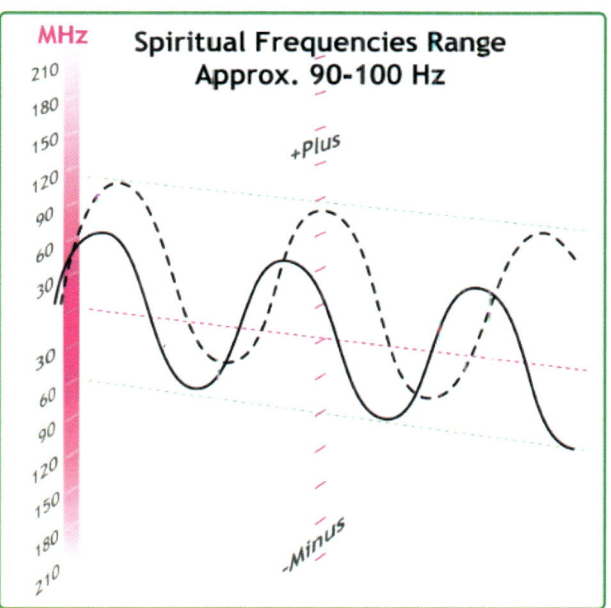

enzyme deficiency and altering the frequency of the food. It appears that heating food containing proteins in the microwave for ten minutes changes the molecular structure of the food, creating a new, harmful type of protein.[70] Surely, the price is just too high in loss of health for this convenience.

Experiments conducted in the 1940s showed some of the dangers of microwave energy. This type of energy was actually discovered in the 1800s but was not considered

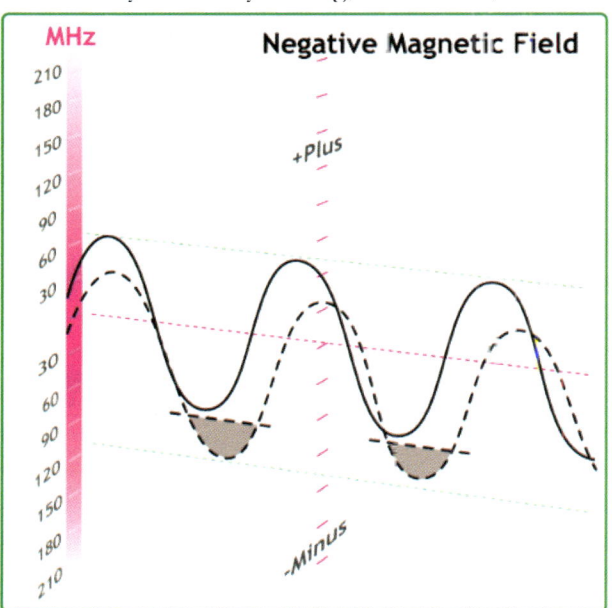

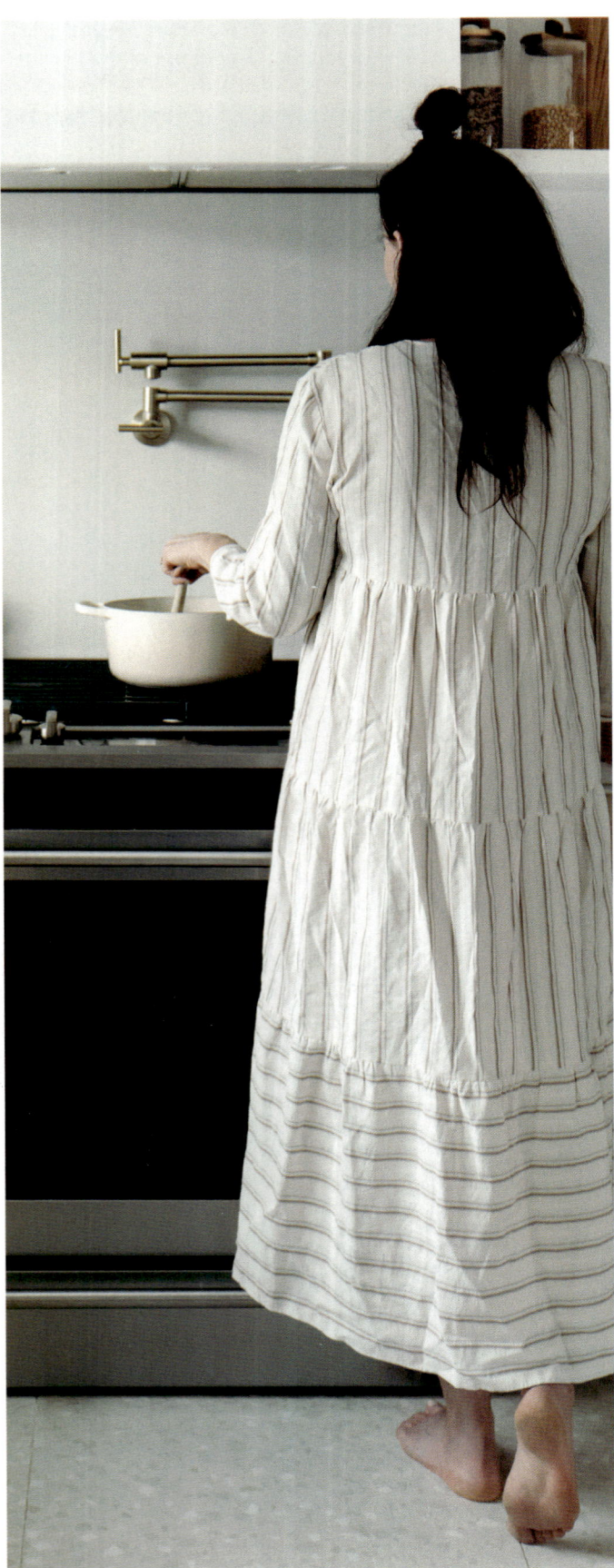

for cooking until the invention of the microwave oven.

Microwaves were first used during World War II for early radar projects. It was during a radar research project in the mid-1940s that Dr. Percy Spencer of Raytheon Corporation noticed the candy bar in his pocket had melted after testing a vacuum. This piqued his curiosity, which gave him the idea to put popcorn kernels near the tube. The popcorn popped all over the office, which brought about the invention of the microwave oven, with Raytheon filing the first microwave cooking patent.

Fact: Hidden Dangers

Microwaves are a form of electromagnetic energy, like radio waves. They are short waves of electromagnetic energy that travel at the speed of light. We have all heard about microwave towers, but what are they? Microwave towers are used to relay long-distance telephone signals, television programs, and computer information across the earth and to satellites in space. But we are most familiar with the microwave as a convenience for cooking food.

Decreased Nutrition: A microwave oven contains a magnetron, which is a tube in which electrons pass through a magnetic field to produce microwave-length radiation, which interacts with the molecules in food. In the microwave oven, the wave energy changes the polarity of molecules from positive to negative millions of times every second. This friction produces extreme heat, and in the food, causes "structural isomerism," or structural damage, of the food molecules.

This decreases the nutritional value of food from 60 to 90 percent. Vitamin B12, which is needed for red blood cell formation, is greatly reduced. In addition, microwave cooking kills 97 percent of the flavonoids in the food, which are some of the body's nutrient soldiers. They fight disease, inflammation, and microbes. Furthermore, vitamins C and E, essential minerals, and enzymes are virtually destroyed.

Decreased Antioxidants: This leaves the cells extremely vulnerable to viruses, fungi, and other micro-organisms. The ability of the cells to repair themselves is suppressed so that rather than producing water and carbon dioxide in the process of cell repair, hydrogen peroxide and carbon monoxide are produced. Imagine eating food filled with carbon monoxide.

A study published in the November 2003 issue of The Journal of the Science of Food and Agriculture found that broccoli cooked in the microwave with a little water lost up to 97 percent of the beneficial antioxidant chemicals it contains. By comparison, steamed broccoli lost only 11 percent or fewer of its antioxidants.[71]

Deadly Blood Changes: In 1991 there was a lawsuit against a hospital in Oklahoma because a microwave was used to warm the blood for a hip-surgery patient, who died after receiving the blood transfusion. Warming blood for a transfusion is routine; unfortunately, using a microwave causes enough changes in the blood to be deadly.

Toxic Milk for Babies: The effects of microwaving breast milk have also been researched. John Kerner, MD, and Richard Quan, MD, from Stanford University, said, "Microwaving human milk, even at a low setting, can destroy some of its important disease-fighting capabilities."

Dr. Kerner subsequently wrote in the April 1992 edition of Pediatrics that "microwaving itself may in fact cause some injury to the milk above and beyond the heating."[72]

In addition, a radio announcement at the University of Minnesota said, "Microwaves are not recommended for heating a baby's bottle. Heating the bottle in a microwave can cause slight changes in the milk, and even though the bottle will feel cool on the outside, the inside could be so hot that it could burn the baby's mouth and throat. In infant formulas, there may be a loss of some vitamins. In expressed milk, some protective properties may be destroyed."

A study using ultra-high-performance liquid chromatography/tandem mass spectrometry discovered chemicals that leached from baby bottles. Low levels of BPA were found in three bottles after they had been heated in a microwave oven. A chemical, 4-n-NP, not reported to be leachable, was found in two brand-name baby-feeding bottles.[73]

Dr. Lita Lee of Hawaii reported in the December 9, 1989, issue of Lancet:

Microwaving baby formulas converted certain trans-amino acids into their synthetic cis-isomers. Synthetic isomers, whether cis-amino acids or trans-fatty acids, are not biologically active. Further, one of the amino acids, L-proline, was converted to its d-isomer, which is known to be neurotoxic (poisonous to the nervous system) and nephrotoxic (poisonous to the kidneys). It's bad enough that many babies are not nursed, but now they are given fake milk (baby formula) made even more toxic via microwaving.[74]

Radiation: Microwave ovens have been known to leak radiation, which can disrupt the delicate balance in cellular growth. Our bodies are regulated by electrical frequencies and electromagnetic fields.

Microwave radiation can disrupt these frequencies and damage normal body functions. Radiation suppresses the immune system, and the constant eating of microwave-cooked food causes memory loss, lowers IQ and mental capacity, and causes emotional problems, most likely due to a disruption in hormone production.

Because the body is electrochemical in nature, any force that disrupts or changes human electrochemical events will affect the physiology of the body. This is further described in Robert O. Becker's book The Body Electric[75] and in Ellen Sugarman's book Warning: The Electricity Around You May Be Hazardous to Your Health.[76]

Another danger to consider is the heating of the plastic in which some food is wrapped, which can increase the carcinogens in the food. Studies have shown that plastic wraps and containers do leak chemicals and toxic agents into the food they are holding. Ethylhexyl, DEHA [Bis(2-ethylhexyl) adipate], and xenoestrogen are all substances that studies have shown migrate into your food from plastic when it is microwaved.

Dr. Edward Fujimoto, the manager of the Wellness Program at the Castle Hospital, said that we should not be heating foods that contain fat in the microwave using plastic containers. He said that the combination of fat, high heat, and plastics releases dioxins into the food and ultimately into the cells of the body. Dioxins are carcinogens and highly toxic to the cells of our bodies.

A Simple Experiment

You can do a simple experiment at home to see for yourself what happens by just using water slightly heated in a microwave oven. Plant some seeds in two pots. Water one pot with water that has been microwaved for just 15 seconds. Water the other with regular tap water. Even with chlorinated tap water, the seeds will germinate and the plants will grow. The seeds that received microwaved water will not sprout. If microwaved water can stop plants from growing, imagine what microwaved food can do to your body.

Several Big Experiments

In 1980 a research project with 20 volunteers was conducted with microwave cooking. Ten volunteers in group A and 10 in group B fasted on liquids for 10 days. Then both groups were fed the same foods for another 10 days with only one exception: the food for group A was steamed, while the food for group B was microwaved. After 10 days, stool samples were taken and analyzed. Group A stools appeared to be normally digested, while group B stools were of a plastic texture. Ultrasound scans showed adhesive food particles stuck to the stomach wall. In the stool sample, altered enzymes were found, as well as protein with altered molecular structures that could not be absorbed.

In test subjects who ate microwaved food, the following changes in blood chemistry were observed:

- Decrease in hemoglobin values
- Decrease in the ratio of HDL cholesterol (good cholesterol) and LDL (bad cholesterol)
- Decrease in lymphocytes (white blood cells, the ones that kill germs)
- Increase in luminous power by luminous bacteria exposed to blood of volunteers. In actuality, radioactive energy was passed on from the microwaved food to the blood cells of those who ate the food.

This implies that a person who eats microwaved food for an extended period could become anemic due to destruction of hemoglobin, could have an increase in heart disease because of a decrease in good cholesterol and an increase in bad cholesterol, and could become subject to a number of contagious diseases due to a weakened immune system.

Swiss biologist Dr. Hans Ulrich Hertel worked as a food scientist for many years with one of the major Swiss food companies that does business on a global scale. In 1989 he was the first scientist to carry out a clinical study on the effects microwaved nutrients have on the blood and physiology of the human body. Because he began questioning certain processing procedures that denatured the food, he was fired from his job.

Hertel's scientific study was conducted with Dr. Bernard H. Blanc of the Swiss Federal Institute of Technology and the University Institute for Biochemistry. Eight people participated in the study for eight weeks. They lived in a controlled environment and intermittently ate raw foods, conventionally cooked foods, and microwaved foods. Blood samples were tested after each meal.

Microwave oven manufacturers insist that microwaved and irradiated foods do not have any significantly higher "radiolytic" compounds than do broiled, baked, or other conventionally cooked foods. However, scientific clinical evidence, such as that provided by Hertel, shows that this is simply a lie.[77]

In America, neither universities nor the federal government have conducted any tests concerning the effects on our bodies from eating microwaved foods. It seems a bit strange that they are more concerned with studies on what happens if the door on a microwave oven doesn't close properly. Since people ingest this altered food, should there not be a concern for how the same damaged molecules will affect our own human biological cell structure?

Hiding the truth seems to be prevalent in the commercial world. At the same time Doctors Hertel and Blanc were publishing their research, an article appeared in the 19th issue of Journal Franz Weber, which stated:

. . . the consumption of food cooked in microwave ovens had cancerous effects on the blood. The violent deformations that can occur in the human body when exposed to microwaves are also seen in the food molecules cooked in microwaves.

Studies conducted on food thawed, cooked, and heated in microwaves showed that many food molecules became carcinogens. The glucoside and galactoside present in frozen foods converted into carcinogenic substances. Plant alkaloids in vegetables were converted into carcinogens. Milk and cereals heated in microwaves also had some of their amino acids converted into carcinogens.[78]

On the cover of the magazine was a picture of the Grim Reaper holding a microwave oven in one of his hands.

The research paper by Doctors Hertel and Blanc followed the article, which must have created a lot of furor with the manufacturers of microwave ovens and those making money from the sale of them. As soon as Doctors Hertel and Blanc's research was published in 1991, a powerful trade organization, the Swiss Association of Dealers for Electro-apparatuses for Households and Industry, known as FEA, struck swiftly in 1992. They forced the president of the Court of Seftigen, Canton of Bern, to issue a "gag order" against Doctors Hertel and Blanc.

In March 1993, Dr. Hertel was convicted for "interfering with commerce" and prohibited from further publishing his results. **However, Dr. Hertel stood his ground and fought this decision over the years.**

Eventually, this decision was reversed in a judgment delivered in Strasbourg on August 25, 1998. The European Court of Human Rights held that there had been a violation of Hertel's rights in the 1993 decision.

The European Court of Human Rights also ruled that the "gag order" issued by the Swiss court in 1992 against Dr. Hertel, prohibiting him from declaring that microwave ovens are dangerous to human health, was contrary to the right of freedom of expression. In addition, Switzerland was ordered to pay Dr. Hertel compensation of 40,000 French Francs.

After World War II, the Russians also experimented

with microwave ovens. Since 1957 their research has been carried out mainly at the Institute of Radio Technology at Klinsk, Belarus.

In 1976 during the Cold War, the Soviet Union banned the use of microwave ovens, based on research they had conducted revealing the damage it does to food. The research was never formally presented, but it became well-known throughout the international community that the Soviets understood the dangers of the microwave oven.

Although controversial, the following effects were said to be observed by Russian forensic teams:

1. Heating prepared meats in a microwave sufficiently for human consumption created:

   - d-Nitrosodiethanolamine (a well-known cancer-causing agent)
   - Destabilization of active protein biomolecular compounds
   - Creation of a binding effect to radioactivity in the atmosphere
   - Creation of cancer-causing agents within protein-hydrolysate compounds in milk and cereal grains

2. Microwave emissions also caused alteration in the catabolic (breakdown) behavior of glucoside- and galactoside-elements within frozen fruits when thawed in this way.

3. Microwaves altered catabolic behavior of plant-alkaloids when raw, cooked, or frozen vegetables were exposed for even very short periods.

4. Cancer-causing free radicals were formed within certain trace-mineral molecular formations in plant substances, especially in raw root vegetables.

5. Ingestion of microwaved foods caused a higher percentage of cancerous cells in blood.

6. Due to chemical alterations within food substances, malfunctions occurred in the lymphatic system, causing degeneration of the immune system's capacity to protect itself against cancerous growth.

7. The unstable catabolism of microwaved foods altered their elemental food substances, leading to disorders in the digestive system.

8. Those ingesting microwaved foods showed a statistically higher incidence of stomach and intestinal cancers, plus a general degeneration of peripheral cellular tissues with a gradual breakdown of digestive and excretory system function.

9. Microwave exposure caused significant decreases in the nutritional value of all foods studied, particularly:

- A decrease in the bioavailability of B-complex vitamins, vitamin C, vitamin E, essential minerals, and lipotropics (such as choline and inositol, which break down fats, necessary for a healthy liver)
- Destruction of the nutritional value of nucleoproteins in meats
- Lowering of the metabolic activity of alkaloids, glucosides, galactosides, and nitrilosides (all basic plant substances in fruits and vegetables)
- Marked acceleration of structural disintegration in all foods

The Russians later lifted the ban, and currently, no countries have a ban on the use of the microwave oven.

No FDA or officially released government studies have proven current microwave usage to be harmful, but we all know that the validity of studies can be—and is sometimes deliberately—limiting, and many of these studies are later proven to be inaccurate.

According to OSHA, the United States Department of Labor's Occupational Safety & Health Administration, adverse effects due to microwave radiation from cellular phones, radio transmissions, and radar traffic devices are topics of controversy and ongoing research. But what does that mean? What keeps the government from conducting studies and releasing their findings to the public? Are they protecting the public or the dollar?

The FDA, Food and Drug Administration, claims that radiation emissions from microwave ovens do not pose a public health risk and that radiation injury is extremely rare. The agency states that unless the microwave oven has a damaged latch, seal, or hinges, there is little concern over leaking microwave radiation. That may be true, but what does that have to do with the effects of the function of a microwave oven?

Over the past few years, manufacturers have certainly improved the technology and design of microwave ovens, but even the most advanced technology cannot change the damaging effects of radiation on our food and subsequently our bodies.

Tests by the U.S. National Institute of Environmental Health Sciences determined that inhaling the artificial butter of microwave popcorn could pose a health risk. According to the Global Health Center, microwave cooking may adversely affect the molecular makeup of certain foods.

According to Robinson, et al., children have been seriously burned after opening a microwave oven, which has the potential of heating liquids to a dangerously hot temperature, which can result in severe burns.[79]

We should all be searching and finding out the facts for ourselves. If you do a Google search for "microwaves," you will find that only good, positive things come up touting the "great value" of microwaves. However, if you search on "dangers of microwaves," you will be astounded at all the research, tests, documentation, and personal stories that come up contrary to the "great value" perceived by the public.

Solution: Essential Oils Counteract Electromagnetic Radiation

Dr. Sabina DeVita, a well-known psychologist from Toronto, Canada, who, for years, has been studying the damaging effects of electromagnetic or radiation poisoning on the human body, says that electromagnetic pollution has become an occupational hazard of our high-tech 21st century and will probably continue to get worse as technology becomes more and more sophisticated the farther we get into the century. We are not only exposed to radiation from microwave ovens but also to that of radios, televisions, computers, cell phones, and electrical appliances that we conveniently use every day.[80]

So, what is the answer to the question of how to avoid radiation? We can avoid some of it, but not all, so what can we do to protect ourselves? There is one possibility that we probably have not thought of, and that is the use of essential oils, which have been used since the beginning of time for beautifying, healing, and protecting, both physically and spiritually.

Their therapeutic qualities have been lost to the synthetic world of perfumes, soaps, lotions, potions, creams, cosmetics, and, of course, the vast food industry. Only in the two decades have essential oils reemerged from their mysterious past as viable products for natural healing and wellness. Studies are being conducted in universities and research laboratories all over the world. Even allopathic medicine is taking notice.

Through all the scientific research, it has been discovered that essential oils are one of the highest-known sources of antioxidants that can prevent free radical damage. They contain bioelectric frequencies that are several times greater than that of herbs and foods, making them profoundly effective in raising the frequencies of the human body and aiding in the prevention of disease.

Dr. DeVita, in her book Electromagnetic Pollution (2000), states that because of their high frequency, high-oxygenating molecules, fast delivery system to the cells, and immune-building and antimicrobial properties, essential oils become a necessary adjunct to protecting ourselves against free radical damage as well as the potential ravages of our electromagnetically polluted environment.

She strongly recommends certain essential oil blends that can be helpful in counteracting the effects of electromagnetic radiation. Many of the essential oils enhance the frequency of the energy field, thus helping to maintain a healthy electrical balance. As with all oils, one has to experiment to see which oils seem to resonate with the body.

Certain essential oil blends to consider are Valor, Harmony, Grounding, Brain Power, Melrose, Clarity, ImmuPower, Present Time, and many others. Single oils such as Royal Hawaiian Sandalwood, Sacred Sandalwood, Tea Tree, Myrtle, Palo Santo, Idaho Grand Fir, Sacred Frankincense, and Frankincense can also help.

In June 2010 Mary Young's blend The Gift, formulated with some of the oils written about in ancient scripture—including Sacred Frankincense from Oman—came on the market. This very special oil blend comes to us with a history from the very center of antiquity. We are learning to deeply appreciate it as we discover more and more about its powerful properties that the people of long ago already knew, and now we can add it to our arsenal of protection. Dr. Sabina's advice is well-founded and can serve us in a most remarkable and gratifying way.

Many people are writing and speaking out about the dangers of microwave usage and the dangers of radiation poisoning, but the information is still suppressed, and the general public is very unaware.

Unfortunately, convenience often takes precedence over common sense, but the price we pay for lack of knowledge can be devastating.

Find out for yourself; the information is there for those who seek it. Inform those around you and in your sphere of influence and let us stop this deception and destruction.

RADIATION: PROTECTING OUR ENVIRONMENT

What Is Radiation?

Radiation is when energy moves away from its source through space, creating two broad types.

1. **Ionizing radiation** comes from radioactive materials and machines, such as x-ray machines, that carry large amounts of energy in each particle. It can hurt and damage anything that it hits and causes chemical changes in people, animals, and vegetation.

Radiation with sufficiently high energy can ionize atoms. That most often occurs when an electron is stripped or knocked out of an electron shell, which leaves the atom with a positive charge. Because cells are made of atoms, this ionization can result in cancer. However, that probability is dependent upon the dose rate of the radiation and the sensitivity of the organism being irradiated.

2. **Nonionizing radiation** comes from other sources and causes effects known as electromagnetic radiation, commonly known as light. Nonionizing radiation does not usually cause damage, although some types can cause chemical changes or make things hotter.

We are exposed to many types of radiations, which we refer to as "natural" or normal radiation, coming from televisions, microwaves, waterbeds, cell phones, and computers, in addition to our visits to the dentist, doctor, or hospital. We're also exposed to other various types of radiation in the atmosphere, particularly when flying.

Energy travels through space in many different ways. One way is in the form of shifting electrical and magnetic fields like a stream of particles of energy called photons. Another way is by traveling in the form of tiny pieces of atoms, like neutrons or protons, and is referred to as particle radiation.

Scientists categorize different kinds of electromagnetic radiation or light based on wavelength and frequency, as follows:

- **Radio waves** have the highest wavelength and are used to send and receive communications.
- **Micro waves** are a type of radio wave used in a microwave oven to warm up food.
- **Radar waves** detect airplanes in the sky, ships in the ocean, and changes in the weather.
- **Infrared waves** are emitted by most objects at room temperature and are not seen by the human eye. Certain types of cameras can take pictures of hot things even on the other side of a wall.
- **Visible light** is the radiation we call "light."
- **Ultraviolet light** is the invisible light that can cause sunburn and is used to kill bacteria and make invisible ink visible.

Environmental Protection Kits

The QuadShield and EndoShield kits each combine four powerful products to help people protect themselves against daily radiation bombardment of cell phones, computers, electrical appliances, and other potential dangers.

The QuadShield kit contains Longevity Softgels, the essential oil blend Melrose, and the nutritional supplements Super C (Tablets or Chewable), and Thyromin.

The EndoShield kit contains Longevity Softgels and the essential oil blends Melrose, EndoFlex, and Citrus Fresh.

To create the kits, purchase products separately.

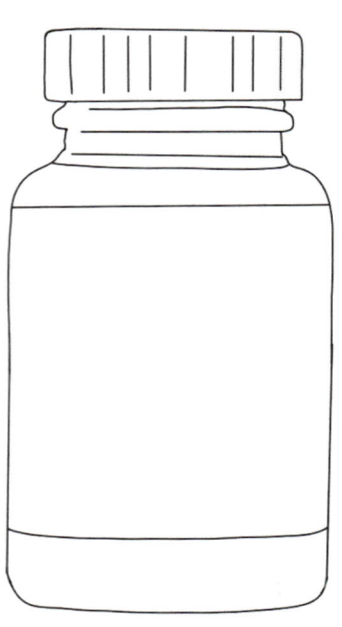

The Japanese earthquake of March 11, 2011, taught the world that nuclear power plants are vulnerable to natural disasters, and years of use have caused deterioration and weakness.

Of the 104 nuclear power plants in the United States, six are identical to the damaged Fukushima plant, 17 others are very similar, and several are close to major earthquake faults.

The "giant" that has been sleeping since the days of the Three Mile Island and Chernobyl disasters has awakened.

- **X-rays and Gamma rays** are extremely strong rays used in medicine to photograph the interior of the body and treat cancer. However, in too large amounts, they are very dangerous to life.

We could say that we live in a world of radiation, if we think specifically about the sun and the light that it gives to our earth. Although the energy from the sun is necessary for our health, too much can be dangerous and even deadly. The pain of a sunburn is excruciating, as those who have had this experience know. Too much of a good thing can turn into something dangerous and unwanted, such as skin cancer.

We are inundated constantly with radiation of various levels. It has been said that those who have been exposed to high levels of radiation could have some allergic reaction in the form of unusual rashes on the skin. We know that radiation is very damaging, because of the many scientific studies and research conducted, besides the stories told by those who have actually had this experience.

However, not only do we have this mild exposure on a daily basis, but now many governments have built nuclear plants for atomic power, national defense, communication, and research. Few of us even understand the use of atomic energy, radiation, and the technical advances that have been made in nuclear energy in the last decade. Sadly, with all this technical advancement comes the threat of even greater radiation exposure and poisoning. Unfortunately, when it comes to risks and toxic exposure levels, the government and medical community will likely downplay the threat.

The last report of the U.S. Nuclear Regulatory Commission, as of September 2018, stated that there are almost 100 nuclear plants in the United States today.[81] Benjamin Sovacool, in The Journal of Contemporary Asia, reported in 2010 that there had been at least 56 accidents at nuclear reactors in the United States (defined as incidents that either resulted in the loss of human life or more than $50,000 of property damage).[82] Also, contaminated, radioactive water was dumped into nearby water supplies, from which many people suffered because of their exposure to an unknown invader.

One independent website listed another incident of nuclear waste. Cited in a May 2013 Scientific American article[83] is the fact that "60 of 177 underground tanks [constructed to contain radioactive waste generated by the ill-fated Hanford plant] have already leaked."

"Controversy surrounding the project," states Allen Lutins, operator of that independent website, "run by contractor Bechtel National, Inc. led to the reassignment

Environmental Protection Kits

QuadShield™

Longevity Softgel—The essential oils in Longevity Softgels increase the oxygen and ATP (adenosine triphosphate) cellular fuel for increasing cell life and immunity for stronger resistance against damage from environmental pollution.
- **Children and teens ages 10–18:** 1-2 capsules daily
- **Adults:** 2–4 capsules daily

Melrose—This blend is formulated with two species of Melaleuca oil: M. alternifolia, also known as Tea Tree, and M. quinquenervia, also known as Niaouli, which were found through research by Daniel Pénoël, MD, and Pierre Franchomme, PhD, to prevent cellular damage from environmental pollution and potential daily radiation exposure.
- **Children ages 1–3:** 1 drop in yogurt or other liquid
- **Children ages 4–7:** 2 drops in yogurt or other liquid
- **Children 8 and older:** 6 drops per capsule 1-3 times daily or in yogurt or other liquid
- **Adults:** 20 drops per capsule, 1-2 capsules, 1-3 times daily or in yogurt or other liquid

Super C (Tablet or Chewable)—Super C provides the body with 2,166 percent of the recommended dietary intake of the powerful antioxidant vitamin C and is enhanced with minerals, bioflavonoids, and pure Orange, Lemon, and other essential oils. It is a natural antioxidant and free-radical scavenger that supports the immune system and protects healthy cells from becoming damaged by the effects of environmental pollution.
- **Children ages 1–3:** 1-2 MightyVites daily
- **Children ages 4–7:** 2-3 MightyVites or Super C Chewables daily
- **Children 8 and older:** 3-4 MightyVites or Super C Chewables daily
- **Adults:** 4-6 tablets daily

Thyromin—Thyromin contains ingredients that give support and nutrition to both the thyroid and adrenal glands for a healthier glandular system.
- **Children:** continue to use MightyVites 2-4 daily
- **Adults:** only 1 capsule, 3 times daily

NingXia Red—Drink 4-6 oz. of NingXia Red for a delicious and healthy addition to your diet

EndoShield™

Longevity Softgel—The essential oils in Longevity Softgels increase the oxygen and ATP (adenosine triphosphate) cellular fuel for increasing cell life and immunity for stronger resistance against damage from environmental pollution.
- **Children and teens ages 10–18:** 1-2 capsules daily
- **Adults:** 2–4 capsules daily

Melrose—This blend is formulated with two species of Melaleuca oil: M. alternifolia, also known as Tea Tree, and M. quinquenervia, also known as Niaouli, which were found through research by Daniel Pénoël, MD, and Pierre Franchomme, PhD, to prevent cellular damage from environmental pollution and potential daily radiation exposure.
- **Children ages 1–3:** 1 drop in yogurt or other liquid
- **Children ages 4–7:** 2 drops in yogurt or other liquid
- **Children 8 and older:** 6 drops per capsule 1-3 times daily or in yogurt or other liquid
- **Adults:** 20 drops per capsule, 1-2 capsules, 1-3 times daily or in yogurt or other liquid

EndoFlex—This blend contains oils very specific to the thyroid while at the same time addressing the entire endocrine system. Myrtle oil stimulates and promotes good thyroid health when combined with Spearmint, encouraging better circulation, stronger metabolism, and production of digestive enzymes. Geranium contains esters that protect the thyroid, which may explain why it is so heralded in French publications as a general tonic for the body. It supports the thyroid in being able to uptake iodine from food.
- **Children ages 1–3:** 1 drop in yogurt or other liquid
- **Children ages 4–7:** 2 drops in yogurt or other liquid
- **Children 8 and older:** 6 drops per capsule 2 times daily or in yogurt or other liquid
- **Adults:** 20 drops per capsule, 1-2 capsules, 1-3 times daily or in yogurt or other liquid

Citrus Fresh—This blend combines six citrus oils that are naturally antioxidant, antibacterial, and increase the uptake of vitamin C.
- **Children ages 1–3:** 1 drop in yogurt or other liquid
- **Children ages 4–7:** 2 drops in yogurt or other liquid
- **Children 8 and older:** 6 drops per capsule 2 times daily or in yogurt or other liquid
- **Adults:** 20 drops per capsule, 1-2 capsules, 1-3 times daily or in yogurt or other liquid

NingXia Red—Drink 4-6 oz. of NingXia Red for a delicious and healthy addition to your diet.

of Chief project engineer Gary Brunson, and the filing of whistleblower complaints alleging that safety concerns were suppressed by Bechtel and were filed by Nuclear and Environmental Safety Manager Donna Busche and former Deputy Chief Process Engineer Walter Tamosaitis."[84]

Also, according to the United Nations and the International Atomic Energy Agency, the former Soviet Union's Chernobyl nuclear plant exploded in 1986, killing 56 and eventually leading to the deaths of more than 4,000 people from radiation exposure. It is impossible to know what other deaths and illnesses were caused by this exposure, but the radiation caused the deaths of thousands of people and damage to thousands of acres of land, contaminating and destroying plants, trees, crops, and other vegetation growing on numerous farms.

We have a more recent example. "Following a major earthquake, a 15-metre tsunami disabled the power supply and cooling of three Fukushima Daiichi reactors, causing a nuclear accident on 11 March 2011. All three cores largely melted in the first three days. The accident was rated 7 on the INES scale, due to high radioactive releases over days 4 to 6, eventually a total of some 940 PBq (I-131 eq). Four reactors were written off due to damage in the accident."[85]

Regardless of the contaminated soil, water we drink, food we eat, or air we breathe, it is virtually impossible to escape the effects of radiation contamination if you are in its silent path. The increase of illness and disease cannot be counted in the case of the Fukushima disaster, but the onset of cancer was measurable to some degree and increased dramatically in those affected areas.

Many experts and scientists talk about how air currents can carry the radioactive material from the point of origination around the world. Based on the history of the 1986 Chernobyl nuclear explosion from which thousands of people died, there is a great concern about the people of the world, especially those directly facing the air pathways carrying radioactive material.

The Power of Essential Oils Against Radiation

D. Gary Young spent two years studying the effects of the Chernobyl disaster and following the path of the radiation in Canada and the United States. He saw the negative effects in his microscopy blood testing, while charting the increased rate of cancer and other related illnesses in those areas.

It is difficult to run and hide from this invisible and odorless danger that can silently fall upon us. What can we do to provide protection for ourselves, families, and loved ones in our homes, work, and outdoor environments?

Diffusing essential oils is a very simple and effective way to help safeguard our homes. You can start with several different essential oil blends such as Purification, Melrose, and Exodus II. These are three distinct essential oil blends that are very effective in cleansing the air of impurities.

The following guidelines show you how to begin diffusing. See additional information in this reference manual about diffusing or go to YoungLiving.com.

There are many different types of diffusers. Some diffuse just with cold air, and others diffuse oil in water that humidifies as well. Some are elaborate, and some are simple.

- Diffusing is a matter of choice, and everyone is different. It is fun to try different oils and see what works best.

- Diffuse different essential oil singles or blends throughout the day.

- If you have two diffusers, in one you can diffuse a single oil such as Sacred Frankincense, and in the other, diffuse the blend of Melrose.

- Later, when you want to change oils, you can diffuse a different combination such as Palo Santo in one and Purification in the other.

- Melrose is a particularly powerful blend because it contains two melaleuca oils that may protect cells from radiation damage, according to Dr. Daniel Pénoël, co-author of the essential oil book l'aromathérapie exactement.[86]

- You can also use other single oils such as Clove, Oregano, Peppermint, Cinnamon Bark, Frankincense, Mountain Savory, etc., and blends such as Exodus II, Raven, and Thieves.

- Another sensible precaution is to wear an inexpensive dust mask while you are outside or traveling. Use Purification, Melrose, Exodus II, or your favorite oil or blend, dilute with water in a small spray bottle, and spray the dust mask. Some oils, if used directly or undiluted, may slightly burn or sting the tender skin of the lips or nose, especially of children. Carrying a small spritzer bottle in your pocket enables you to respray the mask and the area in which you are working.

- Using an incense burner, you will further protect your environment by burning Frankincense Resin—an ancient method of purifying the air—throughout your home and work environment. You can even burn the Frankincense Resin and diffuse the Frankincense oil at the same time or alternate different oils with the resin burning. We cannot protect our homes too much.

Internally, there are also things that you can do to give added protection and strength to your body. Fill a gelatin capsule, 00 size, with the number of oil drops recommended and the rest with V-6 or another vegetable oil and take with water one or two times daily or as you desire. Many people will completely fill the capsule with oil when they know how their body will respond.

Enzyme capsules can be emptied into juice or yogurt, especially for smaller children who have a difficult time swallowing capsules.

Below are some of the products you can choose from, and you must determine how much you can take and what is best suited for your body. You may take more or less according to your desire. Some oils and supplements you may want to take every day, and some you may want to alternate. You be the judge.

PRODUCTS

Allerzyme: 1-2 capsules 3 times a day to digest non-nutritious substances that cause imbalance and irritation

ComforTone: 1 capsule 3 times daily before breakfast and bedtime to support digestive and colon health

Detoxzyme: 1-2 capsules 3 times daily to work at digesting toxins

Digest & Cleanse: 1 softgel 1-3 times daily

DiGize Vitality: Dilute 1 drop with 4 drops of V-6 or other pure carrier oil. Put in a capsule and take 1 daily to help digest and eliminate poisons

EndoFlex Vitality: Dilute 1 drop with 1 drop of V-6 or other pure carrier oil. Put in a capsule and take up to 3 times daily to support the thyroid, often compromised because of radiation

Essentialzyme: 1 caplet 1 hour before meals for best results to keep general digestion continually working for better nutrient absorption and usability

Essentialzymes-4: 2 capsules (1 dual-dose blister pack) 2 times daily with largest meals to aid in the digestion of fats, proteins, fiber, and carbohydrates

Exodus II: 1-2 capsules of oil daily to support the immune system

ICP: 1-2 teaspoons in the morning in at least 8 ounces of water; a good fiber blend that binds with toxins and helps with elimination; high in rutin from buckwheat, helps to protect against radiation, and stimulates new bone marrow production

ImmuPro: 1 tablet before bed to support a healthy immune system

Inner Defense: 1 softgel daily or as needed for immune support

JuvaPower: 1-2 teaspoons at night to help cleanse the colon

KidScents MightyVites, MightyZyme, and MightyPro: Formulated especially for children to provide an all-natural spectrum of critical nutrients for immunity, digestion, protection, and vitality

LavaDerm Cooling Mist: A spray containing Lavender, Northern Lights Black Spruce, and Helichrysum essential oils that is very effective in reducing the burning and pain from the slightest to third-degree burns; spray directly on burn; if no pain, it may be rubbed on the skin with your hand. With any kind of a burn, it can be sprayed directly on the burn every 2 or 3 minutes as necessary.

Life 9: 1 capsule every night or as needed as a probiotic support for a healthy immune system

Longevity Softgels: 1 gel cap 1 times daily for immune and glandular support

Melrose: 6-20 drops per capsule or in kefir or yogurt 1-3 times a day to prevent radiation damage to normal cells; digests toxic material

Mineral Essence: 1 dropper per day; protects from mineral depletion, as minerals work as a catalyst for enzyme conversion

MultiGreens: 2-4 capsules daily, as green vegetables and kelp are a good source of iodine

NingXia Red: 4-6 ounces daily to strengthen body systems

Sulfurzyme: Sulfur helps with metal detoxification and free radical neutralization

Super Vitamin C or Super Vitamin C Chewable: 1-2 tablets daily to strengthen the immune system

Thyromin: 1-2 capsules daily, taken immediately before going to sleep, for thyroid support, which is easily damaged by radiation; capsule may be opened and emptied into yogurt, kefir, or other drink for children who cannot swallow capsules; may have a synergistic, protective effect on your hormonal and immune systems.

General Guidelines

- Foods to eat: Green vegetables and fresh fruits

- Foods to avoid: During a particular time of disaster, do not eat any animal flesh such as red meat, poultry, or fish for 30 days or more to avoid any contamination there may be to this type of food.

- Water: 3 liters of pure water daily, as well as fresh fruit juices

- Superoxide dismutase (SOD) is a very strong intracellular, antioxidant ingredient that helps free radical scavengers as they attack contaminants that try to invade the body.

- Vitamins C and E are very supporting to overall health and protect against whole-body radiation exposure.

- Be sure to eat foods containing antioxidants that offer protection and especially protect your DNA from damage. These foods should be part of your diet. Lipoic acid and the antioxidants from berries have been proven scientifically to protect your body against radiation damage.

  Recent animal research conducted by the United States Department of Agriculture showed that blueberry and strawberry extracts helped prevent brain damage from radiation exposure. The polyphenols of each different fruit protected different areas of the brain—supporting a variety of dietary berry intake.

- NingXia Red is perfect with its many antioxidant berries, which are important for our protection.

- Seaweeds, seaweed extracts, and miso soup are good sources of iodine to help detoxify your body of radiation. Baking soda, iodine, glutathione, and clay work as natural chelators.

- Essential oils such as Patchouli, Hyssop, Ledum or essential oil blends such as GLF, DiGize, JuvaCleanse, Longevity, Melrose, and Thieves digest and chelate toxins naturally.

- ICP, JuvaPower, and ComforTone are very effective for absorbing toxins and digesting waste and help with elimination from the body. Besides that, these natural products have numerous other benefits without toxic overuse and side effects.

- Many people ask about potassium iodide tablets or tinctures to protect the thyroid in an emergency situation where there is a high level of radiation exposure. Potassium iodide floods the thyroid and blocks the uptake of radioactive iodine from inhalation and ingestion. Following the 1986 nuclear disaster among the residents of Belarus, the Russian Federation, and Ukraine, up to 2005, more than 6,000 cases of thyroid cancer had been reported in children and adolescents who were exposed to the radiation.

  Many pros and cons often make decisions difficult. People who have iodine sensitivity, dermatitis herpetiformis, hypocomplementemic vasculitis, and thyroid disorders like Graves' disease should avoid potassium iodide. Therefore, it is better to research the facts in order to make the best choice about whether to take potassium iodide.

- Sodium bicarbonate or baking soda taken internally helps block possible damage to the kidneys from uranium exposure, as this is where it often shows up first. Sodium bicarbonate helps alkalinize the urine. It was used at Los Alamos National Laboratory in New Mexico to clean contaminated soil because it binds with uranium and separates it from the dirt. The United States Army also recommends bicarbonate to protect the kidneys from radiation damage.

- AlkaLime is specifically formulated with the essential oils of Lemon and Lime to help bring the body into proper pH balance. It settles an upset stomach and calms nauseated feelings that are associated with trauma, contamination, and radiation exposure.

- Magnesium salts, magnesium chloride in the form of magnesium bath flakes, or sea salts high in magnesium help to guard against contamination. Keep 5 to 10 pounds of magnesium salts in storage for immediate and emergency use. In 1 cup of salt, mix a few drops of Purification, Melrose, The Gift (which includes Sacred Frankincense), or an oil of choice, and then add to bath water. Soaking in the water for 15 to 30 minutes is enjoyable and relaxing while detoxifying contaminants from daily radiation exposure.

- Chlorella and spirulina powders help flush radioactive substances from the body and were used heavily by the Russians after the Chernobyl nuclear plant disaster.

- MultiGreens is a natural, energizing supplement that contains kelp, spirulina, amino acids, and detoxifying nutrients that synergistically work with the essential oils of Rosemary, Lemon, Lemongrass, and Melissa that cleanses, builds, and stimulates the immune system. The "specific" kelp contains natural iodine that protects the thyroid from daily radiation.

- Cilantro helps move heavy metals and radioactive material out of the brain cells for detoxification and elimination.

- GLF is a gallbladder and liver flush that aids in eliminating the negative effects of toxins in the body.

- Radiation exposure is a real threat to the people of the world, but the responsibility of protection lies with each individual. We are in a time when we must protect ourselves, families, friends, loved ones, and community. We need to help others learn how to protect themselves using natural products that strengthen the immune system, cleanse the body, and protect against daily pollution, contamination, and dangerous radiation.

- Essential oils are simple and easy to use. The benefits are tremendous and can be life-giving and long-lasting. This natural God-given protection that Mother Nature affords us is ours for the taking. It is without risk or side effects and offers immense benefits that only our bodies can determine when given the opportunity.

SECRETS OF LONGEVITY: LIVING TO 100

The study of longevity was a passion of D. Gary Young for over three decades. He traveled the world studying the cultures of different people known for their longevity. In his research, he discovered that these different cultures had two unusual commonalities. The Georgian people in the Caucasus region, in Inner-Mongolia in the Ningxia Province in China, the Hunzakut people in Northern Pakistan, the people of Vilcabamba in southern Ecuador, the people of the Republic of Azerbaijan in the Talish Mountains region in Eurasia, and the Tarahumara natives of Copper Canyon in the southern state of Chihuahua, Mexico, all practiced fasting on a regular basis and lived to be over 120 years of age.

After in-depth studies of the dietary habits of these cultures, he found another common denominator: they lived a very active lifestyle and ate a mineral-rich diet, exceptionally high in antioxidant foods such as wolfberries and apricots. In particular, he found that Chinese wolfberries (Lycium barbarum L.) and the potassium-rich apricots of Hunzaland were two foods routinely consumed by people in these regions who reached 110 to 120 years of age.

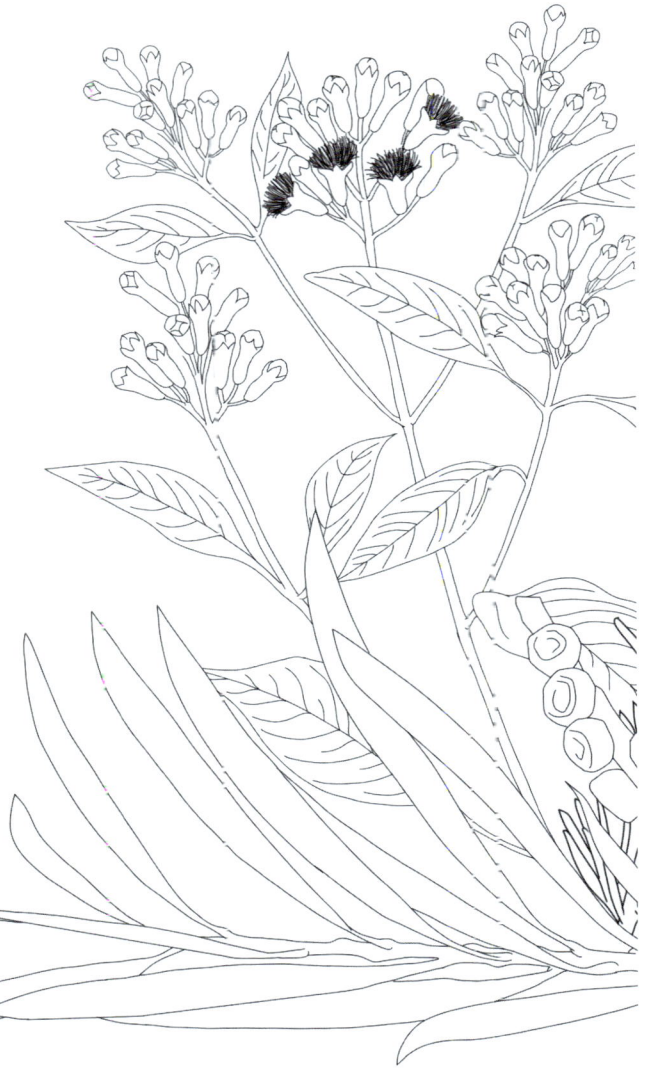

Fasting allows the body to slow down the secretion of digestive enzymes, thereby permitting an increase in metabolic enzymes that help the body to repair and revitalize tissue that has been damaged or destroyed. Fasting, with time, enables the body to rebuild and spurs an increase in human growth hormone, which impedes premature aging.

The human body has the potential to live for 100 years and beyond. However, devitalized and enzyme-deficient foods deplete our enzyme reserves and overly stress the organs and the body's physical processes. As enzymes continue to decrease, the body's resistance to degenerative disease also decreases.

D. Gary Young, in his book Longevity Secrets, discussed important, scientific, antiaging properties found in these foods, which may be due to their extremely high content of important minerals such as magnesium and potassium, as well as their rich supply of potent natural antioxidants. Research indicates that foods high in antioxidants such as wolfberries, blueberries, strawberries, raspberries, and spinach can dramatically increase glutathione levels and actually reverse the signs of aging.

A test developed by USDA researchers at Tufts University in Boston, Massachusetts, has been able to identify the highest-known antioxidant foods. Known as ORAC (oxygen radical absorbance capacity), this test is the first of its kind to measure both time and degree of free-radical inhibition.

The Ningxia wolfberry was documented to have the highest ORAC score of any food tested. A special variety grown on the Yellow River in the Ningxia Province of central China, the Ningxia cultivar is very different from any other type of wolfberry. Among the 17 types of wolfberry identified, the Ningxia wolfberry has by far the highest levels of immune-stimulating polysaccharides. It also possesses over 33 times the antioxidant power of oranges and an amazing 120 times the antioxidant potential of carrots. In addition, the Chinese wolfberry is one of the most nutrient-dense foods known, rich in many vitamins and minerals, including calcium, magnesium, B vitamins, and vitamin C. A diet high in antioxidants can combat the free radical damage in the body associated with premature aging and degenerative diseases.

The limited-calorie intake of the people living in the remote Hunza Valley in northern Pakistan contributes to their longevity. The Hunzakuts, as they call themselves, commonly live past ages 100, 110, and even 120. They also share another remarkable trait: the near absence of degenerative disease.

The diet of the Hunza people is known to be high in potassium and low in sodium. Apricots, barley, millet, and buckwheat are the main staples of their diet, along with mineral-rich water with a pH of 8.5. But there is yet another unusual factor that may protect the health of the Hunza people and increase their longevity: their limited food intake.

Because the land provides just enough food to cover their basic caloric needs, the Hunzakuts rarely indulge in overeating. In fact, prior to the construction of the Karakoram Highway, they annually endured near-fasting conditions for several weeks each spring, a time when the previous year's food supply was depleted, and the current year's harvests had not yet begun.

Restricted caloric intake such as fasting can have powerful effects on longevity because it increases blood levels of growth hormone, which is one of the most significant antiaging hormones to be identified during the last two decades. Secreted by the pituitary gland, growth hormone production steadily declines with age. By age 70, the human body produces less than one tenth of the growth hormone it did at age 20.

Clinical studies have repeatedly shown that growth hormone production is stimulated by low glucose levels. Because fasting depresses glucose levels, it leads to a surge in natural growth hormone production.[87]

A university study showed that older adults are the fastest-growing segment of the U.S. population and a greater proportion of them are entering old age obese. Seven randomized controlled studies revealed that calorie restriction combined with exercise is effective for weight loss.[88] Calorie restriction was tested among healthy non-obese adults and was found to be safe and well tolerated.[89]

Unfortunately, the historical cultures of "longevity and superior health and endurance" are fading away and will only be something we read about in history books. The world is more connected than ever before through the high technology of cell phones, television, media production, and satellite proliferation. The advancement of processed and prepackaged food has infiltrated every country in the world.

The use of synthetic and nature-identical chemicals in the industries of food, body care products, cosmetics, perfumes, household cleaners, drugs, and over-the-counter medicines has gradually brought a decline in health and longevity. Literally every aspect of our lives is contaminated through the food we put in our bodies, the creams and lotions we put on our bodies, the water we drink, and the air we breathe.

We are becoming a world of the sick and obese as the fast-food industry proliferates, we eat frozen dinners, and just "add water" or "pop the pizza in the oven" for a quick meal. We open millions of cans of vegetables and fruits, eat sugar and chemically colored and preserved desserts, and gulp down snacks devoid of nutritional substance.

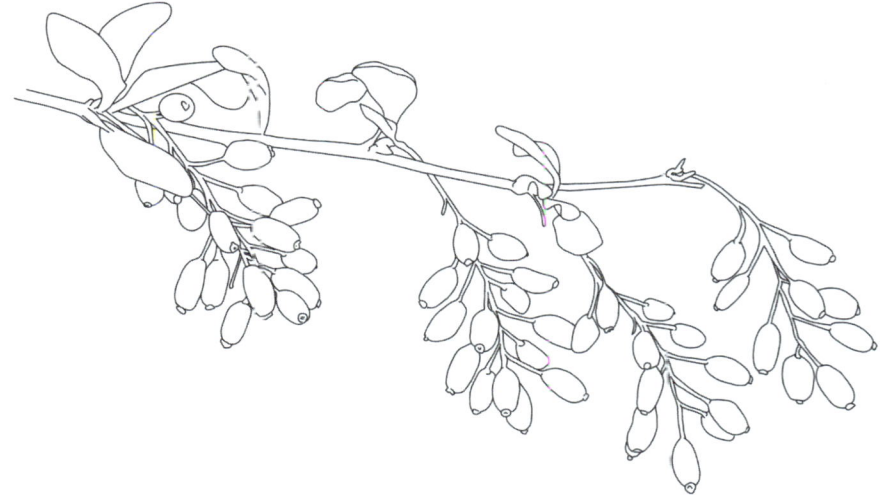

It is sad to see that so many people are content to eat this way and then wonder why they feel awful, have no energy, and are just plain sick.

How sad to see babies and children alike grow with mental and physical deficiencies because society is not teaching anything better to parents, teachers, and those who could have an influence. For those who do see what is happening and want to help change things, the vision is immense. Correct information is the key, and we can all get involved in whatever way is possible. We need to help people become educated, so they can change their habits before they find themselves fighting an unhealthy condition and trying to save the lives of children heading down the wrong path.

It's up to us to choose to become involved. Money talks and if you can become involved with a health-focused company or even build a business in a company that is teaching correct principles, you will have the best of both worlds. Build your business and become the master of your own time and money. You will have the products that you need and the money to educate and disseminate information. After all, word of mouth is one of the most effective ways to spread the news.

Now is the time to act, so join with thousands of others in the world whose mission is to bring health and a better way of life to those in the world they can touch.

SULFUR: AN IMPORTANT MINERAL

Why is sulfur so important to the body? Because sulfur is a mineral which, like vitamin C, is constantly being used up and depleted. When we fail to replenish our reserves of nutritional sulfur, we become more vulnerable to disease and degenerative conditions. Some possible signs of sulfur deficiency are:

- Poor nail and hair growth
- Eczema
- Dermatitis
- Poor muscle tone
- Acne/Pimples
- Gout
- Rheumatism
- Arthritis
- Weakening of the nervous system
- Constipation
- Impairment of mental faculties
- Lowered libido

MSM: A Key to Sulfur

MSM (methylsulfonylmethane) is a natural, sulfur-bearing nutrient that occurs widely in nature (found in everything from mother's breast milk to fresh vegetables). It is an exceptional source of nutritional sulfur—a mineral that is vital to protein synthesis and sound health.

MSM is more than just another essential nutrient. According to research compiled by Ronald Lawrence, PhD, MD, and Stanley Jacob, MD, MSM represents a safe, natural solution for chronic headaches, back pain, tendonitis, fibromyalgia, rheumatism, arthritis, athletic injuries, muscle spasms, asthma, and allergies.

In a book entitled The Miracle of MSM, both Dr. Jacobs and Dr. Lawrence discuss how MSM has benefited hundreds of patients. A UCLA neuropsychiatrist, Dr. Lawrence is convinced that MSM will revolutionize how millions of people deal with inflammatory autoimmune diseases such as rheumatism, asthma, bursitis, and tendonitis, as well as auto-immune diseases like arthritis, lupus, scleroderma, and allergies.

Other doctors have also seen their patients dramatically improve using 2 to 4 grams of MSM daily. According to David Blyweiss, MD, of the Institute of Advanced Medicine in Lauderhill, Florida, many patients experience a 50 percent improvement in their arthritis symptoms, along with less fatigue, better sleep, and better ability to exercise.

Dr. Lawrence has also used MSM to improve the condition of patients who were virtually crippled with arthritis and back pain. One patient was able to get out of bed for the first time after just two weeks on MSM, and after two months of MSM use, he could walk to the grocery store.

Another of Dr. Lawrence's patients was a 70-year-old woman who was suffering from severe arthritis. In this case, MSM actually postponed the need for double knee replacement. In fact, after only two months on oral MSM, she was walking again with much less pain and stiffness.

Numerous other MSM users have experienced results equivalent to cortisone—but without side effects like immune suppression, fluid retention, and weakness.

According to Stanley Jacobs, MD, there may be no pharmaceutical back pain therapy better—or safer—than MSM. "MSM has an important role to play in the nonsurgical treatment of back pain," he said. "I have seen several hundred patients for back pain secondary to osteoarthritis, disc degeneration, spinal misalignments, or accidents. For such pain-related conditions, MSM is usually beneficial."

"I have been recommending MSM for more than six months," said Richard Shaefer, a chiropractor from Wheeling, Illinois. "The results have been excellent. I consistently see major reduction in pain and inflammation in arthritic joints, along with improved range of motion. I can't think of a single individual who isn't getting some kind of positive effect."

MSM may have other benefits aside from its pain and inflammation-reducing properties. Numerous patients have reported a surge in energy levels along with thicker hair, nails, and skin. Some have even reported a softening or disappearance of scar tissue.

One user reported a marked increase in stamina and energy after starting on MSM. "For a long while, I have had the blahs," complained Lou Salyer of Tucson, Arizona. "I had no stamina. I had to force myself to get things done around the house. After two days on MSM, it was like a blast of energy. I am amazed at how much I get done now."

MSM may also do much more than relieve pain. "Prior to taking MSM (30 grams a day for 20 years), I would have a cold or flu two or three times a year," stated Dr. Jacobs. "Since I've been taking MSM, I've not had a single cold or the flu. I can't say that MSM prevented my cold or the flu, but it is a fascinating observation."

MSM contains an exceptionally bioavailable source of sulfur, one of the most neglected minerals needed by the human body. Carl Pfeiffer, MD, PhD, a world-renowned expert on nutritional medicine, agrees: "Sulfur is the forgotten essential element."

Found in such foods as garlic and asparagus, the sulfur within MSM is a critical part of the amino acids cysteine and methionine, which form the building blocks of the nails, hair, and skin. Sulfur is also found in therapeutic mineral baths and hot springs that have brought relief to arthritis sufferers for centuries.

Of particular importance is MSM's ability to equalize water pressure inside the cells—a considerable benefit for those plagued with bursitis, arthritis, and tendonitis. These kinds of inflammatory outbreaks are created when the water pressure inside the cells jumps past the pressure outside the cells, creating pressure and pain. MSM acts as a sort of cellular safety valve, affecting the protein envelope of the cell so that water transfers freely in and out of the cell. The result: rapid relief and less damage to tissues. In addition, because it elasticizes the hold between the cells, MSM can restore flexibility to inflamed tissues.

When our bodies grow older and are chronically shortchanged of key minerals like sulfur and MSM, the bonds between our cells become increasingly rigid and brittle—a condition that can lead to a loss in skin flexibility and contribute to skin wrinkles. The internal manifestations of this cellular brittleness are far less visible but have a far greater negative impact on the body. MSM's ability to reintroduce flexibility into cell structures, therefore, can have widespread, restorative effects.

Sulfurzyme is a unique combination of MSM, protein-building compounds, and Ningxia wolfberry. Together, they create a new concept in balancing the immune system and supporting almost every major function of the body.

SWEETENERS: MAKING THE RIGHT CHOICE

As mentioned, many of today's health concerns are caused by so-called modern conveniences. Increased use of sugars and artificial sweeteners—and some of those "conveniences"—raises the question: what's the difference between sugars, synthetic sweeteners, and natural, low-glycemic sweeteners?

Sugars

Do you remember when "treats" were for special occasions? For many families, eating sweets now begins at breakfast and continues all day long. Instead of a hearty serving of oatmeal, today's children are growing up on bowls of miniature chocolate doughnuts or sugar-coated cereals. Sweet snacks, drinks, and desserts continue until bedtime—and children aren't the only ones guzzling and gulping down sugar. How often have you seen an adult leave a convenience store toting a 64-ounce soft drink?

Nothing stresses the human body as much as refined sugar. Called a "skeletonized food" and a "castrated carbohydrate" by Edward Howell, PhD, and a "metabolic freeloader" by Ralph Golan, MD, sugar actually drains the body of vitamins, minerals, and nutrients in the process of being burned for energy. Sugar also stresses the pancreas, forcing it to pump out a surge of unneeded digestive enzymes.

Sugar also undermines and retards immune response. One study measured the effects of 100 grams of sugar (sucrose) on neutrophils, a form of white blood cell that comprises a central part of immunity. Within one hour of ingestion, neutrophil activity dropped 50 percent and remained below normal for another four hours.[90]

Population studies have also linked sugar consumption with diabetes and heart disease. According to researcher John Yudkin, the reason sugar elevates the risk of heart disease is due to an automatic, built-in safety switch inside the body.[91] To protect itself from being immediately poisoned from excess sugar, the body converts it into fats, like triglycerides. So instead of killing you quickly, the body defends itself by clogging its arteries, thereby killing you on the installment plan.

High-Fructose Corn Syrup

Ever on the lookout for a cheaper sweetener, scientists figured out how to take corn syrup, add genetically modified enzymes, and, in a long chemical process, create a corn sweetener with more fructose than is found in nature (e.g., honey). The high-fructose corn syrup (HFCS) blend that is used in soft drinks, for instance, is 55 percent fructose. For low-calorie "diet" products, a blend has been concocted that has a 90-10 fructose-to-glucose ratio. This refined blend is intensely sweet.

Between 1970, when HFCS was introduced in the U.S., and 2000, consumer consumption jumped from less than 1 pound per person to over 60 pounds yearly. Perhaps not coincidentally, something else jumped during that time frame: obesity.

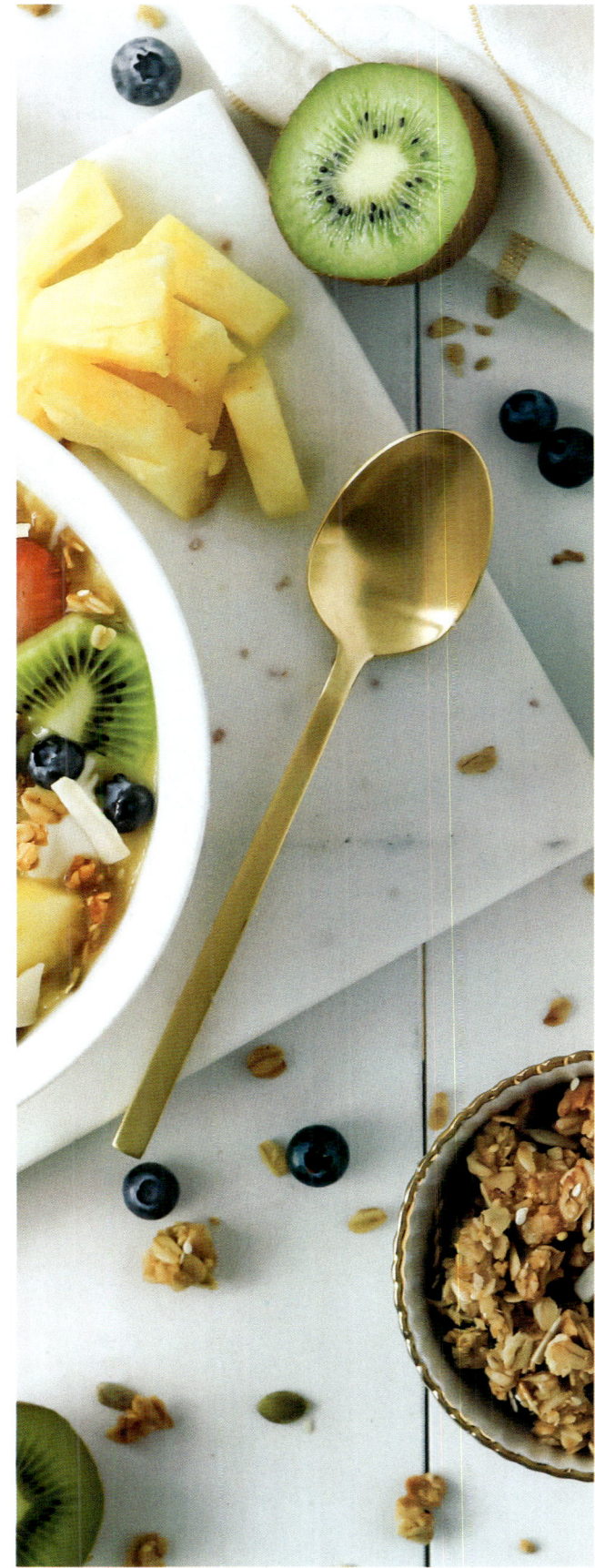

Researchers at Louisiana State University and the University of North Carolina studied food consumption patterns using USDA tables from 1967 to 2000 and found that HFCS consumption increased more than 1,000 percent between 1970 and 1990. They concluded that ". . . overconsumption of HFCS in calorically sweetened beverages may play a role in the epidemic of obesity."[92]

A December 2013 animal study published in the journal Nutrition & Diabetes found that HFCS induced more severe adipose inflammation and insulin resistance than an even higher-calorie-containing 'western' high-fat diet and concluded that "HFCS has detrimental effects on metabolism, suggesting that dietary guidelines on HFCS consumption need to be revisited."[93]

There is yet more bad health news about HFCS. In October 2008 The New York Times reported that in a study tracking over 9,000 people, those who drank two or more sugary sodas a day (a major source of high-fructose corn syrup) were at a 40 percent higher risk for kidney damage, while the risk for women soda drinkers nearly doubled. NYT writer Tara Parker-Pope noted that a study published in the Journal of Hepatology ". . . suggested a link between consumption of high-fructose corn syrup in sodas and fatty liver disease." Parker-Pope also wrote about a smaller study in The Journal of Nutrition that suggested that fructose bypasses the normal regulation of sugar and is turned to fat more quickly than other sugars.

It seems that people are beginning to awaken to the problems with this highly processed sweetener. The same NYT article reported market research showing that ". . . 58 percent of Americans say they are concerned that high-fructose corn syrup poses a health risk."[94] The Corn Refiners Association is fighting back. An advertising blitz in 2008 emphasized that ". . . HFCS is made from corn, has no artificial ingredients, and is fine in moderation."[95] Because HFCS is in a staggering amount of food, the U.S. Time Magazine wryly noted, ". . . unless you're making a concerted effort to avoid it, it's pretty difficult to consume high-fructose corn syrup in moderation."[96]

Petition for a Name Change: Because the public perceives high-fructose corn syrup (HFCS) as dangerous, a backlash has developed. Marion Nestle, a New York University professor of nutrition, said that you have to feel sorry for the corn refiners because ". . . high-fructose corn syrup is the new trans-fat."[97]

Seattle's PCC Natural Markets banned all products containing HFCS. Jason's Deli, a restaurant chain with 200 restaurants in 27 states, replaced all items that contain HFCS, except for some soft drinks. In May 2010, Hunt's ketchup returned to regular sugar because of buyer preference. Snapple, Gatorade, and Starbucks' baked goods also avoid HFCS now. Ocean Spray Cranberry Juice and Wheat Thins crackers also promote "no HFCS."

The backlash is beginning to be significant. After being scolded by a blogger, Chick-Fil-A has removed HFCS and artificial colors from its sauces and dressings, and now, HFCS is gone from its sandwich buns as well.

In September of 2010, The Corn Refiners Association petitioned the FDA to start calling HFCS "corn sugar." The president of the organization believes that HFCS is confusing to consumers and thinks that the "term 'corn sugar' succinctly and accurately describes what this natural ingredient is and where it comes from—corn." HFCS is hardly "natural." We like what one health writer suggested for its new name: "enzymatically altered corn glucose."

In a win for health-conscious consumers, in March of 2012, the FDA rejected the Corn Refiners Association bid to rename HFCS as "corn sugar." Regardless of the failed name change, sales of high fructose corn syrup are in decline. A February 2016 report by the USDA reported: "Domestic use of high-fructose corn syrup (HFCS) declined 0.8 percent in the 2014/15 fiscal year (October 1-September 30) to 7.2 million short tons, continuing a decade-long decline. Since 2004/05, domestic use has fallen by 19.1 percent, and it is down 21.8 percent since its peak in 2001/01."[98]

Synthetic Sweeteners

Health dangers are also found in the use of artificial sweeteners. Seventy-five percent of the adverse reactions reported to the U.S. Food and Drug Administration come from a single substance: the artificial sweetener aspartame. But a newer artificial sweetener, sucralose, may be challenging those numbers with a whole host of new adverse reactions.

Sucralose (Splenda™): Perhaps it is enough to explain that Splenda is chlorinated sugar. The structure of sugar molecules is changed by substituting three chlorine atoms for three hydroxyl groups. How healthy does that sound? However, few human studies have been published. The FDA's "Final Rule" report stated, "Sucralose was weakly mutagenic [capable of causing mutations] in a mouse lymphoma mutation assay," and other reports by the FDA were "inconclusive."[99]

Researchers from North Carolina State University and Avazyme Inc. (an analytical testing company) found, in a recent study on rats, that sucralose is metabolized in the gut, and that the sweetener itself stays in the fatty tissues of the body. "This finding differs from the studies used to garner regulatory approval for sucralose," the researchers said, "which reported that the substance was not broken down in the body."[100] In addition, a study published in the Journal of Food Science Technology in 2014 stated that "11-27% of ingested sucralose is absorbed in the body."[101]

Dr. Joseph Mercola states that, "since Splenda bears more chemical similarity to DDT than it does to sugar," [consumers shouldn't] bet their health on [the weak data provided by the FDA]. He cautions us to remember that fat-soluble substances such as DDT can remain in your fat for decades and devastate your health."[102]

The big news is that in January of 2016, a study was published in the International Journal of Occupational and Environmental Health showing that mice fed sucralose daily throughout their lives developed leukemia and other blood cancers.[103] The nonprofit watchdog group Center for Science in the Public Interest had downgraded Splenda from "safe" to "caution" and now recommends that consumers avoid Splenda.

Helen Kollias of PrecisionNutrition.com says this with regards to a 2008 animal study with Splenda:

[T]here are two major points to take home. First, relatively low amounts of Splenda (100mg/kg/day) may cause weight gain (emphasis added). And second, Splenda at moderate levels (300mg/kg/day and up) has adverse effects on your gut, affecting both levels of gut flora and proteins. Why does this matter? Changes in gut bacteria can lead to problems with your immune system and ability to absorb nutrients.[104]

It is darkly humorous that two makers of artificial sweeteners went to court because the makers of NutraSweet believed that Splenda received an unfair advantage with its sneaky slogan "Made from sugar so it tastes like sugar." McNeil Nutritionals later changed the slogan to "Starts with sugar, tastes like sugar, but is not sugar." But the "unfair" slogan did its job. Between 2000 and 2004, the percentage of U.S. households using Splenda jumped from 3 to 20 percent. In a one-year period, Splenda sales topped $177 million, compared with $62 million spent on aspartame-based Equal and $52 million on saccharin-based Sweet'N Low®.[105]

Is Sucralose natural? Far from it! Is it safe? Science now tells us: NO!

Aspartame: Aspartame is marketed today as NutraSweet®, Equal®, and Equal® Spoonful. With so many Americans on one diet or another, the market for aspartame is simply enormous—and it matters not that aspartame users are suffering from symptoms ranging from headaches, numbness, and seizures to joint pain, chronic fatigue syndrome, multiple sclerosis, and epilepsy.

The 1996 book by Dr. Russell L. Blaylock, professor of neurosurgery at the Medical University of Mississippi, *Excitotoxins: The Taste That Kills*,[06] explains that aspartame is a neurotransmitter, facilitating the transmission of information from one neuron to another. Aspartame allows too much calcium into brain cells, killing certain neurons, earning aspartame the name of "excitotoxin."

With aspartame now in over 9,000 products such as instant breakfasts, breath mints, cereals, frozen desserts, "lite" gelatin desserts, and even multivitamins, it is no surprise that there is a virtual epidemic of memory loss, Alzheimer's disease, and multiple sclerosis. In a move much like a telephone company selling your phone number to telephone solicitors and then charging you to block their calls, G. D. Searle (the Monsanto company that manufactures aspartame) is searching for a drug to combat memory loss caused by excitatory amino acid damage, most often caused by aspartame.

Do you fly the friendly skies? You may be interested to know that both the Air Force's magazine, Flying Safety, and Navy Physiology, the Navy's publication, detailed warnings about pilots being more susceptible to seizures after consuming aspartame. The Aspartame Consumer Safety Network notes that 600 pilots have reported acute reactions to aspartame, including grand mal seizures in the cockpit. Many other publications have warned about aspartame ingestion while flying, including a paper presented at the 57th Annual Meeting of the Aerospace Medical Association.

A final note: The Center for Science in the Public Interest (CSPI) may only currently urge "caution" for Splenda; but for saccharin, aspartame, and acesulfame potassium (Sunett and Sweet One), it says "avoid."

Natural, Low-Glycemic Sweeteners

Natural, low-glycemic sweeteners are excellent alternatives to the sugar dilemma and include the six kinds mentioned below.

Blue Agave Nectar

The blue agave cactus grows in Central America. It produces a sweetener that is about 68 percent fructose, 22 percent glucose, and 4 percent fructooligosaccharides. Because of its heavy fructose concentration, blue agave is 32 percent sweeter than table sugar but has a low glycemic index (about 34). This means that, when consumed, blue agave has a minimal impact on blood sugar levels. It is well suited for people with candida infections.

FOS

FOS is a super nutrient documented to rebuild intestinal flora, improve mineral absorption, and more. Its attributes are shown below:

- Has a minimal impact on blood sugar levels
- Has a glycemic index of 0
- Is an ideal sweetener for diabetics
- Increases populations of beneficial bifidobacteria in the colon
- Reduces populations of harmful bacteria, such as Clostridium perfringens
- Improves calcium and magnesium absorption
- Improves liver function

A naturally sweet, indigestible fiber derived from chicory roots, FOS (fructooligosaccharides) is one of the best-documented classes of natural nutrients for promoting the growth of Lactobacilli and bifidobacteria (beneficial bacteria), a key to sound health. FOS has also been clinically studied for its ability to increase magnesium and calcium absorption; lower blood glucose, cholesterol, and LDL levels; and inhibit production of the reductase enzymes that can contribute to cancer. Because FOS can increase magnesium absorption, it can also lead to lowered blood pressure and better cardiovascular health.

FOS is one of the most powerful prebiotics to be researched in the last decade (a "prebiotic" feeds intestinal flora; a "probiotic" adds more actual cultures to existing intestinal flora). The subject of over 650 clinical studies (as of October 10, 2018), FOS is one of the best-documented, natural nutrients for improving the healthy balance of bacteria in intestines and stimulating the growth of the beneficial bifidobacteria—also called "friendly flora"—that reside in the colon.

How important to good health are these so-called "friendly flora" that populate our intestines? They are our front-line defense against invading, disease-causing organisms, combating premature aging caused by the toxin-producing bacteria and fungi that reside in our intestines.

Seven Reasons Why Bifidobacteria Are Vital to Health

1. They produce substances that stop the growth of harmful, toxic, gram-negative and -positive bacteria in the intestines.[107]
2. They occupy space on the intestinal wall that could be populated by pathogenic organisms. When bifidobacteria increase in numbers, they crowd out invasive, toxin-generating microorganisms.
3. They slow down the production of damaging protein-breakdown products, such as ammonia. This lowers blood ammonia levels that can be toxic to the human body.[108]
4. They produce B vitamins and folic acid.[109,110]
5. They produce digestive enzymes, like phosphatases and lysozymes.[111]
6. They stimulate the immune system to attack cancer cells.[112,113,114]
7. They increase the absorption of essential minerals, magnesium, and calcium. As we age, magnesium levels in the body decline, contributing to high blood pressure and diabetes.

Technically a fiber rather than a sugar, FOS is totally unlike conventional sugars because it feeds the beneficial bifidobacteria while selectively starving the parasitical yeast, fungi, and bacteria that contribute to disease. Most toxin-producing microorganisms in the intestines are unable to use FOS as food. Conventional sugars, like sucrose and lactose, on the other hand, work in just the opposite fashion: they tend to feed harmful bacteria more readily than they feed beneficial bacteria.

FOS Increases Mineral Absorption: Besides building up the beneficial bacteria in the body, FOS has also been shown to improve blood sugar control, liver function, and calcium and magnesium absorption.

A 2010 animal study conducted at the Shandong Centre for Tuberculosis Control in China found that a FOS diet increased magnesium and calcium absorption substantially.[115] A study at the University of Murcia in Spain obtained similar results.[116]

Magnesium is one of the most important nutrients we obtain from our diet, being involved in over 300 enzyme reactions in the body. As we age, our magnesium levels drop markedly, which creates a deficiency that increases the risk of angina, atherosclerosis, cardiac arrhythmias,

FOS Builds Up Friendly Flora

Subjects	Dose g/day	Duration	Fecal Bifidobacteria # bacteria (log) per gram		Reference
			Start of Study	End of Study	
9	1	14	9.8	10.2	Tokunaga, 92
9	3	14	9.9	10.4	Tokunaga, 92
9	5	14	9.7	10.3	Tokunaga, 92
20	12.5	12	7.9	9.1	Bouhnik, 93
38	8	14	5.2	6.2	Rochat, 94
12	4	25	9.5	9.8	Buddington, 96

depression, and diabetes.[117,118,119,120] A Medical University of Ohio study suggested that correcting magnesium deficiencies may prolong life.[121]

FOS also improves liver health. A Louvain Drug Research Institute study at Catholic University in Brussels, Belgium, reported that dietary fructooligosaccharides reduced hepatic triglyceride accumulation and thus provided an advantage in the management of liver disease.[122]

FOS may be the ideal nutrient for diabetics. Because FOS is an indigestible sugar, it triggers no spikes in blood sugar levels the way sucrose and glucose do. About 40 to 60 percent as sweet as sugar, FOS is found in low quantities in many types of foods. However, to obtain just a quarter teaspoon of FOS from foods in your diet, you would have to consume 13 bananas, 16 tomatoes, or 16 onions. Chicory roots have one of the highest amounts of FOS of any plant, and most natural FOS supplements are commercially derived from water-extraction of the roots.

Recommended Usage: To obtain the best results from FOS, daily intake should range between 5 and 10 grams a day. Dosages above 15 grams may cause gas or intestinal cramping from excess bifidobacteria populations.

Fructose

Do NOT confuse fructose with high-fructose corn syrup! Fructose is a natural sweetener that has one of the lowest glycemic indexes of any food. A glycemic index measures the impact that a food has on blood sugar levels two to three hours after ingestion. The lower the glycemic level, the lower the rise in blood sugar levels.

Fructose's low glycemic index of 20 is many times lower than standard breads and processed grains. Its glycemic index is only a third that of glucose, a fourth that of white bread, and a fifth that of boiled potatoes.

Maple Syrup – Grade B

The U.S. and Canada have slightly different grading systems for maple syrup. What is classified as Grade B maple syrup in the U.S. is the same as Grade C maple syrup in Canada. This grade is the best sweetener and the most balanced sugar. It is processed from the last tapping of the maple sap, so it is richer in invert sugars and minerals.

Grade B maple syrup is also a lower-glycemic-index food, resulting in a slow, gradual rise in blood sugar levels. The best maple syrup is currently produced in Vermont because it is strictly regulated for purity and authenticity by government law. Some unscrupulous marketers in other areas have been known to add refined sugars to colored, diluted, genuine maple syrup to produce a cheaper product. Also, a number of years ago, there was a problem with some Canadian and U.S. producers inserting formaldehyde pellets in their sugar maple trees to keep tap holes open longer, increasing yields.

Stevia

For over 1,600 years, the natives of Paraguay in South America have used this intensely sweet herb as a health agent and sweetener. Known as Stevia rebaudiana by botanists and yerba dulce (honey leaf) by the Guarani Indians, stevia has been incorporated into many native medicines, beverages, and foods for centuries. The Guarani used stevia separately or combined with herbs like yerba mate and lapacho.

Fifteen times sweeter than sugar, stevia was introduced to the West in 1899, when M. S. Bertoni discovered natives using it as a sweetener and medicinal herb. However, stevia was very slow to gain popularity in Europe or the United States and was only gradually adopted by several countries throughout Far East Asia.

With Japan's ban on the import of synthetic sweeteners in the 1960s, stevia began to be seriously researched by the Japanese National Institute of Health as a natural sugar substitute. After almost a decade of studies examining the safety and antidiabetic properties of the herb, Japan became a major producer, importer, and user of stevia. Japanese food companies began including stevia in hundreds of products, and eventually stevia use spread through Asia. Stevioside, the super sweet glycoside derived from stevia that is 300 times sweeter than sugar, was even used to sweeten Diet Coke sold in Japan.

Stevia has now gained widespread popularity as a low-calorie sweetener throughout the United States, South America, and Asia. Both the stevia leaf and stevioside are used in Taiwan, China, Korea, and Japan, with many of these same countries growing and harvesting large amounts of the raw herb.

In 1994 the U.S. Food and Drug Administration permitted the importation and use of stevia as a dietary supplement. But the FDA would not approve stevia for use as a food additive until the Coca-Cola Company expressed interest in approval of rebiana, its stevia-derived sweetener. In May 2008 Coca-Cola and Cargill introduced Truvia, a stevia sweetener containing erythritol and rebiana. Now stevia is considered GRAS.

Stevia, however, is more than just a noncaloric sweetener. Several modern clinical studies have documented the ability of stevia to lower and balance blood sugar levels, support the pancreas, protect the liver, and combat infectious microorganisms.[123,124,125,126,127]

Research has also documented stevia's powerful antioxidant and oxidative DNA damage-preventive activity.[128,129]

Regarding stevia and diabetes, one seminal study showed that oral administration of a stevia leaf extract reduced blood sugar levels by over 35 percent.[130] Another study documented similar results.[131] Clearly, these and other clinical evaluations indicate that stevia holds significant promise for the treatment of diabetes.

Yacon

Yacon is a tubular, perennial plant that looks similar to a yam or sweet potato, only with a black skin. It is indigenous to Ecuador and Peru and provides interesting nutritional products such as yacon syrup, yacon tea, and sweet candy-like snacks. These products are very popular, especially among diabetics, because the sugar they contain is not absorbed by humans.

Beyond the healthy sweetening yacon provides are even more health benefits because it contains FOS. According to Wikipedia, this form of sugar, known as FOS (fructooligosaccharide), a special kind of fructose, leaves the body undigested. The syrup is also a prebiotic, which means that it feeds the friendly bacteria in the colon that boost the immune system and help digestion.[132] (See "FOS Increases Mineral Absorption" above.)

Yacon has recently been transplanted to New Zealand and is being studied by the universities there as perhaps the world's greatest-kept secret as a sweetener with a zero glycemic index (a measure to show the impact of sugar on the pancreas), no negative effects on the body, safe for diabetics, safe for hypoglycemics, and safe for people with candida.

A Brazilian university study regarded yacon as a functional food because it "improves the growth of bifidobacteria in the colon, enhances mineral absorption and gastrointestinal metabolism and plays a role in the regulation of serum cholesterol."[133]

Because yacon grows in the ground as a tubular in the Andes Mountains, its roots are able to take advantage of the thousands of years of volcanic ash build-up that has a tremendously high mineral content. As the yacon grows, it takes up many of these minerals and converts them into a usable form within the natural sugars. Besides its high mineral content, it is also high in amino acids and vitamin A, as in carrots, making yacon very similar in profile to the Ningxia wolfberry. Yacon has also been studied as an antidiabetic treatment and is now being studied as a preventive for digestive cancers.

Refined Sugars and Laboratory-made Sweeteners

There is so much research available about them that one cannot deny their dangers, with obesity and heart disease on the top of the list. We have to be responsible, make tough decisions, and discipline ourselves. We must not allow sugar, synthetic sweeteners, or foods made with these substances to be on our "sweet" list anymore.

Unfortunately, sugar and these synthetic sweeteners are used in a great many food recipes. It is impossible to know if these ingredients have been used in the food prepared for us to eat in restaurants, at school or work, as snacks and pastries at parties, or even when invited to dinner in a friend's home. But if we avoid these dangerous and other undesirable ingredients whenever possible and read the labels before buying groceries at stores, including health food stores, the smaller amounts that we do ingest that we cannot detect and avoid will be digested and eliminated by a healthy body.

Is it easy to make any food sweet naturally? Yes. Even certain fruits make tasty, sweet food dishes. Strawberries, boysenberries, peaches, apples, and other fruits can be used as sweeteners in cooking and baking cakes, cookies, breads, and other recipes made at home. Dark-colored fruits mixed with blue agave, yacon syrup, or maple syrup easily color and sweeten cream cheese for a delicious frosting.

The health food industry has used these types of foods for sweetening and coloring for years, but now other food processors and manufacturers outside the health food industry are catching on, and the public is responding positively. We do not need unhealthful sweetening substances. We are so fortunate that Mother Nature has given us so many nutritious alternatives. Let's satisfy our sweet tooth and enjoy our sweets in a naturally sweet way.

ENDNOTES

1. Hayflick L. How and why we age. Reprint ed. New York: Ballantine Books; 1994. 377 p.
2. Harman D. Aging: a theory based on free radical and radiation chemistry. Journal of Gerontology. 1956;11(3):298-300.
3. Harman D. Free radical theory of aging: effect of free radical reaction inhibitors on the mortality rate of male LAF1 mice. Journal of Gerontology. 1968;23(4):476-82.
4. Harman D. Free radical theory of aging: effect of the amount and degree of unsaturation of dietary fat on mortality rate. Journal of Gerontology. 1971;26(4):451-57.
5. Stubbs CD, Smith AD. The modification of mammalian membrane polyunsaturated fatty acid composition in relation to membrane fluidity and function. Biochimica Et Biophysica Acta (BBA) - Reviews on Biomembranes. 1984;779(1):89-137.
6. de Quiroga GB, Barja, Pérez-Campo R, Torres ML. Antioxidant defences and peroxidation in liver and brain of aged rats. Biochemical Journal. 1990;272(1):247-50.

7. Lamptey MS, Walker, BL. A possible essential role for dietary linolenic acid in the development of the young rat. The Journal of Nutrition. 1976;106(1):86-93.

8. Okuyama H. Minimum requirements of n-3 and n-6 essential fatty acids for the function of the central nervous system and for the prevention of chronic disease. Experimental Biology and Medicine. 1992;200(2):174-76.

9. Yamamoto N, Saitoh M, Moriuchi A, Nomura M, Okuyama H. Effects of dietary alpha-linolenate/linolenate balance of brain lipid composition and learning ability of rats. Journal of Lipid Research. 1987;28(2):144-151.

10. Bourre JM, Bonneil M, Clément M, Dumont O, Durand G, Lafont H, Nalbone G, Piciotti M. Function of dietary polyunsaturated fatty acids in the nervous system. Prostaglandins, Leukotrienes and Essential Fatty Acids. 1993;48(1):5-15.

11. Farag RS, Badei AZMA, Hewedi FM, El-Baroty GSA. Antioxidant activity of some spice essential oils on linoleic acid oxidation in aqueous media. Journal of the American Oil Chemists Society. 1989;66(6):792-99.

12. Farag RS, Ali MN, El-Baroty GSA. Inhibitory effects of individual and mixed pairs of essential oils on the oxidation and hydrolysis of cottonseed oil and butter. FASC 1989;40:275-279

13. Farag RS, Abo Raya, GE El-Desoky, El-Baroty GS. Safety evaluation of thyme and clove essential oils as natural antioxidants. African J Sci. 1991;no.18:169-17.

14. Rotstein NP, Ilincheta De Boschero MG, Giusto NM, Aveldaño MI. Effects of aging on the composition and metabolism of docosahexaenoate-containing lipids of retina. Lipids. 1987;22(4):253-60.

15. Neuringer M, Connor WE. n-3 fatty acids in the brain and retina: evidence for their essentiality. Nutrition Reviews. 2009;44(9):285-94.

16. Youdim KA, Deans SG. Effect of thyme oil and thymol dietary supplementation on the antioxidant status and fatty acid composition of the ageing rat brain. Br J Nutr 2000;83(1):87-93.

17. Youdim KA, Deans SG. Dietary supplementation of thyme (Thymus vulgaris L.) essential oil during the lifetime of the rat: its effects on the antioxidant status in liver, kidney and heart tissues. Mechanisms of Ageing and Development. 1999;109(3):163-75.

18. Zheng GQ, Kenney Patrick M, Lam LKT. Sesquiterpenes from clove (Eugenia caryophyllata) as potential anticarcinogenic agents. Journal of Natural Products. 1992;55(7):999-1003.

19. Rompelberg CJM, Steinhuis WH, De Vogel N, Van Osenbruggen WA, Schouten A, Verhagen H. Antimutagenicity of eugenol in the rodent bone marrow micronucleus test. Mutation Research Letters. 1995;346(2):69-75.

20. Sukumaran K, Unnikrishnan MC, Kuttan R. Inhibition of tumour promotion in mice by eugenol. Indian J Physiol Pharmacol. 1994;38(4):306-8.

21. Yokota H, Hoshino J, Yuasa A. 1986. Suppressed mutagenicity of benzo[a]pyrene by the liver S9 fraction and microsomes from eugenol-treated rats. Mutation Research. 1986 Dec;172(3):231-6.

22. Iwano H, Ujita W, Nishikawa M, Ishii S, Inoue H, Yokota H. Effect of dietary eugenol on xenobiotic metabolism and mediation of UDP-glucuronosyltransferase and cytochrome P450 1A1 expression in rat liver. International Journal of Food Science and Nutrition. 2013 Oct 21;64(2):241-244.

23. Grandjean P, Landrigan PJ. Neurobehavioral effects of developmental toxicity. Lancet Neurol. 2014 Mar;13(3):330-8. Epub 204 Feb 17.

24. Woffinden B. Fluoride water 'causes cancer': boys at risk from bone tumours, shock research reveals [Internet]. New York (NY): The Observer; 2005 June 11 [cited 2018 Oct 9]. Available from: https://www.theguardian.com/society/2005/jun/12/medicineandhealth.genderissues.

25. Takahashi K, Akiniwa K, Narita K. Regression analysis of cancer incidence rates and water fluoride in the U.S.A. based on IACR/IARC(WHO) Data(1978-1992). Journal of Epidemiology. 2001;11(4):170-79.

26. Cohn PD. A brief report on the association of drinking water fluoridation and the incidence of osteosarcoma among young males. New Jersey: Department of Health, Environmental Health Services, 1992 Nov.

27. Bassin EB, Wypij D, Davis RB, Mittleman MA. Age-specific fluoride exposure in drinking water and osteosarcoma (United States). Cancer Causes & Control. 2006;17(4):421-28.

28. WebMD.com [Internet]. Does fluoridation up bone cancer risk? New York; WebMD LLC. 2006 Apr 6 [cited 2018 Oct 9]. Available from https://www.webmd.com/cancer/news/20060406/does-fluoridation-up-bone-cancer-risk#1.

29. Fluoride Action Network [Internet]. Binghamton (NY): Fluoride Action Network; c2018. The timeline. Harvard/bone cancer files; [cited October 5, 2018]. Available from http://fluoridealert.org/researchers/harvard/timeline/.

30. Fluoride Action Network [Internet]. Binghamton (NY): Fluoride Action Network; c2018. The conflicts of interest. Harvard/bone cancer files; [cited October 5, 2018]. Available from: http://fluoridealert.org/researchers/harvard/conflicts/.

31. Ibid.

32. Beltrán-Aguilar E, Barker L, Dye BA. National health and nutrition examination survey, 1999-2004 and the 1986-1987 national survey of oral health in U.S. school children. Atlanta (GA): CDC (US). Nov 2010. NCHS Data Brief No. 53 (US). Available at https://www.cdc.gov/nchs/data/databriefs/db53.htm.

33. U.S. Public Health Service Recommendation for Fluoride Concentration in Drinking Water for the Prevention of Dental Caries. Washington (DC): U.S. Department of Health and Human Services Federal Panel on Community Water Fluoridation: Public Health Reports. 2015 July-August 130. 14 p.

34. Washington Action for Safe Water (US). U.S Government Proposed Regulation of Fluoridation Does Not Go Far Enough. News release, 2011 Jan 24.

35. National Research Council (US). Washington, DC: National Academies Press; c2018. Fluoride in drinking water: a scientific review of EPA's standards; 2006.

36. Ibid.

37. Hao P, Ma X, Cheng X, Ba Y, Zhu J, Cui L. [Effect of fluoride on human hypothalamus-hypophysis-testis axis]. Wei Sheng Yan Jiu. 2010 Jan;39(1):53-55. Chinese.

38. Danielson C. Hip fractures and fluoridation in Utah's elderly population. JAMA: The Journal of the American Medical Association. 1992;268(6):746-748.

39. Alarcon-Herrera MT, Martin-Dominguez IR, Trejo-Vazquez R, Dozal SR. Well water fluoride, dental fluorosis, and bone fractures

in the Guadiana Valley of Mexico. Fluoride. 2001 May;34(2):139-49.

40. Karademir S, Akçam M, Kuybulu AE, Olgar S, Öktem F. Effects of fluorosis on QT dispersion, heart rate variability and echocardiographic parameters in children. Anadolu Kardiyol Derg. 2011(1);150-55.

41. Moss AJ, Schwartz PJ, Crampton RS, Tzivoni D, Locati EH, Maccluer J, Hall WJ, Weitkamp L, Vincent GM, Garson A. The Long QT syndrome: prospective longitu-dinal study of 328 families. Circulation. 1991;84(3):1136-144.

42. Canadians Opposed to Fluoridation. Hydrofluorosilicic Acid Origins. COF Blog [Internet]. Ontario Canada: COF. Cited October 08, 2018. Available from: http://cof-cof.ca/hydrofluorosilicic-acid-origins/.

43. The Plant List [Internet]. Richmond UK & Missouri US: [cited 2018 Oct 8]. Available from: http://www.theplantlist.org/1.1/browse/A/Burseraceae/Boswellia/.

44. Hepper H, Nigel F. Arabian and African frankincense trees. The Journal of Egyptian Archaeology. 1969;55(66).

45. Frank MB, Yang Q, Osban J, Azzarello JT, Saban MR, Saban R, Ashley RA, Welter JC, Fung K-M, Lin H-K. Frankincense oil derived from boswellia carteri induces tumor cell specific cytotoxicity. BMC Complementary and Alternative Medicine. 2009;9(1).

46. Ibid.

47. Akihisa T, Keiichi T, Banno N, Tokuda H, Nishihara R, Nakamura Y, Yumiko K, Yasukawa K, Suzuki T. Cancer chemopreventive effects and cytotoxic activities of the triterpene acids from the resin of boswellia carteri. Biological & Pharmaceutical Bulletin. 2006;29(9):1976-979.

48. Chevrier MR, Ryan AE, Lee DWY, Zhongze M, Wu-Yan Z, Via CS. Boswellia carterii extract inhibits TH1 cytokines and promotes TH2 cytokines in vitro. Clinical and Vaccine Immunology. 2005;12(5):575-80.

49. Highet, Juliet. Frankincense: Oman's Gift to the World. Munich (GER): Prestel Publishing; c2006. 66 p.

50. Al-Harrasi A, Al-Saidi A. Phytochemical analysis of the essential oil from botanically certified oleogum resin of boswellia sacra (omani luban). Molecules. 2008;13(9):2181-189.

51. U.S. National Plant Germplasm System [Internet]. Beltsville (Maryland): Taxon. Boswellia Sacra Flueck. Taxonomy - GRIN-Global Web v 1.10.3.6. [Cited 2018 Oct 8]. Available from: https://npgsweb.ars-grin.gov/gringlobal/taxonomydetail.aspx?id=310550.

52. Miller, AG, Morris M, Stuart-Smith S. Plants of Dhofar: the southern region of Oman, traditional, economic and medicinal uses. Oman: The Office of The Advisor for Conservation of The Environment, Diwan of Royal Court, Sultanate of Oman; c1988. 78p.

53. Woolley CL, Suhail MM, Smith BL, Boren KE, Taylor LC, Schreuder MF, Chai JK, Casabianca H, Haq S, Lin H-K, Al-Shahri AA, Al-Hatmi S, Young DG. Chemical differentiation of boswellia sacra and boswellia carterii essential oils by gas chromatography and chiral gas chromatography–mass spectrometry. Journal of Chromatog-raphy. 2012 Oct 26;1261:158-63.

54. Fung KM, Suhail MM, McClendon B, Woolley CL, Young DG, Lin HK. Management of basal cell carcinoma of the skin using frankincense (boswellia sacra) essential oil: a case report. OA Alternative Medicine. 2013;1(2).

55. Ni X, Suhail MM, Yang Q, Cao A, Fung K-M, Postier RG, Woolley C, Young DG, Zhang J, Lin H-K. Frankincense essential oil prepared from hydrodistillation of boswellia sacra gum resins induces human pancreatic cancer cell death in cultures and in a xenograft murine model. BMC Complementary and Alternative Medicine. 2012;12(1).

56. Suhail MM, Weijuan W, Cao A, Mondalek FG, Fung K-M, Shih P-T, Fang Y-T, Woolley C, Young DG, Lin HK. Boswellia sacra essential oil induces tumor cell-specific apoptosis and suppresses tumor aggressiveness in cultured human breast cancer cells. BMC Complementary and Alternative Medicine. 2011;11(1).

57. Moussaieff A, Rimmerman N, Bregman T, Straiker A, Felder CC, Shoham S, Kashman Y, Huang SM, Lee H, Shohami E, Mackie K, Caterina MJ, Walker JM, Fride E, Mechoulam R. Incensole acetate, an incense component, elicits psychoactivity by activating TRPV3 channels in the brain. The FASEB Journal. 2008;22(8):3024-034.

58. Moussaieff A, Shein NA, Tsenter J, Grigoriadis S, Simeonidou C, Alexandrovich AG, Trembovler V, Ben-Neriah Y, Schmitz ML, Fiebich B, Munoz E, Mechoulam R, Shohami E. Incensole acetate: a novel neuroprotective agent isolated from boswellia carterii. Journal of Cerebral Blood Flow & Metabolism. 2008;28(7):1341-352.

59. Weizman Institute of Science. Weizmann Wonder Wander BLOG: Color It Pink {Internet]. Rehovot Israel: Weizman Institute of Science. [Cited 2018 Oct 8]. Availa-ble from: https://wis-wander.weizmann.ac.il/earth-sciences/color-it-pink.

60. Frank A, Unger M. Analysis of frankincense from various boswellia species with inhibitory activity on human drug metabolising cytochrome P450 enzymes using liquid chromatography mass spectrometry after automated on-line extraction. Journal of Chromatography. 2006;1112(1-2):255-62.

61. Blain EJ, Ahmed YA, Duance VC. Boswellia frereana (frankincense) suppresses cytokine-induced matrix metalloproteinase expression and production of pro-inflammatory molecules in articular cartilage. Phytother Res. 2010 Jun;24(6):905-12.

62. Peirce, Penney. Frequency: the power of personal vibration. New York (NY): Atria; c2009. 271 p.

63. Biontology Arizona. Dr. Fritz Albert Popp [Internet]. [Cited 2018 Oct 8]. Available from: https://www.biontologyarizona.com/dr-fritz-albert-popp/.

64. Gnatta JR, Kurebayashi LFS, Turrini RNT, Da Silva MJP. Aromatherapy and nursing: historical and theoretical conception. Rev. Esc. Enferm USP. 2016 Feb;50(1).

65. Becker RO, Selden G. The Body Electric. New York (NY): Morrow; c1985. 368 p.

66. Nordenström BEW. Biologically closed electric circuits. Nordic Medical Publications; c1983. 374 p.

67. Chao SC, Young DG, Oberg CJ. Screening for inhibitory activity of essential oils on selected bacteria, fungi and viruses. Journal of Essential Oil Research. 2000;12(5):639-49.

68. Horne D, Holm M, Oberg C, Chao S, Young DG. Antimicrobial effects of essential oils on streptococcus pneumoniae. Journal of Essential Oil Research. 2001;13(5):387-92.

69. Chao S, Young DG, Oberg C, Nakaoka K. Inhibition of methicillin-resistant staphylococcus aureus (MRSA) by essential

oils. Flavour and Fragrance Journal. 2008;23(6):444-49.

70. Farag RS, Rashed MM, Hgger AAA. Aflatoxin destruction by microwave heating. Int J Food Sci Nutr. 1996 May;47(3):197-208.

71. Vallejo F, Tomás-Barberán F, García-Viguera C. Phenolic compound contents in edible parts of broccoli inflorescences after domestic cooking. Journal of the Science of Food and Agriculture. 2003;83(14):1511-516.

72. Kerner JA, Quan R, Yang C, Rubinstein S, Lewiston NJ, Sunshine P, Stevenson DK. Effects of microwave radiation on anti-infective factors in human milk. Pediatrics. 1992 Apr;89(4 Pt 1):667-69.

73. Wang J, Schnute WC. Direct analysis of trace level bisphenol a, octylphenols and nonylphenol in bottled water and leached from bottles by ultra-high-performance liquid chromatography/ tandem mass spectrometry. Rapid Communications in Mass Spectrometry. 2010;24(17):2605-610.

74. Lubec G, Wolf C, Bartosch B. Aminoacid isomerisation and microwave exposure. The Lancet. 1989 Dec 9;334(8676):1392-393.

75. Becker RO. Selden G. The Body Electric. New York, NY: Morrow; c1985. 368 p.

76. Sugarman, Ellen. Warning: the electricity around you may be hazardous to your health. St. Louis (MO): Miriam Press; c2004. 260 p.

77. Hertel HU, Bernard HB. [Microwaves: danger scientifically proven]. Journal Franz Weber. 1992 Jan-Feb;19. German.

78. Ibid.

79. Robinson MR, O'Connor A, Wallace L, Connell K, Tucker K, Strickland J, Taylor J, Quinlan KF, Gottlieb LJ. Behaviors of young children around microwave ovens. J Trauma. 2011 Nov;71(5 Suppl 2):S534-536.

80. Association for the International Research of Aromatic Science and Education. Sabina M. DeVita, EdD, DNM, DCSJ, IPSP, CBP [Internet]. American Fork: AIRASE [cited 2018 Oct 9].

81. United States Nuclear Regulatory Commission. Map of Power Reactor Sites [Internet]. North Bethesda (MD): USNRC [cited 2018 Oct 9]. Available from: https://www.nrc.gov/reactors/operating/map-power-reactors.html.

82. Sovacool BK. A critical evaluation of nuclear power and renewable electricity in Asia. Journal of Contemporary Asia. 2010 Aug;40(3):379-380.

83. Brown V. Hanford Nuclear Waste Cleanup Plant may be too dangerous. Scientific American. 2013 May 9. Available from: https://www.scientificamerican.com/article/hanford-nuclear-cleanup-problems/.

84. Lutins, Allen. U.S. Nuclear Accidents [Internet]. 2018 Jun 3 Place unknown. [cited 2018 Oct 9]. Available from: http://www.lutins.org/nukes.html.

85. World Nuclear Association [Internet]. London: World Nuclear Association. Fukushima Daiichi accident; 2018 Oct. Available from: http://www.world-nuclear.org/information-library/safety-and-security/safety-of-plants/fukushima-accident.aspx.

86. Franchomme P, Pénoël D. L'aromathérapie exactement. Roger Jollois, editor. Broché: 2001. 490p.

87. Khansari DN, Gustad T. Effects of long-term, low-dose growth hormone therapy on immune function and life expectancy of mice. Mech Ageing Dev. 1991 Jan;57(1):87-100.

88. Locher JL, Goldsby TU, Goss AM, Kilgore ML, Gower B, Ard JD. Calorie restriction in overweight older adults: do benefits exceed potential risks? Exp. Gerontol. 2016 Dec 15;86:4-13.

89. Romashkan SV, Das SK, Villareal DT, Ravussin E, Redman LM, Rochon J, Bhapkar M, Kraus WE, CALERIE Study Group. Safety of two-year caloric restriction in non-obese healthy individuals. Oncotarget. 2016 Apr 12;7(15):19124-33.

90. Sanchez A, Reeser JL, Lau HS, Yahiku PY, Willard RE, McMillan PJ, Cho, SY, Magie AR, U.D. Register. Role of sugars in human neutrophilic phagocytosis. The American Journal of Clinical Nutrition. 1978 Nov;26(11):1180-1184.

91. Kearns CE, Schmidt LA, Glantz ST. Sugar industry and coronary heart disease research: a historical analysis of internal industry documents. JAMA Intern Med. 2016 Nov 1;176(11):1680-1685.

92. Bray GA, Nielsen SJ, Popkim BM. Consumption of high-fructose corn syrup in beverages may play a role in the epidemic of obesity. Am J Clin Nutr. 2004 Apr;79(4):537-43.

93. Ma X, Lin L, Yue J, Pradhan G, Qin G, Minze LJ, Wu H, Sheikh-Hamad D, Smith CW, Sun Y. Ghrelin receptor regulates HFCS-induced adipose inflammation and insulin resistance. Nutr Diabetes. 2013 Dec 23;3(e99). doi. 10.1038/nutd.2013.41.

94. Parker-Pope T. Still spooked by high-fructose corn syrup [Internet]. The New York Times. 2008 Oct 30 [cited 2018 Oct 9] Available from: https://well.blogs.nytimes.com/2008/10/30/still-spooked-by-high-fructose-corn-syrup/.

95. Consumer Report News [Internet]. The whole truth about high-fructose corn syrup. 2008 Oct 28. Available from: https://www.consumerreports.org/cro/news/2008/10/the-whole-truth-about-high-fructose-corn-syrup/index.htm.

96. McLaughlin L. Is high-fructose corn syrup really good for you? [Internet]. Time. 2008 Sep 17. Available from: http://content.time.com/time/health/article/0,8599,1841910,00.html.

97. Parker-Pope T. A new name for high-fructose corn syrup [Internet]. The New York Times. 2010 Sept 14 [cited 2018 Oct 9] Available from: https://well.blogs.nytimes.com/2010/09/14/a-new-name-for-high-fructose-corn-syrup/.

98. Economic Research Service (US). U.S. production and use of high-fructose corn syrup is declining. Washington (DC): United States Department of Agriculture (US); 2016. Available from: https://www.ers.usda.gov/data-products/chart-gallery/gallery/chart-detail/?chartId=78733.

99. Schiffman SS, Rother KI. Sucralose, a synthetic organochlorine sweetener: overview of biological issues. J Toxicol Environ Health B Crit Rev. 2013 Sep;16(7):399-451.

100. Schiffman S, Shipman M. Study finds Sucralose produces previously unidentified metabolites [Internet]. Raleigh (NC): NC State University; 2018 Aug 27 [cited 2018 Oct 18]. Available from: https://news.ncsu.edu/2018/08/sucralose-metabolites/.

101. Chattopadhyay S, Raychaudhuri U, Chakraborty R. Artificial sweeteners - a review. J Food Sci Technol. 2014 Apr;51(4):611-621.

102. Mercola, Joseph. Mercola.com [Internet]. Schaumburg, IL. Joseph Mercola. December 3, 2000 [cited 2018 Oct 10]. Available from: http://articles.mercola.com/sites/articles/archive/2000/12/03/sucralose-dangers.aspx.

103. Soffritti M, Padovani M, Tibaldi E, Falcioni L, Manservisi F, Lauriola M, Bua L, Manservigi M, Belpoggi F. Sucralose administered in feed, beginning prenatally through lifespan, induces hematopoietic neoplasias in male swiss mice. Intl J Occupat Environ Health. 2016;22(1):7-17.

104. Kollias H. Precision Nutrition [Internet]. Research review: is splenda safe? Toronto, Ont, Can.: Precision Nutrition. [cited 2018 Oct 10]. Available from: https://www.precisionnutrition.com/research-review-splenda-is-it-safe.

105. Mercola, Joseph. http://articles.mercola.com/sites/articles/archive/2000/12/03/sucralose-dangers.aspx.

106. Blaylock, Russell L. Excitotoxins: the taste that kills. Santa Fe (NM): Health Press; c1997. 320p.

107. Tejero-Sariñena S, Barlow J, Costabile A, Gibson GR, Rowland I. Antipathogenic activity of probiotics against Salmonella typhimurium and Clostridium difficile in anaerobic batch culture systems: is it due to synergies in probiotic mixtures or the specificity of single strains? Anaerobe. 2013 Dec;24:60-5. Epub 2013 Sep 30.

108. Biagi G, Cipollini I, Bonaldo A, Grandi M, Pompei A, Stefanelli C, Zaghini G. Effect of feeding a selected combination of galacto-oligosaccharides and a strain of Bifidobacterium pseudocatenulatum on the intestinal microbiota of cats. Am J Vet Res. 2013 Jan;74(1):90-5.

109. D'Aimmo MR, Modesto M, Biavati B. Antibiotic resistance of lactic acid bacteria and Bifidobacterium spp. isolated from dairy and pharmaceutical products. International Journal of Food Microbiology. 2017 Apr 1;115(1):35-42.

110. LeBlanc JG, Milani C, de Giori GS, Sesma F, van Sinderen D, Ventura M. Bacteria as vitamin suppliers to their host: a gut microbiota perspective. Curr Opin Biotechnol. 2013 Apr;24(2):160-8.

111. Minagawa K. Significance of lysozyme in infant nutrition. Synthesis of lysozyme by Lactobacillus bifidus. Nihon Shonika Gakkai Zasshi. Acta Paediatrica Japonica. 1970;74(8):761-767.

112. Vitaliti G, Pavone P, Guglielmo F, Spataro G, Falsaperla R. The immunomodulatory effect of probiotics beyond atopy: an update. J Asthma. 2014 Apr;51(3):320-32. Epub 2013 Dec 17.

113. Chong ES. A potential role of probiotics in colorectal cancer prevention: review of possible mechanisms of action. World J Microbiol Biotechnol. 2014 Feb;30(2):351-74. Epub 2013 Sep 26.

114. Harata G, He F, Takahashi K, Hosono A, Kawase M, Kubota A, Hiramatsu M, Kaminogawa S. Bifidobacterium suppresses IgE-mediated degranulation of rat basophilic leukemia (RBL-2H3) cells. Microbiol Immunol. 2010;54(1):54-7.

115. Wang Y, Zeng T, Wang SE, Wang W, Wang Q, Yu HX. Fructo-oligosaccharides enhance the mineral absorption and counteract the adverse effects of phytic acid in mice. Nutrition. 2010 Mar;26(3):305-11. Epub 2009 Aug 8.

116. Sabater-Molina M, Larqué E, Torrella F, Zamora S. Dietary fructooligosaccharides and potential benefits on health. J Physiol Biochem. 2009 Sep;65(3):315-28.

117. González W, Altieri PI, Alvarado S, Banchs HL, Escobales N, Crespo M, Borges W. Magnesium: the forgotten electrolyte. Bol Asoc Med P R. 2013;105(3):17-20.

118. Hruby A, McKeown NM, Song Y, Djoussé L. Dietary magnesium and genetic interactions in diabetes and related risk factors: a brief overview of current knowledge. Nutrients. 2013 Dec 6;5(12):4990-5011.

119. Blaszczyk U, Duda-Chodak A. Magnesium: its role in nutrition and carcinogenesis. Rocz Panstw Zakl Hig. 2013;64(3):165-71.

120. Serefko A, Szopa A, Wlaź P, Nowak G, Radziwoń-Zaleska M, Skalski M, Poleszak E. Magnesium in depression. Pharmacol Rep. 2013;65(3):547-54.

121. Rowe WJ. Correcting magnesium deficiencies may prolong life. Clin Interv Aging. 2012;7:51-4. Epub 2012 Feb 16.

122. Pachikian BD, Essaghir A, Demoulin JB, Catry E, Neyrinck AM, Dewulf EM, Sohet FM, Portois L, Clerbaux LA, Carpentier YA, Possemiers S, Bommer GT, Cani PD, Delzenne NM. Prebiotic approach alleviates hepatic steatosis: implication of fatty acid oxidative and cholesterol synthesis pathways. Mol Nutr Food Res. 2013 Feb;57(2):347-59. Epub 2012 Dec 2.

123. Ritu M, Nandini J. Nutritional composition of Stevia rebaudiana, a sweet herb, and its hypoglycaemic and hypolipidaemic effect on patients with non-insulin depend-ent diabetes mellitus. J Sci Food Agric. 2016 Sep;96(12):4231-4. Epub 2016 Feb 22.

124. Rizzo B, Zambonin L, Angeloni C, Leoncini E, Dalla Sega FV, Prata C, Fiorentini D, Hrelia S. Steviol glycosides modulate glucose transport in different cell types. Oxid Med Cell Longev. 2013;2013:348169. Epub 2013 Nov 12.

125. Chen J, Jeppesen PB, Nordentoft I, Hermansen K. Stevioside counteracts the glyburide-induced desensitization of the pancreatic beta-cell function in mice: studies in vitro. Metabolism. 2006 Dec;55(12):1674-80.

126. Gamboa F, Chaves M. Antimicrobial potential of extracts from Stevia rebaudiana leaves against bacteria of importance in dental caries. Acta Odontol Latinoam. 2012;25(2):171-5.

127. Barba FJ, Criado MN, Belda-Galbis CM, Esteve MJ, Rodrigo D. Stevia rebaudiana Bertoni as a natural antioxidant/antimicrobial for high pressure processed fruit extract: processing parameter optimization. Food Chem. 2014 Apr 1;148:261-7. Epub 2013 Oct 20.

128. Shivanna N, Naika M, Khanum F, Kaul VK. Antioxidant, anti-diabetic and renal protective properties of Stevia rebaudiana. J Diabetes Complications. 2013 Mar-Apr;27(2):103-13. Epub 2012 Nov 7.

129. Ghanta S, Banerjee A, Poddar A, Chattopadhyay S. Oxidative DNA damage preventive activity and antioxidant potential of Stevia rebaudiana (Bertoni) Bertoni, a natural sweetener. J Agric Food Chem. 2007 Dec 26;55(26):10962-7. Epub 2007 Nov 27.

130. Oviedo CA. Accion hipoglicemiante de la Stevia rebaudiana Bertoni (Kaa-he-e). Excerpta Medica. 1971;208:92-93.

131. Suzuki, H. et al. Nippon Nopei Kagaku Kaishi. Influence of oral administration of stevioside on levels of blood glucose & liver glycogen of stevioside on levels of blood glucose & liver glycogen of intact rats. Tokyo. 1977;51(3):171-173.

132. Wikipedia: the free encyclopedia [Internet]. St. Petersburg (FL): Wikimedia Foundation, Inc. 2001 – [cited 2018 Oct 10]. Available from: https://en.wikipedia.org/wiki/Yac%C3%B3n.

133. Delgado GT, Tamashiro WM, Maróstica Junior MR, Pastore GM. Yacon (Smallanthus sonchifolius): a functional food. Plant Foods Hum Nutr. 2013 Sep;68(3):222-8.

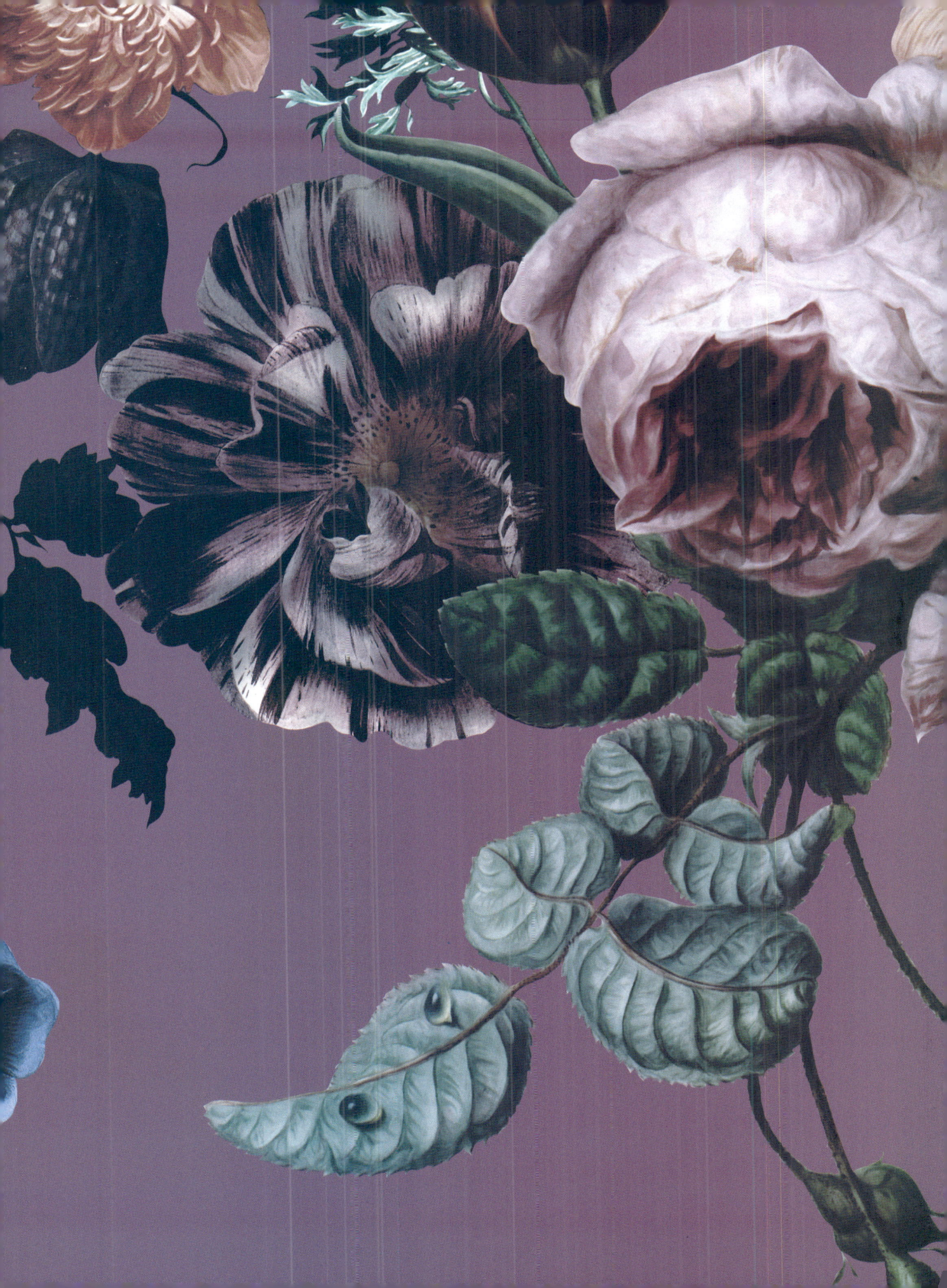

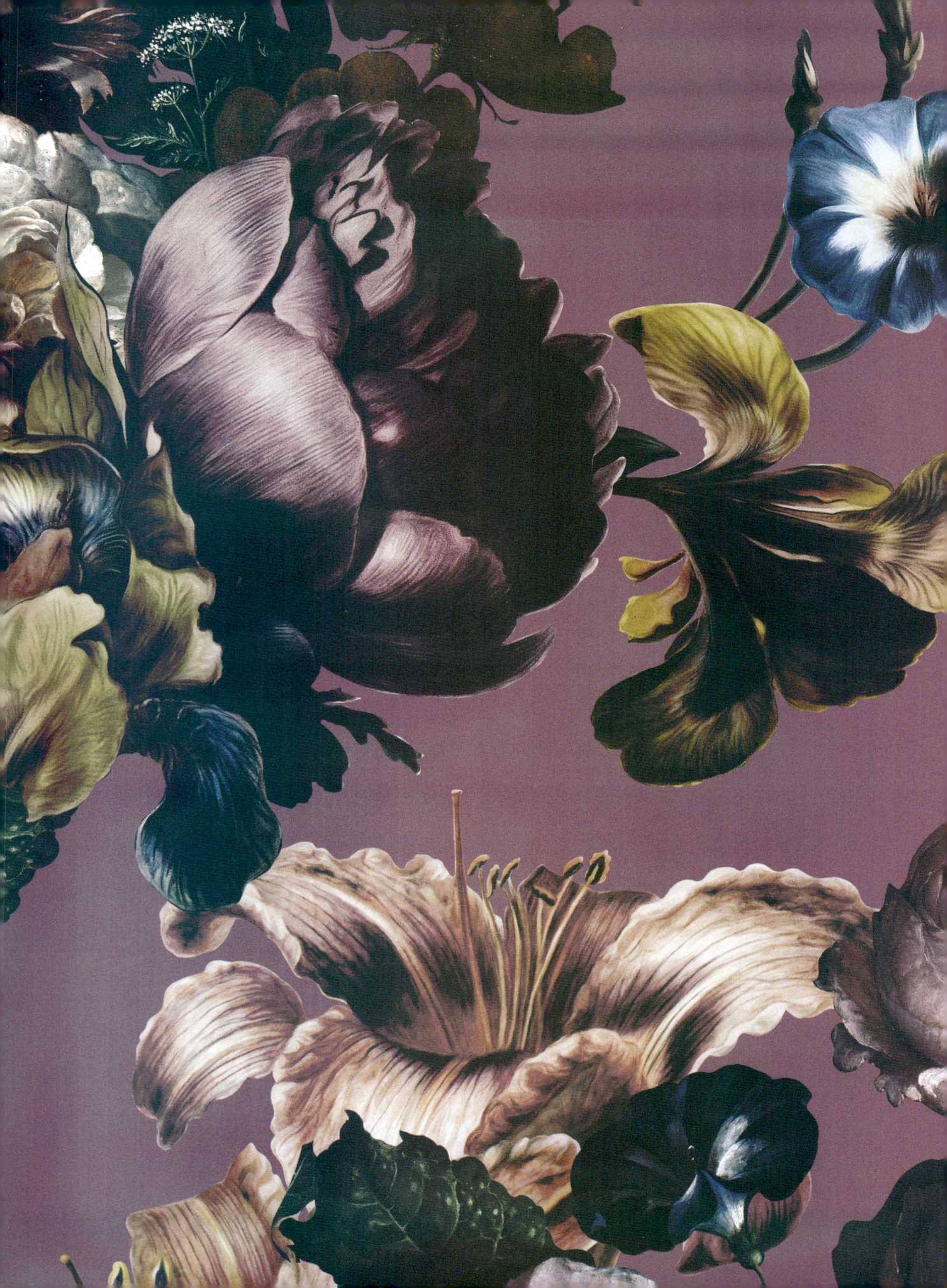

Personal Usage Guide

ABUSE, MENTAL AND PHYSICAL

The trauma from mental and physical abuse can result in self-defeating behaviors that can undermine success later in life. Traumatic memories can be imprinted in DNA. Researchers from Mount Sinai hospital in New York showed epigenetic alterations from Holocaust trauma caused modified genes in the offspring of survivors.[1] Many people believe that powerful memories are stored in the body and that trauma imprinting can be passed from generation to generation.

Through their powerful effect on the limbic system of the brain (the center of stored memories and emotions), essential oils can help release pent-up trauma, emotions, or memories. Always start with Frankincense.

Recommendations

Singles: Sacred Frankincense, Frankincense, Frankincense Vitality, Idaho Grand Fir, Sacred Sandalwood, Royal Hawaiian Sandalwood, Melissa, Cassia, Sage, Sage Vitality

Blends: Freedom, Trauma Life, SARA, Release, Gary's Light, Acceptance, Forgiveness, Amoressence, Surrender, Humility, Reconnect, Journey On, White Angelica, Inner Child, KidScents KidPower, KidScents KidPower Roll-On, Harmony, Hope, Tranquil Roll-On, Valor, Valor Roll-On, Peace & Calming, Peace & Calming II, One Heart, Calm CBD Roll-On, Seedlings Calm, The Gift, Common Sense, Abundance, 3 Wise Men, Present Time, Brain Power

Nutritionals: OmegaGize3, NingXia Red, KidScents Unwind, EndoGize, Mineral Essence, Master Formula, MindWise

Application and Usage
Aromatic: Refer to Application Guidelines.
Topical: Refer to Application Guidelines.

Specific Types of Abuse

Physical Abuse: Apply 2-3 drops of SARA and Forgiveness over the abuse area and around the navel. Follow with 1-2 drops of Release over the Vita Flex points on the feet, especially the liver point of the right foot, under the nose, and directly over the liver. Then apply Trauma Life.

Parental, Sexual, or Ritual Abuse: Apply 1-3 drops of SARA over the area where abuse took place, then Forgiveness, Trauma Life, Release, Joy, Present Time.

Spousal Abuse: Apply SARA, Forgiveness, Trauma Life, Release, Valor, Joy, Amoressence, Envision, Hope.

Feelings of Revenge: Apply 1-2 drops of Surrender on the sternum over the heart, 2-3 drops of Present Time on the thymus, and 2-3 drops of Forgiveness over the navel.

Suicidal: Apply 2 drops of Hope on the rim of the ears. Melissa, Brain Power, Surrender, RutaVaLa, Common Sense, or Present Time may also be beneficial.

Protection and Balance: Apply 1-2 drops of White Angelica on each shoulder and 1-2 drops of Harmony on energy points or chakras. Finish with Valor followed by Sacred Frankincense or Frankincense to set the DNA blueprint.

ACIDOSIS (See also DIGESTIVE PROBLEMS, Heartburn; FUNGAL (YEAST) INFECTIONS)

Acidosis is a condition where the pH of the blood serum becomes excessively acidic. This condition should not be confused with an acid stomach. Acidic blood can stress the liver and eventually lead to many forms of chronic and degenerative diseases. Dietary and oral changes will help in raising the serum pH (making it more alkaline). Cleansing is an essential dietary and oral step in balancing pH.

Recommendations

Singles: Peppermint, Peppermint Vitality, Fennel, Fennel Vitality, Tarragon, Tarragon Vitality, Davana, Jade Lemon, Jade Lemon Vitality, Lemon, Lemon Vitality

Blends: DiGize, DiGize Vitality, EndoFlex, EndoFlex Vitality, KidScents TummyGize, JuvaCleanse, JuvaCleanse Vitality

Nutritionals: AlkaLime, Digest & Cleanse, Essentialzyme, MultiGreens, JuvaPower, Mega Vitamin Cal, Essentialzymes-4, Mineral Essence, Allerzyme

Application and Usage

Dietary and Oral: Refer to Application Guidelines.

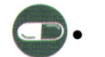 - Take 1 capsule of desired Vitality oil 2 times daily.

 - Take 2-3 drops of desired Vitality oil in a spoonful of syrup or small amount of milk, juice, or water.

 - Take an Essentialzymes-4 yellow capsule with Peppermint Vitality until acid level is balanced, then add Essentialzyme.

 - To reduce acid indigestion and prevent fermentation that can contribute to bad dreams and interrupted sleep, take 1 teaspoon of AlkaLime in water before bedtime.

 - To raise pH, take 2-6 capsules of MultiGreens 3 times daily and take 1 teaspoon of AlkaLime in water 1 hour before or 2 hours after meals each day. For maintenance, take 1 teaspoon of AlkaLime once per week at bedtime.

 - To stimulate enzymatic action in the digestive tract, mix together raw carrot juice, NingXia Red, alfalfa juice, and papaya juice with 1 dropper of Mineral Essence and 1 drop of DiGize Vitality.

Topical: Refer to Application Guidelines.

ADDICTIONS

Many foods and plants—such as tobacco, caffeine, drugs, alcohol, breads, sugar, and other sweeteners—create chemical dependencies.

Cleansing and detoxifying the liver is a crucial first step toward breaking free of these addictions. Alkaline calcium can help bind bile acids and prevent fatty liver. A colon and tissue cleanse is also important.

A body lacking in sufficient enzymes, vitamins, minerals, and other nutrients may also play a part in some addictions. Yacon Syrup, maple syrup, honey, molasses, and other natural sweeteners are good substitutes for sugar, which should be restricted in a diet.

The Thieves oil blend has been very helpful in curbing an addiction. One or two drops on the tongue are sufficient to stop the onset of a craving.

JuvaTone, JuvaPower, and JuvaCleanse may be used long-term to help detoxify the liver. They suppress the addiction and eventually change the addiction blueprint in the cells of the body.

Recommendations

Singles: Orange, Orange Vitality, Ledum, Fennel, Fennel Vitality, Tarragon, Tarragon Vitality, Cassia

Blends: GLF, GLF Vitality, Brain Power, Thieves, Thieves Vitality, Harmony, Reconnect, Gary's Light, Peace & Calming, Peace & Calming II, Calm CBD Roll-On, Seedlings Calm, KidScents KidPower, KidScents KidPower Roll-On, JuvaCleanse, JuvaCleanse Vitality, JuvaFlex, JuvaFlex Vitality

Nutritionals: Detoxzyme, ComforTone, Digest & Cleanse, JuvaPower, MindWise, ICP, JuvaTone, Slique Shake, Slique Bars, Slique CitraSlim, Mega Vitamin Cal, Essentialzyme, Essentialzymes-4, Balance Complete, KidScents Unwind, Yacon Syrup, OmegaGize3, Slique Tea, Slique Bars, Pure Protein Complete, Protein Power Bites

Application and Usage

Aromatic: Refer to Application Guidelines.

Dietary and Oral: Refer to Application Guidelines.

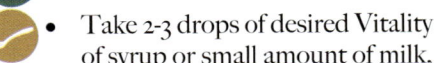 - Take 1 capsule of desired Vitality oil 2 times daily.

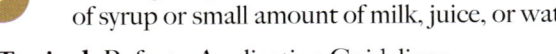 - Take 2-3 drops of desired Vitality oil in a spoonful of syrup or small amount of milk, juice, or water.

Topical: Refer to Application Guidelines.

 - Apply 1-2 drops neat (undiluted) on temples and back of neck 4 times daily or as desired.

 - Place a warm compress with 1-2 drops of chosen oil over the liver.

ADRENAL GLAND DISORDERS

The adrenal glands consist of two sections: an inner part called the medulla, which produces stress hormones, and an outer part called the cortex, which secretes critical hormones called glucocorticoids and aldosterone. Because of these hormones, the cortex has a far greater impact on overall health than the medulla.

Aldosterone and glucocorticoids are very important because they directly affect blood pressure and minerals that help regulate the conversion of carbohydrates into energy.

In cases like Addison's disease, adrenal cortex hormones fail to produce sufficient amounts of or any of the critical hormones, which can lead to life-threatening fluid and mineral loss, unless these hormones are replaced.

On the other hand, Cushing's disease, or syndrome, occurs when the body has too much of the hormone cortisol or other steroid hormones.

Kidneys and Adrenal Glands

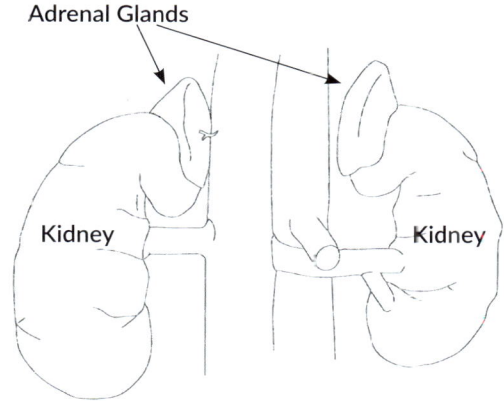

Addison's Disease

Addison's disease is an autoimmune disease in which the body's own immune cells begin to destroy the adrenal glands. Sulfurzyme, an important source of organic sulfur, is known to have positive effects in fighting many types of autoimmune diseases, including lupus, arthritis, and fibromyalgia.

Symptoms associated with Addison's disease
- Severe fatigue
- Lightheadedness when standing
- Nausea
- Depression/irritability
- Craving salty foods
- Loss of appetite
- Muscle spasms
- Dark, tan-colored skin

Some essential oils have chemical components or structures that have adrenal-like action, enabling them to give support to the body's own system, which may help correct those deficiencies by strengthening adrenal cortex function. The EndoFlex oil blend promotes adrenal-like activity that raises energy levels.

Recommendations

Singles: Nutmeg, Nutmeg Vitality, Fennel, Fennel Vitality, German Chamomile, German Chamomile Vitality, Clove, Clove Vitality, Sacred Frankincense, Frankincense, Frankincense Vitality, Bergamot, Bergamot Vitality

Blends: EndoFlex, EndoFlex Vitality, En-R-Gee, KidScents GeneYus, Brain Power, Common Sense, Clarity, 25 Years Young

Nutritionals: Thyromin, Sulfurzyme, EndoGize, MindWise, MultiGreens, Balance Complete, Mega Vitamin Cal, Mineral Essence, Super Vitamin B, Life 9, KidScents MightyPro, NingXia Red

Application and Usage

Aromatic: Refer to Application Guidelines.

Dietary and Oral: Refer to Application Guidelines.

 • Take 1 capsule with Vitality or desired dietary oil 2 times daily.

 • Take 2-3 drops of desired Vitality oil in a spoonful of syrup or small amount of milk, juice, or water.

Topical: Refer to Application Guidelines

Cushing's Syndrome (Disease)

Adrenal gland imbalance is characterized by the overproduction of adrenal cortex hormones such as cortisol. While these hormones are crucial to sound health in normal amounts, their unchecked overproduction can cause as much harm as their underproduction.

This results in the following symptoms:
- Slow wound healing
- Obesity
- Low resistance
- Acne
- Infection
- Moon-shaped face
- Easily bruised skin
- Osteoporosis
- Weak or wasted muscles

Although Cushing's disease can be caused by a malfunction in the pituitary, it is usually triggered by excessive use of immune suppressing corticosteroid medications, such as those used for asthma and arthritis. Once these are stopped, the disease often abates. The key to reducing excess cortisol is often reducing stress.

Support the Adrenal Glands

Add the following amounts of essential oils to ¼ teaspoon of massage oil and apply as a warm compress over the adrenal glands (located on top of the kidneys):

- 3 drops Clove
- 3 drops Nutmeg
- 7 drops Rosemary

Recommendations

Singles: Spearmint, Spearmint Vitality, Dorado Azul, Sacred Frankincense, Frankincense, Frankincense Vitality, Idaho Grand Fir, Lemon Verbena

Blends: EndoFlex, EndoFlex Vitality, Exodus II, Peace & Calming, Peace & Calming II, Acceptance, Release, Grounding, Harmony, DiGize, DiGize Vitality, KidScents TummyGize

Nutritionals: ImmuPro, Inner Defense, PD 80/20, Mineral Essence, CortiStop, Digest & Cleanse, JuvaPower, Omega-Gize3, MindWise

Application and Usage

Aromatic: Refer to Application Guidelines.

Dietary and Oral: Refer to Application Guidelines.

- Take 2 capsules with EndoFlex Vitality or other desired dietary oil 2 times daily.

- Take 2-3 drops of desired Vitality oil in a spoonful of syrup or small amount of milk, juice, or water.

Topical: Refer to Application Guidelines.

- Apply warm compress over adrenal area (on back, over kidneys) with 1-2 drops of recommended oil.

AGITATION

Agitation is caused by a weakened nervous system, lack of sleep, frustration, and is often a result of a congested liver or over-stimulation of the sympathetic nervous system.

Recommendations

Singles: Lavender, Lavender Vitality, Roman Chamomile, Hinoki, Vetiver, Valerian, Idaho Grand Fir, Myrrh, Sacred Frankincense, Frankincense, Frankincense Vitality, Melissa, Helichrysum, Cassia, Marjoram, Marjoram Vitality, Sage, Sage Vitality, Vanilla

Blends: RutaVaLa, RutaVaLa Roll-On, Tranquil Roll-On, Stress Away, Stress Away Roll-On, Forgiveness, Amoressence, Peace & Calming, Peace & Calming II, Gary's Light, One Heart, Calm CBD Roll-On, Seedlings Calm, KidScents KidPower, KidScents KidPower Roll-On, Surrender, Humility, Reconnect, White Angelica

Nutritionals: ImmuPro, KidScents Unwind, Super Vitamin B, JuvaTone, Mega Vitamin Cal, EndoGize, SleepEssence

Application and Usage

Aromatic: Refer to Application Guidelines.

Topical: Refer to Application Guidelines.

- Apply 1-2 drops neat or undiluted on temples and back of neck as desired.
- You may also apply 1-2 drops on the Vita Flex brain and heart points on the bottoms of the feet.
- Applying a single drop under the nose is helpful and refreshing.
- Place a warm compress with 3-4 drops of chosen oil over the back.

AIDS (Acquired Immune Deficiency Syndrome)

The AIDS virus attacks and infects immune cells that are essential for life. Frankincense and Myrrh have immune-building properties. Other oils like Cumin have an inhibitory effect on viral replication.

In May 1994, Dr. Radwan Farag of Cairo University demonstrated that cumin seed oil had an 88 to 92 percent inhibition effect in vitro against HIV, the virus responsible for AIDS. Other antiviral essential oils include Melissa, Oregano, Sacred Sandalwood, and Tea Tree. A study in the journal Retrovirology showed extracts from peppermint, sage, and lemon balm (melissa) also display potent anti-HIV-1 activity.[2]

Recommendations

Singles: Cumin, Cypress, Melissa, Oregano, Oregano Vitality, Ecuadorian Oregano, Sacred Sandalwood, Royal Hawaiian Sandalwood, Tea Tree, Myrrh, Sacred Frankincense, Frankincense, Frankincense Vitality, Sage, Sage Vitality, Northern Lights Black Spruce, Peppermint, Peppermint Vitality, Cistus

Blends: Exodus II, Thieves, Thieves Vitality, Reconnect, Release, Acceptance

Nutritionals: NingXia Red, Inner Defense, Slique Shake, ImmuPro, Longevity Softgels, Essentialzyme, Essentialzymes-4, EndoGize, Pure Protein Complete

Personal Care: Raindrop Technique application

Application and Usage

Aromatic: Refer to Application Guidelines.

Dietary and Oral: Refer to instructions at the beginning of this chapter.

- Take 2 capsules with 50:50 Cistus and Cypress 2 times daily.

- Take 2-3 drops of desired Vitality oil in a spoonful of syrup or small amount of milk, juice, or water.

Topical: Refer to Application Guidelines.

ALCOHOLISM (See also ADDICTIONS)

Alcoholism, also known as alcohol dependence, includes alcohol craving and continued drinking. It includes four symptoms:

1. Craving: A strong compulsion, or need, to drink alcohol
2. Impaired control: The inability to limit drinking
3. Physical dependence: The inability to stop drinking without experiencing withdrawal symptoms such as nausea, shakiness, sweating, and anxiety
4. Tolerance: The need for increasing amounts of alcohol

Recommendations

Singles: Sacred Frankincense, Frankincense, Frankincense Vitality, Lavender, Lavender Vitality, Roman Chamomile, Ledum, Helichrysum, Orange, Orange Vitality

Blends: JuvaCleanse, JuvaCleanse Vitality, GLF, GLF Vitality, Forgiveness, Amoressence, Release, Acceptance, Valor, Valor Roll-On, Motivation, White Angelica, The Gift, KidScents KidPower, KidScents KidPower Roll-On, Common Sense, Reconnect

Nutritionals: JuvaTone, ICP, ComforTone, Super Vitamin B, Slique Shake, Detoxzyme, Master Formula, Mineral Essence, Allerzyme

Application and Usage

Aromatic: Refer to Application Guidelines.

Dietary and Oral: Refer to Application Guidelines.

- Take 1 capsule of desired Vitality oil 2 times daily.

- Take 2-3 drops of desired Vitality oil in a spoonful of syrup or small amount of milk, juice, or water.

Topical: Refer to Application Guidelines.

- Apply 1-2 drops neat on temples and back of neck several times daily.

- Place a warm compress with 6-8 drops of chosen oil over the liver.

ALKALOSIS

Alkalosis is a condition where the pH of the intestinal tract and the blood become excessively alkaline. While moderate alkalinity is essential for good health, excessive alkalinity can cause problems and result in fatigue, depression, irritability, and sickness.

The best way to lower the internal pH of the body from excessive alkalinity is to eat a high protein diet (meat, eggs, dairy, seeds, nuts, legumes, etc.).

Recommendations

Singles: Peppermint, Peppermint Vitality, Jade Lemon, Jade Lemon Vitality, Lemon, Lemon Vitality, Lime, Lime Vitality, Orange, Orange Vitality, Tarragon, Tarragon Vitality, Fennel, Fennel Vitality, Ginger, Ginger Vitality, Patchouli, Lemongrass, Lemongrass Vitality, Bergamot, Bergamot Vitality

Blends: DiGize, DiGize Vitality, GLF, GLF Vitality, EndoFlex, EndoFlex Vitality, KidScents TummyGize

Nutritionals: AlkaLime, Essentialzyme, Essentialzymes-4, ICP, Allerzyme, ComforTone, Digest & Cleanse, Pure Protein Complete, Protein Bites, Slique Shake, Life 9, KidScents MightyPro, Mineral Essence

Application and Usage

Aromatic: Refer to Application Guidelines.

Dietary and Oral: Refer to Application Guidelines.

- Take 1 capsule of desired Vitality oil 2 times daily.

- Take 2-3 drops of desired Vitality oil in a spoonful of syrup or small amount of milk, juice, or water.

- Take 1 teaspoon AlkaLime in 4-6 ounces of water 2 times daily.

Topical: Refer to Application Guidelines.

ALLERGIES

Allergies are a result of the response to many different situations. They can be triggered by food, pollen, environmental chemicals, dander, dust, insect bites, to name just a few, and can affect the following:

- Respiration—wheezing, labored breathing
- Mouth—swelling of the lips or tongue, itching lips
- Digestive tract—diarrhea, vomiting, cramps
- Skin—rashes, dermatitis
- Nose—sneezing, congestion, bloody nose

Food Allergies:

Food allergies are different from food intolerances and sensitivities. Food allergies involve an immune system reaction, whereas food intolerances and sensitivities involve gastrointestinal reactions and are far more common.

For example, peanuts often produce a lifelong allergy due to peanut proteins being targeted by immune system antibodies as foreign invaders. In contrast, intolerance of pasteurized cow's milk that causes cramping and diarrhea may be due to the inability to digest lactose (milk sugar) because of a lack of the enzyme lactase or a reaction to additives included.

Food allergies are often associated with the consumption of peanuts, shellfish, nuts, wheat, cow's milk, eggs, and soy. Infants and children are far more prone to have food allergies than adults, due to the immaturity of their immune and digestive systems.

A thorough intestinal cleansing is one of the best ways to combat most allergies. Start with ICP, ComforTone, Essentialzyme, Essentialzymes-4, JuvaTone, and Life 9 or KidScents MightyPro.

Hay Fever (Allergic Rhinitis):

Hay fever is an allergic reaction triggered by airborne allergens (pollen, animal hair, feathers, dust mites, etc.) that cause the release of histamines and subsequent inflammation of nasal passages and sinus-related areas. A more serious form of respiratory allergy is asthma, which manifests in the chest and lungs.

Symptoms: Inflammation of the nasal passages, sinuses, and eyelids that causes sneezing, runny nose, wheezing, and watery and red, itchy eyes.

Recommendations

Singles: Fennel, Fennel Vitality, Eucalyptus Blue, Lavender, Lavender Vitality, Roman Chamomile, Peppermint, Peppermint Vitality, German Chamomile, German Chamomile Vitality, Marjoram, Marjoram Vitality, Sacred Frankincense, Frankincense, Frankincense Vitality

Blends: DiGize, DiGize Vitality, Harmony, JuvaCleanse, JuvaCleanse Vitality, Valor, Valor Roll-On, R.C., Raven, KidScents TummyGize

Nutritionals: Allerzyme, Mineral Essence, ComforTone, Detoxzyme, Essentialzyme, ICP, JuvaPower, JuvaTone, MultiGreens, Sulfurzyme, Essentialzymes-4 yellow capsule, AlkaLime, Life 9, KidScents MightyPro

Application and Usage

Aromatic: Refer to Application Guidelines.

Dietary and Oral: Refer to Application Guidelines.

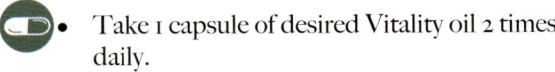

- Take 1 capsule of desired Vitality oil 2 times daily.
- Take 2-3 drops of desired Vitality oil in a spoonful of syrup or small amount of milk, juice, or water.

Topical: Refer to Application Guidelines.

ANALGESIC, NEED FOR

An analgesic is defined as a compound that binds with a number of closely related, specific receptors in the central nervous system to block the perception of pain or affect the emotional response to pain. A number of essential oils have analgesic properties.

Recommendations

Singles: Clove, Clove Vitality, Helichrysum, Dorado Azul, Palo Santo, Copaiba, Copaiba Vitality, Lavender, Lavender Vitality, Eucalyptus Radiata, Elemi, Wintergreen, Geranium, German Chamomile, German Chamomile Vitality, Kunzea

Blends: PanAway, Aroma Siez, Deep Relief Roll-On, Thieves, CBD, Inner Defense, Brain Power, Relieve It, Cool Azul

Nutritionals: PowerGize

Personal Care: Cool Azul Pain Relief Cream, Cool Azul Sports Gel, CBD Muscle Rub, Ortho Sport Massage Oil, Ortho Ease Massage Oil

Application and Usage

Aromatic: Refer to Application Guidelines.

Topical: Refer to Application Guidelines.

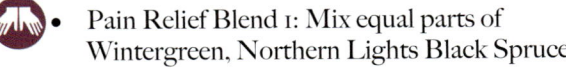

- Pain Relief Blend 1: Mix equal parts of Wintergreen, Northern Lights Black Spruce, and Black Pepper and massage with V-6 Vegetable Oil Complex.

- You may also apply 2-3 drops on the Vita Flex liver point of the right foot.

Dietary and Oral: Refer to Application Guidelines.

- Pain Relief Blend 2: Combine 18 drops Copaiba Vitality with 3 drops Lavender Vitality in a capsule. Take up to 4 times daily with 1-2 droppers of CBD each time.

ANTHRAX

The anthrax bacterium (Bacillus anthracis) is one of the oldest and deadliest diseases known. There are three predominant types:
- External, acquired from contact with infected animal carcasses
- Internal, obtained from breathing airborne anthrax spores
- Battlefield, developed for biological warfare that is a far more lethal variety

When the airborne variety of anthrax invades the lungs, it is 90 percent fatal unless antibiotics are administered at the very beginning of the infection, but anthrax often goes undiagnosed until it is too late for antibiotics.

External varieties of anthrax may be contracted by exposure to animal hides and wool. While vaccinations and antibiotics have stemmed anthrax infection in recent years, new strains have developed that are resistant to all countermeasures.

According to Jean Valnet, MD, Thyme oil may be effective for killing the anthrax bacillus.3 Two highly antimicrobial phenols in Thyme, carvacrol and thymol, are responsible for this action.

Recommendations

Singles: Ravintsara, Thyme, Thyme Vitality, Oregano, Oregano Vitality, Ecuadorian Oregano, Clove, Clove Vitality, Cinnamon Bark, Cinnamon Bark Vitality, Citronella, Lemongrass, Lemongrass Vitality

Blends: Raven, Exodus II, Thieves, Thieves Vitality, The Gift, ImmuPower, Melrose, Longevity, Longevity Vitality

Nutritionals: Inner Defense, ImmuPro, NingXia Red, Super Vitamin C, Super Vitamin C Chewable, Life 9, KidScents MightyPro

Household Care: Thieves Household Cleaner, Thieves Waterless Hand Purifier, Thieves Foaming Hand Soap, Thieves Automatic Dishwasher Powder, Thieves Cleansing Soap, Thieves Dish Soap, Thieves Fruit & Veggie Soak (and Spray), Thieves Laundry Soap, Thieves Spray, Thieves Wipes

Application and Usage

Aromatic: Refer to Application Guidelines.

Dietary and Oral: Refer to Application Guidelines.

- Take 1 capsule 4 times daily, alternating Vitality oils.

- Take 2-3 drops of desired Vitality oil in a spoonful of syrup or small amount of milk, juice, or water.

Topical: Refer to Application Guidelines.

- Use oils neat or dilute 50:50 for hands and other exposed skin areas.

ANTIBIOTIC REACTIONS

Synthetic antibiotic drugs indiscriminately kill both beneficial and harmful bacteria. This can result in yeast infections, including candida, diarrhea, poor nutrient assimilation, fatigue, sulfur toxicity, degenerative diseases, and many other conditions.

Reducing harmful symptoms of antibiotic use with probiotics was the focus of a study in the journal Vaccine.4 A four-strain probiotic was tested in a hospital setting and found to reduce adult patient diarrhea from antibiotic-associated diarrhea (AAD) and C. difficile-associated diarrhea (CDAD).

The average adult has 3-4 pounds of beneficial bacteria or flora constantly in the intestinal tract that support the body in healthy digestion and immune function as follows:
- Constitutes the first line of defense against bacterial and viral infections
- Produces B vitamins
- Maintains pH balance
- Combats yeast and fungus overgrowth
- Aids in the digestive process

Recommendations

Singles: Peppermint, Peppermint Vitality, Spearmint, Spearmint Vitality, Jade Lemon, Jade Lemon Vitality, Lemon, Lemon Vitality, Lime, Lime Vitality, Cassia, Davana

Blends: JuvaCleanse, JuvaCleanse Vitality, DiGize, DiGize Vitality, Purification, Thieves, Thieves Vitality, GLF, GLF Vitality, EndoFlex, EndoFlex Vitality, KidScents TummyGize

Nutritionals: Life 9, KidScents MightyPro, Essentialzyme, Essentialzymes-4, Detoxzyme, Balance Complete, Slique Shake, Mineral Essence, Inner Defense, Digest & Cleanse

Application and Usage
Aromatic: Refer to Application Guidelines.

Dietary and Oral: Refer to Application Guidelines.

- Take 1 capsule of desired Vitality oil 2 times daily.

- Take 2-3 drops of desired Vitality oil in a spoonful of syrup or small amount of milk, juice, or water.

- Life 9: Take 2-3 capsules on an empty stomach before meals during antibiotic treatment.
- KidScents MightyPro: Instead of Life 9, take 1 packet of KidScents MightyPro (a children's pre- and probiotics supplement) on an empty stomach before meals during antibiotic treatment.
- After completing antibiotic treatment, continue using Life 9 or KidScents MightyPro for 10-15 days.
- After a child (2 years of age and older) finishes antibiotic treatment, give 1 packet of KidScents MightyPro daily with food for seven days.

Topical: Refer to Application Guidelines.

ANTISEPTICS AND DISINFECTANTS, NEED FOR

Antiseptics prevent the growth of pathogenic microorganisms. Many essential oils have powerful, antiseptic properties. Clove and Thyme essential oils have been documented to kill over 50 types of bacteria and 10 types of fungi.

Other potent antiseptic essential oils include Cinnamon Bark, Cassia, Tea Tree, Oregano, Mountain Savory, and Dorado Azul.

A September 2018 Canadian study found a connection between household cleaning disinfectants and a higher body mass index (BMI) when the children were three years of age from altering the children's gut microbiota in infancy affected by exposure to those cleaning disinfectants. However, the use of eco-friendly products was associated with decreased odds of overweight or obesity (Kozyrskyj AL, 2018). Thieves essential oil blend or Thieves household cleaning products will not cause this change in children's gut microbiota.

Essential oil expert Kurt Schnaubelt has written that essential oils do not kill beneficial bacteria. He explains that phenylpropanoids such as cinnamic aldehyde, eugenol, and carvacrol are antimicrobial. However, they are also unique in the way that beneficial probiotic bacteria can harmlessly metabolize them.

Recommendations
Singles: Thyme, Thyme Vitality, Clove, Clove Vitality, Dorado Azul, Oregano, Oregano Vitality, Ecuadorian Oregano, Rosemary, Rosemary Vitality, Mountain Savory, Mountain Savory, Eucalyptus Radiata, Eucalyptus Globulus, Cinnamon Bark, Cinnamon Bark Vitality, Cassia, Ravintsara, Tea Tree, Sage, Sage Vitality

Blends: Thieves, Thieves Vitality, Raven, Purification, Melrose, R.C., ImmuPower

Nutritionals: Inner Defense, ImmuPro, Thieves Cough Drops, Thieves Hard Lozenges, Thieves Mints

Oral Care: Thieves AromaBright Toothpaste, Thieves Fresh Essence Plus Mouthwash, Thieves Whitening Toothpaste

Household Care: Thieves Foaming Hand Soap, Thieves Waterless Hand Purifier, Thieves Household Cleaner, Thieves Cleansing Soap, Thieves Automatic Dishwasher Powder, Thieves Dish Soap, Thieves Fruit & Veggie Soak (and Spray), Thieves Laundry Soap, Thieves Spray, Thieves Wipes, Luscious Lemon Foaming Hand Soap

Application and Usage
Aromatic: Refer to Application Guidelines.

Topical: Refer to Application Guidelines.

- Apply 1-2 drops diluted 50:50 and gently rub over affected areas.

APNEA, SLEEP

Apnea is a temporary cessation of breathing during sleep. It can lessen the quality of sleep, resulting in chronic fatigue, lowered immune function, and lack of energy.

Recommendations
Singles: Northern Lights Black Spruce, Idaho Grand Fir, Cedarwood, Ylang Ylang, Lavender, Lavender Vitality, Sacred Frankincense, Frankincense, Frankincense Vitality, Lemon Verbena, Royal Hawaiian Sandalwood, Sacred Sandalwood, Juniper, Vanilla

Blends: Clarity, Valor, Valor Roll-On, Common Sense, Stress Away, Stress Away Roll-On, RutaVaLa, RutaVaLa Roll-On, White Angelica, Sacred Mountain, Present Time, Chivalry, ImmuPower, CBD

Nutritionals: Thyromin, MultiGreens, Super Vitamin B, Inner Defense, ImmuPro, SleepEssence

Application and Usage

Aromatic: Refer to Application Guidelines.

Topical: Refer to Application Guidelines.

- Massage 2-4 drops of oil neat on the bottoms of the feet just before bedtime.

ARTHRITIS

More than 100 different kinds of arthritis have been identified. Two of the most common kinds are osteoarthritis and rheumatoid arthritis.

Osteoarthritis

Osteoarthritis involves the breakdown of the cartilage that forms a cushion between two joints. As this cartilage is eaten away, the two bones of the joint start rubbing together and wearing down.

In contrast, rheumatoid arthritis is caused from a swelling and inflammation of the synovial membrane, the lining of the joint.

Natural anti-inflammatories such as German Chamomile and Wintergreen when combined with cartilage builders (boswellic acid, undenatured collagen, and hyaluronic acid) are powerful, natural cures for arthritis.

The best natural anti-inflammatories include fats rich in omega-3s and essential oils such as Nutmeg, Wintergreen, German Chamomile, and Idaho Grand Fir.

Lemongrass is a well-known anti-inflammatory that can be safely ingested.

Nutmeg, a source of myristicin, has been researched for its anti-inflammatory effects in several studies. It works by inhibiting pro-inflammatory prostaglandins when taken internally or applied topically. Clove exhibits similar action.

Chamazulene, the blue sesquiterpene in German Chamomile, also shows strong anti-inflammatory activity when used both topically and orally. Methyl salicylate is the major compound in Wintergreen, similar to the active agent in aspirin (salicylic acid). PanAway contains nature's natural analgesics from Wintergreen and Clove and is strongly anti-inflammatory. Cool Azul Pain Relief Cream and Cool Azul Sports Gel are also strongly anti-inflammatory.

Type II collagen and hyaluronic acid are the two most powerful natural compounds for rebuilding cartilage and are the key ingredients in the supplement AgilEase.

Recommendations

Singles: Wintergreen, Nutmeg, Nutmeg Vitality, Peppermint, Peppermint Vitality, Lemongrass, Lemongrass Vitality, Vetiver, Valerian, Palo Santo, Idaho Grand Fir, Kunzea, Eucalyptus Globulus, Sacred Frankincense, Frankincense, Frankincense Vitality, German Chamomile, German Chamomile Vitality, Helichrysum, Dorado Azul, Northern Lights Black Spruce, Pine

Blends: Cool Azul, PanAway, Relieve It, Aroma Siez, Deep Relief Roll-On, CBD, Chivalry

Nutritionals: BLM, AgilEase, PowerGize, Essentialzyme, Essentialzymes-4, Sulfurzyme, ImmuPro, ICP, JuvaPower, Juva-Tone, Detoxzyme, Mega Vitamin Cal, Longevity Softgels, Rehemogen, OmegaGize3, EndoGize

Personal Care: Cool Azul Pain Relief Cream, Cool Azul Sports Gel, CBD Muscle Rub, Ortho Sport Massage Oil, Ortho Ease Massage Oil

Application and Usage

Aromatic: Refer to Application Guidelines.

Dietary and Oral: Refer to Application Guidelines.

- Detoxification of the body and strengthening the joints is important. Cleanse the colon and liver.
- Take 1 capsule of desired Vitality oil 2 times daily.
- Take 2-3 drops of desired Vitality oil in a spoonful of syrup or small amount of milk, juice, or water.

BLM, AgilEase: Take 2 capsules daily.

Mega Vitamin Cal: Mix 1 teaspoon in water before going to bed.

ImmuPro: Take 1-2 chewable tablets daily as needed, in the evening. Do not exceed 2 tablets per day.

ComforTone: Take 3 capsules 2 times daily; increase if needed.

ICP: Take 2 scoops in water or juice in the morning.

JuvaPower: Take 2 scoops in water or juice before going to bed.

Rehemogen: Cleans and purifies the blood, which may have toxins that are blocking nutrient and oxygen absorption into the cells (See BLOOD CIRCULATION, POOR).

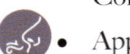**OmegaGize3:** Take 1-3 capsules daily.

Topical: Refer to Application Guidelines.

- Dilute 5-10 drops of oil in 1 teaspoon V-6 Vegetable Oil Complex and apply on location. Essential oils can also be applied neat and then followed by application of V-6 Vegetable Oil Complex.
- Applying a single drop of oil under the nose is helpful and refreshing.
- Cool Azul Pain Relief Cream, Cool Azul Sports Gel, Ortho Sport Massage Oil, or Ortho Ease Massage Oil offer tremendous relief.

Rheumatoid Arthritis

Rheumatoid arthritis is a painful, inflammatory condition of the joints marked by swelling, thickening, and inflammation of the synovial membrane lining the joint. In contrast, osteoarthritis is characterized by a breakdown of the joint cartilage, without any swelling or inflammation.

Rheumatoid arthritis is classified as an autoimmune disease because it is caused by the body's own immune system attacking the joints.

Inflammation from rheumatoid arthritis has been ameliorated by the boswellic acids found in most frankincense species.5

Other factors can aggravate arthritis such as:
- Deficiencies of minerals and other nutrients
- Microbes and toxins
- Lack of water intake
- Eating bread

Essential oils are effective in helping to combat pain and infection. In cases where arthritis is caused by infectious organisms, such as Lyme disease (Borrelia burgdorferi), chlamydia, and salmonella, essential oils may counteract and prevent infection.

Highly antimicrobial essential oils include Mountain Savory, Rosemary, Tea Tree, and Oregano. Essential oils easily pass into the bloodstream when applied topically.

MSM, the main ingredient in the supplement Sulfurzyme, has been documented to be one of the most effective, natural supplements for reducing the pain associated with rheumatism and arthritis.

MSM has been a subject of a number of clinical studies and was used extensively by Ronald Lawrence, MD, in his clinical practice to successfully treat rheumatism and arthritis.

Type II collagen and hyaluronic acid are also powerful, natural compounds for reducing inflammation, halting the progression of arthritis, and rebuilding cartilage. These are the key ingredients in the supplements BLM and AgilEase.

Recommendations

Singles: Wintergreen, Peppermint, Peppermint Vitality, Sacred Frankincense, Frankincense, Frankincense Vitality, Palo Santo, Vetiver, Nutmeg, Nutmeg Vitality, Oregano, Oregano Vitality, Ecuadorian Oregano, Clove, Clove Vitality, Mountain Savory, Mountain Savory Vitality, Rosemary, Rosemary Vitality, Tea Tree, Helichrysum, Kunzea, Idaho Grand Fir, Pine, Eucalyptus Globulus, Copaiba, Copaiba Vitality, Myrrh, Valerian, Dorado Azul, Northern Lights Black Spruce

Blends: PanAway, Relieve It, Aroma Siez, Cool Azul, Deep Relief Roll-On, CBD, Calm CBD Roll-On

Nutritionals: PowerGize, BLM, AgilEase, Detoxzyme, Sulfurzyme, Mega Vitamin Cal, Master Formula, Mineral Essence, Essentialzyme, Essentialzymes-4, Longevity Softgels, ImmuPro, Rehemogen, EndoGize

Personal Care: Cool Azul Pain Relief Cream, Cool Azul Sports Gel, CBD Muscle Rub, Ortho Ease Massage Oil, Ortho Sport Massage Oil

Application and Usage

Aromatic: Refer to Application Guidelines.

Dietary and Oral: Refer to Application Guidelines.

- Take 1 capsule of desired Vitality oil 2 times daily.
- Take 2-3 drops of desired Vitality oil in a spoonful of syrup or small amount of milk, juice, or water.

Topical: Refer to Application Guidelines.

- Dilute 5-10 drops of essential oils in 1 teaspoon of V-6 Vegetable Oil Complex and apply on location. Essential oils can also be applied neat and then followed by V-6 Vegetable Oil Complex.
- Massage 2-4 drops of oil neat on the bottoms of the feet just before bedtime.

• Place a warm compress once daily with oils of your choice on the back.

 • Massage with oils of your choice mixed with V-6 Vegetable Oil Complex, Relaxation Massage Oil, Sensation Massage Oil, Ortho Ease Massage Oil, or Ortho Sport Massage Oil.

• Apply Cool Azul Pain Relief Cream, Cool Azul Sports Gel, or one of the CBD products.

ATTENTION DEFICIT DISORDER (ADD and ADHD)

In 2001 Terry Friedmann, MD, completed pioneering studies using essential oils to combat ADD and ADHD. Using twice a day inhalation of essential oils, including Vetiver, Cedarwood, and Lavender, Dr. Friedmann was able to achieve clinically significant results in 60 days.6

Researchers postulate that essential oils mitigate ADD and ADHD through their stimulation of the limbic system of the brain.

Because attention deficit disorder may be caused by mineral deficiencies in the diet, increasing nutrient intake and absorption of magnesium, potassium, and other trace minerals can also have a significant, beneficial effect in resolving ADD.

Recommendations
Singles: Vetiver, Lavender, Lavender Vitality, Cedarwood, Royal Hawaiian Sandalwood, Sacred Sandalwood, Cardamom, Cardamom Vitality, Cassia, Peppermint, Peppermint Vitality, Sacred Frankincense, Frankincense, Frankincense Vitality

Blends: Brain Power, KidScents GeneYus, Peace & Calming, Peace & Calming II, Calm CBD Roll-On, Seedlings Calm, KidScents KidPower, KidScents KidPower Roll-On, AromaEase, Clarity, Reconnect

Nutritionals: Life 9, KidScents MightyPro, KidScents Unwind, OmegaGize3, MindWise, Mineral Essence, NingXia Red, Slique Shake, Balance Complete, Essentialzyme, Essentialzymes-4, Detoxzyme, MultiGreens, Master Formula, Pure Protein Complete, Protein Power Bites

Application and Usage
Aromatic: Refer to Application Guidelines.

Dietary and Oral: Refer to Application Guidelines.

 • Take 1 capsule of desired Vitality oil 2 times daily.

 • Take 2-3 drops of desired Vitality oil in a spoonful of syrup or small amount of milk, juice, or water.

 • Drink 3-6 ounces of NingXia Red daily.

Topical: Refer to Application Guidelines.

 • Apply 1-2 drops of the oil of your choice neat or diluted 4-8 times daily on the neck, brain stem, and even on the head.

 • Applying a single drop under the nose is helpful and refreshing.

 • Massage 2-4 drops of oil neat on the bottoms of the feet just before bedtime. Children love it.

AUTISM (Autism Spectrum Disorder, ASD)

Improving diet can be the key to reducing the problems associated with autism. Eliminating refined and synthetic sugars and replacing them with natural sweeteners such as Yacon Syrup, natural fruit sweeteners, maple syrup, etc., has produced outstanding results in numerous cases of autism.

Autism is a neurologically based developmental disorder that is four times more common in boys than girls. It is characterized by the following:
- Challenges in social interaction and participation
- Nonverbal and verbal communication difficulties
- Repetitive behavior (rocking, hair twirling)
- Self-injurious behavior (head banging)
- Unconventional or repetitive responses to sensual stimuli
- Reduced or abnormal responses to pain, noises, or other outside stimuli

Although controversial, autism is being increasingly linked to certain vaccinations; and MMR, the one-shot combination for measles, mumps, and rubella, is most often cited by researchers.

At one time, children were receiving, through vaccination, large doses of thimerosal, a vaccine preservative that contains 49.6 percent mercury, which is well above the limit recommended by the EPA. Some success in reversing autism has resulted through mercury detoxification along with nutritional supplementation.

A recent study reports: "There is promising evidence to suggest that probiotic therapy may improve gastrointestinal dysfunction, beneficially alter fecal microbiota, and reduce the severity of ASD symptoms in children with ASD."7 Gastrointestinal disorders may be linked to the brain dysfunctions that cause autism in children.8 In fact, there have been several cases of successful treatment of autism using pancreatic enzymes.

Stimulation of the limbic region of the brain may also help with symptoms of autism. The aromas from essential oils have a powerful ability to stimulate this part of the brain, since the sense of smell (olfaction) is tied directly to the emotional centers. As a result, the aroma of an essential oil has the potential to exert a powerful influence on disorders such as ADD and autism.

Recommendations

Singles: Vetiver, Patchouli, Lavender, Lavender Vitality, Eucalyptus Globulus, Melissa, Myrrh, Peppermint, Peppermint Vitality, Cedarwood, Sacred Sandalwood, Royal Hawaiian Sandalwood, Sacred Frankincense, Frankincense, Frankincense Vitality, Cassia, Idaho Grand Fir

Blends: KidScents GeneYus, Brain Power, KidScents KidPower, KidScents KidPower Roll-On, Release, GLF, GLF Vitality, Valor, Valor Roll-On, Clarity, Peace & Calming, Peace & Calming II, Calm CBD Roll-On, Seedlings Calm, Common Sense, The Gift, Reconnect, SleepyIze

Nutritionals: MightyPro, KidScents Unwind, Essentialzyme, Essentialzymes-4, MindWise, NingXia Red, ½ Super Vitamin B for children, Sulfurzyme, Detoxzyme, Slique Shake, Balance Complete, Pure Protein Complete, Protein Power Bites, AlkaLime

Application and Usage

Aromatic: Refer to Application Guidelines.

Dietary and Oral: Refer to Application Guidelines.

- Take 1 capsule of desired Vitality oil 2 times daily.

- Take 2-3 drops of desired Vitality oil in a spoonful of syrup or small amount of milk, juice, or water.

Topical: Refer to Application Guidelines.

- Apply 1-2 drops neat (undiluted) on temples and back of neck, as desired.

- Applying a single drop under the nose is helpful and refreshing.

- Massage 2-4 drops of oil neat on the bottoms of the feet just before bedtime. Children love it.

Autism Topical Blend
- 15 drops Sacred Frankincense or Frankincense
- 12 drops Myrrh
- 10 drops Idaho Grand Fir
- 10 drops Canadian Fleabane or Orange
- 4 drops Peppermint

Use this blend for Raindrop Technique 2 times daily: morning and night.

Using this regimen, a 7-year-old boy with cerebral palsy and autism, after one month, was able to walk flat-footed without his walker, his test scores in school improved by 28 percent, and his attention span increased 30 percent, his mother reported.

BEDBUGS

Having bedbugs is a very miserable experience. Some bedbugs are so small they just look like specks of dirt that you brush off the sheets. You cannot tell they are alive unless you look at them with a microscope. They thrive in a moist, warm environment, and when you wake up in the morning, you are astounded at all the bites you have in the most unexpected places.

The itching is horrible and lasts for about one week. It is amazing that a tiny, almost microscopic bug can give such an intense bite. Essential oils are the answer to treating those bites and killing the bugs without dreaded chemicals. Some of the oils have a powerful ability to kill on contact. The thought of sleeping with those little, hungry critters is not a pleasant thought, and to some, it's repulsive; but knowing the bugs are dead is a great feeling.

If you suspect bedbugs, wash all of your bedding in hot water and add 10 to 15 drops of Thieves, Palo Santo, Oregano, Thyme, Citrus Fresh, Melrose, etc., and see what works best for you. After you make the bed, spray with a single oil or with one of the **Blends** morning and night to ensure that they do not return.

If you live in a warm or hot, humid environment, then you will probably have to spray at least once every day or perhaps twice. If you see any little specks, make sure they are not biting bugs that have come to visit.

Recommendations

These **Blends** work for most bugs but have been tried and tested with bedbugs.

Bedbug Killer Blend No. 1
- 20 drops Palo Santo
- 20 drops Idaho Tansy

Mix together and spray. Dilute with water as much as you think you can and still have results. You will have to experiment to determine optimum ratio of water to blend. Spray sheets and clothing to kill any insects that might be embedded in the cloth or anywhere else that you might suspect their presence.

Bedbug Killer Blend No. 2
- 20 drops Palo Santo
- 20 drops Idaho Tansy
- 10 drops Eucalyptus Blue

   Apply on bites as needed.

Bedbug Killer Blend No. 3
- Mix 20 drops Thieves with 2-3 cups water, shake well, and spray sheets and pillows.

BLADDER/URINARY TRACT INFECTION (CYSTITIS)

Bladder infections and the inflammation known as cystitis are caused by bacteria that travel up the urethra. This disorder is more common in women than men because of the woman's shorter urethra. If the infection travels up the ureters and reaches the kidneys, kidney infection can result.

Symptoms of infection
- Frequent urge to urinate with only a small amount of urine passing
- Strong smelling urine
- Blood in urine
- Burning or stinging during urination
- Tenderness or chronic pain in bladder and pelvic area
- Pain intensity fluctuates as bladder fills or empties
- Symptoms worsen during menstruation

Recommendations
Singles: Myrrh, Tea Tree, Juniper, Oregano, Oregano Vitality, Ecuadorian Oregano, Jade Lemon, Jade Lemon Vitality, Lemon, Lemon Vitality, Lime, Lime Vitality, Mountain Savory, Mountain Savory Vitality, Davana, Thyme, Thyme Vitality, Cistus, Rosemary, Rosemary Vitality, Frankincense, Frankincense Vitality, Sacred Frankincense, Clove, Clove Vitality, Palo Santo

Blends: Melrose, Thieves, Thieves Vitality, DiGize, DiGize Vitality, EndoFlex, EndoFlex Vitality, R.C., Purification, Inspiration

Nutritionals: K&B, ImmuPro, Inner Defense, AlkaLime

Application and Usage
Dietary and Oral: Refer to Application Guidelines.

- Take 1 capsule of desired Vitality oil 2 times daily.

- Take 2-3 drops of desired Vitality oil in a spoonful of syrup or small amount of milk, juice, or water.

- Use K&B tincture (2-3 droppers in distilled water) 3-6 times daily. K&B helps strengthen and tone weak bladder, kidneys, and urinary tract.

- Take ½ teaspoon of AlkaLime daily, in water only, 1 hour before or after a meal.

- Drink unsweetened cranberry juice and sweeten with honey, Yacon Syrup, or maple syrup.

- Drink 4 liters of purified water daily.

Topical: Refer to Application Guidelines.

- Dilute 50:50 and apply a few drops on location 3-6 times daily.

- Dilute 2-4 drops of Melrose, Purification, or other oil and use in a warm compress over bladder 1-2 times daily.

- Receive a Raindrop Technique 3 times weekly.

- First Week: Use Myrrh, Thyme, Mountain Savory, Palo Santo, and Inspiration and follow with a hot compress.

BLOATING/SWELLING (See also MENSTRUAL AND FEMALE HORMONE CONDITIONS)

Bloating is caused by many imbalances in the body. Bloating during the menstrual cycle or swelling in the lower extremities is caused by pH imbalance and low estrogen. Bloating can also be caused by enzyme deficiencies, resulting in poor digestion and allergies. Swelling in the legs can be from low potassium and poor circulation, which will cause fluid retention.

It is important to determine whether it is bloating or fluid retention; there is a very significant difference.

Recommendations

Singles: Juniper, Tangerine, Tangerine Vitality, Clary Sage, Sage, Sage Vitality, Cypress, Peppermint, Peppermint Vitality, Fennel, Fennel Vitality, Tarragon, Tarragon Vitality, Lemon Verbena, Nutmeg, Nutmeg Vitality

Blends: DiGize, DiGize Vitality, GLF, GLF Vitality, Citrus Fresh, Citrus Fresh Vitality, KidScents TummyGize

Nutritionals: Essentialzyme, Essentialzymes-4, Mineral Essence, AlkaLime, Detoxzyme, Allerzyme, ICP, ComforTone, JuvaPower, Super Vitamin B

Personal Care: Progessence Plus

Application and Usage

Aromatic: Refer to Application Guidelines.

Dietary and Oral: Refer to Application Guidelines.

- Take 1 capsule of desired Vitality oil 2 times daily.

- Take 2-3 drops of desired Vitality oil in a spoonful of syrup or small amount of milk, juice, or water.

- Take 2 capsules of DiGize Vitality 3 times daily.

- Take 1 capsule of Peppermint Vitality 3 times daily.

Topical: Refer to Application Guidelines.

BONE PROBLEMS

Symptoms of bone problems include pain, brittleness, and lumps. Treatment depends on the nature and cause of the problems; unexplained symptoms can be serious and should always receive medical attention.

Broken Bones

A health professional should always be involved in the diagnosis and setting of a broken bone or a suspected broken bone.

Recommendations

Singles: Thyme, Thyme Vitality, Helichrysum, Wintergreen, Peppermint, Peppermint Vitality, Northern Lights Black Spruce, Idaho Grand Fir, Sacred Frankincense, Frankincense, Frankincense Vitality, Pine, Copaiba, Copaiba Vitality, Palo Santo, Myrrh, Lemongrass, Lemongrass Vitality, Ginger, Ginger Vitality, Vetiver

Blends: Cool Azul, Aroma Siez, PanAway, Relieve It, Deep Relief Roll-On, CBD

Nutritionals: PowerGize, BLM, AgilEase, Mega Vitamin Cal, PD 80/20, Super Vitamin Cal Plus, Super Vitamin D, Mineral Essence, OmegaGize3

Personal Care: Cool Azul Pain Relief Cream, Cool Azul Sports Gel, CBD Muscle Rub, Ortho Ease Massage Oil, Ortho Sport Massage Oil, Regenolone, Progessence Plus

The following broken bone **Blends** can also help relieve pain and speed the bone-mending process:

Application and Usage

Topical: Refer to Application Guidelines.

- Dilute 50:50 and apply a few drops on location 3-6 times daily.

- Prior to casting a broken bone, mix one of the above **Blends** and very gently apply 5-10 drops (depending on size) neat to break area. If there are any signs of skin sensitivity or irritation, apply a small amount of V-6 Vegetable Oil Complex.

Note: Apply oils extremely gently if bone break is suspected.

Broken Bone Blend No. 1
- 8 drops Idaho Grand Fir
- 6 drops Helichrysum
- 1 drop Myrrh, Sacred Frankincense, or Frankincense
- 1 drop Wintergreen

Broken Bone Blend No. 1
- 10 drops Wintergreen
- 4 drops Palo Santo
- 4 drops Vetiver
- 3 drops Pine
- 3 drops Helichrysum
- 2 drops Lemongrass

Bone Pain

Bone pain can be caused from injuries, arthritis, or other more serious reasons. See your health care professional for the correct diagnosis and proper treatment.

Recommendations

Singles: Wintergreen, Northern Lights Black Spruce, Copaiba, Copaiba Vitality, Pine, Idaho Grand Fir, Helichrysum

Blends: PanAway, Cool Azul, Aroma Siez, Relieve It, Deep Relief Roll-On, CBD

Nutritionals: Mega Vitamin Cal, BLM, AgilEase, Master Formula, Super Vitamin D, Essentialzyme, Essentialzymes-4

Personal Care: Cool Azul Pain Relief Cream, Cool Azul Sports Gel, CBD Muscle Rub, Ortho Ease Massage Oil, Ortho Sport Massage Oil, Regenolone, Progessence Plus

Application and Usage
Topical: Refer to Application Guidelines.

- Dilute 50:50 and apply a few drops on location 3-6 times daily as needed.
- Poor bone and muscle development can indicate HGH (human growth hormone), potassium, and/or mineral deficiency.

Osteoporosis (Bone Density Loss)
Osteoporosis is primarily caused by six main factors:
- Progesterone deficiency
- Estradiol deficiency
- Testosterone deficiency
- Lack of magnesium and boron in diet
- Lack of vitamin D in diet
- Lack of dietary and oral calcium

Natural progesterone is the single most effective way to increase bone density in women over age 40. Clinical studies by John Lee, MD, showed dramatic increases in bone density using just 20 mg of daily, topically applied progesterone.

Calcium, magnesium, and boron are a few of the most important minerals for bone health and are usually lacking or deficient in most modern diets. Magnesium is especially important for bone strength, but most Americans consume only a fraction of the 400 mg daily value needed for bone health.

Calcium and magnesium may not be adequately metabolized when consumed because of poor intestinal flora and excess phytates in the diet (a problem with vegetarians). Phytates occur in many nuts, grains, and seeds, including rice. Enzymes like phytase are essential for increasing calcium absorption by liberating calcium from insoluble phytate complexes.

Lack of vitamin D (cholecalciferol) has become epidemic among older people and has contributed to a lack of absorption of calcium in the diet.

Mega Vitamin Cal, AlkaLime, and Mineral Essence are all excellent sources of calcium and magnesium, which are essential for strong bones. Mineral Essence is an excellent source of magnesium and other trace minerals.

Avoid drinking anything that is carbonated because it can leach calcium from the bones due to its phosphoric acid content.

Studies show that the majority of women who do resistance training 3-4 times a week do not develop osteoporosis.

Recommendations
Singles: Wintergreen, Idaho Grand Fir, Palo Santo, Sacred Frankincense, Frankincense, Frankincense Vitality, Thyme, Thyme Vitality, Cypress, Peppermint, Peppermint Vitality, Marjoram, Marjoram Vitality, Rosemary, Rosemary Vitality, Basil, Basil Vitality, Elemi, Northern Lights Black Spruce, Pine

Blends: SclarEssence, SclarEssence Vitality, PanAway, Aroma Siez, Purification, Melrose, Sacred Mountain, Relieve It

Nutritionals: FemiGen, EndoGize, BLM, Super Vitamin D, AgilEase, Mega Vitamin Cal, Essentialzyme, Detoxzyme, AlkaLime, Mineral Essence, Essentialzymes-4, Super Vitamin Cal Plus, Sulfurzyme, Thyromin, PowerGize

Personal Care: Prenolone Plus Body Cream, Progessence Plus

Application and Usage
Topical: Refer to Application Guidelines.

- Massage 6-10 drops diluted 50:50 on spine (or area affected) 2-3 times daily.

BRAIN DISORDERS AND PROBLEMS
As the control center of the body, the brain controls speech, movement, thoughts, and memory and regulates the function of many organs. When problems occur, the results can be devastating.

Absentmindedness
Clinical studies on Ningxia wolfberry (Lycium barbarum) have shown that it has an anti-senility effect.9 Clinical studies at Tufts University and the Department of Veterans Affairs Medical Center, Denver, Colorado, and Boston, Massachusetts, found that high antioxidant foods such as spinach, which is found in JuvaPower, and blueberry, which is found in NingXia Red, dramatically improved learning and cognition.10,11

Recommendations

Singles: Peppermint, Peppermint Vitality, Sacred Frankincense, Frankincense, Frankincense Vitality, Rosemary, Rosemary Vitality, Cassia, Cardamom, Cardamom Vitality

Blends: Clarity, M-Grain, Brain Power, KidScents GeneYus, KidScents KidPower, KidScents KidPower Roll-On, Common Sense, Reconnect, One Heart

Nutritionals: MindWise, NingXia Red, PD 80/20, OmegaGize3, NingXia Nitro, NingXia Zyng, Ningxia Wolfberries (Organic, Dried), Master Formula, JuvaPower, Essentialzyme, Essentialzymes-4, Life 9, KidScents MightyPro

Application and Usage

Aromatic: Refer to Application Guidelines.

Topical: Refer to Application Guidelines.

- Apply 1-2 drops neat (undiluted) on temples and back of neck, as desired.

Alzheimer's Disease

Over 5.7 million Americans suffer from Alzheimer's disease, according to the Alzheimer's Association.12 Alzheimer's was found to nearly double in subjects with high levels of homocysteine in the Framingham Study, the longest running prospective study of chronic disease in a population. The Center for Disease Control and Prevention has concluded that the primary cause of Alzheimer's disease is probably not aluminum, although it could be a contributing factor in patients who were already at risk of developing the disease. In spite of this, people are unfortunately still being urged to get yearly flu shots, which contain aluminum as an adjuvant.

Pepper, Grapefruit, and Fennel oils have been found to stimulate brain activity.13 Peppermint oil has been helpful in protecting against stresses and toxins in brain cells.14

Dr. Richard Restick, a leading neurologist in Washington, DC, stated that maintaining normal synaptic firing would forestall many types of neurological deterioration in the body.

Essential oils high in sesquiterpenes such as Cedarwood, Vetiver, Patchouli, German Chamomile, German Chamomile Vitality, Myrrh, Melissa, Sacred Sandalwood, and Royal Hawaiian Sandalwood are known to cross the bloodbrain barrier. Sacred Frankincense, Frankincense, and Frankincense Vitality are general cerebral stimulants.

Recommendations

Singles: Cedarwood, Melissa, Sacred Sandalwood, Royal Hawaiian Sandalwood, Helichrysum, Ginger, Ginger Vitality, Nutmeg, Nutmeg Vitality, German Chamomile, German Chamomile Vitality, Eucalyptus Globulus, Sacred Frankincense, Frankincense, Frankincense Vitality, Cassia, Peppermint, Peppermint Vitality, Patchouli, Myrrh, Black Pepper, Black Pepper Vitality, Grapefruit, Grapefruit Vitality, Fennel, Fennel Vitality, Vetiver

Helichrysum supports neurotransmitter activity and has shown the possibility of chelating aluminum. Nutmeg is a general cerebral stimulant and has adrenal cortex-like activity.

Blends: Brain Power, Common Sense, KidScents GeneYus, Valor, Valor Roll-On, Clarity, KidScents KidPower, KidScents KidPower Roll-On, Harmony, RutaVaLa, RutaVaLa Roll-On, Reconnect, One Heart

Nutritionals: MindWise, MultiGreens, Slique Shake, Sulfurzyme, Essentialzyme, Essentialzymes-4, Mineral Essence, NingXia Red, NingXia Nitro, NingXia Zyng, Ningxia Wolfberries (Organic, Dried), Master Formula, Super Vitamin C, Super Vitamin C Chewable, Mega Vitamin Cal, OmegaGize3

Application and Usage

Aromatic: Refer to Application Guidelines.

Dietary and Oral: Refer to Application Guidelines.

- Take 1 capsule of desired Vitality oil 2 times daily.

- Take 2-3 drops of desired Vitality oil in a spoonful of syrup or small amount of milk, juice, or water.

Topical: Refer to Application Guidelines.

- Apply 1-2 drops directly onto the brain reflex centers. These points include the forehead, temples, and mastoids (the bones just behind the ears). Apply oils and mild, direct pressure to the brainstem area (center top of neck at base of skull) and work down the spine.

- Apply 1-2 drops neat to Vita Flex brain points on feet 1-2 times daily.

- Receive a Raindrop Technique once every 2 weeks.

Concentration Impaired

Impaired concentration is very common and may not always lead to a debilitating condition. Some common reasons why people can't concentrate are lack of sleep, lack of exercise, improper diet, and too much technology. A study in Research in Higher Education showed that students who texted the professor during a lecture scored 42.8 on a test following the lecture while non-texting students had a higher score of 58.67.15

Recommendations

Singles: Peppermint, Peppermint Vitality, Basil, Basil Vitality, Jade Lemon, Jade Lemon Vitality, Lemon, Lemon Vitality, Lime, Lime Vitality, Bergamot, Bergamot Vitality, Rosemary, Rosemary Vitality, Sacred Frankincense, Frankincense, Frankincense Vitality, Cassia, Dorado Azul

Blends: Brain Power, Clarity, KidScents GeneYus, RutaVaLa, RutaVaLa Roll-On, Harmony, KidScents KidPower, KidScents KidPower Roll-On, Valor, Valor Roll-On, Common Sense, 3 Wise Men, Reconnect

Nutritionals: MindWise, Mega Vitamin Cal, Super Vitamin B, OmegaGize3, ImmuPro, Digest & Cleanse, Mineral Essence, NingXia Red, NingXia Nitro, NingXia Zyng, Ningxia Wolfberries (Organic, Dried)

Application and Usage

Aromatic: Refer to Application Guidelines.

Dietary and Oral: Refer to Application Guidelines.

- Take 1 capsule of desired Vitality oil 2 times daily.

- Take 2-3 drops of desired Vitality oil in a spoonful of syrup or small amount of milk, juice, or water.

Topical: Refer to Application Guidelines.

- Apply 1-2 drops neat directly onto the brain reflex centers 2-4 times daily, as needed. These points include the forehead, temples, and mastoids (the bones just behind the ears). Apply oils and mild, direct pressure to the brainstem area (center top of neck at base of skull) and work down the spine.

- Apply 1-2 drops neat to Vita Flex brain points on feet 1-2 times daily.

- Receive a Raindrop Technique once every 2 weeks.

Confusion

Confusion is when a person is not able to think with his or her usual level of clarity. Decision-making ability is reduced, and a feeling of disorientation is common. Confusion may develop gradually or arise suddenly and has multiple causes, including medical conditions, medications, injuries, environmental factors, substance abuse, stress, low hormones, or low thyroid.

Recommendations

Singles: Peppermint, Peppermint Vitality, Jade Lemon, Jade Lemon Vitality, Lemon, Lemon Vitality, Rosemary, Rosemary Vitality, Basil, Basil Vitality, Sacred Frankincense, Frankincense, Frankincense Vitality, Vanilla, Cassia, Cardamom, Cardamom Vitality

Blends: M-Grain, Gathering, Brain Power, Clarity, KidScents GeneYus, Common Sense, Harmony, KidScents KidPower, KidScents KidPower Roll-On, Reconnect, One Heart

Nutritionals: MindWise, Mega Vitamin Cal, Super Vitamin B, OmegaGize3, Digest & Cleanse, Mineral Essence, Thyromin, NingXia Red, EndoGize

Application and Usage

Aromatic: Refer to Application Guidelines.

Topical: Refer to Application Guidelines.

- Applying a single drop under the nose is helpful and refreshing.

- Dilute 50:50 and apply on location 3-6 times daily.

- Massage 2-4 drops of oil neat on the bottoms of the feet just before bedtime.

Convulsions

Convulsions, also called seizures, are involuntary contractions of the voluntary muscles. Monitor diet and discontinue eating sugar, dairy products, and fried and processed foods. A 2018 UCLA study is the first to show a link between lower seizure susceptibility and certain helpful gut bacteria. These gut bacteria play a role in the anti-seizure effect of a high-fat, low-carb ketogenic diet for children who do not respond to anti-epileptic medications.16

Recommendations

Singles: Sacred Frankincense, Frankincense, Frankincense Vitality, Palo Santo, Eucalyptus Blue, Copaiba, Copaiba Vitality, Lemon Verbena, Wintergreen

Blends: Brain Power, KidScents GeneYus, Valor, Valor Roll-On, RutaVaLa, RutaVaLa Roll-On, Tranquil Roll-On, Clarity, KidScents KidPower, KidScents KidPower Roll-On, Common Sense

Nutritionals: MindWise, Detoxzyme, AlkaLime, Mineral Essence, Life 9, KidScents MightyPro

Application and Usage

Aromatic: Refer to Application Guidelines.

Topical: Refer to Application Guidelines.

- Apply 2-4 drops neat at base of skull, across the neck, top of spine (C1-C6 vertebrae), and bottoms of feet.

- Apply 1-2 drops neat on temples and back of neck as desired.

- Place a warm compress with 1-2 drops of chosen oil on the back.

Memory, Impaired/Dementia

Many areas of the brain help create and retrieve memories. Malfunction of or damage to any of these areas can lead to memory loss. Progressive memory loss can lead to dementia.

Recommendations

Singles: Rosemary, Rosemary Vitality, Peppermint, Peppermint Vitality, Cardamom, Cardamom Vitality, Basil, Basil Vitality, Vetiver, Rose, Lemon, Lemon Vitality, Lemongrass, Lemongrass Vitality, Helichrysum, Lavender, Lavender Vitality, Tangerine, Tangerine Vitality, Spearmint, Spearmint Vitality, Palo Santo, Cassia, Geranium

Note: Peppermint improves mental concentration and memory. Dr. William N. Dember conducted a study at the University of Cincinnati in 1994 showing that inhaling peppermint increased mental accuracy by 28 percent.17 The fragrances of diffused oils, such as lemon, have also been reported to increase memory retention and recall.

Blends: Brain Power, Clarity, M-Grain, KidScents GeneYus, KidScents KidPower, KidScents KidPower Roll-On, En-R-Gee, Reconnect, One Heart

Nutritionals: MindWise, Longevity Softgels, MultiGreens, Mineral Essence, Thyromin, NingXia Red

Application and Usage

Aromatic: Refer to Application Guidelines.

Cleansing: Vascular cleansing may improve mental function by supporting improved blood flow, boosting distribution of oxygen and nutrients (See CARDIOVASCULAR CONDITIONS AND PROBLEMS, Vascular Cleansing, Need for)

Dietary and Oral: Refer to Application Guidelines.

- Take 1 capsule of desired Vitality oil 3 times daily.

- Take 2-3 drops of desired Vitality oil in a spoonful of syrup or small amount of milk, juice, or water.

Topical: Refer to Application Guidelines.

- Applying a single drop under the nose is helpful and refreshing.

- Dilute 50:50 and apply 2-3 drops on temples, forehead, mastoids (bone behind ear), and/or brainstem (back of neck) as needed 3-6 times daily.

- Massage 2-4 drops of oil neat on the bottoms of feet just before bedtime.

Memory Blend No. 1

- 5 drops Basil or Basil Vitality
- 10 drops Rosemary or Rosemary Vitality
- 4 drops Helichrysum
- 2 drops Peppermint or Peppermint Vitality
- 2 drops Cardamom or Cardamom Vitality

Memory Blend No. 2

- 4 drops Lavender or Lavender Vitality
- 3 drops Geranium
- 3 drops Palo Santo
- 3 drops Rosemary or Rosemary Vitality
- 2 drops Tangerine or Tangerine Vitality
- 1 drop Spearmint or Spearmint Vitality

Mental Fatigue

Some of the causes of mental fatigue are being overworked, having poor sleep patterns, lacking exercise, and having a poor diet.

Recommendations

Singles: Sacred Frankincense, Frankincense, Frankincense Vitality, Rosemary, Rosemary Vitality, Vetiver, Cedarwood, Peppermint, Peppermint Vitality

Blends: Brain Power, Clarity, KidScents GeneYus, KidScents KidPower, KidScents KidPower Roll-On, Valor, Valor Roll-On, Journey On, One Heart, RutaVaLa, RutaVaLa Roll-On, Tranquil Roll-On, Reconnect, SleepyIze

Nutritionals: MindWise, Thyromin, Super Vitamin B, EndoGize, MultiGreens, ImmuPro, NingXia Red, NingXia Zyng, NingXia Nitro, Ningxia Wolfberries (Organic, Dried), Master Formula, ImmuPro

Application and Usage

Aromatic: Refer to Application Guidelines.

Cleansing: Vascular cleansing may improve mental function by supporting improved blood flow, boosting distribution of oxygen and nutrients (See CARDIOVASCULAR CONDITIONS AND PROBLEMS, Vascular Cleansing, Need for)

Dietary and Oral: Refer to Application Guidelines.

- Take 1 capsule of desired Vitality oil 3 times daily.

- Take 2-3 drops of desired Vitality oil in a spoonful of syrup or small amount of milk, juice, or water.

Topical: Refer to Application Guidelines.

- Applying a single drop under the nose is helpful and refreshing.

- Dilute 50:50 and apply 2-3 drops on temples, forehead, mastoids (bone behind ear), and/or brainstem (back of neck) as needed 3-6 times daily.

- Massage 2-4 drops of oil neat on the bottoms of feet just before bedtime.

Strokes (See STROKES)

BREASTFEEDING PROBLEMS

Dry, Cracked Nipples

The most common causes of sore or cracked nipples are poor breastfeeding technique, dehydration, or infection.

Recommendations

Singles: Myrrh, Vetiver, Royal Hawaiian Sandalwood, Sacred Sandalwood

Blends: Valor, Valor Roll-on, Harmony, Thieves, Thieves Vitality, The Gift, KidScents Owie

Nutritionals: MultiGreens, Master Formula, NingXia Red

Personal Care: Rose Ointment, KidScents Tender Tush, Essential Beauty Serum

Application and Usage

Topical: Refer to Application Guidelines.
- Dilute 50:50 and massage over breast and on Vita Flex points of the feet.
- Wash/cleanse breasts before breast-feeding.

Mastitis (Infected Breast)

Mastitis is an infection of the breast tissue that results in pain, swelling, redness, and warmth of the breast. It most commonly affects women who are breastfeeding.

Recommendations

Singles: Myrrh, Melissa, Tea Tree, Thyme, Thyme Vitality, Patchouli, Roman Chamomile, Rosemary, Rosemary Vitality, Lavender, Lavender Vitality, Lemon, Lemon Vitality, Vetiver, Copaiba, Copaiba Vitality, Idaho Blue Spruce, Mountain Savory, Mountain Savory Vitality

Blends: PanAway, ImmuPower, Thieves, Thieves Vitality

Nutritionals: Longevity Softgels, ImmuPro, Inner Defense

Massage any of these **Singles** or **Blends** on the breasts and under armpits 2 times daily. Wash/cleanse breasts before breast-feeding.

Application and Usage

Topical: Refer to Application Guidelines.

- Dilute 20:80 and massage over breast and on Vita Flex points of the feet.

Breast Blend No. 1
- 3 drops Thyme
- 7 drops PanAway
- 1 teaspoon V-6 Vegetable Oil Complex

Breast Blend No. 2
- 3 drops Myrrh
- 3 drops Vetiver
- 2 drops Copaiba
- 1 drop Idaho Blue Spruce
- ½ teaspoon V-6 Vegetable Oil Complex

Breast Blend No. 3
- 3 drops Lemon
- 4 drops Thyme
- 2 drops Melissa
- 1 teaspoon V-6 Vegetable Oil Complex

Breast Blend No. 4
- 4 drops Melissa
- 10 drops Myrrh
- 1 drop Thyme
- 1 drop Mountain Savory

BURSITIS

Bursitis is an inflammation of the bursa, which are small, fluid-filled sacs located near the joints. Bursa act as shock absorbers when muscles or tendons come into contact with bone. The swelling of the bursa results in pain, particularly when the affected joint is used.

Bursitis can be caused by injury, infection, or arthritis, and usually involves the joints of the knees, elbows, shoulders, and Achilles tendon. Occasionally, bursitis can occur in the base of the big toe. Bursitis may signal the beginning of arthritis.

Recommendations
Singles: Wintergreen, Idaho Blue Spruce, Peppermint, Peppermint Vitality, Copaiba, Copaiba Vitality, Dorado Azul, Palo Santo, Sacred Frankincense, Frankincense, Frankincense Vitality, Idaho Grand Fir, Basil, Basil Vitality, Lavender, Lavender Vitality, Black Pepper, Black Pepper Vitality, Elemi, Oregano, Oregano Vitality, Ecuadorian Oregano, Marjoram, Marjoram Vitality

Blends: PanAway, Relieve It, CBD, Sacred Mountain, Cool Azul, Deep Relief Roll-On, Aroma Siez

Nutritionals: Sulfurzyme, Mega Vitamin Cal, BLM, Super Vitamin D, AgilEase

Personal Care: Cool Azul Pain Relief Cream, Cool Azul Sports Gel, CBD Muscle Rub, Ortho Ease Massage Oil, Ortho Sport Massage Oil

Application and Usage
Aromatic: Refer to Application Guidelines.

Dietary and Oral: Refer to Application Guidelines.

- Take 1 capsule of desired Vitality oil 2 times daily.
- Take 2-3 drops of desired Vitality oil in a spoonful of syrup or small amount of milk, juice, or water.

Topical: Refer to Application Guidelines.

- Apply 2-4 drops neat or diluted 50:50 on affected area or joint 3-5 times daily or as needed to soothe pain.
- Apply a cold compress around affected joint 1-3 times daily.

CANCER

Cancer is among the most complex and difficult of any human disease to treat. A patient diagnosed with cancer should always defer to his or her health care professional for primary care. Keeping this in mind, a number of individuals have achieved successful remission by following a natural regimen and some of the principles outlined in this section.

It is important to note that many natural therapies—especially those using essential oils—work best in the early stages of cancer. In fact, clinical trials are showing that Frankincense is the number one inhibitor of many cancers. Citrus oils, high in d-limonene, including Orange, Grapefruit, Lemon, and Tangerine, work better as cancer preventives than cancer treatments, although they have been tested to have powerful, anticancer properties in all stages of cancer.

A study at Charing Cross Hospital in London, England, published in 1998, documented that close to a 15-percent remission rate was achieved in patients with advanced colon and breast cancer using doses from 1 to 15 grams of d-limonene from Orange oil as their only treatment. In patients with only weeks or months to live, limonene treatment extended patients' lives by up to 18 months in some cases.[18]

The Foundation of Natural Cancer Treatment

The Foundation of Natural Cancer Treatment Natural treatment of cancer or any illness is a highly debated topic, but when you are faced with cancer, finding solutions becomes important.

Emotions and Cancer

Cancer should always be treated first by discovering the underlying emotions that contributed to the onset of the disease. In many cases, negative emotions and trauma not only trigger the beginning of cancer but can further its metastasis. Any kind of negative emotion—anger, fear, rage, hate, helplessness, abandonment—can cause the cancer to spread faster.

When essential oils are used as the basis of an emotional care program, they can have powerfully positive effects in improving the attitude, emotional well-being, and potential outcome of the disease. Essential oil **Blends** such as White Angelica, Release, Grounding, Inner Child, Trauma Life, Forgiveness, Joy, Common Sense, Hope, Believe, Peace & Calming, Peace & Calming II, Calm CBD Roll-On, Seedlings Calm, Valor, and SARA can form the center of any emotional care regimen (See Chapter 16, . . . EMOTIONAL SUPPORT . . .).

Cleansing and Removing Toxins

Industrial pollutants such as benzene and lead, along with lifestyle toxins such as cigarette smoke, chemicals, heterocyclic amines from overcooked meat, and many others contribute to a vast majority of cancers. Even daily radiation from computers, cell phones, and a vast number of electrical appliances may contribute to a toxic overload within the body.

Today's fast-food industry is a major culprit in selling so much of the nutritionally deficient food that we eat. Processed food is fast and convenient, but is eating it worth the threat to our health? A popular children's oat cereal was found in 2018 to have toxic amounts of the RoundUp® chemical glyphosate by the Environmental Working Group.

Cosmetics, hair sprays, dyes, soaps, paints, and household cleaners add to an endless list of pollutants in our environment and toxicity to which we are subjected.

To help lower the risk of cancer, it is important to reduce the exposure to these chemicals and change our diet and the products that we use in our environment. The chemicals should be avoided at all cost, as they can damage DNA, decrease immunity, promote oncogenes (genes that can turn normal cells into cancer cells), and accelerate cancer development.

Cleansing and Chelation

The foundation of any cancer program should begin with a period of cleansing. Cleansing and chelation can help remove some of the toxin- and petrochemical-buildup that may have triggered the cancer initially.

Fasting can be one of the most powerful anticancer tools available, particularly in the early stages. Anyone who is in advanced stages of cancer must cleanse very slowly to see how the body responds. Going without food and drinking only juices immediately could be detrimental to a sick body. Common sense needs to be used in all situations.

Essential oils that improve liver function and promote glutathione can form the center of any detoxification program. Lemon and Orange oils, in studies at Johns Hopkins University, have shown to substantially increase glutathione levels in the liver and colon, which have beneficial effects in detoxification.

Chelation can be particularly important in removing carcinogenic metals from the body. Studies in Germany have shown that transition metals such as iron, mercury, lead, zinc, nickel, and cadmium can accumulate to high levels in tumors, particularly in breast cancer tissue. A series of chelations to eliminate these metals can produce tremendous benefits in the earliest stage of cancer.[19]

Rice bran is a good chelator of metals and contains anticancer phytonutrients such as gamma oryzanol and other compounds. It is also rich in immune-stimulating arabinoxylans that increase cancer cell death.[20]

The Ningxia wolfberry is rich in polysaccharides that similarly amplify immunity. A number of clinical research trials have shown that wolfberry compounds can dramatically improve cancer remission, particularly when combined with immune-stimulating therapies.[21]

Cleansing Products Suitable for Most Cancers

Many products support the body in its cleansing process. You will not be able to take all of the cleansing products, so decide which ones you want to take and how much you want to take of each product. Write down your program so you can follow it consistently. Start slowly so your body can adjust and begin to cleanse.

Cleansing: Essentialzyme, Detoxzyme, Essentialzymes-4, JuvaPower, JuvaTone, ComforTone, KidScents TummyGize, DiGize, DiGize Vitality, GLF, GLF Vitality, JuvaCleanse, JuvaCleanse Vitality, JuvaFlex, JuvaFlex Vitality, NingXia Red

Emotional Support: Release, Freedom, Reconnect, Sacred Frankincense, Frankincense, Frankincense Vitality, Lavender, Lavender Vitality, Palo Santo, Rose, Ylang Ylang, Acceptance, Believe, Brain Power, Common Sense, Dream Catcher, Gathering, Envision, Forgiveness, Gratitude, Harmony, Hope, Joy, Live with Passion, Live Your Passion, Light the Fire, Journey On, Motivation, Present Time, Peace & Calming, Peace & Calming II, Calm CBD Roll-On, Seedlings Calm, RutaVaLa, RutaVaLa Roll-On, The Gift, Transformation, Valor, White Angelica

Enzymes Ramping Regimen

Essentialzyme was formulated in 1984 with this regimen for someone suffering from a degenerative disease.

Phase 1: Take 3 caplets 3 times daily. Increase by 1 caplet every day until you become nauseated and then discontinue Essentialzyme for 24 to 36 hours.

Phase 2: Take 4 caplets 3 times daily. Increase daily by 1 caplet until you become nauseated. Rest (discontinue) again for 24-36 hours.

Phase 4: Take 5 caplets 3 times daily. Increase daily by 1 caplet until you become nauseated. Rest for 24-36 hours.

Phase 4: Start again with the amount you were taking before the nausea occurred the third time. For example: If you were taking 18 caplets, you would have been taking 6 caplets 3 times daily when you became nauseated.

Therefore, start Phase 4 again with 6 caplets 3 times daily and continue with this amount for 6 weeks.

Phase 5: In the 7th week, start the enzyme-ramping program all over again. This means to begin phase 1 again and increase the amount by 1 each day until nausea or vomiting starts again. Repeat and continue for 6 weeks as previously described.

If your doctor determines that you are in remission, you can maintain with 5-10 tablets daily for one year, 6 days a week.

Maintenance: Take 5-10 Essentialzyme caplets 3 times daily.

Caution: This is a very rigorous program, so you should consult with your doctor or health care professional before starting and have that person monitor your progress during the program.

Why Fasting Works

New research has uncovered that numerous insulin receptors make cancer cells different from normal cells. Cancer cells have over 10 times the number of receptors for insulin as a normal cell. Excess insulin can stimulate cancer cells disproportionately compared to well-differentiated cells. Similarly, because cancer cells are fast-growing, they require far more glucose (blood sugar) than normal cells.

The most effective way of lowering both insulin and blood glucose levels is with a fast. Bernard Jensen, ND, used a 180-day fast, made initially of only barley grass juice, to fight and eliminate metastatic prostate cancer. Even a partial fast in which refined carbohydrates are eliminated and caloric intake is reduced to 500-1,000 calories can be potentially very therapeutic.

Determining Hormone Sensitivity

Women dealing with breast, ovarian, uterine, and cervical cancer in most cases can be estrogen receptor sensitive, yet doctors will continue to give and recommend HRT (hormone replacement therapy) made from xenoestrogens that come from petrochemicals, compounds that are known to promote and cause cancer, before determining if a patient has cancer in the early stages of development.

Premarin® is an estrogen-therapy drug created from the urine of pregnant horses. Besides animal cruelty issues, this hormone treatment is not natural to the human body and increases the risks for stroke, heart attack, and breast cancer.

We must understand the mechanism of how natural hormones are synthesized in the body. First, cholesterol cascades down to pregnenolone, to progestogens, and then to androgens that divide and go to the ovaries and testes.

In the ovaries, the androgen called androstenedione crosses the basal membrane, where it is converted to the estradiol sex hormones such as estradiol, estrone, and estriol. The ovaries produce primarily estradiol. Most free-circulating estrone stems from a conversion of estradiol in the liver, even though the ovaries produce small amounts of estrone.

The liver plays a major role as the chemistry laboratory of the body. Because the liver is the body's largest fat-storing organ, it will hold petrochemicals known as xenoestrogens that are cancer-causing agents. Xenoestrogens disrupt the conversion of estradiol and cause a division of the estrone.

This division will be either negative or positive. If estradiol converts to 16-alpha-hydroxyestrone, a cancer-causing agent, this estrone will then bind to the estrogen receptors in female and male reproductive organs. If estradiol converts to 2-hydroxyestrone, a cancer-preventing steroid hormone, it will bind or stick to the receptors, protecting them from the harmful estrone. This has caused a lot of controversy among the natural health and allopathic practitioners for years.

Natural hormones produced in the body are referred to as steroid hormones. Synthetic hormones are called nonsteroidal hormones. Most people do not understand that plant hormones are neither steroid nor nonsteroidal hormones. They are natural phytohormones that encourage the production of 2-hydroxyestrone, the cancer preventive hormone that does not bind or stick to the receptor sites contrary to the nonsteroidal hormones that cause inflammation and cysts on the ovaries.

There is no evidence that phytohormones will stimulate estrogen-sensitive cancer. Phytohormones are the same as the hormone-supporting chemical compounds found in the essential oils of Fennel, Clary Sage, Melissa, Lemongrass, Sage, etc.

There is also no reason to be concerned about food unless it is a GMO food like soy, wheat, or corn. Herbs like black co-hosh do not stimulate estrogen-sensitive cancer. Quite simply they are neither steroidal- nor nonsteroidal-stimulating hormones.

It is also important to understand that metabolic enzymes are required to help facilitate steroid hormone conversion. When the body and liver are toxic, this becomes a serious problem, creating a metabolic enzyme deficiency. In the absence of metabolic enzymes and a toxic liver, estradiol is converted to 16-alpha-hydroxyestrone, the cancer-causing hormone.

The hormones that naturally occur in milk require metabolic hormones to ensure they are converted to 2-hydroxyestrone. When the milk goes through the pasteurization process, it kills the enzymes necessary for the 2-hydroxyestrone conversion and converts to the cancer-causing 16-alpha-hydroxyestrone.

Essentialzyme is the metabolic enzyme, which makes it so important for daily prevention and good health.

Pasteurized milk is also a concern because milk contains steroid hormones fed to cows. When a milk product is pasteurized and homogenized, whether it is milk, cheese, butter, cottage cheese, or any other product containing steroid hormones, the pasteurization destroys the natural enzymes, thus preventing the production of 2-hydroxyestrone, the cancer-preventing steroid, and instead converts it to 16-alpha-hydroxyestrone, the cancer-causing hormone.

This is where the controversy begins and the misunderstanding of estrogen-sensitive cancers becomes a problem. It is easy to see how processed and non-processed foods affect the outcome of our health.

This applies not only to women but also to men as well. Men also have estrogen and will respond the same way to both phytoestrogens and mycoestrogens (estrogens produced by fungi found in stored grain) that stimulate the production of 16-alpha-hydroxyestrone. If there were more focus on eating unprocessed foods; cleansing the liver of toxins, petrochemicals, and undigested pollutants; and improving and building a reserve of metabolic enzymes, there would be much less cancer.

Cancer and Antioxidants

It is recommended to seek the advice of a health care professional before embarking on any antioxidant program. Some studies have reported that certain antioxidants can reduce the effectiveness of some types of chemotherapy, such as cisplatin.

A large number of other studies have found the opposite, showing that antioxidants can improve patient remissions and prognosis. In the case of radiation treatments, a number of well-controlled studies have similarly found that antioxidants can improve patient outcomes dramatically and counter the injury and immune suppression caused by these therapies.

In fact, a 2010 human study by A. Pace and colleagues at the Regina Elena National Cancer Institute in Rome, Italy, found that vitamin E had a neuroprotective effect against the serious, adverse effects of cisplatin.[22]

Similar to DNA-protective essential oils, antioxidants produce their best results as cancer preventives and in the earliest stages of cancer. As cancer progresses, the likelihood of meaningful remissions using only antioxidants declines rapidly.

Research conducted at Brigham Young University in Provo, Utah, and at the UNLV Cancer Research Institute identified some of the most inhibitory essential oils against a variety of cancer cell lines. The oils were also tested for their lack of toxicity to normal cells.

Inflammation and Cancer

The link between cancer and inflammation has become stronger in recent years. It is well known that the salicylates in aspirin have high anti-inflammatory effects and reduce the risk of colon cancer dramatically.

The natural salicylates found in the essential oil of wintergreen are very close in structure to the acetyl salicylic acid found in aspirin. According to Erica Leibert of Harvard University, wintergreen oil is 40 percent stronger than an aspirin equivalent with very similar anti-inflammatory properties. However, it should be ingested only in very small numbers of drops.

Lemongrass oil is a well-known anti-inflammatory (Han X, 2017; Ganjewala D, 2010) that can be safely ingested. But lemongrass is not just an anti-inflammatory. Lemongrass essential oil has shown efficacy against a number of different cancers, particularly lung cancer (Gaonkar R, 2018; Marovka T, 2018; Jiang J, 2017; Sharma PR, 2009).

Clove has been researched as a potential chemopreventive agent for lung cancer because of its powerful anti-inflammatory effects.23 The biochemical alpha-humulene in the oil, also found in Idaho Grand Fir and Copaiba, has been shown to have significant cancer prevention properties through its anti-inflammatory action.24

Frankincense and conifer oils like Idaho Grand Fir containing l-limonene have come to the forefront of attention in cancer research in various cancer-treatment study programs at Oklahoma State University, Wake Forest University, and Virginia-Maryland Regional College of Veterinary Medicine.

The l-limonene found in Frankincense, Idaho Blue Spruce, and Idaho Grand Fir shows a remarkable ability to suppress tumor growth, particularly in melanoma. Boswellic acids found in frankincense gum resin have also been shown to have powerful, anti-inflammatory effects. Myrrh gum has been studied for its ability to combat various cancers, including breast cancer.

Anti-inflammatory Essential Oils Suitable for Most Cancers: Sacred Frankincense, Frankincense, Frankincense Vitality, Clove, Clove Vitality, Idaho Grand Fir, Palo Santo, Ledum, Myrrh, Lemongrass, Lemongrass Vitality, Wintergreen (topically only)

Immunity and Cancer

Enhancing immune function is a vital component of both traditional and complementary approaches to cancer. Typically, chemotherapy and radiation can drastically break down populations of T-cells and NK (natural killer) cells that are responsible for fighting tumor growth. Certain natural compounds can restore levels of these critical immune components.

Singles: Sacred Frankincense, Frankincense, Frankincense Vitality, Idaho Blue Spruce, Idaho Grand Fir, Sacred Sandalwood, Royal Hawaiian Sandalwood, Palo Santo, Hyssop, Thyme, Thyme Vitality, Clove, Clove Vitality, Tea Tree, Blue Cypress

Blends: Citrus Fresh, Citrus Fresh Vitality, Thieves, Thieves Vitality, Exodus II, Melrose, GLF, GLF Vitality, ImmuPower, 3 Wise Men, DiGize, DiGize Vitality, KidScents TummyGize

Immune-Enhancing Supplements Suitable for Most Cancers: ImmuPro, Super Vitamin C, Super Vitamin C Chewable, Master Formula, Essentialzyme, Detoxzyme, Essentialzymes-4, MultiGreens, NingXia Red

Breast Cancer Recommendations

Singles: Sacred Frankincense, Frankincense, Frankincense Vitality, Lemongrass, Lemongrass Vitality, Royal Hawaiian Sandalwood, Sacred Sandalwood, Myrtle, Tsuga, Sage, Sage Vitality

Nutritionals: NingXia Red, Super Vitamin C, Essentialzyme, Essenstialzymes-4, AlkaLime

Cervical Cancer Recommendations

Singles: Patchouli, Royal Hawaiian Sandalwood, Sacred Sandalwood, Lemongrass, Lemongrass Vitality, Valerian, Sacred Frankincense, Frankincense, Frankincense Vitality, Tsuga, Hyssop, Nutmeg, Nutmeg Vitality, Tarragon, Tarragon Vitality, Sage, Sage Vitality

Nutritionals: NingXia Red, Super Vitamin C, Super Vitamin C Chewable, Essentialzyme, Essentialzymes-4, AlkaLime

Leukemia Recommendations

Singles: Clove, Clove Vitality, Hyssop, Idaho Blue Spruce, Sacred Frankincense, Frankincense, Frankincense Vitality, Palo Santo

Nutritionals: NingXia Red, Super Vitamin C, Super Vitamin C Chewable, Essentialzyme, Essentialzymes-4, AlkaLime

Lung Cancer Recommendations

Singles: Sacred Frankincense, Frankincense, Frankincense Vitality, Lemongrass, Lemongrass Vitality, Idaho Blue Spruce, Palo Santo, Royal Hawaiian Sandalwood, Sacred Sandalwood, Clove, Clove Vitality, Thyme, Thyme Vitality, Hyssop

Nutritionals: NingXia Red, Super Vitamin C, Super Vitamin C Chewable, Essentialzyme, Essentialzymes-4, AlkaLime

Prostate Cancer
Recommendations
Singles: Sacred Frankincense, Frankincense, Frankincense Vitality, Sage, Sage Vitality, Thyme, Thyme Vitality, Sacred Sandalwood, Royal Hawaiian Sandalwood, Myrtle, Dill, Dill Vitality, Idaho Blue Spruce

Nutritionals: Prostate Health, NingXia Red, Super Vitamin C, Super Vitamin C Chewable, Essentialzyme, Essentialzymes-4, AlkaLime

Skin Cancer (Melanoma)
Recommendations
Singles: Sacred Frankincense, Frankincense, Frankincense Vitality, Lemongrass, Lemongrass Vitality, Thyme, Thyme Vitality, Sacred Sandalwood, Royal Hawaiian Sandalwood, Grapefruit, Grapefruit Vitality, Hyssop, Tarragon, Tarragon Vitality

Nutritionals: NingXia Red, Super Vitamin C, Super Vitamin C Chewable, Essentialzyme, Essentialzymes-4, AlkaLime

Tumors
Recommendations
Singles: Sacred Frankincense, Frankincense, Frankincense Vitality, Sage, Sage Vitality, Sacred Sandalwood, Royal Hawaiian Sandalwood, Grapefruit, Grapefruit Vitality, Hyssop, Myrtle, Idaho Blue Spruce, Cardamom, Cardamom Vitality, Bergamot, Bergamot Vitality, Blue Cypress

Nutritionals: NingXia Red, Super Vitamin C, Super Vitamin C Chewable, Essentialzyme, Essentialzymes-4, AlkaLime

Uterine Cancer
Recommendations
Singles: Sacred Frankincense, Frankincense, Frankincense Vitality, Sage, Sage Vitality, Thyme, Thyme Vitality, Sacred Sandalwood, Royal Hawaiian Sandalwood, Myrtle, Dill, Dill Vitality, Idaho Blue Spruce

Nutritionals: NingXia Red, Super Vitamin C, Super Vitamin C Chewable, Essentialzyme, Essentialzymes-4, AlkaLime

CANKER SORES
(See also MOUTH SORES)

These are technically known as aphthous ulcers, are not regarded as an infectious disease, and are not caused by the herpes virus.

Canker sores tend to occur because of stress, illness, weakened immune system, or injury caused by such things as hot food, rough brushing of teeth, or dentures. They appear under the tongue more commonly than cold sores.

Recommendations
Singles: Melissa, Clove, Clove Vitality, Lavender, Lavender Vitality, Sacred Sandalwood, Royal Hawaiian Sandalwood, Cypress, Thyme, Thyme Vitality

Blends: Thieves, Thieves Vitality, Melrose

Nutritionals: Inner Defense, ImmuPro, AlkaLime

Oral Care: Thieves Spray, Thieves Fresh Essence Mouthwash

Application and Usage
Dietary and Oral: Refer to Application Guidelines.

- Gargle with Thieves mouthwash 2-4 times daily.
- Take maple syrup 2-4 times daily.

Topical: Refer to Application Guidelines.

- Gently apply 1 drop of oil neat with fingertip to canker sore 4-8 times daily.

CARDIOVASCULAR CONDITIONS AND PROBLEMS

Cardiovascular conditions are those that affect the heart and other circulatory organs.

Anemia

Anemia is a condition caused from insufficient red blood cells. There can be many different causes of anemia, which would suggest that you should see your health care professional for proper diagnosis. Nutritional deficiencies of iron or vitamin B12 can contribute to this disorder as well as to improper liver function. A liver cleanse and nutritional support will certainly help in rebuilding red blood cell counts.

Recommendations
Singles: German Chamomile, German Chamomile Vitality, Thyme, Thyme Vitality, Sacred Frankincense, Frankincense, Frankincense Vitality,

Helichrysum, Lemon, Lemon Vitality, Lime, Lime Vitality, Mountain Savory, Mountain Savory Vitality, Cistus, Rosemary, Rosemary Vitality

Blends: JuvaCleanse, JuvaCleanse Vitality, DiGize, DiGize Vitality, EndoFlex, EndoFlex Vitality, JuvaFlex, JuvaFlex Vitality

Nutritionals: JuvaPower, JuvaTone, MultiGreens, Super Vitamin B, Rehemogen, NingXia Red, Master Formula, Mineral Essence

Application and Usage

Aromatic: Refer to Application Guidelines.

Dietary and Oral: Refer to Application Guidelines.

- Take 2 capsules 2 times daily filled with half Helichrysum and half Cistus.

- Take 2-3 drops of desired Vitality oil in a spoonful of syrup or small amount of milk, juice, or water.

Topical: Refer to Application Guidelines.

Aneurysm

Aneurysms are weak spots on the blood vessel walls that balloon out and may eventually rupture. In cases of brain aneurysms, a bursting blood vessel can cause a stroke, which can result in death or paralysis. (The fatality rate is over 50 percent in the U.S.) Symptoms of a brain aneurysm include a painful headache, nausea, vomiting, or confusion.

Note: Seek medical care immediately if you suspect you have an aneurysm.

Some essential oils and nutritional supplements support the cardiovascular system and help with blood regulation. Cypress strengthens capillary and vascular walls. Helichrysum helps dissolve blood clots.

Recommendations
Singles: Cistus, Helichrysum, Cypress, Jade Lemon, Jade Lemon Vitality, Lemon, Lemon Vitality

Blends: Aroma Life, JuvaCleanse, JuvaCleanse Vitality, Purification

Nutritionals: CardioGize, NingXia Red, Essentialzyme, Essentialzymes-4, Life 9, KidScents MightyPro, Pure Protein Complete, Protein Power Bites, Ningxia Wolfberries (Organic, Dried), Digest & Cleanse, Detoxzyme, MindWise (also supports cardiovascular health), Olive Essentials

Aneurysm Blend
- 5 drops Cistus
- 1 drop Helichrysum
- 1 drop Cypress

Aromatic: Refer to Application Guidelines.

Dietary and Oral: Refer to Application Guidelines.

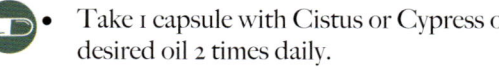
- Take 1 capsule with Cistus or Cypress or other desired oil 2 times daily.

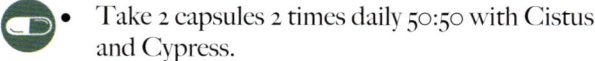
- Take 2 capsules 2 times daily 50:50 with Cistus and Cypress.

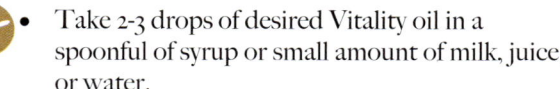
- Take 2-3 drops of desired Vitality oil in a spoonful of syrup or small amount of milk, juice, or water.

Topical: Refer to Application Guidelines.

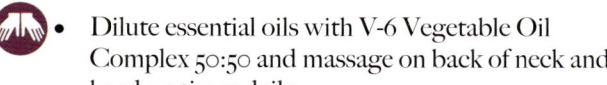
- Dilute essential oils with V-6 Vegetable Oil Complex 50:50 and massage on back of neck and head 3-5 times daily.

Angina

Angina is a severe and crushing chest pain caused by an inadequate supply of oxygen to the heart muscle. It is a symptom of an underlying heart condition. Contact a health care professional for diagnosis.

Recommendations
Singles: Clove, Clove Vitality, Marjoram, Marjoram Vitality, Helichrysum, Goldenrod, Orange, Orange Vitality, Jade Lemon, Jade Lemon Vitality, Lemon, Lemon Vitality, Lavender, Lavender Vitality, Vanilla, Wintergreen

Blends: Aroma Life, Peace & Calming, Peace & Calming II, Stress Away, Stress Away Roll-On, Valor, Valor Roll-On, RutaVaLa, RutaVaLa Roll-On, Longevity, Longevity Vitality, Chivalry

Nutritionals: CardioGize, NingXia Red, Ningxia Wolfberries (Organic, Dried), OmegaGize3, Mega Vitamin Cal, Longevity Softgels, Essentialzyme, Essentialzymes-4, Detoxzyme, MindWise (also supports cardiovascular health), KidScents Unwind, Olive Essentials

Application and Usage

Aromatic: Refer to Application Guidelines.

Dietary and Oral: Refer to Application Guidelines.

- Take 1-2 capsules with desired Vitality oil 2 times daily.

• Take 2-3 drops of desired Vitality oil in a spoonful of syrup or small amount of milk, juice, or water.

Topical: Refer to Application Guidelines.

 • Massage 1-3 drops neat over the heart area 1-3 times daily.

 • Apply on left side of chest, left shoulder, and back of neck.

• Massage 1 drop each of 2 or 3 of the recommended oils on the heart Vita Flex points on foot, hand, and arm, as needed.

Arteriosclerosis (Hardening of the Arteries)

This condition is defined as any one of a group of diseases that causes a thickening and a loss of elasticity of arterial walls. It can be caused by inflammation and is frequently an underlying cause of a heart attack or stroke.

Recommendations

Singles: Clove, Clove Vitality, Helichrysum, Geranium, Lemongrass, Lemongrass Vitality, Frankincense, Frankincense Vitality, Sacred Frankincense, Lavender, Lavender Vitality, German Chamomile, German Chamomile Vitality, Dorado Azul

Blends: Longevity, Longevity Vitality, Aroma Life

Nutritionals: CardioGize, Longevity Softgels, OmegaGize3, Mega Vitamin Cal, Ningxia Wolfberries (Organic, Dried), NingXia Red, Master Formula, MindWise (also supports cardiovascular health), Olive Essentials

Application and Usage

Aromatic: Refer to Application Guidelines.

Dietary and Oral: Refer to Application Guidelines.

 • Take 1 capsule of desired Vitality oil 2 times daily.

• Take 2-3 drops of desired Vitality oil in a spoonful of syrup or small amount of milk, juice, or water.

Topical: Refer to Application Guidelines.

 • Massage 1-3 drops neat over the heart area 2-3 times weekly.

• Apply on left side of chest, left shoulder, and back of neck.

 • Massage 1 drop each of 2 or 3 of the recommended oils on the heart Vita Flex points on foot, hand, and arm, as needed.

Bleeding (Hemorrhaging)

Some essential oils, when topically applied or used on pressure bandages, are excellent for slowing bleeding and initiating healing.

Recommendations

Singles: Helichrysum, Geranium, Cistus, Cypress, Lavender, Lavender Vitality, Myrrh

Blends: Purification, Trauma Life, Deep Relief Roll-On

Nutritionals: JuvaPower, Master Formula

Application and Usage

Topical: Refer to Application Guidelines.

 • Apply 1-2 drops neat (undiluted) on the location of small wounds.

 • You may also apply 2-3 drops on the Vita Flex points of the feet.

 • Place a cold compress diluted with 1-2 drops of Helichrysum, Myrrh, etc.

Blood Circulation, Poor

Essential oils, when used regularly, can improve circulation by as much as 20 percent.

Recommendations

Singles: Helichrysum, Cypress, Clove, Clove Vitality, Idaho Grand Fir, Cistus, Idaho Blue Spruce

Blends: Aroma Life, EndoFlex, EndoFlex Vitality, En-R-Gee, Longevity, Longevity Vitality, Valor, Valor Roll-On

Nutritionals: CardioGize, NingXia Red, Longevity Softgels, Ningxia Wolfberries (Organic, Dried), Mineral Essence, MindWise (also supports cardiovascular health), Olive Essentials

Application and Usage

Dietary and Oral: Refer to Application Guidelines.

 • Take 1 capsule with Helichrysum, Cypress, or other desired oil 2 times daily.

 • Take 2-3 drops of desired Vitality oil in a spoonful of syrup or small amount of milk, juice, or water.

Topical: Refer to Application Guidelines.

 • Apply neat 2-3 drops on Vita Flex points of feet or on inside of wrists 2-3 times daily.

Blood Clots (Embolism, Hematoma, Thrombus)

A blood clot, or hematoma, is a tumor-like mass of coagulated blood, caused by a break in the blood vessel or capillary wall.

Essential oils such as Helichrysum, Geranium, and Cistus are excellent for balancing blood viscosity and dissolving clots. Clove oil and citrus rind oils, such as Lemon and Grapefruit, exert a blood-thinning effect that can help speed the dissolution of the clot.

These oils are also some of the most powerful antioxidants known and can slow the formation of oxidized cholesterol in cells, which contributes to atherosclerosis. Helichrysum is effective in preventing blood clot formation and promoting the dissolution of clots.

As people age, the viscosity or thickness of the blood increases and so does the tendency of the blood to clot excessively.

If blood clots, known as embolisms, occur in the brain, they can cause strokes; if they obstruct a coronary artery, they can cause ischemic heart attacks; if in the lungs, they can cause cardiac arrest.

People with diabetes or high blood pressure are far more likely to die from blood clots.

Foods rich in vitamin E, vitamin A, and omega-3 fats are vital for proper blood viscosity.

Recommendations

Singles: Helichrysum, Cistus, Clove, Clove Vitality, Geranium, Jade Lemon, Jade Lemon Vitality, Lemon, Lemon Vitality, Grapefruit, Grapefruit Vitality, Nutmeg, Nutmeg Vitality, Cypress, Wintergreen

Blends: Aroma Life, PanAway, Relieve It, Longevity, Longevity Vitality, Thieves, Thieves Vitality

Nutritionals: CardioGize, OmegaGize3, Super Vitamin C, Super Vitamin C Chewable, Mineral Essence, Longevity Softgels, Inner Defense, NingXia Red, MindWise (also supports cardiovascular health), Olive Essentials

Oral Care: Thieves toothpastes and mouthwash contain Clove, which has natural blood-thinning properties.

Application and Usage

Aromatic: Refer to Application Guidelines.

Dietary and Oral: Refer to Application Guidelines.

 • Take 1 capsule of desired Vitality oil 2 times daily.

 • Take 2 capsules diluted 50:50 with Helichrysum and Cistus 2 times daily between meals.

 • Take 2-3 drops of desired Vitality oil in a spoonful of syrup or small amount of milk, juice, or water.

Topical: Refer to Application Guidelines.

 • Massage equal parts Lemon, Lavender, and Helichrysum on location with or without hot packs.

 • Massage equal parts Cistus, Lavender, and Helichrysum on location.

• Place a warm compress with 1-2 drops of chosen oil on the back for 15 minutes 2 times daily.

Blood Detoxification

When there are fewer toxins in the blood, it is easier for the blood to function properly and to continually carry the needed nutrients throughout the body and the digested waste and toxins out of the body, which is the key for staying healthy, being able to fight disease, and expelling chemicals and other pollutants.

Recommendations

Singles: Helichrysum, Goldenrod, Geranium, German Chamomile, German Chamomile Vitality, Clove, Clove Vitality, Idaho Grand Fir, Mountain Savory, Mountain Savory Vitality, Rosemary, Rosemary Vitality

Blends: GLF, GLF Vitality, JuvaCleanse, JuvaCleanse Vitality, DiGize, DiGize Vitality

Nutritionals: MultiGreens, Rehemogen, ICP, JuvaPower, JuvaTone, Sulfurzyme, Balance Complete, Slique Tea

MSM (found in Sulfurzyme) purifies the body and blood.

Application and Usage

Dietary and Oral: Refer to Application Guidelines.

• Look up the specific action of these products and decide what best targets your desired results.

 • Take 1 capsule of GLF Vitality or JuvaCleanse Vitality, plus Rosemary Vitality or other desired oil 2 times daily.

 • Take 2-3 drops of desired Vitality oil in a spoonful of syrup or small amount of milk, juice, or water.

Topical: Refer to Application Guidelines.

- Massage 2-3 drops neat (undiluted) on the Vita Flex points of the feet and on the inside of the wrists 2-3 times daily.

Blood Platelets (Low)

Blood platelets (thrombocytes) are necessary for fighting infections and for blood clotting. To avoid a drastic drop in the platelet level, consume leafy vegetables, fruits like bananas and oranges, and dairy products.

Recommendations

Singles: Jade Lemon, Jade Lemon Vitality, Lemon, Lemon Vitality, Thyme, Thyme Vitality, Tea Tree, Davana, Geranium, Cypress

Blends: Aroma Life

Nutritionals: Rehemogen, JuvaTone, JuvaPower

To enhance the effects of Rehemogen, use it with JuvaTone or JuvaPower.

Blood Pressure, High (Hypertension)

One way to help normalize blood pressure is to cleanse the liver and colon for better circulation. Cleansing the colon will help rid the body of wastes and toxins that could be clogging the normal process of digestion. Cleansing and digestion are critical to normal body function.

Recommendations

Singles: Helichrysum, Rosemary, Rosemary Vitality, Clove, Clove Vitality, Lavender, Lavender Vitality, Marjoram, Marjoram Vitality, Ylang Ylang, Cypress, Cinnamon Bark, Cinnamon Bark Vitality, Cardamom, Cardamom Vitality

Blends: Aroma Life, Peace & Calming, Peace & Calming II, AromaEase, Calm CBD Roll-On, Seedlings Calm, Citrus Fresh, Citrus Fresh Vitality, Humility

Nutritionals: Essentialzyme, Detoxzyme, OmegaGize3, ImmuPro, KidScents Unwind, Super Vitamin B, Mineral Essence, Balance Complete, Essentialzymes-4, Mega Vitamin Cal, Ningxia Wolfberries (Organic, Dried), Slique Essence, Slique Tea, MindWise

Application and Usage

Refer to Application Guidelines.

Dietary and Oral: Refer to Application Guidelines.

- Take 1 capsule of desired Vitality oil 2 times daily.

- Take 2-3 drops of desired Vitality oil in a spoonful of syrup or small amount of milk, juice, or water.

Topical: Refer to Application Guidelines.

- Apply 1-3 drops oil diluted 20:80 for a full body massage daily.

- Rub 1-2 drops of oil on the temples and back of neck several times daily.

- Place a warm compress with 1-2 drops of chosen oil on the back.

- For 3 minutes, massage 1-2 drops each of Aroma Life and Ylang Ylang on the heart Vita Flex point and over the heart and carotid arteries along the neck.

- Notice how the blood pressure will begin to drop within 5-20 minutes. Monitor the pressure and reapply as desired.

- Increase the intake of magnesium, which acts as a smooth-muscle relaxant and as a natural calcium channel blocker for the heart, lowering blood pressure and dilating the heart blood vessels.

- Take 1 teaspoon of Mega Vitamin Cal before going to bed.

- Take 1-2 droppers of Mineral Essence 2 times daily.

- Take 1 Super Vitamin B daily with your meal. Vitamin B3 (niacin) 20 mg daily is an excellent vasodilator found in Super Vitamin B.

Bruising (See also MUSCLE PROBLEMS, Bruised Muscles)

Some people bruise easily because the capillary walls are weak and break easily, particularly in the skin. Those who bruise easily may be deficient in vitamin C.

Essential oils can help speed the healing of bruises and reduce the risk of blood clot formation. Oils like Cypress help to strengthen capillary walls, while oils like Helichrysum help speed the reabsorption of the blood that has collected in the tissue.

Recommendations

Singles: Helichrysum, Clove, Clove Vitality, Cistus, Geranium, Lavender, Lavender Vitality, Cypress, Roman Chamomile, Idaho Blue Spruce, Dorado Azul, Peppermint, Peppermint Vitality, Marjoram, Marjoram Vitality, Black Pepper, Black Pepper Vitality

Blends: Deep Relief Roll-On, PanAway, Relieve It, Cool Azul, CBD, KidScents Owie

Nutritionals: MultiGreens, JuvaTone, JuvaPower, Super Vitamin C, Super Vitamin C Chewable, NingXia Red, Slique Tea

Personal Care: Cool Azul Pain Relief Cream, Cool Azul Sports Gel, CBD Muscle Rub, Ortho Sport Massage Oil, Ortho Ease Massage Oil

Application and Usage

Dietary and Oral: Refer to Application Guidelines.

- Take 1 capsule of desired Vitality oil 2 times daily.

- Take 2-3 drops of desired Vitality oil in a spoonful of syrup or small amount of milk, juice, or water.

- Take 1-4 tablets of Super Vitamin C Chewable daily.

- Take 2-3 capsules of MultiGreens 3 times daily.

Topical: Refer to Application Guidelines.

- Apply 2-3 drops neat 2-3 times daily, depending on which oil you choose. Helichrysum is especially beneficial in healing bruises when applied neat on location.

- Dilute the oil you choose 50:50 with V-6 Vegetable Oil Complex and apply 1-3 drops on bruised area 2-5 times daily.

- Apply a cold compress on location 2-4 times daily or as needed.

Bruise Blend No. 1
- 5 drops Helichrysum
- 4 drops Lavender
- 3 drops Cypress
- 3 drops Cistus
- 3 drops Geranium

Bruise Blend No. 2
- 6 drops Clove
- 4 drops Black Pepper
- 3 drops Peppermint
- 2 drops Marjoram
- 2 drops Geranium
- 2 drops Cypress

Cholesterol, High

When fatty cholesterol deposits accumulate in the arteries, physical symptoms like chest pains and heart attacks may take place.

Recommendations

Singles: Lemongrass, Lemongrass Vitality, Helichrysum, Rosemary, Rosemary Vitality, Clove, Clove Vitality, German Chamomile, German Chamomile Vitality, Roman Chamomile

Blends: Aroma Life, Longevity, Longevity Vitality

Nutritionals: OmegaGize3, Essentialzyme, Detoxzyme, Mineral Essence, Mega Vitamin Cal, JuvaPower, MultiGreens, Super Vitamin C, Super Vitamin C Chewable, Super Vitamin Cal Plus, Longevity Softgels, Olive Essentials, ICP, Essentialzymes-4, Balance Complete, Slique Essence, Slique Tea, Slique Shake, Slique CitraSlim, Slique Bars

Application and Usage

Dietary and Oral: Refer to Application Guidelines.

- Take 1 capsule of desired Vitality oil 2 times daily.

- Take 2-3 drops of desired Vitality oil in a spoonful of syrup or small amount of milk, juice, or water.

Topical: Refer to Application Guidelines.

- Apply neat or dilute 50:50, if needed, 2-4 drops at pulse points, where arteries are close to the surface (wrists, inside elbows, base of throat), 2-3 times daily.

- Also rub 6-10 drops along spine 3 times daily.

- Have a body massage 2 times weekly.

Cholesterol-Reducing Blend
- 5 drops Roman Chamomile
- 5 drops Lemongrass or Lemongrass Vitality
- 4 drops Rosemary or Rosemary Vitality
- 3 drops Helichrysum

Supplementation regimens
1. Do a colon and liver cleanse using ICP, ComforTone, Essentialzyme, Digest & Cleanse, JuvaTone, JuvaPower, JuvaFlex Vitality, or JuvaCleanse Vitality. JuvaTone is particularly useful for reducing high cholesterol.
2. Mineral Essence and Mega Vitamin Cal are good sources of magnesium, which acts as a smooth muscle relaxant and supports the cardiovascular system. It acts as a natural calcium channel blocker for the heart, lowering blood pressure and dilating the heart blood vessels (Dr. T. Friedmann).

Congestive Heart Failure
(See also CARDIOVASCULAR CONDITIONS AND PROBLEMS, Heart Attack (Myocardial Infarction))

Congestive heart failure is the inability of the heart to supply enough blood to meet the demands of the body. The most common cause is coronary artery disease, a narrowing of the small blood vessels that supply oxygen and blood to the heart.

Symptoms include shortness of breath, loss of appetite, cough, fatigue, weakness, swollen abdomen, need to urinate at night, weight gain, and swollen feet and ankles.

Gary Young formulated CardioGize with the proper synergistic ratio of CoQ10 and selenium, while deodorized garlic and CoQ10 provide antioxidant properties, and vitamin K supports healthy vascular system function. Gary's formula also includes heart-healthy herbs astragalus, dong quai, motherwort, and hawthorn berry along with natural folic acid.

Knowing that coenzyme Q10 (CoQ10) is one of the most effective supplements for supporting the heart muscle, Young Living also created MindWise nutritional supplement. It contains bio-identical CoQ10, as well as other valuable nutrients that also support cardiovascular health.

Recommendations
Singles: Helichrysum, Goldenrod, Clove, Clove Vitality, Marjoram, Marjoram Vitality, Cypress

Blends: Aroma Life, Longevity, Longevity Vitality

Nutritionals: CardioGize, MindWise, Mega Vitamin Cal, Mineral Essence, Olive Essentials

Personal Care: Thieves Chest Rub

Application and Usage
Dietary and Oral: Refer to Application Guidelines.

- Take 1 capsule of desired Vitality oil 2 times daily.

- Take 2-3 drops of desired Vitality oil in a spoonful of syrup or small amount of milk, juice, or water.

Topical: Refer to Application Guidelines.

- Apply 1-2 drops neat to heart Vita Flex points on foot, hand, and arm, as described under the "Heart Vita Flex" section under the topic Cardiovascular Conditions and Problems.

- Apply neat or dilute 50:50, if needed 2-4 drops at pulse points, where arteries are close to the surface (wrists, inside elbows, base of throat), 2-3 times daily.

- Also rub 6-10 drops along spine 3 times daily.

- Have a body massage 2 times weekly.

Fibrillation
This is a specific form of heart arrhythmia that occurs when the upper heart chambers contract at a rate of over 300 pulsations per minute. The lower chambers cannot keep this pace, so efficiency is reduced, and not enough blood is pumped. Palpitations, a feeling that the heart is beating irregularly, more strongly, or more rapidly than normal, is the most common symptom.

Recommendations
Singles: Ylang Ylang, Valerian, Valerian Vitality, Goldenrod, Marjoram, Marjoram Vitality, Lavender, Lavender Vitality, Rosemary, Rosemary Vitality

Blends: Aroma Life, Peace & Calming, Peace & Calming II, Calm CBD Roll-On, Seedlings Calm

Nutritionals: CardioGize, OmegaGize3, Mineral Essence, Mega Vitamin Cal, Sulfurzyme, Ningxia Wolfberries (Organic, Dried), Master Formula, KidScents Unwind, MindWise (also supports cardiovascular health), Olive Essentials

Application and Usage

Aromatic: Refer to Application Guidelines.

Dietary and Oral: Refer to Application Guidelines.

- Take 1 capsule of desired Vitality oil 2 times daily.

- Take 2-3 drops of desired Vitality oil in a spoonful of syrup or small amount of milk, juice, or water.

Topical: Refer to Application Guidelines.

- Apply 1-3 drops neat 1-3 times daily of 2-3 of the recommended oils on the heart Vita Flex points on foot, hand, and arm as described in CARDIOVASCULAR CONDITIONS AND PROBLEMS, Heart Vita Flex.

- Apply neat or dilute 50:50, if needed, 2-4 drops at pulse points, where arteries are close to the surface (wrists, inside elbows, base of throat), 2-3 times daily.

- Also apply to left chest, left shoulder, and back of neck.

- Also rub 6-10 drops along spine 3 times daily.

- Have a body massage 2 times weekly.

Heart Attack (Myocardial Infarction)

A heart attack is a circulation blockage resulting in an interruption of blood supply to an area of the heart. Depending on the size of the area affected, it can be mild or severe.

Note: Seek medical care immediately if you suspect a heart attack.

Many people do not understand how someone who is relatively healthy, with low cholesterol levels, suffers a heart attack with no explanation. The explanation is actually inflammation, the fundamental cause of heart disease.

Inflammation of the heart is caused when blood vessels leading to the heart are clogged and damaged. This releases a protein into the bloodstream called C-reactive protein. The level of this protein indicates the degree of inflammation in the linings of the arteries. Certain essential oils have been documented to be excellent for reducing inflammation. German Chamomile contains azulene, a blue compound with highly anti-inflammatory properties. Peppermint is also highly anti-inflammatory. Other oils also have anti-inflammatory properties such as Helichrysum, Northern Lights Black Spruce, Wintergreen, and Valerian. Clove, Nutmeg, and Wintergreen are natural blood thinners and help reduce blood clotting.

Magnesium, the most important mineral for the heart, acts as a smooth muscle relaxant and supports the cardiovascular system. Magnesium will act as a natural calcium channel blocker for the heart, lowering blood pressure and dilating the heart blood vessels (according to Terry Friedmann, MD).

Recommendations

Singles: Wintergreen, Peppermint, Peppermint Vitality, Lemongrass, Lemongrass Vitality, Lavender, Lavender Vitality, German Chamomile, German Chamomile Vitality, Helichrysum, Frankincense, Frankincense Vitality, Sacred Frankin-cense, Northern Lights Black Spruce, Valerian, Dorado Azul, Clove, Clove Vitality, Nutmeg, Nutmeg Vitality, Copaiba, Copaiba Vitality, Palo Santo

Blends: Aroma Life, PanAway, Longevity, Longevity Vitality, Peace & Calming, Peace & Calming II, Relieve It, Valor, Valor Roll-On, Chivalry, CBD, Calm CBD Roll-On

Nutritionals: CardioGize, Mega Vitamin Cal, Longevity Softgels, Mineral Essence, OmegaGize3, Sulfurzyme, KidScents Unwind, Rehemogen, NingXia Red, MindWise (also supports cardiovascular health), Olive Essentials

Application and Usage

Aromatic: Refer to Application Guidelines.

Dietary and Oral: Refer to Application Guidelines.

- Take 1 capsule of desired Vitality oil 2 times daily.

- Take 2-3 drops of desired Vitality oil in a spoonful of syrup or small amount of milk, juice, or water.

Topical: Refer to Application Guidelines.

- If there is not enough time to remove shoes to get at the feet, apply the "pumping" action to left hand and arm points. Using 1-2 drops of Aroma Life on each point will increase effectiveness and may even revive an individual having a heart attack while waiting for medical attention.

- Apply 1-3 drops neat 1-3 times daily of 2-3 of the recommended oils on the heart Vita Flex points on foot, hand, and arm as described in CARDIOVASCULAR CONDITIONS AND PROBLEMS, Heart Vita Flex.

- Apply neat or dilute 50:50, if needed, 2-4 drops at pulse points, where arteries are close to the surface (wrists, inside elbows, base of throat), 2-3 times daily.

• Also apply to left chest, left shoulder, and back of neck.

 • Also rub 6-10 drops along spine 3 times daily.

• Have a body massage 2 times weekly.

Heart Disease

Heart disease is the leading cause of death in the United States. Keys to prevention include quitting smoking, controlling high blood pressure, lowering cholesterol, exercising, and maintaining a healthy weight.

Heart Vita Flex

The foot Vita Flex point related to the heart is on the sole of the left foot, below the ring toe (fourth toe) and approximately 1 inch below the base of the toe. Massaging this point is as effective as massaging the hand and arm points together (See Chapter 15, . . . APPLICATION, Vita Flex Foot Chart).

The hand Vita Flex point related to the heart is in the palm of the left hand, 1 inch below the ring finger joint at the life-line (See Chapter 15, . . . APPLICATION, Palm of Left Hand chart). A secondary heart point is on the inside of the lower end of the upper left arm, approximately 2 inches up the arm from the elbow, not on the muscle but up under the muscle. Have another person use his or her thumbs to firmly press these two points alternately for 3 minutes in a kind of pumping action. Work all three points when possible. Start with the foot first; then go to the hand and arm.

Heart Stimulant

The effects of heart stimulants include increased heart rate and blood pressure.

Recommendations

Singles: Rosemary, Rosemary Vitality, Peppermint, Peppermint Vitality, Ylang Ylang, Goldenrod, Mandarin, Thyme, Thyme Vitality, Frankincense, Frankincense Vitality, Sacred Frankincense, Marjoram, Marjoram Vitality

Blends: Aroma Life, Peace & Calming, Peace & Calming II, Release, Joy, Sacred Mountain, RutaVaLa, RutaVaLa Roll-On, Valor, Valor Roll-On, Stress Away, Stress Away Roll-On

Nutritionals: Master Formula, KidScents Unwind, Olive Essentials

Application and Usage

Aromatic: Refer to Application Guidelines.

Dietary and Oral: Refer to Application Guidelines.

 • Take 1 capsule of desired Vitality oil 2 times daily.

 • Take 2-3 drops of desired Vitality oil in a spoonful of syrup or small amount of milk, juice, or water.

Topical: Refer to Application Guidelines.

 • Apply 1-3 drops neat over the heart area 1-3 times daily.

 • Massage the Vita Flex points with one drop each of the 2-3 recommended oils on the heart Vita Flex points along the foot, hand, and arm as needed.

Phlebitis (Inflammation of Veins) (See also EDEMA)

Phlebitis refers to inflammation of a blood vein, usually due to a thrombus or blood clot. Symptoms include pain and tenderness along the course of the vein, discoloration of the skin, inflammatory swelling, joint pain, and acute edema below the inflamed site. Natural progesterone is an effective anti-inflammatory.

Recommendations

Singles: Juniper, Helichrysum, Cistus, Cypress, Wintergreen, Tangerine, Tangerine Vitality, Copaiba, Copaiba Vitality, German Chamomile, German Chamomile Vitality, Geranium, Lavender, Lavender Vitality, Clove, Clove Vitality, Nutmeg, Nutmeg Vitality, Jade Lemon, Jade Lemon Vitality, Lemon, Lemon Vitality, Lemongrass, Lemongrass Vitality, Juniper

Blends: Aroma Life, Longevity, Longevity Vitality

Nutritionals: Longevity Softgels

Personal Care: Progessence Plus, Prenolone Plus Body Cream

Application and Usage

Topical: Refer to Application Guidelines.

• The essential oil of Cypress may help strengthen vascular walls.

• You may apply single oils or **Blends** neat or diluted, depending on the oils that are used.

 • Massage 2-4 drops of oil neat on the bottoms of the feet just before bedtime.

 • Apply 2-4 drops neat on location 2-4 times daily.

 • Apply a cold compress on location 2-4 times daily.

Phlebitis Blend
- 10 drops Tangerine
- 7 drops Lemon
- 5 drops Cypress
- 4 drops Juniper

Plaque
Plaque is a cholesterol build up along the walls of the arteries, which causes the arteries to narrow. This is often when the physical symptoms of high cholesterol are noticed.

Recommendations
Singles: Rosemary, Helichrysum, Cistus, Dorado Azul

Blends: Aroma Life, DiGize, DiGize Vitality

Nutritionals: Detoxzyme, Digest & Cleanse, JuvaPower, Life 9, KidScents MightyPro

Application and Usage
Aromatic: Refer to Application Guidelines.

Dietary and Oral: Whether putting the Vitality oils in a capsule or drinking them in a liquid, please refer to Application Guidelines.

- 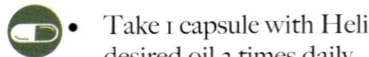 Take 1 capsule with Helichrysum or other desired oil 2 times daily.
- Take 1-2 capsules 50:50 with Helichrysum and Cistus 2 times daily.
- Take 2-3 drops of desired Vitality oil in a spoonful of syrup or small amount of milk, juice, or water.

Topical: Refer to Application Guidelines.

- Apply 1-3 drops, diluted 50:50, on temples, forehead, mastoids, back of neck, and at base of throat just above clavicle notch.
- 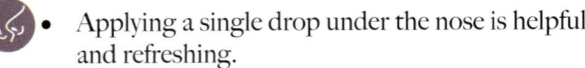 Applying a single drop under the nose is helpful and refreshing.
- 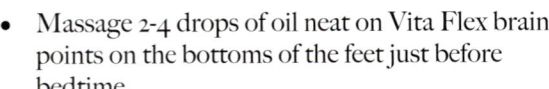 Massage 2-4 drops of oil neat on Vita Flex brain points on the bottoms of the feet just before bedtime.

Strokes (See STROKES)
Tachycardia
Tachycardia is another form of heart arrhythmia in which the heart rate suddenly increases to 160 beats per minute or faster. See your health care professional if you experience this condition. If fainting, difficulty breathing, or chest pain also occur, seek emergency care.

Recommendations
Singles: Ylang Ylang, Rosemary, Rosemary Vitality, Sacred Sandalwood, Royal Hawaiian Sandalwood, Wintergreen, Marjoram, Marjoram Vitality, German Chamomile, German Chamomile Vitality, Lavender, Lavender Vitality, Goldenrod

Blends: Aroma Life, Peace & Calming, Peace & Calming II, Calm CBD Roll-On, Seedlings Calm, Acceptance, Chivalry

Nutritionals: CardioGize, KidScents Unwind, Sulfurzyme, NingXia Red, MindWise (also supports cardiovascular health), Olive Essentials

Application and Usage
Aromatic: Refer to Application Guidelines.

Dietary and Oral: Refer to Application Guidelines.

- 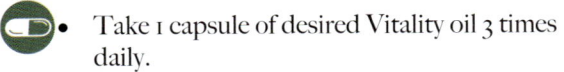 Take 1 capsule of desired Vitality oil 3 times daily.
- Take 2-3 drops of desired Vitality oil in a spoonful of syrup or small amount of milk, juice, or water.

Topical: Refer to Application Guidelines.

- 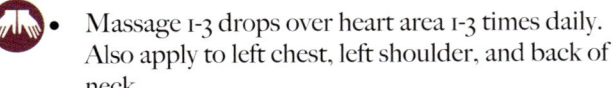 Massage 1-3 drops over heart area 1-3 times daily. Also apply to left chest, left shoulder, and back of neck.
- Massage 1 drop each of 2 or 3 of the recommended oils on heart Vita Flex points on foot, hand, and arm as needed.

Varicose Veins (Spider Veins)
The blue color of varicose veins is coagulated blood in the surrounding tissue from hemorrhaging of capillaries around the veins. This blood has to be dissolved and reabsorbed. Helichrysum helps dissolve the coagulated blood in the surrounding tissue.

Recommendations
Singles: Helichrysum, Cypress, Cistus, Elemi, Geranium, Clove, Clove Vitality, Peppermint, Peppermint Vitality, Jade Lemon, Jade Lemon Vitality, Lemon, Lemon Vitality, Lavender, Lavender Vitality, Tangerine, Tangerine Vitality

Blends: Aroma Life, Citrus Fresh, Aroma Siez, Chivalry

Nutritionals: MultiGreens, Super Vitamin B, Longevity Softgels, PowerGize, Essentialzyme, Essentialzymes-4, Life 9, KidScents MightyPro

Personal Care: Cool Azul Pain Relief Cream, Ortho Ease Massage Oil, Ortho Sport Massage Oil

Application and Usage

Topical: Refer to Application Guidelines.

Varicose Vein Blend
- 3-4 drops Geranium
- 1 drop Cistus
- 1 drop Cypress
- 1 drop Helichrysum

Apply 2-4 drops on location, massaging toward the heart, 3-6 times daily.

Nightly Varicose Vein Regimen (Legs)
1. Apply 1-3 drops of varicose vein blend, neat, on location. Rub very gently toward heart with smooth strokes along the vein, then up and over the vein until the oil is absorbed.
2. Apply 6 drops Tangerine and 6 drops Cypress to the area. Gently massage until absorbed.
3. Do the lymphatic pump procedure as described in Chapter 15.
4. Follow with a soft massage of the whole leg using 10-15 drops of Aroma Life diluted 50:50.
5. Wrap and elevate the leg. It is best to do this at night before retiring and to gradually elevate the foot off the bed, an inch more each night, until it is 4 inches higher than the head.
6. Wear support hose during the daytime. It may take up to a year to achieve desired results.

Vascular Cleansing, Need for
Keeping your blood clean will help you stay healthy.
1. Drink plenty of water.
2. Cleanse the blood by taking blood-cleansing herbs and essential oils.
3. Cleanse the kidneys.
4. Consider fasting for one to three days.
5. Take enzymes.

Recommendations
Singles: Helichrysum, Cistus, Clove, Clove Vitality, Idaho Blue Spruce, Sacred Frankincense, Frankincense, Frankincense Vitality, Dorado Azul

Blends: GLF, GLF Vitality, DiGize, DiGize Vitality, JuvaCleanse, JuvaCleanse Vitality

Nutritionals: Essentialzyme, Essentialzymes-4, Life 9, KidScents MightyPro, JuvaPower, NingXia Red

Application and Usage

Aromatic: Refer to Application Guidelines.

Dietary and Oral: Refer to Application Guidelines.

- Take 1 capsule with Helichrysum or other desired dietary oil 2 times daily.

- Take 1-2 capsules 2 times daily 50:50 with Helichrysum and Cistus.

- Take 2-3 drops of desired Vitality oil in a spoonful of syrup or small amount of milk, juice, or water.

Topical: Refer to Application Guidelines.

- Apply 1-3 drops, diluted 50:50, on temples, forehead, mastoids, back of neck, and at base of throat just above the clavicle notch.

- Applying a single drop under the nose is helpful and refreshing.

- Massage 2-4 drops of oil neat on Vita Flex brain points on the bottoms of the feet just before bedtime.

CELLULITE

Cellulite is one of the harder types of fats to dissolve in the body. It's an accumulation of old fat cell clusters that solidifies and hardens as the surrounding tissue loses its elasticity.

Excess fat is undesirable for two reasons:

1. The extra weight puts an extra load on all body systems, particularly the heart and cardiovascular system, as well as the joints (knees, hips, spine, etc.)

2. Toxins and petrochemicals (pesticides, herbicides, and metals) tend to accumulate in fatty tissue. This can contribute to hormone imbalance, neurological problems, and a higher risk of cancer.

Essential oils such as Ledum, Tangerine, and Grapefruit may help reduce the fat in fat cells. Cypress enhances circulation to support the elimination of fatty deposits. The essential oils of Lemongrass and Spearmint also may help fat metabolism. Cel-Lite Magic Massage Oil contains many of these oils and may help reduce cellulite deposits.

Cellulite is slow to dissolve, so target areas should be worked for a month or more in conjunction with weight training, a weight-loss program, and drinking purified water—one-and-a-half times the body weight in ounces each day. Be patient. You should begin to see results in 4-6 weeks when using the oils in combination with a muscle-building and weight-loss regimen.

Recommendations

Singles: Grapefruit, Grapefruit Vitality, Spearmint, Spearmint Vitality, Ledum, Lavender, Lavender Vitality, Rosemary, Rosemary Vitality, Davana, Helichrysum, Jade Lemon, Jade Lemon Vitality, Patchouli, Lemon, Lemon Vitality, Tangerine, Tangerine Vitality, Cypress, Fennel, Juniper, Orange, Orange Vitality, Lemongrass, Lemongrass Vitality

Blends: Citrus Fresh, Citrus Fresh Vitality, GLF, GLF Vitality, DiGize, DiGize Vitality, Release, Dream Catcher, Into the Future, Live Your Passion, SARA, JuvaFlex, JuvaFlex Vitality

Nutritionals: Thyromin (balances and boosts metabolism), Slique Essence, Slique Shake, Slique Bars, Slique CitraSlim, OmegaGize3, EndoFlex, Digest & Cleanse, Essentialzyme, Essentialzymes-4, Life 9, KidScents MightyPro, Balance Complete, Pure Protein Complete, Protein Power Bites

Personal Care: Cel-Lite Magic Massage Oil

Application and Usage

Topical: Refer to Application Guidelines.

- Dilute 50:50 and massage 3-6 drops vigorously on cellulite locations at least 3 times daily, especially before exercising.

Cellulite Blend No. 1
- 10 drops Grapefruit
- 5 drops Lavender
- 3 drops Helichrysum
- 3 drops Patchouli
- 4 drops Cypress

Use as bath salt 2-4 times weekly.

Cellulite Blend No. 2 (Bath)
- 5 drops Juniper
- 3 drops Orange
- 3 drops Cypress
- 3 drops Rosemary

Mix the above blend together with 2 tablespoons Epsom salts or Bath Gel Base and dissolve in warm bath water. Massage with Cel-Lite Magic after bath.

- Apply 3-5 drops of Grapefruit neat 1-2 times daily to increase fat-reducing action in areas of fat rolls, puckers, and dimples.

The effects of cerebral palsy vary greatly, causing impaired movement associated with exaggerated reflexes or rigidity of the limbs and trunk, abnormal posture, involuntary movements, unsteadiness of walking, or a combination of these.

It is caused most often by abnormal development in the brain before birth or injury during delivery. Individuals stricken with cerebral palsy often have other conditions related to developmental brain abnormalities such as intellectual disabilities, vision and hearing problems, or seizures.

Signs and Symptoms
- Stiff muscles and exaggerated reflexes (spasticity)
- Stiff muscles with normal reflexes (rigidity)
- Lack of muscle coordination, tremors, or involuntary movements
- Slow development of motor skills such as pushing with arms, sitting up, or crawling
- Reaching with only one hand or dragging a leg while crawling
- Difficulty eating and swallowing, excessive drooling
- Slow speech development or difficulty speaking
- Difficulty in picking up toys, spoons, etc.

Medical researchers have not found an answer to the question of specific causes but offer different therapies and medications in an effort to help. Natural medicine offers help with the same desire of seeing improvement. Because essential oils cross the blood-brain barrier, they can stimulate brain activity in a nontoxic way, and one can hope and wait to see what possible benefits will appear.

Different people have tried different things that have resulted in the information below. By investigating further with supplements and natural remedies, many new things will be discovered. The risk is minimal and the gain could be slight to immense.

Recommendations

Singles: Sacred Frankincense, Frankincense, Frankincense Vitality, Myrrh, Idaho Grand Fir, Peppermint, Peppermint Vitality

Blends: PanAway, Aroma Siez, Relieve It, Cool Azul, Deep Relief Roll-On, CBD, Calm CBD Roll-On, Chivalry

Nutritionals: BLM, AgilEase, Sulfurzyme, Essentialzymes-4, Slique Shake, Pure Protein Complete, Protein Power Bites, MultiGreens, Mineral Essence, Essentialzyme, Super Vitamin D, Super Vitamin B, NingXia Red, PowerGize

Personal Care: Cool Azul Pain Relief Cream, Cool Azul Sports Gel, CBD Muscle Rub, Ortho Ease Massage Oil, Ortho Sport Massage Oil

Application and Usage

Aromatic: Refer to Application Guidelines.

Dietary and Oral: Refer to Application Guidelines.

- Take 1 capsule of desired Vitality oil 2 times daily.

- Take 2-3 drops of desired Vitality oil in a spoonful of syrup or small amount of milk, juice, or water.

Topical: Refer to Application Guidelines.

- Use blend for Raindrop Technique 2 times daily: morning and night.

Cerebral Palsy Blend

Take 3 capsules daily: morning, noon, and night:
- 15 drops Frankincense or Frankincense Vitality
- 12 drops Myrrh
- 10 drops Idaho Grand Fir
- 10 drops Canadian Fleabane (Conyza)
- 4 drops Peppermint or Peppermint Vitality

Using this regimen, a 7-year-old boy with cerebral palsy and autism, after one month, was able to walk flat footed without his walker, test scores in school improved by 28 percent, and his attention span increased 30 percent, his mother reported.

CHEMICAL SENSITIVITY REACTION

Environmental poisoning and chemical sensitivity are becoming a major cause of discomfort and disease. Strong chemical compounds, such as insecticides, herbicides, and formaldehyde found in paints, glues, cosmetics, and fingernail polish, enter the body easily. Symptoms include indigestion, upper and lower gas, poor assimilation, poor electrolyte balance, rashes, hypoglycemia, and allergic reaction to foods and other substances, along with mood swings, fatigue, irritability, lack of motivation, and lack of discipline and creativity.

Recommendations

Singles: Wintergreen, Sacred Frankincense, Frankincense, Frankincense Vitality, Jade Lemon, Jade Lemon Vitality, Lemon, Lemon Vitality, Lime, Lime Vitality, Sacred Sandalwood, Davana, Royal Hawaiian Sandalwood, Copaiba, Copaiba Vitality, Eucalyptus Globulus

Blends: PanAway, Citrus Fresh, Citrus Fresh Vitality, Inner Child, Christmas Spirit, M-Grain

Resins: Frankincense Gum Resin

Nutritionals: Detoxzyme, JuvaPower, JuvaTone, Balance Complete, Pure Protein Complete, ICP, ComforTone, Essentialzyme, Essentialzymes-4, Life 9, KidScents MightyPro, Allerzyme

Application and Usage

Aromatic: Refer to Application Guidelines.

Dietary and Oral: Refer to Application Guidelines.

- Take 1 capsule of desired Vitality oil 2 times daily.

- Take 2-3 drops of desired Vitality oil in a spoonful of syrup or small amount of milk, juice, or water.

Topical: Refer to Application Guidelines.

- Dilute oil 50:50 and apply on affected areas 2-4 times daily.

Headache Relief Regimen:
- 4 Essentialzyme
- $1/8$ teaspoon M-Grain diluted 50:50 in vegetable oil

Drink 2-3 large glasses of water immediately after taking these products.

CHICKEN POX (VARICELLA ZOSTER)
(See also COLD SORES (HERPES SIMPLEX TYPE 1); SKIN DISORDERS AND PROBLEMS, Blisters)

The varicella zoster virus causes two distinct syndromes: varicella zoster (chicken pox) and subsequent reactivation of latent varicella zoster in dorsal-root ganglia resulting in "herpes zoster" or "shingles."

What happens is that a childhood bout with chicken pox leaves the virus dormant in the ganglia alongside the spine. If the immune system is taxed by severe emotional stress, illness, or longterm use of cortico-steroids, the dormant viruses may become active and start to infect the pathway of the skin nerves, causing shingles (See SHINGLES (HERPES ZOSTER)).

Recommendations
Singles: Melissa, Lemongrass, Lemongrass Vitality, Lavender, Lavender Vitality, Tea Tree, Sacred Sandalwood, Royal Hawaiian Sandalwood, Clove, Clove Vitality, Cypress, Blue Cypress, Cassia, Geranium, Wintergreen

Blends: Thieves, Thieves Vitality, Australian Blue, Melrose

Nutritionals: Inner Defense, ImmuPro, Balance Complete, Slique Shake, Super Vitamin Cal Plus, PD 80/20

Personal Care: Thieves Spray, Ortho Ease Massage Oil, Ortho Sport Massage Oil, LavaDerm Cooling Mist

Application and Usage
Aromatic: Refer to Application Guidelines.

Dietary and Oral: Refer to Application Guidelines.

- Take 1 capsule of desired Vitality oil 2 times daily.

- Take 2-3 drops of desired Vitality oil in a spoonful of syrup or small amount of milk, juice, or water.

Topical: Refer to Application Guidelines.

- Add 20 drops of essential oils (using any of the above oils) to 1 tablespoon of calamine lotion or V-6 Vegetable Oil Complex and lightly dab on spots (lesions).

CHOLERA

Cholera is an acute diarrheal disease caused by an enterotoxin produced by a gram-negative bacterium called Vibrio cholerae. Severe cases are marked by vomiting, muscle cramps, and constant watery diarrhea, which can result in serious fluid loss, saline depletion, acidosis, and shock. The disease is typically found in India and Southeast Asia and is spread by feces-contaminated water and food. If you suspect cholera, you should immediately seek professional medical advice.

A study done in 2000 shows that "concentrated lemon and [lemon peel] essential oils inhibited V. cholerae completely at all studied dilutions and exposure times." The study stated: "It can be concluded that lemon, a natural product which is easily obtained, acts as a biocide against V. cholerae, and is, therefore, an efficient decontaminant, harmless to humans."[25]

Recommendations
Singles: Jade Lemon, Jade Lemon Vitality, Lemon, Lemon Vitality, Lime, Lime Vitality, Clove, Clove Vitality, Thyme, Thyme Vitality, Rosemary, Rosemary Vitality, Cassia, Oregano, Oregano Vitality

Blends: DiGize, DiGize Vitality, Citrus Fresh, Citrus Fresh Vitality, ImmuPower

Nutritionals: Inner Defense, Digest & Cleanse, ImmuPro

Application and Usage
Aromatic: Refer to Application Guidelines.

Dietary and Oral: Refer to Application Guidelines.

- Take 1 capsule of desired Vitality oil 2 times daily.

- Take 2-3 drops of desired Vitality oil in a spoonful of syrup or small amount of milk, juice, or water.

Topical: Refer to Application Guidelines.

CHRONIC FATIGUE SYNDROME

The cause of chronic fatigue syndrome is somewhat of a mystery, but scientists believe it may be caused by a combination of factors, including immune system problems, hormone imbalances, genetic factors, psychiatric or emotional conditions, brain abnormalities, and viruses, including Epstein-Barr virus, Lyme disease, human herpes virus 6, and mouse leukemia viruses. However, no primary cause has been established.

Recommendations

Singles: Peppermint, Peppermint Vitality, Jade Lemon, Jade Lemon Vitality, Lemon, Lemon Vitality, Cassia, Lime, Lime Vitality, Orange, Orange Vitality

Blends: Awaken, DiGize, DiGize Vitality, Joy, Reconnect, SleepyIze, Citrus Fresh, Citrus Fresh Vitality, KidScents TummyGize

Nutritionals: Detoxzyme, EndoGize, ImmuPro, Inner Defense, PD 80/20, Super Vitamin B, Thyromin, NingXia Red, NingXia Nitro, Olive Essentials, NingXia Zyng

Personal Care: Progessence Plus, PrenoIone Plus Body Cream

Application and Usage

Aromatic: Refer to Application Guidelines.

Dietary and Oral: Refer to Application Guidelines.

- Take 1 capsule of desired Vitality oil 2 times daily.

- Take 2-3 drops of desired Vitality oil in a spoonful of syrup or small amount of milk, juice, or water.

Topical: Refer to Application Guidelines.

COLD SORES
(Herpes Simplex Type 1)

Cold sores are also known as Herpes labialis. Diets high in the amino acid lysine can reduce the incidence of herpes. Conversely, the amino acid arginine can worsen herpes outbreaks.

Studies have shown neat applications of Melissa to be effective against herpes simplex type I and type II. The healing period was shortened, the spread of infection was prevented, and symptoms such as itching, tingling, and burning were lessened.

Also, when lemon balm was used to treat the infection in the very early stages, [by day two] the treatment was the most effective (Wölbling, 1994).

Peppermint and Tea Tree oils have also been studied for positive effects on the pain of herpes.

Recommendations

Singles: Melissa, Peppermint, Peppermint Vitality, Ravintsara, Tea Tree, Lavender, Lavender Vitality, Sacred Sandalwood, Royal Hawaiian Sandalwood, Mountain Savory, Mountain Savory Vitality, Oregano, Oregano Vitality, Ecuadorian Oregano, Thyme, Thyme Vitality, Clove, Clove Vitality

Blends: Thieves, Thieves Vitality, Melrose, Purification

Nutritionals: Inner Defense, ImmuPro, Super Vitamin C, Super Vitamin C Chewable, MultiGreens, ICP, ComforTone, Essentialzyme, JuvaTone, Essentialzymes-4, JuvaPower

Personal Care: Thieves Spray, Rose Ointment

Application and Usage

Topical: Refer to Application Guidelines.

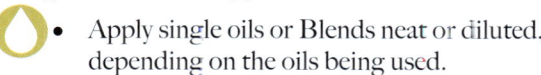
- Apply single oils or Blends neat or diluted, depending on the oils being used.

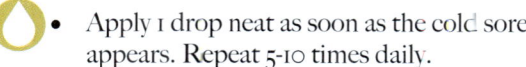
- Apply 1 drop neat as soon as the cold sore appears. Repeat 5-10 times daily.

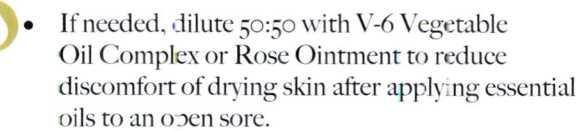
- If needed, dilute 50:50 with V-6 Vegetable Oil Complex or Rose Ointment to reduce discomfort of drying skin after applying essential oils to an open sore.

COLDS
(See also LUNG INFECTIONS AND PROBLEMS, SINUS INFECTIONS AND PROBLEMS, THROAT INFECTIONS AND PROBLEMS)

The best treatment for a cold or flu is prevention. Because many essential oils have strong antimicrobial properties, they can be diffused to prevent the spread of airborne bacteria and viruses. Antiviral and antibacterial essential oils, **Blends**, and supplements are very effective as preventive aids in avoiding colds as well as in helping the body's defenses fight colds once an infection has started. ImmuPro is a powerful immune stimulant that can also increase infection resistance and is best when taken in the evening at bedtime.

Recommendations

Singles: Ravintsara, Cypress, Blue Cypress, Wintergreen, Peppermint, Peppermint Vitality, Thyme, Thyme Vitality, Laurus Nobilis, Laurus Nobilis Vitality, Hyssop, Oregano, Oregano Vitality, Ecuadorian Oregano, Eucalyptus Blue, Northern Lights Black Spruce, Eucalyptus Radiata, Tea Tree, Davana, Sacred Frankincense, Frankincense, Frankincense Vitality, Rosemary, Rosemary Vitality, Clove, Clove Vitality, Cassia, Lemon, Lemon Vitality, Mountain Savory, Mountain Savory Vitality

Blends: Raven, Thieves, Thieves Vitality, Melrose, Australian Blue, Purification, ImmuPower, Sacred Mountain, R.C., Exodus II, Breathe Again, Breathe Again Roll-On, SniffleEase

Nutritionals: Inner Defense, ImmuPro, Thieves Lozenges, Super Vitamin C, Super Vitamin C Chewable, Longevity Softgels, Master Formula, Detoxzyme, AlkaLime

Oral Care: Thieves Spray, Thieves Cough Drops, Thieves Hard Lozenges, Thieves Fresh Essence Mouth Wash

Personal Care: Thieves Chest Rub

Application and Usage

Aromatic: Refer to Application Guidelines.

Dietary and Oral: Refer to Application Guidelines.

- Take 1 capsule of desired Vitality oil 2 times daily.

- Take 2-3 drops of desired Vitality oil in a spoonful of syrup or small amount of milk, juice, or water.

- Take a Cold Blend 3-6 times daily.
- Gargle 3-6 times daily.

Cold Blend No. 1
- 5 drops Rosemary or Rosemary Vitality
- 4 drops Eucalyptus Radiata
- 4 drops Peppermint or Peppermint Vitality
- 3 drops Cypress
- 2 drops Lemon or Lemon Vitality

Cold Blend No. 2
- 5 drops Rosemary or Rosemary Vitality
- 4 drops R.C.
- 4 drops Sacred Frankincense, Frankincense, or Frankincense Vitality
- 2 drops Peppermint or Peppermint Vitality
- 1 drop Oregano or Oregano Vitality

Topical: Refer to Application Guidelines.

- Dilute 50:50 and massage 1-3 drops on each of the following areas: forehead, nose, cheeks, lower throat, chest, and up-per back 1-3 times daily.

- Massage 1-3 drops on Vita Flex points on the feet 1-2 times daily.
- Receive a Raindrop Technique 1-2 times weekly.
- Bath salts (See below)

Bath Blend for Relief of Cold Symptoms
- 15 drops Ravintsara
- 8 drops Wintergreen
- 6 drops Northern Lights Black Spruce
- 6 drops Sacred Frankincense or Frankincense
- 3 drops Laurus Nobilis
- 2 drops Eucalyptus Radiata

Stir essential oils into ½ cup Epsom salt or baking soda and then add the mixture to hot bath water while tub is filling. Soak in hot bath until water cools.

COLITIS
(See also CROHN'S DISEASE; DIGESTIVE PROBLEMS, DIVERTICULOSIS/DIVERTICULITIS)

Also known as ileitis or proctitis, ulcerative colitis is marked by the inflammation of the top layers of the lining of the colon, the large intestine. It is different from both irritable bowel syndrome, which has no inflammation, and Crohn's disease, which usually occurs deeper in the colon wall.

The inflammation and ulcerous sores that are characteristic of ulcerative colitis occur most frequently in the lower colon and rectum and occasionally throughout the entire colon.

Symptoms include fatigue, nausea, weight loss, loss of appetite, bloody diarrhea, loss of body fluids and nutrients, frequent fevers, abdominal cramps, arthritis, liver disease, and skin rash.

Take Essentialzymes-4 along with ComforTone and wait about 2 weeks or more before adding JuvaPower. Start with a small amount and increase slowly. If any discomfort is experienced, reduce the amount taken.

Ulcerative Colitis
Use the remedies below for ulcerative colitis.

Recommendations

Singles: Carrot Seed, Carrot Seed Vitality, Cassia, Spearmint, Spearmint Vitality, Wintergreen, Peppermint, Peppermint Vitality, Tarragon, Tarragon Vitality, Frankincense, Frankincense Vitality, Sacred Frankincense, Fennel, Fennel Vitality

Blends: DiGize, DiGize Vitality, GLF, GLF Vitality, JuvaCleanse, JuvaCleanse Vitality, KidScents TummyGize

Nutritionals: Digest & Cleanse, ComforTone, AlkaLime, Life 9, KidScents MightyPro, JuvaPower, Detoxzyme, ICP, Essentialzyme, Essentialzymes-4, Mega Vitamin Cal

Application and Usage

Aromatic: Refer to Application Guidelines.

Dietary and Oral: Refer to Application Guidelines.

- Take 2 capsules with any 2 of the Vitality oils above 2-3 times daily.

- Take 2-3 drops of desired Vitality oil in a spoonful of syrup or small amount of milk, juice, or water.

Topical: Refer to Application Guidelines.

- Apply 4-6 drops of your choice of oil, diluted 50:50, on lower abdomen 3-6 times daily.

- Massage 2-4 drops of oil neat on the bottoms of the feet just before bedtime.

Viral Colitis

Use the remedies below for colitis that may be caused by a virus rather than bacteria.

Recommendations

Singles: Melissa, Lemongrass, Lemongrass Vitality, Cassia, Clove, Clove Vitality, Melaleuca Quinquenervia (Niaouli), Blue Cypress, Oregano, Oregano Vitality, Ecuadorian Oregano, Helichrysum, Cumin, Tea Tree, Tarragon, Tarragon Vitality, Thyme, Thyme Vitality, Roman Chamomile, German Chamomile, German Chamomile Vitality, Rosemary, Rosemary Vitality, Peppermint, Peppermint Vitality, Cinnamon Bark, Cinnamon Bark Vitality

Blends: Melrose, Thieves, Thieves Roll-On, Thieves Vitality, Purification, DiGize, DiGize Vitality, KidScents TummyGize

Nutritionals: Digest & Cleanse, Inner Defense, Longevity Softgels, Essentialzymes-4, Essentialzyme, Life 9, KidScents MightyPro

Application and Usage

Dietary and Oral: Refer to Application Guidelines.

- Take 1 capsule of desired Vitality oil 2 times daily.

- Take 2-3 drops of desired Vitality oil in a spoonful of syrup or small amount of milk, juice, or water.

Topical: Refer to Application Guidelines

- Apply several drops diluted 50:50 over colon area 4-6 times daily.

- You may also apply 2-3 drops on the Vita Flex colon points.

- Have Raindrop Technique 1-2 times weekly.

- Place a warm compress diluted 20:80 using equal parts Helichrysum and DiGize over the colon area.

- Use the blend below in a rectal implant 3 times weekly.

Colitis-Colon Blend

- 3 drops Melaleuca Quinquenervia (Niaouli)
- 2 drops Oregano Vitality
- 2 drops Thyme Vitality
- 2 drops German Chamomile Vitality
- 2 drops Melissa
- 2 drops Peppermint Vitality

Mix above oils with 1 tablespoon V-6 Vegetable Oil Complex.

COMA

Patients in a coma will likely be in a hospital or care center. Discuss with the patient's health care professional about rubbing essential oils on the bottoms of the patient's feet and diffusing the oils. In one recent case, family members of a patient in a medically induced coma found that the aroma of Sacred Frankincense allowed the unconscious patient to calm down and stop fighting restraints used to prevent dislodging a breathing tube.

After the patient returns home, the oils listed below could be helpful.

Recommendations

Singles: Valerian, Vetiver, Sacred Sandalwood, Royal Hawaiian Sandalwood, Blue Cypress, Black Pepper, Black Pepper Vitality, Peppermint, Peppermint Vitality, Idaho Grand Fir, Copaiba, Copaiba Vitality, Sacred Frankincense, Frankincense, Frankincense Vitality

Blends: Hope, Valor, Valor Roll-On, Surrender, The Gift, Inspiration, Brain Power, KidScents GeneYus, Trauma Life, R.C.

Personal Care: Progessence Plus, Regenolone Moisturizing Cream, Sensation Massage Oil

Application and Usage

Aromatic: Refer to Application Guidelines.

- Diffuse your choice of oils for 15 minutes 4-7 times daily.

Topical: Refer to Application Guidelines.

- Apply 3-5 drops diluted 50:50 on temples, neck, and shoulders.

- Receive a Raindrop Technique with the above-mentioned oils.

CONNECTIVE TISSUE DAMAGE (CARTILAGE, LIGAMENTS, TENDONS)

Tendonitis, often called "tennis elbow" or "golfer's elbow," is a torn or inflamed tendon. Repetitive use or infection may be the cause.

Mega Vitamin Cal, BLM, and AgilEase provide critical nutrients for connective tissue repair. Sulfurzyme, an outstanding source of organic sulfur, equalizes water pressure inside the cells and reduces pain.

PanAway reduces pain and Lemongrass promotes the repair of connective tissue. Lavender with Lemongrass and Marjoram with Lemongrass work well together for inflamed tendons. Deep Relief Roll-On is a convenient way to apply a blend of oils that is both pain-relieving and anti-inflammatory.

When selecting oils for injuries, think through the cause and type of injury and select appropriate oils. For instance, tendonitis could encompass muscle damage, nerve damage, ligament strain/tear, inflammation, infection, and possibly an emotion. Therefore, select an oil or oils for each potential cause and apply in rotation or prepare a blend to address multiple causes. Ortho Sport and Ortho Ease massage oils reduce pain and promote healing. Cool Azul products are also great pain relievers.

Recommendations

Singles: Sacred Frankincense, Frankincense, Frankincense Vitality, Lemongrass, Lemongrass Vitality, Lavender, Lavender Vitality, Marjoram, Marjoram Vitality, Eucalyptus Blue, Dorado Azul

Blends: PanAway, Deep Relief Roll-On, Relieve It, CBD, Aroma Siez, Melrose, Cool Azul, Chivalry

Nutritionals: Mega Vitamin Cal, BLM, AgilEase, Super Vitamin B, Super Vitamin C, Super Vitamin C Chewable, Super Vitamin D, MultiGreens, Mineral Essence, Sulfurzyme, PD 80/20, PowerGize

Personal Care: Cool Azul Pain Relief Cream, Cool Azul Sports Gel, CBD Muscle Rub, Ortho Ease Massage Oil, Ortho Sport Massage Oil, Regenolone Moisturizing Cream

Application and Usage

Topical: Refer to Application Guidelines.

- Apply oils neat or diluted 50:50 on location 3-6 times daily.

- Massage 4-6 drops of oil on affected area. For swelling, elevate and apply ice packs.

- Place a cold compress with 1-2 drops of chosen oil on area 2-4 times daily.

Cartilage Injury on Knee, Elbow, Etc.

People with cartilage damage often experience decreased range of motion, stiffness, joint pain, and/or swelling in the affected area.

Recommendations

Singles: Wintergreen, Copaiba, Copaiba Vitality, Lemongrass, Lemongrass Vitality, Palo Santo, Peppermint, Peppermint Vitality, Idaho Grand Fir, Marjoram, Marjoram Vitality, Eucalyptus Blue, Dorado Azul, Idaho Blue Spruce

Blends: PanAway, Relieve It, Aroma Siez, Deep Relief Roll-On, Cool Azul, CBD

Nutritionals: Mega Vitamin Cal, Super Vitamin B, Super Vitamin C, Super Vitamin C Chewable, MultiGreens, Mineral Essence, BLM, AgilEase, Master Formula, Sulfurzyme, PowerGize

Personal Care: Cool Azul Pain Relief Cream, Cool Azul Sports Gel, CBD Muscle Rub, Ortho Ease Massage Oil, Ortho Sport Massage Oil, Regenolone Moisturizing Cream

Application and Usage
Topical: Refer to Application Guidelines.

- Apply neat or diluted 50:50 on location 3-6 times daily.
- Massage 4-6 drops of oil on affected area. For swelling, elevate and apply ice packs.
- Place a cold compress with 1-2 drops of chosen oil in Ortho Ease or Ortho Sport Massage Oil on area 2-4 times daily.

Cartilage Blend
- 12 drops Wintergreen
- 10 drops Marjoram
- 9 drops Lemongrass

Ligament Sprain or Tear
Note: For sprains, use cold packs. For any serious sprain or constant skeletal pain, always consult a health care professional. Anytime there is tissue damage, there is always inflammation. Reduce this first.

Recommendations
Singles: Lemongrass, Lemongrass Vitality, Helichrysum, Lavender, Lavender Vitality, Cassia, Elemi, Basil, Basil Vitality, Marjoram, Marjoram Vitality, Peppermint, Peppermint Vitality, Palo Santo

Blends: PanAway, Relieve It, Aroma Siez, Deep Relief Roll-On, Cool Azul, CBD

Nutritionals: BLM, AgilEase, AminoWise, Pure Protein Complete, Protein Power Bites, Mega Vitamin Cal, Super Vitamin B, Super Vitamin C, MultiGreens, Essentialzyme, Essentialzymes-4, Life 9, KidScents MightyPro, Mineral Essence, Sulfurzyme, PowerGize

Personal Care: Cool Azul Pain Relief Cream, Cool Azul Sports Gel, CBD Muscle Rub, Ortho Ease Massage Oil, Ortho Sport Massage Oil, Regenolone Moisturizing Cream

Application and Usage
Topical: Refer to Application Guidelines.

- Apply oils neat or diluted 50:50 on location 3-6 times daily.
- Massage 4-6 drops of oil on affected area. For swelling, elevate and apply ice packs.
- Place a cold compress with 1-2 drops of chosen oil on area 2-4 times daily.

Sprain Blend
- 15 drops Aroma Siez
- 5 drops Lemongrass

Scleroderma
Also known as systemic sclerosis, scleroderma is a noninfectious, chronic, autoimmune disease of the connective tissue. Caused by an overproduction of collagen, the disease can involve either the skin or internal organs and can be life threatening.

Scleroderma is far more common among women than men.

Recommendations
Singles: Myrrh, Wintergreen, German Chamomile, German Chamomile Vitality, Sacred Frankincense, Frankincense, Frank-incense Vitality, Copaiba, Copaiba Vitality, Lavender, Lavender Vitality, Cassia, Patchouli, Sacred Sandalwood, Royal Hawaiian Sandalwood

Blends: Melrose, Aroma Siez, Thieves, Thieves Roll-On, Thieves Vitality, Purification, SclarEssence, SclarEssence Vitality

Nutritionals: PD 80/20, ICP, ComforTone, Essentialzyme, JuvaTone, JuvaPower, AminoWise, Thyromin, Pure Protein Complete, Protein Power Bites, Mineral Essence, Slique Shake, Sulfurzyme, Detoxzyme, Longevity Softgels, PowerGize

Personal Care: Prenolone Plus Body Cream, LavaDerm Cooling Mist, Progessence Plus

Application and Usage
Topical: Refer to Application Guidelines.

- Apply 4-6 drops diluted 50:50 on location 3 times daily. Alternate between using Blend No. 1 and Blend No. 2 each day.

Scleroderma Blend No. 1
- 2 drops German Chamomile
- 2 drops Myrrh
- 1 drop Lavender
- 1 drop Patchouli

Scleroderma Blend No. 2
- 3 drops Myrrh
- 2 drops Sacred Sandalwood or Royal Hawaiian Sandalwood

Tendonitis (also Tendinitis)

Tendons are cords of tough, fibrous connective tissue that attach muscles to bones and are found throughout the entire human body. Tendonitis is the irritation and inflammation of those tendons.

Recommendations

Singles: Lemongrass, Lemongrass Vitality, Lemon Verbena, Marjoram, Marjoram Vitality, Copaiba, Copaiba Vitality, Rosemary, Rosemary Vitality, Eucalyptus Radiata, Peppermint, Peppermint Vitality, Frankincense, Frankincense Vitality, Sacred Frankincense, Cassia, Palo Santo, Basil, Basil Vitality, Wintergreen, Vetiver, Valerian, Elemi

Blends: Deep Relief Roll-On, Aroma Siez, PanAway, Relieve It, Cool Azul, CBD

Nutritionals: BLM, AgilEase, AminoWise, Mega Vitamin Cal, Super Vitamin B, Super Vitamin C, Super Vitamin C Chewable, MultiGreens, Mineral Essence, Sulfurzyme, PowerGize, Pure Protein Complete, Protein Power Bites

Personal Care: Cool Azul Pain Relief Cream, Cool Azul Sports Gel, CBD Muscle Rub, Regenolone Moisturizing Cream, Ortho Sport Massage Oil, Ortho Ease Massage Oil

Application and Usage

Topical: Refer to Application Guidelines.

- Apply oils neat or diluted 50:50 on location 3-6 times daily.

- Massage 4-6 drops of oil on affected area. For swelling, elevate and apply ice packs.

- Place a cold compress with 1-2 drops of chosen oil on area 2-4 times daily.

Tendonitis Pain Relief Blend No. 1
- 8 drops Wintergreen
- 4 drops Vetiver
- 4 drops Valerian

Tendonitis Pain Relief Blend No. 2
- 10 drops Rosemary
- 10 drops Eucalyptus Radiata
- 10 drops Peppermint
- 5 drops Palo Santo

CROHN'S DISEASE
(See also COLITIS; DIGESTIVE PROBLEMS, DIVERTICULOSIS/DIVERTICULITIS)

Crohn's disease creates inflammation, sores, and ulcers on the intestinal wall. These sores occur deeper than ulcerative colitis. Unlike other forms of colitis, Crohn's disease can affect the entire digestive tract from the mouth all the way to the rectum.

Symptoms
- Abdominal cramping
- Lower-right abdominal pain
- Diarrhea
- A general sense of feeling ill

Attacks may occur once or twice a day for life. If the disease continues for years, it can cause deterioration of bowel function, leaky gut syndrome, poor absorption of nutrients, loss of appetite and weight, intestinal obstruction, severe bleeding, and increased susceptibility to intestinal cancer.

Most researchers believe that Crohn's disease is caused by an overreacting immune system and is actually an autoimmune disease, where the immune system mistakenly attacks the body's own tissues. MSM has been extensively researched for its ability to treat many autoimmune diseases and is a key ingredient in Sulfurzyme.

Recommendations

Singles: Ginger, Ginger Vitality, Nutmeg, Nutmeg Vitality, Wintergreen, German Chamomile, German Chamomile Vitality, Peppermint, Peppermint Vitality, Copaiba, Copaiba Vitality, Cassia, Fennel, Fennel Vitality, Patchouli

Blends: ImmuPower, DiGize, DiGize Vitality, PanAway, KidScents TummyGize

Nutritionals: Sulfurzyme, OmegaGize3, Life 9, KidScents MightyPro, Detoxzyme, Essentialzyme, Essentialzymes-4, Alka-Lime, AminoWise, ICP, ComforTone, MultiGreens, Digest & Cleanse, NingXia Red, Balance Complete

Application and Usage
Aromatic: Refer to Application Guidelines.

Dietary and Oral: Refer to Application Guidelines.

- Take 1 capsule of desired Vitality oil 2 times daily.

- Take 2-3 drops of desired Vitality oil in a spoonful of syrup or small amount of milk, juice, or water.

Topical: Refer to Application Guidelines.

- Receive a Raindrop Technique 1-2 times weekly incorporating ImmuPower.

- Place a warm compress with 1-2 drops of chosen oil on the back.

Regimen for Crohn's disease

Each phase lasts 3 days and should be added to the previous phase.

- **Phase I:** Essentialzymes-4: Take 1-2 capsules, both white and yellow, 3 times daily.
- **Phase II:** Take the Essentialzymes-4 in yogurt or liquid acidophilus and charcoal tablets. Do not use ICP, ComforTone, or Essentialzyme yet.
- **Phase III:** Drink 6 ounces raw juice (cherry, prune, celery, carrot, or NingXia Red) 2 times daily.
- **Phase IV:** Take 2 scoops Balance Complete in water or juice 2 times daily.
- **Phase V:** (Start only if there is no sign of bleeding.)
- **ComforTone:** Take 1 capsule morning and night until stools loosen.
- **ICP:** Start with 1 level teaspoon 2 times daily and gradually increase.
- **Essentialzyme:** Start with 1 caplet 3 times daily. If irritation occurs, discontinue for a few days and start again.

CYSTS

Cysts are closed, sac-like structures that contain fluid, gas, or semisolid material that is not a normal part of the tissue where it is located. There are hundreds of types that are common, vary in size, and can occur anywhere in the body in people of all ages. Two of the most common types of cysts are ganglion and ovarian.

Ganglion Cysts

Ganglion cysts develop in the tissues near joints and tendons, often in the ankles, in the wrists, and behind the knees. They cause painful swelling and are often filled with a thick fluid.

Recommendations

Singles: Oregano, Thyme, Myrrh, Mountain Savory

Blends: Purification, Thieves, Thieves Roll-On, Deep Relief Roll-On, Cool Azul

Nutritionals: Super Vitamin C, Mineral Essence, Detoxzyme

Personal Care: LavaDerm Cooling Mist, Thieves Spray, Cool Azul Pain Relief Cream, Cool Azul Sports Gel

Application and Usage

Topical: Refer to Application Guidelines.

- Apply 2 drops of chosen oil neat the first day.
- Apply 2 drops of Thyme the second day.
- Apply on location as often as needed.

Ovarian and Uterine Cysts
(See also MENSTRUAL AND FEMALE HORMONE CONDITIONS)

Ovarian cysts can be painless or painful if they grow large and affect the ovary. They may be caused by an egg sac that doesn't properly break open or dissolve as part of the menstrual cycle.

Recommendations

Singles: Myrrh, Geranium, Sacred Frankincense, Frankincense, Frankincense Vitality, Sage, Sage Vitality, Tea Tree, Clary Sage, Thyme, Thyme Vitality, Rosemary, Rosemary Vitality, Oregano, Oregano Vitality

Blends: Dragon Time, SclarEssence, SclarEssence Vitality

Nutritionals: PD 80/20, EndoGize, FemiGen, Mineral Essence, Essentialzyme, Essentialzymes-4

Personal Care: Prenolone Plus Body Cream, Progessence Plus, FemiGen, Regenolone Moisturizing Cream

Application and Usage

Topical: Refer to Application Guidelines.

- Apply 1-3 drops on the reproductive Vita Flex points, located around the anklebone on either side of the foot. Work from the ankle bone down to the arch of the foot.

- Place a warm compress with 1-2 oils of your choice on location as needed.

- Retention: Apply 1-2 drops diluted 50:50 on a tampon and insert nightly for 4 nights. Note: If irritation occurs, dis-continue use for 3 days before resuming.

Female Cyst Blend No. 1
- 9 drops Sacred Frankincense or Frankincense
- 5 drops Clary Sage
- 5 drops Myrrh
- 2 drops Thyme
- 2 drops Rosemary

Female Cyst Blend No. 2
- 4 drops Sacred Frankincense or Frankincense
- 4 drops Geranium
- 2 drops Oregano

DEPRESSION (See also SLEEP DISORDERS, INSOMNIA)

Diffusing or directly inhaling essential oils can have an immediate, positive impact on mood. Olfaction (smell) is the only sense that can have direct effects on the limbic region of the brain. Studies at the University of Vienna have shown that some essential oils and their primary constituents (cineole) can stimulate blood flow and activity in the emotional regions of the brain.26

Clinical studies at the Department of Psychiatry at the Mie University of Medicine showed that lemon not only reduced depression, but it also reduced stress when inhaled.27

Recommendations

Singles: Lavender, Lavender Vitality, Roman Chamomile, Melissa, Jasmine, Sacred Frankincense, Frankincense, Frankincense Vitality, Peppermint, Peppermint Vitality, Ylang Ylang, Cassia, Rosemary, Rosemary Vitality, Jade Lemon, Jade Lemon Vitality, Lemon, Lemon Vitality, Lime, Lime Vitality, Cedarwood, Bergamot, Bergamot Vitality

Blends: Build Your Dream, Release, Freedom, Reconnect, Gary's Light, Valor, Valor Roll-On, Live with Passion, Live Your Passion, Light the Fire, Hope, Joy, One Heart, KidScents KidPower, KidScents KidPower Roll-On, Calm CBD Roll-On, Seedlings Calm, My Destiny, Common Sense, The Gift, RutaVaLa, RutaVaLa Roll-On, Chivalry, SclarEssence, SclarEssence Vitality, Journey On, 25 Years Young

Nutritionals: MultiGreens, Life 9, KidScents MightyPro, Super Vitamin B, Mineral Essence, Balance Complete, Thyromin, EndoGize, Ecuadorian Dark Chocolessence, Slique Bars–Chocolate-Coated, Chocolate-Coated Wolfberry Crisp Bars, NingXia Red, NingXia Zyng, NingXia Nitro

Application and Usage

Aromatic: Refer to Application Guidelines.

Topical: Refer to Application Guidelines.

- Apply 1-2 drops of recommended oil neat on temples and back of neck as desired.

Postpartum Depression

"Baby blues" are normal for a few days after childbirth. Postpartum depression can follow and feel like more of the same or feel worse than before. It can also happen months after childbirth or pregnancy loss.

Recommendations

Singles: Jade Lemon, Jade Lemon Vitality, Lemon, Lemon Vitality, Lime, Lime Vitality, Sage, Sage Vitality, Melissa, Clary Sage, Cedarwood, Sacred Sandalwood, Royal Hawaiian Sandalwood, Sacred Frankincense, Frankincense, Frankincense Vitality, Cassia, Bergamot, Bergamot Vitality

Blends: Joy, Trauma Life, Peace & Calming, Peace & Calming II, One Heart, Tranquility Roll-On, Hope, Gary's Light, KidScents KidPower, KidScents KidPower Roll-On, Calm CBD Roll-On, Seedlings Calm, Loyalty, RutaVaLa, RutaVaLa Roll-On, Transformation, Dragon Time, 25 Years Young

Nutritionals: Super Vitamin B, KidScents Unwind, EndoGize, FemiGen, Ecuadorian Dark Chocolessence, Slique Bars–Chocolate-Coated, Chocolate-Coated Wolfberry Crisp Bars, NingXia Red, NingXia Zyng, NingXia Nitro

Personal Care: Progessence Plus, Prenolone Plus Body Cream

Application and Usage

Aromatic: Refer to Application Guidelines.

Dietary and Oral: Refer to Application Guidelines.

- Take 1 capsule of desired Vitality oil 2 times daily.

- Take 2-3 drops of desired Vitality oil in a spoonful of syrup or small amount of milk, juice, or water.

Topical: Refer to Application Guidelines.

- Apply 2-4 drops neat on temples and back of neck 2-4 times daily or as needed.
- Applying a single drop under the nose is helpful and refreshing.
- Place a warm compress with 1-2 drops of chosen oil on the back.

DIABETES

Diabetes is the leading cause of cardiovascular disease and premature death in westernized countries today. Diabetes causes low energy and persistently high blood glucose. Many other serious complications are also created by diabetes, including damage to the eyes, strokes, foot ulcers, and chronic kidney disease.

Type I diabetes usually manifests by age 30 and is often considered to be genetic. Type II diabetes generally manifests later in life and may have a nutritional origin.

Chromium has been shown to help the body metabolize sugars properly.

Wolfberry (Lycium barbarum) balances the pancreas and is a detoxifier and cleanser. Diabetes is not common in certain regions of China where wolfberry is consumed regularly.

Cinnamon has long been known for balancing blood sugar. Using a cinnamon extract, Chinese researchers found cinnamon improves fasting glucose and glycosylated hemoglobin levels in patients with type 2 diabetes (Lu T, 2012).

Yacon Syrup contains inulin, the complex sugar that slowly breaks down into FOS (fructooligosaccharide). Inulin is not digestible, so it passes through the body, with the result that it is half the calories of other sugars. FOS is well-known for its prebiotic effects and also supports microflora in the large intestine, while it promotes the absorption of calcium.

Recommendations

Singles: Clove, Clove Vitality, Cinnamon, Cinnamon Vitality, Coriander, Coriander Vitality, Davana, Fennel, Fennel Vitality, Dill, Dill Vitality, Cinnamon Bark, Cinnamon Bark Vitality, Cardamom, Cardamom Vitality, Lemongrass, Lemongrass Vitality

Blends: EndoFlex, EndoFlex Vitality, AromaEase, DiGize, DiGize Vitality, Thieves, Thieves Roll-On, Thieves Vitality, 25 Years Young

Nutritionals: MultiGreens, Mega Vitamin Cal, IlluminEyes, Balance Complete, Slique Essence, Essentialzyme, Essen-tialzymes-4, Master Formula, Ningxia Wolfberries (Organic, Dried), NingXia Red, Pure Protein Complete, Protein Power Bites, Olive Essentials, Slique Tea, Yacon Syrup

Application and Usage

Aromatic: Refer to Application Guidelines.

Dietary and Oral: Refer to Application Guidelines.

- Take 2 capsules 50:50 Fennel Vitality and Coriander Vitality 2 times daily.

- Take 2-3 drops of desired Vitality oil in a small amount of milk, juice, or water.

Topical: Refer to Application Guidelines

DIGESTIVE PROBLEMS

Digestive problems often result in symptoms such as stomach pain, constipation, gas, cramps, bloating, and diarrhea.

Constipation (Impacted Bowel)

The principle causes of constipation are inadequate fluid intake and low fiber consumption. Constipation can eventually lead to diverticulosis and diverticulitis, conditions common among older people.

Certain essential oils have demonstrated their ability to improve colon health by supporting intestinal flora, stimulating intestinal motility and peristalsis, fighting infections, and eliminating parasites.

Recommendations

Singles: Ginger, Ginger Vitality, Fennel, Fennel Vitality, Tarragon, Tarragon Vitality, Davana, Peppermint, Peppermint Vitality

Blends: DiGize, DiGize Vitality, JuvaCleanse, JuvaCleanse Vitality, AromaEase, KidScents TummyGize

Nutritionals: Digest & Cleanse, ICP, ComforTone, Detoxzyme, Life 9, KidScents MightyPro, Mega Vitamin Cal, Mineral Essence, Balance Complete, Essentialzyme, Essentialzymes-4, OmegaGize3, JuvaPower

Application and Usage

Aromatic: Refer to Application Guidelines.

Dietary and Oral: Refer to Application Guidelines.

- Take 1 capsule of desired Vitality oil 2 times daily.
- Take 2-3 drops of desired Vitality oil in a spoonful of syrup or small amount of milk, juice, or water.

Topical: Refer to Application Guidelines.

- Apply 6-10 drops neat or diluted 50:50 on stomach area as desired.
- Place a warm compress with 1-3 drops of recommended oil over the stomach area and Vita Flex points of the feet.

Regimen

- Essentialzyme: Take 3-6 tablets 3 times daily.
- ComforTone: Start with 1 capsule and increase the next day to 2 capsules. Continue to increase 1 capsule each day until bowels start moving.
- ICP: 1 week after ComforTone, start with 1 tablespoon ICP 2 times daily and then increase to 3 times daily up to 2 tablespoons 3 times daily.
- Balance Complete: 3 scoops daily or as needed.
- Drink at least ½ cup unsweetened cherry juice, prune juice, pineapple juice, or other raw fruit or vegetable juice each morning.
- Drink 8 glasses of pure water daily.

Cramps, Stomach

Stomach cramps may be caused by constipation, diarrhea, anxiety, gas, bloating, or PMS. Although stomach cramps are fairly common, paying attention to them is important.

Recommendations

Singles: Ginger, Ginger Vitality, Peppermint, Peppermint Vitality, Rosemary, Rosemary Vitality, Lavender, Lavender Vitality, Bergamot, Bergamot Vitality

Blends: DiGize, DiGize Vitality, KidScents TummyGize

Nutritionals: AlkaLime, Digest & Cleanse, Life 9, KidScents MightyPro, Essentialzymes-4, Essentialzyme

Application and Usage

Dietary and Oral: Refer to Application Guidelines.

- Take 1 capsule of desired Vitality oil 2 times daily.
- Take 2-3 drops of desired Vitality oil in a spoonful of syrup or small amount of milk, juice, or water.

Topical: Refer to Application Guidelines.

- Dilute 50:50 and apply 6-10 drops over stomach area 2 times daily.
- Apply a warm compress 1-2 times daily.
- Apply 1-3 drops on stomach Vita Flex points of feet.

Diarrhea

Diarrhea is the second most commonly reported illness in the U.S. and happens to nearly everyone. It may be caused by bacteria, viruses, food, medication, stress, or chronic medical conditions.

Recommendations

Singles: Ginger, Ginger Vitality, Oregano, Oregano Vitality, Ecuadorian Oregano, Mountain Savory, Mountain Savory Vitality, Clove, Clove Vitality, Jade Lemon, Jade Lemon Vitality, Lemon, Lemon Vitality, Lime, Lime Vitality, Peppermint, Peppermint Vitality, Nutmeg, Nutmeg Vitality, Wintergreen

Blends: DiGize, DiGize Vitality, JuvaFlex, JuvaFlex Vitality, Thieves, Thieves Roll-On, Thieves Vitality, AromaEase, KidScents TummyGize

Nutritionals: Life 9, KidScents MightyPro, ComforTone, Essentialzyme, Detoxzyme, Essentialzymes-4, Mega Vitamin Cal, Super Vitamin Cal Plus, Inner Defense, ICP, ImmuPro

Diarrhea Blend

- 4 drops Lemon or Lemon Vitality
- 3 drops Mountain Savory or Mountain Savory Vitality
- 2 drops Wintergreen

Application and Usage

Dietary and Oral: Refer to Application Guidelines.

- Take 1 capsule of desired Vitality oil 2 times daily.

- Take 2-3 drops of desired Vitality oil in a spoonful of syrup or small amount of milk, juice, or water.
- A maintenance dosage of ComforTone has helped to protect travelers going to other countries from diarrhea and other digestive discomforts.
- Nutmeg has been shown to have powerful action against diarrhea in a number of medical studies.

Topical: Refer to Application Guidelines.

- Apply 6-10 drops neat on stomach area as desired.
- Dilute 50:50 and apply on location 3-6 times daily.

- Place a warm compress with 1-2 drops of chosen oil on the back.

Constipation Causes Body Dysfunction

The reason constipation creates diverticulosis is because the muscles of the colon must strain to move an overly hard stool, which puts excess pressure on the colon. Eventually, weak spots in the colon walls form, creating abnormal pockets called diverticula.

These pockets can also be created by parasites that burrow and embed in the lining of the colon wall, lay eggs there, and leave waste matter that hardens on the colon walls, kinking and twisting the colon unnaturally. It is always wise to consider the possibility of parasites and their treatment when diverticula are present.

Enzymes such as Detoxzyme, Essentialzyme, Essentialzymes-4, Allerzyme, and KidScents MightyZyme (for children) are critical to help in the digestion and softening of waste material. ICP and JuvaPower add fiber that help scrub the colon wall, absorb toxins, and help with the elimination process. ParaFree is always a good cleanse at least once a year and certainly when parasites are suspected.

DIVERTICULOSIS/DIVERTICULITIS
(See also COLITIS, CROHN'S DISEASE)

Diverticulosis is one of the most common conditions in the U.S. and is caused by a lack of fiber in the diet. Diverticulosis is characterized by small, abnormal pockets (diverticula) that bulge out through weak spots in the wall of the intestine. It is estimated that half of all Americans from age 60 to 80 have diverticulosis.

Symptoms
- Cramping
- Bloating
- Constipation
- Fever and chills
- Cramping tenderness on lower left side of abdomen

One of the easiest ways to resolve this condition is by increasing fiber intake to 20-30 grams daily. Peppermint oil can also stimulate contractions in the colon.

While diverticulosis involves the condition of merely having colon abnormalities, diverticulitis occurs when these abnormalities or diverticula become infected or inflamed. Diverticulitis is present in 10-25 percent of people with diverticulosis.

Many of these symptoms are similar to those of irritable bowel syndrome.

Recommendations

Singles: Oregano, Oregano Vitality, Ecuadorian Oregano, Patchouli, Tarragon, Tarragon Vitality, Rosemary, Rosemary Vitality, Fennel, Fennel Vitality, Peppermint, Peppermint Vitality, Thyme, Thyme Vitality, Nutmeg, Nutmeg Vitality, Clove, Clove Vitality, Tangerine, Tangerine Vitality, Sacred Frankincense, Frankincense, Frankincense Vitality, Cedarwood

Blends: DiGize, DiGize Vitality, Melrose, Thieves, Thieves Roll-On, Thieves Vitality, Exodus II, ImmuPower

Nutritionals: AlkaLime, Detoxzyme, Inner Defense, Digest & Cleanse, ICP, ComforTone, Essentialzyme, Essentialzymes-4, Balance Complete, JuvaPower

Application and Usage

Aromatic: Refer to Application Guidelines

Dietary and Oral: Refer to Application Guidelines.

- Take 1 capsule of desired Vitality oil 2 times daily.

- Take 2-3 drops of desired Vitality oil in a spoonful of syrup or small amount of milk, juice, or water.

Topical: Refer to Application Guidelines.
- Dilute Diverticulitis Blend 50:50 and apply on lower abdomen 2 times daily.

- Massage 2-4 drops on the intestinal Vita Flex points on the feet 2-3 times daily.
- Retention: Rectal, nightly before retiring, retain overnight.

Diverticulitis Topical Blend
- 15 drops DiGize
- 5 drops Melrose

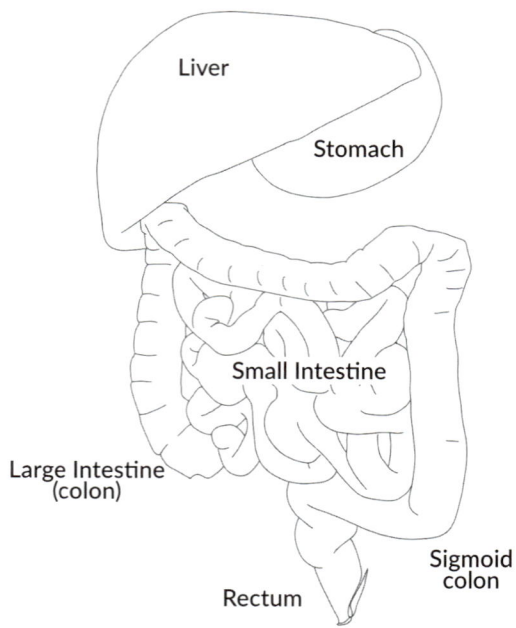

Gastrointestinal System

DYSENTERY

Dysentery is a serious disorder of the digestive tract that commonly occurs throughout the world. It can be caused by viruses, bacteria, protozoa, parasitic worms, or chemical irritation of the intestines.

It is one of the oldest known gastrointestinal disorders, often called the "bloody flux," that frequently occurred in army camps, in walled cities, aboard sailing vessels, and where large groups of people lived together with poor sanitation.

In the modern world, dysentery is most likely to affect people who live in less developed countries and travelers who visit those countries. It also affects immigrants from developing countries, people who live in housing with poor sanitation, military personnel serving in developing countries, people in nursing homes, and children in daycare centers.

Recommendations
Singles: Peppermint, Peppermint Vitality, Jade Lemon, Jade Lemon Vitality, Lemon, Lemon Vitality, Lime, Lime Vitality, Myrrh, Mountain Savory, Mountain Savory Vitality, Oregano, Oregano Vitality

Blends: Thieves, Thieves Roll-On, Thieves Vitality, DiGize, DiGize Vitality, JuvaCleanse, JuvaCleanse Vitality, JuvaFlex, JuvaFlex Vitality, KidScents TummyGize

Nutritionals: Inner Defense, Detoxzyme, ParaFree, Essentialzyme, Essentialzymes-4, ImmuPro, ICP, ComforTone, Mineral Essence, Life 9, KidScents MightyPro

Application and Usage
Aromatic: Refer to Application Guidelines.

Dietary and Oral: Refer to Application Guidelines.

- Take 1 capsule of desired Vitality oil 3 times daily.

- Take 2-3 drops of desired Vitality oil in a spoonful of syrup or small amount of milk, juice, or water.

Dysentery Blend
- 5 drops Thieves or Thieves Vitality
- 5 drops Peppermint or Peppermint Vitality

Topical: Refer to Application Guidelines.

GAS (FLATULENCE)

Gas (flatulence) can be caused by a lack of digestive enzymes and the consumption of indigestible starches and proteins that promote bifid bacteria production in the colon.

Although increasing bifid bacteria production can lead to gas, it is highly beneficial to long-term health, as the increase of beneficial flora crowds out disease-causing microorganisms such as Clostridium perfringens (a common cause of food poisoning).

Consumption of FOS (fructooligosaccharides), an indigestible sugar, can create short-term flatulence, even as it drastically improves bifidobacteria production in the small and large intestines and increases mineral absorption.

Recommendations

Singles: Carrot Seed, Carrot Seed Vitality, Peppermint, Peppermint Vitality, Nutmeg, Nutmeg Vitality, Oregano, Oregano Vitality, Ecuadorian Oregano, Thyme, Thyme Vitality, Clove, Clove Vitality, Ginger, Ginger Vitality, Cumin, Fennel, Fennel Vitality

Blends: DiGize, DiGize Vitality, Thieves, Thieves Roll-On, Thieves Vitality, Longevity, Longevity Vitality, KidScents TummyGize

Nutritionals: AlkaLime, Detoxzyme, Life 9, KidScents MightyPro, Digest & Cleanse, ICP, ComforTone, Essentialzyme, Essentialzymes-4, Inner Defense, JuvaPower, ImmuPro, Longevity Softgels

Application and Usage

Aromatic: Refer to Application Guidelines.

Dietary and Oral: Refer to Application Guidelines.

- Take 1 capsule of desired Vitality oil 2 times daily.

- Take 2-3 drops of desired Vitality oil in a spoonful of syrup or small amount of milk, juice, or water.

Topical: Refer to Application Guidelines.

GIARDIA

Giardia is a microscopic parasite found on surfaces or in soil, water, or food that has been contaminated with feces from infected animals or humans. It is most commonly transmitted in polluted water.

Recommendations

Singles: Basil, Basil Vitality, Patchouli, Peppermint, Peppermint Vitality, Spearmint, Spearmint Vitality

Blends: DiGize, DiGize Vitality, JuvaCleanse, JuvaCleanse Vitality, Melrose, Purification, KidScents TummyGize

Nutritionals: Detoxzyme, ParaFree, Essentialzyme, Digest & Cleanse, Mineral Essence, Essentialzymes-4

Application and Usage

Dietary and Oral: Refer to Application Guidelines.

- Take 1 capsule of desired Vitality oil 2 times daily.

- Take 10 drops of Basil Vitality, Peppermint Vitality, DiGize Vitality, or other oils desired diluted 50:50 in a capsule every 2 hours.

- Take 2-3 drops of desired Vitality oil in a spoonful of syrup or small amount of milk, juice, or water.

HEARTBURN

Heartburn is a burning feeling or pain in the center of the chest that may extend into your back or neck during or after eating.

Lemon juice is one of the best remedies for heartburn. Mix the juice of ½ of a squeezed lemon in 8 ounces of water and sip slowly upon awakening each morning.

Lemon juice helps the stomach stop making digestive acids, therefore alleviating heartburn or other stomach ailments.

Recommendations

Singles: Basil, Basil Vitality, Fennel, Fennel Vitality, Spearmint, Spearmint Vitality, Ginger, Ginger Vitality, Jade Lemon, Jade Lemon Vitality, Lemon, Lemon Vitality, Lime, Lime Vitality, Palo Santo, Cypress, Tarragon, Tarragon Vitality, Sage, Sage Vitality, Royal Hawaiian Sandalwood, Sacred Sandalwood

Blends: DiGize, DiGize Vitality, JuvaCleanse, JuvaCleanse Vitality, Citrus Fresh, Citrus Fresh Vitality, KidScents TummyGize

Nutritionals: AlkaLime, ICP, ComforTone, Essentialzymes-4, Detoxzyme, Allerzyme

Application and Usage

Aromatic: Refer to Application Guidelines.

Dietary and Oral: Refer to Application Guidelines.

- Take 1 capsule of desired Vitality oil 2 times daily.

- Take 2-3 drops of desired Vitality oil in a spoonful of syrup or small amount of milk, juice, or water.

Heartburn Blend
- 8 drops Sage or Sage Vitality
- 3 drops Royal Hawaiian Sandalwood or Sacred Sandalwood
- 2 drops Basil or Basil Vitality
- 1 drop Palo Santo

Topical: Refer to Application Guidelines.
- Dilute 50:50 and apply on location 3-6 times daily.

- Place a warm compress with 1-3 drops of recommended oils over stomach.
- Apply recommended oils to the Vita Flex points of the feet.

INDIGESTION (BLOATING)

Indigestion causes discomfort in the upper abdomen, resulting in bloating, belching, and nausea. It often occurs during or right after eating and is medically known as dyspepsia.

Recommendations
Singles: Peppermint, Peppermint Vitality, Nutmeg, Nutmeg Vitality, Fennel, Fennel Vitality, Ginger, Ginger Vitality, Cumin, Spearmint, Spearmint Vitality, Lemon Verbena, Grapefruit, Grapefruit Vitality, Davana, Copaiba, Copaiba Vitality, Wintergreen

Blends: DiGize, DiGize Vitality, JuvaCleanse, JuvaCleanse Vitality, KidScents TummyGize

Nutritionals: AlkaLime, Detoxzyme, ICP, ComforTone, JuvaPower, Essentialzyme, Essentialzymes-4, Mineral Essence, Allerzyme

Application and Usage
Dietary and Oral: Refer to Application Guidelines.

- Take 1 capsule of desired Vitality oil 2 times daily.

- Take 2-3 drops of desired Vitality oil in a spoonful of syrup or small amount of milk, juice, or water.

- Take 2-4 capsules of Essentialzymes-4, Essentialzyme, or Detoxzyme before eating to help with digestion and upset stomach.

- When the stomach feels "heavy" from eating meat, Essentialzymes-4 is a beneficial companion to DiGize Vitality (See Chapter 18, . . . BUILDING BLOCKS . . .).

Topical: Refer to Application Guidelines.
- Dilute 50:50 and apply on location 3-6 times daily.

- Place a warm compress with 1-3 drops of recommended oil over the stomach.

SPASTIC COLON SYNDROME/ IRRITABLE BOWEL SYNDROME

Spastic colon syndrome, often called irritable bowel syndrome, is a functional disorder where the bowel does not work as it should. It is characterized by constipation, diarrhea, gas, bloating, lower abdominal pain or discomfort, and nausea.

Singles: Fennel, Fennel Vitality

Blends: DiGize, DiGize Vitality, AromaEase

Nutritionals: AlkaLime, Essentialzymes-4, Life 9, KidScents MightyPro, Mineral Essence, NingXia Red, Slique Tea

Application and Usage
Aromatic: Refer to Application Guidelines.

Dietary and Oral: Refer to Application Guidelines.

- Take 1 capsule of desired Vitality oil 2 times daily.

- Take 2-3 drops of desired Vitality oil in a spoonful of syrup or small amount of milk, juice, or water.

Topical: Refer to Application Guidelines.
- Dilute 50:50 and apply on location 3-6 times daily.

- Place a warm compress with 1-3 drops of recommended oils over stomach.
- Apply recommended oils to the Vita Flex points of the feet.

STOMACHACHE

The term "stomachache" is used for many types of stomach or other abdominal discomfort. Some of the following symptoms may occur: pain before or after eating, bloating, heartburn, flatulence, feeling full, vomiting, loss of appetite, etc.

Personal Usage Guide | Chapter 15

Recommendations

Singles: Peppermint, Peppermint Vitality, Roman Chamomile, Lavender, Lavender Vitality, Blue Tansy, Cedarwood, Marjoram, Marjoram Vitality, Rose, Royal Hawaiian Sandalwood, Sacred Sandalwood, Sacred Frankincense, Frankincense, Frankincense Vitality, Valerian

Blends: DiGize, DiGize Vitality, KidScents TummyGize, Trauma Life, Humility, Harmony, RutaVaLa, RutaVaLa Roll-On, Valor, Valor Roll-On, Peace & Calming, Peace & Calming II, Calm CBD Roll-On, Seedlings Calm, Tranquil Roll-On

Nutritionals: Super Vitamin B, Super Vitamin C, MultiGreens, Mega Vitamin Cal, Mineral Essence, OmegaGize3, Alka-Lime, Life 9, KidScents MightyPro

Application and Usage

Aromatic: Refer to Application Guidelines.

Dietary and Oral: Refer to Application Guidelines.

 • Take 1 capsule of desired Vitality oil 2 times daily.

 • Take 2-3 drops of desired Vitality oil in a spoonful of syrup or small amount of milk, juice, or water.

Topical: Refer to Application Guidelines.

- Apply any of the desired oils diluted 50:50 on stomach area 2 times daily or as needed.
- Add desired oil to bath salts and incorporate into daily bathing.

STOMACH ULCERS

Ulcers may be caused by several gastroduodenal diseases such as gastritis or gastric or peptic ulcers caused by the Helicobacter pylori bacteria. While antibiotics are prescribed, plant sources will also kill these bacteria. Regarding phytochemicals against Helicobacter pylori infections, a 2018 study28 in the International Journal of Molecular Sciences stated, "in this critical review, plant sources used as effective antibacterial agents are carefully described." Myrtle essential oil has been shown to be effective against H. pylori.29

Recommendations

Singles: Lemongrass, Lemongrass Vitality, Copaiba, Copaiba Vitality, Jade Lemon, Jade Lemon Vitality, Lemon, Lemon Vitality, Lime, Lime Vitality, Myrtle, German Chamomile, German Chamomile Vitality, Davana, Myrrh, Patchouli, Peppermint, Peppermint Vitality

Blends: Thieves, Thieves Roll-On, Thieves Vitality, DiGize, DiGize Vitality, Melrose

Nutritionals: Digest & Cleanse, Inner Defense, ICP, JuvaPower, AlkaLime, Essentialzymes-4, Essentialzyme

Application and Usage

Aromatic: Refer to Application Guidelines.

Dietary and Oral: Refer to Application Guidelines.

 • Take 1 capsule of desired Vitality oil 3 times daily for 20 days.

 • Take 2-3 drops of desired Vitality oil in a spoonful of syrup or small amount of milk, juice, or water.

Topical: Refer to Application Guidelines.

Any calming oil or blend applied through massage may help to decrease stress and bring a relaxing atmosphere: Lavender, Tranquil Roll-On, Dream Catcher, Gathering, Egyptian Gold, The Gift, Peace & Calming, Peace & Calming II, Calm CBD Roll-On, Seedlings Calm, Stress Away, Stress Away Roll-On, Harmony, Inner Child, White Angelica, etc.

DIPHTHERIA

Diphtheria is an acute infectious disease caused by toxigenic strains of Corynebacterium diphtheriae, acquired by contact with an infected person or carrier. It is usually confined to the upper respiratory tract and characterized by the formation of a tough, false membrane attached firmly to the underlying tissue that will bleed if forcibly removed.

In the most serious infections, the membrane begins in the tonsil area and may spread to the uvula, soft palate, and pharyngeal wall, followed by the larynx, trachea, and bronchial tree, where it may cause life-threatening bronchial obstructions. See your health care professional.

Recommendations

Singles: Oregano, Oregano Vitality, Ecuadorian Oregano, Thyme, Thyme Vitality, Clove, Clove Vitality, Mountain Savory, Mountain Savory Vitality, Eucalyptus Radiata, Palo Santo, Northern Lights Black Spruce, Sacred Frankincense, Frankincense, Frankincense Vitality, Eucalyptus Blue, Spearmint, Spearmint Vitality, Ravintsara,

Cassia, Peppermint, Peppermint Vitality, Dorado Azul

Blends: Thieves, Thieves Roll-On, Thieves Vitality, Melrose, Exodus II, Raven, R.C.

Nutritionals: Inner Defense, ImmuPro, NingXia Red

Oral Care: Thieves Fresh Essence Plus Mouthwash, Thieves Cough Drops, Thieves Spray, Thieves Hard Lozenges

Personal Care: Thieves Chest Rub

Household Care: Thieves Household Cleaner, Thieves Waterless Hand Purifier, Thieves Foaming Hand Soap, Thieves Automatic Dishwasher Powder, Thieves Cleansing Soap, Thieves Dish Soap, Thieves Fruit & Veggie Soak (and Spray), Thieves Laundry Soap, Thieves Spray, Thieves Wipes

Application and Usage

Aromatic: Refer to Application Guidelines.

Dietary and Oral: Refer to Application Guidelines.

- Take 1 capsule of desired Vitality oil 2 times daily.

- Take 2-3 drops of desired Vitality oil in a spoonful of syrup or small amount of milk, juice, or water.

- Gargle with Thieves Fresh Essence Plus Mouthwash several times daily.
- Spray throat as desired with Thieves Spray.
- Use Thieves Cough Drops and/or Thieves Hard Lozenges as desired.

Topical: Refer to Application Guidelines.

- Applying a single drop under the nose is helpful and refreshing.

- Apply 2-3 drops over neck and lung areas several times daily.

DIZZINESS

Feeling dizzy is not an illness but a symptom of something else. Light headedness is often caused by a decrease in blood supply to the brain, while vertigo may be caused by an imbalance in the inner ear or brain. Dizziness may also be caused by dehydration or heat stroke.

Recommendations

Singles: Peppermint, Peppermint Vitality, Eucalyptus Blue, Dorado Azul, Tangerine, Tangerine Vitality, Basil, Basil Vitality, Cardamom, Cardamom Vitality, Melaleuca Quinquenervia (Niaouli), Sacred Sandalwood, Royal Hawaiian Sandal-wood, Sacred Frankincense, Frankincense, Frankincense Vitality, Idaho Blue Spruce

Blends: Clarity, R.C., Brain Power, Common Sense, KidScents GeneYus, M-Grain, Grounding, Citrus Fresh, Citrus Fresh Vitality, Harmony

Nutritionals: MindWise, NingXia Red, MultiGreens, Master Formula, Mega Vitamin Cal, Mineral Essence

Application and Usage

Aromatic: Refer to Application Guidelines.

Dietary and Oral: Refer to Application Guidelines.

- Take 1 capsule of desired Vitality oil 2 times daily.

- Take 2-3 drops of desired Vitality oil in a spoonful of syrup or small amount of milk, juice, or water.

Topical: Refer to Application Guidelines.

- Apply 1-2 drops neat (undiluted) on temples and back of neck, as desired.

- Applying a single drop under the nose is helpful.

- Massage 2-4 drops of oil neat on the bottoms of the feet.

EAR PROBLEMS

Although ear problems are often caused by infections, other conditions may also cause ear pain or discomfort.

Earache

Earaches result from inflammation and swelling of the structures that make up the ear and have a multitude of causes and a variety of symptoms.

Recommendations

Singles: Helichrysum, Lavender, Lavender Vitality, Tea Tree, Roman Chamomile, Ravintsara, Peppermint, Peppermint Vitality, Eucalyptus Radiata, Frankincense, Frankincense Vitality, Sacred Frankincense, Basil, Basil Vitality

Blends: Purification, PanAway, ImmuPower, Melrose

Nutritionals: ImmuPro, Super Vitamin C, Super Vitamin C Chewable, Inner Defense, Thieves Spray

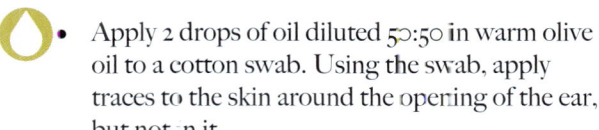

Application and Usage

Aromatic: Refer to Application Guidelines.

Dietary and Oral: Refer to Application Guidelines.

- Take 1 capsule of desired Vitality oil 2 times daily.

- Take 2-3 drops of desired Vitality oil in a spoonful of syrup or small amount of milk, juice, or water.

- Gargle up to 8 times daily with Thieves Fresh Essence Plus Mouthwash.

- Spray Thieves Spray into the throat up to 5 times daily.

Topical: Refer to Application Guidelines.

- Apply 2 drops of oil diluted 50:50 in warm olive or fractionated coconut oil to a cotton swab. Using the swab, apply traces to the skin around the opening of the ear, but not in it. Put 2-3 drops of the diluted essential oil on a piece of cotton and place it carefully over the ear opening. Leave in overnight.

- Additional relief may be obtained by placing a warm compress over the ear.

- Massage 1-2 drops on ears and earlobes using the Vita Flex Technique and on the Vita Flex points for the ear on the feet.

CAUTION: Never put essential oils directly into the ear canal. Ear pain can be very serious. Always seek medical attention if pain persists.

Ear Infection

An ear infection often occurs in conjunction with other symptoms, which may vary in character and intensity in different individuals. The bacteria Pseudomonas aeruginosa is a common cause of ear infections with biofilm production that stops most antibiotics. A 2016 study30 showed sage essential oil caused 81.8 percent lower P. aeruginosa biofilm production, while basil essential oil showed a reduction of 63.6 percent.

Recommendations

Singles: Sage, Sage Vitality, Basil, Basil Vitality, Myrrh, Thyme, Thyme Vitality, Wintergreen, Helichrysum, Davana, Mountain Savory, Mountain Savory Vitality

Blends: ImmuPower, Melrose, Thieves, Thieves Roll-On, Thieves Vitality, Purification, Exodus II

Nutritionals: ImmuPro, Inner Defense

Application and Usage

Aromatic: Refer to Application Guidelines.

Topical: Refer to Application Guidelines.

- Put Basil on the outer ear when you feel an ear infection coming on. Just the aromatic fumes will kill an ear infection.

- Apply 2 drops of oil diluted 50:50 in warm olive oil to a cotton swab. Using the swab, apply traces to the skin around the opening of the ear, but not in it.

- Put 2-3 drops of the diluted essential oil on a piece of cotton and place it carefully over the ear opening. Leave on overnight.

CAUTION: Never put essential oils directly into the ear. Ear pain can be very serious. Always seek medical attention if pain persists.

Hearing Impairment

Hearing impairment refers to people with either partial or full hearing loss.

Recommendations

Singles: Helichrysum, Juniper, Geranium, Peppermint, Lavender, Basil

Blends: Purification, Surrender, Awaken, Magnify Your Purpose

Application and Usage

Aromatic: Refer to Application Guidelines.

Topical: Refer to Application Guidelines

- Apply single oils or Blends neat or diluted, depending on the oils that are used.

- Apply 1 drop neat on a cotton ball and place it carefully in the opening of the ear canal. Retain overnight. DO NOT place oils directly in the ear canal.

- Massage 1-2 drops of oil neat on each earlobe, behind the ears, and down the jaw line along the Eustachian tube.

Hearing Vita Flex Regimen

- Apply 1-2 drops neat of Helichrysum on the area outside the opening to the ear canal with fingertip or cotton swab. DO NOT put oil inside the ear canal.

- After applying the Helichrysum, hold earlobes firmly and pull in a circular motion 10 times to help stimulate absorption and circulation in the ear canal.

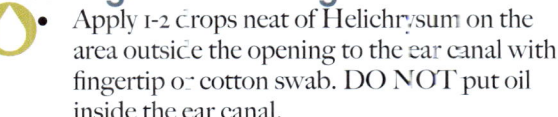

Ear

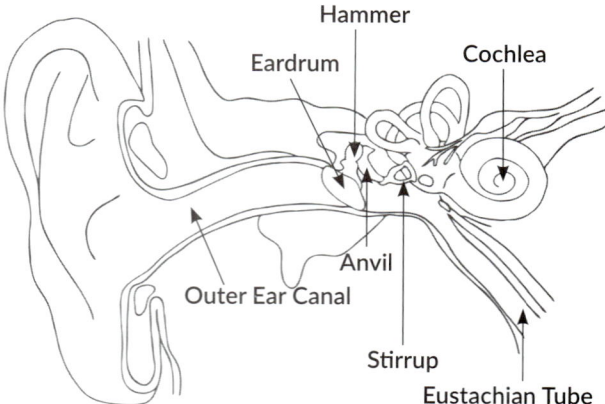

Tinnitus (Ringing in the Ears)

Tinnitus is a sound in one or both ears like buzzing, whistling, or ringing and occurs without an external stimulus, although it may be caused or partially caused by a buildup of earwax.

Recommendations

Singles: Helichrysum, Juniper, Geranium, Rose, Peppermint, Peppermint Vitality, Lavender, Lavender Vitality, Basil, Basil Vitality

Blends: Purification

Nutritionals: NingXia Red, Detoxzyme, Sulfurzyme

Application and Usage

Aromatic: Refer to Application Guidelines.

Topical: Refer to Application Guidelines.

- Massage 1-2 drops neat on temples, forehead, and back of neck.

- Apply 1 drop each on tips of the toes and fingers so that the oils get into the Vita Flex pathways.

Hearing Vita Flex Regimen:

- Apply 1-2 drops neat of Helichrysum to the area outside the opening to the ear canal with fingertip or cotton swab. DO NOT put oil inside the ear canal.
- After applying Helichrysum, hold earlobes firmly and pull in a circular motion 10 times to help stimulate absorption and circulation in the ear canal.

EATING DISORDERS (See also ADDICTIONS)

Eating disorders are serious psychological conditions that generally involve negative, self-critical feelings and thoughts about body weight, size, and shape. They involve eating habits that disrupt daily activities and normal body functions.

Anorexia Nervosa

Anorexia nervosa is an eating disorder characterized by total avoidance of food and virtual self-starvation. It may or may not be accompanied by bulimia (binge-purge behavior).

While psychotherapy remains indispensable, the aroma of essential oils may alter emotions enough to effect a change in the underlying psychology or disturbed-thinking patterns that support this self-destructive behavior. This is accomplished by the ability of aroma to directly stimulate the amygdala gland, which is part of the emotional center of the brain known as the limbic system.

Many essential oils such as Lemon and Ginger when inhaled regularly can combat the emotional addiction that leads anorexics to premature death.

Many people with anorexia believe they do not deserve to be healthy or loved unless they are "slender."

Many people who are anorexic suffer life-threatening nutrient and mineral deficiencies. The lack of magnesium and potassium can actually trigger heart rhythm abnormalities and cardiac arrest. It is absolutely essential that calcium, magnesium, potassium, and other mineral deficiencies are replenished.

Recommendations

Singles: Lemon, Lemon Vitality, Jade Lemon, Jade Lemon Vitality, Ginger, Ginger Vitality, Lime, Lime Vitality, Tangerine, Tangerine Vitality, Cassia, Vanilla, Mandarin

Blends: Release, Freedom, Reconnect, Gary's Light, Valor, Valor Roll-On, Motivation, Journey On, Brain Power, Stress Away, Stress Away Roll-On, One Heart, KidScents KidPower, KidScents KidPower Roll-On

Nutritionals: Mineral Essence, Balance Complete, Mega Vitamin Cal, MindWise, Slique Shake, Slique Bars, Essentialzyme, Essentialzymes-4, OmegaGize3, Slique Bars–Chocolate-Coated, Chocolate-Coated Wolfberry Crisp Bars

Application and Usage

Aromatic: Refer to Application Guidelines.

Dietary and Oral

- Refer to Application Guidelines.
- Take 1 capsule of desired Vitality oil 2 times daily.

- Take 2-3 drops of desired Vitality oil in a spoonful of syrup or small amount of milk, juice, or water.

Topical: Refer to Application Guidelines.

Appetite, Loss of

Ginger has been shown to stimulate digestion and improve appetite.

Recommendations

Singles: Ginger, Ginger Vitality, Spearmint, Spearmint Vitality, Orange, Orange Vitality, Nutmeg, Nutmeg Vitality, Peppermint, Peppermint Vitality, Cassia, Lemon Verbena

Blends: Gary's Light, One Heart, Citrus Fresh, Citrus Fresh Vitality, Christmas Spirit, RutaVaLa, RutaVaLa Roll-On, KidScents TummyGize, DiGize, DiGize Vitality

Nutritionals: Essentialzyme, Essentialzymes-4, ComforTone, Mega Vitamin Cal, Mineral Essence, NingXia Red, Slique Bars, Wolfberry Crisp Bars

Application and Usage

Aromatic: Refer to Application Guidelines.

Dietary and Oral: Refer to Application Guidelines.

- Take 1 capsule with DiGize Vitality or other desired oil 2 times daily.

- Take 2-3 drops of desired Vitality oil in a spoonful of syrup or small amount of milk, juice, or water.

Topical: Refer to Application Guidelines.

- Apply 5-6 drops with massage oil 3-5 times daily or as needed.
- You may also apply 2-3 drops on the Vita Flex points on the feet.

- Applying a single drop under the nose is helpful and refreshing.

Binge Eating Disorder

Binge eating disorder is characterized by the binge eater consuming unnaturally large amounts of food in a short period of time, which acts as a psychological release for excessive emotional stress. However, unlike a bulimic, the binge eater does not usually engage in excessive exercise, vomiting, or taking laxatives to reduce weight.

Singles: Sacred Frankincense, Frankincense, Frankincense Vitality, Cassia, Peppermint, Peppermint Vitality, Vanilla

Blends: Release, Freedom, Reconnect, Gary's Light, One Heart, 3 Wise Men, KidScents KidPower, KidScents KidPower Roll-On

Nutritionals: Slique Tea, Slique Bars, Slique Bars-Chocolate-Coated, Chocolate-Coated Wolfberry Crisp Bars, Slique Essence, Slique Gum, NingXia Red

Application and Usage

Aromatic: Refer to Application Guidelines.

Dietary and Oral: Refer to Application Guidelines.

- Take 1 capsule of desired Vitality oil 2 times daily.

- Take 2-3 drops of desired Vitality oil in a spoonful of syrup or small amount of milk, juice, or water.

Topical: Refer to Application Guidelines.

Bulimia

Bulimia is characterized by habitual binge eating and then purging.

Singles: Idaho Grand Fir, Fennel, Fennel Vitality, Nutmeg, Nutmeg Vitality, Cassia

Blends: Gary's Light, Common Sense, One Heart, DiGize, DiGize Vitality, Forgiveness, KidScents KidPower, KidScents KidPower Roll-On

Nutritionals: Slique Tea, Slique CitraSlim Caps, Slique Essence, Slique Bars, Slique Bars-Chocolate-Coated, NingXia Red

Chocolate-Coated Wolfberry Crisp Bars, Slique Gum

Application and Usage

Aromatic: Refer to Application Guidelines.

Dietary and Oral: Refer to Application Guidelines.

- Take 1 capsule of desired Vitality oil 2 times daily.

- Take 2-3 drops of desired Vitality oil in a spoonful of syrup or small amount of milk, juice, or water.

Topical: Refer to Application Guidelines.

EDEMA (SWELLING) (See also CARDIOVASCULAR CONDITIONS and PROBLEMS, PHLEBITIS . . .)

Swelling, particularly around the ankles, is noticeable when fluids accumulate in the tissue. This puffiness under the skin and around the ankles is more apparent at the end of the day when fluids settle to the lowest part of the body. A potassium deficiency can make swelling worse, so the first recourse is to increase potassium intake.

Recommendations

Singles: Fennel, Fennel Vitality, Juniper, German Chamomile, German Chamomile Vitality, Peppermint, Peppermint Vitality, Lavender, Lavender Vitality, Grapefruit, Grapefruit Vitality, Helichrysum, Cassia, Tangerine, Tangerine Vitality, Patchouli, Geranium, Cypress, Wintergreen

Blends: Aroma Life, EndoFlex, EndoFlex Vitality, DiGize, DiGize Vitality, CBD

Nutritionals: Digest & Cleanse, Super Vitamin C, Super Vitamin C Chewable, ICP, JuvaPower, Essentialzyme, Essentialzymes-4, Olive Essentials, Detoxzyme, Life 9, KidScents MightyPro, Mega Vitamin Cal, Balance Complete

Application and Usage

Dietary and Oral: Refer to Application Guidelines.

- Take 1 capsule of desired Vitality oil 2 times daily.

- Take 2-3 drops of desired Vitality oil in a spoonful of syrup or small amount of milk, juice, or water.

Topical: Refer to Application Guidelines.

- Apply 1-3 drops diluted 50:50 on affected area 2-3 times daily.

- Place a cold compress with 1-2 drops of chosen oil 1-2 times daily on the area.

- Massage 1-3 drops on bladder Vita Flex point on foot.

- Massage 15-20 drops of the Topical Edema Blend diluted 60:40 in V-6 Vegetable Oil Complex or other massage oil on legs, working from the feet up to the thighs. Do this for 1 week.

- Massage 15-20 drops of Morning Edema Blend diluted 60:40 in V-6 Vegetable Oil Complex or other massage oil on legs, working from the feet up to the thighs. Do this in the morning for 1 week. Repeat the same process in the evening with the Evening Edema Blend.

Edema Topical Blend (General)
- 10 drops Wintergreen
- 8 drops Tangerine
- 6 drops Fennel
- 4 drops Juniper
- 3 drops Patchouli

Edema Topical Blend (Morning)
- 10 drops Tangerine
- 10 drops Cypress

Edema Topical Blend (Evening)
- 8 drops Geranium
- 5 drops Cypress
- 5 drops Helichrysum or Grapefruit

EMOTIONAL TRAUMA

The effect of heavy emotional trauma can disrupt the stomach and digestive system.

Recommendations

Singles: Sacred Frankincense, Frankincense, Frankincense Vitality, Idaho Blue Spruce, Idaho Grand Fir, Jade Lemon, Jade Lemon Vitality, Lemon, Lemon Vitality, Lime, Lime Vitality, Cassia, German Chamomile, German Chamomile Vitality, Rose, Lavender, Lavender Vitality, Marjoram, Marjoram Vitality, Spearmint, Spearmint Vitality, Peppermint, Peppermint Vitality, Vanilla, Valerian, Vetiver

Blends: Release, Freedom, Reconnect, Gary's Light, Fulfill Your Destiny, Trauma Life, Hope, Build Your Dream, Inner Child, Present Time, Valor, Valor Roll-On, Sacred Mountain, Christmas Spirit, 3 Wise Men, Tranquil Roll-On, Stress Away, Stress Away Roll-On, One Heart, Harmony, KidScents KidPower, KidScents KidPower Roll-On, Forgiveness, Amoressence, Peace & Calming, Peace & Calming II, Calm CBD Roll-On, Seedlings Calm, White Angelica, The Gift, Grounding

Nutritionals: Thyromin, KidScents Unwind, Master Formula, EndoGize, PD 80/20

Application and Usage

Aromatic: Refer to Application Guidelines.

Dietary and Oral: Refer to Application Guidelines.

- Take 1 capsule of desired Vitality oil 2 times daily.

- Take 2-3 drops of oil in a spoonful of syrup or small amount of milk, juice, or water.

Topical: Refer to Application Guidelines.

- Place 1-3 drops of Release over the thymus and rub in gently. Apply up to 3 times daily as needed.

- Blend equal parts Frankincense and Valor and apply 1-2 drops neat on temples, forehead, crown, and back of neck before retiring. Use for 3 nights.

- Apply 1-2 drops neat to the crown of head and forehead as needed. It is best if it is applied in a quiet, darkened room.

- Massage 1-3 drops on heart Vita Flex points 2-3 times daily.

- Rub 1-2 drops of oil on the temples and back of neck several times daily.

ENDOCRINE SYSTEM PROBLEMS
(See also THYROID PROBLEMS; ADRENAL GLAND DISORDERS; CUSHING'S SYNDROME (DISEASE); MALE HORMONE IMBALANCE; MENSTRUAL AND FEMALE HORMONE CONDITIONS)

The endocrine system encompasses the hormone-producing glands of the body. These glands cluster around blood vessels and release their hormones directly into the bloodstream. The pituitary gland exerts a wide range of control over the hormonal (endocrine) system and is often called the master gland. Other glands include the pancreas, adrenals, thyroid, parathyroid, ovaries, and testes.

The limbic system lies along the margin of the cerebral cortex (brain) and is the hormone-producing system of the brain. It includes the amygdala, hippocampus, pineal, pituitary, thalamus, and hypothalamus.

Essential oils increase circulation to the brain and enable the pituitary and other glands to better secrete neural transmitters and hormones that support the endocrine and immune systems.

The thyroid is one of the most important glands for regulating the body systems. The hypothalamus plays an even more important role, since it regulates not only the thyroid but also the adrenals and the pituitary gland.

Recommendations
Singles: Myrtle, Sacred Frankincense, Frankincense, Frankincense Vitality, Fennel, Fennel Vitality, Idaho Blue Spruce, Sage, Sage Vitality

Blends: EndoFlex, EndoFlex Vitality, Harmony, The Gift, Shutran

Nutritionals: Thyromin, CortiStop, Super Vitamin B, NingXia Red, Master Formula

Application and Usage
Aromatic: Refer to Application Guidelines.

Topical: Refer to Application Guidelines.

- Massage 2-4 drops on brain Vita Flex points on feet 2-3 times daily.

EPILEPSY

Note: Epileptics should consult their health care professional before using essential oils. Use extreme caution with high ketone oils such as Basil, Rosemary, and Sage.

Recommendations
Singles: Clary Sage, Royal Hawaiian Sandalwood, Sacred Sandalwood, Cedarwood, Sacred Frankincense, Frankincense, Frankincense Vitality, Lavender, Lavender Vitality

Blends: Valor, Valor Roll-On, Brain Power, KidScents GeneYus, RutaVaLa, RutaVaLa Roll-On, Common Sense, Peace & Calming, Peace & Calming II, Calm CBD Roll-On, Seedlings Calm

Nutritionals: MindWise, ICP, ComforTone, Essentialzyme, Essentialzymes-4, Life 9, KidScents MightyPro, NingXia Red, JuvaPower, KidScents Unwind, Master Formula, Super Vitamin B

Application and Usage
Aromatic: Refer to Application Guidelines

Topical: Refer to Application Guidelines.

- Massage 2-4 drops on brain Vita Flex points on feet 2-3 times daily.

EPSTEIN-BARR VIRUS

Epstein-Barr virus is a type of herpes virus that also causes mononucleosis.

Symptoms include indigestion, upper and lower gas, poor assimilation, poor electrolyte balance, allergic reaction to foods and other substances, emotional mood swings, fatigue, irritability, and a lack of motivation, discipline, and creativity.

Hypoglycemia is a precursor and can render the body susceptible to the Epstein-Barr virus. Treat the hypoglycemia, and the symptoms of the Epstein-Barr virus may begin to disappear.

Recommendations

Singles: Melissa, Palo Santo, Mountain Savory, Mountain Savory Vitality, Oregano, Oregano Vitality, Ecuadorian Oregano, Rosemary, Rosemary Vitality, Thyme, Thyme Vitality, Clove, Clove Vitality, Sacred Sandalwood, Royal Hawaiian Sandal-wood, Northern Lights Black Spruce, Grapefruit, Grapefruit Vitality, Nutmeg, Nutmeg Vitality, Tea Tree, Lemon Verbena, Cassia, Sage, Sage Vitality

Blends: Exodus II, Melrose, Thieves, Thieves Roll-On, Thieves Vitality, ImmuPower, EndoFlex, EndoFlex Vitality, Longevity, Longevity Vitality, KidScents TummyGize, DiGize, DiGize Vitality

Nutritionals: Inner Defense, Super Vitamin C, Super Vitamin C Chewable, ImmuPro, Thyromin, Detoxzyme, Digest & Cleanse, ICP, JuvaPower, ComforTone, Essentialzyme, Allerzyme, Life 9, KidScents MightyPro, Essentialzymes-4, Master Formula

Application and Usage

Aromatic: Refer to Application Guidelines.

Dietary and Oral: Whether putting the Vitality oils in a capsule or drinking them in a liquid, please refer to Application Guidelines.

- Take 1 capsule of desired Vitality oil 3 times daily.

- Take 2-3 drops of desired Vitality oil in a spoonful of syrup or small amount of milk, juice, or water.

Epstein Barr Regimen

- 1 capsule Exodus II 3 times a day, preferably with food
- 1 capsule Melrose 3 times a day, preferably with food
- 3 Life 9 or 3 MightyPro 1 time a day
- 5-day Nutritive Cleanse (2 or 3 times)

Diet:
- Absolutely no sugar. Fruit, honey, and stevia are fine.
- No white flour. No GMO whole wheat flour. Use Einkorn products.
- Drink veggie juices
- Drink lots of water
- Follow for 3 to 4 months.

Topical: Refer to Application Guidelines.

- Receive a Raindrop Technique weekly with ImmuPower, Thieves, Thieves Roll-On, Exodus II, and the oils of Raindrop Technique.

- Massage 2-4 drops of oil neat on the bottoms of the feet just before bedtime.

MONONUCLEOSIS

Infectious mononucleosis is a disease caused by the Epstein-Barr virus (EBV), which is a type of herpes virus. The symptoms usually last for four weeks or more. The spleen enlarges and may even rupture in severe cases.

Recommendations

Singles: Ravintsara, Hyssop, Clove, Clove Vitality, Melissa, Thyme, Thyme Vitality, Sacred Frankincense, Northern Lights Black Spruce, Frankincense, Frankincense Vitality, Cassia, Palo Santo, Mountain Savory, Mountain Savory Vitality

Blends: Thieves, Thieves Roll-On, Thieves Vitality, Inner Defense, R.C., Breathe Again, Breathe Again Roll-On, Raven, Exodus II, ImmuPower

Nutritionals: ImmuPro, Super Vitamin C, Super Vitamin C Chewable, Longevity Softgels, ICP, ComforTone, Essentialzyme, Essentialzymes-4, Detoxzyme, Life 9, KidScents MightyPro

Application and Usage

Aromatic: Refer to Application Guidelines.

Dietary and Oral: Refer to Application Guidelines.

- Take 1 capsule of desired Vitality oil 3 times daily.

- Take 2-3 drops of desired Vitality oil in a spoonful of syrup or small amount of milk, juice, or water.

Mononucleosis Blend
- 3 drops Thieves or Thieves Vitality
- 3 drops Thyme or Thyme Vitality
- 3 drops Mountain Savory or Mountain Savory Vitality
- 2 drops Ravintsara

Topical: Refer to Application Guidelines.
- Receive a Raindrop Technique 2 times weekly.

- Massage 3-6 drops using the Vita Flex technique on the bottoms of feet 2 times daily

Endocrine System

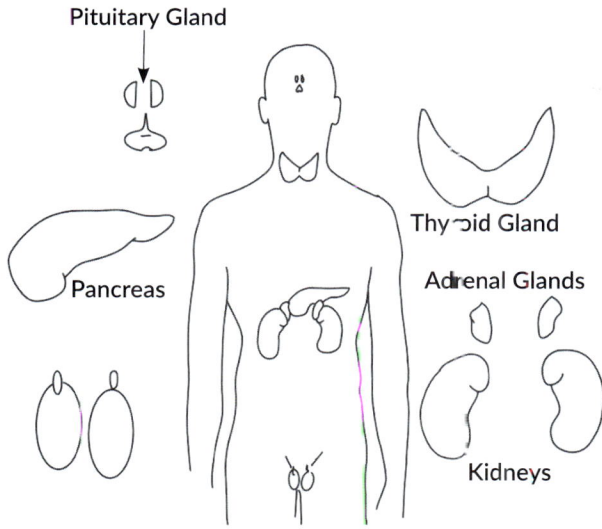

EYE DISORDERS

In 1997 Dr. Terry Friedmann, MD, eliminated his need for glasses after applying Sandalwood and Juniper on the areas around his eyes, above the eyebrows, and on the cheeks, being careful never to get oil into his eyes. He also used the supplements of MultiGreens, ICP, ComforTone, Essentialzyme, JuvaTone, and JuvaPower for a complete colon and liver cleanse.

Caution: Never put any essential oils in the eyes or on the eyelids.

Age-Related Macular Degeneration (AMD)

AMD is one of the most common causes of blindness among people over 60 years of age. In fact, 30 percent of all people over 70 years of age suffer to some degree from this disease. The most common form of the disease is called "dry" because this form doesn't involve leakage of blood or serum.

The "wet" form of the disease is when there is abnormal blood vessel growth that results in macula-damaging blood leaks. The disease results in a steady loss of central vision until eyesight is totally impaired.

For dry AMD, the best prevention will be foods rich in antioxidants and carotenoids. The Ningxia wolfberry, the highest known antioxidant food, is also extremely high in lutein and zeaxanthin, which are vital for preserving eye health. Other foods rich in carotenoids that are also powerful antioxidants include blueberries and spinach.

For dry AMD, Lemon Vitality may be helpful as a Dietary and Oral supplement.

Clove Vitality, one of the highest known antioxidant nutrients, may be a good nutritional defense for wet AMD only.

Recommendations
Singles: Sacred Frankincense, Lemon, Lemon Vitality (dry AMD only) as a Dietary and Oral supplement, Cassia, Clove, Clove Vitality (wet AMD only) as a Dietary and Oral supplement

Blends: Longevity, Longevity Vitality

Nutritionals: NingXia Red, IlluminEyes, OmegaGize3, Longevity Softgels, Slique Shake, Slique Bars, Slique Bars—Chocolate-Coated, Slique CitraSlim, MultiGreens, Essentialzyme, Essentialzymes-4, Super Vitamin C, Super Vitamin C Chewable, Ningxia Wolfberries (Organic, Dried), Master Formula, MindWise

Application and Usage
Aromatic: Refer to Application Guidelines.

Dietary and Oral: Refer to Application Guidelines.

- Take 1 capsule of desired Vitality oil 2 times daily.

- Take 2-3 drops of desired Vitality oil in a spoonful of syrup or small amount of milk, juice, or water.

Topical: Refer to Application Guidelines.

- Receive a Raindrop Technique 2 times weekly.

- Massage 3-6 drops using the Vita Flex technique on the bottoms of feet 2 times daily.

Blocked Tear Ducts

A blocked tear duct is a partial or complete blockage in the system that carries tears away from the eye into the nose.

Recommendations

Singles: Lavender, Lavender Vitality, Sacred Frankincense, Frankincense, Frankincense Vitality, Cypress, Idaho Blue Spruce

Blends: Inner Child, Sacred Mountain

Nutritionals: NingXia Red, OmegaGize3, Longevity Softgels, Essentialzyme, Essentialzymes-4, Master Formula

Application and Usage

Aromatic: Refer to Application Guidelines.

Topical: Refer to Application Guidelines.

- Rubbing 1 drop of Lavender oil over the bridge of the nose 2 times daily has been reported to help in some cases.
- Receive a Raindrop Technique 2 times weekly.

- Massage 3-6 drops using the Vita Flex technique on the bottoms of feet 2 times daily.

Cataracts

Cataracts are a clouding of the eye lens that often comes with aging.

Recommendations

Singles: Lavender, Lavender Vitality, Cassia, Lemongrass, Lemongrass Vitality, Cypress, Sacred Frankincense, Frankincense, Frankincense Vitality, Eucalyptus Radiata, Jade Lemon, Jade Lemon Vitality, Lemon, Lemon Vitality, Clove, Clove Vitality

Blends: Longevity, Melrose, En-R-Gee, Purification

Nutritionals: JuvaPower, OmegaGize3, Mineral Essence, Essentialzyme, Essentialzymes-4, IlluminEyes, ImmuPro, NingXia Red, Ningxia Wolfberries (Organic, Dried)

Application and Usage

Aromatic: Refer to Application Guidelines.

Dietary and Oral:

- Clove Vitality is a powerful antioxidant, and when taken internally, it can slow or prevent both cataracts and AMD.
- Drink 2-6 ounces of NingXia Red daily or more if desired.

Topical: Refer to Application Guidelines.

- Apply 2-4 drops diluted 20:80 in a wide circle around the eye 1-3 times daily. being careful not to get any oil in the eyes or on the eyelids. This may also help with puffiness.
- Apply on temples and eye Vita Flex points on the feet and hands (the undersides of your two largest toes and your index and middle fingers).

Eye Blend

- 10 drops Lemongrass
- 5 drops Cypress
- 3 drops Eucalyptus Radiata
- 2 drops Sacred Frankincense or Frankincense

Mix this blend with a little V-6 Vegetable Oil Complex and apply around the eyes, being careful not to touch the eyes. It is best at night because the eyes could water, just like when you cut onions.

Note: If essential oils should ever accidentally get into the eyes, dilute with V-6 Vegetable Oil Complex or other pure vegetable oil. Never rinse with water. However, the essential oils will not cause any damage and will slowly stop burning.

Conjunctivitis/Pink Eye

Conjunctivitis (also called pink eye) is inflammation of the outermost layer of the eye and the inner surface of the eyelids. It has many causes, which may be infectious or noninfectious.

Recommendations

Singles: Myrrh, Lavender, Lavender Vitality, Vetiver

Blend: Exodus II

Nutritionals: NingXia Red, Ningxia Wolfberries (Organic, Dried), OmegaGize3, ImmuPro

Application and Usage

Aromatic: Refer to Application Guidelines.

Eye

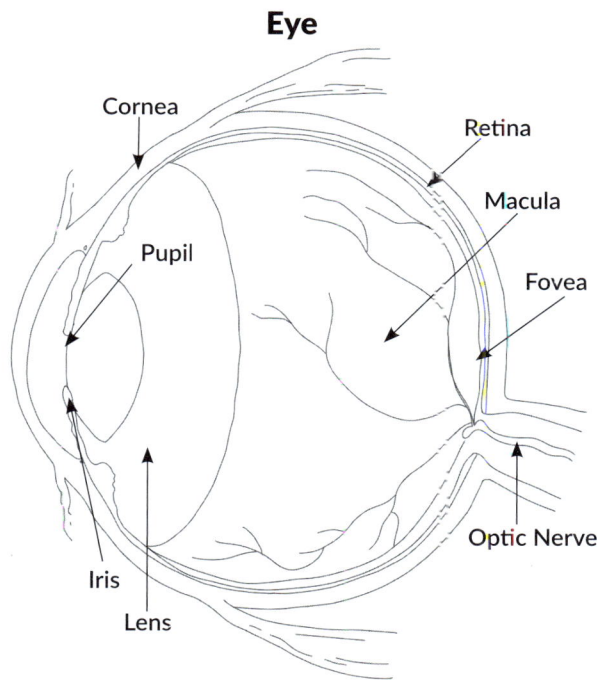

Topical: Refer to Application Guidelines.

- Apply 2-4 drops diluted 20:80 in a wide circle around the eye 1-3 times daily, being careful not to get any oil in the eyes or on the eyelids. This may also help with puffiness.
- Apply on temples and eye Vita Flex points on the feet and hands (the undersides of your two largest toes and your index and middle fingers).

Note: If essential oils should ever accidentally get into the eyes, dilute with V-6 Vegetable Oil Complex or other pure vegetable oil. Never rinse with water. The essential oils will not cause any damage and will slowly stop burning.

FAINTING (See also SHOCK)

Fainting happens when your brain does not get enough oxygen and you lose consciousness for a brief time. It can be caused by many different things. See your health care professional.

Recommendations
Singles: Idaho Blue Spruce, Peppermint, Peppermint Vitality, Sacred Sandalwood, Royal Hawaiian Sandalwood, Cardamom, Cardamom Vitality, Spearmint, Spearmint Vitality, Sacred Frankincense, Frankincense, Frankincense Vitality

Blends: Clarity, Trauma Life, Brain Power, KidScents GeneYus, R.C., Awaken

Application and Usage
Aromatic:
- Open an oil bottle and wave it under the nose of the person who fainted.
- If you are feeling faint, open the oil bottle and inhale or put 2-3 drops of your chosen oil in your hands, rub them together, cup your hands over your nose, and inhale.

Topical: Refer to Application Guidelines.

FATIGUE

Hormone imbalances may play a large role in fatigue as well as in latent viral infections (herpes virus and/or Epstein-Barr virus). Also, mineral deficiencies (especially magnesium) can play a large part in low energy.

Natural progesterone for women and DHEA for men can be instrumental in helping combat the fatigue that comes with age and declining hormone levels. Because pregnenolone is a precursor for all male and female hormones, both men and women can benefit from its supplementation.

Mental Fatigue
Mental fatigue is excessive mental tiredness and may manifest itself in difficulty concentrating and solving problems, irritability, loss of passion for work, anxiety, sleeplessness, confusion, or frustration. A 2013 study by Jane Buckle showed that a group of people who received personal inhalers of peppermint, basil, and helichrysum had a much larger reduction in mental exhaustion and moderate burnout than the placebo group.

Recommendations
Singles: Idaho Blue Spruce, Peppermint, Peppermint Vitality, Spearmint, Spearmint Vitality, Idaho Grand Fir, Sacred Frankincense, Frankincense, Frankincense Vitality, Basil, Basil Vitality, Helichrysum, Black Pepper, Black Pepper Vitality, Sage, Sage Vitality, Nutmeg, Nutmeg Vitality, Pine

Blends: Envision, Valor, Motivation, Gary's Light, En-R-Gee, Clarity, Common Sense, Shutran, Chivalry

Nutritionals: Slique Shake, Slique Bars, Slique Bars-Chocolate-Coated, Protein Power Bites, Chocolate-Coated Wolfberry Crisp Bars, Slique CitraSlim, Balance Complete, MultiGreens, Mineral Essence, Longevity Softgels, NingXia Red, NingXia Nitro, NingXia Zyng, Pure Protein Complete, One Heart, Essentialzyme, Essentialzymes-4, Super Vitamin B, EndoGize, ImmuPro, Sleep Essence

Application and Usage

Aromatic: Refer to Application Guidelines.

Dietary and Oral: Refer to Application Guidelines.

- Take 1 capsule of desired Vitality oil 2 times daily.

- Take 2-3 drops of desired Vitality oil in a spoonful of syrup or small amount of milk, juice, or water.

Topical: Refer to Application Guidelines.

- Apply 2-4 drops diluted 50:50 at base of throat, temples, and back of neck as needed.

- Massage 1-3 drops on corresponding Vita Flex points on feet 1-3 times daily.

Physical Fatigue

Physical fatigue is a lack of energy that can be caused by a host of factors, including poor thyroid function, adrenal imbalance, diabetes, cancer, and other conditions.

MultiGreens is a plant-derived, high-protein energy formula that athletes use to boost endurance. AminoWise helps reduce muscle fatigue. Longevity Softgels increase energy and endurance. Digestion and colon problems may cause fatigue. A colon and liver cleanse unburdens the digestive system and increases energy.

Recommendations

Singles: Peppermint, Peppermint Vitality, Nutmeg, Nutmeg Vitality, Lemongrass, Lemongrass Vitality, Eucalyptus Blue, Dorado Azul, Juniper, Basil, Basil Vitality, Jade Lemon, Jade Lemon Vitality, Lemon, Lemon Vitality, Lemon Verbena, Lime, Lime Vitality, Rosemary, Rosemary Vitality, Thyme, Thyme Vitality, Cypress

Blends: Awaken, Motivation, GLF, Valor, Valor Roll-On, En-R-Gee, Hope, Gary's Light, EndoFlex, EndoFlex Vitality, 25 Years Young

Nutritionals: Thyromin, MultiGreens, AminoWise, Slique Shake, Slique Bars, Slique Bars-Chocolate-Coated, Protein Pow-er Bites, Wolfberry Crisp Bars-Chocolate-Coated, Slique CitraSlim, EndoGize, Longevity Softgels, Super Vitamin B, NingXia Red, Ningxia Wolfberries (Organic, Dried), Digest & Cleanse, Life 9, KidScents MightyPro, NingXia Nitro, NingXia Zyng, ImmuPro

Application and Usage

Aromatic: Refer to Application Guidelines.

Dietary and Oral: Refer to Application Guidelines.

- Take 1 capsule of desired Vitality oil 3 times daily.

- Take 2-3 drops of desired Vitality oil in a spoonful of syrup or small amount of milk, juice, or water.

Topical: Refer to Application Guidelines.

- Apply 2-4 drops diluted 50:50 on temples, in clavicle notch (over thyroid), and behind ears 2-4 times daily as needed.

- Place a warm compress with 1-2 drops of chosen oil on the back.

FEVER

Fevers are one of the most powerful healing responses of the human body and are an indication that the body is fighting an infectious disease. However, if the fever raises body temperature excessively (over 104°F), then neurological damage can occur.

Reducing the fever is best accomplished by using anti-inflammatory essential oils internally and topically.

Recommendations

Singles: Peppermint, Peppermint Vitality, Eucalyptus Blue, Nutmeg, Nutmeg Vitality, German Chamomile, German Chamomile Vitality, Idaho Grand Fir, Copaiba, Copaiba Vitality, Myrrh, Dorado Azul, Lemongrass, Lemongrass Vitality

Blends: ImmuPower, Melrose, Raven, Clarity, M-Grain, RutaVaLa, RutaVaLa Roll-On

Nutritionals: Super Vitamin C, Super Vitamin C Chewable, ImmuPro, Longevity Softgels, Thieves Spray

Personal Care: Cinnamint Lip Balm, Lavender Lip Balm, Grapefruit Lip Balm

Application and Usage

Aromatic: Refer to Application Guidelines.

Dietary and Oral: Refer to Application Guidelines.

- Take 1 capsule of desired Vitality oil 2 times daily.

- Take 2-3 drops of desired Vitality oil in a spoonful of syrup or small amount of milk, juice, or water.

Topical: Refer to Application Guidelines.

- Apply 2-3 drops diluted 50:50 to forehead, temples, and back of neck.

- You may also apply 2-3 drops on the Vita Flex liver point of the right foot.

FIBROIDS
(See also MENSTRUAL AND FEMALE HORMONE CONDITIONS)

Fibroids are fairly common benign tumors of the female pelvis that are composed of smooth muscle cells and fibrous connective tissue. Fibroids are not cancerous and neither develop into cancer nor increase a woman's risk of uterine cancer.

Fibroids can have a diameter as small as 1 mm or as large as 8 inches. They can develop in clusters or alone as a single knot or nodule.

Fibroids frequently occur in premenopausal women and are seldom seen in young women who have not begun menstruation. Fibroids usually stabilize or even regress in women who have been through menopause.

Recommendations
Singles: Sacred Frankincense, Frankincense, Frankincense Vitality, Oregano, Oregano Vitality, Ecuadorian Oregano, Pine, Cistus, Helichrysum, Lavender, Lavender Vitality, Davana, Geranium

Blends: Valor, Valor Roll-On, EndoFlex, EndoFlex Vitality

Nutritionals: MultiGreens, Slique Shake, AminoWise, Balance Complete, Pure Protein Complete, PD 80/20, Essentialzyme, Essentialzymes-4, Life 9, KidScents MightyPro, Protein Power Bites

Personal Care: Cel-Lite Magic Massage Oil

Application and Usage
Aromatic: Refer to Application Guidelines.

Topical: Refer to Application Guidelines.

- Place a warm compress with 1-2 drops of chosen oil on the pelvic area.

- Applying a single drop under the nose is helpful and refreshing.

- Dilute 50:50 and apply on location 3-6 times daily.

- Massage 2-4 drops of oil neat on the bottoms of the feet just before bedtime.

FIBROMYALGIA

Fibromyalgia is an autoimmune disorder of the soft tissues and appears to include problems within the pain-signaling pathways of the brain and the spinal cord. By contrast, arthritis occurs in the joints.

The symptoms of fibromyalgia include general body pain, in some places worse than others, and are usually brought on by short periods of exercise or low levels of stimulation. Diagnosis includes tenderness or pain in at least 11 of 18 specific points in muscles, tendons, and bones.

The pain is generally continuous, and interrupts sleep patterns so that the fourth stage of sleep is never attained, and the body cannot rejuvenate and heal. Fibromyalgia is an acid condition in which the liver is toxic (See LIVER DISEASES AND DISORDERS).

The best natural remedy for fibromyalgia is to consume supplements such as flax seed and omegas, proteolytic enzymes such as bromelain and pancreatin, and MSM.

According to UCLA researcher Ronald Lawrence, MD, PhD, supplementation with MSM often offers a breakthrough in the treatment of fibromyalgia. Sulfurzyme combines MSM with Ningxia Wolfberry.

Recommendations
Singles: Sacred Frankincense, Frankincense, Frankincense Vitality, Wintergreen, Idaho Blue Spruce, Copaiba, Copaiba Vitality, German Chamomile, German Chamomile Vitality, Nutmeg, Nutmeg Vitality, Idaho Grand Fir

Blends: PanAway, Relieve It, Cool Azul, ImmuPower, Deep Relief Roll-On, CBD, Stress Away, Stress Away Roll-On, Chivalry, EndoFlex, EndoFlex Vitality

Nutritionals: AlkaLime, AminoWise, BLM, AgilEase, Sulfurzyme, Life 9, KidScents MightyPro, Essentialzyme, Super Vitamin C, Super Vitamin C Chewable, MultiGreens, ICP, ComforTone, Super Vitamin Cal Plus, Super Vitamin D, Thy-romin, SleepEssence, Essentialzymes-4, OmegaGize3, EndoGize

Personal Care: Cool Azul Pain Relief Cream, Cool Azul Sports Gel, CBD Muscle Rub, Ortho Ease Massage Oil, Ortho Sport Massage Oil

Application and Usage
Aromatic: Refer to Application Guidelines.

Dietary and Oral: Refer to Application Guidelines.

- Take 1-2 capsules with desired Vitality oil 2 times daily.

- Take 2-3 drops of desired Vitality oil in a spoonful of syrup or small amount of milk, juice, or water.

Topical: Refer to Application Guidelines.

- Apply a warm compress on location 3 times weekly.

- Massage into muscle tissue in a full-body massage weekly.

- Receive a Raindrop Technique and add an immune blend weekly.

FOOD POISONING
(See also DIGESTIVE PROBLEMS, GIARDIA)

Food poisoning symptoms vary with the source and type of contamination and may include nausea, diarrhea, vomiting, congestion, coughing, abdominal pain, cramps, sore throat, and fever.

Recommendations

Singles: Oregano, Oregano Vitality, Ecuadorian Oregano, Thyme, Thyme Vitality, Clove, Clove Vitality, Ginger, Ginger Vitality

Blends: Thieves, Thieves Roll-On, Thieves Vitality, DiGize, DiGize Vitality, KidScents TummyGize

Nutritionals: Essentialzymes-4, Inner Defense, ComforTone, Digest & Cleanse, Detoxzyme, Essentialzyme, AlkaLime

Oral Care: Thieves Cough Drops, Thieves Hard Lozenges, Thieves Mints

Personal Care: Thieves Chest Rub

Application and Usage

Dietary and Oral: Refer to Application Guidelines.

- Take 2 capsules with desired Vitality oil 2-3 times daily.

- Take 2-3 drops of desired Vitality oil in a spoonful of syrup or small amount of milk, juice, or water.

FOOT CONDITIONS AND PROBLEMS

Foot problems can occur due to a variety of reasons such as injuries, medical conditions such as fungal and bacterial conditions, or bone spurs, poorly fit shoes, or age.

Athlete's Foot

Athlete's foot (Tinea pedis) is a fungal infection of the feet. It is identical to ringworm that infects the skin elsewhere on the body (See FUNGAL (YEAST) INFECTIONS, Ringworm and Skin Candida). This fungus thrives in a warm, moist environment.

The best remedy is to keep feet cool and dry and avoid wearing tight-fitting shoes or heavy, natural-fiber socks such as cotton or wool, as they hold moisture next to the feet. It is helpful to wear sandals, shoes, and socks woven from a light, breathable fabric.

Essential oils with antifungal properties such as Tea Tree, Melaleuca Ericifolia, and Melaleuca Quinquenervia, or Melrose (a blend of Tea Tree, Melaleuca Quinquenervia, Clove, and Rosemary) can be added to bath water or Epsom salts and used in specially designed showerheads to help add antifungal protection to the water.

Recommendations

Singles: Patchouli, Tea Tree, Cassia, Davana, Melaleuca Ericifolia, Melaleuca Quinquenervia, Blue Cypress, Lemongrass or Lemongrass Vitality (usually diluted), Lavender, Lavender Vitality, Peppermint, Peppermint Vitality, Thyme, Thyme Vitality, Mountain Savory, Mountain Savory Vitality, Melissa, Myrrh, Hinoki, Rosemary, Rosemary Vitality, Laurus Nobilis

Blends: Melrose, Thieves, Thieves Roll-On, Thieves Vitality, Purification

Nutritionals: Detoxzyme, Digest & Cleanse

Personal Care: ClaraDerm, Thieves Spray, Ortho Ease Massage Oil, Ortho Sport Massage Oil, Thieves Fresh Essence Plus Mouthwash on the feet

Application and Usage

Topical: Refer to Application Guidelines.

- Pour ½ cup of Thieves Fresh Essence Plus Mouthwash into a pan of water for soaking the feet. It works amazingly well.

Athlete's Foot Blend
- 8 drops Tea Tree
- 4 drops Peppermint
- 2 drops Mountain Savory
- 1 drop Myrrh

Blisters (See SKIN DISORDERS AND PROBLEMS, Blisters)
Bunions (See also BURSITIS)

Bunions are caused from bursitis at the base of a toe and develop when the joints in the big toe no longer fit together as they should and become tender and swollen.

Recommendations
Singles: Eucalyptus Radiata, Raven, Lemon, Wintergreen, Vetiver, Idaho Blue Spruce, Hinoki

Blends: PanAway, Cool Azul, Deep Relief Roll-On, CBD, Relieve It, Aroma Siez

Personal Care: Cool Azul Pain Relief Cream, Cool Azul Sports Gel, CBD Muscle Rub, Ortho Sport Massage Oil, Ortho Ease Massage Oil

Application and Usage
Topical: Refer to Application Guidelines.
- Apply 2-4 drops neat or diluted 50:50 over bunion area 2-3 times daily.

Bunion Blend
- 6 drops Eucalyptus Radiata
- 4 drops Raven
- 3 drops Lemon
- 1 drop Wintergreen
- 1 drop Vetiver

Corns and Calluses
Corns and calluses are caused by friction and pressure when the bony parts of the feet rub against the shoes.

Recommendations
Singles: Lavender, Helichrysum, Basil, Idaho Blue Spruce, Myrrh, Cypress, Oregano, Hinoki

Blends: PanAway, Deep Relief Roll-On, Cool Azul, Relieve It, CBD

Personal Care: Cool Azul Pain Relief Cream, Cool Azul Sports Gel, CBD Muscle Rub, Ortho Sport Massage Oil, Ortho Ease Massage Oil

Application and Usage
Topical: Refer to Application Guidelines.
- Apply 1 drop neat directly on the corn 2-3 times daily.

Corns Blend
- 4 drops Basil
- 2 drops Myrrh
- 2 drops Cypress
- 1 drop Oregano
- 1 drop Hinoki

Sore Feet
Having sore feet is very common and is usually a symptom of an underlying problem or condition. Some causes are simple and require simple fixes, while others are more complicated and require more complex treatment.

Recommendations
Single Oils: Peppermint, Lavender, Patchouli, Myrrh, Sacred Frankincense, Frankincense, Royal Hawaiian Sandalwood, Sacred Sandalwood, Vetiver, Wintergreen, German Chamomile, Idaho Blue Spruce, Copaiba

Blends: Melrose, PanAway, Deep Relief Roll-On, Cool Azul, Relieve It, CBD

Personal Care: Cool Azul Pain Relief Cream, Cool Azul Sports Gel, CBD Muscle Rub, Ortho Sport Massage Oil, Ortho Ease Massage Oil

Application and Usage
Topical: Refer to Application Guidelines.
- Dilute Sore Feet Blend 50:50 and massage 6-9 drops onto each foot at night.

- Apply a warm compress for added effect and penetration.

- Mix 10 drops essential oils in 1 tablespoon Epsom salts and add to hot water in a basin large enough for a footbath.

Sore Feet Blend
- 5 drops Wintergreen
- 3 drops Peppermint
- 2 drops German Chamomile
- 2 drops Idaho Blue Spruce
- 1 drop Copaiba
- 1 drop Royal Hawaiian Sandalwood or Sacred Sandalwood

FUNGAL (YEAST) INFECTIONS

Fungi and yeast feed on decomposing or dead tissues and exist inside our stomachs, on our skin, out on the lawn, and just about everywhere. When kept under control, the yeast and fungi populating our bodies are harmless and digest what our bodies cannot or do not use.

When we feed the naturally occurring fungi in our body too many simple sugars, the fungal populations can grow out of control. This condition is known as systemic candidiasis and is marked by fungi invading the blood, gastrointestinal tract, and tissues.

Reducing or eliminating simple sugars from the diet is essential to combating all fungal infections. Antibiotics should also be avoided, and alcohol is deadly.

Fungal cultures such as candida excrete large amounts of poisons called mycotoxins as part of their life cycles. These poisons in the blood flow through the liver and hopefully are digested and eliminated from the body. If there is too much poison creating a toxic overload, the body eventually weakens. These toxins can wreak enormous damage on the tissues and organs and can be an aggravating factor in many degenerative diseases such as cancer, arteriosclerosis, and diabetes.

Insufficient intake of minerals and trace minerals like magnesium, potassium, and zinc may also stimulate candida and fungal overgrowth in the body.

Three Fungi Go Rogue

On April 17, 2019, the New York Times reported a deadly U.S. outbreak of pan-resistant Candida auris. By November the U.S. Centers for Disease Control stated, "Candida auris is an emerging fungus that presents a serious global health threat."1

The Times stated that nearly ". . . 600 cases of C. auris have been reported in the United States, the majority of them in New York, New Jersey and Illinois." Unfortunately, the Times reported, ". . . nearly half the people who contract the illness die within 90 days."2

An earlier Times article discussed the outbreak of this deadly fungus at the Royal Brompton Hospital in London. A man infected with Candida auris died. Efforts to decontaminate his hospital room were surprising. The April 6, 2019, Times article reported that at the Royal Brompton ". . . hospital workers used a special device to spray aerosolized hydrogen peroxide around the room used for a patient with C. auris." After a week's treatment, a "settle plate" in the middle of the room showed that only one organism survived: Candida auris.3

A 2016 European C. auris outbreak was the focus of a study by Schelenz et al. The conclusion was worrisome. "Despite a comprehensive review of modern technologies for environmental decontamination, there is currently no published data in the literature on the effectiveness of cleaning agents or decontamination of the environment for C. auris specifically."4

Thankfully, a 2014 study in Acta Biochem Pol. is just one of many showing antifungal effects of essential oils. In this study, Budzyńska et al. found ". . . the influence of Clove oil, Geranium oil, Lemon balm and Citronella oil on possible mechanisms reported to be relevant for Candida pathogenesis, namely germ tube and mycelium formation, adhesive and invasive properties and extracellular production of various enzymes."5

Drunk Driver? No, Yeast in His Gut Makes Beer!

A North Carolina man was arrested for an alcohol level 2.5 times the legal limit. No one would believe his claim that he did not drink. The man's aunt heard of people becoming inebriated even though they drank no alcohol. She heard of a doctor in Ohio who had treated a similar case. So, the man traveled to see this doctor.

There was yeast in his gut that was converting carbohydrates in his food to alcohol. A CNN article told how the man got in touch with researchers at the Richmond University Medical Center. They told him that ". . . antibiotics he took years ago altered his gut microbiome and allowed fungi to grow in his gastrointestinal tract."

The man's "auto-brewery syndrome (ABS)" was treated with an antifungal (itraconazole). The CNN article states, "Early signs of gut fermentation syndrome can include mood changes, delirium and brain fog."6 There is even a study on PubMed about ABS.7 The study explains the six-week therapy of a single-strain probiotic. The ". . . single-strain L. acidophilus (probiotic) with 3 billion colony-forming units per capsule" was administered. The man's alcohol-making fungus, Saccharomyces cerevisiae, was wiped out. Happily, the man's gut biome was returned to normal.

Common Fungi May Drive Cancer in Pancreas

On October 3, 2019, the New York Times published an article showing the surprising presence of Malassezia species yeast in pancreatic cancer.8 Dr. Mercola wrote about this important find. "Research shows fungi can migrate from your gut to your pancreas, where it can contribute to the development of pancreatic cancer. . .

. In summary, the fungi trapped in the pancreas appears to drive tumor growth by activating MBL (mannose-binding lectin), a liver protein.... When MBL activation was inhibited, tumor growth was also inhibited."9

Dangerous bacteria and viruses seem to get all the attention. Perhaps we need to take the fungal realm a little more seriously.

Endnotes

1. https://www.cdc.gov/fungal/candida-auris/index.html

2. Richtel M, New York Times, April 17, 2019. How a Chicago Woman Fell Victim to Candida Auris, a Drug-Resistant Fungus. https://www.nytimes.com/2019/04/17/health/candida-auris-fungus-chicago.html.

3. Richtel M and Jacobs A, New York Times, April 6, 2019, A Mysterious Infection, Spanning the Globe in a Climate of Secrecy. https://www.nytimes.com/2019/04/06/health/drug-resistant-candida-auris.html.

4. Schelenz S, Hagen F, Rhods JL, Abdolrasouli A, Chowdhary A, Hall A, Ryan L, Shackleton J, Trimlett R, Meis JF, Armstrong-Jones D. First Hospital Outbreak of the globally emerging Candida auris in a European Hospital. Antimicr Resist Infect Control. 2016 Oct 19; 5:35 eCollection 2016. https://www.ncbi.nlm.nih.gov/pmc/articles/PMC5069812/

5. Budzyńska A, Sadowska B, Więckowska-Szakiel M, Różalska B. Ezymatic profile, adhesive and invasive properties of Candida albicans under the influence of selected plant essential oils. Acta Biochim Pol. 2014;61(1):115-21. Epub 2014 Mar 19.

6. Kaur H, CNN, No one believed him when he said he hadn't been drinking. Then researchers found his body was producing alcohol. Oct 26, 2019.

7. Malik F, Wickremesinghe P. Saverimuttu J. Case Report and literature review of auto-brewer syndrome: probably an underdiagnosed medical condition. BMJ Open Gastroenterology. 2019;6:e000325.

8. https://www.nytimes.com/2019/10/03/health/pancreatic-cancer-fungi.html

9. https://articles.mercola.com/sites/articles/archive/2019/10/23/tumor-fungus-baking-soda.aspx

Symptoms of Systemic Fungal Infection
- Fatigue/low energy
- Overweight
- Low resistance to illness
- Allergies
- Unbalanced blood sugar
- Headaches
- Irritability
- Mood swings
- Indigestion
- Colitis and ulcers
- Diarrhea/constipation
- Urinary tract infections
- Rectal or vaginal itch

ATHLETE'S FOOT
(See also FOOT CONDITIONS and PROBLEMS, ATHLETE'S FOOT; See also RINGWORM AND SKIN CANDIDA in this section)

Candida Albicans (Candidiasis)

Two of the most powerful weapons for fighting intestinal fungal (yeast) infections such as candida are FOS (fructooligosac-charides) and L. acidophilus cultures.

FOS has been clinically documented in dozens of peer-reviewed studies for its ability to build up the healthy intestinal flora in the colon and combat the overgrowth of negative bacteria and fungi.

Acidophilus cultures have also been shown to combat fungus overgrowth in the gastrointestinal tract.

Recommendations

Singles: Lemongrass, Lemongrass Vitality, Geranium, Tea Tree, Cassia, Thyme, Thyme Vitality, Peppermint, Peppermint Vitality, Lavender, Lavender Vitality, Rosemary, Rosemary Vitality, Davana, Palmarosa

Blends: Thieves, Thieves Roll-On, Thieves Vitality

Nutritionals: Detoxzyme, Life 9, KidScents MightyPro, Essentialzyme, Essentialzymes-4, ImmuPro, MultiGreens, Digest & Cleanse, Super Vitamin C, Super Vitamin C Chewable, AlkaLime

Application and Usage
Aromatic: Refer to Application Guidelines.

Dietary and Oral: Refer to Application Guidelines.

- Take 1 capsule of desired Vitality oil 2 times daily.

- Take 2-3 drops of desired Vitality oil in a spoonful of syrup or small amount of milk, juice, or water.

Candida Blend
- 5 drops Lemongrass or Lemongrass Vitality
- 4 drops Thyme or Thyme Vitality
- 4 drops Tea Tree
- 2 drops Geranium

(Note: This blend is not recommended for those with estrogen-sensitive cancers.)

Topical: Refer to Application Guidelines.
- Dilute 50:50 or 20:80, as needed, and massage 3-4 drops on thymus (at clavicle notch, center of collarbone at base of throat) to stimulate the immune system. Also apply 3-6 drops on bottoms of the feet and on the chest. Also apply 5-10 drops on stomach. Do these applications 2 times daily.

- Massage 2-4 drops on relevant Vita Flex points on feet 2-4 times daily.
- Use bath salts daily.

Ringworm and Skin Candida

The ringworm fungus infects the skin, causing scaly, round, itchy patches. It is infectious and can be spread from either an animal or human host.

Skin candida is a fungal infection that can erupt almost anywhere on the skin. It shows up in various places such as behind the knees, inside the elbows, behind the ears, on the temple area, and between the breasts.

Recommendations
Singles: Geranium, Tea Tree, Cassia, Melaleuca Quinquenervia, Cypress, Lavender, Rosemary, Mastrante, Lemongrass, Lemon Myrtle, Oregano, Spearmint, Peppermint, Laurus Nobilis

Blends: Melrose, Raven, R.C., Thieves, Thieves Roll-On, Purification

Personal Care: Thieves Spray, Ortho Sport Massage Oil, Ortho Ease Massage Oil

Application and Usage
Topical: Refer to Application Guidelines.
- Dilute 50:50 and massage 2-4 drops over affected area 2-4 times daily. In severe cases, use 35 percent food-grade hydrogen peroxide to clean infected areas before applying essential oils. Saturate a gauze pad with essential oils, apply to affected area, and wrap to hold in place.

Ringworm Blend
- 3 drops Tea Tree
- 3 drops Spearmint
- 1 drop Peppermint
- 1 drop Rosemary

Skin Candida Blend
- 10 drops Tea Tree
- 4 drops Lavender
- 2 drops Geranium
- 1 drop Oregano

Thrush

Thrush is a fungal infection of the mouth and throat marked by creamy, curd-like patches in the oral cavity. Even though it appears in the mouth, thrush is usually a sign of systemic fungal overgrowth throughout the body. Thrush can usually be treated locally through the use of antifungal essential oils such as Clove Vitality, Cinnamon Bark Vitality, Rosemary Vitality, or Peppermint Vitality.

Recommendations
Singles: Clove, Clove Vitality, Cinnamon Bark, Cinnamon Bark Vitality, Peppermint, Peppermint Vitality, Rosemary, Rosemary Vitality, Geranium, Orange, Orange Vitality, Cassia, Lavender, Lavender Vitality, Tea Tree

Blends: Melrose, Thieves, Thieves Roll-On, Thieves Vitality, Inner Defense, Purification

Oral Care: Thieves Hard Lozenges, Thieves Cough Drops, Thieves Fresh Essence Plus Mouthwash, Thieves Spray

Personal Care: Thieves Chest Rub

Application and Usage
Aromatic: Refer to Application Guidelines.

Dietary and Oral: Refer to Application Guidelines.

- Take 1 capsule of desired Vitality oil 2-3 times daily between meals.

- Take 2-3 drops of desired Vitality oil in a spoonful of syrup or small amount of milk, juice, or water.
- Gargle 3-5 times daily with Thieves Fresh Essence Plus Mouthwash.

Thrush (Mouth) Tea Tree
- Mix 5 drops of Tea Tree with 2 teaspoons water. Swish around in mouth, then spit out; do 3 times a day.

Thrush (Throat) Tea Tree
- Mix 5 drops Tea Tree with 2 teaspoons water. Gargle, then spit out; do 3 times a day.

Note: These applications are for adults, not infants. In cases of infants with thrush, consult a medical professional first.

Topical: Refer to Application Guidelines.

- Dilute 50:50 or 20:80 as needed and massage 3-4 drops on the thymus (at clavicle notch, center of collarbone at base of throat) to stimulate the immune system. Also apply 3-6 drops on the bottoms of the feet and on the chest. Also apply 5-10 drops on the stomach. Do these applications 2 times daily.

- Massage 2-4 drops on relevant Vita Flex points on the bottoms of the feet 2-4 times daily.

Vaginal Yeast Infection

Vaginal yeast infections are usually caused from overgrowth of fungi like Candida albicans. These naturally occurring intestinal yeast and fungi are normally kept under control by the immune system, but when excess sucrose is consumed or antibiotics are used, these organisms convert from relatively harmless yeast into an invasive, harmful fungus that secretes toxins as part of its life cycle.

Vaginal yeast infections are just one symptom of systemic fungal infestation. While the yeast infection can be treated locally, the underlying problem of systemic candidiasis may still remain, unless specific dietary, oral, and health practices are used.

Diet and cleansing are two major factors in overcoming this problem. Sugar, milk products, breads, and medications such as antibiotics all contribute to the growth of candida. A cleansing program should be considered with various supplements and essential oils (See Chapter 17, CLEANSING AND DIET).

Recommendations
Singles: Tea Tree, Myrrh, Melissa, Cassia, Oregano, Oregano Vitality, Ecuadorian Oregano, Thyme, Thyme Vitality, Mastrante, Rosemary, Rosemary Vitality, Palo Santo, Davana, Mountain Savory, Mountain Savory Vitality, Idaho Blue Spruce, Hinoki

Blends: Melrose, Thieves, Thieves Roll-On, Thieves Vitality, Exodus II, Purification, 3 Wise Men, Inspiration

Nutritionals: ICP (a.m.), JuvaPower (p.m.), ComforTone, Detoxzyme, Essentialzyme, Essentialzymes-4, Life 9 or KidScents MightyPro (for 60 days)

Personal Care: ClaraDerm

Application and Usage
Dietary and Oral: Refer to Application Guidelines.

- Take 1 capsule of desired Vitality oil 2-3 times daily between meals.

- Take 2-3 drops of desired Vitality oil in a spoonful of syrup or small amount of milk, juice, or water.
- Stop eating sugar.

Retention
- Mix an 80:20 ratio (8 parts chosen essential oil to 2 parts V-6 Vegetable Oil Complex), put 1-2 tablespoons on a tampon, and insert into the vagina daily for internal infection.
- Alternate approach: Douche with 1 tablespoon Thieves Fresh Essence Plus Mouthwash overnight 3 times a week. If it stings a little, dilute with a little V-6 Vegetable Oil Complex.

Vaginal Yeast Infection Blend
- 7 drops Tea Tree
- 5 drops Mountain Savory
- 2 drops Myrrh

GALLSTONES (CHOLECYSTITIS)

The gallbladder stores the bile created by the liver and releases it through the biliary ducts into the duodenum to promote digestion. Bile is extremely important for fat digestion and the absorption of vitamins A, D, and E.

When bile contains excessive cholesterol, bilirubin, or bile salts, gallstones can form. Stones made from hardened cholesterol account for the vast majority of gallstones, while stones made from bilirubin, the brownish pigment in bile, constitute only about 20 percent of gallstones.

When the bile flow is obstructed due to gallstones, serious consequences can ensue, including poor digestion, jaundice, and severe abdominal pain.

Gallstones can block both bile flow and the passage of pancreatic enzymes. This can result in inflammation in the gallbladder (cholecystitis), pancreas (pancreatitis), and jaundice. In some cases, gallstones can be life threatening, depending on where they are lodged.

Several Japanese studies show that limonene, a key constituent in orange, lemon, and tangerine oils, can effectively dissolve gallstones with no negative side effects.31,32

Note: Extreme pain may necessitate removal of the gallbladder surgically. See your health care professional.

Recommendations

Singles: Carrot Seed, Carrot Seed Vitality, Jade Lemon, Jade Lemon Vitality, Lemon, Lemon Vitality, Lime, Lime Vitality, Helichrysum, Sacred Frankincense, Frankincense, Frankincense Vitality, Orange, Orange Vitality, Grapefruit, Grapefruit Vitality, Mandarin, Tangerine, Tangerine Vitality, Juniper, Rosemary, Rosemary Vitality, Idaho Grand Fir

Blends: GLF, GLF Vitality, Citrus Fresh, Citrus Fresh Vitality, JuvaCleanse, JuvaCleanse Vitality

Nutritionals: Essentialzyme, Essentialzymes-4, Life 9, KidScents MightyPro, JuvaPower, ComforTone, ICP, JuvaTone

Application and Usage

Dietary and Oral: Refer to Application Guidelines.

- Take 1 capsule of desired Vitality oil 2 times daily for 2 weeks.

- Take 2-3 drops of desired Vitality oil in a spoonful of syrup or small amount of milk, juice, or water.

Topical: Refer to Application Guidelines.
- Dilute 50:50 and massage 6-10 drops over gallbladder 2 times daily.

- Apply a compress 2-3 times daily.

- You may also apply 1-3 drops on the Vita Flex liver and digestive points of the right foot 2-3 times daily.

GANGRENE

Gangrene is the death or decay of living tissue caused by a lack of blood supply. A shortage of blood can result from a blood clot, arteriosclerosis, frostbite, diabetes, infection, or some other obstruction in the arterial blood supply. Gas gangrene, also known as acute or moist gangrene, occurs when tissues are infected with clostridium bacteria. Unless the body is given antibiotics to treat the disease or the limb is amputated, gangrene can be fatal.

Note: As with all serious medical conditions, consult your health care professional immediately if you suspect gangrene.

The part of the body affected by gangrene displays the following symptoms:
- Coldness
- Dark in color or even black
- Looks rotten or decomposed
- Putrid smell
- Fever
- Anemia

Dr. René Gattefossé suffered gas gangrene as a result of burns from a chemical explosion at the turn of the century. He successfully engineered his own recovery solely with the use of pure lavender oil.

Recommendations

Singles: Myrrh, Lavender, Lavender Vitality, Thyme, Thyme Vitality, Peppermint, Peppermint Vitality, Oregano, Oregano Vitality, Ecuadorian Oregano, Rosemary, Rosemary Vitality, Sacred Frankincense, Frankincense, Frankincense Vitality, Mountain Savory, Mountain Savory Vitality, Cistus, Cassia, Cypress, Vetiver, Copaiba, Copaiba Vitality

Blends: Exodus II, Thieves, Thieves Roll-On, Thieves Vitality, ImmuPower, Melrose

Nutritionals: Super Vitamin C, Super Vitamin C Chewable, Inner Defense, ImmuPro, Mineral Essence, Essentialzyme, Essentialzymes-4, MultiGreens, AminoWise, Pure Protein Complete, Balance Complete, Protein Power Bites, Detoxzyme

Application and Usage

Topical: Refer to Application Guidelines.

- Apply 2-4 drops diluted 20:80 on the affected area 3-5 times daily.

- Apply a warm compress 3 times daily every other day.

GASTRITIS

Gastritis occurs when the stomach's mucosal lining becomes inflamed and the cells become eroded. This can lead to bleeding ulcers and severe digestive disturbances. Gastritis is caused by excess acid production in the stomach, alcohol consumption, stress, and fungal or bacterial infections.

Symptoms of gastritis are weight loss, abdominal pain, and cramping.

Recommendations

Singles: Peppermint, Peppermint Vitality, Jade Lemon, Jade Lemon Vitality, Lemon, Lemon Vitality, Lime, Lime Vitality, Fennel, Fennel Vitality, Patchouli, Tarragon, Tarragon Vitality, Cassia, Davana, Spearmint, Spearmint Vitality

Blends: DiGize, DiGize Vitality, Purification, JuvaCleanse, JuvaCleanse Vitality

Nutritionals: AlkaLime, Essentialzymes-4, Essentialzyme, Detoxzyme, Life 9, KidScents MightyPro, Slique Essence, Digest & Cleanse, Balance Complete

Application and Usage

Dietary and Oral: Refer to Application Guidelines.

- Take 1 capsule of desired Vitality oil 2 times daily.

- Take 2-3 drops of desired Vitality oil in a spoonful of syrup or small amount of milk, juice, or water.

Supplementation regimen for gastritis:

- AlkaLime: Take ½ teaspoon each morning.
- Essentialzymes-4: Take 3-4 yellow capsules 3 times daily.
- ComforTone and ICP: Begin after 2 weeks of using the products listed above.
- Mega Vitamin Cal: Take 1 tablespoon each morning in 8 ounces of warm water.

GOUT (See also JOINT STIFFNESS OR PAIN)

Gout is a disease marked by abrupt, temporary bouts of joint pain and swelling that are most evident in the joint of the big toe. It can also affect the wrist, elbow, knee, ankle, hand, and foot. As the disease progresses, pain and swelling in the joints become more frequent and chronic, with deposits called tophi appearing over many joints, including on the elbows and strangely on the ears. Ears are a body extremity, colder, with slower blood circulation. All are factors to attract gout attacks. If you have ear tophi, you almost certainly have chronic gout.

Gout is characterized by accumulation of uric acid crystals in the joints caused by excess uric acid in the blood. Uric acid is a byproduct of the breakdown of protein that is normally excreted by the kidneys into the urine. To reduce uric acid concentrations, it is necessary to support the kidneys, adrenals, and immune functions. It is also necessary to detoxify by cleansing and drinking plenty of fluids.

Excess alcohol, allergy-producing foods, or strict diets can cause outbreaks of gout. Foods rich in purines such as wine, anchovies, and animal liver can also cause gout.

Recommendations

Singles: Juniper, Helichrysum, Jade Lemon, Jade Lemon Vitality, Lemon, Lemon Vitality, Lime, Lime Vitality, Idaho Blue Spruce, Roman Chamomile, Tea Tree, Sacred Frankincense, Frankincense, Frankincense Vitality

Blend: GLF, GLF Vitality, JuvaCleanse, JuvaCleanse Vitality, Cool Azul, Deep Relief Roll-On, CBD

Nutritionals: AlkaLime, BLM, AgilEase, MultiGreens, ICP (a.m.), ComforTone, Essentialzyme, JuvaPower (p.m.), Juva-Tone

Personal Care: Cool Azul Pain Relief Cream, Cool Azul Sports Gel, CBD Muscle Rub, Ortho Ease Massage Oil, Ortho Sport Massage Oil

Application and Usage

Dietary and Oral: Refer to Application Guidelines.

- Take 1 capsule of desired Vitality oil 1 time daily for 10 days, rest 4 days, repeat as needed.

- Take 2-3 drops of desired Vitality oil in a spoonful of syrup or small amount of milk, juice, or water.

Topical: Refer to Application Guidelines.

- Gently massage 1-3 drops neat on affected joints 2-3 times daily.

Gout Blend

- 10 drops Lemon
- 5 drops Idaho Blue Spruce
- 4 drops Juniper
- 3 drops Tea Tree
- 2 drops Roman Chamomile

HAIR AND SCALP PROBLEMS

Sulfur is the single most important mineral for maintaining the strength and integrity of the hair and hair follicle.

Recommendations

Singles: Lavender, Lavender Vitality, Cedarwood (dry scalp), Peppermint (oily scalp), Peppermint Vitality, Rosemary, Rosemary Vitality, Clary Sage, Sage, Sage Vitality, Basil, Basil Vitality, Juniper, Ylang Ylang, Royal Hawaiian Sandalwood, Sacred Sandalwood, Geranium, Lemon, Lemon Vitality, Cypress, Patchouli

Blends: Melrose, Thieves, Thieves Roll-On, Thieves Vitality, Citrus Fresh, Citrus Fresh Vitality, Purification, Inspiration, The Gift

Nutritionals: Sulfurzyme, AlkaLime, Super Vitamin B, Pure Protein Complete, Essentialzymes-4, Essentialzyme, Balance Complete

Hair Care: Lavender Mint Daily Shampoo, Lavender Mint Daily Conditioner, Copaiba Vanilla Moisturizing Shampoo, Copaiba Vanilla Moisturizing Conditioner, Lavender Shampoo, Lavender Conditioner

Application and Usage

Topical: Refer to Application Guidelines.

- Apply 1 teaspoon diluted 20:80 onto the scalp and rub vigorously for 2-3 minutes. Leave on scalp for 60-90 minutes.
- Mix 2-4 drops of essential oils with 1-2 teaspoons of shampoo to wash hair after exercising.

Dry Scalp Blend
- 6 drops Cedarwood
- 4 drops Lavender
- 2 drops Royal Hawaiian Sandalwood, Sacred Sandalwood, or Geranium
- 2 drops Patchouli

Oily Scalp Blend
- 6 drops Peppermint
- 4 drops Lemon
- 2 drops Lavender

Scalp Rinse Blend to Restore Acid Mantle
- 1 drop Rosemary
- 1 teaspoon pure apple cider vinegar
- 8 ounces water

Rub 1-2 drops of oil on hair to prevent static electricity.

Baldness/Hair Loss (Alopecia Areata)

Male pattern baldness is often a result of hormonal imbalances such as excess conversion of testosterone to dihydrotestosterone through the enzyme 5-alpha reductase. It can also be caused by an inflammatory condition called alopecia areata.

Alopecia is an inflammatory hair loss disease that is the second-leading cause of baldness in the U.S. A double-blind study conducted at the Aberdeen Royal Infirmary in Scotland found that the essential oils of thyme, rosemary, lavender, and cedarwood were effective in combating this disease.[33]

Essential oils are excellent for cleansing, nourishing, and strengthening the hair follicle and shaft. Rosemary (cineole chemotype) encourages hair growth. The Arabian people for centuries have used frankincense resin water to rinse their hair and massage their scalp to maintain a healthy head of hair and stimulate regrowth.

Thyroid balance also prevents hair loss.

Recommendations

Singles: Lavender, Lavender Vitality, Cypress, Sacred Frankincense, Frankincense, Frankincense Vitality, Peppermint, Peppermint Vitality, Sacred Sandalwood, Royal Hawaiian Sandalwood, Black Pepper, Black Pepper Vitality, Rosemary, Rosemary Vitality, Thyme, Thyme Vitality, Cedarwood, Juniper, Eucalyptus Blue, Palo Santo, Clary Sage

Blends: Melrose, Longevity, Longevity Vitality, Mister, M-Grain, Transformation, JuvaCleanse, JuvaCleanse Vitality

Nutritionals: PD 80/20, EndoGize, Master Formula, Sulfurzyme, Balance Complete, Mineral Essence, Essentialzyme, Essentialzymes-4, Allerzyme, Thyromin

Application and Usage
Topical: Refer to Application Guidelines.

- Dilute 50:50 oil of choice and V-6 Vegetable Oil Complex and massage 1 teaspoon into scalp vigorously and thoroughly for 2-3 minutes before retiring.

- Dilute 5 drops of your essential oil in 20 drops of V-6 Vegetable Oil Complex, grape seed oil, or coconut oil and massage into scalp before going to bed.
- Add 10 drops of any of the above Blends to 1 teaspoon of coconut oil and massage into the scalp where it is balding; then rub gently into the remainder of the scalp. This works best when done at night. It may also help to alternate Blends.

- Mix 2-4 drops of essential oils with 1-2 teaspoons of shampoo. Massage into the scalp vigorously and thoroughly for 2-3 minutes and then leave the shampoo on the scalp for 15 minutes.

This is an excellent time to do an exercise routine. Rinse hair afterward.

Hair Loss Prevention Blend No. 1
- 10 drops Cedarwood
- 10 drops Sacred Sandalwood or Royal Hawaiian Sandalwood
- 10 drops Lavender
- 8 drops Rosemary
- 1 drop Juniper

Hair Loss Prevention Blend No. 2
- 5 drops Lavender
- 4 drops Cypress
- 3 drops Rosemary
- 2 drops Clary Sage
- 2 drops Palo Santo

Hair Loss Prevention Blend No. 3
- 5 drops Lavender
- 5 drops Sacred Frankincense or Frankincense
- 2 drops Clary Sage
- 3 drops Eucalyptus Blue
- 1 drop Peppermint

Hair Loss Prevention Blend No. 4
- 4 drops Rosemary
- 4 drops Thyme
- 4 drops Lavender
- 4 drops Cedarwood
- 2 drops Sacred Frankincense or Frankincense

Dandruff
Dandruff may be caused by allergies, parasites (fungal), and/or chemicals. The mineral selenium has been shown to help prevent dandruff.

Tea Tree has been shown to be effective in treating dandruff and other fungal infections.34

Recommendations
Singles: Tea Tree, Lemon, Lemon Vitality, Cedarwood, Lavender, Lavender Vitality, Rosemary, Rosemary Vitality, Peppermint, Peppermint Vitality, Copaiba, Copaiba Vitality, Eucalyptus Blue, Sacred Frankincense, Frankincense, Frankincense Vitality, Vetiver, Dorado Azul, Davana

Blends: Citrus Fresh, Citrus Fresh Vitality, Melrose, Thieves, Thieves Roll-On, Thieves Vitality, The Gift

Nutritionals: Mineral Essence, NingXia Red

Hair Care: Lavender Mint Daily Shampoo, Lavender Mint Daily Conditioner, Copaiba Vanilla Moisturizing Shampoo, Copaiba Vanilla Moisturizing Conditioner, Lavender Shampoo, Lavender Conditioner

Application and Usage
Dietary and Oral: Refer to Application Guidelines.
- Take 1 dropper of Mineral Essence and 2 ounces of NingXia Red in water in the morning.

Topical: Refer to Application Guidelines.

- Add a few drops of a single oil or blend to your shampoo and massage it into your scalp or add a few drops of the oils of your choice to the Bath & Shower Gel Base for your own custom shampoo.
- Apply 1 teaspoon of the shampoo mixture to the scalp and rub vigorously for 2-3 minutes and then leave shampoo on scalp for 15 minutes. Mix 2-4 drops of the essential oils with 1 teaspoon shampoo to wash hair afterward.

Dandruff Blend No. 1
- 5 drops Lemon
- 2 drops Lavender
- 2 drops Peppermint
- 1 drop Rosemary

Dandruff Blend No. 2
- 5 drops Tea Tree
- 2 drops Lavender
- 2 drops Peppermint
- 1 drop Rosemary

HALITOSIS (BAD BREATH)
(See also ORAL CARE PROBLEMS, TEETH AND GUMS; FUNGAL (YEAST) INFECTIONS, CANDIDA ALBICANS (CANDIDIASIS))

Persistent bad breath or gum disease may be a sign of poor digestion, candida, yeast infestation, or other health problems.

Recommendations
Singles: Clove, Clove Vitality, Peppermint, Peppermint Vitality, Jade Lemon, Jade Lemon Vitality, Lemon, Lemon Vitality, Lime, Lime Vitality, Tea Tree, Spearmint, Spearmint Vitality, Mandarin, Cinnamon Bark, Cinnamon Bark Vitality, Rosemary, Rosemary Vitality, Wintergreen

Blends: Thieves, Thieves Roll-On, Thieves Vitality, Melrose, Purification, KidScents TummyGize, DiGize, DiGize Vitality, AromaEase

Nutritionals: Detoxzyme, Allerzyme, Digest & Cleanse, Mineral Essence, Life 9, KidScents MightyPro, ICP, ComforTone, Slique Essence, Slique Gum

Oral Care: Thieves AromaBright Toothpaste, Thieves Spray, Thieves Hard Lozenges, Thieves Cough Drops, Thieves Mints, YL Vitality Drops, KidScents Toothpaste, Thieves Whitening Toothpaste, Thieves Dental Floss

Personal Care: Thieves Chest Rub

Application and Usage
Dietary and Oral: Refer to Application Guidelines.

- Take 1 capsule of desired Vitality oil 2 times daily.

- Take 2-3 drops of desired Vitality oil in a spoonful of syrup or small amount of milk, juice, or water.
- Dilute essential oils and Blends in 2 teaspoons of Yacon and 4 ounces of hot water. Gargle as needed (2-4 times daily).

Bad Breath Blend No. 1
- 3 drops Peppermint Vitality
- 2 drops Lemon Vitality
- 2 drops Clove Vitality
- 1 drop Tea Tree

Bad Breath Blend No. 2
- 4 drops Spearmint Vitality
- 2 drops Mandarin
- 2 drops Cinnamon Bark Vitality

Topical: Refer to Application Guidelines.
- Swab 4-8 drops of the Singles or Blends above diluted 50:50 inside cheeks and on tongue, gums, and teeth 2-4 times daily as needed.

HEADACHE
(See STRESS; THYROID PROBLEMS, HYPOGLYCEMIA; LIVER DISEASES AND DISORDERS; MENSTRUAL and FEMALE HORMONE CONDITIONS)

Headaches are usually caused by hormone imbalances, circulatory problems, stress, sugar imbalance (hypoglycemia), structural (spinal) misalignments, and blood pressure concerns.

Placebo-controlled, double-blind, crossover studies at the Christian-Albrecht University in Kiel, Germany, found that essential oils (particularly peppermint alone and in combination with eucalyptus) were just as effective in blocking pain from tension-type headaches as acetaminophen (i.e., Tylenol®).[35, 36]

Essential oils also promote circulation, reduce muscle spasms, and decrease inflammatory response.

Recommendations
Singles: Peppermint, Peppermint Vitality, Clove, Clove Vitality, Copaiba, Copaiba Vitality, Eucalyptus Globulus, Eucalyptus Blue, Dorado Azul, Mastrante, German Chamomile, German Chamomile Vitality, Lavender, Lavender Vitality,

Myrrh, Roman Chamomile, Rosemary, Rosemary Vitality, Spearmint, Spearmint Vitality, Valerian, Vanilla, Wintergreen

Blends: Brain Power, Clarity, KidScents GeneYus, Deep Relief Roll-On, M-Grain, PanAway, Stress Away, Stress Away Roll-On, Relieve It, R.C., Raven, Tranquil Roll-On

Personal Care: Prenolone Plus Body Cream, Progessence Plus

Application and Usage

Aromatic: Refer to Application Guidelines.

Dietary and Oral: Refer to Application Guidelines.

 Take 1 capsule of desired Vitality oil 2 times daily.

 Place 1 drop on the tongue and then push it against the roof of the mouth.

 Take 2-3 drops of desired Vitality oil in a spoonful of syrup or small amount of milk, juice, or water.

Topical: Refer to Application Guidelines.

- Dilute 50:50 and apply 1-3 drops on the back of the neck, behind the ears, on the temples, on the forehead, and under the nose. Be careful to keep away from eyes and eyelids.

 Massage 2-4 drops of oil neat on the bottoms of the feet just before bedtime.

 Place a warm compress with 1-2 drops of chosen oil on the back.

General Headache Blend No. 1
- 4 drops Wintergreen
- 3 drops German Chamomile or German Chamomile Vitality
- 2 drops Lavender or Lavender Vitality
- 2 drops Copaiba or Copaiba Vitality
- 1 drop Clove or Clove Vitality

General Headache Blend No. 2
- 6 drops Peppermint or Peppermint Vitality
- 4 drops Eucalyptus Globulus
- 2 drops Myrrh

Migraine (Vascular-type Headache)

The vast majority of migraine headaches may be due to colon congestion or poor digestion. They are much more severe than regular headaches. The combination of ICP, ComforTone, and Essentialzyme is most important for cleansing the colon. Eyestrain and decreased vision can accompany migraine headaches. Dried wolfberries contain large amounts of lutein and zeaxanthin, which are vital for healthy vision.

Recommendations
Singles: Basil, Basil Vitality, Copaiba, Copaiba Vitality, Eucalyptus Globulus, Mastrante, German Chamomile, German Chamomile Vitality, Helichrysum, Lavender, Lavender Vitality, Marjoram, Marjoram Vitality, Peppermint, Peppermint Vitality, Rosemary, Rosemary Vitality, Wintergreen

Blends: M-Grain, Thieves, Thieves Roll-On, Thieves Vitality, Clarity, PanAway, Relieve It, The Gift, R.C., Raven, AromaEase, CBD, Stress Away, Stress Away Roll-On, Tranquil Roll-On

Nutritionals: Essentialzyme, Essentialzymes-4, NingXia Red, IlluminEyes, Balance Complete, ComforTone, Ningxia Wolf-berries (Organic, Dried), ICP, Mega Vitamin Cal

Application and Usage
Aromatic: Refer to Application Guidelines.

Topical: Refer to Application Guidelines.

 Apply 1-2 drops neat to temples, at the base of the neck, in the center of the forehead, and at the nostril openings. Also massage on thumbs and big toes.

 Place a warm compress with 1-2 drops of chosen oil on the back of the neck or on the back.

Sinus Headache (See also SINUS INFECTIONS AND PROBLEMS)

Signs and symptoms of migraines and sinus headaches can be confused with each other. With both kinds, the pain often gets worse when you bend forward and can be accompanied by various nasal signs and symptoms. However, sinus headaches are usually not associated with nausea or vomiting or aggravated by bright light or noise, which are common features of migraines.

Recommendations
Singles: Dorado Azul, Peppermint, Peppermint Vitality, Eucalyptus Blue, Eucalyptus Radiata, Tea Tree, Davana, Mastrante, Geranium, Lavender, Lavender Vitality, Rosemary, Rosemary Vitality

Blends: R.C., Breathe Again, Breathe Again Roll-On, SniffleEase, Melrose, Purification, Raven,

RutaVaLa, RutaVaLa Roll-On, Stress Away, Stress Away Roll-On, CBD, Chivalry

Nutritionals: Super Vitamin C, Super Vitamin C Chewable, ImmuPro, Mineral Essence, Detoxzyme

Application and Usage
Aromatic: Refer to Application Guidelines.

Topical: Refer to Application Guidelines.

- Apply 1-2 drops neat or diluted 2-5 times daily or as needed.

- Massage 2-4 drops neat on the bottoms of the feet just before bedtime

Sinus Headache Blend
- 9 drops Rosemary
- 5 drops Tea Tree
- 4 drops Geranium
- 3 drops Peppermint
- 2 drops Eucalyptus Blue
- 2 drops Lavender

Tension (Stress) Headache (See also STRESS)

Tension headaches are the most common type of headaches among adults and are commonly referred to as stress headaches. They are usually triggered by some type of internal or environmental stress. In some people, tension headaches are caused by tightened muscles in the scalp and in the back of the neck and may be caused by anxiety, fatigue, overexertion, hunger, inadequate rest, poor posture, mental or emotional stress, or depression.

Recommendations
Singles: Valerian, Cardamom, Cardamom Vitality, Tangerine, Tangerine Vitality, Jasmine, Palmarosa, Mastrante, Geranium, Sacred Frankincense, Frankincense, Frankincense Vitality, Peppermint, Peppermint Vitality, Davana, Lavender, Lavender Vitality, Roman Chamomile, Vanilla, Bergamot, Bergamot Vitality

Blends: Release, Freedom, Valor, Valor Roll-On, Deep Relief Roll-On, Aroma Siez, PanAway, M-Grain, Peace & Calming, Peace & Calming II, CBD, Calm CBD Roll-On, Seedlings Calm, Hope, Gary's Light, Sacred Mountain, Trauma Life, Reconnect, SleepyIze, PanAway, Stress Away, Stress Away Roll-On, RutaVaLa, RutaVaLa Roll-On, Tranquil Roll-On, AromaEase

Nutritionals: Mega Vitamin Cal, Essentialzyme, Essentialzymes-4, Balance Complete, KidScents Unwind, NingXia Red, Mineral Essence, IlluminEyes, ICP, ComforTone, SleepEssence, PowerGize

Application and Usage
Aromatic: Refer to Application Guidelines.

Topical: Refer to Application Guidelines.

- Apply 1-2 drops diluted 50:50 around the hairline, on the back of the neck, and across the forehead. Be careful not to use too much, as it will burn if any oil drips near the eyes. If this should occur, dilute with a pure vegetable oil—never with water.

HEAVY METAL ABSORPTION

We absorb heavy metals from air, water, food, skin care products, and mercury fillings in teeth, etc. These chemicals lodge in the fatty tissues of the body, which, in turn, give off toxic gases that may cause allergic symptoms. Cleansing the body of these heavy metals is extremely important to have a healthy immune function, especially if one has amalgam fillings. Drink at least 64 ounces of distilled water daily to flush toxins and chemicals out of the body (See CARDIOVASCULAR CONDITIONS AND PROBLEMS, Blood Circulation, Poor).

Recommendations
Singles: Helichrysum, Jade Lemon, Jade Lemon Vitality, Lemon, Lemon Vitality, Lime, Lime Vitality, Orange, Orange Vitality, Tangerine, Tangerine Vitality, Clove, Clove Vitality, Patchouli

Blends: GLF, GLF Vitality, Thieves, Thieves Roll-On, Thieves Vitality, JuvaCleanse, JuvaCleanse Vitality, DiGize, DiGize Vitality

Nutritionals: MultiGreens, Detoxzyme, Essentialzyme, ComforTone, Mega Vitamin Cal, JuvaPower, Super Vitamin C, Super Vitamin C Chewable, Mineral Essence, Olive Essentials, Life 9, KidScents MightyPro, ICP

Aluminum Toxicity

Aluminum is a very toxic metal that can cause serious neurological damage in the human body—even in minute amounts. Aluminum has been implicated as a possible cause of many maladies in the body, especially Alzheimer's disease.

People unwittingly ingest aluminum from their cookware, beverage cans, antacids, and even deodorants and other cosmetic compounds. The first step toward reducing aluminum toxicity in the body is to avoid these types of aluminum-based products. Read the labels and see for yourself.

Recommendations

Singles: Helichrysum, Jade Lemon, Jade Lemon Vitality, Lemon, Lemon Vitality, Lime, Lime Vitality, Orange, Orange Vitality, Tangerine, Tangerine Vitality, Clove, Clove Vitality, Patchouli

Blends: GLF, GLF Vitality, Thieves, Thieves Roll-On, Thieves Vitality, JuvaCleanse, JuvaCleanse Vitality, DiGize, DiGize Vitality

Nutritionals: JuvaTone, ICP (a.m.), Detoxzyme, Essentialzyme, Mega Vitamin Cal, ComforTone, JuvaPower (p.m.)

Application and Usage

Aromatic: Refer to Application Guidelines.

Dietary and Oral: Refer to Application Guidelines.

- Begin by cleansing the liver, blood, and colon to rid the body of toxins and waste.

- Take 1 capsule of desired Vitality oil 2 times daily.
- Take 2-3 drops of desired Vitality oil in a spoonful of syrup or small amount of milk, juice, or water.

Topical: Refer to Application Guidelines.

HEMORRHOIDS

Symptoms of hemorrhoids are bleeding during bowel movements, rectal pain, and itching.

Recommendations

Singles: Myrrh, Helichrysum, Cypress, Cistus, Basil, Basil Vitality, Jade Lemon, Jade Lemon Vitality, Lemon, Lemon Vitality, Lime, Lime Vitality, Peppermint, Peppermint Vitality

Blends: Melrose, Purification, Aroma Siez, Aroma Life, PanAway

Nutritionals: Essentialzymes-4, Essentialzyme, MultiGreens, Longevity Softgels, Mega Vitamin Cal, Digest & Cleanse, ICP, ComforTone, JuvaPower

Personal Care: Rose Ointment, KidScents Tender Tush, Seedlings Diaper Rash Cream

Application and Usage

Topical: Refer to Application Guidelines.

- Apply single oils or Blends neat or diluted, depending on the oils that are used.
- Use a rectal implant of your choice of the Blends below; place in rectum with a small syringe 1 time every other day for 6 days. It is best done at night to be able to retain as long as possible.
- Apply 3-5 drops diluted 50:50 on location. This may sting but usually brings relief with 1 or 2 applications.

Hemorrhoid Blend No. 1
- 4 drops Basil
- 1 drop Cistus
- 1 drop Cypress
- 1 drop Helichrysum

Mix with Rose Ointment for dilution and easier application.

Hemorrhoid Blend No. 2
- 4 drops Myrrh
- 3 drops Cypress
- 2 drops Helichrysum

Mix with Rose Ointment for dilution and easier application.

HICCUPS

People have been curious about the cause of hiccups for years. There are many ideas, but scientifically, everyone is still waiting for an explanation. Some say hiccups are caused by irritated nerves of the diaphragm, possibly from eating too much or from indigestion.

One technique that often works for stopping hiccups is to put 1 drop of Cypress and 1 drop of Tarragon on the end of the index finger and then place that finger on the neck against the esophagus in the clavicle notch in the center, curl inward and down like you are curling down inside the throat, and release.

Tarragon or Cypress applied topically or taken as a Dietary and Oral supplement may relax intestinal spasms, nervous digestion, and hiccups. It's worth a try.

Recommendations

Singles: Carrot Seed, Carrot Seed Vitality, Tarragon, Tarragon Vitality, Cypress, Spearmint, Spearmint Vitality, Peppermint, Peppermint Vitality

Blends: DiGize, DiGize Vitality, JuvaFlex, JuvaFlex Vitality, KidScents TummyGize

Nutritionals: AlkaLime, Digest & Cleanse, Mega Vitamin Cal

Application and Usage
Dietary and Oral: Refer to Application Guidelines.

- Take 1 capsule of desired Vitality oil 2 times daily.

- Take 2-3 drops of desired Vitality oil in a spoonful of syrup or small amount of milk, juice, or water.

Topical: Refer to Application Guidelines.

- Apply 3-5 drops diluted 50:50 to chest and stomach areas.

HIVES

Hives are a generalized itching or dermatitis that can be due to allergies, damaged liver, chemicals, emotions, or other factors.

Recommendations
Singles: Myrrh, German Chamomile, German Chamomile Vitality, Roman Chamomile, Ravintsara, Lavender, Lavender Vitality, Eucalyptus Radiata, Tea Tree, Peppermint, Peppermint Vitality, Vanilla

Blends: RutaVaLa, RutaVaLa Roll-On, Stress Away, Stress Away Roll-On, Tranquil Roll-On, Gary's Light, Peace & Calming, Peace & Calming II, Calm CBD Roll-On, Seedlings Calm

Nutritionals: Super Vitamin Cal Plus, Mega Vitamin Cal, Mineral Essence, Sulfurzyme, Master Formula, KidScents Unwind, MultiGreens, Super Vitamin B

Personal Care: Rose Ointment, KidScents Tender Tush

Application and Usage
Topical: Refer to Application Guidelines.

- Apply 2-4 drops diluted 50:50 on location as needed.

- Place a cold compress on location as needed.

HYPERACTIVITY
(See also ATTENTION DEFICIT DISORDER)

Hyperactivity behavior usually refers to a group of characteristics, including inability to concentrate, being easily distracted, impulsive, or aggressive; fidgeting; moving constantly, talking too much, and having difficulty participating in quiet activities.

Recommendations
Singles: Lavender, Lavender Vitality, Vetiver, Hinoki, Idaho Blue Spruce, Roman Chamomile, Peppermint, Peppermint Vitality, Valerian, Vanilla, Cedarwood

Blends: RutaVaLa, RutaVaLa Roll-On, Gary's Light, Peace & Calming, Peace & Calming II, Stress Away, Stress Away Roll-On, Calm CBD Roll-On, Seedlings Calm, KidScents KidPower, KidScents KidPower Roll-On, Tranquil Roll-On, Sacred Mountain, Grounding, Gathering

Nutritionals: Super Vitamin B, Master Formula, KidScents Unwind, Mega Vitamin Cal

Application and Usage
Aromatic: Refer to Application Guidelines.

- Diffuse 5 times daily for up to 30 days, stop for 5 days, and then repeat, if necessary.

Topical: Refer to Application Guidelines.

- Apply 2-4 drops neat on toes and balls of feet as needed.

INFECTIONS, BACTERIAL AND VIRAL

Diffusing essential oils is one of the best ways to prevent the spread of airborne bacteria and viruses. Many essential oils, such as Oregano, Mountain Savory, and Rosemary, exert highly antimicrobial effects and can effectively eliminate many kinds of pathogens.

Viruses and bacteria have a tendency to hibernate along the spine. The body may hold a virus in a suspended state for a long period of time. When the immune system is compromised, these viruses may be released and then manifest as illness.

Raindrop Technique along the spine using Oregano and Thyme helps reduce inflammation and kills the microorganisms. However, other oils may also be used, which also have strong antiviral and antibacterial properties. ImmuPower, R.C., and Purification all work well in the Raindrop Technique application method.

Mountain Savory, Ravintsara, Eucalyptus Blue, Palo Santo, Sacred Frankincense, Frankincense, and Thyme, etc., applied along the spine through the Raindrop Technique application, may be beneficial for many infections, particularly chest-related (See COLDS, LUNG INFECTIONS AND PROBLEMS, SINUS INFECTIONS, THROAT INFECTIONS AND PROBLEMS).

Recommendations

Singles: Palo Santo, Sacred Frankincense, Frankincense, Frankincense Vitality, Mountain Savory, Mountain Savory Vitality, Ravintsara, Eucalyptus Blue, Rosemary, Rosemary Vitality, Lemongrass, Lemongrass Vitality, Clove, Clove Vitality, Melissa, Tea Tree, Oregano, Oregano Vitality, Ecuadorian Oregano, Thyme, Thyme Vitality, Geranium, Cassia, Dorado Azul, Northern Lights Black Spruce, Cardamom, Cardamom Vitality, Davana

Blends: Thieves, Thieves Roll-On, Thieves Vitality, Purification, Melrose, R.C., ImmuPower, Exodus II, Raven, The Gift, AromaEase, Breathe Again, Breathe Again Roll-On, SniffleEase

Nutritionals: Inner Defense, Super Vitamin C, Super Vitamin C Chewable, NingXia Red, Longevity Softgels, MultiGreens, ImmuPro, OmegaGize3, Life 9, KidScents MightyPro, Ningxia Wolfberries (Organic, Dried)

Application and Usage

Aromatic: Refer to Application Guidelines.

Dietary and Oral: Refer to Application Guidelines.

- Take 1 capsule of desired Vitality oil 2 times daily.

- Take 2-3 drops of desired Vitality oil in a spoonful of syrup or small amount of milk, juice, or water.

Topical: Refer to Application Guidelines.

- Apply 4-6 drops on location diluted 20:80 2-3 times daily.

- Receive a Raindrop Technique treatment 1-2 times weekly.

INFLAMMATION (See also MUSCLE PROBLEMS)

Inflammation can be caused by a variety of conditions, including bacterial infection, poor diet, chemicals, hormonal imbalance, and physical injury.

Certain essential oils have been documented to be excellent for reducing inflammation such as German Chamomile, which contains azulene, a blue compound with highly anti-inflammatory properties. Other oils with anti-inflammatory properties include Peppermint, Tea Tree, Clove, Lemongrass, Mountain Savory, Palo Santo, Dorado Azul, and Wintergreen.

Some oils are better suited for certain types of inflammation, for example:

- Myrrh, Vetiver, Cistus, and Helichrysum work well for inflammation due to tissue and capillary damage and bruising.
- German Chamomile and Tea Tree are helpful with inflammation due to bacterial infection.
- Ravintsara, Hyssop, Myrrh, Thyme are appropriate for inflammation caused by viral infection.

Recommendations

Singles: Wintergreen, Vetiver, German Chamomile, German Chamomile Vitality, Tea Tree, Idaho Blue Spruce, Myrrh, Ravintsara, Hinoki, Copaiba, Copaiba Vitality, Palo Santo, Helichrysum, Cistus, Clove, Clove Vitality, Lemongrass, Lemongrass Vitality, Nutmeg, Nutmeg Vitality, Lavender, Lavender Vitality, Thyme, Thyme Vitality, Frankincense, Frankincense Vitality, Roman Chamomile, Sacred Frankincense, Frankincense, Frankincense Vitality, Cassia, Hyssop, Peppermint, Peppermint Vitality, Eucalyptus Blue, Eucalyptus Globulus, Mountain Savory, Mountain Savory Vitality, Dorado Azul

Blends: Purification, PanAway, Cool Azul, Aroma Siez, Melrose, Relieve It, Deep Relief Roll-On, CBD

Nutritionals: PowerGize, ImmuPro, Super Vitamin C, Super Vitamin C Chewable, Super Vitamin D, Slique Shake, Slique CitraSlim

Personal Care: Cool Azul Pain Relief Cream, Cool Azul Sports Gel, CBD Muscle Rub, Ortho Ease Massage Oil, Ortho Sport Massage Oil

Application and Usage

Dietary and Oral: Refer to Application Guidelines.

- Take 1 capsule of desired Vitality oil 2 times daily.

- Take 2-3 drops of desired Vitality oil in a spoonful of syrup or small amount of milk, juice, or water.

Topical: Refer to Application Guidelines.

- Apply 2-4 drops diluted 50:50 2 times daily.

- Place a cold compress 1-3 times daily as needed.

Anti-inflammation Blend No. 1
- 6 drops Eucalyptus Blue
- 6 drops Tea Tree
- 4 drops German Chamomile or German Chamomile Vitality
- 2 drops Peppermint or Peppermint Vitality
- 2 drops Idaho Blue Spruce

Anti-inflammation Blend No. 2
- 6 drops Myrrh
- 6 drops Eucalyptus Globulus
- 4 drops Clove or Clove Vitality
- 3 drops Palo Santo
- 1 drop Vetiver

INFLUENZA

Having the flu may seem like just having a cold with a sore throat, runny nose, and sneezing. However, colds usually develop slowly, whereas the flu generally comes on suddenly. Although a cold can be a nuisance, you usually feel much worse with the flu.

Common symptoms of the flu include nasal congestion, headache, dry cough, fatigue and weakness, aching muscles, chills and sweats, and high fever. Stomach flu may cause cramps, nausea, vomiting, and diarrhea.

Recommendations

Singles: Mountain Savory, Mountain Savory Vitality, Oregano, Oregano Vitality, Ecuadorian Oregano, Eucalyptus Radiata, Peppermint, Peppermint Vitality, Clove, Clove Vitality, Tea Tree, Eucalyptus Blue, Dorado Azul, Sacred Frankincense, Frankincense, Frankincense Vitality, Idaho Blue Spruce, Cassia, Ravintsara, Wintergreen

Blends: ImmuPower, Exodus II, Thieves, Thieves Roll-On, Thieves Vitality, Raven, R.C., Breathe Again, Breathe Again Roll-On, SniffleEase, DiGize, DiGize Vitality, KidScents TummyGize

Nutritionals: Digest & Cleanse, Inner Defense, AlkaLime, Life 9, KidScents MightyPro, Essentialzyme, Essentialzymes-4, Detoxzyme, ICP, JuvaPower

Oral Care: Thieves Cough Drops, Thieves Hard Lozenges, Thieves Spray, Thieves Mints

Personal Care: Thieves Chest Rub

Application and Usage

Aromatic: Refer to Application Guidelines.

Dietary and Oral: Refer to Application Guidelines.

- Take 1 capsule of desired Vitality oil 3 times daily.

- Take 2-3 drops of desired Vitality oil in a spoonful of syrup or small amount of milk, juice, or water.

Topical: Refer to Application Guidelines.
- Apply 2-4 drops diluted 50:50 on chest, stomach, or lower back 2 times daily or as needed.
- Receive Raindrop Technique 1-2 times weekly.
- Place a warm compress on lower abdomen 1-2 times daily.
- Take a warm bath with custom bath salts, using the following influenza blend:

Blend for Influenza or Colds
- 15 drops Ravintsara
- 6 drops Sacred Frankincense or Frankincense
- 6 drops Idaho Blue Spruce
- 3 drops Dorado Azul
- 2 drops Eucalyptus Radiata
- 1 drop Wintergreen

Stir the above essential oils thoroughly into $\frac{1}{4}$ cup Epsom salt or baking soda and then add salt and oil mixture to hot bath water while tub is filling. Soak in hot bath for 20 to 30 minutes or until water cools.

INSECT BITES AND STINGS

Essential oils are ideal for treating most kinds of insect bites because of their outstanding antiseptic and oil-soluble properties. Essential oils and Blends such as Purification, Lavender, and Peppermint reduce insect bite-induced itching and infection.

Recommendations

Singles: Lavender, Citronella, Eucalyptus Globulus, Eucalyptus Radiata, Eucalyptus Blue, Tea Tree, Peppermint, Rosemary, Copaiba, Dorado Azul, Palo Santo, Idaho Tansy, German Chamomile, Thyme

Blends: Purification, PanAway, Melrose, Thieves

Personal Care: YL Insect Repellant

Application and Usage

Topical: Refer to Application Guidelines.

- Apply 1-2 drops of the sting and bite Blends neat or diluted 50:50 on location 2-4 times daily.

Stings and Bites Blend No. 1
- 10 drops Lavender
- 4 drops Eucalyptus Radiata
- 3 drops German Chamomile
- 2 drops Thyme

Spray sheets and clothing to kill any insects that might be embedded in the cloth.

Insect Bite Blend No. 2
- 20 drops Palo Santo
- 20 drops Idaho Tansy
- 10 drops Eucalyptus Blue

 Rub a small amount on skin or use in spray bottle.

Bee Stings

Bee stings can be painful and annoying, but they rarely cause serious problems, unless you are allergic to the venom—then they can be fatal.

Recommendations

Singles: Lavender, Peppermint, Palo Santo, German Chamomile, Idaho Grand Fir, Vetiver

Blends: Purification, PanAway, Melrose, Deep Relief Roll-On

Application and Usage

Topical: Refer to Application Guidelines.
- Apply 1-2 drops of the Bee Sting Blend neat or diluted 50:50 on location 2-4 times daily.

Bee Sting Blend
- 2 drops Lavender
- 1 drop Peppermint
- 1 drop German Chamomile
- 1 drop Vetiver

Bee Sting Regimen
- Flick or scrape stinger out with a knife or hard plastic like a credit card, taking care not to squeeze the venom sac.
- Apply 1-2 drops of the Bee Sting Blend on location. Repeat every 15 minutes for 1 hour.
- Apply any of the recommended Blends 2-3 times daily until redness abates.

Bites

Essential oils are ideal for treating most kinds of insect bites because of their outstanding antiseptic and oil-soluble properties. Essential oils such as Lavender and Peppermint reduce insect bite-induced itching and infection.

Recommendations

Singles: Lavender, Eucalyptus Radiata, German Chamomile, Citronella, Thyme, Eucalyptus Globulus, Tea Tree, Pepper-mint, Rosemary, Idaho Tansy, Palo Santo, Copaiba, Dorado Azul

Blends: Purification, PanAway, Melrose

Personal Care: YL Insect Repellent

Application and Usage

Topical: Refer to Application Guidelines.
- Apply 1-2 drops of either Stings and Bites Blends neat or diluted 50:50 on location 2-4 times daily.

Stings and Bites Blend No. 1
- 10 drops Lavender
- 4 drops Eucalyptus Radiata
- 3 drops German Chamomile
- 2 drops Thyme

Stings and Bites Blend No. 2
- 20 drops Palo Santo
- 20 drops Idaho Tansy
- 10 drops Eucalyptus Blue

Bedbug Bites
Bedbug bites can be difficult to distinguish from other insect bites. However, bedbug bites are usually:
- Found on the face, neck, arms, and hands
- Arranged in a rough line or in a cluster
- Itchy
- Red, often with a darker red spot in the middle

Singles: Palo Santo, Eucalyptus Blue, Idaho Tansy

Blends: Purification, Thieves

Personal Care: YL Insect Repellent

Application and Usage
Topical: Refer to Application Guidelines.

- Apply 1-2 drops of a Stings and Bites blend neat or diluted 50:50 on location 2-4 times daily.

Stings and Bites Blend No. 1
- 10 drops Lavender
- 4 drops Eucalyptus Radiata
- 3 drops German Chamomile
- 2 drops Thyme

Insect Bite Blend No. 2
- 20 drops Palo Santo
- 20 drops Idaho Tansy
- 10 drops Eucalyptus Blue

Black Widow Spider Bite
A bite from a female black widow spider can cause pain and affect the victim's nervous system, but it is rarely fatal. If you know you have been bitten by a black widow spider, seek emergency medical treatment immediately.

Recommendations
Singles: Myrrh, Lemon

Blends: Purification, Thieves, Thieves Roll-On, Melrose, PanAway, The Gift

Nutritionals: Inner Defense

Application and Usage
Topical: Refer to Application Guidelines.

- Put on 1 drop of any oil you have such as Purification, Melrose, The Gift, Lemon, etc.

Brown Recluse Spider Bite
The bite of this spider causes a painful redness and blistering, which progresses to a gangrenous slough of the affected area. Seek immediate medical attention.

Recommendations
Singles: Myrrh, Sacred Frankincense, Frankincense, Rosemary, Lemon

Blends: Purification, Thieves, Thieves Roll-On, Melrose, PanAway, The Gift

Nutritionals: Inner Defense

Application and Usage
Topical: Refer to Application Guidelines.

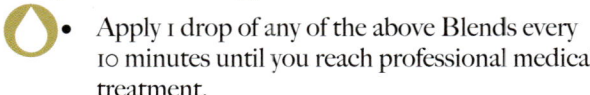
- Apply 1 drop of any of the above Blends every 10 minutes until you reach professional medical treatment.

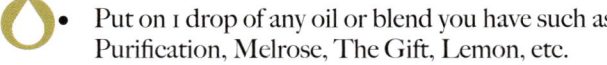
- Put on 1 drop of any oil or blend you have such as Purification, Melrose, The Gift, Lemon, etc.

Spider Bite Blend
- 1 drop Sacred Frankincense or Frankincense
- 1 drop Myrrh
- 1 drop Melrose

Chigger and Tick Bites
It is important that ticks and chiggers be removed before treating the bite. People have tried many different ways of getting rid of these invaders. Sometimes chiggers can be removed or killed by covering the bite with clear fingernail polish.

A common method for removing ticks is to touch them gently with a recently blown-out match head. The heat often causes ticks to let go so that they can just be brushed off and killed.

Essential oils work quickly to remove ticks and chiggers. Mix Thyme or Oregano in a 50:50 dilution and apply 1-2 drops on the bite area. The phenols in these oils will usually cause them to let go and squirm to get away from the oil. When they do, they can be brushed off and killed.

Applying a single drop of Peppermint, Abundance, Exodus II, Thieves, or any other oil or blend that is considered to be "hot" will cause the tick or chigger to come out of the skin. A "hot" oil is one that is high in phenols that can burn the skin when applied neat. In this case, the objective is to "get the critter out."

For most people, a little stinging does not matter. After the tick or chigger is removed, apply 1-2 drops of any of the oils listed below on the bite location.

Recommendations

Singles: Peppermint, Oregano, Clove, Tea Tree, Lavender, Rosemary, Myrrh, Sacred Frankincense, Frankincense, Thyme, Idaho Grand Fir

Blends: Purification, Exodus II, Abundance, Melrose, Thieves, R.C., The Gift

Personal Care: YL Insect Repellent

Application and Usage
Topical: Refer to Application Guidelines.

- Apply 1-6 drops neat or diluted, depending on size of affected area, 3-5 times daily.

Mosquito Bites

For most people, a mosquito bite causes minor irritation. For those who are allergic to bites, their skin breaks out in hives, the chest and throat feel tight, they develop a dry cough, their eyes itch, and they often have nausea, vomiting, abdominal pain, and dizziness.

If you suspect you have a mosquito bite allergy, let your health care professional see your red, swollen bite.

Recommendations

Singles: Peppermint, Tea Tree, Lavender, Rosemary, Myrrh, Sacred Frankincense, Frankincense, Idaho Grand Fir, Laurus Nobilis

Blends: Purification, Melrose, Thieves, Thieves Roll-On, R.C., The Gift, KidScents Owie

Personal Care: YL Insect Repellent, Thieves Chest Rub

Application and Usage
Topical: Refer to Application Guidelines.

- Apply 1-6 drops neat or diluted, depending on size of affected area, 3-5 times daily.

West Nile Virus

Most people infected with West Nile virus have no signs or symptoms, and mild symptoms usually go away in a few days. However, if you experience symptoms or signs of a serious infection like a high fever, severe headache, stiff neck, or an altered mental state, see your health care professional immediately. A serious West Nile virus infection generally requires hospitalization.

Recommendations

Singles: Peppermint, Tea Tree, Melissa, Melaleuca Quinquenervia, Lavender, Rosemary, Myrrh, Sacred Frankincense, Frankincense, Idaho Grand Fir, Oregano, Thyme, Northern Lights Black Spruce, Laurus Nobilis

Blends: Purification, Melrose, Thieves, Thieves Roll-On, R.C., The Gift

Personal Care: YL Insect Repellent (for prevention)

Application and Usage
Topical: Refer to Application Guidelines.

- Apply 1-6 drops neat or diluted, depending on size of affected area, 3-5 times daily.

Scorpion Sting

Several species of scorpions are found in the United States and Canada, but most do not produce a significant toxicity by stinging and are not as toxic as those found in South America and other parts of the world. A sting may cause swelling and a lot of discomfort but is rarely fatal. However, a person who has been stung by a scorpion should see a doctor as soon as possible. Follow these first-aid measures:

- If breathing and heartbeat stop, start CPR immediately.
- Apply an ice pack or cold water to the bite area to help slow the spread of the venom.
- Seek medical care.

Recommendations

Singles: Lemongrass, Sacred Frankincense, Frankincense

Blends: Purification

Application and Usage
Topical: Refer to Application Guidelines.

- Apply 1-6 drops neat or diluted 50:50, depending on size of affected area, 3-5 times daily.

INSECT REPELLENT, NEED FOR

An insect repellent is a substance applied to skin, clothing, or other surfaces that discourages insects from landing on those surfaces. Repellents help prevent the outbreak of insect-borne diseases such as West Nile virus, Lyme disease, dengue fever, bubonic plague, and malaria.

Recommendations

Singles: Palo Santo, Idaho Tansy, Peppermint, Tea Tree, Geranium, Lemon, Rosemary, Lemongrass, Thyme, Spearmint, Citronella, Oregano, Basil

Blends: Purification, Melrose, Thieves, Thieves Roll-On, DiGize

Personal Care: YL Insect Repellent

Application and Usage

Topical: Refer to Application Guidelines.

 • Apply 1-6 drops neat or diluted, depending on size of affected area, 3-5 times daily.

Insect Repellent Blend No. 1
- 9 drops Idaho Tansy or Palo Santo
- 6 drops Peppermint
- 6 drops Citronella

Insect Repellent Blend No. 2
- 6 drops Idaho Tansy
- 6 drops Palo Santo

Mix together and use undiluted or diluted with a little water.

Ed & Steven Geiger's Bug Spray
- 1 gallon distilled water
- 1 ounce organic catnip made into a tea, strained, and cooled
- 1 teaspoon Bath Gel Base
- 40 drops Purification
- 40 drops Idaho Tansy or Palo Santo
- 40 drops DiGize
- 20 drops Rosemary
- 8 drops Peppermint

Optional: Add Lemongrass and/or Oregano

Chérie Ross's Formula for Flea, Tick, and Insect Repellent
- 1 gallon distilled or pure water
- 4 heaping tablespoons organic dried catnip
- $2\frac{1}{2}$ tablespoons organic Neem oil
- 2 teaspoons Thieves Household Cleaner or Bath Gel Base
- 80 drops Purification
- 80 drops Lemongrass
- 40 drops Idaho Tansy
- 40 drops Palo Santo
- 40 drops Basil
- 20 drops Peppermint (optional for high temperatures)

Steep the catnip in the gallon of water for 20-30 minutes. Cool to room temperature. Strain if needed. Add all remaining ingredients into Thieves Household Cleaner or Bath Gel Base. Then mix together and put into spray bottle. Use as needed.

Insect Repellent

Mosquito repellent: Palo Santo, Lemon, Idaho Tansy, Citronella

Moth repellent: Patchouli, Palo Santo

Horsefly repellent: Idaho Tansy, Citronella

Aphids repellent: Mix 10 drops Spearmint and 15 drops Orange essential oils in 2 quarts salt water, shake well, and spray on plants.

Cockroach repellent: Mix 10 drops Peppermint and 5 drops Cypress in $\frac{1}{2}$ cup salt water. Shake well and spray where roaches live.

Silverfish repellent: Eucalyptus Radiata, Thieves, To repel insects, essential oils can be diffused or put on cotton balls or cedar chips (for use in closets or drawers). Experiment with your own combination of oils and make new discoveries

INSOMNIA
(See also SLEEP DISORDERS, INSOMNIA; DEPRESSION; THYROID PROBLEMS)

After age 40, sleep quality and quantity deteriorate noticeably as melatonin production in the brain declines. Supple-mental melatonin has been researched to dramatically improve sleep/wake cycles and combat age-related insomnia.

Insomnia may also be caused by bowel or liver toxicity, poor heart function, negative memories and trauma, depression, mineral deficiencies, hormone imbalance, or underactive thyroid.

The fragrance of many essential oils can exert a powerful, calming effect on the mind through their influence on the limbic region of the brain. Historically, lavender sachets or pillows were used for babies, children, and adults alike.

Recommendations
Singles: Lavender, Lavender Vitality, Valerian, Lemon Verbena, Cedarwood, Orange, Orange Vitality, Roman Chamomile, Dorado Azul, Vanilla

Blends: RutaVaLa, RutaVaLa Roll-On, Gary's Light, Peace & Calming, Peace & Calming II, Calm CBD Roll-On, Seed-lings Calm, Harmony, Dream Catcher, Valor, Valor Roll-On, Gentle Baby, Tranquil Roll-On, Trauma Life, Stress Away, Stress Away Roll-On

Nutritionals: ImmuPro, Mega Vitamin Cal, PD 80/20, Life 9, KidScents MightyPro, KidScents Unwind, OmegaGize3, SleepEssence, MindWise

Personal Care: Progessence Plus, Prenolone Plus Body Cream

Application and Usage
Aromatic: Refer to Application Guidelines.

Dietary and Oral: Refer to Application Guidelines.

- Take 1 capsule of desired Vitality oil 2 times daily.

- Take 1 capsule of Lavender Vitality oil or any desired oil undiluted or diluted 50:50 1 hour before bedtime.

- Take 2-3 drops of desired Vitality oil in a spoonful of syrup or small amount of milk, juice, or water.

Insomnia Blend
- 12 drops Orange or Orange Vitality
- 8 drops Lavender or Lavender Vitality
- 4 drops Dorado Azul
- 3 drops Valerian
- 2 drops Roman Chamomile

Topical: Refer to Application Guidelines.

- Apply 1-3 drops neat to shoulders, stomach, and on bottoms of feet.

- Mix 6-8 drops of oils with ¼ cup Epsom salt or baking soda in hot water and add to hot bath water while tub is filling. Soak in bathtub for 20 to 30 minutes or until water cools.

- Rub 1-2 drops of oil on the temples and back of neck several times daily.

- Place a warm compress with 1-2 drops of chosen oil on the back.

IRRITABLE BOWEL SYNDROME

Irritable bowel syndrome (IBS) is a common disorder of the intestines marked by the following symptoms:
- Cramps
- Gas and bloating
- Constipation
- Diarrhea and loose stools

It may be caused by a combination of stress and a high-fat diet. Fatty foods increase the intensity of the contractions in the colon, thereby increasing symptoms. Chocolate and milk products, in particular, seem to have the most negative effects on those suffering.

Irritable bowel syndrome is not the same as colitis, mucus colitis, spastic colon, and spastic bowel. Unlike colitis, it does not involve any inflammation and is actually called "functional disorder" because it presents no obvious, outward signs of disease.

A number of medical studies have documented that peppermint oil, in capsules, is beneficial in treating irritable bowel syndrome and decreasing pain.37, 38, 39

Recommendations
Singles: Tarragon, Tarragon Vitality, Peppermint, Peppermint Vitality, Fennel, Fennel Vitality, Nutmeg, Nutmeg Vitality, Frankincense, Frankincense Vitality, Sacred Frankincense, Juniper

Blends: DiGize, DiGize Vitality, JuvaFlex, JuvaFlex Vitality, AromaEase, KidScents TummyGize

Nutritionals: Detoxzyme, OmegaGize3, Digest & Cleanse, Life 9, KidScents MightyPro, AlkaLime, JuvaPower. After symptoms stop, then start Essentialzymes-4, Essentialzyme, and ICP.

Application and Usage

Aromatic: Refer to Application Guidelines.

Dietary and Oral: Refer to Application Guidelines.

- Take 1 capsule of desired Vitality oil 3 times daily.

- Take 2-3 drops of desired Vitality oil in a spoonful of syrup or small amount of milk, juice, or water.

Topical: Refer to Application Guidelines.

JOINT STIFFNESS OR PAIN

Joint stiffness is caused by inflammation in the lining of the joint. Specific causes may be rheumatoid arthritis, osteoarthritis, bone diseases, cancer, joint trauma, or overuse of the joint. However, no matter what causes it, joint pain and stiffness can be very bothersome.

Recommendations

Singles: Wintergreen, Lemongrass, Lemongrass Vitality, Palo Santo, Idaho Blue Spruce, Elemi, Idaho Grand Fir, German Chamomile, German Chamomile Vitality, Peppermint, Peppermint Vitality, Pine, Vetiver, Black Pepper, Black Pepper Vitality, Marjoram, Marjoram Vitality, Frankincense, Frankincense Vitality, Sacred Frankincense, Rosemary, Rosemary Vitality

Blends: PanAway, Aroma Siez, Cool Azul, Relieve It, Deep Relief Roll-On, CBD, Chivalry

Nutritionals: BLM, AgilEase, PowerGize, Mega Vitamin Cal, Super Vitamin D, Sulfurzyme, OmegaGize3, MultiGreens

Resins: Myrrh or Frankincense Gum Resin (ingest 2 crystals 2 times daily)

Personal Care: Cool Azul Pain Relief Cream, Cool Azul Sports Gel, CBD Muscle Rub, Regenolone Moisturizing Cream, Ortho Ease Massage Oil, Ortho Sport Massage Oil

Application and Usage

Topical: Refer to Application Guidelines.

- Massage 3-6 drops diluted 50:50 on location. Repeat as needed to control pain.

- Apply to appropriate Vita Flex points on the feet. Repeat as needed.

Joint Pain Blend No. 1
- 10 drops Black Pepper
- 5 drops Marjoram
- 5 drops Idaho Blue Spruce
- 2 drops Rosemary

Joint Pain Blend No. 2
- 7 drops Idaho Grand Fir
- 4 drops Wintergreen
- 3 drops Vetiver
- 2 drops German Chamomile

KIDNEY DISORDERS

The kidneys remove waste products from the blood and help control blood pressure. They filter over 200 quarts of blood each day and remove over 2 quarts of waste products and water that flow into the bladder as urine through tubes called ureters.

Strong kidneys are essential for good health. Inefficient or damaged kidneys can result in waste accumulating in the blood and causing serious damage.

High blood pressure can be a cause and a result of chronic kidney failure, since kidneys are central to blood regulation (See CARDIOVASCULAR CONDITIONS AND PROBLEMS, Blood Pressure, High).

Symptoms of poor kidney function:
- Infrequent or inefficient urinations
- Swelling, especially around the ankles
- Labored breathing due to fluid accumulation in the chest

Recommendations

Singles: Grapefruit, Grapefruit Vitality, Jade Lemon, Jade Lemon Vitality, Lemon, Lemon Vitality, Geranium, Juniper

Blends: DiGize, DiGize Vitality, GLF, GLF Vitality, JuvaFlex, JuvaFlex Vitality, Citrus Fresh, Citrus Fresh Vitality

Nutritionals: K&B, Digest & Cleanse

Application and Usage

Aromatic: Refer to Application Guidelines.

Dietary and Oral: Refer to Application Guidelines.

- Take 1 capsule of desired Vitality oil 2 times daily.

- Take 2-3 drops of desired Vitality oil in a spoonful of syrup or small amount of milk, juice, or water.

Topical: Refer to Application Guidelines.

- Apply 6-8 drops diluted 50:50 on the back over the kidney area as needed.

- Applying a single drop under the nose is helpful and refreshing.

- Massage 2-4 drops of oil neat on the bottoms of the feet just before bedtime. Children with kidney disorders may especially benefit from this application.

- Place a warm compress with 1-2 drops of chosen oil on the back 1-2 times daily.

Kidney Inflammation/Infection (Nephritis)

Kidney inflammation can be caused by structural defects, poor diet, or bacterial infection, including Escherichia coli, Staphylococcus aureus, Enterobacter, and Klebsiella bacteria. Abnormal proteins trapped in the glomeruli (tiny filtering units in the kidneys), called glomerulonephritis, can also cause inflammation and damage to these tiny filtering units.

This disease can be acute (flaring up in a few days) or chronic (taking months or years to develop). The mildest forms may not show any symptoms except through a urine test. At more advanced stages, urine appears smoky as small amounts of blood are passed and eventually turn red as more blood is excreted—the signs of impending kidney failure.

As with all serious conditions, you should immediately consult a health care professional if you suspect a kidney infection of any kind.

Symptoms may include the following:
- Feeling of discomfort in lower back
- Drowsiness
- Nausea
- Smokey or red-colored urine

Damage to the glomeruli caused by bacterial infections is called pyelonephritis. To reduce infection, drink a gallon of water mixed with 8 ounces of unsweetened cranberry juice daily and use the products listed below.

Kidneys

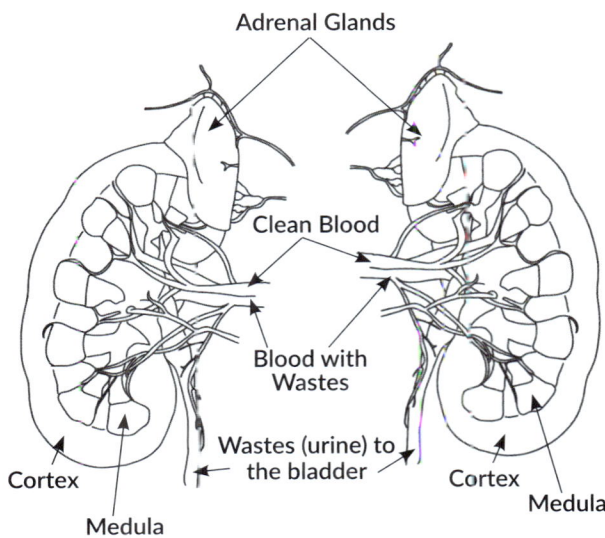

Recommendations

Singles: Cumin, Cistus, Sacred Frankincense, Frankincense, Frankincense Vitality, Juniper, Myrrh, Helichrysum, Lemongrass, Lemongrass Vitality, Rosemary, Rosemary Vitality, Cassia, Davana, Geranium, Thyme, Thyme Vitality

Blends: Melrose, Purification, Longevity, Longevity Vitality, Thieves, Thieves Roll-On, Thieves Vitality, 3 Wise Men

Nutritionals: K&B, Mineral Essence, ICP, JuvaPower, Inner Defense, Super Vitamin C, Super Vitamin C Chewable, Super Vitamin D, Life 9, KidScents MightyPro, Digest & Cleanse

Application and Usage

Aromatic: Refer to Application Guidelines.

Dietary and Oral: Refer to Application Guidelines.

- Take 2 capsules with desired Vitality oil 2 times daily for 10 days.

- Take 2-3 drops of desired Vitality oil in a spoonful of syrup or small amount of milk, juice, or water.

Topical: Refer to Application Guidelines.

- Massage 2-4 drops of oil neat on the bottoms of the feet Vita Flex points just before bedtime.

- Place a cold compress with 1-2 drops of chosen oil over the kidney area 1-2 times daily.

A Simple Way to Strengthen the Kidneys

- Take 3 droppers of K&B in 4 oz. distilled water 3 times daily.
- Drink 89 oz. water with about 10 perecent unsweetned cranberry juice and the fresh juice of 1/2 lemon
- Drink plenty of other liukds, preferably distilled water.

Kidney Stones
(See also BLADDER/URINARY TRACT INFECTION (CYSTITIS))

Kidney stones can create intense pain and dangerous infection. You should always consult a qualified health care professional before beginning any treatment for kidney stones.

A kidney stone is a solid piece of material that forms in the kidney from mineral or protein-breakdown products in the urine. Occasionally, larger stones can become trapped in the ureter, bladder, or urethra, which can block urine flow, causing intense pain.

There are four types of kidney stones:
- Stones made from calcium (the most common type)
- Stones made from magnesium and ammonia (struvite stones)
- Stones made from uric acid
- Stones made from cystine (the rarest)

Symptoms may include the following:
- Persistent, penetrating pain in side or lower back
- Blood in the urine
- Fainting

It is important to drink plenty of water (at least six 8-ounce glasses daily) to help pass a kidney stone. Also, the high acidity of apple cider vinegar helps break down the tissues of a kidney stone, even dissolving smaller kidney stones.

Recommendations
Singles: Carrot Seed, Carrot Seed Vitality, Helichrysum, Jade Lemon, Jade Lemon Vitality, Lemon, Lemon Vitality, Sacred Frankincense, Frankincense, Frankincense Vitality, Geranium, Juniper, Orange, Orange Vitality

Detoxifying the Kidneys

The Chinese wolfberry has been used in China for centuries as a kidney tonic and detoxifier. Essential oils can also assist in the detoxification due to various chemical constituents and unique, lipid-soluble properties.

Kidney Detoxifying Recipe:
- 6 drops German Chamomile
- 6 drops Juniper
- 2 drops Fennel

Put 5 drops of the recipe in a gel capsule and then fill the capsule with V-6 Vegetable Oil Complex; take 2 times daily. You may also apply the recipe neat in a compress over the kidneys.

Supplements: K&B, MultiGreens, Sulfurzyme, Detoxzyme, Essentialzyme, ICP, JuvaPower

Blends: Citrus Fresh, Citrus Fresh Vitality, Purification

Nutritionals: K&B, Essentialzymes-4, Essentialzyme, Detoxzyme

Application and Usage
Aromatic: Refer to Application Guidelines.

Dietary and Oral: Refer to Application Guidelines.

- Take 2 capsules with desired Vitality oil 2 times daily.

- Take 2-3 drops of desired Vitality oil in a spoonful of syrup or small amount of milk, juice, or water.

Topical: Refer to Application Guidelines.

- Massage 2-4 drops neat to the kidney Vita Flex points of the feet just before bedtime.

- Apply 6-10 drops of recommended oils neat over kidney area 1-2 times daily.

- Place a warm compress with 1-2 drops of chosen oil over the back.

LEUKEMIA
(See CANCER, LEUKEMIA)

LICE

The most commonly recommended remedy for lice (pediculosis) and their eggs (nits) is lindane (gamma benzene hexachloride), a highly toxic polychlorinated chemical that is structurally very similar to hazardous banned pesticides such as DDT and chlordane. It is so dangerous that Dr. Guy Sansfacon, head of the Quebec Poison Control Centre in Canada, requested that lindane be banned.

Essential oils offer a safe, effective alternative. A 1996 study by researchers in Iceland showed the effectiveness against head lice of the essential oils of anise seed, cinnamon leaf, thyme, tea tree, peppermint, and nutmeg in shampoo and rinse solutions.40

Recommendations
Singles: Tea Tree, Anise, Palo Santo, Lavender, Peppermint, Thyme, Geranium, Nutmeg, Rosemary, Cinnamon Bark

Blends: Purification, Thieves

Application and Usage
Topical: Refer to Application Guidelines.

- You may apply single oils or Blends neat or diluted, depending on the oils that are used. Add 1 teaspoon of oil diluted 50:50 to shampoo and massage onto entire scalp.
- Cover with a disposable shower cap and leave on for at least ½ hour.
- Rinse well using 1 cup of Thieves Fresh Essence Plus Mouthwash massaged into hair and scalp. Leave on for 10 minutes before rinsing out.

Head Lice Blend
- 4 drops Thyme
- 2 drops Lavender
- 2 drops Geranium

LIVER DISEASES AND DISORDERS

The liver is one of the most important organs, playing a major role in detoxifying the body. When the liver is damaged, frequently due to excess alcohol consumption, viral hepatitis, or poor diet, an excess of toxins can build up in the blood and tissues that can result in degenerative disease and death.

Jaundice (abnormal yellow color of the skin), may be the only visible sign of liver disease.

Symptoms of a stressed or diseased liver:
- Nausea
- Loss of appetite
- Dark-colored urine
- Yellowish or gray-colored bowel movements
- Abdominal pain or ascites, an unusual swelling of the abdomen caused by an accumulation of fluid, itching, dermatitis, or hives
- Disturbed sleep caused by the buildup of unfiltered toxins in the blood
- General fatigue and loss of energy
- Lack of sex drive

Hepatitis
Viral hepatitis is a serious, life-threatening disease of the liver that can result in scarring (cirrhosis) and eventual organ destruction and death. A qualified health professional should be seen immediately if you suspect hepatitis.

There are several different kinds of hepatitis: Hepatitis A (spread by contaminated food, water, or feces) and Hepatitis B and C (spread by contaminated blood or semen).

An unpublished 2003 study conducted by Roger Lewis, MD, at the Young Life Research Clinic in Springville, Utah, evaluated the efficacy of Helichrysum, Ledum, and Celery Seed in treating cases of advanced Hepatitis C. In one case, a 20-year-old male diagnosed with Hepatitis C had a viral count of 13,200. After taking 2 capsules (approximately 750 milligrams each) of GLF, a blend of Helichrysum, Ledum, Celery Seed, and JuvaCleanse daily for one month with no other intervention, the patient's viral count dropped more than 80 percent to 2,580.

Hepatitis symptoms include jaundice, weakness, loss of appetite, nausea, brownish or tea colored urine, abdominal discomfort, fever, and whitish bowel movements.

Recommendations
Singles: Carrot Seed, Carrot Seed Vitality, German Chamomile, German Chamomile Vitality, Helichrysum, Ledum, Celery Seed, Celery Seed Vitality, Ravintsara, Peppermint, Peppermint Vitality, Cassia, Myrrh

Blends: GLF, GLF Vitality, JuvaCleanse, JuvaCleanse Vitality, JuvaFlex, JuvaFlex Vitality

Nutritionals: ImmuPro, MultiGreens, JuvaPower, JuvaTone, Essentialzymes-4, Detoxzyme, Life 9, KidScents MightyPro, ICP, ComforTone, Essentialzyme, Master Formula

Note: Avoid grapefruit juice and any medications that stress the liver.

Liver

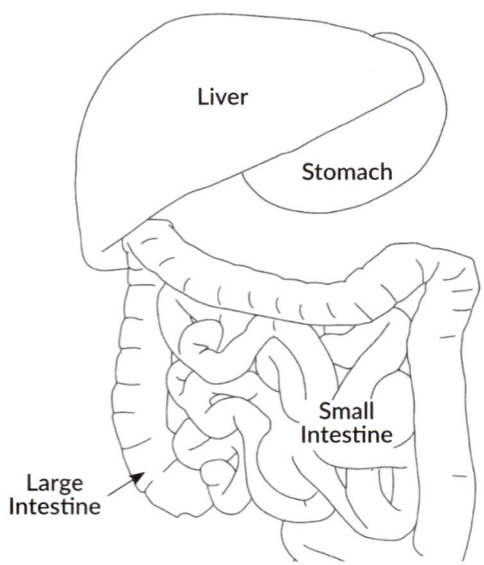

Application and Usage
Aromatic: Refer to Application Guidelines.

Dietary and Oral: Refer to Application Guidelines.

 • Take 2 capsules with desired Vitality oil 3 times daily.

 • Take 2-3 drops of desired Vitality oil in a spoonful of syrup or small amount of milk, juice, or water.

Topical: Refer to Application Guidelines.

 • Apply 1-3 drops diluted 50:50 on carotid arteries on the right and left side of the throat just under the jawbone on either side 2-5 times daily. Carotid arteries are an excellent place to apply oils for fast absorption.

 • Apply 1-3 drops on the Vita Flex liver point of the right foot 1-3 times daily.

• Receive a Raindrop Technique 2-3 times weekly.

 • Place a warm compress with 1-2 drops of chosen oil over the liver 1-2 times daily.

Daily hepatitis regimen
- Begin with a colon cleanse using ICP, ComforTone, and Essentialzyme.
- After 3 days, add 1-2 tablets of JuvaTone 3 times daily.
- ImmuPro: Take 1-2 tablets before going to bed. Do not exceed 2 daily.
- MultiGreens: Take 1-3 capsules 3 times daily.

Jaundice
Jaundice is the yellowish staining of the skin and the whites of the eyes that is caused by too much bilirubin being produced for the liver to remove it from the blood.

Recommendations
Singles: Carrot Seed, Carrot Seed Vitality, German Chamomile, German Chamomile Vitality, Ledum, Celery Seed, Celery Seed Vitality, Ravintsara, Peppermint, Peppermint Vitality, Myrrh

Blends: JuvaCleanse, JuvaCleanse Vitality, JuvaFlex, JuvaFlex Vitality, GLF, GLF Vitality

Nutritionals: JuvaPower, MultiGreens, JuvaTone, ImmuPro, Essentialzymes-4, Detoxzyme, Life 9, KidScents MightyPro, ICP, ComforTone, Essentialzyme, Master Formula

Note: Avoid grapefruit juice and any medications that stress the liver.

Application and Usage
Aromatic: Refer to Application Guidelines.

Dietary and Oral: Refer to Application Guidelines.

 • Take 2 capsules with desired Vitality oil 3 times daily.

Protecting Your Liver
- Avoid alcoholic beverages.
- Avoid unnecessary use of prescription drugs. Even over-the-counter pain relievers can have toxic effects on the liver in moderately high doses.
- Consume a diet high in selenium found in plant food, Brazil nuts, tuna, meat, eggs, etc. Selenium helps proteins make important antioxidant enzymes that prevent cellular damage from free radicals
- Avoid mixing pharmaceutical drugs, especially with alcohol.
- Avoid exposure to industrial chemicals whenever possible.
- Eat a healthy diet of vegetables and fruits; fruits are naturally cleansing.
- Nutritionals: Detoxzyme, Essentialzyme, and Ningxia wolfberry, which is widely used in China as a liver tonic and detoxifier

Personal Usage Guide | Chapter 15

- Take 2-3 drops of desired Vitality oil in a spoonful of syrup or small amount of milk, juice, or water.

Topical: Refer to Application Guidelines.

- Apply 1-3 drops diluted 50:50 on carotid arteries on the right and left side of the throat just under the jawbone on either side 2-5 times daily. Carotid arteries are an excellent place to apply oils for fast absorption.
- Apply 1-3 drops on the Vita Flex liver point of the right foot 1-3 times daily.
- Receive a Raindrop Technique 2-3 times weekly.

- Place a warm compress with 1-2 drops of chosen oil over the liver 1-2 times daily.

Toxic Liver
The liver is important in transforming and eliminating chemicals and is susceptible to becoming toxic from these substances.

Recommendations
Singles: Carrot Seed, Carrot Seed Vitality, Orange, Orange Vitality, Ledum, Celery Seed, Celery Seed Vitality, Jade Lemon, Jade Lemon Vitality, Lemon, Lemon Vitality, Lime, Lime Vitality, Cardamom, Cardamom Vitality, Geranium, German Chamomile, German Chamomile Vitality, Rosemary, Rosemary Vitality

Blends: GLF, GLF Vitality, JuvaFlex, JuvaFlex Vitality, Release, JuvaCleanse, JuvaCleanse Vitality, Citrus Fresh, Citrus Fresh Vitality

Nutritionals: JuvaTone, JuvaPower, Longevity Softgels, Sulfurzyme, Digest & Cleanse, ICP, ComforTone, Essentialzyme, Life 9, KidScents MightyPro, K&B

Application and Usage
Aromatic: Refer to Application Guidelines.

Dietary and Oral: Refer to Application Guidelines.

- Take 1 capsule of desired Vitality oil 2 times daily.

- Take 2-3 drops of desired Vitality oil in a spoonful of syrup or small amount of milk, juice, or water.

Liver Support Blend
- 10 drops Orange or Orange Vitality
- 5 drops Rosemary or Rosemary Vitality
- 3 drops Celery Seed or Celery Seed Vitality
- 2 drops German Chamomile or German Chamomile Vitality

Topical: Refer to Application Guidelines.

- Apply 1-3 drops on the liver Vita Flex point of the right foot.

- Massage 2-4 drops of oil neat on the bottoms of the feet just before bedtime.

- Place a warm compress with 1-2 drops of chosen oil over the liver 1-2 times daily.
- Have Raindrop Technique 1-2 times weekly.

LUNG INFECTIONS AND PROBLEMS
The lungs provide us with oxygen and remove carbon dioxide through respiration. Breathing brings irritants and contaminants into the lungs, making them susceptible to damage and infection.

Asthma (See also ALLERGIES)
During an asthma attack, the bronchial air tubes in the lungs become swollen and clogged with thick, sticky mucus. The muscles of the air tubes will also begin to constrict or tighten.

This results in very difficult or labored breathing. If an attack is severe, it can be life-threatening, so seek medical attention immediately.

Many asthma attacks are triggered by an allergic reaction to pollen, skin particles, dandruff, cat and dog dander, dust mites, as well as from foods such as eggs, milk, flavorings, dyes, preservatives, and other chemicals. Asthma can also be triggered by respiratory infection, exercise, stress, and psychological factors.

Recommendations
Singles: Dorado Azul, Eucalyptus Radiata, Sacred Frankincense, Frankincense, Frankincense Vitality, Eucalyptus Blue, Ravintsara, Davana, Palo Santo

Blends: R.C., Breathe Again, Breathe Again Roll-On, Valor, Raven, Inspiration, Sacred Mountain, SniffleEase

Nutritionals: Detoxzyme, ICP, JuvaPower, MultiGreens, ImmuPro, Essentialzyme, Essentialzymes-4, KidScents MightyZyme

Personal Care: Ortho Ease Massage Oil, Ortho Sport Massage Oil, Relaxation Massage Oil, Sensation Massage Oil

First Edition | Essential Oils Complete Home Reference | 861

Application and Usage

Aromatic: Refer to Application Guidelines.

Dietary and Oral: Refer to Application Guidelines.

 • Take 1-2 capsules of Dorado Azul, Palo Santo, or other Vitality oil 2 times daily.

 • Take 2-3 drops of desired Vitality oil in a spoonful of syrup or small amount of milk, juice, or water.

Topical: Refer to Application Guidelines.

 • Apply 1-2 drops mixed with Ortho Ease, Ortho Sport Massage Oil, Relaxation, or Sensation massage oils on temples and back of neck as desired.

 • You may also apply 2-3 drops on the Vita Flex points on the feet.

Bronchitis (See also ALLERGIES; ASTHMA)

Bronchitis is characterized by inflammation of the bronchial tube lining accompanied by a heavy mucus discharge. Bronchitis can be caused by an infection or exposure to dust, chemicals, air pollution, or cigarette smoke.

When bronchitis occurs regularly over long periods (i.e., three months out of the year for several years), it is known as chronic bronchitis. It can eventually lead to emphysema.

Symptoms may include the following:
- Persistent, hacking cough
- Mucus discharge from the lungs
- Difficulty breathing

Avoiding air pollution is an easy way to reduce bronchitis symptoms. In cases where bronchitis is caused by a bacteria or virus, the aroma of high antimicrobial essential oils may help combat the infection. Heavy mucus may increase after eating foods containing processed sugar or flour or high levels of fat.

Recommendations

Singles: Northern Lights Black Spruce, Dorado Azul, Myrtle, Ravintsara, Eucalyptus Blue, Palo Santo, Rosemary, Rosemary Vitality, Eucalyptus Radiata, Eucalyptus Globulus, Lavender, Lavender Vitality, Myrrh, Thyme, Thyme Vitality, Wintergreen, Pine, Oregano, Oregano Vitality, Ecuadorian Oregano, Tea Tree, Idaho Grand Fir, Copaiba, Copaiba Vitality, Clove, Clove Vitality, Frankincense, Frankincense Vitality, Sacred Frankincense, Peppermint, Peppermint Vitality, Laurus Nobilis, Laurus Nobilis Vitality

Blends: Raven, R.C., Melrose, Purification, PanAway, Thieves, Thieves Roll-On, Thieves Vitality, Breathe Again, Breathe Again Roll-On, SniffleEase, Exodus II

Nutritionals: Super Vitamin C, Super Vitamin C Chewable, Life 9, KidScents MightyPro, Longevity Softgels, Digest & Cleanse, Inner Defense

Oral Care: Thieves Cough Drops, Thieves Hard Lozenges, Thieves Fresh Essence Plus Mouthwash, Thieves Spray

Personal Care: Thieves Chest Rub

Application and Usage

Aromatic: Refer to Application Guidelines.

Dietary and Oral: Refer to Application Guidelines.

 • Take 1 capsule of desired Vitality oil 2 times daily.

 • Take 2-3 drops of desired Vitality oil in a spoonful of syrup or small amount of milk, juice, or water.

Topical: Refer to Application Guidelines.

 • Apply 2-6 drops neat or diluted 50:50 to the neck and chest as needed.

 • Massage 2-3 drops on the lung Vita Flex points of the feet 2-4 times daily.

 • Place a warm compress with 1-2 drops of chosen oil on the neck, chest, and upper back areas 1-3 times daily.

- Rectal: Using any of the recommended Blends, combine 20 drops with 1 tablespoon olive oil. Insert into rectum with bulb syringe and retain throughout the night. Repeat nightly for 2-3 days.

- Gargle a mixture of essential oils and water 4-8 times daily.

Bronchitis Topical Blend No. 1

- 6 drops Ravintsara
- 5 drops Clove or Clove Vitality
- 4 drops Myrrh
- 2 drops Palo Santo

Bronchitis Topical Blend No. 2

- 10 drops Dorado Azul
- 6 drops Eucalyptus Blue
- 5 drops Lavender or Lavender Vitality
- 3 drops Eucalyptus Globulus

Note: Essential oil Blends work especially well in respiratory applications.

Coughs, Congestive and Dry

Coughs are classified into two categories: acute and chronic. An acute cough is one that has been present for less than three weeks and is divided into infectious and noninfectious causes.

Chronic coughs are those that have been present for more than three weeks and are categorized as conditions within the lungs, conditions within the chest cavity but outside of the lungs, and conditions along the passages that transmit air from the lungs to the environment.

Recommendations
Singles: Eucalyptus Blue, Eucalyptus Globulus, Peppermint, Peppermint Vitality, Tea Tree, Eucalyptus Radiata, Myrrh, Goldenrod, Ledum, Lemon, Lemon Vitality, Mastrante, Northern Lights Black Spruce, Ravintsara, Cedarwood, Marjoram, Marjoram Vitality, Hyssop, Copaiba, Copaiba Vitality, Idaho Grand Fir, Cypress, Melissa, Wintergreen

Blends: Raven, R.C., Breathe Again, Breathe Again Roll-On, SniffleEase, Thieves, Thieves Roll-On, Thieves Vitality, Melrose, Peace & Calming, Peace & Calming II, Calm CBD Roll-On, Seedlings Calm, CBD, Exodus II

Nutritionals: Inner Defense, Life 9, KidScents MightyPro, ImmuPro, Super Vitamin C, Super Vitamin C Chewable,

Oral Care: Thieves Cough Drops, Thieves Fresh Essence Mouthwash, Thieves Hard Lozenges, Thieves Mints, Thieves Spray

Personal Care: Thieves Chest Rub

Application and Usage
Aromatic: Refer to Application Guidelines

Dietary and Oral: Refer to Application Guidelines.

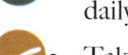

- Take 1 capsule with Vitality or desired oil 2 times daily.
- Take 2-3 drops of desired Vitality oil in a spoonful of syrup or small amount of milk, juice, or water.
- Gargle with Thieves Fresh Essence Plus Mouthwash throughout the day as desired.
- Use Thieves Spray as desired.
- Dissolve Thieves Cough Drops in your mouth as desired.

Dry Cough Tea Blend
- 3 drops Marjoram Vitality
- 2 drops Lemon Vitality
- 1 teaspoon Yacon or maple syrup
- 4 ounces heated distilled or purified water

Sip slowly. Repeat as often as needed for relief.

Topical: Refer to Application Guidelines.

- Place a warm compress with 1-2 drops of chosen oil on the chest, throat, and upper back 2 times daily.
- Apply 1-3 drops to lung Vita Flex points 1-3 times daily.
- Receive a Raindrop Technique 1-2 times weekly.

Cough Blend
- 10 drops Eucalyptus Globulus
- 1 drop Wintergreen
- 1 drop Peppermint Vitality

The Cough Blend may be applied topically and/or diffused as you wish.

Pleurisy

This is an inflammation of the pleura, the outer membranes covering the lungs and the thoracic cavity.

Recommendations
Singles: Ravintsara, Eucalyptus Blue, Dorado Azul, Eucalyptus Radiata, Wintergreen, Myrrh, German Chamomile, German Chamomile Vitality

Blends: PanAway, Raven, Exodus II, Thieves, Thieves Roll-On, Thieves Vitality

Nutritionals: Sulfurzyme, Super Vitamin C, Super Vitamin C Chewable, OmegaGize3, Mineral Essence, Essentialzyme, Essentialzymes-4, Digest & Cleanse, ICP, JuvaPower

Oral Care: Thieves Cough Drops, Thieves Hard Lozenges, Thieves Fresh Essence Plus Mouthwash, Thieves Spray

Personal Care: Thieves Chest Rub

Application and Usage
Aromatic: Refer to Application Guidelines.

Topical: Refer to Application Guidelines.

- Massage 5-7 drops of oil diluted 20:80 on neck and chest 2-3 times daily.

- Place a warm compress with 1-2 drops of oil on the neck, chest, and upper back areas daily.
- Apply 1-3 drops on the lung Vita Flex points on the feet daily.
- Receive a Raindrop Technique 1-2 times weekly.

Pneumonia

Pneumonia is a lung infection caused by bacteria or viruses. It starts when you breathe germs into your lungs and is likely to occur after having a cold or the flu.

Recommendations

Singles: Thyme, Thyme Vitality, Ravintsara, Eucalyptus Radiata, Eucalyptus Globulus, Mountain Savory, Mountain Savory Vitality, Clove, Clove Vitality, Oregano, Oregano Vitality, Ecuadorian Oregano, Tea Tree, Eucalyptus Blue, Dorado Azul, Peppermint, Peppermint Vitality, Northern Lights Black Spruce

Blends: Raven, Melrose, R.C., Thieves, Thieves Roll-On, Thieves Vitality, Breathe Again, Breathe Again Roll-On, SniffleEase

Nutritionals: Inner Defense, Super Vitamin C, Super Vitamin C Chewable, Longevity Softgels, MultiGreens, ImmuPro, Digest & Cleanse, Life 9, KidScents MightyPro

Oral Care: Thieves Spray, Thieves Cough Drops, Thieves Hard Lozenges, Thieves Fresh Essence Plus Mouthwash

Personal Care: Thieves Chest Rub

Application and Usage

Aromatic: Refer to Application Guidelines.

Dietary and Oral: Refer to Application Guidelines.

- Take 1 capsule of desired Vitality oil 2 times daily.
- Take 2-3 drops of desired Vitality oil in a spoonful of syrup or small amount of milk, juice, or water.
- Gargle a mixture of essential oils and water 4-8 times daily.

Topical: Refer to Application Guidelines.

- Apply 2-6 drops neat or diluted 50:50 to the neck and chest as needed.
- Massage 2-3 drops on the lung Vita Flex points of the feet 2-4 times daily.
- Place a warm compress with 1-2 drops of chosen oil on the neck, chest, and upper back areas 1-3 times daily.
- Rectal: Using any of the recommended Blends, combine 20 drops with 1 tablespoon olive oil. Insert into rectum with bulb syringe and retain throughout the night. Repeat nightly for 5-6 days.

Pneumonia Topical Blend
- 10 drops Eucalyptus Globulus
- 8 drops Ravintsara
- 2 drops Oregano
- 2 drops Dorado Azul

Tuberculosis

Tuberculosis (TB) is a highly contagious lung disease caused by Mycobacterium tuberculosis. The germs are spread via coughs, sneezes, and physical contact. A 2014 study41 at the University of Illinois found that a mixture of constituents from Eucalyptus citriodora, including citronellol, monoterpenes, and eugenol, showed efficacy against airborne multi- and extremely drug-resistant tuberculosis, with inhibition greater than 90 percent.

The most worrisome aspect of this disease is its latency. Those infected may harbor the germ for years yet display no outward or visible signs of infection. However, when the immune system becomes challenged or weakened due to stress, candida, diabetes, corticosteroid use, or other factors, the bacteria can become activated and develop into full-blown TB.

Because many essential oils have broad-spectrum, antimicrobial properties, they can be diffused to prevent the spread of airborne bacteria like Mycobacterium tuberculosis. Essential oils and **Blends** like Thieves, Purification, Raven, R.C., and Sacred Mountain are extremely effective for killing these bacteria.

Many essential oils have also been shown to stimulate the immune system. Lemon oil has been shown to increase lymphocyte production—a pivotal part of the immune system.

Recommendations

Singles: Lemon, Lemon Vitality, Oregano, Oregano Vitality, Ecuadorian Oregano, Thyme, Thyme Vitality, Eucalyptus Blue, Dorado Azul, Sacred Frankincense, Frankincense, Frankincense Vitality, Palo Santo, Ravintsara, Rosemary, Rosemary Vitality, Cinnamon Bark, Cinnamon Bark Vitality, Eucalyptus Radiata, Eucalyptus Globulus, Clove, Clove Vitality, Mountain Savory, Mountain Savory Vitality, Peppermint, Peppermint Vitality, Spearmint, Spearmint Vitality, Myrtle, Idaho Grand Fir, Myrrh

Blends: Exodus II, Thieves, Thieves Roll-On, Thieves Vitality, Raven, Melrose, R.C., ImmuPower, Purification, Sacred Mountain, Breathe Again, Breathe Again Roll-On, SniffleEase

Nutritionals: Inner Defense, ImmuPro, Super Vitamin C, Super Vitamin C Chewable, Longevity Softgels, MultiGreens, ICP, ComforTone, Essentialzyme, Essentialzymes-4, Life 9, KidScents MightyPro, Olive Essentials, NingXia Red

Oral Care: Thieves Cough Drops, Thieves Hard Lozenges, Thieves Fresh Essence Plus Mouthwash, Thieves Spray

Personal Care: Thieves Chest Rub

Application and Usage

Aromatic: Refer to Application Guidelines.

Dietary and Oral: Refer to Application Guidelines.

- Take 1 capsule of desired Vitality oil 2 times daily.

- Take 2-3 drops of desired Vitality oil in a spoonful of syrup or small amount of milk, juice, or water.

Topical: Refer to Application Guidelines.

- Apply 6-10 drops of oil, diluted 50:50, on chest and upper back 1-3 times daily.

- Apply a warm compress with chosen oils on chest and upper back 2 times daily.

Tuberculosis-Specific Regimen
- Alternate diffusing Raven and R.C. combined with Eucalyptus Globulus as often as possible during the day.

Retention Blend No. 1
- 15 drops Frankincense or Sacred Frankincense
- 5 drops Clove
- 4 drops Myrrh
- 2 drops Oregano

Retention Blend No. 2
- 10 drops Dorado Azul
- 5 drops Eucalyptus Blue
- 5 drops Myrrh
- 2 drops Oregano

Mix blend with 2 tablespoons of V-6 Vegetable Oil Complex. Using a bulb syringe, insert into rectum and retain overnight. Do this nightly for 7 nights, rest for 4 nights, and then repeat.

- Take 2 Inner Defense 3 times daily for 10 days.
- Rub 4-6 drops Thieves on the bottoms of the feet nightly.
- Massage Melrose (15 drops) up the spine daily. Apply compress on back and chest 2 times daily.
- Receive a Raindrop Technique weekly.
- For cough: Mix 10 drops Myrrh and 1 drop Peppermint Vitality in water and gargle; dissolve Thieves Cough Drops in mouth as needed.

Whooping Cough

Whooping cough is a contagious disease affecting the respiratory system, particularly in children. The lungs become infected as the air passages become clogged with thick mucus. Over the course of several days, the condition worsens, resulting in long coughing bouts (up to 1 minute). The continual coughing makes breathing difficult and labored. Watch carefully and seek medical attention if needed.

Whooping cough usually affects children, so always dilute the essential oils in V-6 Vegetable Oil Complex or other cold-pressed vegetable oil before topically applying. Start with low concentrations until response is observed. Diffuse intermittently and observe reaction.

Recommendations

Singles: Rosemary, Rosemary Vitality, Lavender, Lavender Vitality, Basil, Basil Vitality, Wintergreen, Thyme, Thyme Vitality, Oregano, Oregano Vitality, Ecuadorian Oregano, Mastrante, Tea Tree, Northern Lights Black Spruce, Nutmeg, Nutmeg Vitality, Peppermint, Peppermint Vitality, Eucalyptus Blue, Dorado Azul

Blends: Thieves, Thieves Roll-On, Thieves Vitality, Melrose, Raven, R.C., Breathe Again, Breathe Again Roll-On, SniffleEase

Nutritionals: Super Vitamin C, Super Vitamin C Chewable, Longevity Softgels, Essentialzyme, Essentialzymes-4, Detoxzyme, MultiGreens, ImmuPro, Sulfurzyme, Digest & Cleanse, Inner Defense, Master Formula

Oral Care: Thieves Cough Drops, Thieves Spray, Thieves Fresh Essence Plus Mouthwash, Thieves Hard Lozenges, Thieves Mints

Personal Care: Thieves Chest Rub

Application and Usage

Aromatic: Refer to Application Guidelines.

Topical: Refer to Application Guidelines.

- Apply 2-4 drops diluted 50:50 on neck and chest as needed.

- Massage 2-4 drops of oil neat on the bottoms of the feet and on Vita Flex points just before bedtime. Children may especially benefit from this application.

- Place a warm compress with 1-2 drops of chosen oil on the neck, chest, and upper back area 1-3 times daily.

LUPUS
(See also MIXED CONNECTIVE TISSUE DISEASE)

Lupus is an autoimmune disease that has several different varieties:

Lupus vulgaris is characterized by brownish lesions that may form on the skin and/or face and become ulcerous and form scars.

Discoid Lupus erythematosus is characterized by scaly, red patches on the skin or butterfly-shaped lesions on the face. It is milder than the systemic type.

Systemic Lupus erythematosus is more serious—and more common—than discoid lupus. It inflames the connective tissue in any part of the body, including the joints, muscles, skin, blood vessels, membranes surrounding the lungs and heart, and occasionally the kidneys and brain.

Because lupus is an autoimmune disease, it has been successfully treated using MSM, a form of organic sulfur, which can be found in Sulfurzyme.

Recommendations

Singles: Myrrh, Wintergreen, Lavender, Lavender Vitality, Basil, Basil Vitality, Eucalyptus Globulus, Thyme, Thyme Vitality, Nutmeg, Nutmeg Vitality

Blends: Valor, Valor Roll-On, PanAway, R.C., Breathe Again, Breathe Again Roll-On, EndoFlex, EndoFlex Vitality

Nutritionals: AminoWise, Thyromin, Sulfurzyme, Essentialzyme, Essentialzymes-4, MultiGreens, Master Formula

Application and Usage

Aromatic: Refer to Application Guidelines.

Dietary and Oral: Refer to Application Guidelines.

- Take 1 capsule with 5 drops of desired Vitality oil 2 times daily.

- Take 2-3 drops of desired Vitality oil in a spoonful of syrup or small amount of milk, juice, or water.

Topical: Refer to Application Guidelines.

- Apply 1-2 drops neat on temples and back of neck as desired.
- Have Raindrop Technique 1-2 times weekly.

- Have body massage using desired essential oils once every other day.

Lupus Blend
- 10 drops Lavender
- 4 drops Eucalyptus Globulus
- 3 drops Myrrh
- 3 drops Nutmeg

Lupus Daily Regimen

1. **Bath Salts:** Using lupus blend above, add 30 drops to ½ cup Epsom salt or baking soda and add to hot bath. Soak for 20-30 minutes or until water cools.
2. **Vita Flex:** Massage PanAway on bottoms of the feet and follow 2 hours later with a foot massage using Thieves.
3. **Topical:** Massage 10-15 drops Basil over liver and on bottoms of the feet 2-3 times daily.
4. **Sulfurzyme:** Take 1-2 tablespoons of powder or 5 capsules 1-2 times daily.
5. **Essentialzyme:** Take 2-6 caplets 2 times daily.
6. **MultiGreens:** Take 2-4 capsules 2 times daily.

LYME DISEASE/ROCKY MOUNTAIN SPOTTED FEVER

Lyme disease is a bacterial infection caused by the bite of an infected tick. It is caused by the microorganism Borrelia burgdorferi. This microorganism is neither gram-positive nor gram-negative but diderm (a double-membrane) bacteria, which makes it difficult to kill. Some researchers believe that "stealth viruses" may also be involved in Lyme disease. While the suggested oils of Eucalyptus Blue and Dorado Azul are antibacterial, except for Melissa (antiviral), all other oils listed are both antibacterial and antiviral, which will fight either type of infection.

Rocky Mountain Spotted Fever is caused by the bacterium Rickettsia rickettsii and is also transmitted to humans by the bite of an infected tick.

Typical symptoms are headache, fever, muscle pain, abdominal pain, and vomiting. A rash may develop after a few days. Both illnesses can be severe or even fatal if not treated in the first few days of symptoms. Seek medical attention as soon as possible after being bitten by a tick.

Recommendations

Singles: Melissa, Oregano, Oregano Vitality, Ecuadorian Oregano, Myrrh, Eucalyptus Blue, Dorado Azul, Thyme, Thyme Vitality, Clove, Clove Vitality, Northern Lights Black Spruce, Melaleuca Quinquenervia

Blends: PanAway, Melrose, Thieves, Thieves Roll-On, Thieves Vitality, Exodus II

Nutritionals: Inner Defense, Slique Shake, Essentialzyme, Essentialzymes-4, Life 9, KidScents MightyPro, Detoxzyme

Application and Usage

Aromatic: Refer to Application Guidelines

Dietary and Oral: Refer to Application Guidelines.

- Take 1 capsule of desired Vitality oil 3 times daily.

- Take 2-3 drops of desired Vitality oil in a spoonful of syrup or small amount of milk, juice, or water.

Topical: Refer to Application Guidelines.

- Apply 1-2 drops of oil neat on temples and back of neck, as desired.

- Massage 2-4 drops of oil neat on bottoms of the feet just before bedtime.

LYMPHATIC SYSTEM

Essential oils have long been known to aid in stimulating and detoxifying the lymphatic system, which filters lymph, fights infection, recycles plasma proteins, and drains fluid back into the circulatory system from the tissues in order to prevent dehydration. It plays a crucial role in maintaining good health.

Recommendations

Singles: Ginger, Ginger Vitality, Myrtle, Grapefruit, Grapefruit Vitality, Lemongrass, Lemongrass Vitality, Tangerine, Tangerine Vitality, Orange, Orange Vitality, Rosemary, Rosemary Vitality, Peppermint, Peppermint Vitality, Cypress, Hyssop, Myrrh

Blends: DiGize, DiGize Vitality, Aroma Life, En-R-Gee, Citrus Fresh, Citrus Fresh Vitality

Nutritionals: ImmuPro, Super Vitamin C, Super Vitamin C Chewable, Longevity Softgels, MultiGreens, Digest & Cleanse, Life 9, KidScents MightyPro

Personal Care: Cel-Lite Magic Massage Oil, Regenolone Moisturizing Cream

Application and Usage

Aromatic: Refer to Application Guidelines.

Dietary and Oral: Refer to Application Guidelines.

- Take 1 capsule with 5 drops of Lymphatic System Blend 2 times daily.

- Take 2-3 drops of desired Vitality oil in a spoonful of syrup or small amount of milk, juice, or water.

Topical: Refer to Application Guidelines.

- Apply 2-4 drops of lymphatic system blend below or other recommended oils diluted 50:50 on sore lymph glands and under arms 2-3 times daily.

- Have Raindrop Technique weekly or as needed.

- Place a warm compress with 1-2 drops of chosen oil over affected areas 1-2 times daily.

- Massage lymphatic system blend above over lymph gland areas and then apply Cel-Lite Magic Massage Oil and Grapefruit or Cypress oil that help detoxify chemicals stored in body fat.

Lymphatic System Blend
- 3 drops Cypress
- 2 drops Grapefruit
- 1 drop Orange

MCT (MIXED CONNECTIVE TISSUE DISEASE) (SEE ALSO LUPUS)

MCT is an autoimmune disease similar to lupus in which the connective tissue in the body becomes inflamed and painful. This condition is usually due to poor assimilation of protein and mineral deficiencies.

Recommendations
Singles: Rosemary, Rosemary Vitality, Nutmeg, Nutmeg Vitality, Clove, Clove Vitality, Basil, Basil Vitality, Marjoram, Marjoram Vitality, Peppermint, Peppermint Vitality, Cypress, Wintergreen

Blends: Relieve It, Valor, Valor Roll-On, ImmuPower, PanAway, Cool Azul, Deep Relief Roll-On, CBD

Nutritionals: Sulfurzyme, Essentialzyme, Detoxzyme, AminoWise, Super Vitamin D, Pure Protein Complete, Protein Power Bites, Mineral Essence, JuvaPower, ICP, MultiGreens, Mega Vitamin Cal, OmegaGize3

Personal Care: Cool Azul Pain Relief Cream, Cool Azul Sports Gel, CBD Muscle Rub, Ortho Ease Massage Oil, Ortho Sport Massage Oil

Application and Usage
Aromatic: Refer to Application Guidelines.

Topical: Refer to Application Guidelines.

- Massage 4-8 drops diluted 50:50 on affected locations 2-3 times daily.

- Apply 1-3 drops on the Vita Flex points of the feet.

- Have Raindrop Technique weekly or as needed.

MCT Blend for Aches and Discomfort
- 10 drops Basil
- 8 drops Wintergreen
- 6 drops Cypress
- 3 drops Peppermint

MCT/Lupus Regimen
- Rub 2-4 drops of ImmuPower over the liver and on the liver Vita Flex Points on the bottom of the right foot 2-3 times daily. This has been reported to help fight lupus, which is similar to MCT.

MALARIA

Malaria is a serious disease contracted from several species of Anopheles mosquitoes. While malaria is largely confined to the continents of Asia and Africa, an increasing number of cases have arisen in North and South America. If not treated, malaria can be fatal. If malaria is suspected, seek medical attention. Symptoms are fever, chills, and anemia.

The best defense against malaria is to use insect repellents effective against Anopheles mosquitoes. Once a person has contracted the disease, one of the few natural aids to healing it is natural quinine. Essential oils such as Melaleuca Quinquenervia (Niaouli) can help amplify immune response.

Recommendations
Singles: Melaleuca Quinquenervia (Niaouli), Jade Lemon, Jade Lemon Vitality, Lemon, Lemon Vitality, Lime, Lime Vitality, Thyme, Thyme Vitality, Sacred Frankincense, Frankincense, Frankincense Vitality, Rosemary, Rosemary Vitality, Sage, Sage Vitality, Fennel, Fennel Vitality, Geranium

Blends: Thieves, Thieves Roll-On, Thieves Vitality, Melrose, ImmuPower

Nutritionals: Inner Defense, Digest & Cleanse, MultiGreens, JuvaPower

Personal Care: YL Insect Repellent, Prenolone Plus Body Cream, Thieves Spray (for protection from nerve damage)

Application and Usage
Aromatic: Refer to Application Guidelines.

Dietary and Oral: Refer to Application Guidelines.

- Take 1 capsule of desired Vitality oil 2 times daily.

- Take 2-3 drops of desired Vitality oil in a spoonful of syrup or small amount of milk, juice, or water.

- Mix 3-6 drops Lemon Vitality in 1 teaspoon Yacon Syrup and 8 ounces of water, shake, and sip regularly to build the immune system.

Topical: Refer to Application Guidelines.

- Apply 1-2 drops neat or diluted 50:50 on temples and back of neck, as desired.

- Applying a single drop under the nose is helpful and refreshing.

- Massage 2-4 drops of oil neat on the bottoms of the feet just before bedtime.

MALE HORMONE IMBALANCE

As men age, their DHEA and testosterone levels decline. Conversely, levels of dihydrotestosterone (DHT) increase, contributing to prostate enlargement and hair loss.

Because pregnenolone is the master hormone from which all hormones are created, men can directly benefit from transdermal pregnenolone creams as a way of jump-starting sagging DHEA levels.

Herbs such as saw palmetto and Pygeum africanum can prevent the conversion of testosterone into DHT (dihydrotestosterone, the male hormone thought to contribute to male-pattern hair loss), thereby reducing prostate enlargement and slowing hair loss.

Recommendations
Singles: Idaho Blue Spruce, Rosemary, Rosemary Vitality, Sage, Sage Vitality, Fennel, Fennel Vitality, Geranium, Clary Sage, Yarrow, Sacred Frankincense, Frankincense, Frankincense Vitality

Blends: Shutran, Mister, SclarEssence, SclarEssence Vitality

Nutritionals: Prostate Health, EndoGize

Personal Care: Prenolone Plus Body Cream

Application and Usage
Aromatic: Refer to Application Guidelines.

Dietary and Oral: Refer to Application Guidelines.

- Take 1 capsule of desired Vitality oil 1 time daily only.

- Take 2-3 drops of desired Vitality oil in a spoonful of syrup or small amount of milk, juice, or water.

Topical: Refer to Application Guidelines.

- Dilute 50:50 and apply on location 3-6 times daily.

- Massage 2-4 drops of oil neat on the bottoms of the feet just before bedtime.

MEASLES

Measles, also called rubella, is a highly contagious respiratory infection caused by a virus. The U.S. had 100 cases develop in 21 states in 2018. It causes a total-body skin rash and flu-like symptoms, including a fever, cough, and runny nose.

Since measles is caused by a virus, symptoms typically go away on their own without medical treatment once the virus has run its course. A person with measles should get plenty of fluids and rest and avoid spreading the infection to others.

The first symptoms of the infection are sometimes a hacking cough, runny nose, high fever, and watery, red eyes. Another indicator is Koplik's spots, small red spots with blue-white centers inside the mouth.

The measles rash typically has a red or reddish brown, blotchy appearance and first usually shows up on the forehead, then spreads downward over the face, neck, and body and then down to the feet.

Recommendations
Singles: Lavender, Lavender Vitality, Roman Chamomile, Tea Tree, Clove, Clove Vitality, Northern Lights Black Spruce, Thyme, Thyme Vitality, German Chamomile, German Chamomile Vitality, Ravintsara, Laurus Nobilis, Laurus Nobilis Vitality

Blends: Thieves, Thieves Roll-On, Thieves Vitality, Melrose

Nutritionals: ImmuPro, Super Vitamin C, Super Vitamin C Chewable, Longevity Softgels, Life 9, KidScents MightyPro, Digest & Cleanse, Inner Defense

Personal Care: Thieves Chest Rub

Application and Usage
Aromatic: Refer to Application Guidelines.

Dietary and Oral: Refer to Application Guidelines.

- Take 1 capsule with 5 drops of desired Vitality oil 2-3 times daily.

- Take 2-3 drops of desired Vitality oil in a spoonful of syrup or small amount of milk, juice, or water.

Topical: Refer to Application Guidelines.

- Apply 2-3 drops diluted 50:50 on location 3-5 times daily or as needed.
- Mix 6-9 drops of any of the recommended oils in bath salts and soak at least 30 minutes daily.
- Mix 6-9 drops of any of the recommended oils in 8 ounces water, shake well, and use to sponge down the patient 1-2 times daily.

Measles Topical Blend
- 10 drops Lavender
- 10 drops German Chamomile
- 5 drops Ravintsara
- 5 drops Tea Tree

MENSTRUAL AND FEMALE HORMONE CONDITIONS
(See also CYSTS, OVARIAN and UTERINE CYSTS)

Natural hormones such as natural progesterone and pregnenolone are the most effective treatment for menstrual difficulties and irregularities. The most effective method of administration is transdermal delivery in a cream. Just 20 mg applied to the skin twice daily is equivalent to 1,000 mg taken internally.

As women reach menopause, progesterone production declines, and a state of estrogen dominance often arises. The most commonly prescribed drugs are conjugated estrogens (from horse urine) or synthetic medroxyprogesterone. The molecules in these animal and synthetic hormones are foreign to the human body and can dramatically increase the risk for ovarian and breast cancer with time.

Endometriosis

Endometriosis occurs when the uterine lining develops on the outer wall of the uterus, ovaries, fallopian tubes, vagina, intestines, or on the abdominal wall. These fragments cannot escape like the normal uterine lining that is shed during menstruation.

Because of this, fibrous cysts often form around the misplaced uterine tissue. Symptoms can include abdominal or back pain during menstruation or pain that often increases after the period is over. Other symptoms may include heavy periods and pain during intercourse.

Recommendations
Singles: Fennel, Fennel Vitality, Clary Sage, Sage, Sage Vitality, Helichrysum

Blends: Thieves, Thieves Roll-On, Thieves Vitality, Melrose, SclarEssence, SclarEssence Vitality, Lady Sclareol

Nutritionals: ImmuPro, EndoGize, FemiGen, Super Vitamin C, Super Vitamin C Chewable, PD 80/20, ICP, ComforTone, Essentialzyme, Essentialzymes-4

Personal Care: Prenolone Plus Body Cream, Progessence Plus

Application and Usage
Aromatic: Refer to Application Guidelines.

Dietary and Oral: Refer to Application Guidelines.

- Take 1 capsule with Vitality desired oil 2 times daily.

- Take 2-3 drops of desired Vitality oil in a spoonful of syrup or small amount of milk, juice, or water.
- Colon and liver cleanse: ICP, ComforTone, Detoxzyme, Essentialzyme, JuvaPower

Topical: Refer to Application Guidelines.

- Apply a hot compress containing Melrose on the stomach.
- Massage 2-4 drops of Thieves blend neat on the bottoms of the feet.

Excessive Bleeding

The most common causes of heavy menstrual bleeding are hormonal imbalances, uterine fibroids or polyps, lack of ovulation, use of an intrauterine device, miscarriage, use of anticoagulants, or endometriosis.

Recommendations
Singles: Helichrysum, Cypress, Cistus

Blends: PanAway, Deep Relief Roll-On, Relieve It, Cool Azul

Nutritionals: OmegaGize3, JuvaTone, Rehemogen

Personal Care: Progessence Plus, Prenolone Plus Body Cream, Cool Azul Pain Relief Cream

Application and Usage
Aromatic: Refer to Application Guidelines.

Dietary and Oral: Refer to Application Guidelines.

- Take 1 capsule of desired Vitality oil 2 times daily.

- Take 2-3 drops of desired Vitality oil in a spoonful of syrup or small amount of milk, juice, or water.
- Drink 1/10 teaspoon cayenne in 8 ounces warm water to help regulate bleeding during periods.

Topical: Refer to Application Guidelines.

- Apply 4-6 drops diluted 50:50 to the forehead, crown of the head, bottoms of the feet, lower abdomen, and lower back 1-3 times daily.

- Place a warm compress with 1-2 drops of chosen oil on lower back and abdomen.

Excessive Bleeding Blend
- 10 drops Cypress
- 5 drops Helichrysum
- 5 drops Cistus

Hormonal Edema (Cyclic)

This type of edema usually fluctuates with the female menstrual cycle. A good progesterone hormone cream might be the way to begin; however, before starting any hormone therapy, you should see your doctor or health care professional and ask for a hormone blood panel to evaluate your needs.

Recommendations

Singles: Clary Sage, Sage, Sage Vitality, Geranium, Tangerine, Tangerine Vitality

Blends: SclarEssence, SclarEssence Vitality, Lady Sclareol, Dragon Time, EndoFlex, EndoFlex Vitality

Nutritionals: Thyromin, PD 80/20, FemiGen, EndoGize

Personal Care: Progessence Plus, Prenolone Plus Body Cream

Application and Usage

Aromatic: Refer to Application Guidelines.

Topical: Refer to Application Guidelines.

- Massage 2-4 drops of oil neat on the bottoms of the feet just before bedtime.
- Place a warm compress with 1-2 drops of chosen oil over the lower back and abdomen.

Hysterectomy

A hysterectomy is the surgical removal of a woman's uterus and may also include removal of ovaries and fallopian tubes.

Recommendations

Singles: Sage, Sage Vitality, Clary Sage

Blends: Dragon Time, Lady Sclareol, SclarEssence, SclarEssence Vitality

Nutritionals: PD 80/20, EndoGize, FemiGen

Personal Care: Progessence Plus, Prenolone Plus Body Cream

Application and Usage

Aromatic: Refer to Application Guidelines.

Topical: Refer to Application Guidelines.

- Massage 2-4 drops of oil neat on the bottoms of the feet just before bedtime.

- Place a warm compress with 1-2 drops of chosen oil over the lower back and abdomen.

Irregular Periods

Menstrual cycles that vary more than a few days in length from month to month are considered to be irregular. All women have variations occasionally, but true irregularity persists over several months.

Recommendations

Singles: Peppermint, Peppermint Vitality, Clary Sage, Sage, Sage Vitality, Roman Chamomile, Fennel, Fennel Vitality, Jasmine

Blends: EndoFlex, SclarEssence, SclarEssence Vitality, Inner Child, Peace & Calming, Peace & Calming II, Calm CBD Roll-On, Seedlings Calm

Personal Care: Progessence Plus, Prenolone Plus Body Cream

Application and Usage

Aromatic: Refer to Application Guidelines.

Topical: Refer to Application Guidelines.

- Apply 4-6 drops diluted 50:50 to forehead, crown of the head, bottoms of the feet, lower abdomen, and lower back 1-3 times daily.
- Massage 3-5 drops on the reproductive Vita Flex points of the feet 2-3 times daily.
- Place a warm compress on the lower back and lower abdomen daily.

Period Regulator Blend No. 1

- 16 drops Clary Sage
- 11 drops Sage
- 9 drops Canadian Fleabane (Conyza)
- 5 drops Peppermint
- 5 drops Jasmine

Period Regulator Blend No. 2

- 10 drops Roman Chamomile
- 10 drops Fennel

Menopause

As women age, their levels of progesterone decline and contribute to osteoporosis, increased risk of breast and uterine cancers, mood swings, depression, and many other conditions. Estrogen levels can also decline and increase women's risk of heart disease.

Between the ages of 45 and 55, these hormones decline to a point where menstruation ceases. Replacing these declining levels using topically applied progesterone or pregnenolone creams may be the most effective way to replace and boost declining hormone levels.

Pregnenolone may be especially effective as it is the precursor hormone from which the body creates both progesterone and estrogens.

Recommendations

Singles: Geranium, Clary Sage, Sage, Sage Vitality, Bergamot, Bergamot Vitality, Davana

Blends: Dragon Time, Lady Sclareol, Transformation, SclarEssence, SclarEssence Vitality

Nutritionals: PD 80/20, EndoGize

Personal Care: Progessence Plus, Prenolone Plus Body Cream

Application and Usage

Aromatic: Refer to Application Guidelines.

Topical: Refer to Application Guidelines.

- Apply 4-6 drops diluted 50:50 to forehead, crown of the head, bottoms of the feet, lower abdomen, and lower back 1-3 times daily.

- Massage 3-6 drops on the reproductive Vita Flex points of the feet.

- Place a warm compress on the lower back and lower abdomen daily.

Menstrual Cramps

Menstrual cramps (dysmenorrhea) are throbbing, dull, or cramping pains in the lower abdomen that many women experience just before and during their menstrual periods. The pain may be just annoying, or it may be severe enough to interfere with daily activities. Treating the underlying cause is important to reducing pain.

Recommendations

Singles: Valerian, Lavender, Lavender Vitality, Clary Sage, Basil, Basil Vitality, Rosemary, Rosemary Vitality, Sage, Sage Vitality, Roman Chamomile, Cypress, Tarragon, Tarragon Vitality, Vetiver, Idaho Blue Spruce

Blends: Dragon Time, EndoFlex, EndoFlex Vitality

Nutritionals: PD 80/20, EndoGize, Deep Relief Roll-On, Relieve It, PanAway

Personal Care: Prenolone Plus Body Cream, Regenolone Moisturizing Cream

Application and Usage

Aromatic: Refer to Application Guidelines.

Dietary and Oral: Refer to Application Guidelines.

- Take 1 capsule of desired Vitality oil 2 times daily for 2 weeks prior to menses.

- Take 2-3 drops of desired Vitality oil in a spoonful of syrup or small amount of milk, juice, or water.

- If migraine headaches accompany periods, a colon and liver cleanse may reduce symptoms.

Topical: Refer to Application Guidelines.

- Place a warm compress over the uterus area 2-3 times weekly.

- Massage 2-4 drops on the reproductive Vita Flex points of the feet.

- Apply 2-3 drops of the recommended oils above to the lower back and stomach area several times daily as needed.

Premenstrual Syndrome (PMS)

PMS is one of the most common hormone-related conditions in otherwise healthy women.

Women can experience a wide range of symptoms for 10 to 14 days before menstruation and even 2 to 3 days into menstruation. These symptoms include mood swings, fatigue, headaches, breast tenderness, abdominal bloating, anxiety, depression, confusion, memory loss, sugar cravings, cramps, low back pain, irritability, weight gain, acne, and oily skin and hair.

Causes are hormonal, nutritional, and psychological. The stress of the western culture can also be a cause.

Recommendations

Singles: Rose, Clary Sage, Idaho Blue Spruce, Sage, Sage Vitality, Fennel, Fennel Vitality, Ylang Ylang, Neroli, Bergamot, Bergamot Vitality

Blends: SclarEssence, SclarEssence Vitality, Dragon Time, EndoFlex, EndoFlex Vitality, Acceptance, Aroma Siez, Lady Sclareol, Transformation

Nutritionals: PowerGize, MultiGreens, Super Vitamin B, Sulfurzyme, Mineral Essence, ImmuPro, PD 80/20, Thyromin, EndoGize

Personal Care: Prenolone Plus Body Cream, Progessence Plus

Application and Usage

Aromatic: Refer to Application Guidelines.

Dietary and Oral: Refer to Application Guidelines.

- Take 1 capsule of desired Vitality oil 2 times daily.

- Take 2-3 drops of desired Vitality oil in a spoonful of syrup or small amount of milk, juice, or water.
- Place 1 drop of EndoFlex Vitality on the tongue and then hold the tongue on the roof of the mouth 2-4 times daily.

Topical: Refer to Application Guidelines.

- Apply 4-6 drops diluted 50:50 to forehead, crown of the head, bottoms of the feet, lower abdomen, and lower back 1-3 times daily.

- Massage 2-4 drops on reproductive Vita Flex points of the feet.

- Place a warm compress on the lower back and lower abdomen daily.

MENTAL ILLNESS

Many categories or types of mental illness can be found in literature and on the internet. They are all complex issues and consist of many subtypes. In addition, many people don't know they have a mental illness, and many mental illnesses are misdiagnosed.

A few mental illnesses are included in this chapter, but not all. As you become familiar with the different aspects of the many mental illnesses that are experienced, you will find similarities that can help you identify which products to use to help the systems that are being affected.

Some of the main groups of mental illnesses are:
- Anxiety disorders (including panic disorder, phobias, obsessive-compulsive disorder
- Dementia
- Developmental disorders (including autism)
- Eating disorders
- Mood disorders (such as depression and bipolar affective disorder)
- Personality disorders
- Schizophrenia and other psychoses
- Substance abuse disorders
- Trauma-related disorders (such as post-traumatic stress disorder)
  A few of the symptoms and signs include:
- Withdrawal from friends and activities
- Confused thinking or reduced ability to concentrate
- Feeling consistently sad
- Significant tiredness, low energy, or problems sleeping
- Extreme high and low mood changes
- Excessive fears or worries
- Extreme feelings of guilt
- Problems with eating or not wanting to eat

MIGRAINES
(See HEADACHES, MIGRAINES)

MUCUS (EXCESS)

Many oils are natural expectorants, helping tissues discharge mucus, soft and hard plaque, and toxins.

Recommendations

Singles: Lavender, Lavender Vitality, Jade Lemon, Jade Lemon Vitality, Lemon, Lemon Vitality, Lime, Lime Vitality, Cypress, Peppermint, Peppermint Vitality, Tea Tree, Pine, Thyme, Thyme Vitality, Eucalyptus Globulus, Rosemary, Rosemary Vitality

Blends: DiGize, DiGize Vitality, Raven, 3 Wise Men, Purification, R.C., Breathe Again, Breathe Again Roll-On, SniffleEase

Nutritionals: Allerzyme, Detoxzyme, Essentialzyme, Essentialzymes-4, ImmuPro, Inner Defense, Life 9, KidScents Mighty-Pro

Application and Usage

Aromatic: Refer to Application Guidelines.

Note: Some studies conclude that the expectorant effect of essential oils is obtained faster and stronger through aroma than through ingestion.

Dietary and Oral: Refer to Application Guidelines.

- Take 1 capsule of desired Vitality oil 2 times daily.

- Take 2-3 drops of desired Vitality oil in a spoonful of syrup or small amount of milk, juice, or water.

Expectorant Blend
- 3 drops Lemon
- 3 drops Eucalyptus Globulus
- 2 drops Pine

Topical: Refer to Application Guidelines.

- Apply 2-4 drops, diluted 50:50, on the T4 and T5 thoracic vertebrae at the neck to the shoulder intersection 3-5 times daily.

- Massage recommended oils on Vita Flex points of the feet 2-4 times daily.

MUMPS (INFECTIOUS PAROTITIS)

Mumps is an acute, contagious, viral disease marked by painful swelling and inflammation of the salivary glands. The causative agent is a paramyxovirus that is spread by direct contact, airborne droplets, and urine. The incidence of mumps has increased to the point that 5,000 cases were reported in the U.S. in 2016. Health officials are calling for a third measles vaccine injection.

Recommendations

Singles: Dorado Azul, Thyme, Thyme Vitality, Tea Tree, Ravintsara, Melissa, Myrrh, Blue Cypress, Northern Lights Black Spruce, Wintergreen

Blends: R.C., Raven, Breathe Again, Breathe Again Roll-On, SniffleEase, Thieves, Thieves Roll-On, Thieves Vitality, Deep Relief Roll-On, PanAway, Relieve It, Cool Azul, CBD, JuvaCleanse, JuvaCleanse Vitality

Nutritionals: ImmuPro, Super Vitamin C, Super Vitamin C Chewable, Exodus II, Inner Defense, Essentialzyme, Detoxzyme, JuvaPower, Sulfurzyme, Slique Shake, Balance Complete, Pure Protein Complete

Personal Care: Cool Azul Pain Relief Cream, CBD Muscle Rub

Application and Usage

Aromatic: Refer to Application Guidelines.

Dietary and Oral: Refer to Application Guidelines.

- Take 1 capsule of desired Vitality oil 2 times daily.

- Take 2-3 drops of desired Vitality oil in a spoonful of syrup or small amount of milk, juice, or water.

Topical: Refer to Application Guidelines.

- Apply 2-4 drops diluted 50:50 behind the ears 4 times daily.

- Receive a Raindrop Technique 1-2 times weekly.

- Place a warm compress 1-3 times daily around the throat and jaw.

The body has more than 600 muscles that are grouped into three categories—smooth, cardiac, and skeletal—and are all made of a type of elastic tissue.

Bruised Muscles (See also CARDIOVASCULAR CONDITIONS AND PROBLEMS, Bruising)

A bruise is a skin discoloration and occurs when small blood vessels break and leak their contents into the tissue beneath the skin. The main symptoms of a bruise are pain, skin discoloration, and swelling.

Recommendations

Singles: Helichrysum, Copaiba, Copaiba Vitality, Geranium, German Chamomile, German Chamomile Vitality, Winter-green, Cypress, Basil, Basil Vitality, Peppermint, Peppermint Vitality, Lemon Verbena, Lavender, Lavender Vitality

Blends: Cool Azul, Aroma Siez, PanAway, Deep Relief Roll-On, CBD, Relieve It

Nutritionals: AminoWise, PowerGize, Pure Protein Complete, Protein Power Bites, Mega Vitamin Cal, Mineral Essence, NingXia Red, Sulfurzyme, BLM, Super Vitamin D, AgilEase, Super Vitamin B

Personal Care: Cool Azul Pain Relief Cream, Cool Azul Sports Gel, CBD Muscle Rub, Ortho Ease Massage Oil, Ortho Sport Massage Oil, Relaxation Massage Oil

Application and Usage

Topical: Refer to Application Guidelines.

- Apply 2-4 drops diluted 50:50 to bruised area 3 times daily.

- Sequence of application for bruising:

- When a bruise displays black and blue discoloration and pain, start with Helichrysum, Geranium, or Wintergreen.

- When the pain and inflammation decrease, use Cypress, then Basil, and then Aroma Siez to help the muscle relax.

- Follow with Peppermint to stimulate nerve response and reduce inflammation.

- Finish with cold packs.

Inflammation Due to Infection

Inflammation is the first response of the immune system to irritation or infection and is characterized by swelling, heat, redness, pain, and dysfunction of the organs involved. Treatment depends on the type of infection.

Recommendations

Singles: Ravintsara, German Chamomile, German Chamomile Vitality, Tea Tree, Thyme, Thyme Vitality, Myrrh, Hyssop, Blue Cypress, Lemongrass, Lemongrass Vitality

Blends: Melrose, Purification, Longevity, Longevity Vitality, Thieves, Thieves Roll-On, Thieves Vitality, 3 Wise Men

Nutritionals: AminoWise, BLM, AgilEase, Longevity Softgels, ImmuPro, Detoxzyme, Essentialzyme, Essentialzymes-4, Digest & Cleanse, Olive Essentials

Personal Care: Cool Azul Pain Relief Cream, Cool Azul Sports Gel, CBD Muscle Rub

Application and Usage

Topical: Refer to Application Guidelines.

- Massage 2-4 drops diluted 50:50 on inflamed muscle 3 times daily.

- Place a cold compress on location up to 1-3 times daily.

Inflammation Due to Injury

Tissue damage is usually accompanied by inflammation. Reduce inflammation by massaging with anti-inflammatory oils to minimize further tissue damage and speed healing.

Recommendations

Singles: Wintergreen, German Chamomile, German Chamomile Vitality, Nutmeg, Nutmeg Vitality, Palo Santo, Peppermint, Peppermint Vitality, Lavender, Lavender Vitality, Cassia, Myrrh, Marjoram, Marjoram Vitality, Clove, Clove Vitality, Thyme, Thyme Vitality, Copaiba, Copaiba Vitality, Lemongrass, Lemongrass Vitality, Vetiver

Blends: PanAway, Aroma Siez, Deep Relief Roll-On, Relieve It, Cool Azul, CBD, Calm CBD Roll-On

Nutritionals: AminoWise, BLM, AgilEase, PowerGize, Mineral Essence, Mega Vitamin Cal, Super Vitamin D, Sulfurzyme, Detoxzyme, Allerzyme, MultiGreens, Life 9, KidScents MightyPro, Pure Protein Complete, Protein Power Bites

Personal Care: Cool Azul Pain Relief Cream, Cool Azul Sports Gel, CBD Muscle Rub, Ortho Ease Massage Oil, Ortho Sport Massage Oil, Relaxation Massage Oil

Application and Usage

Topical: Refer to Application Guidelines.
- Massage 2-4 drops diluted 50:50 on inflamed muscle 3 times daily.

Muscle Injury Blend
- 10 drops German Chamomile
- 8 drops Lavender
- 6 drops Marjoram
- 2 drops Peppermint

Muscle Spasms, Cramps, and Charley Horses

Magnesium and calcium deficiency may contribute to muscle cramps.

Recommendations

Singles: Idaho Blue Spruce, Idaho Grand Fir, Dorado Azul, Wintergreen, Ravintsara, Basil, Basil Vitality, Rosemary, Rosemary Vitality, Fennel, Fennel Vitality, Marjoram, Marjoram Vitality, Elemi, Nutmeg, Nutmeg Vitality, Copaiba, Copaiba Vitality, Black Pepper, Black Pepper Vitality, Palo Santo

Blends: PanAway, Cool Azul, Relieve It, Aroma Siez, Deep Relief Roll-On, CBD

Nutritionals: AminoWise, PowerGize, Mega Vitamin Cal, Mineral Essence, BLM, AgilEase, Sulfurzyme, Life 9, KidScents MightyPro

Personal Care: Cool Azul Pain Relief Cream, Ortho Sport Massage Oil, CBD Muscle Rub, Ortho Ease Massage Oil, Cool Azul Sports Gel, Relaxation Massage Oil, Regenolone Moisturizing Cream

Application and Usage

Aromatic: Refer to Application Guidelines.

Topical: Refer to Application Guidelines.

Blend for Muscle Spasms
- 2 drops Ravintsara
- 5 drops Aroma Siez
- 2 drops Black Pepper
- Apply 2-4 drops diluted 50:50 on cramped muscle 3 times daily. Alternate with cold and hot packs when applying the blend for muscle spasms.

Muscle Weakness

To overcome temporary muscle weakness, eat a balanced diet, replace lost fluids, engage in only light activities, and slowly start exercising again. However, muscles that slowly become weaker for no apparent reason could indicate a disease or condition in the body. Check with your health care professional.

Recommendations
Singles: Idaho Grand Fir, Ravintsara, Dorado Azul, Palo Santo, Northern Lights Black Spruce, Juniper, Nutmeg, Nutmeg Vitality, Lemongrass, Lemongrass Vitality, Lemon Verbena

Blends: En-R-Gee, The Gift, Sacred Mountain

Nutritionals: AminoWise, BLM, AgilEase, Super Vitamin D, Slique Shake, MultiGreens, Balance Complete, Pure Protein Complete, Protein Power Bites, Mega Vitamin Cal, JuvaPower, PowerGize

Application and Usage
Topical: Refer to Application Guidelines.

- Massage 4-6 drops diluted 50:50 into weak muscles 3 times daily.

Sore Muscles

Whenever you engage in a more strenuous activity than you normally do, you may create microscopic tears (micro-trauma) in your muscle tissue. The more tears you create, the more soreness you feel later on as the muscles are being repaired. The soreness is a result of both the damage to the muscles and the chemical waste products produced by the muscles when they are being used.

Recommendations
Singles: Rosemary, Rosemary Vitality, Wintergreen, Black Pepper, Black Pepper Vitality, Eucalyptus Blue, Ginger, Ginger Vitality, Northern Lights Black Spruce, Pine, Marjoram, Marjoram Vitality, Peppermint, Peppermint Vitality, Lemongrass, Lemongrass Vitality, Helichrysum, Idaho Grand Fir, Basil, Basil Vitality, Vetiver, Elemi, Cypress, Dorado Azul, Eucalyptus Radiata, Lemon Verbena

Blends: PanAway, Deep Relief Roll-On, Cool Azul, CBD, Peace & Calming, Peace & Calming II, Calm CBD Roll-On, Seedlings Calm, M-Grain, Aroma Siez

Nutritionals: PowerGize, AminoWise, Pure Protein Complete, Protein Power Bites, Mega Vitamin Cal, Mineral Essence, Slique Shake, Sulfurzyme

Personal Care: Cool Azul Pain Relief Cream, Cool Azul Sports Gel, CBD Muscle Rub, Ortho Sport Massage Oil, Ortho Ease Massage Oil

Application and Usage
Topical: Refer to Application Guidelines.

- Massage 4-6 drops diluted 50:50 into sore muscles up to 3 times daily.

- Place a warm compress on location up to 1-3 times daily.

Sore Muscle Blend No. 1
- 5 drops Idaho Grand Fir
- 4 drops Marjoram
- 4 drops Basil
- 2 drops Rosemary

Sore Muscle Blend No. 2
- 5 drops Pine
- 4 drops Rosemary
- 4 drops Ginger
- 1 drop Vetiver

Make Your Own High-powered Massage Oil

Add either of these recipes to 4 ounces of V-6 Vegetable Oil Complex to create a custom, muscle-toning formula.

Massage Oil Recipe No. 1:
- 10 drops Eucalyptus Blue
- 10 drops Idaho Balsam Fir
- 10 drops Marjoram
- 8 drops Elemi
- 8 drops Vetiver
- 5 drops Helichrysum
- 5 drops Cypress
- 5 drops Peppermint

Massage Oil Recipe No. 2:
- 20 drops Eucalyptus Blue
- 15 drops Marjoram
- 10 drops Juniper
- 10 drops Cypress
- 6 drops Dorado Azul

MUSCULAR DYSTROPHY

Muscular dystrophy is a group of disorders that involve loss of muscle tissue and muscle weakness that get progressively worse. All or only specific groups of muscles may be affected.

Recommendations

Singles: Palo Santo, Pine, Lavender, Lavender Vitality, Marjoram, Marjoram Vitality, Lemongrass, Lemongrass Vitality, Vetiver, Idaho Grand Fir

Blends: PanAway, Aroma Siez, Relieve It, Deep Relief Roll-On, Cool Azul, CBD

Nutritionals: BLM, AgilEase, Super Vitamin D, PowerGize, AminoWise, Sulfurzyme, Essentialzymes-4, Slique Shake, Pure Protein Complete, Protein Power Bites, MultiGreens, Mineral Essence, Essentialzyme, Super Vitamin B

Personal Care: Cool Azul Pain Relief Cream, Cool Azul Sports Gel, CBD Muscle Rub, Ortho Ease Massage Oil, Ortho Sport Massage Oil

Application and Usage

Topical: Refer to Application Guidelines.

- Massage 4-6 drops diluted 50:50 along spine 3 times daily.

> **Tired and Fatigued Muscles**
>
> Tired muscles may be lacking in minerals such as calcium and magnesium. Mega Cal and Mineral Essence are excellent sources of both trace and macro minerals and are good for all muscle conditions. Enzymes including Essentialzyme, Essentialzymes-4, and Allerzyme all help with the needed enzymatic conversion of minerals for absorption.

NAILS, BRITTLE OR WEAK

Poor or weak nails, often containing ridges, indicate a sulfur, calcium, and/or vitamin A deficiency, disease, infection, trauma, unhealthy diet, use of nail polish and remover, use of detergents, or excessive exposure to water.

Recommendations

Singles: Myrrh, Lemon, Lemon Vitality, Sacred Frankincense, Frankincense, Frankincense Vitality, Wintergreen, Idaho Grand Fir

Blends: Citrus Fresh, Citrus Fresh Vitality, DiGize, DiGize Vitality, GLF, GLF Vitality

Nutritionals: Sulfurzyme, Mega Vitamin Cal, Mineral Essence, Master Formula, Essentialzyme, Essentialzymes-4, NingXia Red, NingXia Wolfberries (Organic, Dried)

Application and Usage

Dietary and Oral: Refer to Application Guidelines.

- Take 1 capsule of desired Vitality oil 2 times daily.
- Place a few drops of oil on the tongue 1-4 times as needed.
- Take 2-3 drops of desired Vitality oil in a spoonful of syrup or small amount of milk, juice, or water.

Topical: Refer to Application Guidelines.

- Apply 1-3 drops of oil neat on nails and at base of nails daily for 30 days.
- Apply 1 drop of the Nail Strengthening Blend on each nail 2-3 times daily for 30 days.

Nail Strengthening Blend
- 4 drops Wheat Germ Oil
- 2 drops Sacred Frankincense or Frankincense
- 2 drops Myrrh
- 2 drops Lemon
- 1 drop Wintergreen

NARCOLEPSY (See also THYROID)

Narcolepsy is a chronic ailment consisting of uncontrollable, recurrent attacks of drowsiness and sleep during the daytime. Narcolepsy may be aggravated by hypothalamus dysregulation or thyroid hormone deficiency.

Recommendations

Singles: Peppermint, Peppermint Vitality, Lemon, Lemon Vitality, Rosemary, Rosemary Vitality, Black Pepper, Black Pepper Vitality

Blends: Clarity, Brain Power, Awaken, Common Sense, KidScents GeneYus, Motivation, M-Grain

Nutritionals: Thyromin, MultiGreens, Mineral Essence, MindWise, Essentialzyme, Essentialzymes-4, Life 9, KidScents MightyPro, Sulfurzyme, JuvaPower, Slique Shake

Application and Usage
Aromatic: Refer to Application Guidelines.

Topical: Refer to Application Guidelines.

- Apply 1-2 drops diluted 50:50 on temples, behind ears, back of neck, on forehead, and under nostrils as needed.

NAUSEA

Patchouli oil contains compounds that are extremely effective in preventing vomiting due to their ability to reduce the gastrointestinal muscle contractions associated with vomiting.42 Peppermint has also been found to be effective in many kinds of stomach upset, including nausea.

Recommendations
Singles: Patchouli, Peppermint, Peppermint Vitality, Ginger, Ginger Vitality, Nutmeg, Nutmeg Vitality, Cardamom, Cardamom Vitality, JuvaFlex, JuvaFlex Vitality

Blends: DiGize, DiGize Vitality, KidScents TummyGize, JuvaCleanse, JuvaCleanse Vitality, GLF, GLF Vitality, AromaEase, Aroma Life, Citrus Fresh, Citrus Fresh Vitality, Forgiveness

Nutritionals: AlkaLime, Detoxzyme, Essentialzymes-4, Essentialzyme, Digest & Cleanse, ComforTone, ICP, Mega Vitamin Cal, Life 9, KidScents MightyPro, Allerzyme, AminoWise

Application and Usage
Aromatic: Refer to Application Guidelines.

Dietary and Oral: Refer to Application Guidelines.

- Take 1 capsule of desired Vitality oil 2 times daily.

- Place a few drops of oil on the tongue 1-4 times as needed.

- Take 2-3 drops of desired Vitality oil in a spoonful of syrup or small amount of milk, juice, or water.

Topical: Refer to Application Guidelines.

- Massage 1-3 drops diluted 50:50 behind each ear (mastoids) and over navel 2-3 times hourly.

- Place a warm compress with 1-2 drops of chosen oil over the back or the stomach as needed.

- Rub 1-2 drops of oil on the temples and back of neck several times daily.

Morning Sickness

The medical definition for "morning sickness" is "nausea and vomiting of pregnancy." Sometimes the symptoms are worse in the morning, but they can strike at any time; and for many women, they last all day. The intensity varies from woman to woman. An extreme form of morning sickness is called hyperemesis gravidarum, which may require hospitalization to receive intravenous fluids after constant vomiting.

Recommendations
Singles: Peppermint, Peppermint Vitality, Ginger, Ginger Vitality, Spearmint, Spearmint Vitality, Lavender, Lavender Vitality, Jade Lemon, Jade Lemon Vitality, Lemon, Lemon Vitality, Lime, Lime Vitality, Patchouli

Blends: DiGize, DiGize Vitality, Gentle Baby

Nutritionals: Essentialzymes-4, Essentialzyme, Life 9, KidScents MightyPro, Detoxzyme, AlkaLime, Slique Shake, Mega Vitamin Cal

Application and Usage
Aromatic: Refer to Application Guidelines.

Dietary and Oral: Refer to Application Guidelines.

- Take 1 capsule of desired Vitality oil 2 times daily.

- Place a few drops of oil on the tongue 1-4 times as needed.

- Take 2-3 drops of desired Vitality oil in a spoonful of syrup or small amount of milk, juice, or water.

Topical: Refer to Application Guidelines.

- Massage 1-3 drops diluted 50:50 behind each ear (mastoids) and over navel 2-3 times hourly.

- Place a warm compress on stomach as needed.

Motion Sickness

Motion sickness is a bodily response to real or perceived movement. The inner ear senses movement, while your eyes tell you that you are standing still. This confuses the brain and causes dopamine levels to increase, which causes motion sickness. Common symptoms are nausea, vomiting, dizziness, and fatigue.

Recommendations
Singles: Peppermint, Peppermint Vitality, Ginger, Ginger Vitality, Patchouli, Spearmint, Spearmint Vitality, Lavender, Lavender Vitality, Rose, Sacred Frankincense, Frankincense, Frankincense Vitality, Palo Santo

Blends: Valor, Valor Roll-On, Harmony, DiGize, DiGize Vitality, KidScents TummyGize, Tranquil Roll-On, Peace & Calming, Peace & Calming II, Calm CBD Roll-On, Seedlings Calm

Nutritionals: Essentialzymes-4, Essentialzyme, Detoxzyme, Mega Vitamin Cal, Mineral Essence, EndoGize

Application and Usage

Aromatic: Refer to Application Guidelines.

Dietary and Oral: Refer to Application Guidelines.

- Take 1 capsule of desired Vitality oil 2 times daily.

- Place a few drops of desired Vitality oil on the tongue 1-4 times as needed.

- Take 2-3 drops of desired Vitality oil in a spoonful of syrup or small amount of milk, juice, or water.

Topical: Refer to Application Guidelines.

- Massage 1-3 drops diluted 50:50 behind each ear (mastoids) and over navel 2-3 times hourly.

- Place a warm compress on stomach as needed.
- Rub 6-10 drops of the following blend on chest and stomach 1 hour before traveling:

Motion Sickness Preventive Blend
- 2 drops Peppermint
- 2 drops Ginger
- 2 drops Patchouli
- 5 drops V-6 Vegetable Oil Complex

NERVE DISORDERS
(See also NEUROLOGICAL DISEASES)

Nerve disorders usually involve peripheral or surface nerves and include Bell's palsy, carpal tunnel syndrome, neuralgia, neuritis, and neuropathy. In contrast, neurological diseases are usually associated with deep neurological disturbances in the brain. These conditions include ALS (Lou Gehrig's disease), MS, and Parkinson's disease.

Mega Vitamin Cal, Super Vitamin D, and Mineral Essence used with OmegaGize3 and MindWise help provide calcium, magnesium, and natural lipids, including healthy omega-3 fatty acids, necessary to maintain nerve signal transmissions along neurological pathways.

Sulfur deficiency is often present in nerve problems. Sulfur requires calcium and vitamins B and C for the body to metabolize. Super Vitamin B, Super Vitamin C, and Sulfurzyme work well together to help repair nerve damage and the myelin sheath.

CAUTION: Never use hot packs for neurological problems. Always use cold packs to reduce pain and inflammation.

Bell's Palsy

This is a type of neuritis, marked by paralysis on one side of the face and inability to open or close the eyelid.

Recommendations

Singles: Peppermint, Peppermint Vitality, Rosemary, Rosemary Vitality, Vetiver, Cypress, Sacred Sandalwood, Royal Hawaiian Sandalwood, Helichrysum, Pine

Blends: Aroma Siez, Cool Azul, RutaVaLa, RutaVaLa Roll-On, Deep Relief Roll-On, PanAway, Relieve It, CBD

Nutritionals: MultiGreens, Sulfurzyme, PowerGize, Super Vitamin B, Super Vitamin C, Super Vitamin C Chewables, Mega Vitamin Cal, Mineral Essence, MindWise, OmegaGize3

Personal Care: Cool Azul Pain Relief Cream, Cool Azul Sports Gel, CBD Muscle Rub, Ortho Ease Massage Oil, Ortho Sport Massage Oil

Application and Usage

Aromatic: Refer to Application Guidelines.

Topical: Refer to Application Guidelines.

- Use 1-2 drops neat to massage on the facial nerve in front and behind the ears and on any areas of pain 3-5 times daily until symptoms end.

Carpal Tunnel Syndrome

Nerves pass through a tunnel formed by wrist bones (known as carpals) and a tough membrane on the underside of the wrist that binds the bones together. The tunnel is rigid, so if the tissues within it swell, they press and pinch the nerves and create a painful condition known as carpal tunnel syndrome, which is often the result of a combination of factors that increase pressure on the median nerve and tendons in the carpal tunnel, rather than a problem with the nerve itself.

Often the problem is due to a genetic factor in which the carpal tunnel is smaller in some people than in others. Other possible factors are trauma or injury to the wrist that causes swelling, such as a fracture or sprain; overactivity of the pituitary gland; work stress; hypothyroidism; rheumatoid arthritis; repeated use of vibrating hand tools; fluid retention during pregnancy or menopause; mechanical problems in the wrist joint; or the development of a cyst or tumor in the canal. Sometimes other causes or no causes can be identified.

Repeated motions can result in repetitive motion disorders such as tendonitis or bursitis, but there is little clinical data to prove that such repetitive or forceful movements of the hand and wrist during leisure activities or work can cause carpal tunnel syndrome.

A similar but less common condition can occur in the ankle (tarsal tunnel syndrome) or elbow.

Recommendations

Singles: Wintergreen, Helichrysum, Marjoram, Marjoram Vitality, Peppermint, Peppermint Vitality, Vetiver, Basil, Basil Vitality, Cypress, Lemongrass, Lemongrass Vitality, Myrrh

Blends: PanAway, Cool Azul, Relieve It, Aroma Siez, Deep Relief Roll-On, CBD

Nutritionals: Sulfurzyme, Mega Vitamin Cal, Mineral Essence, PD 80/20, BLM, AgilEase, PowerGize

Personal Care: Cool Azul Pain Relief Cream, Cool Azul Sports Gel, CBD Muscle Rub, Regenolone Moisturizing Cream, Ortho Ease Massage Oil, Ortho Sport Massage Oil

Application and Usage

Topical: Refer to Application Guidelines.

- Apply 2-4 drops neat or diluted 50:50 to affected area 3-5 times daily, as needed.

- Place a cold compress on location 2-3 times daily.

Carpal Tunnel Blend
- 5 drops Wintergreen
- 3 drops Cypress
- 3 drops Myrrh
- 2 drops Marjoram
- 1 drop Peppermint

Neuralgia

Neuralgia is pain from a damaged nerve. It can occur in the face, spine, or elsewhere. This recurring pain can be traced along a nerve pathway. Carpal tunnel syndrome is a specific type of neuralgia. The primary symptom is temporary sharp pain in the peripheral nerve(s).

Recommendations

Singles: Wintergreen, Helichrysum, Peppermint, Peppermint Vitality, Marjoram, Marjoram Vitality, Nutmeg, Nutmeg Vitality, Tea Tree, Roman Chamomile, Rosemary, Rosemary Vitality

Blends: Cool Azul, RutaVaLa, RutaVaLa Roll-On, Relieve It, Peace & Calming, Peace & Calming II, Deep Relief Roll-On, CBD, PanAway, Calm CBD Roll-On, Seedlings Calm, Relieve It

Nutritionals: PD 80/20, BLM, AgilEase, Super Vitamin D, Sulfurzyme, Super Vitamin B, Super Vitamin C, Super Vita-min C Chewable, MindWise, OmegaGize3

Personal Care: Cool Azul Pain Relief Cream, Cool Azul Sports Gel, CBD Muscle Rub, Regenolone Moisturizing Cream, Prenolone Plus Body Cream, Ortho Ease Massage Oil, Ortho Sport Massage Oil

Application and Usage

Topical: Refer to Application Guidelines.

- Apply 2-4 oil drops neat or diluted 50:50 to affected area 3-5 times daily, as needed.

- Place a cold compress on location 2-3 times daily.

Neuritis

Neuritis is a painful inflammation of the peripheral nerves. It is usually caused by prolonged exposure to cold temperature, heavy-metal poisoning, diabetes, vitamin deficiencies (beriberi and pellagra), or infectious diseases such as typhoid fever and malaria.

Symptoms may include pain, burning, numbness, tingling, muscle weakness, or paralysis.

Recommendations

Singles: Lavender, Lavender Vitality, Nutmeg, Nutmeg Vitality, Copaiba, Copaiba Vitality, Helichrysum, Juniper, Vetiver, Frankincense, Frankincense Vitality, Sacred Frankincense, Valerian, Thyme, Thyme Vitality, Clove, Clove Vitality

Blends: Cool Azul, PanAway, Relieve It, Valor, Valor Roll-On, Aroma Siez, Deep Relief Roll-On, CBD, RutaVaLa, RutaVaLa Roll-On, Light the Fire

Nutritionals: PowerGize, Sulfurzyme, AminoWise, Super Vitamin D, EndoGize, CortiStop, Super Vitamin B, Super Vita-min C, Super Vitamin C Chewable, PD 80/20, OmegaGize3, MindWise

Personal Care: Cool Azul Pain Relief Cream, Cool Azul Sports Gel, CBD Muscle Rub, Regenolone Moisturizing Cream, Prenolone Plus Body Cream

Application and Usage

Aromatic: Refer to Application Guidelines.

Topical: Refer to Application Guidelines.

- Apply 2-4 drops neat or diluted 50:50 to affected area 3-5 times daily as required.

- Place a cold compress on location 2-3 times daily.

Neuropathy

Neuropathy refers to actual damage to the peripheral nerves, usually from an autoimmune condition.

Damage to these peripheral nerves (other than spinal or those in the brain) generally starts as tingling in hands and feet and slowly spreads along limbs to the trunk.

Numbness, sensitive skin, neuralgic pain, and weakening of muscle power can all develop in varying degrees. Most common causes include complications from diabetes (diabetic neuropathy), alcoholism, vitamin B12 deficiency, tumors, too many painkillers, exposure to and absorption of chemicals, metals, pesticides, etc.

B vitamins and minerals such as magnesium, calcium, potassium, and organic sulfur are important in repairing nerve damage and quenching pain from inflamed nerves.

Canadian Fleabane (Conyza) may boost production of pregnenolone and human growth hormone. Pregnenolone aids in repairing damage to the myelin sheath.[43]

Juniper also may help in supporting nerve repair.

If paralysis is a problem, a regeneration of up to 60 percent may be possible. If, however, the nerve damage is too severe, treatment may not help. If the damage starts to reverse, there will be pain. Apply a few drops of PanAway neat on location.

Symptoms can include a prickling or burning sensation, increased sensitivity to touch, tingling, or numbness.

Recommendations

Singles: Sacred Frankincense, Frankincense, Frankincense Vitality, Lavender, Lavender Vitality, Cedarwood, Idaho Blue Spruce, Peppermint, Peppermint Vitality, Roman Chamomile, Vetiver, Valerian, Geranium, Goldenrod, Helichrysum, Nutmeg, Nutmeg Vitality

Blends: Cool Azul, Aroma Siez, Peace & Calming, Peace & Calming II, PanAway, RutaVaLa, RutaVaLa Roll-On, Deep Relief Roll-On, CBD Calm CBD Roll-On, Seedlings Calm

Nutritionals: PowerGize, AminoWise, Super Vitamin D, Super Vitamin B, OmegaGize3, Sulfurzyme, Longevity Softgels, Mineral Essence, Mega Vitamin Cal, Super Vitamin B, Super Vitamin C, Super Vitamin C Chewable, MultiGreens, PD 80/20, MindWise

Personal Care: Prenolone Plus Body Cream, Regenolone Moisturizing Cream, Cool Azul Pain Relief Cream, Cool Azul Sports Gel, CBD Muscle Rub, Ortho Ease Massage Oil, Ortho Sport Massage Oil

Application and Usage

Aromatic: Refer to Application Guidelines.

Topical: Refer to Application Guidelines.

- Apply 2-4 drops neat or diluted 50:50 to affected area 3-5 times daily, as required.

- Place a cold compress on location 2-3 times daily.

Neuropathy Blend No. 1
- 3 drops Sacred Frankincense or Frankincense
- 3 drops Geranium
- 3 drops Lavender

Neuropathy Blend No. 2
- 3 drops Geranium
- 3 drops Helichrysum
- 3 drops Cedarwood
- 2 drops Peppermint

NERVOUS SYSTEM, AUTONOMIC

The autonomic nervous system controls involuntary activities such as heartbeat, breathing, digestion, glandular activity, and contraction and dilation of blood vessels.

The autonomic nervous system is composed of two parts that balance and complement each other: the parasympathetic and sympathetic nervous systems. More simply, the sympathetic nervous system is "fight or flight" or excitatory while the parasympathetic system is "rest and digest" or inhibitory.

To Stimulate Parasympathetic Nervous System

The parasympathetic nervous system has relaxing effects and is responsible for secreting acetylcholine, which slows the heart and speeds digestion.

Recommendations
Singles: Lavender, Lavender Vitality, Lemon Verbena, Valerian, Patchouli, Marjoram, Marjoram Vitality, Ylang Ylang, Rose, Vetiver, Idaho Blue Spruce, Sage, Sage Vitality

Blends: Peace & Calming, Peace & Calming II, Harmony, Valor, Valor Roll-On, CBD, Calm CBD Roll-On, Seedlings Calm, RutaVaLa, RutaVaLa Roll-On

Nutritionals: NingXia Red, Mega Vitamin Cal, MindWise, Sulfurzyme, Super Vitamin D, Mineral Essence, Super Vitamin B, Super Vitamin C, Super Vitamin C Chewable

Application and Usage
Aromatic: Refer to Application Guidelines.

Dietary and Oral: Refer to Application Guidelines.

- Take 1 capsule of desired Vitality oil 2 times daily.

- Take 2-3 drops of desired Vitality oil in a spoonful of syrup or small amount of milk, juice, or water.

Topical: Refer to Application Guidelines.
- Have Raindrop Technique 2 times a week.

To Stimulate Sympathetic Nervous System
The sympathetic nervous system has stimulatory effects and is responsible for secreting stress hormones like adrenaline and noradrenaline.

Recommendations
Singles: Fennel, Fennel Vitality, Ginger, Ginger Vitality, Eucalyptus Radiata, Peppermint, Peppermint Vitality, Rosemary, Rosemary Vitality, Black Pepper, Black Pepper Vitality

Blends: Clarity, Brain Power, KidScents GeneYus

Nutritionals: Super Vitamin D, Super Vitamin B, Super Vitamin C, Super Vitamin C Chewable, Sulfurzyme, Mineral Essence, MindWise, Essentialzymes-4, Essentialzyme, Mega Vitamin Cal

Application and Usage
Aromatic: Refer to Application Guidelines.

Dietary and Oral: Refer to Application Guidelines.

- Take 1 capsule of desired Vitality oil 2 times daily.

- Take 2-3 drops of desired Vitality oil in a spoonful of syrup or small amount of milk, juice, or water.

Topical: Refer to Application Guidelines.
- Have Raindrop Technique 2 times a week.

NEUROLOGICAL DISEASES
(See also NERVE DISORDERS)

Neurologic diseases are disorders of the spinal cord, brain, and nerves throughout your body. Together they control all the functions of the body. There are more than 600 neurological diseases.

CAUTION: Never use hot packs for neurological problems. Always use cold packs to reduce pain and inflammation. In other words, reduce the temperature of the damaged site.

ALS (Lou Gehrig's Disease)
Lou Gehrig's disease is another name for Amyotrophic Lateral Sclerosis (ALS), a degenerative nerve disorder. ALS affects the nerve fibers in the spinal cord that control voluntary movement.

Muscles require continuous stimulation by their associated nerves to maintain their tone. Removal or deadening of these nerves results in muscular atrophy. The lack of control forces the muscles to spasm, resulting in twitching and cramps. The sensory pathways are unaffected, so feeling is never lost in the afflicted muscles.

Juniper may support nerve function. Frankincense may help clear the emotions of fear and anger, which is common with people who have these neurologic diseases. When these diseases are contracted, people often become suicidal.

Hope, Joy, Gathering, and Forgiveness will help individuals work through the psychological and emotional aspects of the disease.

Sulfur deficiency is often prevalent in neurological diseases. Sulfur requires calcium and vitamin C for the body to metabolize. Super Vitamin B and Sulfurzyme work well together to help repair nerve damage and the myelin sheath.

Recommendations
Singles: Rosemary, Rosemary Vitality, Royal Hawaiian Sandalwood, Sacred Sandalwood, Sacred Frankincense, Frankincense, Frankincense Vitality, Helichrysum, Cypress, Sage, Sage Vitality, Juniper, Clove, Clove Vitality, Cardamom, Cardamom Vitality, Eucalyptus Blue, Ylang Ylang

Blends: Hope, Joy, Gathering, Brain Power, Clarity, KidScents GeneYus, Forgiveness, Common Sense

Nutritionals: PD 80/20, BLM, AgilEase, AminoWise, Super Vitamin D, Sulfurzyme, MindWise, MultiGreens, Mega Vitamin Cal, Super Vitamin C, Super Vitamin C Chewable, Super Vitamin B, Longevity Softgels, OmegaGize3

Personal Care: Prenolone Plus Body Cream, Cool Azul Pain Relief Cream

Application and Usage
Aromatic: Refer to Application Guidelines.

Dietary and Oral: Refer to Application Guidelines.

- Take 1 capsule of desired Vitality oil 2 times daily.

- Take 2-3 drops of desired Vitality oil in a spoonful of syrup or small amount of milk, juice, or water.

ALS Blend
- 3 drops Rosemary or Rosemary Vitality
- 2 drops Clove or Clove Vitality
- 1 drop Eucalyptus Blue
- 1 drop Ylang Ylang
- 1 drop Sacred Frankincense, Frankincense, or Frankincense Vitality

Topical: Refer to Application Guidelines.
- Apply 1-3 drops diluted 50:50 on the brain reflex points on the forehead, temples, and mastoids (just behind ears).

- Use a direct pressure application and massage 6-10 drops diluted 50:50 from the base of the skull, down the neck, and down the spine.
- Place a few drops of oil on a loofah brush and rub along the spine vigorously. Always use a natural bristle brush, since the oils may dissolve plastic bristles.
- Receive a Raindrop Technique 3 times monthly.

Huntington's Chorea
Huntington's chorea is a degenerative nerve disease that generally becomes manifest in middle age. It is marked by uncontrollable body movements, which are followed—and occasionally preceded—by mental deterioration.

Note: Huntington's chorea should not be confused with Sydenham's chorea, often called St. Vitus Dance, chorea minor, or juvenile chorea that affects children, especially females, usually appearing between the ages of 7 and 14. The jerking symptoms eventually disappear.

Recommendations
Singles: Peppermint, Peppermint Vitality, Juniper, Basil, Basil Vitality, Royal Hawaiian Sandalwood, Sacred Sandalwood, Sacred Frankincense, Frankincense, Frankincense Vitality, Geranium, Palo Santo, Eucalyptus Blue

Blends: Aroma Siez, RutaVaLa, RutaVaLa Roll-On, EndoFlex, EndoFlex Vitality, Awaken, Christmas Spirit, Citrus Fresh, Citrus Fresh Vitality, Tranquil Roll-On

Nutritionals: PowerGize, Sulfurzyme, Super Vitamin D, BLM, AgilEase, MultiGreens, NingXia Red, Ningxia Wolfberries (Organic, Dried), Slique Shake, Super Vitamin C, Super Vitamin C Chewable, Super Vitamin B, Mega Vitamin Cal, MindWise, OmegaGize3, Master Formula, Balance Complete, Mineral Essence, Essentialzyme, Allerzyme

Application and Usage
Aromatic: Refer to Application Guidelines.

Dietary and Oral: Refer to Application Guidelines.

- Take 1 capsule of desired Vitality oil 2 times daily.

- Take 2-3 drops of desired Vitality oil in a spoonful of syrup or small amount of milk, juice, or water.

Topical: Refer to Application Guidelines.
- Apply 1-3 drops diluted 50:50 on the brain reflex points on the forehead, temples, and mastoids just behind ears.

- Use a direct pressure application and massage 6-10 drops diluted 50:50 from the base of the skull, down the neck, and down the spine.
- Place a few drops of oil on a loofah brush and rub along the spine vigorously. Always use a natural bristle brush, since the oils may dissolve plastic bristles.
- Receive a Raindrop Technique 3 times monthly.

Nerve Blend
- 5 drops Juniper
- 3 drops Aroma Siez
- 2 drops Peppermint or Peppermint Vitality
- 1 drop Basil or Basil Vitality

Multiple Sclerosis (MS)

Multiple sclerosis is a progressive, disabling autoimmune disease of the nervous system, brain, and spinal cord in which inflammation occurs in the central nervous system. Eventually, the myelin sheaths protecting the nerves are destroyed, resulting in a slowing or blocking of nerve transmission.

MS is an autoimmune disease in which the body's own immune system attacks the nerves. Some researchers believe that MS is triggered by a virus, while others make a case that it has a strong genetic or environmental component.

Symptoms
- Muscle weakness in extremities
- Deteriorating coordination and balance
- Numbness or prickling sensations
- Poor attention or memory
- Speech impediments
- Incontinence
- Tremors
- Dizziness
- Hearing loss

Recommendations

Singles: Juniper, Geranium, Sacred Frankincense, Frankincense, Frankincense Vitality, Rosemary, Rosemary Vitality, Basil, Basil Vitality, Helichrysum, Sacred Sandalwood, Royal Hawaiian Sandalwood, Peppermint, Peppermint Vitality, Thyme, Thyme Vitality, Marjoram, Marjoram Vitality, Cypress

Blends: PanAway, Cool Azul, Valor, Valor Roll-On, Aroma Siez, Deep Relief Roll-On, CBD, RutaVaLa, RutaVaLa Roll-On, Acceptance, Awaken

Nutritionals: BLM, AgilEase, PowerGize, OmegaGize3, Sulfurzyme, Super Vitamin D, MultiGreens, Slique Shake, Essentialzyme, Essentialzymes-4, Mineral Essence, Mega Vitamin Cal, Super Vitamin C, Super Vitamin C Chewable, Super Vitamin B, NingXia Red, MindWise

Personal Care: Cool Azul Pain Relief Cream, Cool Azul Sports Gel, CBD Muscle Rub, Progessence Plus, Regenolone Moisturizing Cream, Ortho Sport Massage Oil, Ortho Ease Massage Oil

Application and Usage

Aromatic: Refer to Application Guidelines.

Dietary and Oral: Refer to Application Guidelines.

- Take 1 capsule of desired Vitality oil 2 times daily.

- Take 2-3 drops of desired Vitality oil in a spoonful of syrup or small amount of milk, juice, or water.

Topical: Refer to Application Guidelines.

- Apply 1-3 drops diluted 50:50 on the brain reflex points on the forehead, temples, and mastoids just behind the ears.

- Apply direct pressure and massage 6-10 drops diluted 50:50 from the base of the skull, down the neck, and down the spine.

- Place a few drops of oil on a loofah brush and rub along the spine vigorously. Always use a natural bristle brush, since the oils may dissolve plastic bristles.

- Receive a Raindrop Technique 3-4 times monthly.

MS Blend
- 4 drops Geranium
- 4 drops Rosemary or Rosemary Vitality
- 2 drops Helichrysum
- 2 drops Juniper

MS Daily Regimen

1. Apply neat 4-6 drops of Helichrysum, Geranium, Juniper, Sacred Sandalwood, Royal Hawaiian Sandalwood, Rosemary, and Peppermint Raindrop-style along the spine. Lightly massage oils in the direction of the MS paralysis. For example, if it is in the lower part of the spine, massage down; if it is in the upper part of the spine, massage up. Follow the application with 30 minutes of cold packs (change cold packs as needed).

2. Apply 4-6 drops of Valor on the spine. If the MS affects the legs, rub down the spine; if it affects the neck, rub up the spine.

3. Apply 2-3 drops each of Cypress, Sacred Sandalwood, Royal Hawaiian Sandalwood, and Marjoram to the back of the neck and then cover with 2-3 drops of Aroma Siez.

To give additional emotional support to the person with MS symptoms, use Acceptance and Awaken. Be patient. Overcoming MS is a long-term endeavor.

Maintaining Multiple Sclerosis (MS) Status Quo

One of the simplest ways to keep MS symptoms from progressing or becoming more severe is to keep the body cool and avoid any locations or physical activities that heat the body (including hot showers or exercise). Cold baths and relaxed swimming are two of the best activities for relieving symptoms.

Applying heat is the worst thing to do for MS. If an MS patient is experiencing increasingly severe symptoms, lower the patient's body temperature (by up to 3 degrees F) by having the patient lie on a table, covering the patient with a sheet, ice, shower curtain, and blankets (in that order) for 10 to 15 minutes or longer if possible. The individual can tell you how he or she feels. Work the feet with oils and watch for benefits.

Parkinson's Disease

Parkinson's disease is a deterioration of specific nerve centers in the brain that affects more men than women by a ratio of 3:2.

Symptoms
- Tremors, an involuntary shaking of hands, head, or both
- Rigidity, slowed movement, and loss of balance
- Stooped posture
- Continuous rubbing together of thumb and forefinger
- Mask-like face
- Trouble swallowing
- Depression
- Difficulty performing simple tasks

These symptoms may all be seen at different stages of the disease. The tremors are most severe when the affected part of the body is not in use. There is no pain or other sensation, other than a decreased ability to move. Symptoms appear slowly in no particular order and may end before they interfere with normal activities.

Restoring dopamine levels in the brain can reduce symptoms of Parkinson's. Sulfurzyme provides a source of organic sulfur, a vital nutrient for nerve and myelin sheath formation.

Recommendations

Singles: Helichrysum, Lavender, Lavender Vitality, Peppermint, Peppermint Vitality, Cedarwood, Myrrh, Basil, Basil Vitality, Sacred Sandalwood, Royal Hawaiian Sandalwood

Blends: GLF, GLF Vitality, Peace & Calming, Peace & Calming II, Calm CBD Roll-On, Seedlings Calm, Valor, Valor Roll-On, 25 Years Young, Brain Power, Shutran

Nutritionals: PowerGize, Sulfurzyme, Super Vitamin B, PD 80/20, BLM, AgilEase, MindWise, Mineral Essence, Slique Shake, JuvaPower, Super Vitamin C, Super Vitamin C Chewable, Life 9, KidScents MightyPro, OmegaGize3, Essentialzyme, Essentialzymes-4

Application and Usage

Aromatic: Refer to Application Guidelines.

Dietary and Oral: Refer to Application Guidelines.

- Take 1 capsule of desired Vitality oil 2 times daily.

- Take 2-3 drops of desired Vitality oil in a spoonful of syrup or small amount of milk, juice, or water.

Topical: Refer to Application Guidelines.

- Apply 1-3 drops diluted 50:50 on the brain reflex points on the forehead, temples, and mastoids just behind the ears.

- Use a direct pressure application and massage 6-10 drops diluted 50:50 from the base of the skull, down the neck, and down the spine.

- Place a few drops of oil on a loofah brush and rub along the spine vigorously. Always use a natural bristle brush, since the oils may dissolve plastic bristles.

- Receive a Raindrop Technique 3 times monthly.

CAUTION: Never use hot packs for neurological problems. Always use cold packs to reduce pain and inflammation. In other words, reduce the temperature of the affected area.

Restless Legs Syndrome (See also ATTENTION DEFICIT DISORDER)

Restless legs syndrome (Willis-Ekbom disease) is a neurological disorder characterized by an irresistible urge to move the body to stop odd or uncomfortable sensations. It commonly affects the legs but can also affect the torso, arms, and even phantom limbs. For many people, Peace & Calming on the bottoms of the feet at night is the solution for this problem.

Recommendations

Singles: Valerian, Lavender, Lavender Vitality, Basil, Basil Vitality, Marjoram, Marjoram Vitality, Cypress, Roman Chamomile

Blends: RutaVaLa, RutaVaLa Roll-On, Aroma Siez, Peace & Calming, Peace & Calming II, Tranquil Roll-On, Stress Away, Stress Away Roll-On, Valor, Valor Roll-On, CBD, Calm CBD Roll-On, Seedlings Calm

Nutritionals: ImmuPro, Mineral Essence, MultiGreens, Mega Vitamin Cal, OmegaGize3, SleepEssence, KidScents Unwind, Thyromin, MindWise, PowerGize, BLM, AgilEase

Personal Care: Cool Azul Pain Relief Cream, Cool Azul Sports Gel, CBD Muscle Rub, Progessence Plus, Regenolone Moisturizing Cream, Ortho Sport Massage Oil, Ortho Ease Massage Oil

Application and Usage

Aromatic: Refer to Application Guidelines.

Dietary and Oral: Whether putting the Vitality oils in a capsule or drinking them in a liquid, please refer to Application Guidelines.

- Take 1 capsule of desired Vitality oil 2 times daily.

- Take 2-3 drops of desired Vitality oil in a spoonful of syrup or small amount of milk, juice, or water.

Topical: Refer to Application Guidelines.

- Apply 2-4 drops neat as desired.

- Massage 2-4 drops of oil on the Vita Flex points of the feet before retiring.
- Receive a Raindrop Technique 1 time a week.

Schizophrenia

Schizophrenia is a complex mental illness and has many possible causes. The term means roughly "splitting of the mind" and has more recently been called "integration-dysregulation syndrome" to reduce the stigma attached to the term "schizophrenia."

Negative symptoms are a challenge to treat, as they are generally not improved by medication. Some cases are believed to be caused by viral infection. Sometimes it is considered to be a neurologic disease that involves identity confusion.

Onset is typically between the late teens and early 30's. Abnormal neurological findings may show a broad range of dysfunction, including slow reaction time, poor coordination, abnormalities in eye tracking, violence, and impaired sensory gating.

Typically, schizophrenia involves dysfunction in many areas such as interpersonal relations, work, education, or self-care.

Recommendations

Singles: Cardamom, Cardamom Vitality, Cedarwood, Vetiver, Melissa, Rosemary, Rosemary Vitality, Valerian, Peppermint, Peppermint Vitality, Sacred Frankincense, Frankincense, Frankincense Vitality

Blends: Brain Power, Gary's Light, KidScents GeneYus, Valor, Valor Roll-On, KidScents KidPower, KidScents KidPower Roll-On, Seedlings Calm, M-Grain, Clarity, One Heart, Common Sense

Nutritionals: Mineral Essence, Mega Vitamin Cal, MindWise, NingXia Red, Super Vitamin B, Slique Shake, JuvaPower, Master Formula, Ningxia Wolfberries (Organic, Dried)

Application and Usage

Aromatic: Refer to Application Guidelines.

- Diffuse your choice of oils for ½ hour every 4-6 hours or as desired.

Dietary and Oral: Refer to Application Guidelines.

- Take 1 capsule of desired Vitality oil 2 times daily.

- Take 2-3 drops of desired Vitality oil in a spoonful of syrup or small amount of milk, juice, or water.

Topical: Refer to Application Guidelines.

- Receive a Raindrop Technique treatment 1 time a week.

NOSE AND SINUS PROBLEMS

Millions of people have chronic sinus troubles, and millions more suffer from rhinitis, a term for stuffy nose. One of the most effective treatments for nasal and sinus problems is a saltwater nose rinse.

Dry Nose

Dry nose refers to a lack of moisture in the nasal passage, which can occasionally cause the skin inside the nose to itch, crack, and bleed.

Recommendations

Singles: Myrrh, Lavender, Lemon, Peppermint

Blends: R.C., Raven, Breathe Again, Breathe Again Roll-On, SniffleEase

Personal Care: Rose Ointment, Boswellia Wrinkle Cream, Sandalwood Moisturizing Cream

Application and Usage
Aromatic: Refer to Application Guidelines.

Topical: Refer to Application Guidelines.

- Apply 1-2 drops diluted 50:50 to the nostril walls with a cotton swab 2 times daily.

- Massage 2-4 drops of oil neat on the bottoms of the feet on the Vita Flex points just before bedtime.

Dry Nose Blend
- 2 drops Lavender
- 1 drop Myrrh

Loss of Smell
The senses of smell and taste are strongly connected. Some of the common causes of loss of smell and taste are cigarette smoke, medications like antibiotics and blood pressure medicines, the common cold, pollutants, allergies, blocked nasal passages, tooth and gum diseases, chemotherapy, Alzheimer's disease, surgery, tumors, Parkinson's disease, polyps, or even a head injury.

Recommendations
Singles: Peppermint, Peppermint Vitality, Thyme, Thyme Vitality, Myrtle, Eucalyptus Globulus

Blends: R.C., Raven, Exodus II, Joy, Highest Potential, The Gift, Sensation

Nutritionals: NingXia Red

Application and Usage
Aromatic: Refer to Application Guidelines.

Topical: Refer to Application Guidelines.

Nosebleeds
Nosebleeds usually are not serious. However, if bleeding does not stop in a short time or is excessive or frequent, consult your health care professional.

Recommendations
Singles: Cistus, Helichrysum, Cypress, Dorado Azul, Geranium

Blends: GLF, GLF Vitality, JuvaCleanse, JuvaCleanse Vitality

Nutritionals: Mineral Essence, Sulfurzyme, Master Formula

Application and Usage
Topical: Refer to Application Guidelines.

- Apply 2-4 drops neat to the bridge and sides of the nose and back of the neck. Repeat as needed.
- Applying a single drop under the nose is helpful and refreshing.
- Dilute 50:50 and apply on location 3-6 times daily.

- Massage 2-4 drops of oil neat on the bottoms of the feet on the Vita Flex points just before bedtime. Children love it.

Nosebleed Blend
- 3 drops Geranium or Helichrysum
- 2 drops Cistus
- 2 drops Cypress

Nosebleed Regimen
Put 1 drop of Geranium on a tissue paper and wrap the paper around a chip of ice about the size of a thumb nail, push it up under the top lip in the center to the base of the nose. Hold from the outside with lip pressure. This usually will stop bleeding in a very short time.

Polyps, Nasal
Nasal polyps are soft, painless, noncancerous growths on the lining of the nasal passages or sinuses. They hang down like grapes or teardrops and result from chronic inflammation due to allergies, asthma, recurring infection, drug sensitivity, or certain immune disorders.

Small polyps may not cause problems, but larger growths or groups of polyps can block the nasal passages, lead to breathing problems, cause frequent infections, or cause a lost sense of smell.

Recommendations
Singles: Citronella, Helichrysum, Sacred Frankincense, Frankincense, Frankincense Vitality

Blend: Purification, Citrus Fresh, Melrose

Application and Usage
Topical: Refer to Application Guidelines.

- Apply 1-2 drops diluted 50:50 on a cotton swab and carefully apply on the inside nostrils 1-3 times daily.

Nasal Irrigation Regimen

Essential oils can be used in a saline solution for very effective nasal irrigation that clears and decongests sinuses. As recommended by Daniel Pénoël, MD, the saline solution is prepared as follows:

- 10 drops Rosemary
- 6 drops Tea Tree
- 8 tablespoons ultra-fine sea salt

Also very effective is the following:

- 10 drops Rosemary
- 6 drops Thyme
- 2 drops Cypress
- 8 tablespoons ultra-fine sea salt

The essential oils are mixed thoroughly in the fine salt and stored in a sealed container. For each nasal irrigation session, 1 teaspoon of this salt mixture is dissolved into 1½ cups of distilled water.

This solution is then placed in the tank of an oral irrigator or neti pot to irrigate the nasal cavities, which is done while bending over a sink. This application has brought surprisingly positive results in treating latent sinusitis and other nasal congestion problems.

OBESITY (See also DEPRESSION)

Hormone treatments using natural progesterone (for women) and testosterone (for men) may be one of the most powerful treatments for obesity. In women, progesterone levels drop dramatically after menopause, and this can result in substantial weight gain, particularly around the hips and thighs. Using transdermal creams or serums to replace declining progesterone can result in a substantial decline in body fat.

Diffusing or directly inhaling essential oils can have an immediate positive impact on moods and appetites. Olfaction is the only sense that can have a direct effect on the limbic region of the brain. Studies at the University of Vienna have shown that some essential oils and their primary constituents can stimulate blood flow and activity in the emotional centers of the brain.44

Fragrance influences can penetrate the amygdala in the center of the brain in such a manner that frequent smelling of pleasing aromas can significantly reduce appetite. Dr. Alan Hirsch, in his landmark studies, showed dramatic weight loss in research subjects using aromas from peppermint oil and vanilla absolute to curb food cravings.45

Recommendations

Singles: Peppermint, Peppermint Vitality, Roman Chamomile, Nutmeg, Nutmeg Vitality, Clove, Clove Vitality, Grapefruit, Grapefruit Vitality, Fennel, Fennel Vitality, Cinnamon Bark, Cinnamon Bark Vitality, Lavender, Lavender Vitality, Sacred Frankincense, Frankincense, Frankincense Vitality, Davana, Bergamot, Bergamot Vitality

Blends: Build Your Dream, Gary's Light, Valor, Valor Roll-On, JuvaCleanse, JuvaCleanse Vitality, Joy, The Gift, 3 Wise Men, Sacred Mountain, White Angelica, One Heart, Gathering, Freedom, My Destiny, Fulfill Your Destiny, 25 Years Young

Nutritionals: JuvaPower, Thyromin, Detoxzyme, OmegaGize3, Slique Shake, Slique Essence, Slique CitraSlim, Slique Bars, Slique Bars–Chocolate-Coated, Slique Gum, Balance Complete, Digest & Cleanse, Pure Protein Complete, Chocolate-Coated Wolfberry Crisp Bars

Personal Care: Progessence Plus, Prenolone Plus Body Cream, Cel-Lite Magic Massage Oil

Application and Usage

Aromatic: Refer to Application Guidelines.

Dietary and Oral: Refer to Application Guidelines.

 • Take 1 capsule of desired Vitality oil 2 times daily.

 • Take 2-3 drops of desired Vitality oil in a spoonful of syrup or small amount of milk, juice, or water.

Topical: Refer to Application Guidelines.

 • Applying a single drop under the nose is helpful and refreshing.

 • Massage 2-4 drops of oil neat on the bottoms of the feet just before bedtime.

ORAL CARE PROBLEMS, TEETH AND GUMS

Poor oral hygiene has not only been linked to bad breath (halitosis) but also to cardiovascular disease. Some of the same bacteria that populate the mouth have now been implicated in arteriosclerosis.

Essential oils make excellent oral antiseptics, analgesics, and anti-inflammatories. Clove essential oil has been used in mainstream dentistry for decades to numb the gums and help prevent infections. Similarly, menthol (found in Peppermint essential oil), methyl salycilate (found in Wintergreen essential oil), thymol (found in Thyme essential oil), and eucalyptol (found in Eucalyptus and Rosemary essential oils) are in approved OTC drug products for combating gingivitis and periodontal disease.

Bleeding Gums

Bleeding gums can be a sign that you have, or are at risk for, gum disease. However, persistent gum bleeding may be caused by serious medical conditions such as leukemia or bleeding and platelet disorders. Bleeding gums are mainly due to inadequate plaque removal from the teeth at the gum line, which will lead to gingivitis, or inflamed gums.

Recommendations

Singles: Clove, Clove Vitality, Eucalyptus Globulus, Sacred Frankincense, Frankincense, Frankincense Vitality, Rosemary, Rosemary Vitality, Helichrysum, Wintergreen, Cinnamon Bark, Cinnamon Bark Vitality, Mountain Savory, Mountain Savory Vitality, Myrrh, Peppermint, Peppermint Vitality, Thyme, Thyme Vitality

Blends: Thieves, Thieves Roll-On, Thieves Vitality, Melrose, PanAway, Relieve It

Nutritionals: Super Vitamin C, Super Vitamin C Chewable, Slique Essence

Oral Care: Thieves AromaBright Toothpaste, Thieves Fresh Essence Plus Mouthwash, KidScents Toothpaste, Thieves Whitening Toothpaste, Thieves Dental Floss, Thieves Hard Lozenges, Thieves Mints, Slique Gum

Application and Usage

Dietary and Oral: Refer to Application Guidelines.

- Take 1 capsule of desired Vitality oil 2 times daily.

- Take 2-3 drops of desired Vitality oil in a spoonful of syrup or small amount of milk, juice, or water.

- Gargle 3-10 times daily with Thieves Fresh Essence Plus Mouthwash or as needed.

- Brush teeth and gums after every meal with a Thieves Toothpaste.

Blend for Combating Gum Bleeding
- 2 drops Myrrh
- 2 drops Helichrysum
- 1 drop Thieves Vitality or Thieves
- 1 drop Frankincense Vitality, Frankincense, or Sacred Frankincense

Topical: Refer to Application Guidelines

- Apply 1-2 drops diluted 50:50 on gums 2-3 times daily.

Gingivitis and Periodontitis

Periodontal diseases are infections of the gum and bone that hold the teeth in place. Gingivitis affects the upper areas of the gum where it bonds to the visible enamel, while periodontitis is a more internal infection affecting the gum at the root level of the tooth. In advanced stages, these diseases can lead to painful chewing problems and even tooth loss.

Oils such as Peppermint, Wintergreen, Clove, Thyme, and all eucalyptus varieties can kill bacteria and effectively combat a variety of gum infections.

Recommendations

Singles: Clove, Clove Vitality, Tea Tree, Thyme, Thyme Vitality, Mountain Savory, Mountain Savory Vitality, Wintergreen, Peppermint, Peppermint Vitality, Oregano, Oregano Vitality, Ecuadorian Oregano, Helichrysum, Eucalyptus Globulus, Eucalyptus Radiata

Blends: Thieves, Thieves Roll-On, Thieves Vitality, Exodus II, PanAway, ImmuPower

Nutritionals: Super Vitamin C, Super Vitamin C Chewable, Longevity Softgels, OmegaGize3, Slique Essence, Inner Defense, ImmuPro

Oral Care: Thieves AromaBright Toothpaste, Thieves Fresh Essence Plus Mouthwash, Thieves Hard Lozenges, Thieves Mints, Thieves Spray, Thieves Dental Floss, Slique Gum

Application and Usage

Dietary and Oral: Whether putting the Vitality oils in a capsule or drinking them in a liquid, please refer to Application Guidelines.

- Take 1 capsule of desired Vitality oil 2 times daily.

- Take 2-3 drops of desired Vitality oil in a spoonful of syrup or small amount of milk, juice, or water.

- Gargle 3-10 times daily with Thieves Fresh Essence Plus Mouthwash or as needed.

- Brush teeth and gums after every meal with a Thieves Toothpaste.

Topical: Refer to Application Guidelines.

Oral Infection

Dental Visits: Prior to visiting the dentist, rub 1 drop each of Clove or Clove Vitality and PanAway on gums and jaw. Clove may interfere with bonding of crowns, so keep it off the teeth if this procedure is planned.

General Oral Infection: For general oral infection of any kind, roll a piece of gauze tightly into a string about ¼ inch thick. Put drops of Thieves blend on it; if it feels too "hot," add V-6. Put the string between the teeth and the lip near the tooth and leave it all night, allowing it to "wick up," or absorb, the infection. Change as often as needed.

MOUTH ULCERS (See CANKER SORES)

Mouth ulcers are sores or open lesions in the mouth and are caused by many disorders such as canker sores, oral cancer, thrush, fever blisters, or gingivostomatitis.

Recommendations

Singles: Carrot Seed, Carrot Seed Vitality, Tea Tree, Thyme, Thyme Vitality, Myrrh, Lavender, Lavender Vitality, Peppermint, Peppermint Vitality, Oregano, Oregano Vitality

Blends: Thieves, Thieves Roll-On, Thieves Vitality, Exodus II, ImmuPower

Nutritionals: AlkaLime, ImmuPro, Inner Defense, Slique Essence

Oral Care: Thieves AromaBright Toothpaste, KidScents Toothpaste, Thieves Whitening Toothpaste, Thieves Fresh Essence Plus Mouthwash, Thieves Spray, Thieves Hard Lozenges, Thieves Mints, Slique Gum

Application and Usage

Dietary and Oral: Refer to Application Guidelines.

- Take 1 capsule of desired Vitality oil 2 times daily.

- Take 2-3 drops of desired Vitality oil in a spoonful of syrup or small amount of milk, juice, or water.
- Gargle 3-10 times daily with Thieves Fresh Essence Plus Mouthwash or as needed.
- Brush teeth and gums after every meal with a Thieves Toothpaste.
- Gargle with Thieves Fresh Essence Plus Mouthwash or Thieves Spray and add 1-2 drops of Thieves Vitality, Clove Vitality, and Exodus II to strengthen the therapeutic action.

Topical: Refer to Application Guidelines.

- Apply 1-2 drops diluted 50:50 on gums 2 times daily.

Oral Infection Control

Oral infection control procedures are precautions taken in dental offices and other health care settings to prevent the spread of disease.

Recommendations

Singles: Clove, Clove Vitality, Myrrh, Oregano, Oregano Vitality, Ecuadorian Oregano, Thyme, Thyme Vitality, Helichrysum, Eucalyptus Radiata

Blends: PanAway, Thieves, Thieves Roll-On, Thieves Vitality, R.C., ImmuPower

Nutritionals: Inner Defense, ImmuPro, Mineral Essence, Essentialzyme, Essentialzymes-4, Life 9, KidScents MightyPro, Slique Essence, Detoxzyme, Mega Vitamin Cal, Slique Shake

Oral Care: Thieves Fresh Essence Plus Mouthwash, Thieves Spray, Thieves AromaBright Toothpaste, KidScents Toothpaste, Thieves Whitening Toothpaste, Thieves Hard Lozenges, Thieves Cough Drops, Thieves Mints, Slique Gum

Application and Usage

Topical: Refer to Application Guidelines.

- Apply 1-2 drops diluted 50:50 on gums and around teeth. Repeat as needed.
- Just before a tooth extraction, rub 1-2 drops of Helichrysum, Thieves or Thieves Vitality, and R.C. around the gum area.
- Rubbing R.C. on gums may also help to bring back feeling after numbness from anesthesia.

Pyorrhea

Essential oils are some of the best treatments against gum diseases such as gingivitis and pyorrhea. For example: the active constituent in Clove oil is eugenol, which is used as a dental disinfectant and is one of the best-studied germ killers available.

Recommendations

Singles: Clove, Clove Vitality, Thyme, Thyme Vitality, Oregano, Oregano Vitality, Ecuadorian Oregano, Wintergreen (dilute all 50:50)

Blends: Thieves, Thieves Roll-On, Thieves Vitality, Exodus II, ImmuPower (dilute all if desired)

Nutritionals: Mineral Essence, Essentialzyme, Essentialzymes-4, Detoxzyme, Mega Vitamin Cal, Slique Shake, Inner Defense, ImmuPro

Oral Care: Thieves Fresh Essence Plus Mouthwash, Thieves Spray, Thieves AromaBright Toothpaste, KidScents Toothpaste, Thieves Whitening Toothpaste, Thieves Hard Lozenges, Thieves Cough Drops, Thieves Mints, Thieves Dental Floss

Application and Usage

Dietary and Oral: Use any of the recommended single oils or **Blends** with toothpaste on toothbrush or alone. Generally, 1-2 drops are enough. For some people, the recommended oils will seem very "hot." Even one drop mixed with toothpaste may seem strong, but within a minute the "hot" sensation is gone, and the mouth feels very clean and refreshed. Many people like using one drop of Slique Essence or Thieves directly on the toothbrush without using any toothpaste.

- Gargle 4-6 times daily with Thieves Fresh Essence Plus Mouthwash or as needed.
- Mix 1-2 drops of Clove Vitality or any other recommended oil of choice in a glass of water and gargle.
- Spray mouth several times daily with Thieves Spray.

Topical: Refer to Application Guidelines.

- Put 1-2 drops of Thieves on your toothbrush directly or put 1-2 drops of Thieves on your Thieves toothpaste.
- Put 1 drop of Thieves directly on affected tooth and gum area, as needed.

Teeth Grinding

Teeth grinding (bruxism) is a condition in which you grind, clench, or gnash your teeth, consciously or unconsciously. If it is frequent and severe enough, it can lead to jaw disorders, headaches, damaged teeth, and other problems.

Recommendations

Singles: Valerian, Lavender, Lavender Vitality, Roman Chamomile

Blends: Peace & Calming, Peace & Calming II, RutaVaLa, RutaVaLa Roll-On, Stress Away, Stress Away Roll-On, Calm CBD Roll-On, Seedlings Calm, Tranquil Roll-On, ImmuPower

Nutritionals: Mineral Essence, Mega Vitamin Cal, ImmuPro, SleepEssence, KidScents Unwind, Inner Defense

Oral Care: Thieves Spray, Thieves AromaBright Toothpaste, KidScents Toothpaste, Thieves Whitening Toothpaste, Thieves Fresh Essence Plus Mouthwash, Slique Gum

Application and Usage

Aromatic: Refer to Application Guidelines.

Topical: Refer to Application Guidelines.

- Massage 1-3 drops neat of Lavender, RutaVaLa, and Valerian on bottoms of feet each night before retiring.

Toothache and Teething Pain

A toothache is a pain in or around a tooth, and treatment for a toothache depends on the cause.

Recommendations

Singles: Clove, Clove Vitality, Sacred Frankincense, Frankincense, Frankincense Vitality, German Chamomile, German Chamomile Vitality, Tea Tree

Blends: Thieves, Thieves Roll-On, Thieves Vitality, PanAway, Cool Azul

Oral Care: Thieves Spray, Thieves AromaBright Toothpaste, KidScents Toothpaste, Thieves Whitening Toothpaste, Thieves Fresh Essence Plus Mouthwash, Slique Essence, Slique Gum

Application and Usage

Dietary and Oral: Refer to Application Guidelines.

- Take 1 capsule of desired Vitality oil 2 times daily.

- Take 2-3 drops of desired Vitality oil in a spoonful of syrup or small amount of milk, juice, or water.
- Gargle 4-6 times daily or as needed with Thieves Fresh Essence Plus Mouthwash.

Note: All essential oils should be diluted 20:80 before being used orally on small children.

Topical: Refer to Application Guidelines.

- Apply oil neat or diluted 50:50 on affected tooth and gum area as needed.

PAIN

One of the most effective essential oils for blocking pain is Helichrysum. A study in 1994 showed that Peppermint is extremely effective in blocking calcium channels and substance P, important factors in the transmission of pain signals.46 Other essential oils also have unique pain-relieving and anti-inflammatory properties, including Sacred Frankincense, Frankincense, Eucalyptus Blue, Vetiver, Dorado Azul, Copaiba, Palo Santo, Valerian, and Idaho Grand Fir.

MSM, a source of organic sulfur, has also been proven to be extremely effective for alleviating pain, especially tissue and joint pain. The subject of a best-selling book by Dr. Ronald Lawrence and Dr. Stanley Jacobs, MSM has redefined the treatment of pain, especially associated with arthritis and fibromyalgia. Sulfurzyme is an excellent source of MSM.

Natural pregnenolone can also blunt pain.

Smart Spectrum CBD products interact with your body's endocannabinoid system receptors, which are found in places such as your brain, connective tissues, immune cells, organs, and glands. They help regulate critical processes throughout your body, including pain, memory, appetite, mood, and peripheral nervous system. CBD is especially effective when combined with essential oils, including Copaiba, Lavender, Frankincense, Lemon, Peppermint, Spearmint, Grapefruit, Orange, and Cinnamon Bark

Bone-related Pain

Bone pain emanates from the bone tissue and occurs as a result of disease and/or physical conditions. Each type of bone pain has many potential sources or causes.

Recommendations

Singles: Helichrysum, Wintergreen, Idaho Grand Fir, Copaiba, Copaiba Vitality, Peppermint, Peppermint Vitality, Vetiver, Dorado Azul, Palo Santo, Idaho Blue Spruce, Pine, Cypress

Blends: PanAway, Relieve It, Deep Relief Roll-On, Cool Azul, CBD

Nutritionals: Sulfurzyme, Mega Vitamin Cal, BLM, AgilEase, Mineral Essence, Master Formula, MultiGreens, Super Vitamin B, Super Vitamin C, Super Vitamin C Chewable

Personal Care: Cool Azul Pain Relief, Cool Azul Sports Gel, CBD Muscle Rub, Ortho Ease Massage Oil, Ortho Sport Massage Oil, Regenolone Moisturizing Cream

Application and Usage

Dietary and Oral: Refer to Application Guidelines.

- Take 1 capsule of desired Vitality oil 2 times daily.

- Take 2-3 drops of desired Vitality oil in a spoonful of syrup or small amount of milk, juice, or water.

Topical: Refer to Application Guidelines.

- Apply 2-4 drops diluted 50:50 on location, as needed.

- Massage several drops onto the Vita Flex points of the feet and repeat as needed.

Chronic Pain

To pinpoint the most effective essential oil single, blend, or product for quenching pain, it may be necessary to try each of the products in these categories to find those that are most effective for your particular pain situation.

Recommendations

Singles: Helichrysum, Wintergreen, Clove, Clove Vitality, Peppermint, Peppermint Vitality, Dorado Azul, Palo Santo, Idaho Blue Spruce, Elemi, Oregano, Oregano Vitality, Ecuadorian Oregano, Idaho Grand Fir, Copaiba, Copaiba Vitality, Sacred Frankincense, Frankincense, Frankincense Vitality, Northern Lights Black Spruce

Blends: PanAway, Deep Relief Roll-On, Cool Azul, Relieve It, CBD, Aroma Siez, Release, Sacred Mountain

Nutritionals: PowerGize, Sulfurzyme, Super Vitamin Cal Plus, Mega Vitamin Cal, BLM, AgilEase

Personal Care: Cool Azul Pain Relief Cream, Cool Azul Sports Gel, CBD Muscle Rub, Ortho Sport Massage Oil, Ortho Ease Massage Oil, Regenolone Moisturizing Cream

Application and Usage

Dietary and Oral: Refer to Application Guidelines.

- Take 1 capsule of desired Vitality oil 2 times daily.

- Take 2-3 drops of desired Vitality oil in a spoonful of syrup or small amount of milk, juice, or water.

Pain Blend
- 18 drops Copaiba Vitality
- 3 drops Lavender Vitality

Take up to 4 times a day in a capsule.

Note: All Vitality essential oils should be diluted 20:80 before being used orally in small children.

Topical: Refer to Application Guidelines.

- Apply 2-4 drops diluted 50:50 on location, as needed.

- Place 1-2 drops oil with a warm compress on location, as needed.

Essential Oils for Pain Control

PanAway, Cool Azul, and Relieve It blends are powerful for pain reduction. When applied on location or to the Vita Flex points on the feet, they can act within seconds. Alternate them. These blends are powerful for deep-tissue pain as well as for bone-related pain. Deep Relief Roll-On is extremely helpful and handy to use at home, at work, or when traveling.

PANCREATITIS

Pancreatitis is an inflammation of the pancreas that can be either acute or chronic.

Acute pancreatitis can be brought on by a sudden blockage in the main pancreatic duct caused by enzymes unable to function properly with the pancreas. They literally begin digesting the pancreas unless remedied. If there is not good flow of the enzymatic process whereby nutrients are able to be absorbed and waste eliminated, the enzymes begin to fight against that blockage.

Chronic pancreatitis occurs more gradually, with attacks recurring over weeks or months.

Symptoms
- Abdominal pain
- Abdominal swelling
- Sudden hypertension
- Rapid weight loss
- Fever
- Muscle aches
- Vomiting
- Jaundice

In the case of acute pancreatitis, a total fast for at least 4-5 days is one of the safest and most effective methods of alleviating the problem. In the case of infection, fasting should be combined with immune stimulation by using Thieves combined with vitamin C and Super Vitamin B vitamin complex.

Recommendations
Singles: Geranium, Peppermint, Peppermint Vitality, Oregano, Oregano Vitality, Ecuadorian Oregano, Vetiver, Mountain Savory, Mountain Savory Vitality, Frankincense, Frankincense Vitality, Sacred Frankincense, Orange, Orange Vitality

Blends: DiGize, DiGize Vitality, Exodus II, Thieves, Thieves Roll-On, Thieves Vitality, ImmuPower

How MSM Works to Control Pain

When fluid pressure inside cells is higher than outside, pain is experienced. MSM, found in Sulfurzyme, equalizes fluid pressure inside cells and helps balance the protein envelope of the cell so that water transfers freely in and out.

Nutritionals: MultiGreens, Super Vitamin B, Digest & Cleanse, OmegaGize3, Super Vitamin C, Super Vitamin C Chewable, Essentialzyme, Essentialzymes-4, Detoxzyme, ImmuPro, Inner Defense

Application and Usage
Dietary and Oral: Refer to Application Guidelines.

- Take 1 capsule of desired Vitality oil 3 times weekly.

- Take 2-3 drops of desired Vitality oil in a spoonful of syrup or small amount of milk, juice, or water.

Topical: Refer to Application Guidelines.
- Receive a Raindrop Technique 2 times a week.
- Retention: Use an enema with the recommended oils 3 times per week.

PARASITES, INTESTINAL (WORMS)

Many types of parasites use up nutrients while giving off toxins; this can leave the body depleted, nutritionally deficient, and susceptible to infectious disease.

Occasionally, parasites can lie dormant in the body and then become active due to ingestion of a particular food or drink. This can result in the appearance and disappearance of symptoms, even though parasites are always present.

The parasite Cryptosporidium parvum may be present in many municipal or tap waters. To remove this parasite, the water must be distilled or filtered using a 0.3-micron filter.

Symptoms
- Fatigue
- Weakness
- Diarrhea
- Blood in stools
- Chronic pain
- Weight loss
- Gas and bloating

- Cramping
- Nausea
- Irregular bowel movements

The first step to controlling parasites is beginning a fasting and cleansing program. A colon cleanse is particularly important.

Recommendations

Singles: Tarragon, Tarragon Vitality, Cassia, Davana, Fennel, Fennel Vitality, Basil, Basil Vitality, Peppermint, Peppermint Vitality, Ginger, Ginger Vitality, Nutmeg, Nutmeg Vitality, Tea Tree, Rosemary, Rosemary Vitality

Blends: Thieves, Thieves Roll-On, Thieves Vitality, DiGize, DiGize Vitality, JuvaFlex, JuvaFlex Vitality, JuvaCleanse, JuvaCleanse Vitality, AromaEase

Nutritionals: ParaFree, Digest & Cleanse, Inner Defense, Life 9, KidScents MightyPro, ICP, ComforTone, Detoxzyme, JuvaPower, Essentialzyme, Essentialzymes-4

Application and Usage

Dietary and Oral: Refer to Application Guidelines.

 • Take 1 capsule of desired Vitality oil 2 times daily.

 • Take 2-3 drops of desired Vitality oil in a spoonful of syrup or small amount of milk, juice, or water.

Topical: Refer to Application Guidelines.

 • Place a warm compress with recommended oils over intestinal area 2 times weekly.

 • Massage up to 6 drops on the small intestine and colon Vita Flex points of the feet daily (instep area on both feet).

Retention Blend for Parasite Killing

- 4 drops Ginger
- 4 drops DiGize
- 16 drops V-6 Vegetable Oil Complex

Retention: Add the blend for parasite killing to an enema and insert nightly for 7 nights, then rest for 7 nights. Repeat this cycle 3 times to eliminate all stages of parasite development.

Polio (poliomyelitis) is an acute, infectious disease, usually manifested in epidemics and caused by a virus. It creates an inflammation of the gray matter of the spinal cord and is characterized by fever, sore throat, headache, vomiting, and sometimes stiffness of the neck and back. If it develops into the major illness, it can involve paralysis and atrophy of groups of muscles, ending in contraction and permanent deformity.

If polio is suspected, seek medical attention.

Recommendations

Singles: Sacred Frankincense, Frankincense, Frankincense Vitality, Ravintsara, Blue Cypress, Wintergreen, Tea Tree, Melissa, Northern Lights Black Spruce, Peppermint, Peppermint Vitality, Royal Hawaiian Sandalwood, Sacred Sandalwood, Palo Santo, Oregano, Oregano Vitality, Ecuadorian Oregano, Thyme, Thyme Vitality, Cassia, Myrrh, Lemon, Lemon Vitality, Mountain Savory, Mountain Savory Vitality

Blends: The Gift, Aroma Siez, ImmuPower, Valor, Valor Roll-On

Nutritionals: ImmuPro, PowerGize, Inner Defense, Super Vitamin D

Oral Care: Thieves Cough Drops, Thieves Hard Lozenges, Thieves Spray, Thieves Mints

Personal Care: Thieves Chest Rub

Application and Usage

Aromatic: Refer to Application Guidelines.

Dietary and Oral: Refer to Application Guidelines.

 • Take 1 capsule of desired Vitality oil 2 times daily.

 • Take 2-3 drops of desired Vitality oil in a spoonful of syrup or small amount of milk, juice, or water.

Topical: Refer to Application Guidelines.

 • Apply 1-2 drops neat or undiluted as desired.

 • Applying a single drop under the nose is helpful and refreshing.

- Receive a Raindrop Technique 3 times a week.

Polio Topical Blend

- 15 drops Myrrh
- 10 drops Ravintsara
- 10 drops Wintergreen
- 7 drops Sacred Frankincense or Frankincense
- 8 drops Blue Cypress
- 6 drops Lemon

DiGize and ParaFree for Parasite Control

The essential oil blend DiGize and ParaFree softgel capsules are excellent for parasite removal.

DiGize: Add 6 drops to 1 teaspoon V-6 Vegetable Oil Complex or to 4 ounces of rice, almond, or goat milk and take as a dietary supplement 2 times a day for 14 days or take 15 drops in a capsule 3 times a day for 7 days. DiGize can also be diluted in massage oil and applied on abdomen.

ParaFree: Take 5 softgels, 2-3 times daily for 21 days, then rest for 7 days. Repeat up to 3 times to achieve desired results

PREGNANCY PROBLEMS

Essential oils can be invaluable companions during pregnancy. Oils like Lavender and Myrrh may help reduce stretch marks and improve the elasticity of the skin. Geranium and Gentle Baby have similar effects and can be massaged on the perineum (tissue between the vagina and rectum) to lower the risk of tearing or the need for an episiotomy (an incision in the perineum) during birth.

Recommendations
Singles: Lavender, Myrrh, Rose, Geranium, Helichrysum, German Chamomile, Neroli, Royal Hawaiian Sandalwood, Sacred Sandalwood, Frankincense, Sacred Frankincense

Blends: Gentle Baby, Amoressence, Forgiveness, Valor, Valor Roll-On, Grounding, Peace & Calming, Peace & Calming II, Highest Potential, Joy, Calm CBD Roll-On, Seedlings Calm, Sacred Mountain, White Angelica

Personal Care: ClaraDerm, Tender Tush

Application and Usage
Aromatic: Refer to Application Guidelines.

- Diffuse Gentle Baby, Joy, or Valor to reduce stress before and after the birth. Expectant fathers will also find this helps to reduce anxiety during delivery.

Topical: Refer to Application Guidelines.

- Massage 2-4 drops Labor Blend 50:50 on reproductive Vita Flex points on the sides of the ankles. Apply ONLY after labor has started.

- Massage 2-4 drops Labor Blend on lower stomach and lower back.

Labor Blend (Use only after labor has started.)
- 5 drops Ylang Ylang
- 4 drops Helichrysum
- 2 drops Fennel
- 2 drops Peppermint
- 2 drops Clary Sage

PROSTATE PROBLEMS

Natural progesterone is one of the best natural remedies for prostate inflammation (BPH) that can obstruct urinary flow and lead to impotence. Transdermal creams are the most effective means of hormone delivery.

Scientists are tracing the higher incidence of hormone-dependent cancers, including cancer of the breast, prostate, and testes, to exposure to endocrine disrupters in the environment. Contamination from 39 petrochemicals like DDT, PCB, pesticides, the phthalate DBP, recombinant bovine growth hormone (rBGH) in milk and synthetic steroids in meat, are all implicated in interfering with hormone receptors, rendering them unable to function properly, eventually leading to cancer.

For prostate problems, Peppermint acts as an anti-inflammatory to the prostate. Saw palmetto, Pygeum africanum, and pumpkin seed oil also help reduce prostate swelling.

Recommendations
Singles: Peppermint, Peppermint Vitality, Myrrh, Idaho Grand Fir, Oregano, Oregano Vitality, Ecuadorian Oregano, Sage, Sage Vitality, Thyme, Thyme Vitality, Wintergreen

Blends: Mister, EndoFlex, EndoFlex Vitality, Australian Blue, Chivalry

Nutritionals: Prostate Health, Master Formula, Longevity Softgels, PD 80/20

Personal Care: Prenolone Plus Body Cream

Application and Usage
Aromatic: Refer to Application Guidelines

Topical: Refer to Application Guidelines.

- Apply 2-4 drops diluted 20:80 between the rectum and scrotum 2 times daily. Mister works especially well applied there.

- Massage 4-6 drops on the Vita Flex reproductive points on the feet 2 times daily.

- Retention: Rectal, nightly for 7 days, rest 7 days, then repeat.

Benign Prostate Hyperplasia (BPH)

Almost all males over age 50 have some degree of benign prostate hyperplasia, a condition that worsens with age. BPH (prostate enlargement) can severely restrict urine flow and result in frequent, small urinations.

Two herbs that are extremely effective for treating this condition are saw palmetto and pumpkin seed oil. The hormone-like activity of some essential oils can support a nutritional regimen to reduce BPH swelling.

Recommendations

Singles: Sacred Frankincense, Frankincense, Frankincense Vitality, Myrrh, Idaho Grand Fir, Blue Cypress

Blends: Mister, EndoFlex, EndoFlex Vitality, Australian Blue

Nutritionals: Prostate Health, Master Formula, Longevity Softgels, Mineral Essence

Personal Care: Prenolone Plus Body

Essential Oils and Pregnancy

As always, when using essential oils, common sense is most important when deciding how to use them. During pregnancy, most oils are safe and bring peace and contentment. When rubbing them over the stomach, many women have said that they have felt a positive response from the unborn infant. Energy sensitivity is very high during this time and is something to be aware of and enjoyed. Gentle Baby, Valor, White Angelica, RutaVaLa, Magnify Your Purpose, Joy, Harmony, Highest Potential, Gathering, DiGize, and Dream Catcher are just a few that are enjoyable for both mother and baby throughout the pregnancy.

During pregnancy, some essential oils are contra-indicated. Be sure you read all cautions and only use oils that are safe for your unborn child.

Some essential oils, such as Fennel and Clary Sage, may help to accelerate labor once it has begun. Take 1-2 capsules 2 times daily when labor is imminent. Always consult a health professional before using essential oils during pregnancy, other than the ones recommended in this book.

A few drops of Vetiver and Valerian mixed together with 1 tablespoon of V-6 Vegetable Oil Complex may help reduce the pain of contractions when applied on the lower back.

Application and Usage

Aromatic: Refer to Application Guidelines.

Topical: Refer to Application Guidelines.

- PSA counts typically rise when BPH occurs. The following regimen reduced PSA (prostate specific antigen) counts 70 percent in 2 months. Use the following applications simultaneously:
- Mix the BPH Retention Blend with 1 tablespoon olive oil and use 3 times weekly as an overnight rectal retention enema.
- Apply 2-4 drops of the BPH Retention Blend diluted 50:50 between the rectum and scrotum 1-3 times daily.
- Massage 1-3 drops of the BPH Retention Blend on the reproductive Vita Flex points on the feet 2 times daily

BPH Retention Blend

- 10 drops Frankincense or Sacred Frankincense
- 5 drops Myrrh
- 3 drops Sage

Prostatitis

Prostatitis is an inflammation of the prostate that can present symptoms similar to benign prostate hyperplasia: frequent urinations, restricted flow, etc.

Recommendations

Singles: Peppermint, Peppermint Vitality, Clary Sage, Palo Santo, German Chamomile, German Chamomile Vitality, Wintergreen, Rosemary, Rosemary Vitality, Myrtle, Thyme, Thyme Vitality, Tsuga, Blue Cypress

Blends: Australian Blue, Mister, Aroma Siez, DiGize, DiGize Vitality

Nutritionals: Prostate Health, PowerGize, Longevity Softgels, ImmuPro, Mineral Essence, JuvaPower, ICP

Personal Care: Prenolone Plus Body Cream

Application and Usage

Topical: Refer to Application Guidelines.

- Apply 1-3 drops diluted 20:80 to the area between the rectum and the scrotum daily.

- Massage 4-6 drops on the reproductive Vita Flex points on the feet daily.

- Retention: Rectal 3 times per week at night.

RADIATION EXPOSURE DAMAGE

Many cancer treatments use radiation therapy that can severely damage both the skin and vital organs. Using gentle, antioxidant essential oils topically, as well as proper nutrients internally, is helpful in minimizing radiation damage.

Daily radiation from cell phones, computers, air travel, televisions, all types of electronic equipment, and kitchen appliances bombards us constantly. The more we can do to protect ourselves as well as cleanse on a regular basis, the better health we can maintain.

Recommendations

Singles: Sacred Frankincense, Frankincense, Frankincense Vitality, Idaho Grand Fir, Blue Cypress, Royal Hawaiian Sandalwood, Sacred Sandalwood, Hyssop, Oregano, Oregano Vitality, Ecuadorian Oregano, Tea Tree, Melaleuca Quinquenervia

Blends: Melrose (also in QuadShield and EndoShield Environmental Protection Kits), Longevity (also in QuadShield and EndoShield Environmental Protection Kits), Longevity Vitality, Valor, Valor Roll-On, Stress Away, Stress Away Roll-On

Nutritionals: QuadShield or EndoShield Environmental Protection Kits, Super Vitamin C, Super Vitamin C Chewable, Slique Shake, Slique Bars, Slique CitraSlim, ImmuPro, NingXia Red, Mineral Essence, Essentialzyme, Longevity Softgels, Pure Protein Complete, Protein Power Bites, OmegaGize3, Ningxia Wolfberries (Organic, Dried)

Application and Usage

Aromatic: Refer to Application Guidelines.

Dietary and Oral: Refer to Application Guidelines.

- Take 1 capsule of desired Vitality oil 2 times daily.

- Take 2-3 drops of desired Vitality oil in a spoonful of syrup or small amount of milk, juice, or water.

Topical: Refer to Application Guidelines.

- Apply 1-2 drops diluted 50:50 on affected area 1-2 times daily.

- Massage 2-4 drops of oil neat on the bottoms of the feet just before bedtime.

Environmental Protection Kits
(See Chapters 17 and 19, QuadShield and EndoShield)

RHEUMATIC FEVER

Rheumatic fever results from a streptococcus infection that primarily strikes children (usually before age 12). It can lead to inflammation that damages the heart muscle and valve.

Rheumatic fever is caused by the same genus of bacteria that causes strep throat and scarlet fever. Diffusing essential oils can help reduce the likelihood of contracting the disease. Essential oils such as Mountain Savory, Rosemary, Tea Tree, Thyme, Palo Santo, Sacred Frankincense, Frankincense, Eucalyptus Blue, and Oregano have powerful antimicrobial effects.

In cases where a person is already infected, the use of essential oils in the Raindrop Technique may be appropriate.

Recommendations

Singles: Oregano, Oregano Vitality, Ecuadorian Oregano, Clove, Clove Vitality, Tea Tree, Mountain Savory, Mountain Savory Vitality, Peppermint, Peppermint Vitality, Thyme, Thyme Vitality, Rosemary, Rosemary Vitality, Black Pepper, Black Pepper Vitality, Eucalyptus Blue, Sacred Frankincense, Frankincense, Frankincense Vitality, Palo Santo, Cistus

Blends: Thieves, Thieves Roll-On, Thieves Vitality, Melrose, Exodus II, ImmuPower

Nutritionals: Inner Defense, ImmuPro, Super Vitamin C, Super Vitamin C Chewable, SulFurzyme, Longevity Softgels, Master Formula, NingXia Red, Essentialzyme, Essentialzymes-4, Life 9, KidScents MightyPro, Mineral Essence

Application and Usage

Aromatic: Refer to Application Guidelines.

Topical: Refer to Application Guidelines.

- Apply 3-5 drops diluted 50:50 on the bottoms of the feet and on carotid artery spots under the earlobes.

- Receive a Raindrop Technique 1 time weekly.

ROCKY MOUNTAIN SPOTTED FEVER
(See LYME DISEASE/ROCKY MOUNTAIN SPOTTED FEVER)

SCAR TISSUE

Scar tissue is the fibrous connective tissue that forms a scar and can be found on any tissue on the body where an injury, surgery, cut, or disease has taken place and then has healed. It is thicker, paler, and denser than the surrounding tissue because it has a limited blood supply.

Recommendations
Singles: Sacred Frankincense, Frankincense, Frankincense Vitality, Sacred Sandalwood, Helichrysum, Royal Hawaiian Sandalwood, Cypress, Elemi, Rose, Cistus, Myrrh, Geranium, Lavender, Lavender Vitality

Blends: Gentle Baby, Australian Blue, 3 Wise Men

Nutritionals: Super Vitamin C, Super Vitamin C Chewable, Sulfurzyme, Slique Shake, Mega Vitamin Cal, Mineral Essence, Essentialzyme, Essentialzymes-4, Life 9, KidScents MightyPro

Personal Care: Sacred Sandalwood Moisturizing Cream, Boswellia Wrinkle Cream, KidScents Tender Tush, Regenolone Body Cream, Rose Ointment

Application and Usage
Topical: Refer to Application Guidelines.

- Apply 2-6 drops neat of the scar prevention blend around and over the wound daily until healed.

Scar Prevention Blend
- 4 drops Myrrh
- 3 drops Lavender
- 2 drops Helichrysum
- 1 drop Sacred Sandalwood or Royal Hawaiian Sandalwood

This condition is due to a deficiency of vitamin C in the diet and marked by weakness, anemia, spongy gums, bleeding of the gums and nose, tooth loss, and pain in the limbs and joints.

Note: Vitamin C is water soluble and destroyed at temperatures above 70°F. Thus, it is not found in citrus essential oils.

Recommendations
Singles: Wintergreen, Helichrysum, Dorado Azul, Idaho Blue Spruce

Blends: Cool Azul, Deep Relief Roll-On, PanAway, Relieve It, Aroma Siez

Nutritionals: Super Vitamin C Chewable, Super Vitamin C, Sulfurzyme, Super Vitamin Cal Plus, Mega Vitamin Cal, BLM, AgilEase

Personal Care: Thieves Fresh Essence Plus Mouthwash, Thieves Spray, Thieves AromaBright Toothpaste, KidScents Tooth-paste, Thieves Whitening Toothpaste, Thieves Hard Lozenges, Thieves Cough Drops, Thieves Mints, Thieves Dental Floss, Cool Azul Pain Relief Cream, Cool Azul Sports Gel, Ortho Sport Massage Oil, Ortho Ease Massage Oil

SEIZURES

Many seizures can be reduced or alleviated by removing all forms of sugar, artificial colors and flavors, processed foods from the diet, and chemicals of all types. Avoid using personal care products with ammonia-based compounds such as quaterniums and polyquaterniums.

Recommendations
Singles: Peppermint, Peppermint Vitality, Sacred Frankincense, Frankincense, Frankincense Vitality, Sacred Sandalwood, Royal Hawaiian Sandalwood, Melissa, Jasmine, Basil, Basil Vitality

Blends: RutaVaLa, RutaVaLa Roll-On, R.C., Valor, Valor Roll-On, Breathe Again, Breathe Again Roll-On, Aroma Siez, Exodus II, Peace & Calming, Peace & Calming II, Calm CBD Roll-On, Seedlings Calm, CBD, Trauma Life, Stress Away, Stress Away Roll-On

Nutritionals: Mineral Essence, MultiGreens, Essentialzyme, Essentialzymes-4, Life 9, KidScents MightyPro, BLM, AgilEase, PowerGize, Super Vitamin B, Longevity Softgels, Slique Shake, Sulfurzyme, OmegaGize3, Balance Complete, MindWise, KidScents Unwind, Master Formula, Yacon Syrup in place of sugars

Application and Usage
Aromatic: Refer to Application Guidelines.

Topical: Refer to Application Guidelines.

- Massage 10 drops of chosen oils into scalp diluted 50:50 up to 3 times daily to help reduce risk of seizure.
- Supplement with Seizure Regimen below:

Seizure Regimen (do all the following)

- Diffuse Peace & Calming or Peace & Calming II for 30 minutes 3-4 times daily.

- Massage 4-6 drops Valor on bottoms of feet daily.

- Massage 4-6 drops Joy over heart daily.

- Receive a Raindrop Technique 2 times monthly.

SEXUAL DYSFUNCTION

There is an extensive, historical basis that fragrance may amplify desire and create a mood that can overcome frigidity or impotence. In fact, aromas such as rose and jasmine have been used since antiquity to attract the opposite sex and create a romantic atmosphere.

Modern research has shown that the aroma of some essential oils can stimulate the emotional center of the brain. This may explain why essential oils have the potential to help people overcome impotence or frigidity based on emotional factors or inhibitions.

Dysfunction (Men)
Sexual dysfunction can be a result of physical or psychological problems.

Impotence (Men)
Impotence, the inability to perform sexually, may be caused by physical limitations due to an accident or injury or by psychological factors such as inhibitions, trauma, stress, etc.

Male impotence is often linked to problems with the prostate or prostate surgery.

If impotence is related to psychological trauma or unresolved emotional issues, it may be necessary to deal with these issues before any meaningful progress can be made.

Recommendations
Singles: Idaho Blue Spruce, Goldenrod, Sacred Frankincense, Frankincense, Frankincense Vitality, Myrrh, Ginger, Ginger Vitality, Nutmeg, Nutmeg Vitality, Jasmine, Ylang Ylang

Blends: Shutran, Build Your Dream, Freedom, Reconnect, Valor, Valor Roll-On, Mister, SclarEssence, SclarEssence Vitality, One Heart

Nutritionals: EndoGize, Prostate Health, PowerGize

Application and Usage
Aromatic: Refer to Application Guidelines.

Topical: Refer to Application Guidelines.

- Apply 2-3 drops neat to Vita Flex points on feet or lower abdomen. Do not apply on sensitive skin in crotch area.

Infertility (Men)
Male infertility is the inability of a male to achieve pregnancy in a fertile female. It is commonly due to deficiencies in the semen.

Recommendations
Singles: Idaho Blue Spruce, Sage, Sage Vitality, Sacred Frankincense, Frankincense, Frankincense Vitality, Clary Sage, Goldenrod

Blends: Mister, SclarEssence, SclarEssence Vitality, One Heart, Shutran, Valor, Valor Roll-On

Nutritionals: Prostate Health, EndoGize, MultiGreens, Prostate Health, Sulfurzyme, Essentialzyme, Essentialzymes-4, Life 9, KidScents MightyPro, Super Vitamin B, Mineral Essence, Thyromin

Personal Care: Prenolone Plus Body Cream

Application and Usage
Topical: Refer to Application Guidelines.

- Apply 2-4 drops neat or diluted on the reproductive Vita Flex points of hands and feet inside of wrists, around the front of the ankles in line with the anklebone, on the lower sides of the anklebone, and along the Achilles tendon 1-3 times daily.

Lack of Libido (Men)
Lack of libido in men is a much more common complaint than our culture would seem to indicate. The leading reasons men don't want to have sex are medications, usually antidepressants and antihypertensive drugs, drug or alcohol abuse, or low testosterone.

Recommendations
Singles: Idaho Blue Spruce, Pine, Myrrh, Black Pepper, Black Pepper Vitality, Ylang Ylang, Ginger, Ginger Vitality, Nutmeg, Nutmeg Vitality

Blends: Light the Fire, SclarEssence, SclarEssence Vitality, Valor, Valor Roll-On, Mister, Live with Passion, Live Your Passion, Transformation, The Gift, En-R-Gee, Shutran, Fulfill Your Destiny, Joy, One Heart, 25 Years Young

Nutritionals: EndoGize, MultiGreens, Prostate Health, Sulfurzyme, Essentialzyme, Essentialzymes-4, Life 9, KidScents MightyPro, Super Vitamin B, Mineral Essence, Thyromin

Personal Care: Prenolone Plus Body Cream

Application and Usage
Aromatic: Refer to Application Guidelines.

Topical: Refer to Application Guidelines.

- Massage 4-6 drops diluted 50:50 on neck, shoulders, and lower abdomen 1-3 times daily.

Dysfunction (Women)
Sexual dysfunction can be a result of physical or psychological problems.

Frigidity (Women)
Frigidity is a condition in which women have a lack of libido and tend to become unresponsive to sexual intercourse or are unable to achieve an orgasm. It may leave a woman unhappy, unsatisfied, and depressed.

Recommendations
Singles: Jasmine, Rose, Ylang Ylang, Clary Sage, Nutmeg, Nutmeg Vitality

Blends: En-R-Gee, The Gift, Joy, One Heart, Fulfill Your Destiny, Valor, Valor Roll-On, Joy, 25 Years Young

Nutritionals: EndoGize, Thyromin, Mineral Essence, Super Vitamin B, PD 80/20, Mega Vitamin Cal, ImmuPro

Personal Care: Progessence Plus, Prenolone Plus Body Cream

- Ylang Ylang helps balance sexual emotion and sex drive problems. Its aromatic influence elevates sexual energy and enhances relationships.
- Clary Sage can help with lack of sexual desire, particularly in women, by regulating and balancing hormones.
- Nutmeg supports the nervous system to help overcome frigidity.

Application and Usage
Aromatic: Refer to Application Guidelines.

Topical: Refer to Application Guidelines.

- Massage 4-6 drops diluted 50:50 on neck, shoulders, and lower abdomen up to 1-3 times daily.

Infertility (Women)
Natural progesterone creams, when used from the middle to the end of the cycle starting on the day after ovulation (usually day 15 or later), may improve fertility. Some essential oils have hormone-like qualities that can support or improve fertility processes.

Recommendations
Singles: Clary Sage, Ylang Ylang, Sage, Sage Vitality, Fennel, Fennel Vitality, Geranium

Blends: Dragon Time, Acceptance, Mister, SclarEssence, SclarEssence Vitality, One Heart, Lady Sclareol, EndoFlex, EndoFlex Vitality

Nutritionals: PD 80/20, MultiGreens (take 3-8 capsules 2-3 times daily), Mineral Essence, Super Vitamin Cal Plus, Thyromin, EndoGize, FemiGen

Personal Care: Progessence Plus, Prenolone Plus Body Cream

Application and Usage
Dietary and Oral: Refer to Application Guidelines.

- Take 1 capsule of desired Vitality oil 2 times daily.
- Take 2-3 drops of desired Vitality oil in a spoonful of syrup or small amount of milk, juice, or water.

Topical: Refer to Application Guidelines.

- Apply 2-4 drops neat or diluted 50:50 on the lower back and lower abdomen areas 2-3 times daily.

- Apply 2-4 drops on the reproductive Vita Flex points of hands and feet, inside of wrists, around the front of the ankles in line with the anklebones, on the lower sides of the anklebones, and along the Achilles tendons 1-3 times daily.

- Rub daily 10 drops Progessence Plus or ½ teaspoon Prenolone Plus Body Cream on lower back area and the lower bowel area near the pubic bone.

Lack of Libido/Desire (Women)
A woman's sexual desires naturally fluctuate over the years and are affected by a range of physical and emotional factors. Most physical causes of low libido are a result of hormonal imbalance.

Recommendations

Singles: Clary Sage, Nutmeg, Nutmeg Vitality, Geranium, Ylang Ylang, Rose, Idaho Grand Fir, Lemongrass, Lemongrass Vitality, Jasmine, Sacred Frankincense, Frankincense, Frankincense Vitality, Sage, Sage Vitality

Blends: Light the Fire, SclarEssence, SclarEssence Vitality, Sensation, Lady Sclareol, Joy, Build Your Dream, Fulfill Your Destiny, Valor, Valor Roll-On, Live with Passion, Live Your Passion, One Heart, 25 Years Young

Nutritionals: EndoGize, MultiGreens, Sulfurzyme, PD 80/20, Thyromin, FemiGen

Personal Care: Progessence Plus, Prenolone Plus Body Cream

- Ylang Ylang helps balance sexual emotions and sex-drive problems. Its aromatic influence elevates sexual energy and enhances relationships.
- Clary Sage can help with lack of sexual desire, particularly with women, by regulating and balancing hormones.
- Nutmeg supports the nervous system to help overcome frigidity.

Application and Usage

Aromatic: Refer to Application Guidelines

Dietary and Oral: Refer to Application Guidelines.

- Take 1 capsule of desired Vitality oil diluted 50:50 2 times daily.

- Take 2-3 drops of desired Vitality oil in a spoonful of syrup or small amount of milk, juice, or water.

Topical: Refer to Application Guidelines.

- Massage 4-6 drops diluted 50:50 on neck, shoulders, and lower abdomen up to 1-3 times daily or apply 2-3 drops neat to Vita Flex points on the bottoms of the feet.

Excessive Sexual Desire (Both Sexes)

Excessive sexual desire is a psychological disorder in which the person is unable to manage his or her sex life and may feel compelled to continually seek sexual activity. Some professionals speculate that it is a form of obsessive-compulsive disorder or a manifestation of the manic phase of bipolar disorder. Excessive sexual desire is best diagnosed and treated by a health care professional.

Recommendations

Singles: Rose, Myrrh, Marjoram, Marjoram Vitality, Valerian, Lavender, Lavender Vitality

Blends: Peace & Calming, Peace & Calming II, Acceptance, Surrender, Joy, Calm CBD Roll-On, Seedlings Calm, Harmony, Gathering, One Heart, Loyalty

Application and Usage

Aromatic: Refer to Application Guidelines.

Topical: Refer to Application Guidelines.

- Massage 4-6 drops diluted 50:50 on neck, shoulders, and lower abdomen up to 1-3 times daily.

SEXUALLY TRANSMITTED DISEASES (See also INFECTIONS . . .)

Sexually transmitted diseases are infections that you can get from having sex with someone who has an infection, which can be caused by bacteria or viruses.

Genital Human Papillomavirus (HPV)

Infection by genital HPV is very common. At least half of the people who are sexually active will contract the virus, yet many will not know it because they will not have any symptoms. There are more than 100 types of HPV, and some types are associated with genital warts, although the warts are not always visible. The longer the virus is in the body, the higher the risk of developing health problems such as cervical cancer or oral cancer.

Recommendations

Singles: Melissa, Dorado Azul, Ravintsara, Palo Santo, Tea Tree, Davana, Lavender, Lavender Vitality, Royal Hawaiian Sandalwood, Sacred Sandalwood

Blends: Melrose, Thieves, Thieves Roll-On, Thieves Vitality, ImmuPower, Hope

Nutritionals: ImmuPro, Inner Defense, Life 9, KidScents MightyPro

Personal Care: Thieves Spray

Application and Usage

Aromatic: Refer to Application Guidelines.

Dietary and Oral: Refer to Application Guidelines.

- Take 1 capsule of desired Vitality oil diluted 50:50 2 times daily.

- Take 2-3 drops of desired Vitality oil in a spoonful of syrup or small amount of milk, juice, or water.

Topical: Refer to Application Guidelines.

- Apply 1-3 drops neat or dilute 50:50 and apply on location 3-6 times daily.

- Massage 2-4 drops of oil neat on the bottoms of the feet or on the Vita Flex points of the feet just before bedtime.

- Use Thieves Spray on location.

Retention: Put 2-3 drops of oil of your choice on a tampon and insert nightly.

Genital Warts/Blisters (Herpes Simplex Type 2)

Genital warts are a form of viral infection caused by the human papillomavirus (HPV), of which there are more than 100 different types.

One type of HPV is among the most common sexually transmitted diseases. Up to 24 million Americans may currently be infected with HPV, which is usually spread through sexual contact. HPV lives only in genital tissue and can later lead to cervical cancer in women.

Recommendations

Singles: Melissa, Dorado Azul, Ravintsara, Palo Santo, Tea Tree, Lavender, Lavender Vitality, Sacred Sandalwood, Royal Hawaiian Sandalwood

Blends: Melrose, Thieves, Thieves Roll-On, Thieves Vitality, ImmuPower, Hope

Nutritionals: ImmuPro, Inner Defense, Life 9, KidScents MightyPro

Personal Care: Thieves Spray

Application and Usage

Aromatic: Refer to Application Guidelines.

Dietary and Oral: Refer to Application Guidelines.

- Take 1 capsule of desired Vitality oil diluted 50:50 2 times daily.

- Put 2-3 drops of desired Vitality oil in a spoonful of Yacon Syrup, maple syrup, coconut oil, milk, etc.

- Put the desired amount of desired Vitality oil in a glass of rice milk, almond milk, goat milk, carrot juice, NingXia Red, or even water and then drink it.

Topical: Refer to Application Guidelines.

- Apply 1-3 drops neat or dilute 50:50 and apply on location 3-6 times daily.

- Massage 2-4 drops of oil neat on the Vita Flex points on the bottoms of the feet just before bedtime.

- Use Thieves Spray on location.

Retention: Put 2-3 drops of the oil or blend of your choice on a tampon and insert nightly.

Gonorrhea and Syphilis

Gonorrhea is a very common sexually transmitted disease caused by a bacterium (Neisseria gonorrhoeae) that can grow and multiply easily in the warm, moist areas of the reproductive tract. It can also grow in the eyes, mouth, throat, and anus.

Syphilis, also a common sexually transmitted disease, is caused by a bacterium (Treponema pallidum), and has often been called "the great imitator" because so many of the signs and symptoms are the same as those of other diseases. Sores occur mainly on the external genitals, vagina, anus, or in the rectum. Sores can also occur on the lips and in the mouth.

Note: Seek immediate professional medical attention if you suspect you may have either of these diseases.

Recommendations

Singles: Thyme, Thyme Vitality, Mountain Savory, Mountain Savory Vitality, Cinnamon Bark, Cinnamon Bark Vitality, Oregano, Oregano Vitality, Ecuadorian Oregano, Tea Tree

Blends: Melrose, Exodus II, Thieves, Thieves Roll-On, Thieves Vitality, ImmuPower

Nutritionals: Inner Defense, ImmuPro, Life 9, KidScents MightyPro

Personal Care: Thieves Spray

Application and Usage

Dietary and Oral: Refer to Application Guidelines.

- Take 1 capsule of desired Vitality oil 2 times daily for 15 days.

- Take 2-3 drops of desired Vitality oil in a spoonful of syrup or small amount of milk, juice, or water.

Topical: Refer to Application Guidelines.

Herpes Simplex Type 2

Herpes genitalis is transmitted by sexual contact and results in sores or lesions. Four to seven days after contact with an infected partner, tingling, burning, or persistent itching usually heralds an outbreak. One or two days later, small pimple-like bumps appear over reddened skin. The itching and tingling continue, and the pimples turn into painful blisters, which burst, bleeding with yellowish pus. Five to seven days after the first tingling, scabs form, and healing begins.

Antiviral essential oils have generally been very effective in treating herpes lesions and reducing their onset. Oils such as Melissa, Tea Tree, and Rosemary have been successfully used for this purpose by Daniel Pénoël, MD, in his clinical practice. A study at the University of Buenos Aires found that sandalwood essential oil inhibited the replication of herpes simplex vi-ruses 1 and 2.47

Those with herpes should avoid diets high in the amino acid l-arginine, substituting with l-lysine. Lysine retards the growth of the virus. Foods such as amaranth and plain yogurt are good sources of lysine.

Recommendations

Singles: Melissa, Royal Hawaiian Sandalwood, Sacred Sandalwood, Ravintsara, Dorado Azul, Tea Tree, Blue Cypress, Rosemary, Rosemary Vitality, Northern Lights Black Spruce, Sage, Sage Vitality, Lavender, Lavender Vitality

Blends: Melrose, Thieves, Thieves Roll-On, Thieves Vitality, Exodus II, Purification

Nutritionals: ImmuPro, Sulfurzyme, Super Vitamin C, Super Vitamin C Chewable, ICP, Essentialzyme, Essentialzymes-4, Life 9, KidScents MightyPro, Mineral Essence, ComforTone

Personal Care: Thieves Spray, Rose Ointment

Application and Usage

Aromatic: Refer to Application Guidelines.

Topical: Refer to Application Guidelines.

- Apply single oils or Blends neat or diluted, depending on the oils that are used.
- Use Herpes Blend No. 2 diluted 20:80 and put a few drops on a tampon or sanitary pad for nightly applications. If it continues to sting after 5 minutes, remove and change the dilution to 10:90.
- Apply Herpes Blend No. 1 on lesions as soon as they appear. Apply 1-2 drops neat 2-3 times daily, alternating between Herpes Blend No. 1 and Melrose each day.

- Receive a Raindrop Technique 1-2 times monthly, as needed.

Herpes Blend No. 1 (Topical)
- 4 drops Dorado Azul
- 2 drops Tea Tree
- 1 drop Melissa

Herpes Blend No. 2 (Vaginal)
- 4 drops Dorado Azul
- 3 drops Ravintsara
- 2 drops Sage
- 1 drop Lavender

SHINGLES (HERPES ZOSTER)

Caused by the virus Varicella zoster (which causes chicken pox), shingles is a viral infection of the nervous system that can start with fatigue, fever, and headaches. Presenting as a painful skin rash that blisters, most people will have just one occurrence. Shingles results in a wide stripe of red rash around the left or right side of the torso.

Most older people were infected with the chicken pox as children. The virus then goes into hiding in the ganglia alongside the spine where stress may trigger an attack. Approximately half of shingles cases occur in those 50 years of age or older. The pain can be mild or extreme, ranging from tingling or aching up to piercing stabs of pain.

Note: Occurrences of shingles around the eye are called herpes zoster ophthalmicus and can cause blindness. Consult an ophthalmologist (eye doctor) immediately if such outbreaks occur.

Recommendations

Singles: Melissa, Blue Cypress, Elemi, Tea Tree, Oregano, Oregano Vitality, Ecuadorian Oregano, Geranium, German Chamomile, German Chamomile Vitality, Mountain Savory, Mountain Savory Vitality, Sacred Sandalwood, Royal Hawaiian Sandalwood, Thyme, Thyme Vitality, Peppermint, Peppermint Vitality, Ravintsara, Northern Lights Black Spruce, Laurus Nobilis, Sage, Sage Vitality, Vanilla

Blends: Thieves, Thieves Roll-On, Thieves Vitality, Australian Blue, Exodus II

Nutritionals: Super Vitamin Cal Plus, Sulfurzyme, PD 80/20, Mega Vitamin Cal, Mineral Essence, Essentialzyme

Application and Usage

Aromatic: Refer to Application Guidelines.

Topical: Refer to Application Guidelines.

- Apply 6-10 drops neat or diluted 50:50 on affected area, back of the neck, and down the spine 1-3 times daily.

- Apply a compress alternating warm and cold on the spine 1-3 times daily.

- Layering in Raindrop Technique style, apply 3-4 drops each of Oregano, Mountain Savory, and Thyme along the spine.

- Apply 15-20 drops V-6 Vegetable Oil Complex to the spine, massage briefly over the other oils, cover the skin with a dry towel, and apply a warm pack for 15-20 minutes.

Note: Be cautious about warming. If the back becomes too hot, remove the warm pack immediately and add V-6 Vegetable Oil Complex to cool.

- Remove the warm pack and towel, and then layer 4-8 drops each of Tea Tree, Elemi, and Peppermint along the spine.

- Put the dry towel back over the skin and apply an ice pack for 30 minutes.

Shingles Blend No. 1
- 10 drops German Chamomile
- 5 drops Lavender
- 4 drops Sacred Sandalwood or Royal Hawaiian Sandalwood
- 2 drops Geranium

Shingles Blend No. 2
- 10 drops Sacred Sandalwood or Royal Hawaiian Sandalwood
- 5 drops Blue Cypress
- 4 drops Peppermint
- 2 drops Ravintsara

Shingles Blend No. 3
- 5 drops Melissa
- 4 drops Geranium
- 10 drops V-6 Vegetable Oil Complex

SHOCK (See also FAINTING; SKIN DISORDERS AND PROBLEMS, BURNS)

Shock can be described as a state of profound depression of the vital processes associated with reduced blood volume and pressure. The blood rushes to the vital organs after trauma.

It may be caused by the sudden stimulation of the nerves and convulsive contraction of the muscles caused by the discharge of electricity. Other causes include sudden trauma, terror, surprise, horror, or disgust.

Symptoms or signs
- Irregular breathing
- Low blood pressure
- Dilated pupils
- Cold and sweaty skin
- Weak and rapid pulse
- Dry mouth
- Muscle weakness
- Dizziness or fainting

Any injury that results in the sudden loss of substantial amounts of fluids can trigger shock.

Shock can also be caused by allergic reactions (anaphylactic shock), infections in the blood (septic shock), or emotional trauma (neurogenic shock).

To help someone in shock while waiting for first responders, first cover the victim with a blanket and elevate the feet, unless there is a head or upper torso injury. Inhaling any one of many different essential oils can also help—especially in cases of emotional shock.

Recommendations

Singles: Peppermint, Idaho Grand Fir, Basil, Sacred Frankincense, Frankincense, Eucalyptus Blue, Dorado Azul, Cardamom, Rosemary, Melissa

Blends: Trauma Life, Gary's Light, Freedom, Clarity, 3 Wise Men, Build Your Dream, Valor, Valor Roll-On, R.C., Harmony, Reconnect, Present Time

Application and Usage

Aromatic: Refer to Application Guidelines.

Topical: Refer to Application Guidelines.

- When applying essential oil to the temples, be careful to not get the oil too close to the eyes.

- Apply 1-2 drops diluted 50:50 on temples, back of the neck, and under the nose neat as desired.

- You may also apply 2-3 drops on the Vita Flex points of the feet.
- Applying a single drop under the nose is helpful and stimulating.

SINUS INFECTIONS AND PROBLEMS

A sinus infection is an inflammation of the sinuses and nasal passages. Sinus problems are among the most common chronic ailments.

Nasopharyngitis

Nasopharyngitis is an inflammatory condition of the mucus membranes of the back of the nasal cavity where it connects to the throat and the Eustachian tubes.

Recommendations

Singles: Peppermint, Peppermint Vitality, Ravintsara, Eucalyptus Blue, Thyme, Thyme Vitality, Rosemary, Rosemary Vitality, Blue Cypress, Dorado Azul, Eucalyptus Radiata, Tea Tree

Blends: Raven, R.C., Exodus II, Thieves, Thieves Roll-On, Thieves Vitality, Breathe Again, Breathe Again Roll-On

Nutritionals: Super Vitamin C, Super Vitamin C Chewable, ImmuPro, Digest & Cleanse, Inner Defense

Oral Care: Thieves AromaBright Toothpaste, KidScents Toothpaste, Thieves Whitening Toothpaste, Thieves Hard Lozenges, Thieves Cough Drops, Thieves Mints, Thieves Fresh Essence Plus Mouthwash, Thieves Spray

Personal Care: Thieves Chest Rub

Application and Usage

Aromatic: Refer to Application Guidelines.

Dietary and Oral: Refer to Application Guidelines.

- Take 1 capsule of desired Vitality oil 2 times daily.

- Take 2-3 drops of desired Vitality oil in a spoonful of syrup or small amount of milk, juice, or water.

- Gargle 2-5 times daily with Thieves Fresh Essence Plus Mouthwash or with water that contains 1-2 drops of another oil.

- Put 1 drop of Thieves at the very back of the tongue and hold it in the mouth, mixing it with saliva for several minutes, and then swallow. This can be very effective if started at the very first indication of infection and repeated 3-4 times for the first hour, then once an hour until symptoms subside.

- Spray inside mouth with Thieves Spray as often as desired.

- Put 1 drop of Exodus II on tongue and swish it around in your mouth before swallowing.

Special Note: In most sinus infections, including nasopharyngitis, rhinitis, sinus congestion, and sinusitis, the nasal irrigation regimen can be extremely effective.

Topical: Refer to Application Guidelines.

- Apply 1-2 drops diluted 50:50 just under jawbone on right and left sides 4-8 times daily.

- You may also apply 2-3 drops on the Vita Flex points of the feet.

Sinus Congestion

Sinus congestion is extremely annoying, and symptoms can last for several days. The most common symptom is difficulty breathing because of blocked nasal passages due to excessive mucus. As a result, the sinuses become inflamed and produce other symptoms such as headaches, fatigue, coughing, sinus pressure or pain, and loss of smell.

Recommendations

Singles: Eucalyptus Blue, Peppermint, Peppermint Vitality, Dorado Azul, Eucalyptus Globulus, Palo Santo, Eucalyptus Radiata, Ravintsara, Myrrh, Idaho Grand Fir, Thyme, Thyme Vitality, Fennel, Fennel Vitality, Rosemary, Rosemary Vitality

Blends: Raven, DiGize, DiGize Vitality, Thieves, Thieves Roll-On, Thieves Vitality, Exodus II, Breathe Again, Breathe Again Roll-On, SniffleEase, Melrose, R.C., Christmas Spirit

Nutritionals: Super Vitamin C, Super Vitamin C Chewable, ImmuPro, Inner Defense

Oral Care: Thieves AromaBright Toothpaste, KidScents Toothpaste, Thieves Whitening Toothpaste, Thieves Hard Lozenges, Thieves Cough Drops, Thieves Mints, Thieves Fresh Essence Plus Mouthwash, Thieves Spray

Personal Care: Thieves Chest Rub

Application and Usage

Aromatic: Refer to Application Guidelines.

Dietary and Oral: Refer to Application Guidelines.

- Take 1 capsule of desired Vitality oil 2 times daily.
- Take 2-3 drops of desired Vitality oil in a spoonful of syrup or small amount of milk, juice, or water.
- Gargle with Thieves Fresh Essence Plus Mouthwash 4-6 times daily, as desired.

Topical: Refer to Application Guidelines.

- Apply 1-2 drops neat on the temples and back of the neck, as desired.
- Apply a single drop of chosen oil or a swipe of Breathe Again or Breathe Again Roll-On under the nose, which is helpful and refreshing.
- Dilute 50:50 and apply on location 3-6 times daily.
- Massage 2-4 drops of oil neat on the bottoms of the feet just before bedtime. Children love it.

Nasal Irrigation Regimen (See box above)

- Place a warm compress with 1-2 drops of chosen oil on the back.

Sinusitis/Rhinitis

Sinusitis is an inflammation of the sinuses and nasal passages. It can cause pressure in the eyes, cheek area, nose, or on one side of the head. A person with a sinus infection may also have a headache, cough, fever, bad breath, and nasal congestion.

Essential oils such as Eucalyptus Radiata and Ravintsara strengthen the respiratory system, open the pulmonary tract, and fight respiratory infection.

Recommendations

Singles: Eucalyptus Blue, Peppermint, Peppermint Vitality, Eucalyptus Radiata, Ravintsara, Tea Tree, Idaho Grand Fir, Thyme, Thyme Vitality, Northern Lights Black Spruce, Fennel, Fennel Vitality, Rosemary, Rosemary Vitality

Blends: R.C., Melrose, Raven, Thieves, Thieves Roll-On, Thieves Vitality, Exodus II, Breathe Again, Breathe Again Roll-On, SniffleEase

Nutritionals: Super Vitamin C, Super Vitamin C Chewable, ImmuPro, Inner Defense, IlluminEyes

Oral Care: Thieves AromaBright Toothpaste, Thieves Whitening Toothpaste, Thieves Fresh Essence Mouthwash, Thieves Hard Lozenges, Thieves Cough Drops, Thieves Mints, Thieves Spray

Personal Care: Thieves Chest Rub

Application and Usage

Aromatic: Refer to Application Guidelines.

Dietary and Oral: Refer to Application Guidelines.

- Take 1 capsule of desired Vitality oil 2 times daily.
- Take 2-3 drops of desired Vitality oil in a spoonful of syrup or small amount of milk, juice, or water.
- Gargle 2-6 times daily with Thieves Fresh Essence Plus Mouthwash.

Topical: Refer to Application Guidelines.

- Massage 1-3 drops neat on forehead, nose, cheeks, lower throat, chest, and upper back 3-5 times daily. Be careful not to get oils in or near eyes or eyelids.
- Apply 1-2 drops neat on temples and back of neck as desired.
- Apply 1-3 drops on the Vita Flex points of feet 2-4 times daily.
- Use the Raindrop Technique 1-2 times weekly.
- Bath salts: Mix 4-5 drops of oil with 1 cup of salt in hot water to dissolve salts. Pour into bathtub and then soak for 15-20 minutes or until water cools.
- Place a warm compress with 1-2 drops of chosen oil on the back.

Nasal Irrigation Regimen (See box on next page)

SKIN DISORDERS AND PROBLEMS

Essential oils can have powerful antioxidant and antibacterial benefits for the skin. Essential oils used on the skin are often combined with a vegetable carrier oil to:

- Slow evaporation. allowing more time for the oils to penetrate the skin.
- Maintain the lipid barrier of the skin because most essential oils will tend to dry the skin.

Nasal Irrigation Regimen

Essential oils can be used in a saline solution for very effective nasal irrigation that clears and decongests sinuses. As recommended by Daniel Pénoël, MD, the saline solution is prepared as follows:

- 10 drops Rosemary
- 6 drops Tea Tree
- 8 tablespoons ultra-fine sea salt

Also very effective is the following:

- 10 drops Rosemary
- 6 drops Thyme
- 2 drops Cypress
- 8 tablespoons ultra-fine sea salt

The essential oils are mixed thoroughly in the fine salt and stored in a sealed container. For each nasal irrigation session, 1 teaspoon of this salt mixture is dissolved into 1½ cups of distilled water.

This solution is then placed in the tank of an oral irrigator or neti pot to irrigate the nasal cavities, which is done while bending over a sink. This application has brought surprisingly positive results in treating latent sinusitis and other nasal congestion problems.

- Enhance the effect of the essential oils because many oils work well synergistically in a vegetable oil. Many skin conditions are related to dysfunctions of the liver. It may be necessary to cleanse, stimulate, and condition the liver and colon for 30-90 days before the skin begins to improve.

Abscesses and Boils

Skin abscesses are small pockets of pus that collect under the skin, usually caused by a bacterial or fungal infection.

Any number of essential oils may help reduce inflammation and combat infection, helping to bring an abscess or boil to a head, so the pus will come out and the healing can begin.

Recommendations

Singles: Oregano, Oregano Vitality, Ecuadorian Oregano, Clove, Clove Vitality, Myrrh, Tea Tree, Sacred Frankincense, Frankincense, Frankincense Vitality, Lavender, Lavender Vitality, Rosemary, Rosemary Vitality, Thyme, Thyme Vitality, Cassia, Patchouli, Laurus Nobilis

Blends: Melrose, Purification, Thieves, Thieves Roll-On, Thieves Vitality

Nutritionals: JuvaTone, ComforTone, Essentialzyme, Essentialzymes-4, Life 9, KidScents MightyPro, Digest & Cleanse, Inner Defense

Application and Usage

Topical: Refer to Application Guidelines.

 - Apply 2-3 drops neat (undiluted), depending on which oil you choose.

 - Dilute the oil you choose 50:50 with V-6 Vegetable Oil Complex and apply on location 3-6 times daily or as needed.

Acne and Blemishes

Acne results from an excess accumulation of dirt and sebum (oil) produced in the follicles and pores of the skin. As the pores and hair follicles become congested, bacteria begin to feed on the sebum. This leads to inflammation, infection, and the formation of a pimple or a blackhead around the hair follicle.

One of the most common forms of acne, Acne vulgaris, occurs primarily in adolescents due to hormone imbalances that stimulate the production of sebum.

Acne may be caused by a hormone imbalance, poor diet, and the use of chemicals found in cleaning products, soaps, cosmetics, lotions, and creams.

Essential oils are outstanding for treating acne because of their ability to dissolve sebum, kill bacteria, and preserve the acid mantle of the skin. Natural hormone creams such as Prenolone Plus Body Cream or the gentle Progessence Plus may help with hormone imbalance problems directly affecting the skin.

Stress may also play a role. According to research conducted by Dr. M. Toyoda in Japan, acne and other skin problems are a direct result of physical and emotional stress.48 Essential oils are also great to use to release emotions and deal with stress.

Recommendations

Singles: Tea Tree, Geranium, Vetiver, Royal Hawaiian Sandalwood, Sacred Sandalwood, Patchouli, Lavender, Lavender Vitality, German Chamomile, German Chamomile Vitality, Roman Chamomile, Cassia, Cedarwood, Eucalyptus Radiata, Melaleuca Quinquenervia (Niaouli)

Blends: Melrose, Purification, Thieves, Thieves Roll-On, Thieves Vitality, Harmony, Shutran, Peace & Calming, Peace & Calming II, Calm CBD Roll-On, Seedlings Calm, CBD, Stress Away, Stress Away Roll-On

Nutritionals: Mineral Essence, Detoxzyme, MultiGreens, ICP, ComforTone, Essentialzyme, Essentialzymes-4, Life 9, KidScents MightyPro, Ningxia Wolfberries (Organic, Dried), NingXia Red, OmegaGize3, Digest & Cleanse, Balance Complete

Personal Care: Boswellia Wrinkle Cream, Sandalwood Moisturizing Cream, ART Gentle Cleanser, ART Refreshing Toner, Satin Facial Scrub (Mint), Progessence Plus, Prenolone Plus Body Cream, Lemon-Sandalwood Cleansing Soap, Shutran Bar Soap, Melaleuca-Geranium Moisturizing Soap

Application and Usage

Dietary and Oral: Remove sugar and dairy from your diet.

Topical: Refer to Application Guidelines.

- Gently massage 3-5 drops of chosen oil or blend neat or diluted with V-6 Vegetable Oil Complex into the oily areas 1-3 times daily. Alternate the oils daily for maximum effect.

Blisters

Blisters happen when fluid is trapped under the skin. They can be caused by pressure (e.g., tight or ill-fitting shoes), physical injury, chemical burns, toxins, sunburns, or allergies. They can also be caused by microbial infestations from fungal and viral diseases, such as herpes simplex, athlete's foot, shingles, etc.

Recommendations

Singles: Tea Tree, Myrrh, Lavender, Roman or German Chamomile, Helichrysum, Cassia, Laurus Nobilis

Blends: Melrose, Purification, Valor, KidScents Owie, CBD

Personal Care: LavaDerm Cooling Mist, Rose Ointment, CBD Muscle Rub, Genesis Hand & Body Lotion, Lavender Hand & Body Lotion

Application and Usage

Topical: Refer to Application Guidelines.

- Dilute chosen oil 50:50 and apply to blistered area 3-6 times daily.

- Spray LavaDerm as often as every 30 minutes or as desired.

- Gently apply a little Rose Ointment or lotion to keep skin soft and moist.

Boils

Boils and carbuncles (a group of boils) are caused by a bacterial infection that creates a pus-filled hair follicle. They can be easily treated with antiseptic essential oils, including Tea Tree and Clove.

Recommendations

Singles: Tea Tree, Myrrh, Clove, Thyme, Cassia, Oregano

Blends: Melrose, Purification, Thieves, Thieves Roll-On, CBD

Application and Usage

Topical: Refer to Application Guidelines.

- Dilute 2-3 drops of any oil above 50:50 and apply on location 3-6 times daily.

Burns (See also SHOCK)

There are three types of burns:

First-degree burns damage only the outer layer of the skin. Sunburn is typically a first-degree burn.

Second-degree burns damage both the outer layer and the underlying layer, known as the dermis, and are manifested by blisters.

Third-degree burns not only destroy or damage skin but can even damage underlying tissues.

Burns can be caused by sunlight, chemicals, electricity, radiation, and heat. Thermal burns are the most common type.

Aloe vera gel (contained in LavaDerm) is used extensively in the treatment of burns and has been studied for its anti-inflammatory and tissue-regenerating properties.

Helichrysum, Lavender, Idaho Grand Fir, and Frankincense oils support tissue regeneration and reduce scarring and skin discoloration.

Severe burns can result in dehydration and mineral loss. Inflammation often accompanies burns, so Dietary and Oral regimen should be used to lessen inflammation.

If the burn is large or severe, the individual may go into shock. Inhaling oils may help reduce the shock.

After a burn has started to heal and is drying and cracking, use Rose Ointment or a body lotion with a few drops of Lavender oil to keep skin soft and to promote faster healing.

Seek medical attention for serious burns as necessary.

First-Degree Burns (Sunburn)

The best prevention for sunburn is to avoid prolonged exposure to the sun. When you do go outdoors, always wear sunscreen or lotion with a SPF greater than 15—especially during the summer and when you expect to be outdoors for a prolonged period of time.

Certain natural vegetable oils and essential oils have been found to provide some protection against the sun. Sesame oil can screen or reduce about 30 percent of the burning rays, coconut and olive oils can reduce about 20 percent, and aloe vera inhibits about 20 percent. Helichrysum essential oil has been researched for its ability to effectively screen out some of the sun's rays.

Young Living's chemical-free sunscreen products are formulated with naturally derived plant- and mineral-based ingredients. Mineral Sunscreen Lotion SPF 50 offers 80 minutes of sun protection.

Recommendations

Singles: Lavender, Idaho Grand Fir, Helichrysum, Rose, Melaleuca Quinquenervia (Niaouli), German Chamomile, Vetiver

Blends: Gentle Baby, Australian Blue, Melrose, Valor, Valor Roll-On

Nutritionals: Longevity Softgels, Sulfurzyme, Mega Vitamin Cal, OmegaGize3, AminoWise, Pure Protein Complete, Protein Power Bites

Personal Care: Mineral Sunscreen Lotion SPF 50, LavaDerm After Sun Spray, LavaDerm Cooling Mist, Rose Ointment

---

Tips for Clearing Acne

- Eliminate dairy products, fried foods, chemical additives, and sugar from diet
- Avoid using makeup or chlorinated water
- Avoid using plastics that may exude estrogenic chemicals
- Topically apply essential oils such as Tea Tree to problem areas. It was shown to be equal to benzoyl peroxide in the treatment of acne, according to research published in the Medical Journal of Australia .49
- Begin a cleansing program with the Cleansing Trio, Sulfurzyme, Detoxzyme, Essentialzyme, ICP, and JuvaPower.

Application and Usage

Topical: Refer to Application Guidelines.

- Mineral Sunscreen Lotion SPF 50: Apply liberally 15 minutes before sun exposure. Reapply after 80 minutes of swimming or sweating, immediately after towel drying, or at least every 2 hours.
- For fast relief of first-degree burns, spray burn immediately with LavaDerm After Sun Spray or LavaDerm Cooling Mist and continue misting as necessary to cool the area. Spray as often as needed for the first several hours and follow with 2-3 drops of Lavender or Idaho Grand Fir.

💧 Apply 1-3 drops neat or diluted 50:50 on burn location to cool tissue and reduce inflammation.

💧 Apply 3-6 times daily or as needed.

Chérie Ross's Sunscreen Blend No. 1

- 10 drops Helichrysum
- 5 drops Lavender
- 3 drops Roman Chamomile
- 1 ounce Sesame Oil
- ½ ounce Coconut Oil
- ½ ounce Olive Oil

Mix and apply before going out in the sun.

Chérie Ross's Sunscreen Blend No. 2

- 30 drops Lavender
- 4 ounces Avocado Oil

Mix and apply before going out in the sun.

In the event of a sunburn, LavaDerm Cooling Mist, and Lavender and Idaho Grand Fir essential oils can offer excellent pain-relieving and healing benefits.

Second-Degree Burns (Blisters)

- Spray burn immediately with LavaDerm After Sun Spray or LavaDerm Cooling Mist and continue misting when necessary to cool the area. Spray as often as needed for the first several hours and follow with 2-3 drops of Lavender or Idaho Grand Fir.
- Thereafter, apply LavaDerm every 15-30 minutes during the first day. Apply 2-4 drops of Lavender or Melaleuca Quinquenervia as needed immediately after each LavaDerm misting.
- On days 2 through 5, mist every hour and follow with 2-4 drops Lavender or Melaleuca Quinquenervia.

- Continue using LavaDerm 3 to 6 times daily until healed. Apply Rose Ointment to keep tissue soft.
- Mineral Essence: Put 2 droppers full in 3 liters of water and drink throughout the day.

Third-Degree Burns
- Spray LavaDerm After Sun Spray or LavaDerm Cooling Mist to hydrate the skin, then seek medical attention immediately.

Chapped, Cracked, or Dry Skin
Dry skin results from loss of the protective lipid layer on the skin surface. It results from exposure to low humidity environments and is often more prevalent during the winter. Dry skin may also crack, creating an opportunity for infection.

Recommendations
Singles: Neroli, Rose, Cedarwood, Roman Chamomile, Palmarosa, Geranium, Lavender, Myrrh, Sacred Sandalwood, Royal Hawaiian Sandalwood

Blends: Gentle Baby, KidScents Owie

Personal Care: LavaDerm Cooling Mist, Essential Beauty Serum for Dry Skin, Sandalwood Moisturizing Cream, Boswellia Wrinkle Cream, Rose Ointment, KidScents Lotion, KidScents Tender Tush, Genesis Hand & Body Lotion, Lavender Hand & Body Lotion, ART Light Moisturizer, ART Intensive Moisturizer, Lemon-Sandalwood Cleansing Soap, Shutran Bar Soap, Melaleuca-Geranium Moisturizing Soap, Evening Peace Bath and Shower Gel, Morning Start Bath and Shower Gel, Sensation Bath and Shower Gel

Lip Care: Lavender Lip Balm, Cinnamint Lip Balm, Grapefruit Lip Balm, Vanillamint Lip Balm

The Deadly Dehydration of Burns
Burns tend to swell and blister because of fluid loss from the damaged blood vessels. This is why it is im-portant to keep the burn well-hydrated and to drink plenty of water. In cases of serious burns, fluid loss can become so severe that it sends the victim into shock and requires intravenous transfusions of saline solution to bring up blood pressure.

Application and Usage
Topical: Refer to Application Guidelines.

- Apply 2-3 drops of oil diluted 20:80 in a natural, unperfumed lotion base (V-6 Vegetable Oil Complex or avocado oil) or other high-grade, emollient oil. Apply on location as often as needed.

- Combine 3-5 drops of essential oils with 1 teaspoon of KidScents Lotion, Lavender Hand & Body Lotion, or Genesis Hand & Body Lotion to create a very effective lotion for rehydrating the skin of chapped hands and maintaining the natural pH balance of the skin.

- Bath and shower gels, such as Evening Peace, Morning Start, and Sensation are formulated to help balance the acid mantle of the skin. The bar soaps are rich in moisturizers.

Clogged Pores
Most skin blemishes begin as clogged pores. To have clean pores, you should maintain a regular skin care routine. If you keep your pores unclogged and clean, you will have fewer breakouts and more beautiful skin.

Recommendations
Singles: Lemon, Orange, Geranium, Cypress, Lavender

Blends: Melrose, Purification, Inner Child

Skin Care: ART Gentle Cleanser, ART Refreshing Toner, Satin Facial Scrub - Mint, Orange Blossom Facial Wash, Boswel-lia Wrinkle Cream, Sandalwood Moisturizing Cream

Application and Usage
Topical: Refer to Application Guidelines.

- Apply 2-4 drops neat to affected area and gently remove with cotton ball.
- Use ART Refreshing Toner and moisturizing bar soaps.
- Satin Facial Scrub - Mint is a gentle exfoliator designed to clarify skin and reduce acne. If its texture is too abrasive for your skin, mix it with Orange Blossom Facial Wash. This is excellent for those with severe or mild acne.
- Spread scrub over face and let dry for perhaps five minutes to draw out impurities, purifying and toning the skin at the same time. Put a hot towel over face for greater penetration.

- Wash off with warm water by gently patting skin with warm face cloth. If you do not have time to let the mask dry, gently massage in a circular motion for 30 seconds, then rinse.
- Afterward, apply Rose Ointment, Orange Blossom Moisturizer, Sandalwood Moisturizing Cream, or Boswellia Wrinkle Cream. This also works well underneath foundation makeup.

Cuts, Scrapes, and Wounds

When selecting essential oils for surface injuries, determine the needs of the entire body, not just of the cut. Think through the cause and type of injury and select oils for each aspect of the trauma. For instance, a wound could encompass muscle damage, nerve damage, ligament damage, inflammation, infection, bone injury, fever, and possibly an emotion. Therefore, select an oil or blend that is specific to each need.

Recommendations

Single Oils: Tea Tree, Lavender, Helichrysum, Rosemary, Eucalyptus Globulus, Dorado Azul, Cypress, Wintergreen, Thyme, Oregano, German Chamomile, Mountain Savory, Sacred Frankincense, Frankincense, Cassia, Myrrh, Eucalyptus Blue, Eucalyptus Radiata, Cistus

Blends: Melrose, Thieves, Thieves Roll-On, The Gift, 3 Wise Men, Aroma Siez, Aroma Life, Purification, Trauma Life, Peace & Calming, Peace & Calming II, R.C., RutaVaLa, RutaVaLa Roll-On, Stress Away, Stress Away Roll-On, Tranquil Roll-On, KidScents Owie, Calm CBD Roll-On, Seedlings Calm

Personal Care: Thieves Spray, LavaDerm After Sun Spray, LavaDerm Cooling Mist, Boswellia Wrinkle Cream, Sandalwood Moisturizing Cream, Genesis Hand & Body Lotion, Lavender Hand & Body Lotion, ART Light Moisturizer, ART Intensive Moisturizer,

Application and Usage

Topical: Refer to Application Guidelines.

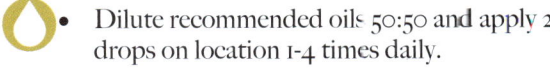
- Dilute recommended oils 50:50 and apply 2-6 drops on location 1-4 times daily.
- Apply LavaDerm After Sun Spray or LavaDerm Cooling Mist to the affected area.

Note: Peppermint can be helpful in treating wounds but may sting when applied to an open wound. To reduce discomfort, dilute with Lavender or mix in a sealing ointment before applying. When applied to a wound or cut that has a scab, a diluted Peppermint blend will soothe, cool, and reduce inflammation in damaged tissue.

Bruise and Scrape Blend
(May be used on infants and children)
- 4 drops Lavender
- 1 drop Cistus
- 1 drop Myrrh

Infected Cut Blend
- 7 drops Geranium
- 5 drops Myrrh
- 3 drops Tea Tree

TO DISINFECT
Recommendations

Singles: Tea Tree, Oregano, Lemongrass, Melissa, Thyme, Mountain Savory, Lemon, Rosemary, Eucalyptus Radiata, Cinnamon Bark, Cassia, Clove

Blends: Thieves, Thieves Roll-On, Melrose, Purification, Citrus Fresh

Personal Care: Thieves Spray

Application and Usage
Topical: Refer to Application Guidelines.

- Apply Thieves Spray.

- Dilute recommended oils 50:50 and apply 2-4 drops on the wound 2-5 times daily.

TO PROMOTE HEALING
Recommendations

Singles: Sacred Frankincense, Frankincense, Royal Hawaiian Sandalwood, Sacred Sandalwood, Melissa, Lavender, Idaho Grand Fir, Palo Santo, Patchouli, Melaleuca Quinquenervia, Myrrh, Helichrysum

Blends: Melrose, Purification, Gentle Baby, Valor, KidScents Owie

Personal Care: Genesis Hand & Body Lotion, Lavender Hand & Body Lotion, ART Light Moisturizer, ART Intensive Moisturizer, Sandalwood Moisturizing Cream, Boswellia Wrinkle Cream

Application and Usage
Topical: Refer to Application Guidelines.

- Dilute recommended oils 50:50 and apply 2-4 drops on the wound 2-5 times daily.

TO REDUCE BLEEDING
Recommendations
Singles: Helichrysum, Cistus, Cypress, Lemon, Geranium, Vetiver, Valerian, Sacred Frankincense, Frankincense, Myrrh, German Chamomile

Blends: PanAway, Relieve It, Aroma Siez

Application and Usage
Topical: Refer to Application Guidelines.

- Apply a cold compress to the affected area 1-2 times until bleeding stops.

Wound Compress Blend
- 5 drops Geranium
- 5 drops Lemon
- 5 drops German Chamomile
- 2 drops Helichrysum

First Aid Spray

First Aid Recipe:
- 5 drops Lavender
- 3 drops Tea Tree
- 2 drops Dorado Azul

Mix the recipe above thoroughly in ½ teaspoon of salt. Add this to 8 ounces of distilled water, shake vigorously, and pour into a spray bottle. Spray minor cuts and wounds before applying a bandage. Repeat 2-3 times a day for 3 days. Continue the healing process by applying 1-2 drops of Tea Tree oil to the wound daily for the next few days. Apply Rose Ointment or Tender Tush to keep the scab soft and help prevent scarring.

Animal Scents works extremely well for any animal, and it is also very effective for any person who wishes to cover a large area such as the bottoms of the feet. When working in rough conditions such as the cold outdoors, doing construction or building, or anything that is abrasive to the hands, add a few drops of the recipe to a tablespoon of Animal Scents or Rose Ointment and use it throughout the day to relieve the pain and ache of small cuts and scrapes on the skin.

TO REDUCE SCARRING
Recommendations
Singles: Sacred Frankincense, Frankincense, Lavender, Royal Hawaiian Sandalwood, Sacred Sandalwood, Cistus, Geranium, Helichrysum, Myrrh, Vetiver, Patchouli

Blends: Gentle Baby, Valor, Melrose, KidScents Owie

Application and Usage
Topical: Refer to Application Guidelines.
- Dilute recommended oils 50:50 and apply 2-4 drops on the wound 2-5 times daily.

Scar Prevention Blend No. 1
- 3 drops Royal Hawaiian Sandalwood or Sacred Sandalwood
- 3 drops Sacred Frankincense or Frankincense
- 1 drop Vetiver

Scar Prevention Blend No. 2
- 10 drops Geranium
- 8 drops Helichrysum
- 6 drops Lavender
- 4 drops Patchouli

Diaper Rash
Dilute all oils when used for babies. Just 1-2 drops mixed in Tender Tush or Rose Ointment are sufficient for using on diaper rash. Seedlings Diaper Rash Cream's nine vegetable oils, which include coconut, sunflower, and olive, seal out moisture and soothe baby's tender skin.

Recommendations
Singles: Lavender, Helichrysum, German Chamomile, Cypress

Blends: Gentle Baby, Purification, Valor, KidScents Owie

Personal Care: Seedlings Diaper Rash Cream, Tender Tush, Rose Ointment, ClaraDerm, LavaDerm Cooling Mist

Application and Usage
Topical: Refer to Application Guidelines.
- Apply Seedlings Diaper Rash Cream liberally with each diaper change.
- Apply 1-2 drops diluted 50:50 and/or ointments on location 2-4 times daily during diaper changes.

Eczema/Dermatitis

Eczema and dermatitis are both inflammations of the skin and are most often due to allergies, including gluten (wheat) and dairy, but they also can be a sign of liver disease.

Dermatitis usually results from external factors such as sunburn or contact with poison ivy, metals from wristwatches, earrings, jewelry, etc.; internal factors such as irritant chemicals, soaps, and shampoos; or from gluten and lactose allergies or intolerance.

In both dermatitis and eczema, the skin can become red, flaky, and itchy. Small blisters may form, and if they are broken by scratching, they can become infected.

Recommendations
Singles: Lavender, Lavender Vitality, German Chamomile, German Chamomile Vitality, Cassia, Myrrh, Blue Cypress, Roman Chamomile, Geranium, Laurus Nobilis, Laurus Nobilis Vitality

Blends: JuvaCleanse, JuvaCleanse Vitality, Purification, Melrose, Australian Blue

Nutritionals: Detoxzyme, ICP, ComforTone, Essentialzyme, JuvaTone, JuvaPower, Essentialzymes-4, KidScents MightyZyme, Life 9

Personal Care: Rose Ointment, Regenolone Moisturizing Cream, Sandalwood Moisturizing Cream, Boswellia Wrinkle Cream, Orange Blossom Moisturizer, Genesis Hand & Body Lotion, Lavender Hand & Body Lotion, ART Light Moisturizer, ART Intensive Moisturizer

Application and Usage
Topical: Refer to Application Guidelines

- Apply 1-2 drops diluted 50:50 on location as needed.

Fungal Skin Infections

Fungi and yeast feed on decomposing or dead tissues that exist everywhere, such as in our stomachs, on our skin, on food, outside in the lawn, in the garden, on pets, etc. When kept under control, the yeast and fungi populating our bodies are harmless and digest what our bodies cannot or do not use.

When we feed the naturally occurring fungi in our bodies with simple sugars, the fungi are more likely to grow out of control. This condition is known as systemic candidiasis, which invades the blood, gastrointestinal tract, and tissues.

Recommendations
Singles: Tea Tree, Lemongrass, Lemongrass Vitality, Oregano, Oregano Vitality, Ecuadorian Oregano, Lavender, Lavender Vitality, Northern Lights Black Spruce, Cassia, Patchouli, Davana, Melaleuca Quinquenervia

Blends: Melrose, Purification, Thieves, Thieves Roll-On, Thieves Vitality

Nutritionals: Life 9, KidScents MightyPro, Digest & Cleanse, ICP, ComforTone, Essentialzyme, Mineral Essence

Skin Care: ClaraDerm

Application and Usage
Topical: Refer to Application Guidelines.

- Apply 2-4 drops of oil diluted 50:50 on location 3-5 times daily.

Antifungal Skin Blend
- 10 drops Patchouli
- 5 drops Lemongrass
- 4 drops Melaleuca Quinquenervia
- 2 drops Tea Tree

Itching

Itching can be due to dry skin, impaired liver function, insects, allergies, toxins, or overexposure to chemicals or sunlight.

Recommendations
Singles: Peppermint, Peppermint Vitality, Patchouli, Lavender, Lavender Vitality, Oregano, Oregano Vitality, Ecuadorian Oregano, Vetiver, Nutmeg, Nutmeg Vitality, German Chamomile, German Chamomile Vitality

Blends: Aroma Siez, Purification, Melrose, Thieves, Thieves Roll-On, Thieves Vitality, DiGize, DiGize Vitality, KidScents Owie, JuvaFlex, JuvaFlex Vitality, JuvaCleanse, JuvaCleanse Vitality

Nutritionals: Digest & Cleanse, Life 9, KidScents MightyPro, JuvaTone, ComforTone, Essentialzyme, Essentialzymes-4, Detoxzyme, ICP, JuvaPower, PowerGize

Personal Care: KidScents Tender Tush, Rose Ointment, Regenolone Moisturizing Cream, Sandalwood Moisturizing Cream, Boswellia

Wrinkle Cream, Orange Blossom Moisturizer, LavaDerm Cooling Mist, LavaDerm After Sun Spray, ClaraDerm, Genesis Hand & Body Lotion, Lavender Hand & Body Lotion, ART Light Moisturizer, ART Intensive Moisturizer

Application and Usage

Topical: Refer to Application Guidelines.

- Apply 1-2 drops neat on location several times daily as needed.
- Dilute 50/50 and apply on location 3-6 times daily.
- Spray LavaDerm Cooling Mist, LavaDerm After Sun Spray, or any Young Living personal care products if condition is evident on the skin.

Liver Spots (Solar Lentigines)

Mistakenly called liver spots, these "sun" or "age" spots are actually solar lentigines, which are caused by exposure to the sun over time. These flat sunspots are brown, gray, or black and vary in size. They usually are found on the face, arms, shoulders, and hands—the areas that receive the greatest sun exposure.

Recommendations

Singles: Frankincense, Sacred Frankincense, Myrrh, Sacred Sandalwood, Royal Hawaiian Sandalwood, Geranium, Lavender, Helichrysum

Personal Care: Mineral Sunscreen Lotion SPF 50, LavaDerm After-Sun Spray

Application and Usage

Topical: Refer to Application Guidelines.

- Apply 2-4 drops neat of the sunspot blend over affected area 3 times daily for 2 weeks. The oils from the blend can be applied on individual sunspots with a cotton swab.

Sunspot Blend

- 20 drops V-6 Vegetable Oil Complex
- 6 drops Frankincense or Sacred Frankincense
- 4 drops Sacred Sandalwood or Royal Hawaiian Sandalwood
- 4 drops Lavender
- 4 drops Myrrh

Moles

Moles appear often as small, dark brown spots; come in many colors; and can develop virtually anywhere on your body. Most moles are harmless but monitoring them is important in detecting skin cancer.

Recommendations

Singles: Oregano, Thyme, Tea Tree, Frankincense, Sacred Frankincense

Blends: Melrose, Purification

Application and Usage

Topical: Refer to Application Guidelines.

- To dry up moles, apply 1-2 drops of Oregano neat (undiluted) on the mole 2-3 times daily.
- Other oils may be used that may also show benefit.

Poison Oak/Poison Ivy/Poison Sumac

Poison ivy, poison oak, and poison sumac are plants that contain an irritating, oily sap called urushiol, which triggers an allergic reaction when it comes in contact with skin. An itchy rash can appear within hours of exposure or several days later and usually develops into oozing blisters.

Recommendations

Singles: Peppermint, Peppermint Vitality, Myrrh, Patchouli, Vetiver, Eucalyptus Blue, German Chamomile, German Chamomile Vitality, Roman Chamomile, Rose, Lemon, Lemon Vitality, Palo Santo, Tea Tree, Rosemary, Rosemary Vitality, Geranium, Idaho Tansy, Basil, Basil Vitality

Blends: Melrose, Purification, R.C., JuvaCleanse, JuvaCleanse Vitality, KidScents Owie

Nutritionals: Detoxzyme, ComforTone, Mineral Essence, Digest & Cleanse, ICP, JuvaPower, OmegaGize3

Tea Tree (Melaleuca alternifolia)

During World War II, tea tree oil (Melaleuca alternifolia) was found to have very strong antibacterial properties and worked well in preventing infection in open wounds.

Melrose is a blend containing two types of Melaleuca oil: Tea Tree (M. alternifolia) and Niaouli (M. quinquenervia), plus Rosemary and Clove, making it an exceptional antiseptic and tissue regenerator.

The pH Balance Makes a Difference

Psoriasis, eczema, dermatitis, dry skin, allergies, and similar problems indicate an excessive acidic pH in the body. The more acid that is in the blood and skin, the less therapeutic effect the oils will have.

People who have a negative reaction to essential oils are usually highly acidic. An alkaline balance must be maintained in the blood and skin for the oils to work the best. AlkaLime and MultiGreens are both helpful for this balancing (See Fungus).

Personal Care: Rose Ointment, KidScents Tender Tush, Boswellia Wrinkle Cream, Sandalwood Moisturizing Cream, ART Light Moisturizer, Thieves Spray, LavaDerm Cooling Mist, ClaraDerm

Application and Usage
Topical: Refer to Application Guidelines

- Apply 4-6 drops of oil diluted 50:50 to affected areas 2 times daily.

- Apply a cold compress on affected area 2 times daily.

Psoriasis

Psoriasis is a noninfectious skin disorder that is marked by skin patches or flaking skin that can occur in limited areas such as the scalp or that can cover up to 80-90 percent of the body. This disorder is believed to be an immune-mediated disease, and genetics may play a role.

The overly rapid growth of skin cells is the primary cause of psoriasis. In some cases, skin cells grow four times faster than normal, resulting in the formation of silvery layers that flake off. However, silvery layers of skin may also be a result of the body being overly acidic.

Symptoms
- It occurs on elbows, chest, knees, and scalp.
- Slightly elevated reddish lesions are covered with silver-white scales.
- The disease can be limited to one small patch or can cover the entire body.
- Rashes subside after exposure to sunlight.
- Rashes recur over a period of years.

Stop eating sugar and junk food! Psoriasis is an inflammatory condition. Junk foods contain saturated and trans fats, refined starches and sugars, which can promote inflammation.

Recommendations

Singles: Roman Chamomile, Tea Tree, Patchouli, Helichrysum, Rose, Melissa, German Chamomile, German Chamomile Vitality, Lavender, Lavender Vitality, Vetiver, Royal Hawaiian Sandalwood, Sacred Sandalwood

Blends: Melrose, Gentle Baby, JuvaCleanse, JuvaCleanse Vitality, JuvaFlex, JuvaFlex Vitality

Nutritionals: ICP, ComforTone, Essentialzyme, Essentialzymes-4, Life 9, KidScents MightyPro, Balance Complete, Alka-Lime, JuvaTone, JuvaPower, Sulfurzyme

Personal Care: KidScents Tender Tush, Rose Ointment, Boswellia Wrinkle Cream, Sandalwood Moisturizing Cream, Genesis Hand & Body Lotion, Lavender Hand & Body Lotion, ART Light Moisturizer, ART Intensive Moisturizer

Application and Usage
Topical: Refer to Application Guidelines.

- Apply 2-4 drops neat to affected area 2 times daily.
- Add 6-10 drops to 1 teaspoon of regular skin lotion and apply daily or as needed.

- Place a warm compress with 1-2 drops of chosen oil on the back 3 times weekly.

Psoriasis Blend
- 4 drops Palo Santo
- 2 drops Patchouli
- 2 drops Roman Chamomile
- 2 drops Vetiver
- 2 drops Royal Hawaiian Sandalwood or Sacred Sandalwood

Sagging Skin

Sagging skin is a common problem for many people, especially as they get older. It occurs as the skin loses its elasticity over time.

Recommendations

Singles: Lavender, Lavender Vitality, Helichrysum, Patchouli, Cypress, Tangerine, Tangerine Vitality, Sacred Sandalwood, Royal Hawaiian Sandalwood, Geranium

Blends: Humility, Inspiration, Joy

Nutritionals: Super Vitamin C, Super Vitamin C Chewable, ICP, ComforTone, Essentialzyme, Essentialzymes-4, Life 9, KidScents MightyPro, Mineral Essence, JuvaPower

Personal Care: ART Refreshing Toner, Sandalwood Moisturizing Cream, Boswellia Wrinkle Cream, Cel-Lite Magic Mas-sage Oil, Genesis Hand & Body Lotion, Lavender Hand & Body Lotion, ART Light Moisturizer, ART Intensive Moisturizer

Application and Usage
Topical: Refer to Application Guidelines.

- Apply 4-6 drops neat or diluted 50:50 on affected area 2 times daily. Use the morning blend before dressing in the morning and the evening blend before bed at night.
- Strength training with weights can also help tighten sagging skin.

Skin Firming Blend (Morning)
- 3 drops Tangerine
- 3 drops Cypress

Skin Firming Blend (Evening)
- 8 drops Patchouli
- 5 drops Cypress
- 5 drops Geranium
- 1 drop Sacred Sandalwood or Royal Hawaiian Sandalwood

Scabies

Scabies are caused by eight-legged insects known as itch mites—tiny parasites that burrow into the skin, usually in the fingers and genital areas. The most common variety, Sarcoptes scabiei, can quickly infest other people. Although it lives for only one to two months, the female continually lays eggs once it digs into the skin.

The most common remedy for scabies and lice is lindane (gamma benzene hexachloride), a highly toxic polychlorinated chemical that is structurally very similar to hazardous banned pesticides such as DDT and chlordane. It is so dangerous that Dr. Guy Sansfacon, head of the Quebec Poison Control Centre in Canada, requested that lindane be banned.

Natural, plant-derived essential oils have the same activity as commercial pesticides but are far safer. Essential oils have been studied for their ability to not only repel insects but also to kill them and their eggs as well. Because most oils are non-toxic to humans, they make excellent treatments to combat scabies infestations.

Recommendations
Singles: Palo Santo, Peppermint, Citronella, Rosemary, Davana, Palmarosa, Eucalyptus Globulus, Black Pepper, Ginger, Oregano, Thyme, Mountain Savory

Blends: Purification, Melrose, Thieves, Thieves Roll-On, Exodus II, ImmuPower

Application and Usage
Topical: Refer to Application Guidelines.

- Apply 2-4 drops of recommended oils neat or diluted 50:50 if needed on location 3 times daily.
- To treat hair or scalp, add 3-5 drops of essential oil to 1 teaspoon of shampoo and massage into wet hair. Leave for 5 minutes, then rinse.

Skin Ulcers

Skin ulcers are open sores that are often accompanied by the sloughing-off of inflamed tissue. They can be caused by problems with blood circulation, irritation from exposure to corrosive material, or exposure to heat, cold, or trauma.

Recommendations
Singles: Helichrysum, Roman Chamomile, Patchouli, Lavender, Lavender Vitality, Clove, Clove Vitality, Myrrh, Sacred Sandalwood, Royal Hawaiian Sandalwood

Blends: Thieves, Thieves Roll-On, Thieves Vitality, Purification, Relieve It, Melrose

Nutritionals: Super Vitamin C, Super Vitamin C Chewable, ICP, ComforTone, Essentialzyme, Essentialzymes-4, Life 9, KidScents MightyPro, NingXia Red, Inner Defense, AminoWise, Pure Protein Complete, Protein Power Bites, Digest & Cleanse, Slique Shake, ImmuPro

Personal Care: Rose Ointment, KidScents Tender Tush, Boswellia Wrinkle Cream, Sandalwood Moisturizing Cream, Genesis Hand & Body Lotion, Lavender Hand & Body Lotion, ART Light Moisturizer, ART Intensive Moisturizer

Application and Usage
Topical: Refer to Application Guidelines.

- Apply 4-6 drops neat or diluted 50:50 on affected area 2 times daily.

Essential Oils Skin Rejuvenation

Rejuvenate and heal
- Rose, Sacred Sandalwood, Myrrh, Frankincense, Vetiver

Prevent and retard wrinkles
- Lavender, Myrrh, Frankincense, Sacred Sandalwood

Regenerate
- Geranium, Helichrysum, Melrose, Sacred Sandalwood

Restore skin elasticity
- Sacred Sandalwood with Lavender
- Ylang Ylang with Lavender
- Patchouli with Ylang Ylang

Combat premature aging of the skin
Mix the following recipe into 1 tablespoon of V-6 Vegetable Oil Complex, any high-grade vegetable oil, or unscented skin lotion, and apply on location 2 times daily.

Skin Rejuvenating Recipe
- 6 drops Sacred Sandalwood
- 4 drops Geranium
- 3 drops Lavender
- 2 drops Sacred Frankincense

Stretch Marks

Stretch marks are most commonly associated with pregnancy but can also occur during growth spurts and periods of weight gain.

Singles: Sacred Frankincense, Frankincense, Frankincense Vitality, Elemi, Geranium, Lavender, Lavender Vitality, Myrrh, Spearmint, Spearmint Vitality

Blends: Gentle Baby, Sensation, Valor, White Angelica

Nutritionals: Sulfurzyme, Mega Vitamin Cal, Super Vitamin B, Super Vitamin C, Super Vitamin C Chewable, Essentialzyme, Essentialzymes-4, Life 9, KidScents MightyPro, Master Formula

Personal Care: Rose Ointment, KidScents Tender Tush, Boswellia Wrinkle Cream, Sandalwood Moisturizing Cream, Gen-esis Hand & Body Lotion, Lavender Hand & Body Lotion, ART Light Moisturizer, ART Intensive Moisturizer

Application and Usage
Topical: Refer to Application Guidelines.

- Apply 3-6 drops of oil neat or diluted 50:50 2 times daily.

Vitiligo

Vitiligo is a condition in which your skin loses melanin, the pigment that determines the color of your skin, hair, and eyes and occurs when the cells that produce melanin die or no longer form melanin, causing slowly enlarging white patches of irregular shapes to appear on your skin.

The cause has not yet been determined, but there are theories that it may be due to an immune system disorder, heredity possibilities, nutritional deficiencies, overuse of chemicals, and perhaps environmental pollution that affects the proper function of the body that produces melanin.

Some people have reported a single event such as sunburn or emotional distress that triggered the condition. However, none of these theories has been proved to be a definite cause of vitiligo.

Recommendations

Singles: Sacred Sandalwood, Royal Hawaiian Sandalwood, Myrrh, Vetiver, Patchouli

Blends: Brain Power, Dream Catcher, Humility

Nutritionals: Essentialzyme, Essentialzymes-4, Life 9, KidScents MightyPro, Detoxzyme, ICP, JuvaPower, Mineral Essence, MindWise, Digest & Cleanse, Inner Defense

Application and Usage
Topical: Refer to Application Guidelines.

- Apply 2-4 drops of desired oil neat 2 times daily.
- A cleansing diet might be helpful. Cleansing the liver and digestive system facilitates greater nutritional absorption and waste elimination for proper body function and vibrant health.

Essential Oils and Skin Vitality

Tea Tree, Dorado Azul, and Lemongrass can help clear acne and balance oily skin conditions. Lemongrass is the predominant ingredient in Morning Start Bath and Shower Gel, which can be used to balance the pH of the skin, decongest the lymphatics, and stimulate circulation.

Wrinkles

Although wrinkles are a natural part of aging, sun exposure is the major cause. Exposure to heat, wind, and dust, as well as smoking, may also contribute to wrinkling.

Recommendations

Singles: Sacred Frankincense, Frankincense, Frankincense Vitality, Myrrh, Vetiver, Helichrysum, Cypress, Rose, Lavender, Lavender Vitality, Patchouli, Geranium, Sacred Sandalwood, Royal Hawaiian Sandalwood, Neroli, Palmarosa

Blends: Gentle Baby, Sensation, 3 Wise Men, White Angelica, Highest Potential

Nutritionals: Mega Vitamin Cal, Longevity Softgels, NingXia Red, OmegaGize3, Master Formula, Sulfurzyme, Super Vitamin B, Ningxia Wolfberries (Organic, Dried), MindWise

Personal Care: Boswellia Wrinkle Cream, Wolfberry Eye Cream, BLOOM Brightening Cleanser, BLOOM Brightening Essence, BLOOM Brightening Lotion, ART Sheerlumé Brightening Cream, ART Gentle Cleanser, ART Refreshing Toner, Rose Ointment, ART Light Moisturizer, Genesis Hand & Body Lotion, Lavender Hand & Body Lotion, ART Inten-sive Moisturizer

Application and Usage

Topical: Refer to Application Guidelines.

- Mix 3-4 drops of oil 50:50 in V-6 Vegetable Oil Complex or add to the ART skin care lotions or moisturizing creams, especially Boswellia Wrinkle Cream, and apply as needed.
- Rose Ointment was developed to keep the skin soft and moist and to supply healing nutrients. It is a natural emollient and contains no chemicals or synthetic ingredients that can cause skin irritation.

Note: Be careful not to get lotion or oils near the eyes.

Wrinkle-Reducing Blend

- 6 drops Sacred Frankincense or Frankincense
- 5 drops Sacred Sandalwood or Royal Hawaiian Sandalwood
- 4 drops Geranium
- 3 drops Lavender

SLEEP DISORDERS

Melatonin is the most powerful natural remedy for restoring both quality and quantity of sleep. It improves the length of time the body sustains deep, stage 4 sleep, the time when the immune system and growth hormone production reaches its maximum.

ImmuPro not only contains melatonin but also mineral and polysaccharide complexes to restore natural sleep rhythm and eliminate insomnia.

Valerian has been shown to be effective in calming the mind, enabling one to fall asleep easier.

Recommendations

Singles: Lavender, Lavender Vitality, Goldenrod, Valerian, Roman Chamomile, Orange, Orange Vitality, Mandarin

Blends: RutaVaLa, RutaVaLa Roll-On, Tranquil Roll-On, Peace & Calming, Peace & Calming II, Calm CBD Roll-On, Seedlings Calm, Gary's Light, Surrender, Trauma Life, Hope, Humility, Stress Away, Stress Away Roll-On, SleepyIze, Chivalry

Nutritionals: SleepEssence, ImmuPro, Essentialzyme, Mega Vitamin Cal, Mineral Essence, OmegaGize3, Life 9, KidScents MightyPro, KidScents Unwind, Thyromin (take just before getting into bed), MindWise

Application and Usage

Aromatic: Refer to Application Guidelines.

Topical: Refer to Application Guidelines.

- Apply 1-2 drops neat on temples and back of neck, as desired.
- Applying a single drop under the nose is helpful.
- Dilute 50:50 and apply on location 3-6 times daily.
- Massage 2-4 drops of oil neat on the bottoms of the feet just before bedtime. Children love it.

SMOKING CESSATION PROBLEMS
(See also ADDICTIONS)

Smoking is a difficult habit to break because it involves many aspects of a person's emotions and social life as well as a physical addiction to nicotine. Smoking cessation (quitting smoking) is a vital part of cancer prevention.

Recommendations

Singles: Cinnamon Bark, Cinnamon Bark Vitality, Clove, Clove Vitality, Nutmeg, Nutmeg Vitality, Peppermint, Peppermint Vitality, Roman Chamomile, Clary Sage, Sage, Sage Vitality

Blends: Thieves, Thieves Roll-On, Thieves Vitality, Gary's Light, Harmony, JuvaCleanse, JuvaCleanse Vitality, Peace & Calming, Peace & Calming II, GLF, GLF Vitality, Calm CBD Roll-On, Seedlings Calm

Nutritionals: ICP, ComforTone, Essentialzyme, Essentialzymes-4, Life 9, KidScents MightyPro, KidScents Unwind, JuvaTone, JuvaPower

Application and Usage

Aromatic: Refer to Application Guidelines.

- Inhale the oils that work best for you whenever the urge for a cigarette arises.

Dietary and Oral: Refer to Application Guidelines.

- Take 1 capsule of desired Vitality oil 2 times daily.

- Take 2-3 drops of desired Vitality oil in a spoonful of syrup or small amount of milk, juice, or water.

- Cleanse colon and liver with ICP, ComforTone, Essentialzyme, and JuvaTone.

- Put 1 drop of Thieves on the tongue every time you have the urge to smoke.

- JuvaTone and JuvaPower detoxify the liver, which in turn helps to reduce cravings for nicotine and caffeine

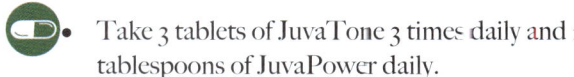
- Take 3 tablets of JuvaTone 3 times daily and 2 tablespoons of JuvaPower daily.

Topical: Refer to Application Guidelines.

CAUTION: Seek medical attention immediately if you are bitten by a poisonous snake.

Recommendations

Singles: Clove, Eucalyptus Blue, Idaho Grand Fir, Copaiba, Lemon, Patchouli, Sacred Frankincense, Frankincense, Thyme, Tea Tree

Blends: Purification, Melrose, Thieves

Personal Care: Thieves Spray

Application and Usage

Topical: Refer to Application Guidelines.

- Apply 2-3 drops diluted 50:50 on location every 15 minutes until professional medical help is available.

SNORING (See also APNEA, SLEEP; SLEEP DISORDERS)

Just about everyone snores occasionally, but it can affect the quantity and quality of your sleep, which can lead to fatigue, irritability, and increased health problems, in addition to relationship problems with your partner.

Recommendations

Singles: Idaho Grand Fir, Sacred Sandalwood, Royal Hawaiian Sandalwood, Rose, Lavender, Lavender Vitality, Valerian, Ylang Ylang

Blends: RutaVaLa, RutaVaLa Roll-On, Stress Away, Stress Away Roll-On, The Gift, Harmony, Sacred Mountain, Transfor-mation, Chivalry

Nutritionals: SleepEssence, ImmuPro, Mega Vitamin Cal, Mineral Essence, Detoxzyme, Essentialzyme, Essentialzymes-4, Life 9, KidScents MightyPro

Application and Usage

Dietary and Oral: Refer to Application Guidelines.

- Take 1 capsule of desired Vitality oil 2 times daily.

- Take 2-3 drops of desired Vitality oil in a spoonful of syrup or small amount of milk, juice, or water.

Topical: Refer to Application Guidelines.

- Rub 4-6 drops diluted 50:50 on the bottoms of both feet at bedtime.

Spina bifida (SB) is a defect in which the spinal cord of the fetus fails to close during the first month of pregnancy. This results in varying degrees of permanent nerve damage, paralysis in lower limbs, and incomplete brain development. The exact cause is unknown, but scientists suspect that nutritional, genetic, and environmental factors such as exposure to harmful substances may play a role in its cause. Having enough folate (found in multivitamins as the B-vitamin folic acid) during the mother's pregnancy reduces the risk of spina bifida, as well as other neural tube disorders, up to 70 percent.50

Spina bifida has three different variations:

The most severe form is myelomeningocele, when the spinal cord and its protective sheath (known as the meninges) protrude from an opening in the spine.

Meningocele is when only the meninges protrude from the opening in the spine. The mildest form is occulta, characterized by malformed vertebrae.

Symptoms of this condition range from bowel and bladder dysfunctions to excess buildup of cerebrospinal fluid in the brain.

The easiest way to possibly prevent spina bifida is with folic acid supplementation (at least 400 mcg daily, found in Super Vitamin B) by all women of child-bearing ages.

Recommendations
Singles: Mountain Savory, Mountain Savory Vitality, Helichrysum, Thyme, Thyme Vitality, Tea Tree, Idaho Grand Fir, Sacred Frankincense, Frankincense, Frankincense Vitality

Blends: Melrose, Exodus II, The Gift, Peace & Calming, Peace & Calming II, Deep Relief Roll-On, Tranquil Roll-On, Aroma Siez, Calm CBD Roll-On, Seedlings Calm, Cool Azul

Nutritionals: Super Vitamin B, Balance Complete, Sulfurzyme, PowerGize, Mega Vitamin Cal, JuvaPower, Master Formula, OmegaGize3, Essentialzyme, Essentialzymes-4, Life 9, KidScents MightyPro, MindWise, Slique Shake

Application and Usage
- Receive a Raindrop Technique weekly.

SPINAL INJURIES AND PAIN

According to numerous chiropractors, the Raindrop Technique using therapeutic-grade essential oils is revolutionizing the treatment of many types of back pain, spine inflammation, and vertebral misalignments.

The following essential oils, Blends, and supplements are for supporting the structural integrity of the spine and reducing discomfort:

Recommendations
Singles: Idaho Blue Spruce, Dorado Azul, Wintergreen, Kunzea, Marjoram, Marjoram Vitality, Idaho Grand Fir, Helichrysum, Palo Santo, Peppermint, Peppermint Vitality, Basil, Basil Vitality, Copaiba, Copaiba Vitality

Blends: PanAway, Cool Azul, Aroma Siez, Relieve It, Valor, Valor Roll-On, Deep Relief Roll-On, CBD

Nutritionals: PowerGize, Mega Vitamin Cal, Super Vitamin Cal Plus, Super Vitamin D, Longevity Softgels, BLM, AgilEase, Essentialzyme, Mineral Essence, Slique Shake, AminoWise, Pure Protein Complete, Power Protein Bites, Sulfurzyme

Personal Care: Cool Azul Pain Relief Cream, Cool Azul Sports Gel, CBD Muscle Rub, Ortho Sport Massage Oil, Ortho Ease Massage Oil

Application and Usage
Dietary and Oral: Refer to Application Guidelines.

- Take 1 capsule of desired Vitality oil 2 times daily.

- Take 2-3 drops of desired Vitality oil in a spoonful of syrup or small amount of milk, juice, or water.

Topical: Refer to Application Guidelines.

- Apply 6-10 drops diluted 50:50 on location 2 times daily or as needed.

- Place a warm compress with 1-2 drops of desired oil daily (if area is not inflamed).

- Receive a Raindrop Technique 3 times a month.

Back Injuries and Pain (Backache) (See also MUSCLE PROBLEMS)

According to numerous chiropractors, the Raindrop Technique, which uses therapeutic-grade essential oils, has added tremendous benefit to the treatment of many types of back pain, inflammation, and vertebral misalignments.

Recommendations
Singles: Lavender, Lavender Vitality, Idaho Grand Fir, Kunzea, Helichrysum, Wintergreen, German Chamomile, German Chamomile Vitality, Basil, Basil Vitality, Frankincense, Frankincense Vitality, Sacred Frankincense, Copaiba, Copaiba Vitality, Marjoram, Marjoram Vitality, Peppermint, Peppermint Vitality

Blends: Cool Azul, Aroma Siez, PanAway, Relieve It, Deep Relief Roll-On, CBD, Valor, Valor Roll-On

Nutritionals: BLM, AgilEase, Super Vitamin D, PowerGize, Mega Vitamin Cal, Master Formula, Slique Shake, Multi-Greens, AminoWise, Pure Protein Complete, Protein Power Bites, NingXia Red

Personal Care: Cool Azul Pain Relief Cream, Cool Azul Sports Gel, CBD Muscle Rub, Regenolone Moisturizing Cream, Ortho Sport Massage Oil, Ortho Ease Massage Oil

Application and Usage
Topical: Refer to Application Guidelines.

- Apply 2-4 drops neat on specific area 1-3 times daily or as needed.

- Apply 2-4 drops on Vita Flex area of foot.

- Use warm compress with 1-2 drops of chosen oil on the back daily.

- Apply Raindrop Technique 2 times weekly for 3 weeks.

- Massage with Ortho Ease or Ortho Sport Massage Oil.

Backache Blend
- 5 drops Wintergreen
- 3 drops Lavender
- 3 drops Idaho Grand Fir
- 2 drops Marjoram

Herniated Disc/Disc Deterioration
A herniated disc is an abnormal rupture of the central portion of a disc of the spine. For this situation, it is best to consult a specialist.

However, many essential oils can give temporary pain relief.

Recommendations
Singles: Basil, Basil Vitality, Tarragon, Tarragon Vitality, Idaho Blue Spruce, Kunzea, Sacred Frankincense, Frankincense, Frankincense Vitality, Idaho Grand Fir, Helichrysum, Wintergreen, Vetiver, Valerian

Blends: PanAway, Cool Azul, Relieve It, Aroma Siez, Deep Relief Roll-On, CBD

Nutritionals: Sulfurzyme, Super Vitamin D, BLM, AgilEase, PowerGize, Mega Vitamin Cal, Slique Shake, Master Formula, Essentialzyme, Mineral Essence, AminoWise, Pure Protein Complete, Protein Power Bites, OmegaGize3

> Chiropractors have found that by applying Valor on the bottoms of the feet, spinal manipulations are easier to do and last 75% longer.

Personal Care: Cool Azul Pain Relief Cream, Cool Azul Sports Gel, CBD Muscle Rub, Regenolone Moisturizing Cream, Ortho Sport Massage Oil, Ortho Ease Massage Oil

Application and Usage
Topical: Refer to Application Guidelines.

- Dilute 50:50 and apply on location for pain relief.

- Place a cold compress on location as needed.
- Receive a Raindrop Technique 2 times weekly.
- Stimulate vertebrae with "pointer technique."

(See box with explanation)

Lumbago (Lower Back Pain)
Chronic lower back pain can have many causes, including a damaged or pinched nerve (neuralgia) or a congested colon.

Recommendations
Singles: Basil, Basil Vitality, Helichrysum, German Chamomile, German Chamomile Vitality, Elemi, Peppermint, Peppermint Vitality, Kunzea, Copaiba, Copaiba Vitality, Marjoram, Marjoram Vitality, Wintergreen

Blends: Relieve It, Cool Azul, PanAway, Aroma Siez, Deep Relief Roll-On, CBD, Stress Away, Stress Away Roll-On

Nutritionals: Mega Vitamin Cal, BLM, AgilEase, ICP, ComforTone, Essentialzyme, Essentialzymes-4, Life 9, KidScents MightyPro, OmegaGize3, AminoWise, Pure Protein Complete, Protein Power Bites, PowerGize

Personal Care: Cool Azul Pain Relief Cream, Cool Azul Sports Gel, CBD Muscle Rub, Regenolone Moisturizing Cream, Ortho Sport Massage Oil, Ortho Ease Massage Oil

Application and Usage
Topical: Refer to Application Guidelines.

- Apply 6-10 drops of oil diluted 50:50 on location 2 times daily. Also apply around navel.

- Apply 2-3 drops of desired oil on stomach and intestine and on Vita Flex points of the feet.

- Place a warm compress on lower back 1-2 times daily. If inflamed, use a cool compress.

- Receive a complete Raindrop Technique 3 times each month.

Neck Pain and Stiffness

Neck pain and stiffness can be caused by a variety of factors, including stress, injury, tension, everyday activities, or other health problems, some of which may have serious consequences.

Recommendations

Singles: Basil, Basil Vitality, Marjoram, Marjoram Vitality, Idaho Blue Spruce, Helichrysum, Idaho Grand Fir, Peppermint, Peppermint Vitality, Wintergreen, Cypress, Nutmeg, Nutmeg Vitality, Copaiba, Copaiba Vitality, Kunzea, Elemi, Dora-do Azul

Blends: Cool Azul, Relieve It, PanAway, Aroma Siez, Deep Relief Roll-On, CBD

Nutritionals: Mineral Essence, Mega Vitamin Cal, Master Formula, Balance Complete, BLM, AgilEase, AminoWise, Pure Protein Complete, Protein Power Bites, OmegaGize3

Personal Care: Cool Azul Pain Relief Cream, Cool Azul Sports Gel, CBD Muscle Rub, Regenolone Moisturizing Cream, Ortho Sport Massage Oil, Ortho Ease Massage Oil

Application and Usage

Topical: Refer to Application Guidelines.

- Apply 4-6 drops diluted 50:50 to neck area and massage 1-3 times daily as needed.

- Place a warm compress on neck area daily or as needed. With inflammation, use a cool compress.

Neck Stiffness Blend
- 5 drops PanAway
- 5 drops Marjoram
- 3 drops Peppermint

Neck Pain Blend
- 7 drops Basil
- 5 drops Wintergreen
- 4 drops Cypress
- 2 drops Peppermint

Sciatica

Sciatica is characterized by pain in the buttocks and down the back of the thigh. The pain worsens during coughing, sneezing, or while flexing and stretching the back. The pain is caused by pressure on the sciatic nerve as it leaves the spine in the lower pelvic region due to spinal misalignment and/or nerve inflammation.

The sciatic nerve is the largest in the body, with branches throughout the legs and feet; sciatic pain can be intense and immobilizing. Acute sciatica has a sudden onset and is usually triggered by compressed or herniated lumbar discs, as well as misaligned vertebra pressing against the sciatic nerve due to accident, injury, pregnancy, or inflammation.

Symptoms
- Lower back pain
- Swelling or stiffness in a leg
- Loss of sensation in a leg
- Muscle wasting in a leg

Recommendations

Singles: Helichrysum, Tarragon, Tarragon Vitality, Vetiver, Peppermint, Peppermint Vitality, Nutmeg, Nutmeg Vitality, Thyme, Thyme Vitality, Idaho Blue Spruce, Basil, Basil Vitality, Frankincense, Frankincense Vitality, Sacred Frankin-cense, Rosemary, Rosemary Vitality, Copaiba, Copaiba Vitality

Blends: Cool Azul, Aroma Siez, Relieve It, PanAway, Deep Relief Roll-On, CBD

Nutritionals: Sulfurzyme, PowerGize, Super Vitamin B, Essentialzyme, Master Formula, OmegaGize3, Mega Vitamin Cal, Mineral Essence

Note: Sulfurzyme, Super Vitamin B, and OmegaGize3 work well together to help rebuild nerve damage and the myelin sheath.

Personal Care: Cool Azul Pain Relief Cream, Cool Azul Sports Gel, CBD Muscle Rub, Regenolone Moisturizing Cream, Ortho Sport Massage Oil, Ortho Ease Massage Oil

Application and Usage

Topical: Refer to Application Guidelines.

- Apply 6-10 drops diluted 50:50 on location 2 times daily or as needed.

- Place a warm compress on affected area 1-2 times daily; cold compress if inflamed.

- Massage 2-3 drops into Vita Flex points of the feet 2-4 times daily.

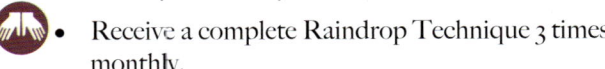
- Receive a complete Raindrop Technique 3 times monthly.

- Walk backwards for 20 minutes daily with no shoes.

Scoliosis

Scoliosis is an abnormal lateral or side-to-side curvature or twist in the spine. It is different from hyperkyphosis (hunch-back) or hyperlordosis (swayback), which involve excessive front-to-back accentuation of existing spine curvatures.

While some cases of scoliosis can be attributed to congenital deformities such as MS, cerebral palsy, Down syndrome, or Marfan syndrome, the vast majority of scoliosis types are of unknown origin.

Some medical professionals believe that scoliosis may be caused by persistent muscle spasms that pull the vertebrae of the spine out of alignment. Others feel—and there is a growing body of research documenting this hypothesis—that it begins with hard-to-detect inflammation along the spine caused by latent viruses.

> ### Pointer Technique for Nerve Damage
>
> The Pointer Technique uses a small, pen-shaped instrument with a rounded end to stimulate specific locations on the skin after the essential oils have been applied to the area. It works very well on the Vita Flex points of the foot but may cause quite a tickling sensation. The pointer stimulation promotes greater blood flow to a particular area, increasing the nutrient supply and healing properties.
>
> If there is nerve damage, apply 4-6 drops of Peppermint, or other desired oil, along the spine. Use a gentle rocking motion on the tissue between each vertebra, between each rib on the vertebra, with knuckles starting at the base of the spine and working all the way up on each side of the spine to the neck. Use medium pressure with the rocking motion for 1-10 seconds at each location. Then follow the same procedure once more along the spine next to each vertebra.

Symptoms
- When bending forward, the left side of the back is higher or lower than the right side (the patient must be viewed from the rear).
- One hip may appear to be higher or more prominent than the other.
- Shoulders or scapulas (shoulder blades) appear uneven.
- When the arms are hanging loosely, the distance between the left arm and left side is different than the distance between the right arm and right side.

The Raindrop Technique is proving to be an effective therapy for helping scoliosis, easing pain, and reducing misalignment.

Recommendations

Singles: Oregano, Oregano Vitality, Ecuadorian Oregano, Thyme, Thyme Vitality, Basil, Basil Vitality, Melissa, Winter-green, Frankincense, Frankincense Vitality, Sacred Frankincense, Cypress, Marjoram, Marjoram Vitality, Peppermint, Peppermint Vitality

Blends: Valor, Valor Roll-On, Aroma Siez, PanAway, Cool Azul, Deep Relief Roll-On, CBD

Nutritionals: PowerGize, Mineral Essence, Mega Vitamin Cal, Super Vitamin D, AminoWise, Pure Protein Complete, Protein Power Bites, Slique Shake, Sulfurzyme, BLM, AgilEase, Master Formula, NingXia Red

Personal Care: Cool Azul Pain Relief Cream, Cool Azul Sports Gel, CBD Muscle Rub, Ortho Ease Massage Oil, Ortho Sport Massage Oil

Application and Usage
Topical: Refer to Application Guidelines

 • Apply 3-6 drops diluted 50:50 along the spine daily or as needed.

 • Receive a Raindrop Technique 2-3 times a week.

SPRAIN

A sprain is an injury to a ligament caused by excessive stretching. The ligament can have a partial tear or be completely torn apart. Sprained ligaments swell rapidly and are painful. Usually, the greater the pain, the more severe the injury is.

Recommendations

Singles: Basil, Basil Vitality, Dorado Azul, Idaho Blue Spruce, Peppermint, Peppermint Vitality, Copaiba, Copaiba Vitality, Idaho Grand Fir, Helichrysum, Wintergreen, Kunzea

Blends: PanAway, Cool Azul, Relieve It, Aroma Siez, Deep Relief Roll-On, CBD

Nutritionals: PowerGize, BLM, AgilEase, Super Vitamin D, AminoWise, Pure Protein Complete, Protein Power Bites, Sulfurzyme, Mineral Essence, Mega Vitamin Cal, Essentialzyme, Super Vitamin C, Slique Shake, Super Vitamin B

Personal Care: Cool Azul Pain Relief Cream, Cool Azul Sports Gel, CBD Muscle Rub, Prenolone Plus Body Cream, Ortho Sport Massage Oil, Ortho Ease Massage Oil

Application and Usage

Topical: Refer to Application Guidelines.

- Apply 4-6 drops diluted 50:50 on location 3-5 times daily.

- Place a cold compress on location 2 times daily.

STRESS

Stress can be either good or bad. However, long-term stressful situations can produce a lasting, low-level stress that's hard on people. The nervous system pumps out extra stress hormones over an extended period, which can wear out the body's reserves and the adrenals, leaving a person feeling depleted or overwhelmed, weakening the body's immune system, and causing other problems. Getting plenty of sleep should help ease negative stress.

Recommendations

Singles: Lavender, Lavender Vitality, Roman Chamomile, Blue Tansy, Cedarwood, Marjoram, Marjoram Vitality, Rose, Sa-cred Sandalwood, Royal Hawaiian Sandalwood, Sacred Frankincense, Frankincense, Frankincense Vitality, Davana, Valerian, Bergamot, Vanilla, Sage, Sage Vitality

Blends: Valor, Valor Roll-On, Gary's Light, Peace & Calming, Peace & Calming II, KidScents KidPower, KidScents KidPower Roll-On, One Heart, Tranquil Roll-On, Trauma Life, Calm CBD Roll-On, Seedlings Calm, Humility, Har-mony, RutaVaLa, RutaVaLa Roll-On, The Gift, Common Sense

Nutritionals: Super Vitamin B, Super Vitamin C, MultiGreens, ImmuPro, SleepEssence, Master Formula, Mega Vitamin Cal, OmegaGize3, MindWise, CortiStop Women's

Application and Usage

Aromatic: Refer to Application Guidelines.

Dietary and Oral: Refer to Application Guidelines.

- Take 1 capsule of desired Vitality oil 2 times daily.

- Take 2-3 drops of desired Vitality oil in a spoonful of syrup or small amount of milk, juice, or water.

Topical: Refer to Application Guidelines.

- Dilute 50:50 and apply on temples, neck, and shoulders 2 times daily or as needed.
- Use bath salts daily.

STROKES

Two principal kinds of strokes can damage the brain: hemorrhagic strokes and thrombotic strokes.

Some essential oils can be used topically to help strengthen the integrity of capillary walls. In particular, the essential oils of Helichrysum, Cistus, and Nutmeg are known to have anticlotting properties and can be used as a preventive measure to reduce the risk of thrombotic stroke.

Hemorrhagic Strokes

A hemorrhagic stroke is caused by an aneurysm or a weakness in the blood vessel wall that balloons out and ruptures, spilling blood into the surrounding brain tissue. Strokes are very serious events, and if you suspect that you may be susceptible, immediately see a health care professional.

Recommendations

Singles: Cypress, Cistus, Helichrysum, Nutmeg, Nutmeg Vitality, Royal Hawaiian Sandalwood, Sacred Sandalwood

Blends: Brain Power, Common Sense, Clarity, KidScents GeneYus, Longevity, Longevity Vitality, Stress Away, Stress Away Roll-On, Peace & Calming, Peace & Calming II, Calm CBD Roll-On, Seedlings Calm

Nutritionals: Sulfurzyme, MindWise, Mega Vitamin Cal, Mineral Essence, Essentialzyme, Rehemogen, Master Formula, NingXia Red

Application and Usage

Aromatic: Refer to Application Guidelines.

Dietary and Oral: Refer to Application Guidelines.

- Take 1 capsule with Helichrysum or other desired Vitality oil 2 times daily.

- Take 1-2 capsules 50:50 with Helichrysum and Cistus 2 times daily.

- Take 2-3 drops of desired Vitality oil in a spoonful of syrup or small amount of milk, juice, or water.

Topical: Refer to Application Guidelines.

- Apply 1-3 drops, diluted 50:50, on temples,

forehead, mastoids, back of neck, and at base of throat just above clavicle notch.

- Applying a single drop under the nose is helpful and refreshing.

- Massage 2-4 drops of oil neat on Vita Flex brain points on the bottoms of the feet just before bedtime.

Thrombotic Strokes

Thrombotic strokes are caused by a blood clot lodging in a cerebral blood vessel and cutting blood supply to a part of the brain.

Recommendations

Singles: Helichrysum, Cistus, Nutmeg, Nutmeg Vitality, Cypress, Royal Hawaiian Sandalwood, Sacred Sandalwood, Juniper, Grapefruit, Grapefruit Vitality, Orange, Orange Vitality, Clove, Clove Vitality

Blends: Longevity, Aroma Life, JuvaCleanse, JuvaCleanse Vitality

Nutritionals: Sulfurzyme, Mega Vitamin Cal, OmegaGize3, MindWise, Essentialzyme, AminoWise, Pure Protein Complete, Protein Power Bites, Master Formula, Mineral Essence, Essentialzymes-4, Slique Shake, Slique Bars, Slique CitraSlim, NingXia Red

These supplements are rich in essential minerals, fatty acids, and nutrients necessary for regenerating and rebuilding damaged nerve tissues.

Application and Usage

Aromatic: Refer to Application Guidelines.

Topical: Refer to Application Guidelines.

- Applying the essential oil of Cypress may help strengthen vascular walls.

- You may apply single oils or Blends neat or diluted, depending on the oils that are used.

- Apply 1-2 drops neat on temples and back of neck as desired.

- Applying a single drop under the nose is helpful and refreshing.

- Massage 2-4 drops of oil neat on the bottoms of the feet just before bedtime.

> ### See the Whole Picture to Product the Best Results
>
> When selecting oils, particularly for injuries, think through the cause and type of injury and then select oils for each segment. For instance, a broken bone could encompass muscle damage, nerve damage, ligament strain or tear, inflammation, infection, and bone injury. The emotion of shock, anger, guilt, or suffering from long-time pain is another dimension of the injury that needs to be dealt with through understanding and help on an emotional level. All factors of the injury need to be considered in order to choose the oils that would offer the most benefits. Select the single oils for each perceived problem, or select a blend that may address all of the needs, and then apply gently in a rotating motion. It would be best to apply the oils first to the feet using the Vita Flex Technique, if that is possible.

THROAT INFECTIONS AND PROBLEMS
(See also COLDS; INFECTIONS . . .; LUNG INFECTIONS AND PROBLEMS, COUGHS, CONGESTIVE and DRY)

Throat infection is one of the most common conditions in the world. It is broadly divided into two types, viral and bacterial.

Laryngitis

Laryngitis is inflammation and swelling of the larynx, also known as the voice box. Laryngitis is usually caused by a virus, sometimes caused by a bacterial infection, or occurs in people who overuse their voice. While Longevity contains oils that protect DNA, it also has two highly antibacterial oils: Thyme and Clove, making it valuable for bacterial infections.

Recommendations

Singles: Eucalyptus Radiata, Jade Lemon, Jade Lemon Vitality, Lemon, Lemon Vitality, Lime, Lime Vitality, Eucalyptus Blue, Palo Santo, Oregano, Oregano Vitality, Ecuadorian Oregano, Sacred Frankincense, Frankincense, Frankincense Vitality, Ravintsara, Thyme, Thyme Vitality, Clove, Clove Vitality, Myrrh, Cedarwood, Eucalyptus Globulus, Davana, Northern Lights Black Spruce, Peppermint, Peppermint Vitality, Davana

Blends: R.C., Thieves, Thieves Roll-On, Thieves Vitality, Longevity, Longevity Vitality, Melrose, Raven, Purification, Exodus II, Breathe Again, Breathe Again Roll-On

Nutritionals: Longevity Softgels, Super Vitamin C, Super Vitamin C Chewable, MultiGreens, ImmuPro, OmegaGize3

Oral Care: Thieves Cough Drops, Thieves Spray, Thieves Fresh Essence Plus Mouthwash, Thieves Hard Lozenges, Thieves Mints

Personal Care: Thieves Chest Rub

Application and Usage

Aromatic: Refer to Application Guidelines.

- Receive a Raindrop Technique 2-3 times weekly.

Dietary and Oral: Refer to Application Guidelines.

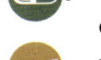
- Take 1 capsule of desired Vitality oil 2 times daily.

- Take 2-3 drops of desired Vitality oil in a spoonful of syrup or small amount of milk, juice, or water.

- Put 2 drops of Longevity Vitality and 1 drop of Lemon Vitality in ½ teaspoon of Yacon Syrup, maple syrup, etc., hold in the back of the mouth for 1-2 minutes, and then swallow. Repeat as needed.

- Place a few drops on or under your tongue 2-6 times daily or as often as needed.

- Gargle with a mixture of Vitality essential oils and water 4-8 times daily.

- Spray throat with Thieves Spray as often as desired.

- Gargle with Thieves Fresh Essence Plus Mouthwash as needed.

- Dissolve Thieves Cough Drops or Thieves Hard Lozenges in your mouth as desired.

Topical: Refer to Application Guidelines.

- Apply 1-3 drops diluted 50:50 to throat, chest, and back of neck 2-4 times daily.

- Apply 1-3 drops of selected oil to lung Vita Flex points of the feet 1-3 times daily.

Sore Throat

Sore throats are caused by many things, such as viruses, bacteria, smoking, polluted air, and allergies to pet dander, pollens, and molds.

Recommendations

Singles: Tea Tree, Ravintsara, Cypress, Eucalyptus Radiata, Eucalyptus Globulus, Jade Lemon, Jade Lemon Vitality, Lemon, Lemon Vitality, Lime, Lime Vitality, Sacred Frankincense, Frankincense, Frankincense Vitality, Thyme, Thyme Vitality, Oregano, Oregano Vitality, Ecuadorian Oregano, Northern Lights Black Spruce, Peppermint, Peppermint Vitality, Myrrh, Wintergreen

Blends: Thieves, Thieves Roll-On, Thieves Vitality, Longevity, Longevity Vitality, Melrose, Raven, ImmuPower, R.C.

Nutritionals: Inner Defense, Super Vitamin C, Super Vitamin C Chewable, ImmuPro, Longevity Softgels, OmegaGize3

Oral Care: Thieves Cough Drops, Thieves Hard Lozenges, Thieves Fresh Essence Mouthwash, Thieves Spray, Thieves Mints

Personal Care: Thieves Chest Rub

Application and Usage

Aromatic: Refer to Application Guidelines.

Dietary and Oral: Refer to Application Guidelines.

- Take 1 capsule of desired Vitality oil 2 times daily.

- Take 2-3 drops of desired Vitality oil in a spoonful of syrup or small amount of milk, juice, or water.

- Place a drop of desired Vitality on or under the tongue 2-6 times daily or as often as needed.

- Gargle 4-8 times daily with a mixture of essential oils and water.

- Dissolve Thieves Cough Drops or Thieves Hard Lozenges in your mouth as desired.

Topical: Refer to Application Guidelines.

- Apply 1-3 drops diluted 50:50 to the throat, chest, and back of the neck 2-4 times daily.

- Apply 1-3 drops on the lung Vita Flex points of the foot 1-3 times daily.

- Receive a Raindrop Technique weekly.

- Place a warm compress with 1-2 drops of chosen oil on the throat and chest area 2-3 times daily

Sore Throat Blend No. 1
- 2 drops Thyme Vitality
- 2 drops Cypress
- 1 drop Eucalyptus Radiata
- 1 drop Peppermint Vitality
- 1 drop Myrrh
- 1 teaspoon honey

Sore Throat Blend No. 1
- 5 drops Lemon Vitality
- 2 drops Eucalyptus Globulus
- 2 drops Wintergreen
- 1 drop Peppermint Vitality

Strep Throat
Strep throat is a bacterial throat infection caused by Group A streptococcus and is generally more severe than a viral throat infection. If left untreated, strep throat can lead to kidney inflammation and rheumatic fever.

Recommendations
Singles: Oregano, Oregano Vitality, Ecuadorian Oregano, Thyme, Thyme Vitality, Eucalyptus Globulus, Sacred Frankincense, Frankincense, Frankincense Vitality, Lavender, Lavender Vitality, Myrrh, Dorado Azul, Eucalyptus Blue, Mountain Savory, Mountain Savory Vitality, Clove, Clove Vitality, Cinnamon Bark, Cinnamon Bark Vitality

Blends: Thieves, Thieves Roll-On, Thieves Vitality, Exodus II, Melrose, Longevity, Longevity Vitality, Raven, R.C., ImmuPower

Nutritionals: Inner Defense, ImmuPro, Super Vitamin C, Longevity Softgels, Super Vitamin C Chewable, MultiGreens, ICP, ComforTone, Essentialzyme, Life 9, KidScents MightyPro, OmegaGize3

Oral: Thieves Spray, Thieves Cough Drops, Thieves Hard Lozenges, Thieves Fresh Essence Mouthwash, Thieves Mints

Personal Care: Thieves Chest Rub

Application and Usage
Aromatic: Refer to Application Guidelines.

Dietary and Oral: Refer to Application Guidelines.

- Take 1 capsule of desired Vitality oil 2 times daily.

- Take 2-3 drops of desired Vitality oil in a spoonful of syrup or small amount of milk, juice, or water.

- Place a drop of desired Vitality oil on or under the tongue 2-6 times daily or as often as needed.

- Gargle with a mixture of essential oils and water 4-8 times daily.
- Spray throat with Thieves Spray as often as desired.
- Dissolve Thieves Cough Drops or Thieves Hard Lozenges in your mouth as desired.

Topical: Refer to Application Guidelines.

- Apply 1-3 drops diluted 50:50 to the throat, chest, and back of the neck 2-4 times daily.

- You may also apply 1-3 drops on the lung Vita Flex points of the foot 1-3 times daily.

- Place a warm compress with 1-2 drops of chosen oil on the throat and chest area 2-3 times daily.

- Receive a Raindrop Technique weekly.

Strep Throat Blend
- 6 drops Lavender Vitality
- 2 drops Oregano Vitality
- 1 drop Cinnamon Bark Vitality
- 1 drop Thyme Vitality

Regimen for Strep Throat
- ImmuPro: Take 1-2 before going to bed. Do not exceed 2 daily.
- Longevity Softgels: Take 2-4 softgels daily.
- Super Vitamin C: Take 2-3 tablets 2 times daily or chew Super Vitamin C Chewable as desired.
- Receive a Raindrop Technique with ImmuPower and/or Exodus II along sides of spine weekly.
- Spray throat with Thieves Spray every 2 hours.

Tonsillitis
The tonsils are infection-fighting lymphatic tissues at the back of the throat. When they become infected with streptococcal bacteria, they become inflamed, causing a condition known as tonsillitis.

It became popular in the 1960's and 1970's to have the tonsils removed when they became infected. However, tonsillectomies have become much less frequent, as researchers have discovered the important role tonsils play in protecting and fighting infectious diseases and optimizing immune response.

The pharyngeal tonsils located at the back of the throat (known as the adenoids) can also become infected—a condition known as adenoiditis.

Recommendations

Singles: Clove, Clove Vitality, Tea Tree, Myrrh, Dorado Azul, Cassia, Goldenrod, Oregano, Oregano Vitality, Ecuadorian Oregano, Mountain Savory, Mountain Savory Vitality, Ravintsara, Thyme, Thyme Vitality

Blends: Thieves, Thieves Roll-On, Thieves Vitality, Melrose, Exodus II, Longevity, Longevity Vitality, ImmuPower

Nutritionals: Inner Defense, ImmuPro, Super Vitamin C Chewable, Super Vitamin C, Detoxzyme, Mineral Essence

Oral Care: Thieves Spray, Thieves Cough Drops, Thieves Fresh Essence Mouthwash, Thieves Hard Lozenges, Thieves Mints

Personal Care: Thieves Chest Rub

Application and Usage

Aromatic: Refer to Application Guidelines.

Dietary and Oral: Refer to Application Guidelines.

- Take 1 capsule of desired Vitality oil 2 times daily.

- Take 2-3 drops of desired Vitality oil in a spoonful of syrup or small amount of milk, juice, or water.

- Place a drop of desired Vitality oil on or under the tongue 2-6 times daily or as often as needed.
- Gargle a mixture of Vitality essential oils and water 4-8 times daily.
- Dissolve Thieves Cough Drops or Thieves Hard Lozenges in your mouth as desired.

Topical: Refer to Application Guidelines.

- Apply 1-3 drops diluted 50:50 to the throat, chest, and back of the neck 2-4 times daily.

- You may also apply 1-3 drops on the lung Vita Flex points of the feet 1-3 times daily.

- Place a warm compress with 1-2 drops of chosen oil on the throat and chest area 2-3 times daily.
- Use the Raindrop Technique weekly.

NARCOLEPSY, MALE HORMONE IMBALANCE, MENSTRUAL AND FEMALE HORMONE CONDITIONS)

The thyroid is the energy gland of the human body and produces T_3 and T_4 thyroid hormones that control the body's metabolism. The thyroid also controls other vital functions such as digestion, circulation, immune function, hormone bal-ance, and emotions.

The thyroid gland is controlled by the pituitary gland, which signals the thyroid when to produce the thyroid hormone.

The hypothalamus gland sends chemical signals to the pituitary gland to monitor hormone levels in the blood stream.

A lack of the thyroid hormone does not necessarily mean that the thyroid is not functioning properly. In some instances, the pituitary gland may be malfunctioning because of its failure to release sufficient TSH (thyroid stimulating hormone) to stimulate the thyroid to make thyroid hormones.

Other cases of thyroid hormone deficiency may be due to the hypothalamus failing to release sufficient TRH (thyrotropin-releasing hormone).

In cases where thyroid hormone deficiency is caused by a malfunctioning pituitary or hypothalamus, supplements or essential oils such as Cedarwood may help stimulate the pituitary or hypothalamus.

People with type-A blood have more of a tendency to have weak thyroid function.

Hyperthyroid (Graves' Disease)

When the thyroid becomes overactive and produces excess thyroid hormone, the following symptoms may occur:
- Anxiety
- Restlessness
- Insomnia
- Premature gray hair
- Diabetes mellitus
- Arthritis
- Vitiligo (loss of skin pigment)

Graves' disease, unlike Hashimoto's disease, is an autoimmune disease that results in an excess of thyroid hormone production. MSM has been studied for its ability to reverse many kinds of autoimmune diseases. MSM is a key component of Sulfurzyme.

Recommendations

Singles: Myrrh, Idaho Blue Spruce, Lemongrass, Lemongrass Vitality, Wintergreen, German Chamomile, German Chamomile Vitality, Bergamot, Bergamot Vitality, Cedarwood, 25 Years Young

Blends: EndoFlex, EndoFlex Vitality, Brain Power, Clarity, Common Sense

Nutritionals: Sulfurzyme, MultiGreens, Mineral Essence, Mega Vitamin Cal, MindWise, Essentialzyme, Detoxzyme, Essentialzymes-4, Life 9, KidScents MightyPro, OmegaGize3, Thyromin (only in the morning)

Application and Usage

Aromatic: Refer to Application Guidelines.

Dietary and Oral: Refer to Application Guidelines.

- Take 1 capsule of desired Vitality oil 2 times daily.

- Take 2-3 drops of desired Vitality oil in a spoonful of syrup or small amount of milk, juice, or water.

Topical: Refer to Application Guidelines.

Hypoglycemia

Hypoglycemia may be caused by low thyroid function. Excessive consumption of sugar or honey will also cause reactive hypoglycemia, in which a rapid rise in blood sugar is followed by a steep drop to abnormally low levels.

In some cases, hypoglycemia may be a precursor to candida, allergies, chronic fatigue syndrome, depression, or chemical sensitivities.

Signs of hypoglycemia (low blood sugar) include:
- Fatigue, drowsiness, and sleepiness after meals
- Headache or dizziness if times between meals are too long
- Craving for sweets
- Allergic reaction to foods
- Palpitations, tremors, sweats, rapid heartbeat
- Inattentiveness, mood swings, irritability, anxiety, nervousness, inability to cope with stress, and feelings of emotional depression
- Lack of motivation, discipline, and creativity
- Hunger that cannot be satisfied

Often people with some of these symptoms are misdiagnosed as suffering either chronic fatigue or neurosis. Instead, they may be hypoglycemic.

To treat chronic hypoglycemia, it is important to treat the underlying cause, such as candida or yeast overgrowth (See also FUNGAL (YEAST) INFECTIONS).

Essential oils may reduce hypoglycemic symptoms by helping to normalize sugar cravings, supporting and stabilizing sugar metabolism in the body.

Recommendations

Singles: Lavender, Lavender Vitality, Coriander, Coriander Vitality, Dill, Dill Vitality, Fennel, Fennel Vitality, Cinnamon Bark, Cinnamon Bark Vitality, Davana

Nutritionals: MultiGreens, NingXia Red, Life 9, KidScents MightyPro, Digest & Cleanse, Essentialzyme, Essentialzymes-4, ICP, JuvaPower, Ningxia Wolfberries (Organic, Dried)

Application and Usage

Aromatic: Refer to Application Guidelines.

Dietary and Oral: Refer to Application Guidelines.

- Take 1 capsule of desired oil 1 time daily (Coriander Vitality, Dill Vitality, and Fennel Vitality work best through ingestion).

- Take 2-3 drops of desired Vitality oil in a spoonful of syrup or small amount of milk, juice, or water.

Topical: Refer to Application Guidelines.

- Rub 1-2 drops of oil on the temples and back of neck several times daily.

- Place a warm compress with 1-2 drops of chosen oil on the back.

Hypothyroid (Hashimoto's Disease)

This condition occurs when the thyroid is underactive and produces insufficient thyroid hormone. Approximately 40 percent of the U.S. population suffers from milder forms of this disorder to some degree, and these people tend to suffer from hypoglycemia (low blood sugar). In its severe form, it is referred to as Hashimoto's disease.

Hashimoto's disease, like Graves' disease, is an autoimmune condition that affects the thyroid differently, however, by limiting its ability to produce thyroid hormone.

The following symptoms may occur:
- Fatigue
- Yeast infections (candida)
- Lack of energy
- Reduced immune function
- Poor resistance to disease
- Recurring infections
- Low sex hormones

Recommendations

Singles: Lemongrass, Lemongrass Vitality, Spearmint, Spearmint Vitality, Ledum, Myrtle, Peppermint, Peppermint Vitality, Myrrh, Clove, Clove Vitality

Blends: EndoFlex, EndoFlex Vitality, Brain Power, Clarity, 25 Years Young

Nutritionals: Thyromin, MultiGreens, Sulfurzyme, Essentialzyme, Essentialzymes-4, Life 9, KidScents MightyPro, De-toxzyme, Mega Vitamin Cal, MindWise

Application and Usage

Aromatic: Refer to Application Guidelines.

Dietary and Oral: Refer to Application Guidelines.

- Take 1 capsule of desired Vitality oil 2 times daily.

- Take 2-3 drops of desired Vitality oil in a spoonful of syrup or small amount of milk, juice, or water.

Topical: Refer to Application Guidelines.

- Apply 3-5 drops neat or diluted 50:50 over the thyroid, the front of the neck, and on both sides of the trachea 1-3 times daily.

- Apply 1-3 drops on the thyroid Vita Flex points of the feet located on the inside edge of the ball of the foot just below the base of the big toe.

TOXEMIA

Toxins or bacteria that accumulate in the bloodstream create a condition called toxemia.

Recommendations

Singles: Clove, Clove Vitality, Tangerine, Tangerine Vitality, Jade Lemon, Jade Lemon Vitality, Lemon, Lemon Vitality, Lime, Lime Vitality, Cypress, Orange, Orange Vitality, Patchouli

Blends: Purification, Thieves, Thieves Roll-On, Thieves Vitality, Melrose, Citrus Fresh, Citrus Fresh Vitality

Nutritionals: Rehemogen, ICP, ComforTone, Essentialzyme, Essentialzymes-4, Life 9, KidScents MightyPro, Super Vitamin C, JuvaTone, JuvaPower, Detoxzyme, Super Vitamin C Chewable

Application and Usage

Aromatic: Refer to Application Guidelines.

Dietary and Oral: Refer to Application Guidelines.

- Take 1 capsule of desired Vitality oil 3 times daily.

- Take 2-3 drops of desired Vitality oil in a spoonful of syrup or small amount of milk, juice, or water.

- Best results may be achieved by eliminating certain foods, such as all sugar, white flour, breads, pasta, fried foods, and chlorinated water.

Topical: Refer to Application Guidelines.

- Dilute 50:50 and apply on location 2-3 times daily or as needed.

- Massage 2-4 drops of oil neat on the bottoms of the feet just before bedtime.

TRAUMA, EMOTIONAL

Emotional trauma can be generated from events that involve loss, abuse, bereavement, accidents, or misfortunes. The volatile aromatic compounds of essential oils have the ability to cross the blood-brain barrier, simulating the amygdala that controls the emotional and memory center of the brain. Certain essential oils help facilitate the processing and release of emotional trauma in a simple way that minimizes psychological turmoil.

Recommendations

Singles: Sacred Frankincense, Frankincense, Frankincense Vitality, Idaho Blue Spruce, Idaho Grand Fir, Northern Lights Black Spruce, Royal Hawaiian Sandalwood, Sacred Sandalwood, Lemon Verbena, Rose, Cassia, Palo Santo, Cedarwood

Blends: Freedom, The Gift, Trauma Life, Gary's Light, One Heart, Peace & Calming, Peace & Calming II, Calm CBD Roll-On, Seedlings Calm, KidScents KidPower, KidScents KidPower Roll-On, Hope, RutaVaLa, RutaVaLa Roll-On, Harmony, Reconnect, Gathering, Amoressence, Forgiveness, Release, Envision, My Destiny, Build Your Dream, Valor, Valor Roll-On, Joy, Fulfill Your Destiny, Highest Potential, 3 Wise Men, Sacred Mountain

Nutritionals: Super Vitamin C, Super Vitamin C Chewable, Mineral Essence, KidScents Unwind, Mega Vitamin Cal, Es-sentialzyme, Essentialzymes-4, Life 9, KidScents MightyPro, OmegaGize3, Balance Complete, Pure Protein Complete, NingXia Red

Application and Usage

Aromatic: Refer to Application Guidelines.

Topical: Refer to Application Guidelines.

- Apply 2-4 drops of oil diluted 50:50 or neat to the temples, forehead, crown, and shoulders 1-3 times daily.

TRIGGER FINGER (STENOSING TENOSYNOVITIS)

Tendonitis, often called "tennis elbow" and "golfer's elbow," is a torn or inflamed tendon. Tenosynovitis, sometimes called "trigger finger," is an inflamed tendon being restricted by its sheath (particularly in thumbs and fingers). Repetitive use or infection may be the cause.

When selecting oils for injuries, think through the cause and type of injury and select appropriate oils. For instance, tendonitis could encompass muscle damage, nerve damage, ligament strain/tear, inflammation, infection, and possibly an emotion. The emotional distress may be anger or guilt.

Therefore, select a single oil or blend for each potential cause or to address multiple causes.

Recommendations

Singles: Lemongrass (promotes the repair of connective tissue), Lemongrass Vitality. Royal Hawaiian Sandalwood, Sacred Sandalwood, Helichrysum, Frankincense, Frankincense Vitality, Lavender, Lavender Vitality, Marjoram, Marjoram Vitality

Blends: Cool Azul, PanAway, Relieve It, Aroma Siez, Deep Relief Roll-On, CBD

Nutritionals: Mega Vitamin Cal, BLM, AgilEase, Super Vitamin D, Sulfurzyme, AminoWise, Pure Protein Complete, Protein Power Bites

- Mega Vitamin Cal builds and strengthens bones. Mix 1 teaspoon in water and drink. Taken at night, Mega Vitamin Cal promotes peaceful sleep.
- BLM and AgilEase provide critical nutrients for connective tissue and muscle repair and strengthens the bones. Take 1 capsule 1-3 times daily.
- Sulfurzyme equalizes water pressure inside the cells and reduces pain. Mix 1-2 teaspoons in water and drink 2 times daily.

Personal Care: Cool Azul Pain Relief Cream, Cool Azul Sports Gel, CBD Muscle Rub, Ortho Sport Massage Oil, Ortho Ease Massage Oil

The oils in the Personal Care products reduce pain and promote healing.

Application and Usage

Aromatic: Refer to Application Guidelines.

Topical: Refer to Application Guidelines.

- Massage finger with Lavender and Lemongrass.
- Massage Marjoram with Lemongrass for inflamed tendons.
- Single oils or Blends may be used singularly or together.

TYPHOID FEVER

Typhoid fever is an infectious disease caused by a bacterium known as Salmonella typhi. Usually contracted through infected food or water, typhoid is common in lesser-developed countries.

Some people infected with typhoid fever display no visible symptoms of disease, while others become seriously ill. Both people who recover from typhoid fever and those who remain symptomless are carriers for the disease and can infect others through the bacteria they shed in their feces.

To avoid contracting typhoid fever—especially when traveling overseas—it is essential to drink purified or distilled water and to thoroughly cook foods. Fresh vegetables can be carriers of the bacteria, especially if they have been irrigated with water that has come into contact with human waste.

Symptoms:
- Sustained, high fever (101° to 104°F)
- Stomach pains
- Headache
- Rash of reddish spots
- Impaired appetite
- Weakness

Recommendations

Singles: Clove, Clove Vitality, Thyme, Thyme Vitality, Ravintsara, Cinnamon Bark, Cinnamon Bark Vitality, Cassia, Pep-permint, Peppermint Vitality, Black Pepper, Black Pepper Vitality, Mountain Savory, Mountain Savory Vitality, Oregano, Oregano Vitality, Ecuadorian Oregano, Tea Tree

Blends: Thieves, Thieves Roll-On, Thieves Vitality, Melrose, Exodus II

Nutritionals: Inner Defense, ImmuPro, Super Vitamin C, Super Vitamin C Chewable, NingXia Red

Application and Usage

Aromatic: Refer to Application Guidelines.

Dietary and Oral: Refer to Application Guidelines.

 • Take 1 capsule of desired Vitality oil 2 times daily for 10 days.

 • Take 2-3 drops of desired Vitality oil in a spoonful of syrup or small amount of milk, juice, or water.

Topical: Refer to Application Guidelines.

 • Apply 4-6 drops of oil diluted 50:50 on lower abdomen 2-4 times daily.

YEAST INFECTIONS
(See FUNGAL (YEAST) INFECTIONS)

Appendix A
Common and Botanical Plant Names

Botanical Name First

Abies balsamea .... Idaho Balsam Fir (Balsam Canada)
Abies concolor .... White Fir
Achillea millefolium .... Yarrow
Acorus calamus .... Calamus
Anethum graveolens .... Dill
Anethum graveolens .... Dill Vitality
Angelica archangelica .... Angelica
Anthemis nobilis .... Roman Chamomile
Apium graveolens .... Celery Seed
Apium graveolens .... Celery Seed Vitality
Artemisia dracunculus .... Tarragon
Artemisia dracunculus .... Tarragon Vitality
Artemisia pallens .... Davana
Backhousia citriodora .... Lemon Myrtle
Boswellia carterii .... Frankincense
Boswellia carterii .... Frankincense Vitality
Boswellia frereana .... Frereana Frankincense
Boswellia sacra .... Sacred Frankincense
Bursera graveolens .... Palo Santo
Callitris columellaris .... White Cypress Pine
Callitris intratropica .... Blue Cypress
Cananga odorata .... Ylang Ylang
Cananga odorata Equitoriana .... Amazonian Ylang Ylang
Canarium luzonicum .... Elemi
Cedrus atlantica .... Cedarwood
Chamaecyparis formosensis .... Hong Kuai
Chamaecyparis obtusa .... Hinoki
Chamaemelum nobile .... Roman Chamomile
Chamomilla recutita .... German Chamomile (Matricaria)
Cinnamomum aromaticum .... Cassia
Cinnamomum camphora .... Ravintsara
Cinnamomum verum .... Cinnamon Bark Vitality
Cinnamomum zeylanicum (Syn. *C. verum*) ...... Cinnamon Bark
Cistus ladanifer (Syn. *C. ladaniferus*) .... Cistus
Cistus ladaniferus .... Rose of Sharon (Cistus)
Citrus aurantifolia .... Lime
Citrus aurantifolia .... Lime Vitality
Citrus aurantium amara .... Neroli (Bitter Orange)
Citrus aurantium amara .... Petitgrain
Citrus aurantium bergamia .... Bergamot
Citrus aurantium bergamia .... Bergamot Vitality
Citrus aurantium dulcis .... Sweet Orange
Citrus hystrix .... Citrus Hystrix
Citrus junos .... Yuzu
Citrus limon .... Lemon
Citrus limon .... Lemon Vitality
Citrus limon eureka var. *formosensis* .... Jade Lemon
Citrus limon eureka var. *formosensis* .... Jade Lemon Vitality
Citrus paradisi .... Grapefruit

Citrus paradisi .... Grapefruit Vitality
Citrus reticulata .... Mandarin
Citrus reticulata .... Tangerine
Citrus reticulata .... Tangerine Vitality
Citrus sinensis .... Orange
Commiphora erythraea .... Biblical Sweet Myrrh
Commiphora gileadensis .... Balm of Gilead
Commiphora myrrha .... Myrrh
Conyza canadensis .... Canadian Fleabane
Copaifera officinalis .... Copaiba (Balsam Copaiba)
Copaifera officinalis .... Copaiba Vitality
Coriandrum sativum .... Coriander
Coriandrum sativum .... Coriander Vitality
Cuminum cyminum .... Cumin
Cupressus sempervirens .... Cypress
Cymbopogon citratus .... Xiang Mao
Cymbopogon flexuosus .... Lemongrass
Cymbopogon flexuosus .... Lemongrass Vitality
Cymbopogon martini .... Palmarosa
Cymbopogon nardus .... Citronella
Cymbopogon winterianus, Java Type .... Citronella
Daucus carota .... Carrot Seed
Daucus carota .... Carrot Seed Vitality
Dorado Azul Guayfolius officinalis ...... Dorado Azul (Ecuador)
Elettaria cardamomum .... Cardamom
Elettaria cardamomum .... Cardamom Vitality
Eucalyptus bicostata .... Eucalyptus Blue
Eucalyptus citriodora .... Eucalyptus Citriodora
Eucalyptus globulus .... Eucalyptus Globulus
Eucalyptus radiata .... Eucalyptus Radiata
Eucalyptus staigeriana .... Eucalyptus Staigeriana
Eugenia caryophyllus .... Clove
Ferula galbaniflua .... Galbanum
Foeniculum vulgare .... Fennel
Foeniculum vulgare .... Fennel Vitality
Gaultheria procumbens .... Wintergreen
Helichrysum italicum .... Helichrysum
Hyptis suaveolens .... Dorado Azul
Hyssopus officinalis .... Hyssop
Jasminum officinale .... Jasmine
Juniperus osteosperma .... Juniper
Laurus nobilis .... Laurus Nobilis (Bay Laurel)
Laurus nobilis .... Laurus Nobilis Vitality
Lavandula angustifolia .... Lavender
Lavandula angustifolia .... Lavender Vitality
Lavandula intermedia .... Lavandin
Leptospermum scoparium .... Manuka
Lippia alba .... Mastrante
Matricaria recutita .... German Chamomile (Matricaria)

Matricaria recutita .... German Chamomile Vitality
Melaleuca alternifolia .... Tea Tree
Melaleuca ericifolia .... Melaleuca Ericifolia
Melaleuca viridiflora .... Melaleuca Quinquenervia (Niaouli)
Melissa officinalis .... Melissa
Mentha piperita .... Peppermint
Mentha piperita .... Peppermint Vitality
Mentha spicata .... Spearmint
Mentha spicata .... Spearmint Vitality
Mesosphaerum suaveolens .... Hyptis
Micromeria fruticosa .... Micromeria
Myristica fragrans .... Nutmeg
Myristica fragrans .... Nutmeg Vitality
Myrtus communis .... Myrtle
Nardostachys jatamansi .... Spikenard
Nymphaea lotus .... White Lotus
Ocimum basilicum .... Basil
Ocimum basilicum .... Basil Vitality
Ocotea quixos .... Ocotea
Ocotea quixos .... Ishpingo
Origanum majorana .... Marjoram
Origanum majorana .... Marjoram Vitality
Origanum majorana (Syn. *O. vulgare*) .... Oregano
Origanum vulgare .... Oregano Vitality
Pelargonium graveolens .... Geranium
Picea mariana .... Black Spruce
Picea mariana .... Northern Lights Black Spruce
Picea pungens .... Idaho Blue Spruce
Pimpinella anisum .... Anise
Pinus ponderosa .... Idaho Ponderosa Pine
Pinus sylvestris .... Pine
Piper nigrum .... Black Pepper
Piper nigrum .... Black Pepper Vitality
Plectranthus amboinicus .... Plectranthus Oregano

Pogostemon cablin .... Patchouli
Pseudotsuga menziesii .... Douglas Fir
Rhododendrum groenlandicum .... Ledum
Rosa damascena .... Rose
Rosmarinus officinalis .... Rosemary
Rosmarinus officinalis .... Rosemary Vitality
Ruta graveolens .... Rue
Salvia lavandulaefolia .... Spanish Sage
Salvia officinalis .... Sage
Salvia sclarea .... Clary Sage
Santalum album .... Sacred Sandalwood
Santalum paniculatum .... Royal Hawaiian Sandalwood™*
Satureja montana .... Mountain Savory
Satureja montana .... Mountain Savory Vitality
Solidago canadensis .... Goldenrod
Styrax benzoin .... Onycha
Syzygium aromaticum .... Clove
Syzygium aromaticum .... Clove Vitality
Tanacetum annuum .... Blue Tansy
Tanacetum vulgare .... Idaho Tansy
Thuja plicata .... Western Red Cedar
Thymus vulgaris .... Thyme
Thymus vulgaris .... Thyme Vitality
Tsuga canadensis .... Tsuga
Valeriana officinalis .... Valerian
Vanilla planifolia .... Vanilla
Vetiveria zizanoides (Syn. *Vetiveria zizanioides*) .... Vetiver
Zingiber officinale .... Ginger
Zingiber officinale .... Ginger Vitality

*Registered trademark of Jawmin, LLC

Common Name First

Common Name	Scientific Name
Amazonian Ylang Ylang	Cananga odorata Equitoriana
Angelica	Angelica archangelica
Anise	Pimpinella anisum
Balsam Canada (Idaho Balsam Fir)	Abies balsamea
Balsam Copaiba (Copaiba)	Copaifera officinalis
Balm of Gilead	Commiphora gileadensis
Basil	Ocimum basilicum
Basil Vitality	Ocimum basilicum
Bay Laurel (Laurus Nobilis)	Laurus nobilis
Bergamot	Citrus aurantium bergamia
Bergamot Vitality	Citrus aurantium bergamia
Biblical Sweet Myrrh	Commiphora erythraea
Black Pepper	Piper nigrum
Black Pepper Vitality	Piper nigrum
Black Spruce	Picea mariana
Blue Cypress	Callitris intratropica
Blue Tansy	Tanacetum annuum
Calamus	Acorus calamus
Canadian Fleabane	Conyza canadensis
Cardamom	Elettaria cardamomum
Cardamom Vitality	Elettaria cardamomum
Carrot Seed	Daucus carota
Carrot Seed Vitality	Daucus carota
Cassia	Cinnamomum aromaticum
Cedarwood	Cedrus atlantica
Celery Seed	Apium graveolens
Celery Seed Vitality	Apium graveolens
Cinnamon Bark	Cinnamomum zeylanicum (Syn. C. verum)
Cinnamon Bark Vitality	Cinnamomum verum
Cistus	Cistus ladanifer (Syn. C. ladaniferus)
Citronella	Cymbopogon nardus
Citronella	Cymbopogon winterianus, Java Type
Citrus Hystrix	Citrus hystrix
Clary Sage	Salvia sclarea
Clove	Syzygium aromaticum (Syn. Eugenia caryophyllus)
Clove Vitality	Syzygium aromaticum (Syn. E. caryophyllus)
Copaiba (Balsam Copaiba)	Copaifera officinalis
Copaiba Vitality	Copaifera officinalis
Coriander	Coriandrum sativum
Coriander Vitality	Coriandrum sativum
Cumin	Cuminum cyminum
Cypress	Cupressus sempervirens
Davana	Artemesia pallens
Dill	Anethum graveolens
Dill Vitality	Anethum graveolens
Dorado Azul	Hyptis suaveolens
Dorado Azul (Ecuador)	Dorado Azul Guayfolius officinalis
Douglas Fir	Pseudotsuga menziesii
Elemi	Canarium luzonicum
Eucalyptus Blue	Eucalyptus bicostata
Eucalyptus Citriodora	Eucalyptus citriodora
Eucalyptus Globulus	Eucalyptus globulus
Eucalyptus Radiata	Eucalyptus radiata
Eucalyptus Staigeriana	Eucalyptus staigeriana
Fennel	Foeniculum vulgare
Fennel Vitality	Foeniculum vulgare
Frankincense	Boswellia carterii
Frankincense Vitality	Boswellia carterii
Frereana Frankincense	Boswellia frereana
Galbanum	Ferula galbaniflua
Geranium	Pelargonium graveolens
German Chamomile (Matricaria)	Chamomilla recutita (Syn. Matricaria recutita)
German Chamomile Vitality	Matricaria recutita
Ginger	Zingiber officinale
Ginger Vitality	Zingiber officinale
Goldenrod	Solidago canadensis
Grapefruit	Citrus paradisi
Grapefruit Vitality	Citrus paradisi
Helichrysum	Helichrysum italicum
Hinoki	Chamaecyparis obtusa
Hong Kuai	Chamaecyparis formosensis
Hyptis	Mesosphaerum suaveolens
Hyssop	Hyssopus officinalis
Idaho Balsam Fir (Balsam Canada)	Abies balsamea
Idaho Blue Spruce	Picea pungens
Idaho Ponderosa Pine	Pinus ponderosa
Idaho Tansy	Tanacetum vulgare
Ishpingo	Ocotea quixos
Jade Lemon	Citrus limon eureka var. formosensis
Jade Lemon Vitality	Citrus limon eureka var. formosensis
Jasmine	Jasminum officinale
Juniper	Juniperus osteosperma
Laurus Nobilis (Bay Laurel)	Laurus nobilis
Laurus Nobilis Vitality	Laurus nobilis
Lavandin	Lavandula intermedia
Lavender	Lavandula angustifolia
Lavender Vitality	Lavandula angustifolia
Ledum	Rhododendrum groenlandicum
Lemon	Citrus limon
Lemon Vitality	Citrus limon
Lemon Myrtle	Backhousia citriodora
Lemongrass	Cymbopogon flexuosus
Lemongrass Vitality	Cymbopogon flexuosus
Lime	Citrus latifolia (Syn. C. aurantifolia)
Lime Vitality	Citrus aurantifolia
Mandarin	Citrus reticulata
Manuka	Leptospermum scoparium
Marjoram	Origanum majorana
Marjoram Vitality	Origanum majorana
Mastrante	Lippia alba
Matricaria (German Chamomile)	Chamomilla recutita (Syn. Matricaria recutita)
Melaleuca Ericifolia	Melaleuca ericifolia
Melaleuca Quinquenervia (Niaouli)	Melaleuca viridiflora
Melissa	Melissa officinalis
Micromeria	Micromeria fruticosa
Mountain Savory	Satureja montana
Mountain Savory Vitality	Satureja montana
Myrrh	Commiphora myrrha

Common Name	Botanical Name
Myrtle	*Myrtus communis*
Neroli (Bitter Orange)	*Citrus aurantium amara*
Niaouli (Melaleuca Quinquenervia)	*Melaleuca viridiflora*
Northern Lights Black Spruce	*Picea mariana*
Nutmeg	*Myristica fragrans*
Nutmeg Vitality	*Myristica fragrans*
Ocotea	*Ocotea quixos*
Onycha	*Styrax benzoin*
Orange	*Citrus sinensis*
Orange Vitality	*Citrus sinensis*
Oregano	*Origanum vulgare* (Syn. *O. majorana*)
Oregano Vitality	*Origanum vulgare*
Palmarosa	*Cymbopogon martini*
Palo Santo	*Bursera graveolens*
Patchouli	*Pogostemon cablin*
Peppermint	*Mentha piperita*
Peppermint Vitality	*Mentha piperita*
Petitgrain	*Citrus aurantium amara* (Syn. *Citrus sinensis*)
Pine	*Pinus sylvestris*
Plectranthus Oregano	*Plectranthus amboinicus*
Ravintsara	*Cinnamomum camphora*
Roman Chamomile	*Anthemis nobilis* (Syn. *Chamaemelum nobile*)
Rose	*Rosa damascena*
Rose of Sharon (Cistus)	*Cistus ladaniferus*
Rosemary	*Rosmarinus officinalis*
Rosemary Vitality	*Rosmarinus officinalis*
Royal Hawaiian Sandalwood™*	*Santalum paniculatum*
Rue	*Ruta graveolens*
Sacred Frankincense	*Boswellia sacra*
Sage	*Salvia officinalis*
Sandalwood	*Santalum album*
Spanish Sage (Sage Lavender)	*Salvia lavandulifolia*
Spearmint	*Mentha spicata*
Spearmint Vitality	*Mentha spicata*
Spikenard	*Nardostachys jatamansi*
Sweet Orange	*Citrus aurantium dulcis*
Tangerine	*Citrus reticulata*
Tangerine Vitality	*Citrus reticulata*
Tarragon	*Artemisia dracunculus*
Tarragon Vitality	*Artemisia dracunculus*
Tea Tree	*Melaleuca alternifolia*
Thyme	*Thymus vulgaris*
Thyme Vitality	*Thymus vulgaris*
Tsuga	*Tsuga canadensis*
Valerian	*Valeriana officinalis*
Vanilla	*Vanilla planifolia*
Vetiver	*Vetiveria zizanoides* (Syn. *V. zizanioides*)
Western Red Cedar	*Thuja plicata*
White Cypress Pine	*Callitris columellaris*
White Fir	*Abies concolor*
White Lotus	*Nymphaea lotus*
Wintergreen	*Gaultheria procumbens*
Xiang Mao	*Cymbopogon citratus*
Yarrow/Blue Yarrow	*Achillea millefolium*
Ylang Ylang	*Cananga odorata*
Yuzu	*Citrus junos*

*Registered trademark of Jawmin, LLC

Appendix B
Single Oil Data

Single Oil Name	Botanical Name	Products Containing Single Oil
Amazonian Ylang Ylang	*Cananga odorata Equitoriana*	
Angelica	*Angelica archangelica*	Angelica, Awaken, CardioGize, Divine Release, Forgiveness, Friends, Grounding, Harmony, Inner Harmony, Live with Passion, Loyalty, Oola Balance, Surrender, T-Away, T.R. Care
Anise	*Pimpinella anisum*	Allerzyme, Animal Scents Dental Pet Chews, Animal Scents ParaGize, Anise, Awaken, Build Your Dream, ComforTone, Detoxzyme, Digest & Cleanse, DiGize, DiGize Vitality, Dream Catcher, Essentialzyme, Essentialzymes-4, ICP, Journey On, JuvaPower, MindWise, ParaFree, Thieves Fruit & Veggie Soak, TummyGize
Basil	*Ocimum basilicum*	Aroma Siez, Basil, Basil Vitality, Clarity, Finance, Fitness, M-Grain
Basil Vitality		
Bergamot	*Citrus aurantium bergamia*	Acceptance, Animal Scents Ointment, AromaGuard Meadow Mist Deodorant, Aroma Sleep, ART Renewal Serum, Awaken, Believe, Bergamot, Bergamot Vitality, Build Your Dream, Clarity, Divine Release, Dragon Time Bath & Shower Gel, Dream Catcher, Evening Peace Bath & Shower Gel, Faith, Family, Field, Finance, Forgiveness, Friends, Genesis Hand & Body Lotion, GeneYus, Gentle Baby, Gratitude, Harmony, Humility, Inspiration, Journey On, Joy, KidScents Lotion, KidScents Tender Tush, Lady Sclareol, Lavender-Oatmeal Bar Soap, Magnify Your Purpose, Mirah Luminous Cleansing Oil, Oola Balance, Oola Grow, Peace & Calming II, Prenolone Plus Body Cream, Progessence Plus, Reconnect, Relaxation Massage Oil, Rose Ointment, Sandalwood Moisture Cream, Savvy Minerals - Misting Spray, Seedlings Baby Lotion, Seedlings Baby Oil, Seedlings Baby Wash & Shampoo, Seedlings Baby Wipes, Seedlings Linen Spray, Sensation, Sensation Bath & Shower Gel, Sensation Hand & Body Lotion, Sensation Massage Oil, SleepyIze, T-Away, Thieves Dish Soap, Thieves Laundry Soap, T.R. Care, Valor Moisturizing Soap, White Angelica, Wolfberry Eye Cream
Bergamot Vitality		
Biblical Sweet Myrrh	*Commiphora erythraea*	
Bitter Orange (See Neroli)	*Citrus aurantium amara*	Fulfill Your Destiny
Black Pepper	*Piper nigrum*	Awaken, Black Pepper, Black Pepper Vitality, Build Your Dream, Dream Catcher, En-R-Gee, Fitness, Fulfill Your Destiny, Journey On, Light the Fire, NingXia Nitro, NingXia Zyng, Relieve It
Black Pepper Vitality		

Single Oil Name	Botanical Name	Products Containing Single Oil
Black Spruce	*Picea mariana*	3 Wise Men, Abundance, Awaken, Christmas Spirit, Family, Field, Friends, GeneYus, Grounding, Harmony, Hope, Inner Child, Inspiration, Journey On, Mirah Lustrous Hair Oil, Motivation, Northern Lights Black Spruce, Present Time, R.C., Relieve It, Sacred Mountain, Sacred Mountain Moisturizing Soap, Savvy Minerals - Misting Spray, Seedlings Diaper Cream, SniffleEase, Super Cal Plus, Surrender, T-Away, Trauma Life, T.R. Care, Valor, Valor Roll-On, White Angelica
Blue Cypress	*Callitris intratropica*	Acceptance, ART Sheerlumé Brightening Cream, Australian Blue, Australian Kuranya, Awaken, Blue Cypress, Brain Power, Breathe Again Roll-On, Build Your Dream, Cool Azul, Cool Azul Pain Relief Cream, Cool Azul Sports Gel, Divine Release, Dream Catcher, Essential Beauty Serum (Dry Skin), Friends, GeneYus, Highest Potential, Journey On, Oola Grow, Reconnect, Release, SARA, T.R. Care
Blue Tansy	*Tanacetum annuum*	Australian Blue, Awaken, Blue Tansy, Build Your Dream, Dragon Time Bath & Shower Gel, Dream Catcher, Evening Peace Bath & Shower Gel, Highest Potential, Journey On, JuvaFlex, JuvaFlex Vitality, JuvaTone, Peace & Calming, Release, SARA, T-Away, T.R. Care, Valor, Valor Roll-On
Calamus	*Acorus calamus*	Exodus II
Canadian Fleabane	*Conyza canadensis*	CortiStop, EndoGize, Light the Fire
Cardamom	*Elettaria cardamomum*	AromaEase, Cardamom, Cardamom Vitality, CardioGize, Clarity, Family, Field, Finance, Fulfill Your Destiny, Loyalty, Master Formula Liquid Vitamin Capsule, Transformation, TummyGize
Cardamom Vitality		
Carrot Seed	*Daucus carota*	Animal Scents Ointment, ART Sheerlumé Brightening Cream, Carrot Seed, Carrot Seed Vitality, Mineral Sunscreen Lotion, Rose Ointment
Carrot Seed Vitality		
Cassia	*Cinnamomum aromaticum*	EndoGize, Exodus II, Fulfill Your Destiny, Light the Fire, Loyalty, Peace & Calming II, PowerGize, Red Shot, Slique CitraSlim Powder Capsule, Valor Moisturizing Soap
Cedarwood	*Cedrus atlantica*	ART Beauty Masque, ART Intensive Moisturizer, Australian Blue, Brain Power, Cedarwood, Cel-Lite Magic Massage Oil, Egyptian Gold, Essential Beauty Serum (Dry Skin), Faith, Family, Fun, GeneYus, Grounding, Highest Potential, Inspiration, Into the Future, InTouch, KidScents Bath Gel, KidScents Lotion, Live with Passion, Mirah Shave Oil, Oola Grow, Peppermint-Cedarwood Moisturizing Soap, Progessence Plus, Reconnect, Sacred Mountain, Sacred Mountain Moisturizing Soap, SARA, Savvy Minerals - Misting Spray, Shutran, Shutran 3-in-1 Men's Wash, Shutran Aftershave Lotion, Shutran Bar Soap, Shutran Beard Oil, Shutran Shave Cream, Stress Away, Stress Away Relaxing Bath Bomb, Stress Away Roll-On, T.R. Care, Tranquil Roll-On
Celery Seed	*Apium graveolens*	Celery Seed Vitality, GLF, GLF Vitality, JuvaCleanse, JuvaCleanse Vitality
Celery Seed Vitality		

Single Oil Name	Botanical Name	Products Containing Single Oil
Cinnamon Bark Cinnamon Bark Vitality	Cinnamomum zeylanicum (Syn. C. verum)	Abundance, CardioGize, Christmas Spirit, Cinnamint Lip Balm, Cinnamon Bark, Cinnamon Bark Vitality, Egyptian Gold, Exodus II, Finance, Gathering, Highest Potential, Inner Defense, Journey On, KidScents Slique Toothpaste, Magnify Your Purpose, Mineral Essence, Oola Grow, Slique Bars, Slique Bars-Chocolate-Coated, Thieves, Thieves AromaBright Toothpaste, Thieves Automatic Dishwasher Powder, Thieves Cleansing Soap, Thieves Cough Drops, Thieves Dental Floss, Thieves Dentarome Plus Toothpaste, Thieves Dentarome Ultra Toothpaste, Thieves Dish Soap, Thieves Foaming Hand Soap, Thieves Fresh Essence Plus Mouthwash, Thieves Fruit & Veggie Soak, Thieves Fruit & Veggie Spray, Thieves Hard Lozenges, Thieves Household Cleaner, Thieves Laundry Soap, Thieves Mints, Thieves Spray, Thieves Vitality, Thieves Waterless Hand Purifier, Thieves Wipes, T.R. Care, Treasure of the Season
Cistus	Cistus ladanifer (Syn. C. ladaniferus)	Animal Scents PuriClean, Cistus, Fitness, ImmuPower, Journey On, KidScents Tender Tush, Mineral Sunscreen Lotion, Oola Balance, Owie, Peace & Calming II, The Gift, Valor Moisturizing Soap
Citronella	Cymbopogon nardus	Animal Scents PuriClean, Animal Scents Shampoo, Citronella, Finance, Insect Repellent, Purification, Thieves Fruit & Veggie Soak
Citrus Hystrix/ Combava (see also Kaffir lime)	Citrus hystrix	Acceptance, Awaken, Dream Catcher, Highest Potential, Journey On, Oola Grow, SARA, T-Away, Trauma Life, T.R. Care
Clary Sage	Salvia sclarea	Cel-Lite Magic Massage Oil, Clary Sage, CortiStop, Dragon Time, Dragon Time Bath & Shower Gel, Dragon Time Massage Oil, EndoGize, Evening Peace Bath & Shower Gel, FemiGen, Fitness, Fulfill Your Destiny, Into the Future, Lady Sclareol, Lavender Conditioner, Lavender Shampoo, Live with Passion, Oola Grow, Prenolone Plus Body Cream, SclarEssence, SclarEssence Vitality, Transformation
Clove Clove Vitality	Syzygium aromaticum (Syn. Eugenia caryophyllus)	Abundance, AgilEase, AromaGuard Meadow Mist Deodorant, AromaGuard Mountain Mint Deodorant, ART Sheerlumé Brightening Cream, BLM Capsules, Clove, Clove Vitality, Deep Relief Roll-On, En-R-Gee, Essential Beauty Serum (Dry Skin), Essentialzyme, ImmuPower, Inner Defense, Insect Repellent, Journey On, K&B, KidScents Slique Toothpaste, Longevity, Longevity Softgels, Longevity Vitality, Master Formula Liquid Vitamin Capsule, Melrose, My Destiny, OmegaGize³, Owie, PanAway, ParaFree, Progessence Plus, Thieves, Thieves AromaBright Toothpaste, Thieves Automatic Dishwashing Powder, Thieves Cleansing Soap, Thieves Cough Drops, Thieves Dental Floss, Thieves Dentarome Plus Toothpaste, Thieves Dentarome Ultra Toothpaste, Thieves Dish Soap, Thieves Foaming Hand Soap, Thieves Fresh Essence Plus Mouthwash, Thieves Fruit & Veggie Soak, Thieves Fruit & Veggie Spray, Thieves Hard Lozenges, Thieves Household Cleaner, Thieves Laundry Soap, Thieves Mints, Thieves Spray, Thieves Vitality, Thieves Waterless Hand Purifier, Thieves Wipes
Copaiba (Balsam Copaiba) Copaiba Vitality	Copaifera officinalis	AgilEase, ART Beauty Masque, Breathe Again Roll-On, Cool Azul, Cool Azul Pain Relief Cream, Cool Azul Sports Gel, Copaiba, Copaiba Vanilla Moisturizing Conditioner, Copaiba Vanilla Moisturizing Shampoo, Copaiba Vitality, Deep Relief Roll-On, Fitness, Freedom, Journey On, My Destiny, Progessence Plus, Stress Away, Stress Away Relaxing Bath Bomb, Stress Away Roll-On, Super Cal Plus

Single Oil Name	Botanical Name	Products Containing Single Oil
Coriander Coriander Vitality	*Coriandrum sativum*	Acceptance, Animal Scents Ointment, AromaGuard Meadow Mist Deodorant, ART Renewal Serum, Awaken, Believe, Build Your Dream, Clarity, Coriander, Coriander Vitality, Dragon Time Bath & Shower Gel, Evening Peace Bath & Shower Gel, Faith, Family, Field, Finance, Forgiveness, Friends, Genesis Hand & Body Lotion, GeneYus, Gentle Baby, Gratitude, Harmony, Humility, Inspiration, Joy, KidScents Lotion, KidScents Tender Tush, Lady Sclareol, Lavender-Oatmeal Bar Soap, Magnify Your Purpose, Mirah Luminous Cleansing Oil, Mirah Shave Oil, Oola Balance, Oola Grow, Reconnect, Relaxation Massage Oil, Rose Ointment, Sandalwood Moisture Cream, Seedlings Baby Lotion, Seedlings Baby Oil, Seedlings Baby Wash & Shampoo, Seedlings Baby Wipes, Seedlings Linen Spray, Sensation, Sensation Bath & Shower Gel, Sensation Hand & Body Lotion, Sensation Massage Oil, Shutran, Shutran 3-in-1 Men's Wash, Shutran Aftershave Lotion, Shutran Bar Soap, Shutran Beard Oil, Shutran Shave Cream, T-Away, T.R. Care, Valor Moisturizing Soap, White Angelica, Wolfberry Eye Cream
Cumin	*Cuminum cyminum*	Animal Scents ParaGize, Detoxzyme, ImmuPower, Journey On, ParaFree, Protec
Cypress	*Cupressus sempervirens*	Aroma Life, Aroma Siez, CardioGize, Cel-Lite Magic Massage Oil, Cypress, Fitness, My Destiny, R.C., SniffleEase
Davana	*Artemisia pallens*	Acceptance, Amoressence, ART Creme Masque, ART Sheerlumé Brightening Cream, Australian Blue, Awaken, Dream Catcher, Highest Potential, Journey On, Lavender Bath & Shower Gel, Lavender Hand & Body Lotion, Mirah Shave Oil, Peace & Calming II, Release, SARA, Shutran, Shutran 3-in-1 Men's Wash, Shutran Aftershave Lotion, Shutran Bar Soap, Shutran Beard Oil, Shutran Shave Cream, T-Away, T.R. Care, Trauma Life, Valor Moisturizing Soap
Dill Dill Vitality	*Anethum graveolens*	Dill, Dill Vitality
Dorado Azul	*Hyptis suaveolens*	Animal Scents Infect Away, Common Sense, Cool Azul, Cool Azul Pain Relief Cream, Cool Azul Sports Gel, Deep Relief Roll-On, Dorado Azul, ImmuPower, Journey On, My Destiny, ParaFree, SniffleEase
Douglas Fir	*Pseudotsuga menziesii*	Regenolone Moisturizing Cream
Elemi	*Canarium luzonicum*	Cool Azul, Cool Azul Pain Relief Cream, Cool Azul Sports Gel, Elemi, Ortho Sport Massage Oil, Owie
Eucalyptus Blue	*Eucalyptus bicostata*	Breathe Again Roll-On, Eucalyptus Blue, SniffleEase
Eucalyptus Citriodora	*Eucalyptus citriodora*	My Destiny, R.C., SniffleEase
Eucalyptus Globulus	*Eucalyptus globulus*	Breathe Again Roll-On, Eucalyptus Globulus, My Destiny, Ortho Ease Massage Oil, Ortho Sport Massage Oil, R.C., SniffleEase

Single Oil Name	Botanical Name	Products Containing Single Oil
Eucalyptus Radiata	*Eucalyptus radiata*	AromaGuard Mountain Mint Deodorant, Australian Kuranya, Breathe Again Roll-On, Eucalyptus Radiata, Inner Defense, KidScents Slique Toothpaste, My Destiny, Ortho Ease Massage Oil, Raven, R.C., SniffleEase, Thieves, Thieves AromaBright Toothpaste, Thieves Automatic Dishwasher Powder, Thieves Cleansing Soap, Thieves Cough Drops, Thieves Dental Floss, Thieves Dentarome Plus Toothpaste, Thieves Dentarome Ultra Toothpaste, Thieves Dish Soap, Thieves Foaming Hand Soap, Thieves Fresh Essence Plus Mouthwash, Thieves Fruit & Veggie Soak, Thieves Fruit & Veggie Spray, Thieves Hard Lozenges, Thieves Household Cleaner, Thieves Laundry Soap, Thieves Mints, Thieves Spray, Thieves Vitality, Thieves Waterless Hand Purifier, Thieves Wipes
Eucalyptus Staigeriana	*E. staigeriana*	Breathe Again Roll-On
Fennel / Fennel Vitality	*Foeniculum vulgare*	Allerzyme, Animal Scents ParaGize, AromaEase, Australian Kuranya, CortiStop, Detoxzyme, Digest & Cleanse, DiGize, DiGize Vitality, Dragon Time, Dragon Time Bath & Shower Gel, Dragon Time Massage Oil, Essentialzyme, Essentialzymes-4, FemiGen, Fennel, Fennel Vitality, ICP, JuvaFlex, JuvaFlex Vitality, JuvaPower, K&B, Master Formula Liquid Vitamin Capsule, MindWise, Mister, ParaFree, Prenolone Plus Body Cream, Prostate Health, SclarEssence, SclarEssence Vitality, Slique CitraSlim Powder Capsule, Thieves Fruit & Veggie Soak, TummyGize
Frankincense / Frankincense Vitality	*Boswellia carterii*	3 Wise Men, Abundance, Acceptance, Acne Treatment - Maximum Strength, Animal Scents Mendwell, ART Chocolate Masque, ART Gentle Cleanser, ART Intensive Moisturizer, ART Light Moisturizer, ART Refreshing Toner, Awaken, Believe, Boswellia Wrinkle Cream, Brain Power, Build Your Dream, ClaraDerm, Common Sense, CortiStop, Divine Release, Egyptian Gold, Exodus II, Family, Field, Finance, Forgiveness, Frankincense, Frankincense Vitality, Friends, Fulfill Your Destiny, Gratitude, Harmony, Highest Potential, Humility, ImmuPower, Inspiration, Into the Future, Journey On, KidScents Tender Tush, Live Your Passion, Longevity, Longevity Softgels, Longevity Vitality, My Destiny, Oola Balance, Oola Grow, Progessence Plus, Protec, T-Away, T.R. Care, Trauma Life, Treasure of the Season, Valor, Valor Moisturizing Soap, Valor Roll-On, Wolfberry Eye Cream
Frereana Frankincense	*Boswellia frereana*	Slique Gum, Treasure of the Season
Geranium	*Pelargonium graveolens*	Acceptance, Acne Treatment - Maximum Strength, Amoressence, Animal Scents Mendwell, Animal Scents Ointment, Animal Scents Shampoo, AromaGuard Meadow Mist Deodorant, Aroma Sleep, ART Chocolate Masque, ART Creme Masque, ART Renewal Serum, ART Sheerlumé Brightening Cream, Australian Blue, Awaken, Believe, Boswellia Wrinkle Cream, Build Your Dream, Clarity, Copaiba Vanilla Moisturizing Conditioner, Copaiba Vanilla Moisturizing Shampoo, Divine Release, Dragon Time Bath & Shower Gel, Dream Catcher, EndoFlex, EndoFlex Vitality, Envision, Evening Peace Bath & Shower Gel, Faith, Family, Field, Finance, Forgiveness, Friends, Gathering, Genesis Hand & Body Lotion, GeneYus, Gentle Baby, Geranium, Gratitude, Harmony, Highest Potential,

Single Oil Name	Botanical Name	Products Containing Single Oil
Geranium (continued)		Humility, Inner Harmony, Insect Repellent, Inspiration, Journey On, Joy, JuvaFlex, JuvaFlex Vitality, JuvaTone, K&B, KidScents Lotion, KidScents Tender Tush, Lady Sclareol, Lavender-Oatmeal Bar Soap, Loyalty, Magnify Your Purpose, Melaleuca-Geranium Moisturizing Soap, Mirah Luminous Cleansing Oil, Mirah Lustrous Hair Oil, Oola Balance, Oola Grow, Prenolone Plus Body Cream, Prostate Health, Reconnect, Relaxation Massage Oil, Release, Rose Ointment, Sandalwood Moisture Cream, SARA, Savvy Minerals - Misting Spray, Seedlings Baby Lotion, Seedlings Baby Oil, Seedlings Baby Wash & Shampoo, Seedlings Baby Wipes, Seedlings Linen Spray, Sensation, Sensation Bath & Shower Gel, Sensation Hand & Body Lotion, Sensation Massage Oil, SleepyIze, T-Away, T.R. Care, Trauma Life, Valor, Valor Moisturizing Soap, Valor Roll-On, White Angelica, Wolfberry Eye Cream
German Chamomile (Matricaria) German Chamomile Vitality	*Chamomilla recutita* (Syn. *Matricaria recutita*)	Acceptance, Australian Blue, Awaken, ComforTone, Cool Azul, Cool Azul Pain Relief Cream, Cool Azul Sports Gel, Dream Catcher, EndoFlex, EndoFlex Vitality, German Chamomile, German Chamomile Vitality, Highest Potential, Journey On, JuvaTone, OmegaGize^3, Orange Blossom Facial Wash, Peace & Calming II, Release, SARA, T-Away, T.R. Care, Valor Moisturizing Soap
Ginger Ginger Vitality	*Zingiber officinale*	Abundance, Allerzyme, Animal Scents Cat Treats, Animal Scents ParaGize, AromaEase, ComforTone, Digest & Cleanse, DiGize, DiGize Vitality, EndoGize, Essentialzymes-4, Field, Ginger, Ginger Vitality, ICP, Live with Passion, Magnify Your Purpose, Master Formula Liquid Vitamin Capsule, ParaFree, Thieves Fruit & Veggie Soak, TummyGize
Goldenrod	*Solidago canadensis*	Common Sense, Goldenrod, PowerGize
Grapefruit Grapefruit Vitality	*Citrus paradisi*	Acceptance, Australian Blue, Awaken, Cel-Lite Magic Massage Oil, Citrus Fresh, Citrus Fresh Vitality, Coconut-Lime Replenishing Body Butter, Divine Release, Dream Catcher, Fun, GLF, GLF Vitality, Grapefruit, Grapefruit Lip Balm, Grapefruit Vitality, Highest Potential, Journey On, KidScents Slique Toothpaste, Oola Grow, Red Shot, Release, SARA, Savvy Minerals - Poppy Seed Lip Scrub, Slique Essence, Slique Shake, Super C, T.R. Care
Helichrysum	*Helichrysum italicum*	Aroma Life, Awaken, Brain Power, CardioGize, ClaraDerm, Deep Relief Roll-On, Divine Release, Forgiveness, GLF, GLF Vitality, Helichrysum, JuvaCleanse, JuvaCleanse Vitality, JuvaFlex, JuvaFlex Vitality, LavaDerm After-Sun Spray, LavaDerm Cooling Mist, Live with Passion, M-Grain, Mineral Sunscreen Lotion, My Destiny, Owie, PanAway, Seedlings Diaper Cream, T-Away, T.R. Care, Trauma Life
Hinoki	*Chamaecyparis obtusa*	Animal Scents Mendwell, ART Intensive Moisturizer, Divine Release, Hinoki, Owie, Shutran, Shutran 3-in-1 Men's Wash, Shutran Aftershave Lotion, Shutran Bar Soap, Shutran Beard Oil, Shutran Shave Cream
Hong Kuai	*Chamaecyparis formosensis*	Build Your Dream, Hong Kuai
Ho Wood	*Cinnamomum camphora CT linalool*	Valor
Hyptis	*Mesosphaerum suaveolens*	Cool Azul Pain Relief Cream

Single Oil Name	Botanical Name	Products Containing Single Oil
Hyssop	Hyssopus officinalis	Animal Scents Mendwell, Egyptian Gold, Exodus II, Faith, Friends, GeneYus, GLF, GLF Vitality, Harmony, Hyssop, ImmuPower, Journey On, Oola Balance, Reconnect, Relieve It, T-Away, T.R. Care, White Angelica
Idaho Balsam Fir (Balsam Canada)	Abies balsamea	Animal Scents Ointment, Believe, BLM Capsules, Deep Relief Roll-On, Egyptian Gold, En-R-Gee, Faith, Field, Finance, Fitness, Gratitude, Idaho Balsam Fir, My Destiny, Oola Balance, Owie, Sacred Mountain, Sacred Mountain Moisturizing Soap, Slique CitraSlim Liquid Capsule, The Gift, Treasure of the Season
Idaho Blue Spruce	Picea pungens	Amoressence, Believe, Build Your Dream, Field, Fitness, Freedom, Fulfill Your Destiny, GeneYus, Idaho Blue Spruce, Inner Harmony, Into the Future, InTouch, Lady Sclareol, Live Your Passion, Loyalty, Mirah Shave Oil, My Destiny, Oola Balance, Oola Grow, PowerGize, Reconnect, Shutran, Shutran 3-in-1 Men's Wash, Shutran Aftershave Lotion, Shutran Bar Soap, Shutran Beard Oil, Shutran Shave Cream, Super Cal Plus, Transformation, Valor Moisturizing Soap
Idaho Tansy	Tanacetum vulgare	
Ishpingo	Ocotea quixos	
Jade Lemon	Citrus limon Eureka var. formosensis	Jade Lemon, Jade Lemon Vitality
Jade Lemon Vitality		
Jasmine	Jasminum officinale	Acceptance, Amoressence, ART Crème Masque, ART Renewal Serum, ART Sheerlumé Brightening Cream, Australian Blue, Awaken, Clarity, Dragon Time, Dragon Time Bath & Shower Gel, Dragon Time Massage Oil, Dream Catcher, Evening Peace Bath & Shower Gel, Faith, Finance, Forgiveness, Fun, Genesis Hand & Body Lotion, Gentle Baby, Harmony, Highest Potential, Inner Child, Into the Future, Jasmine, Journey On, Joy, Lady Sclareol, Lavender Conditioner, Lavender Shampoo, Live with Passion, Mirah Luminous Cleansing Oil, Mirah Shave Oil, Oola Balance, Oola Grow, Release, SARA, Sensation, Sensation Bath & Shower Gel, Sensation Hand & Body Lotion, Sensation Massage Oil, The Gift, T.R. Care, T-Away
Juniper	Juniperus osteosperma	3 Wise Men, Allerzyme, Awaken, Build Your Dream, Cel-Lite Magic Massage Oil, DiGize, DiGize Vitality, Dream Catcher, En-R-Gee, Faith, Grounding, Hope, Into the Future, Journey On, Juniper, K&B, Morning Start Bath & Shower Gel, Morning Start Moisturizing Soap, Oola Grow, Ortho Ease Massage Oil, ParaFree, Animal Scents ParaGize, Thieves Fruit & Veggie Soak
Kaffir Lime (see Citrus Hystrix)	Citrus Hystrix	Acceptance, Australian Blue, Release, T-Away
Kunzea	Kunzea ambigua	Australian Kuranya, Kunzea
Laurus Nobilis (Bay Laurel)	Laurus nobilis	Breathe Again Roll-On, Laurus Nobilis, Laurus Nobilis Vitality, ParaFree
Laurus Nobilis Vitality		
Lavandin	Lavandula intermedia	Animal Scents PuriClean, Animal Scents Shampoo, Purification, Release, Thieves Fruit & Veggie Soak

Single Oil Name	Botanical Name	Products Containing Single Oil
Lavender Lavender Vitality	*Lavandula angustifolia*	Acne Treatment - Maximum Strength, Animal Scents PuriClean, AromaGuard Meadow Mist Deodorant, Aroma Siez, Aroma Sleep, ART Beauty Masque, ART Gentle Cleanser, ART Refreshing Toner, Awaken, Brain Power, Build Your Dream, CardioGize, Charcoal Bar Soap, ClaraDerm, Cool Azul, Cool Azul Pain Relief Cream, Cool Azul Sports Gel, Copaiba Vanilla Moisturizing Conditioner, Copaiba Vanilla Moisturizing Shampoo, Dragon Time, Dragon Time Bath & Shower Gel, Dragon Time Massage Oil, Egyptian Gold, Envision, Essential Beauty Serum (Dry Skin), Family, Finance, Forgiveness, Freedom, Friends, Gathering, Gentle Baby, Harmony, Highest Potential, Inner Harmony, Journey On, KidScents Tender Tush, LavaDerm After-Sun Spray, LavaDerm Cooling Mist, Lavender, Lavender Bath & Shower Gel, Lavender Calming Bath Bombs, Lavender Conditioner, Lavender Foaming Hand Soap, Lavender Hand & Body Lotion, Lavender Lip Balm, Lavender Mint Daily Conditioner, Lavender Mint Daily Shampoo, Lavender-Oatmeal Bar Soap, Lavender Shampoo, Lavender Vitality, Loyalty, Mendwell, M-Grain, Mineral Sunscreen Lotion, Mirah Lustrous Hair Oil, Mirah Shave Oil, Mister, Motivation, My Destiny, Oola Balance, Oola Grow, Orange Blossom Facial Wash, Orange Blossom Moisturizer, Prostate Health, R.C., Reconnect, Relaxation Massage Oil, RutaVaLa, RutaVaLa Roll-On, Sandalwood Moisture Cream, SARA, Savvy Minerals - Misting Spray, Seedlings Baby Lotion, Seedlings Baby Oil, Seedlings Baby Wash & Shampoo, Seedlings Diaper Cream, Seedlings Linen Spray, Shutran, Shutran 3-in-1 Men's Wash, Shutran Aftershave Lotion, Shutran Bar Soap, Shutran Beard Oil, Shutran Shave Cream, SleepEssence, SleepyIze, SniffleEase, Stress Away, Stress Away Relaxing Bath Bomb, Stress Away Roll-On, Surrender, T-Away, T.R. Care, Tranquil Roll-On, Trauma Life, Wolfberry Eye Cream
Ledum	*Rhododendrum groenlandicum*	Divine Release, GLF, GLF Vitality, JuvaCleanse, JuvaCleanse Vitality, Ledum
Lemon Lemon Vitality	*Citrus limon*	Acceptance, AlkaLime, AminoWise, Animal Scents Shampoo, AromaGuard Meadow Mist Deodorant, AromaGuard Mountain Mint Deodorant, ART Gentle Cleanser, ART Refreshing Toner, Australian Blue, Awaken, Charcoal Bar Soap, Citrus Fresh, Citrus Fresh Vitality, Clarity, Coconut-Lime Replenishing Body Butter, Digest & Cleanse, Deep Relief Roll-On, Dragon Time Bath & Shower Gel, Evening Peace Bath & Shower Gel, Faith, Family, Finance, Forgiveness, Friends, Fun, Gary's True Grit NingXia Berry Syrup, Genesis Hand & Body Lotion, Gentle Baby, Harmony, Highest Potential, Inner Defense, Journey On, Joy, JuvaTone, KidScents Shampoo, KidScents Slique Toothpaste, Lavender Bath & Shower Gel, Lavender Conditioner, Lavender Foaming Hand Soap, Lavender Hand & Body Lotion, Lavender Shampoo, Lemon, Lemon Vitality, Lemon-Sandalwood Cleansing Soap, Light the Fire, MegaCal, MindWise, Mineral Essence, Mirah Luminous Cleansing Oil, Mirah Shave Oil, MultiGreens, My Destiny, NingXia Red, Oola Balance, Oola Grow, Orange Blossom Facial Wash, Orange Blossom Moisturizer, Raven, Release, SARA, Savvy Minerals - Poppy Seed Lip Scrub, Shutran, Shutran 3-in-1 Men's Wash,

Single Oil Name	Botanical Name	Products Containing Single Oil
Lemon Vitality (continued)		Shutran Aftershave Lotion, Shutran Bar Soap, Shutran Beard Oil, Shutran Shave Cream, Slique Essence, Slique Shake, Super C, Surrender, T-Away, Thieves, Thieves AromaBright Toothpaste, Thieves Automatic Dishwasher Powder, Thieves Cleansing Soap, Thieves Cough Drops, Thieves Dental Floss, Thieves Dentarome Plus Toothpaste, Thieves Dentarome Ultra Toothpaste, Thieves Dish Soap, Thieves Foaming Hand Soap, Thieves Fresh Essence Plus Mouthwash, Thieves Fruit & Veggie Soak, Thieves Fruit & Veggie Spray, Thieves Household Cleaner, Thieves Hard Lozenges, Thieves Laundry Soap, Thieves Mints, Thieves Spray, Thieves Vitality, Thieves Waterless Hand Purifier, Thieves Wipes, Transformation, T.R. Care
Lemongrass Lemongrass Vitality	*Cymbopogon flexuosus*	Allerzyme, DiGize, DiGize Vitality, En-R-Gee, Essentialzymes-4, Family, Friends, ICP, Inner Child, Inner Defense, Insect Repellent, Lemongrass, Lemongrass Vitality, Morning Start Bath & Shower Gel, Morning Start Moisturizing Soap, MultiGreens, Ortho Ease Massage Oil, Ortho Sport Massage Oil, ParaFree, Animal Scents ParaGize, Animal Scents PuriClean, Purification, Slique CitraSlim, Super C, Thieves Automatic Dishwasher Powder, Thieves Fruit & Veggie Soak
Lemon Myrtle	*Backhousia citriodora*	Australian Kuranya, Coconut-Lime Replenishing Body Butter, Lemon Myrtle, Slique CitraSlim Liquid Capsule
Lime Lime Vitality	*Citrus latifolia* (Syn. *C. aurantifolia*)	AlkaLime, AminoWise, ART Beauty Masque, Coconut-Lime Replenishing Body Butter, Common Sense, Copaiba Vanilla Moisturizing Conditioner, Copaiba Vanilla Moisturizing Shampoo, Family, Lime, Lime Vitality, Live Your Passion, MindWise, My Destiny, NingXia Zyng, Red Shot, Savvy Minerals - Misting Spray, Stress Away, Stress Away Relaxing Bath Bomb, Stress Away Roll-On, Thieves Fruit & Veggie Spray
Mandarin	*Citrus reticulata*	Citrus Fresh, Citrus Fresh Vitality, Coconut-Lime Replenishing Body Butter, Friends, Red Shot, Savvy Minerals - Poppy Seed Lip Scrub
Manuka	*Leptospermum scoparium*	Acne Treatment - Maximum Strength, Manuka
Marjoram Marjoram Vitality	*Origanum majorana*	Aroma Life, Aroma Siez, Dragon Time, Dragon Time Bath & Shower Gel, Fitness, Marjoram, Marjoram Vitality, M-Grain, My Destiny, Ortho Ease Massage Oil, R.C., SniffleEase
Mastrante	*Lippia alba*	Light the Fire, Loyalty, Mastrante
Melaleuca Ericifolia	*Melaleuca ericifolia*	Australian Kuranya, Melaleuca-Geranium Moisturizing Soap
Melaleuca Quinquenervia (Niaouli)	*Melaleuca viridiflora*	AromaGuard Meadow Mist Deodorant, Cool Azul, Cool Azul Pain Relief Cream, Cool Azul Sports Gel, Melaleuca Quinquenervia, Melrose
Melissa	*Melissa officinalis*	ART Gentle Cleanser, ART Refreshing Toner, Awaken, Brain Power, Build Your Dream, Divine Release, Finance, Forgiveness, GeneYus, Hope, Humility, Inner Harmony, InTouch, Live with Passion, Loyalty, Melissa, MultiGreens, Reconnect, White Angelica
Micromeria	*Micromeria fruticosa*	

Single Oil Name	Botanical Name	Products Containing Single Oil
Mountain Savory	*Satureja montana*	Animal Scents PuriClean, ImmuPower, Journey On, Mountain Savory, Mountain Savory Vitality, Surrender
Mountain Savory Vitality		
Myrrh	*Commiphora myrrha*	3 Wise Men, Abundance, Animal Scents Mendwell, Animal Scents Ointment, Boswellia Wrinkle Cream, ClaraDerm, Egyptian Gold, EndoGize, Essential Beauty Serum (Dry Skin), Exodus II, Faith, Finance, GeneYus, Gratitude, Hope, Humility, Infect Away, Inner Harmony, Lavender Bath & Shower Gel, Lavender Foaming Hand Soap, Lavender Hand & Body Lotion, Mineral Sunscreen Lotion, Myrrh, Oola Balance, Protec, Reconnect, Rose Ointment, Sandalwood Moisture Cream, The Gift, Thyromin, White Angelica
Myrtle	*Myrtus communis*	Animal Scents PuriClean, Breathe Again Roll-On, EndoFlex, EndoFlex Vitality, Fun, Inspiration, JuvaTone, Mister, My Destiny, Prostate Health, Purification, R.C., SniffleEase, Thieves Fruit & Veggie Soak, Thyromin
Neroli (Bitter Orange)	*Citrus aurantium amara*	Acceptance, Australian Blue, Awaken, Field, Finance, Friends, Fulfill Your Destiny, Humility, Inner Child, Live with Passion, Neroli, Oola Grow, Present Time
Niaouli (See Melaleuca Quinquenervia)	*Melaleuca viridiflora*	
Northern Lights Black Spruce	*Picea mariana*	AgilEase, Animal Scents Shampoo, Egyptian Gold, Exodus II, Finance, Gathering, GeneYus, Gratitude, Highest Potential, Humility, Inner Harmony, LavaDerm After-Sun Spray, LavaDerm Cooling Mist, Light the Fire, Live Your Passion, Mineral Sunscreen Lotion - SPF 10, My Destiny, Northern Lights Black Spruce, Oola Balance, Oola Grow, Peace & Calming II, Reconnect, Shutran, Shutran 3-in-1 Men's Wash, Shutran Aftershave Lotion, Shutran Bar Soap, Shutran Beard Oil, Shutran Shave Cream, The Gift, T.R. Care
Nutmeg	*Myristica fragrans*	EndoFlex, EndoFlex Vitality, En-R-Gee, Field, Fitness, Fulfill Your Destiny, Fun, Light the Fire, Live Your Passion, Magnify Your Purpose, My Destiny, NingXia Nitro, Nutmeg, Nutmeg Vitality, ParaFree, Super B
Nutmeg Vitality		
Ocotea	*Ocotea quixos*	Acceptance, Amoressence, Animal Scents Infect Away, ART Beauty Masque, ART Creme Masque, Australian Blue, ComforTone, Common Sense, Finance, Highest Potential, Journey On, KidScents Slique Toothpaste, Light the Fire, Mirah Shave Oil, Oola Balance, Oola Grow, ParaFree, Release, SARA, Savvy Minerals - Misting Spray, Shutran, Shutran 3-in-1 Men's Wash, Shutran Aftershave Lotion, Shutran Bar Soap, Shutran Beard Oil, Shutran Shave Cream, Slique CitraSlim Powder Capsule, Slique Essence, Slique Shake, Stress Away, Stress Away Relaxing Bath Bombs, Stress Away Roll-On, Thieves AromaBright Toothpaste, Transformation, T.R. Care

Single Oil Name	Botanical Name	Products Containing Single Oil
Orange Orange Vitality	*Citrus sinensis*	Abundance, Balance Complete, Christmas Spirit, Cinnamint Lip Balm, Citrus Fresh, Citrus Fresh Vitality, Coconut-Lime Replenishing Body Butter, Envision, Family, Finance, Friends, Gary's True Grit NingXia Berry Syrup, Harmony, ImmuPro, Inner Child, Inner Harmony, Into the Future, Lady Sclareol, Live Your Passion, Longevity, Longevity Softgels, Longevity Vitality, Mirah Lustrous Hair Oil, My Destiny, NingXia Red, Oola Balance, Oola Grow, Orange, Orange Blossom Facial Wash, Orange Vitality, Peace & Calming, Peace & Calming II, Pure Protein Complete (Vanilla), Pure Protein Complete (Chocolate), SARA, Savvy Minerals - Misting Spray, Savvy Minerals - Poppy Seed Lip Scrub, Slique Bars, Slique Bars-Chocolate-Coated, Super C, Super C Chewable, T-Away, Thieves Automatic Dishwasher Powder, Thieves Foaming Hand Soap, T.R. Care
Oregano Oregano Vitality	*Origanum vulgare* (Syn. *O. majorana*)	Cool Azul, ImmuPower, Inner Defense, Journey On, Oregano, Oregano Vitality, Ortho Sport Massage Oil, Regenolone Moisturizing Cream
Palmarosa	*Cymbopogon martini*	Animal Scents Ointment, Awaken, Clarity, Dragon Time Bath & Shower Gel, Evening Peace Bath & Shower Gel, Faith, Family, Finance, Forgiveness, Friends, Genesis Hand & Body Lotion, Gentle Baby, Harmony, Joy, Mirah Luminous Cleansing Oil, Oola Balance, Palmarosa, Rose Ointment, T-Away, T.R. Care
Palo Santo	*Bursera graveolens*	Animal Scents Infect Away, Animal Scents PuriClean, Faith, Freedom, Friends, GeneYus, Palo Santo, Reconnect, SniffleEase, Transformation
Patchouli	*Pogostemon cablin*	Abundance, Allerzyme, Animal Scents Infect Away, Animal Scents Ointment, Animal Scents ParaGize, Animal Scents PuriClean, Charcoal Bar Soap, DiGize, DiGize Vitality, Live with Passion, Loyalty, Magnify Your Purpose, Orange Blossom Facial Wash, Orange Blossom Moisturizer, ParaFree, Patchouli, Peace & Calming, Peace & Calming II, Rose Ointment, T-Away, Thieves Fruit & Veggie Soak, T.R. Care
Peppermint Peppermint Vitality	*Mentha piperita*	Allerzyme, Animal Scents ParaGize, AromaEase, Aroma Siez, AromaGuard Mountain Mint Deodorant, ART Refreshing Toner, ART Sheerlumé Brightening Cream, Breathe Again Roll-On, Chocolessence Peppermint Almond Bar, Cinnamint Lip Balm, Clarity, ComforTone, Cool Azul, Cool Azul Pain Relief Cream, Cool Azul Sports Gel, CortiStop, Deep Relief Roll-On, Digest & Cleanse, DiGize, DiGize Vitality, Essentialzyme, Finance, Fitness, Freedom, Journey On, KidScents MightyZyme, Lavender Mint Daily Conditioner, Lavender Mint Daily Shampoo, Live Your Passion, Loyalty, M-Grain, MightyZyme, MindWise, Mineral Essence, Mister, Morning Start Bath & Shower Gel, Morning Start Moisturizing Soap, My Destiny, NingXia Nitro, Ortho Ease Massage Oil, Ortho Sport Massage Oil, PanAway, ParaFree, Peppermint, Peppermint-Cedarwood Moisturizing Soap, Peppermint Vitality, Progessence Plus, Prostate Health, R.C., Raven, Regenolone Moisturizing Cream, Relaxation Massage Oil, Relieve It, Satin Facial Scrub–Mint, Savvy Minerals - Lip Gloss (Colors: Abundant, Anchors Aweigh, Embrace, Headliner, Journey, Maven), Savvy Minerals Lip Gloss (Sets: Let It Glow, Sleigh Ride), SclarEssence, SclarEssence Vitality,

Single Oil Name	Botanical Name	Products Containing Single Oil
Peppermint Vitality (continued)		Slique Gum, SniffleEase, Super Cal Plus, Thieves AromaBright Toothpaste, Thieves Cough Drops, Thieves Dental Floss, Thieves Dentarome Plus Toothpaste, Thieves Dentarome Ultra Toothpaste, Thieves Fresh Essence Plus Mouthwash, Thieves Fruit & Veggie Soak, Thieves Hard Lozenges, Thieves Mints, Thieves Waterless Hand Purifier, Thyromin, Transformation, TummyGize
Petitgrain	*Citrus aurantium amara (Syn. C. sinensis)*	Petitgrain
Pine	*Pinus sylvestris*	Family, Grounding, My Destiny, Pine, R.C., SniffleEase
Plectranthus Oregano	*Plectranthus amboinicus*	Animal Scents Infect Away, Cool Azul, Cool Azul Pain Relief Cream, Cool Azul Sports Gel
Ravintsara	*Cinnamomum camphora*	ImmuPower, Journey On, My Destiny, Raven, Ravintsara, SniffleEase
Roman Chamomile	*Anthemis nobilis (Syn. Chamaemelum nobile)*	Amoressence, Aroma Sleep, ART Creme Masque, Awaken, ClaraDerm, Clarity, Divine Release, Dragon Time Bath & Shower Gel, Evening Peace Bath & Shower Gel, Faith, Family, Finance, Forgiveness, Friends, Genesis Hand & Body Lotion, Gentle Baby, Harmony, Inner Harmony, Journey On, Joy, JuvaFlex, JuvaFlex Vitality, K&B, KidScents Tender Tush, M-Grain, Mirah Luminous Cleansing Oil, Motivation, Oola Balance, Oola Grow, Rehemogen, Roman Chamomile, Satin Facial Scrub - Mint, SleepyIze, Surrender, T-Away, T.R. Care, Tranquil Roll-On, Wolfberry Eye Cream
Rose	*Rosa damascena*	Australian Blue, Awaken, Divine Release, Dream Catcher, Egyptian Gold, Envision, Faith, Finance, Forgiveness, Friends, Gathering, GeneYus, Gentle Baby, Harmony, Highest Potential, Humility, Inner Harmony, Journey On, Joy, Loyalty, Mirah Luminous Cleansing Oil, Mirah Lustrous Hair Oil, Mirah Shave Oil, Oola Balance. Oola Grow, Reconnect, Release, Rose, Rose Ointment, SARA, Savvy Minerals - Misting Spray, T-Away, T.R. Care, Trauma Life, White Angelica
Rose of Sharon (see Cistus)	*Cistus ladaniferus*	Rose of Sharon
Rosemary / Rosemary Vitality	*Rosmarinus officinalis*	Acne Treatment - Maximum Strength, Animal Scents ParaGize, Animal Scents PuriClean, AromaGuard Meadow Mist Deodorant, AromaGuard Mountain Mint Deodorant, CardioGize, Charcoal Bar Soap, Clarity, ComforTone, En-R-Gee, Essentialzymes-4, Finance, ICP, Inner Defense, Insect Repellent, JuvaFlex, JuvaFlex Vitality, JuvaTone, KidScents Slique Toothpaste, Melrose, Mirah Luminous Cleansing Oil, Morning Start Bath & Shower Gel, Morning Start Moisturizing Soap, MultiGreens, Orange Blossom Facial Wash, Orange Blossom Moisturizer, Purification, Rehemogen, Rosemary, Rosemary Vitality, Sandalwood Moisture Cream, Satin Facial Scrub - Mint, Shutran Bar Soap, Thieves, Thieves AromaBright Toothpaste, Thieves Automatic Dishwasher Powder, Thieves Cleansing Soap, Thieves Cough Drops, Thieves Dental Floss, Thieves Dentarome Plus Toothpaste,

Single Oil Name	Botanical Name	Products Containing Single Oil
Rosemary Vitality (continued)		Thieves Dish Soap, Thieves Foaming Hand Soap, Thieves Fresh Essence Plus Mouthwash, Thieves Fruit & Veggie Soak, Thieves Fruit & Veggie Spray, Thieves Hard Lozenges, Thieves Household Cleaner, Thieves Laundry Soap, Thieves Mints, Thieves Spray, Thieves Vitality, Thieves Waterless Hand Purifier, Thieves Wipes, Valor Moisturizing Soap
Royal Hawaiian Sandalwood	Santalum paniculatum	3 Wise Men, Acceptance, ART Gentle Cleanser, ART Intensive Moisturizer, ART Light Moisturizer, ART Refreshing Toner, ART Sheerlumé Brightening Cream, Awaken, Boswellia Wrinkle Cream, Divine Release, Essential Beauty Serum (Dry Skin), Evening Peace Bath & Shower Gel, Family, Finance, Forgiveness, Gathering, Highest Potential, Inner Child, Inner Harmony, Inspiration, InTouch, Lady Sclareol, Lemon-Sandalwood Cleansing Soap, Live with Passion, Live Your Passion, Mirah Shave Oil, Oola Grow, Reconnect, Release, Royal Hawaiian Sandalwood, Sandalwood Moisture Cream, Transformation, Trauma Life, T.R. Care
Rue	Ruta graveolens	Aroma Sleep, Common Sense, Freedom, RutaVaLa, RutaVaLa Roll-On, SleepEssence, SleepyIze, T-Away, T.R. Care
Sacred Frankincense	Boswellia sacra	Aroma Sleep, ART Sheerlumé Brightening Cream, Build Your Dream, Faith, Freedom, GeneYus, Inner Harmony, Loyalty, Mineral Sunscreen Lotion, Oola Balance, Progessence Plus, Reconnect, Sacred Frankincense, SleepyIze, The Gift, Transformation
Sacred Sandalwood	Santalum album	ART Chocolate Masque, Australian Kuranya, Awaken, Brain Power, Build Your Dream, Dream Catcher, Friends, GeneYus, Harmony, Journey On, Loyalty, Magnify Your Purpose, Mirah Luminous Cleansing Oil, My Destiny, Oola Balance, Sacred Sandalwood, T.R. Care, White Angelica
Sage Sage Vitality	Salvia officinalis	Cool Azul, Cool Azul Pain Relief Cream, Cool Azul Sports Gel, Dragon Time Bath & Shower Gel, Dragon Time Massage Oil, EndoFlex, EndoFlex Vitality, Envision, Faith, FemiGen, K&B, Magnify Your Purpose, Mirah Lustrous Hair Oil, Mister, Prenolone Plus Body Cream, Protec, Sage, Sage Vitality, Savvy Minerals - Misting Spray
Spanish Sage (Sage Lavender)	Salvia lavandulifolia	Friends, Harmony, Lady Sclareol, Oola Balance, SclarEssence, SclarEssence Vitality, T-Away, T.R. Care
Spearmint Spearmint Vitality	Mentha spicata	Acceptance, Animal Scents Dental Pet Chews, Animal Scents ParaGize, AromaEase, ART Sheerlumé Brightening Cream, Australian Blue, Awaken, Cinnamint Lip Balm, Citrus Fresh, Citrus Fresh Vitality, Coconut-Lime Replenishing Body Butter, Dream Catcher, EndoFlex, EndoFlex Vitality, Fun, GLF, GLF Vitality, Highest Potential, Insect Repellent, Journey On, KidScents Slique Toothpaste, Lady Sclareol, Lavender Mint Daily Conditioner, Lavender Mint Daily Shampoo, NingXia Nitro, OmegaGize³, Oola Grow, Red Shot, Relaxation Massage Oil, Release, SARA, Savvy Minerals - Poppy Seed Lip Scrub, Slique CitraSlim Powder Capsule, Slique Essence, Slique Shake, Slique Gum, Spearmint, Spearmint Vitality, Thieves AromaBright Toothpaste, Thieves Fresh Essence Plus Mouthwash, Thyromin, T.R. Care, TummyGize

Single Oil Name	Botanical Name	Products Containing Single Oil
Tangerine Tangerine Vitality	*Citrus reticulata*	Acceptance, Aroma Sleep, Australian Blue, Awaken, Build Your Dream, Citrus Fresh, Citrus Fresh Vitality, Coconut-Lime Replenishing Body Butter, ComforTone, Dragon Time Bath & Shower Gel, Dream Catcher, Family, Fulfill Your Destiny, Fun, Highest Potential, Inner Child, Inner Harmony, Journey On, Joy, KidScents Shampoo, KidScents Slique Toothpaste, Mirah Luminous Cleansing Oil, NingXia Red, Oola Grow, Peace & Calming, Peace & Calming II, Red Shot, Relaxation Massage Oil, Release, SARA, Savvy Minerals - Lipstick (Colors: Bedazzled, I Dare You, It Girl, Mic Drop, Miss Congeniality, Sweet Life), Savvy Minerals - Poppy Seed Lip Scrub, SleepEssence, SleepyIze, Slique Essence, Slique Shake, Super C, Tangerine, Tangerine Vitality, T-Away, T.R. Care, TummyGize
Tarragon Tarragon Vitality	*Artemisia dracunculus*	Allerzyme, ComforTone, DiGize, DiGize Vitality, Essentialzyme, Essentialzymes-4, ICP, ParaFree, Tarragon Vitality, Thieves Fruit & Veggie Soak
Tea Tree	*Melaleuca alternifolia*	Acne Treatment - Maximum Strength, Animal Scents Ointment, Animal Scents PuriClean, AromaGuard Meadow Mist Deodorant, Australian Kuranya, ClaraDerm, Melaleuca-Geranium Moisturizing Soap, Melrose, Owie, ParaFree, Purification, Rehemogen, Rose Ointment, Shutran Shave Cream, Tea Tree, Thieves Fruit & Veggie Soak
Thyme Thyme Vitality	*Thymus vulgaris*	Inner Defense, Insect Repellent, Longevity, Longevity Softgels, Longevity Vitality, Ortho Ease Massage Oil, Ortho Sport Massage Oil, ParaFree, Rehemogen, Thyme, Thyme Vitality
Tsuga	*Tsuga canadensis*	Tsuga
Valerian	*Valeriana officinalis*	Aroma Sleep, Freedom, RutaVaLa, RutaVaLa Roll-On, SleepEssence, SleepyIze, T-Away, T.R. Care, Trauma Life, Valerian
Vanilla	*Vanilla planifolia*	Amoressence, NingXia Nitro, Slique Bars, Slique Bars–Chocolate-Coated, Slique Tea, Stress Away, Stress Away Roll-On
Vetiver	*Vetiveria zizanoides* (Syn. *V. zizanioides*)	Amoressence, Animal Scents Shampoo, ART Creme Masque, ART Sheerlumé Brightening Cream, Cool Azul, Cool Azul Pain Relief Cream, Cool Azul Sports Gel, Deep Relief Roll-On, Egyptian Gold, Exodus II, Finance, Freedom, Gathering, GeneYus, Gratitude, Highest Potential, Humility, Inner Harmony, Inspiration, InTouch, Lady Sclareol, Loyalty, Melaleuca-Geranium Moisturizing Soap, My Destiny, Oola Balance, Oola Grow, Ortho Ease Massage Oil, Ortho Sport Massage Oil, ParaFree, Peace & Calming II, Reconnect, SleepEssence, Super Cal Plus, The Gift, Thieves Fresh Essence Plus Mouthwash, T.R. Care, Valor Moisturizing Soap, Vetiver
Western Red Cedar	*Thuja plicata*	KidScents Lotion
White Cypress Pine	*Callitris columellaris*	Cool Azul Pain Relief Cream
White Fir	*Abies concolor*	AromaGuard Mountain Mint Deodorant, Australian Blue, Grounding, Highest Potential, Into the Future, Oola Grow, T.R. Care, White Light
White Lotus	*Nymphaea lotus*	Into the Future, Oola Grow, SARA

Single Oil Name	Botanical Name	Products Containing Single Oil
Wintergreen	*Gaultheria procumbens*	AgilEase, BLM Capsules, Cool Azul, Cool Azul Sports Gel, Deep Relief Roll-On, My Destiny, Ortho Ease Massage Oil, Ortho Sport Massage Oil, PanAway, Raven, Regenolone Moisturizing Cream, Thieves Dentarome Plus Toothpaste, Thieves Dentarome Ultra Toothpaste, Wintergreen
Xiang Mao	*Cymbopogon citratus*	Family, Friends, Xiang Mao
Yarrow/Blue Yarrow	*Achillea millefolium*	Dragon Time, Dragon Time Massage Oil, Mister, Prenolone Plus Body Cream
Ylang Ylang (Also, Amazonian/Ecuadorian Ylang Ylang)	*Cananga odorata* (*Cananga odorata Equitoriana*)	Amoressence, Animal Scents Ointment, Aroma Life, AromaGuard Meadow Mist Deodorant, ART Creme Masque, ART Chocolate Masque, ART Intensive Moisturizer, ART Renewal Serum, Australian Blue, Awaken, Believe, Boswellia Wrinkle Cream, Build Your Dream, Clarity, Common Sense, Dragon Time Bath & Shower Gel, Dragon Time Massage Oil, Dream Catcher, Evening Peace Bath & Shower Gel, Faith, Family, FemiGen, Field, Finance, Forgiveness, Friends, Gathering, Genesis Hand & Body Lotion, GeneYus, Gentle Baby, Gratitude, Grounding, Harmony, Highest Potential, Humility, Inner Child, Inner Harmony, Inspiration, Into the Future, Journey On, Joy, KidScents Lotion, KidScents Tender Tush, Lady Sclareol, Lavender-Oatmeal Bar Soap, Live Your Passion, Loyalty, Magnify Your Purpose, Mineral Sunscreen Lotion, Mirah Luminous Cleansing Oil, Mirah Lustrous Hair Oil, Mirah Shave Oil, Motivation, My Destiny, Oola Balance, Oola Grow, Peace & Calming, Peace & Calming II, Prenolone Plus Body Cream, Present Time, Reconnect, Relaxation Massage Oil, Release, Rose Ointment, Sacred Mountain, Sacred Mountain Moisturizing Soap, Sandalwood Moisture Cream, SARA, Seedlings Baby Lotion, Seedlings Baby Wash & Shampoo, Seedlings Baby Wipes, Seedlings Linen Spray, Sensation, Sensation Bath & Shower Gel, Sensation Hand & Body Lotion, Sensation Massage Oil, Shutran, Shutran 3-in-1 Men's Wash, Shutran Aftershave Lotion, Shutran Bar Soap, Shutran Beard Oil, Shutran Shave Cream, T-Away, T R. Care, Valor Moisturizing Soap, White Angelica, Wolfberry Eye Cream, Ylang Ylang
Yuzu	*Citrus junos*	NingXia Red

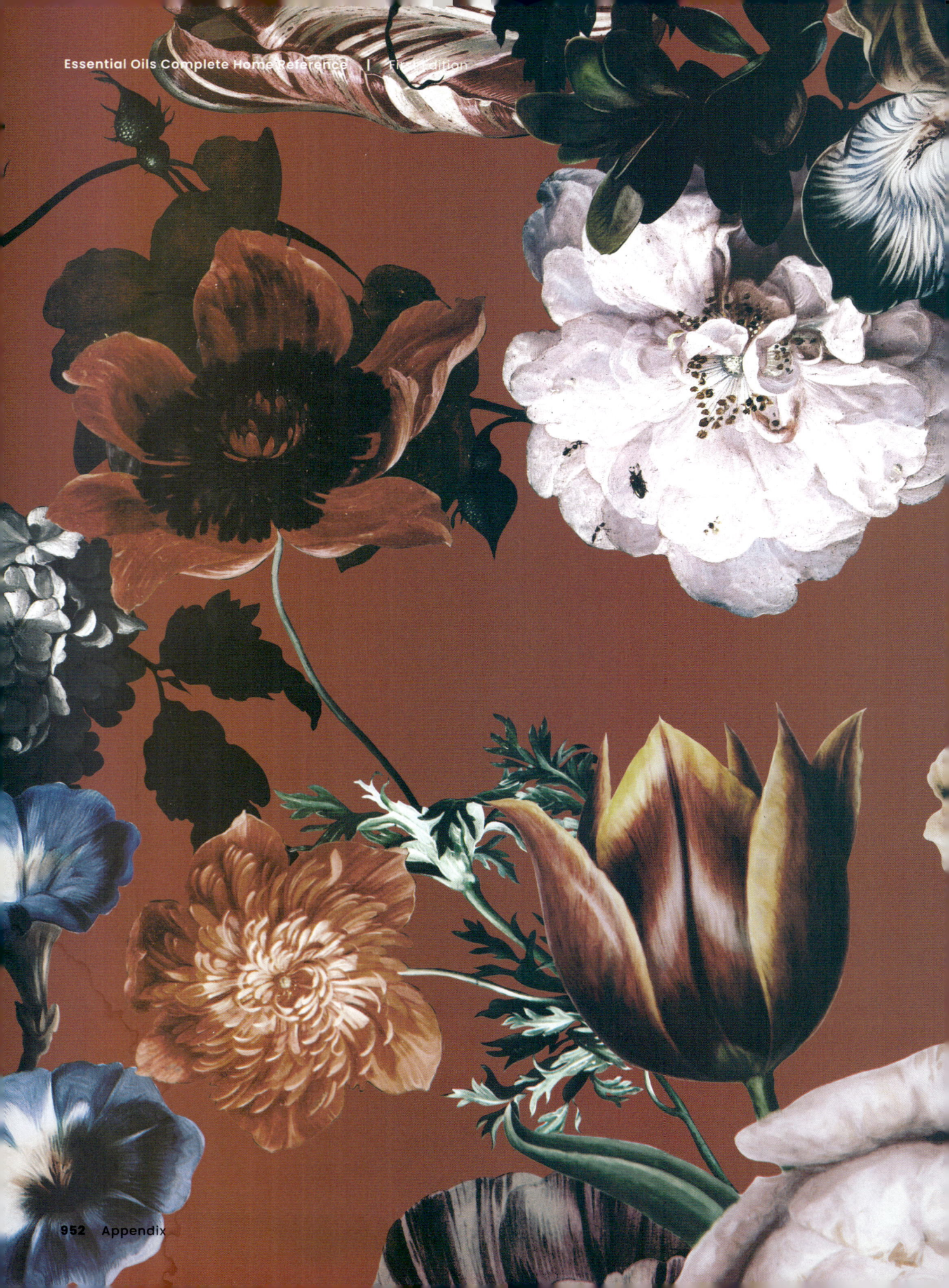

Appendix C
Essential Oil Blends Data

Blend Name	Ingredients
3 Wise Men	Sweet almond oil, Royal Hawaiian Sandalwood, Juniper, Frankincense, Black Spruce, Myrrh
Abundance	Orange, Frankincense, Patchouli, Clove, Ginger, Myrrh, Cinnamon Bark, Black Spruce
Acceptance	Sweet almond oil, Coriander, Geranium, Bergamot, Frankincense, Royal Hawaiian Sandalwood, Bitter Orange (Neroli), Grapefruit, Tangerine, Spearmint, Lemon, Blue Cypress, Davana, Kaffir Lime, Ocotea, Jasmine, Matricaria (German Chamomile)
Amoressence	Vetiver, Idaho Blue Spruce, Jasmine, Davana, Ocotea, Ylang Ylang, Roman Chamomile, Vanilla, Geranium
Aroma Ease	Peppermint, Spearmint, Ginger, Cardamom, Fennel
Aroma Life	Sesame seed oil, Cypress, Marjoram, Ylang Ylang, Helichrysum
Aroma Siez	Basil, Marjoram, Lavender, Peppermint, Cypress
AromaSleep	Lavender, Geranium, Roman Chamomile, Bergamot, Tangerine, Sacred Frankincense, Valerian, Rue
Australian Blue	Blue Cypress, Ylang Ylang, Cedarwood, White Fir, Geranium, Grapefruit, Tangerine, Spearmint, Davana, Kaffir Lime, Lemon, Ocotea, Jasmine, Matricaria (German Chamomile), Blue Tansy, Rose
Australian Kuranya	Lemon Myrtle, Kunzea, Blue Cypress, Sacred Sandalwood, Fennel, Melaleuca Ericifolia, Eucalyptus Radiata, Tea Tree
Awaken	Joy, Forgiveness, Present Time, Dream Catcher, Harmony
Believe	Balsam Canada (Idaho Balsam Fir), Coriander, Bergamot, Frankincense, Idaho Blue Spruce, Ylang Ylang, Geranium
Brain Power	Sacred Sandalwood, Cedarwood, Frankincense, Melissa, Blue Cypress, Lavender, Helichrysum
Breathe Again Roll-On	Caprylic/capric triglyceride, Eucalyptus Staigeriana, Eucalyptus Globulus, Laurus Nobilis (Bay Laurel), Rose Hip Seed Oil, Peppermint, Eucalyptus Radiata, Copaiba, Myrtle, Blue Cypress, Eucalyptus Blue
Build Your Dream	Lavender, Ylang Ylang, Blue Cypress, Sacred Frankincense, Hong Kuai, Melissa, Idaho Blue Spruce, Balsam Canada, Sacred Sandalwood, Coriander, Tangerine, Black Pepper, Bergamot, Frankincense, Juniper, Anise, Blue Tansy, Geranium, Blue Lotus,
Christmas Spirit	Orange, Cinnamon Bark, Black Spruce
Citrus Fresh	Orange, Tangerine, Grapefruit, Lemon, Mandarin, Spearmint
Citrus Fresh Vitality	Orange, Tangerine, Grapefruit, Lemon, Mandarin, Spearmint
Clarity	Basil, Cardamom, Rosemary, Peppermint, Coriander, Geranium, Bergamot, Lemon, Ylang Ylang, Jasmine, Roman Chamomile, Palmarosa
Common Sense	Frankincense, Ylang Ylang, Ocotea, Goldenrod, Rue, Dorado Azul, Lime

Blend Name	Ingredients
Cool Azul	Wintergreen, Peppermint, Sage, Copaiba, Oregano, Melaleuca Quinquenervia (Niaouli), Plectranthus Oregano, Lavender, Blue Cypress, Elemi, Vetiver, Caraway, Dorado Azul, Matricaria (German Chamomile)
Deep Relief Roll-On	Peppermint, caprylic/capric triglyceride, Lemon, Balsam Canada (Idaho Balsam Fir), Clove, Copaiba, coconut oil, Wintergreen, Helichrysum, Vetiver, Dorado Azul
DiGize	Tarragon, Ginger, Peppermint, Juniper, Fennel, Lemongrass, Anise, Patchouli
DiGize Vitality	Tarragon, Ginger, Peppermint, Juniper, Fennel, Lemongrass, Anise, Patchouli
Divine Release	Royal Hawaiian Sandalwood, Roman Chamomile, Frankincense, Melissa, Geranium, Grapefruit, Blue Cypress, Hinoki, Helichrysum, Bergamot, Rose, Ledum, Angelica
Dragon Time	Fennel, Clary Sage, Marjoram, Lavender, Yarrow, Jasmine
Dream Catcher	Sacred Sandalwood, Tangerine, Ylang Ylang, Black Pepper, Bergamot, Anise, Juniper, Geranium, Blue Cypress, Davana, Citrus Hystrix, Jasmine, Matricaria (German Chamomile), Blue Tansy, Rose, Grapefruit, Spearmint
Egyptian Gold	Frankincense, Balsam Canada (Idaho Balsam Fir), Lavender, Myrrh, Hyssop, Northern Lights Black Spruce, Cedarwood, Vetiver, Rose, Cinnamon Bark
EndoFlex	Spearmint, Sesame Seed oil, Sage, Geranium, Myrtle, Matricaria (German Chamomile), Nutmeg
EndoFlex Vitality	Spearmint, sesame seed oil, Sage, Geranium, Myrtle, Matricaria (German Chamomile), Nutmeg
En-R-Gee	Rosemary, Juniper, Lemongrass, Nutmeg, Balsam Canada (Idaho Balsam Fir), Clove, Black Pepper
Envision	Black Spruce, Geranium, Orange, Lavender, Sage, Rose
Exodus II	Olive oil, Myrrh, Cassia, Cinnamon Bark, Calamus, Northern Lights Black Spruce, Hyssop, Vetiver, Frankincense
Faith	Caprylic/capric triglyceride, Sacred Frankincense, Balsam Canada (Idaho Balsam Fir), Myrrh, Juniper, Hyssop, Cedarwood, Sage, Rose, Geranium, Palo Santo, Coriander, Bergamot, Lemon, Ylang Ylang, Jasmine, Roman Chamomile, Palmarosa
Family	Caprylic/capric triglyceride, Ylang Ylang, Lavender, Orange, Geranium, Cardamom, Tangerine, Frankincense, Cedarwood, Coriander, Pine, Royal Hawaiian Sandalwood, Lemongrass, Bergamot, Xiang Mao, Lemon, Black Spruce, Lime, Roman Chamomile, Palmarosa
Field	Caprylic/capric triglyceride, Cardamom, Frankincense, Ylang Ylang, sweet almond oil, Nutmeg, Ginger, Bitter Orange (Neroli), Balsam Canada (Idaho Balsam Fir), Coriander, Black Spruce, Bergamot, Idaho Blue Spruce, Geranium
Finance	Fractionated coconut oil, Frankincense, Orange, Ocotea, Balsam Canada (Idaho Balsam Fir), Royal Hawaiian Sandalwood, Basil, Geranium, Lavender, Cardamom, Coriander, Ylang Ylang, Northern Lights Black Spruce, Rosemary, Citronella (nardus), Citronella (winterianus), Bergamot (furocoumarin-free), Vetiver, Peppermint, Melissa, Myrrh, Cinnamon Bark, Lemon, Jasmine, Roman Chamomile, Palmarosa, Bitter Orange (Neroli), Rose
Fitness	Caprylic/capric triglyceride, Cypress, Copaiba, Basil, Cistus, Marjoram, Peppermint, Clary Sage, Idaho Blue Spruce, Balsam Canada (Idaho Balsam Fir), Nutmeg, Black Pepper
Friends	Caprylic/capric triglyceride, Lavender, Frankincense, Blue Cypress, Orange, Palo Santo, Xiang Mao, Ylang Ylang, Sacred Sandalwood, Mandarin, Angelica, Geranium, Black Spruce, Hyssop, Spanish Sage, Lemongrass, Bitter Orange (Neroli), Coriander, Bergamot (Furocoumarin-free), Lemon, Roman Chamomile, Palmarosa, Rose
Fun	Caprylic/capric triglyceride, Spearmint, Cedarwood, Myrtle, Lemon, Grapefruit, Tangerine, Jasmine, Nutmeg

Blend Name	Ingredients
Forgiveness	Sesame seed oil, Melissa, Geranium, Frankincense, Royal Hawaiian Sandalwood, Coriander, Angelica, Lavender, Bergamot, Lemon, Ylang Ylang, Jasmine, Helichrysum, Roman Chamomile, Palmarosa, Rose
Freedom	Caprylic/capric triglyceride, Copaiba, Lavender, Sacred Frankincense, Vetiver, Idaho Blue Spruce, Palo Santo, Valerian, Rue
Fulfill Your Destiny	Tangerine, Frankincense, Nutmeg, Cassia, Cardamom, Clary Sage, Black Pepper, Idaho Blue Spruce, Bitter Orange (Neroli)
Gathering	Lavender, Northern Lights Black Spruce, Geranium, Royal Hawaiian Sandalwood, Ylang Ylang, Vetiver, Cinnamon Bark, Rose
GeneYus	Cocus nucifera oil, Sacred Frankincense, Blue Cypress, Cedarwood, Idaho Blue Spruce, Melissa, Palo Santo, Northern Lights Black Spruce, sweet almond oil, Vetiver, Bergamot, Myrrh, Geranium, Sacred Sandalwood, Ylang Ylang, Hyssop, Rose
Gentle Baby	Coriander, Geranium, Palmarosa, Lavender, Ylang Ylang, Roman Chamomile, Bergamot (furocoumarin-free), Lemon, Jasmine, Rose
GLF	Grapefruit, Ledum, Helichrysum, Celery Seed, Hyssop, Spearmint
GLF Vitality	Grapefruit, Ledum, Helichrysum, Celery Seed, Hyssop, Spearmint
Gratitude	Balsam Canada (Idaho Balsam Fir), Frankincense, Coriander, Myrrh, Ylang Ylang, Bergamot (furocoumarin-free), Northern Lights Black Spruce, Vetiver, Geranium
Grounding	White Fir, Black Spruce, Ylang Ylang, Pine, Cedarwood, Angelica, Juniper
Harmony	Sacred Sandalwood, Lavender, Ylang Ylang, Frankincense, Orange, Angelica, Geranium, Hyssop, Spanish Sage, Black Spruce, Coriander, Bergamot, Lemon, Jasmine, Roman Chamomile, Palmarosa, Rose
Highest Potential	Blue Cypress, Ylang Ylang, Jasmine, Cedarwood, Geranium, Lavender, Northern Lights Black Spruce, Frankincense, Royal Hawaiian Sandalwood, White Fir, Vetiver, Cinnamon Bark, Davana, Citrus Hystrix, Rose, German Chamomile, Blue Tansy, Grapefruit, Tangerine, Spearmint, Lemon, Ocotea
Hope	Sweet almond oil, Melissa, Juniper, Myrrh, Black Spruce
Humility	Caprylic/capric triglyceride, Coriander, Ylang Ylang, Bergamot (furocoumarin-free), Geranium, Melissa, Frankincense, Myrrh, Northern Lights Black Spruce, Vetiver, Bitter Orange (Neroli), Rose
ImmuPower	Hyssop, Mountain Savory, Cistus, Camphor (Ravintsara), Frankincense, Oregano, Clove, Cumin, Dorado Azul
Inner Child	Orange, Tangerine, Ylang Ylang, Royal Hawaiian Sandalwood, Jasmine, Lemongrass, Black Spruce, Bitter Orange (Neroli)
Inner Harmony	Geranium, Lavender, Royal Hawaiian Sandalwood, Ylang Ylang, Idaho Blue Spruce, Sacred Frankincense, Roman Chamomile, Tangerine, Orange, Northern Lights Black Spruce, Myrrh, Rose, Angelica, Vetiver, Melissa
Inspiration	Cedarwood, Black Spruce, Myrtle, Coriander, Royal Hawaiian Sandalwood, Frankincense, Bergamot (furocoumarin-free), Vetiver, Ylang Ylang, Geranium
Into the Future	Sweet almond oil, Clary Sage, Ylang Ylang, White Fir, Idaho Blue Spruce, Jasmine, Juniper, Frankincense, Orange, Cedarwood, White Lotus
InTouch	Caprylic/capric triglyceride, Vetiver, Melissa, Royal Hawaiian Sandalwood, Cedarwood, Idaho Blue Spruce

Blend Name	Ingredients
Journey On	Peppermint, Copaiba, Hyssop, Mountain Savory, Cistus, Ravintsara, Frankincense, Oregano, Sacred Sandalwood, Tangerine, Ylang Ylang, Cinnamon, Clove, Cumin, Black Pepper, Roman Chamomile, Bergamot, Anise, Juniper, Black Spruce, Geranium, Lavender, German Chamomile, Dorado Azul, Blue Cypress, Davana, Citrus Hystrix, Jasmine, Blue Tansy, Rose, Grapefruit, Spearmint, Lemon, Ocotea
Joy	Bergamot, Ylang Ylang, Geranium, Lemon, Coriander, Tangerine, Jasmine, Roman Chamomile, Palmarosa, Rose
JuvaCleanse	Helichrysum, Ledum, Celery Seed
JuvaCleanse Vitality	Helichrysum, Ledum, Celery Seed
JuvaFlex	Sesame seed oil, Fennel, Geranium, Rosemary, Roman Chamomile, Blue Tansy, Helichrysum
JuvaFlex Vitality	Sesame seed oil, Fennel, Geranium, Rosemary, Roman Chamomile, Blue Tansy, Helichrysum
Lady Sclareol	Geranium, Coriander, Vetiver, Orange, Clary Sage, Bergamot, Ylang Ylang, Royal Hawaiian Sandalwood, Spanish Sage, Jasmine, Idaho Blue Spruce, Spearmint
Light the Fire	Nutmeg, Cassia, Mastrante, Ocotea, Canadian Fleabane, Lemon, Black Pepper, Northern Lights Black Spruce
Live with Passion	Royal Hawaiian Sandalwood, Clary Sage, Ginger, Jasmine, Angelica, Patchouli, Cedarwood, Helichrysum, Melissa, Bitter Orange (Neroli)
Live Your Passion	Orange, Royal Hawaiian Sandalwood, Nutmeg, Lime, Idaho Blue Spruce, Northern Lights Black Spruce, Ylang Ylang, Frankincense, Peppermint
Longevity	Thyme, Orange, Clove, Frankincense
Longevity Vitality	Thyme, Orange, Clove, Frankincense
Loyalty	Caprylic/capric triglyceride, Angelica, Ylang Ylang, Lavender, Idaho Blue Spruce, Cassia, Vetiver, Sacred Sandalwood, Geranium, Sacred Frankincense, Patchouli, Cardamom, Mastrante, Peppermint, Melissa, Rose
Magnify Your Purpose	Sacred Sandalwood, Sage, Coriander, Patchouli, Nutmeg, Bergamot, Cinnamon Bark, Ginger, Ylang Ylang, Geranium
Melrose	Rosemary, Tea Tree, Clove, Niaouli, Melaleuca Quinquenervia (Niaouli)
M-Grain	Basil, Marjoram, Lavender, Roman Chamomile, Peppermint, Helichrysum
Mister	Sesame seed oil, Sage, Fennel, Lavender, Myrtle, Yarrow, Peppermint
Motivation	Roman Chamomile, Black Spruce, Ylang Ylang, Lavender
My Destiny	Wintergreen, Peppermint, Helichrysum, Clove, Myrtle, Lemon, Ravintsara, Lavender, caprylic/capric triglyceride, Idaho Balsam Fir, Eucalyptus Globulus, Copaiba, Pine, Marjoram, coconut oil, Eucalyptus Radiata, Eucalyptus Citriodora, Cypress, Northern Lights Black Spruce, Vetiver, Orange, Sacred Sandalwood, Nutmeg, Ylang Ylang, Lime, Idaho Blue Spruce, Frankincense, Dorado Azul
Oola Balance	Caprylic/capric triglyceride, Lavender, Ylang Ylang, Frankincense, Ocotea, Idaho Blue Spruce, Sacred Sandalwood, Balsam Canada (Idaho Balsam Fir), Sacred Frankincense, Jasmine, Northern Lights Black Spruce, Orange, Angelica, Geranium, Hyssop, Spanish Sage, Myrrh, Vetiver, Cistus, Coriander, Bergamot, Lemon, Roman Chamomile, Palmarosa, Rose
Oola Grow	Fractionated coconut oil, White Fir, Blue Cypress, Ylang Ylang, Roman Chamomile, sweet almond oil, Northern Lights Black Spruce, Coriander, Geranium, Jasmine, Cedarwood, Lavender, Frankincense, Bergamot (furocoumarin-free), Clary Sage, Royal Hawaiian Sandalwood, Grapefruit, Tangerine, Spearmint, Vetiver, Lemon, Neroli, Idaho Blue Spruce, Ocotea, Juniper, Orange, Cinnamon Bark, Citrus Hystrix, Rose, White Lotus

Blend Name	Ingredients
Owie	Caprylic/capric glycerides, Balsam Canada (Idaho Balsam Fir), Tea Tree, Helichrysum, Elemi, Cistus, Hinoki, Clove
PanAway	Wintergreen, Helichrysum, Clove, Peppermint
Peace & Calming	Tangerine, Orange, Ylang Ylang, Patchouli, Blue Tansy
Peace & Calming II	Tangerine, Orange, Ylang Ylang, Patchouli, Northern Lights Black Spruce, Matricaria (German Chamomile), Vetiver, Cistus, Bergamot, Cassia, Davana
Present Time	Sweet almond oil, Bitter Orange (Neroli), Black Spruce, Ylang Ylang
Purification	Citronella, Rosemary, Lemongrass, Tea Tree, Lavandin, Myrtle
Raven	Camphor (Ravintsara), Lemon, Wintergreen, Peppermint, Eucalyptus Radiata
R.C.	Eucalyptus Globulus, Myrtle, Marjoram, Pine, Eucalyptus Radiata, Eucalyptus Citriodora, Lavender, Cypress, Black Spruce, Peppermint
Reconnect	Caprylic/capric triglyceride, Sacred Frankincense, Lavender, Blue Cypress, Cedarwood, Melissa, Idaho Blue Spruce, Palo Santo, Northern Lights Black Spruce, sweet almond oil, Bergamot, Myrrh, Vetiver, Geranium, Royal Hawaiian Sandalwood, Ylang Ylang, Hyssop, Coriander, Rose
Red Shot	Tangerine, Mandarin, Lime, Grapefruit, Cassia, Spearmint
Release	Ylang Ylang, olive oil, Lavandin, Geranium, Royal Hawaiian Sandalwood, Grapefruit, Tangerine, Spearmint, Lemon, Blue Cypress, Davana, Kaffir Lime, Ocotea, Jasmine, Matricaria (German Chamomile), Blue Tansy, Rose
Relieve It	Black Spruce, Black Pepper, Hyssop, Peppermint
RutaVaLa	Lavender, Valerian, Rue
RutaVaLa Roll-On	Caprylic/capric triglyceride, Lavender, Valerian, Rue
Sacred Mountain	Black Spruce, Ylang Ylang, Balsam Canada (Idaho Balsam Fir), Cedarwood
SARA	Sweet almond oil, Ylang Ylang, Geranium, Lavender, Orange, Cedarwood, Blue Cypress, Davana, Citrus Hystrix, Jasmine, Rose, Matricaria (German Chamomile), Blue Tansy, Grapefruit, Tangerine, Spearmint, Lemon, Ocotea, White Lotus
SclarEssence	Clary Sage, Peppermint, Spanish Sage, Fennel
SclarEssence Vitality	Clary Sage, Peppermint, Spanish Sage, Fennel
Sensation	Coriander, Ylang Ylang, Bergamot (furocoumarin-free), Jasmine, Geranium
Shutran	Idaho Blue Spruce, Ylang Ylang, Ocotea, Hinoki, Davana, Cedarwood, Lavender, Coriander, Lemon, Northern Lights Black Spruce
SleepyIze	Caprylic/capric glycerides, Lavender, Geranium, Roman Chamomile, Tangerine, Bergamot, Sacred Frankincense, Valerian, Rue
Slique Essence	Grapefruit, Tangerine, Spearmint, Lemon, Ocotea, Stevia Extract
SniffleEase	Caprylic/capric glycerides, Eucalyptus Blue, Palo Santo, Lavender, Dorado Azul, Ravintsara, Myrtle, Eucalyptus Globulus, Marjoram, Pine, Eucalyptus Citriodora, Cypress, Eucalyptus Radiata, Black Spruce, Peppermint
Stress Away	Copaiba, Lime, Cedarwood, Vanilla, Ocotea, Lavender
Stress Away Roll-On	Copaiba, Lime, Cedarwood, Vanilla, Ocotea, Lavender
Surrender	Lavender, Lemon, Black Spruce, Roman Chamomile, Angelica, Mountain Savory
The Gift	Balsam Canada (Idaho Balsam Fir), Sacred Frankincense, Jasmine, Northern Lights Black Spruce, Myrrh, Vetiver, Cistus

Blend Name	Ingredients
Thieves	Clove, Lemon, Cinnamon Bark, Eucalyptus Radiata, Rosemary
Thieves Vitality	Clove, Lemon, Cinnamon Bark, Eucalyptus Radiata, Rosemary
Tranquil Roll-On	Lavender, Cedarwood, caprylic/capric triglyceride, Roman Chamomile, coconut oil
Transformation	Lemon, Peppermint, Royal Hawaiian Sandalwood, Clary Sage, Sacred Frankincense, Idaho Blue Spruce, Cardamom, Ocotea, Palo Santo
Trauma Life	Royal Hawaiian Sandalwood, Frankincense, Valerian, Black Spruce, Davana, Lavender, Geranium, Helichrysum, Citrus Hystrix, Rose
T.R. Care	Roman Chamomile, Tangerine, Lavender, Bergamot, Ylang Ylang, Frankincense, Valerian, Blue Cypress, Orange, Royal Hawaiian Sandalwood, Sacred Sandalwood, Geranium, Black Spruce, Davana, Rue, Jasmine, Angelica, Cedarwood, Helichrysum, Hyssop, Spanish Sage, Patchouli, Citrus Hystrix, Northern Lights Black Spruce, White Fir, Blue Tansy, Vetiver, Coriander, Bergamot (Furocoumarin-free), Rose, Lemon, Cinnamon Bark, Palmarosa, Matricaria (German Chamomile), Grapefruit, Spearmint, Ocotea
Treasure of the Season	Frankincense, Frereana Frankincense, Cinnamon, Idaho Balsam Fir
TummyGize	Caprylic/capric glycerides, Spearmint, Peppermint, Tangerine, Fennel, Anise, Ginger, Cardamom
Valor	Caprylic/capric triglyceride, Black Spruce, Ho Wood, Blue Tansy, Frankincense, Geranium
Valor Roll-On	Caprylic/capric triglyceride, Black Spruce, Camphor, Blue Tansy, Frankincense, Geranium
White Angelica	Sweet almond oil, Bergamot, Myrrh, Geranium, Sacred Sandalwood, Ylang Ylang, Coriander, Black Spruce, Melissa, Hyssop, Rose
White Light	White Fir, White Cedar, White Spruce, White Pine

Appendix D
Flash Points for Essential Oils

Single Oils

Angelica	111°F
Anise	>200°F
Basil/Basil Vitality	177°F
Bergamot/Bergamot Vitality	149°F
Black Pepper/Black Pepper Vitality	112°F
Black Spruce	102°F
Blue Cypress	>200°F
Blue Tansy	137°F
Calamus	194°F
Canadian Fleabane (Conyza)	118°F
Cardamom/Cardamom Vitality	154°F
Carrot Seed/Carrot Seed Vitality	144°F
Cassia	152°F
Cedarwood	>200°F
Celery Seed/Celery Seed Vitality	123.1°F
Cinnamon Bark/Cinnamon Bark Vitality	179°F
Cistus	114°F
Citronella	147°F
Clary Sage	190°F
Clove/Clove Vitality	>200°F
Coriander/Coriander Vitality	153°F
Cumin	142°F
Cypress	103°F
Davana	>200°F
Dill/Dill Vitality	150°F
Dorado Azul	121.5°F
Elemi	114°F
Eucalyptus Blue	114.8°F
Eucalyptus Citriodora	176°F
Eucalyptus Globulus	114°F
Eucalyptus Radiata	130°F
Fennel/Fennel Vitality	168°F
Frankincense/Frankincense Vitality	102°F
Geranium	181°F
German Chamomile/G. Chamomile Vitality	>200°F
Ginger/Ginger Vitality	168°F
Goldenrod	118°F
Grapefruit/Grapefruit Vitality	133°F
Helichrysum	150°F
Hinoki	110.9°F
Hong Kuai	291°F
Hyssop	158°F
Idaho Balsam Fir	118°F
Idaho Blue Spruce	111°F
Idaho Tansy	168°F
Jade Lemon/Jade Lemon Vitality	127.3°F
Jasmine	>200°F
Juniper	104°F
Laurus Nobilis/Laurus Nobilis Vitality	142°F
Lavandin	168°F
Lavender/Lavender Vitality	157°F
Ledum	147°F
Lemon/Lemon Vitality	109°F
Lemon Myrtle	256.8°F
Lemongrass/Lemongrass Vitality	181°F
Lime/Lime Vitality	109°F
Mandarin	113°F
Manuka	208.4°F
Marjoram/Marjoram Vitality	149°F
Mastrante	>252°F
Melaleuca Ericifolia	127°F
Melaleuca Quinquenervia (Niaouli)	168°F

Melissa	189°F
Micromeria	>293°F
Mountain Savory/Mountain Savory Vitality	170°F
Myrrh	>200°F
Myrtle	100°F
Neroli	143.1°F
Northern Lights Black Spruce	102°F
Nutmeg/Nutmeg Vitality	110°F
Ocotea	138.7°F
Orange/Orange Vitality	142°F
Oregano/Oregano Vitality	168°F
Palmarosa	199°F
Palo Santo	140.1°F
Patchouli	>200°F
Peppermint/Peppermint Vitality	172°F
Petitgrain	150°F
Pine	103°F
Ravintsara	124°F
Roman Chamomile	150°F
Rose	156°F
Rosemary/Rosemary Vitality	116°F
Royal Hawaiian Sandalwood	>284
Rue	159.3°F
Sacred Frankincense	101.9°F
Sage/Sage Vitality	146°F
Spanish Sage	108°F
Spearmint/Spearmint Vitality	149°F
Tangerine/Tangerine Vitality	115°F
Tarragon/Tarragon Vitality	148°F
Tea Tree	157°F
Thyme/Thyme Vitality	162°F
Tsuga	103°F
Valerian	112°F
Vetiver	>200°F
White Fir	107°F
Wintergreen	191°F
Xiang Mao	188.7°F
Yarrow	172°F
Ylang Ylang	>200°F
Yuzu	114.2°F

Blends

Abundance	144°F
Acceptance	166°F
Amoressence	116.1°F
Aroma Ease	155.6°F
Aroma Life	142°F
Aroma Siez	157°F
AromaSleep	141°F
Australian Blue	150°F
Awaken	164°F
Believe	129°F
Brain Power	152°F
Breathe Again Roll-On	135.2°F
Build Your Dream	134°F
Christmas Spirit	125°F
Citrus Fresh/Citrus Fresh Vitality	125°F
Clarity	156°F
Common Sense	100.4°F
Deep Relief Roll-On	133.4°F
DiGize/DiGize Vitality	163°F
Divine Release	126.5°F
Dragon Time	171°F
Dream Catcher	142°F
Egyptian Gold	125.1°F
En-R-Gee	121°F
EndoFlex/EndoFlex Vitality	149°F
Envision	122°F
Exodus II	165°F
Faith	133.8°F
Family	159.2°F
Field	148.6°F
Finance	139.1°F
Fitness	148.1°F
Forgiveness	172°F
Freedom	130.2°F

Friends	160.7°F	Oola Balance	168.9°F
Fun	149.9°F	PanAway	187°F
Gathering	142°F	Peace & Calming	128°F
Gentle Baby	170°F	Present Time	142°F
GLF/GLF Vitality	134°F	Purification	132°F
Gratitude	115°F	Raven	127°F
Grounding	134°F	R.C.	119°F
Harmony	144°F	Reconnect	125.9°F
Highest Potential	155°F	Red Shot	132.6°F
Hope	142°F	Release	209°F
Humility	194°F	Relieve It	123°F
ImmuPower	132°F	RutaVaLa Roll-On	159.3°F
Inner Child	131°F	Sacred Mountain	124°F
Inner Harmony	128.3°F	SARA	185°F
Inspiration	153°F	SclarEssence/SclarEssence Vitality	169°F
Into the Future	152°F	Sensation	181°F
InTouch	168°F	Shutran	125°F
Joy	146°F	Slique Essence	134.6°F
JuvaCleanse/JuvaCleanse Vitality	135°F	Stress Away	73.4°F
JuvaFlex/JuvaFlex Vitality	165°F	Stress Away Roll-On	74.5°F
Lady Sclareol	150.8°F	Surrender	131°F
Light the Fire	126.6°F	The Gift	109.3°F
Live with Passion	160.7°F	Thieves/Thieves Vitality	144°F
Live Your Passion	126.9°F	T.R. Care	130.6°F
Longevity/Longevity Vitality	137°F	Tranquil Roll-On	158.4 °F
M-Grain	159°F	Transformation	125.1 °F
Magnify Your Purpose	163°F	Trauma Life	133°F
Melrose	137°F	Valor	143°F
Mister	155°F	Valor Roll-On	117.2 °F
Motivation	131°F	White Angelica	180°F

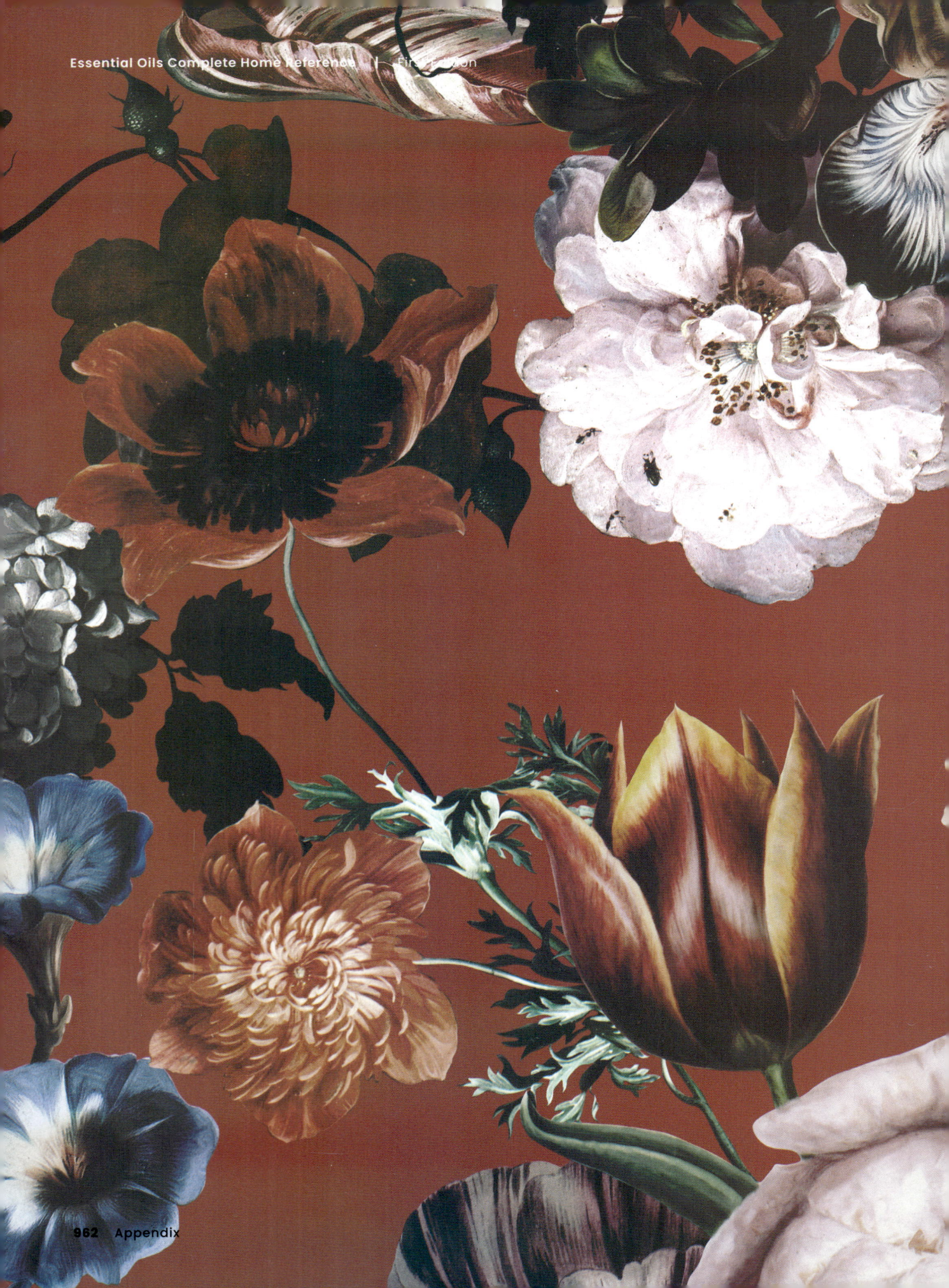

Appendix E

Product Usage for Body Systems

Product Type Key:
- S Essential Oil Single
- B Essential Oil Blend
- D Dietary Supplement
- P Personal Care/Hair and Skin
- L Lotions/Creams/Massage Oils
- G Bath and Shower Gels/Soaps
- A Antiseptic/Sanitizing
- O Oral Care

Product	Product Type	Antiaging	Anti-inflammatory	Cardiovascular System	Digestive / Elimination	Emotional Balance	Glandular / Hormonal	Immune / Anti-infectious	Muscle and Bone	Nervous System	Oral Hygiene	Respiratory System	Skin and Hair
3 Wise Men	B					■							
Abundance	B					■							
Acceptance	B					■							
Acne Treatment, Maximum Strength	P												■
AgilEase	D		■					■	■				
AlkaLime	D				■								
Allerzyme	D				■								
Amazonian Ylang Ylang	S					■							
AminoWise	D									■			
Amoressence	B					■							
Angelica	S				■	■	■					■	■
Animal Scents Cat Treats	D				■								
Animal Scents Dental Pet Chews	O										■		
Animal Scents Infect Away	A												■
Animal Scents Mendwell	B												■
Animal Scents Ointment	L												■
Animal Scents ParaGize	B				■								
Animal Scents PuriClean	B												■
Animal Scents Shampoo	G												■
Animal Scents T-Away	B					■							
Anise	S	■			■								
AromaEase	B				■								
AromaGuard Meadow Mist Deodorant	P												■
AromaGuard Mountain Mint Deodorant	P												■
Aroma Life	B			■		■							
Aroma Siez	B		■						■	■			
AromaSleep	B					■							

Essential Oils Complete Home Reference | First Edition

Product Type Key:
- S Essential Oil Single
- B Essential Oil Blend
- D Dietary Supplement
- P Personal Care/Hair and Skin
- L Lotions/Creams/Massage Oils
- G Bath and Shower Gels/Soaps
- A Antiseptic/Sanitizing
- O Oral Care

Product

Product	Product Type	Antiaging	Anti-inflammatory	Cardiovascular System	Digestive / Elimination	Emotional Balance	Glandular / Hormonal	Immune / Anti-infectious	Muscle and Bone	Nervous System	Oral Hygiene	Respiratory System	Skin and Hair
ART Beauty Masque	P												■
ART Chocolate Masque	P												■
ART Creme Masque	P												■
ART Gentle Cleanser	P												■
ART Intensive Moisturizer	P												■
ART Light Moisturizer	P												■
ART Refreshing Toner	P												■
ART Renewal Serum	P												■
ART Sheerlumé Brightening Cream	P												■
Australian Blue	B					■		■					
Australian Kuranya	B					■							
Awaken	B					■	■						
Balance Complete	D				■			■					
Basil	S		■		■			■	■			■	■
Basil Vitality	D				■								
Bath & Shower Gel Base	G												■
Believe	B					■							
Bergamot	S				■	■							
Bergamot Vitality	D				■	■							
Black Pepper	S				■				■	■			
Black Pepper Vitality	D				■				■	■			
Black Spruce	S		■			■		■				■	
BLM Capsules	D		■						■				
Blue Cypress	S		■					■					
Blue Tansy	S		■				■	■		■			■
Boswellia Wrinkle Cream	L	■											■
Brain Power	B	■				■	■						
Breathe Again Roll-On	B		■					■				■	
Build Your Dream	B					■							
Calamus	S					■		■				■	
Canadian Fleabane (Conyza)	S	■		■			■	■					
Cardamom	S				■			■	■			■	
Cardamom Vitality	D				■			■				■	
CardioGize	D			■									
Carrot Seed	S				■								■
Carrot Seed Vitality	D				■								
Cassia	S		■					■					
Cedarwood	S							■		■			■
Celery Seed	S				■			■					

Product Type Key:
- S Essential Oil Single
- B Essential Oil Blend
- D Dietary Supplement
- P Personal Care/Hair and Skin
- L Lotions/Creams/Massage Oils
- G Bath and Shower Gels/Soaps
- A Antiseptic/Sanitizing
- O Oral Care

Product	Product Type	Antiaging	Anti-inflammatory	Cardiovascular System	Digestive / Elimination	Emotional Balance	Glandular / Hormonal	Immune / Anti-infectious	Muscle and Bone	Nervous System	Oral Hygiene	Respiratory System	Skin and Hair
Celery Seed Vitality	D				■		■						
Cel-Lite Magic Massage Oil	L					■							■
Charcoal Bar Soap	A												■
Christmas Spirit	B					■							
Cinnamint Lip Balm	P												■
Cinnamon Bark	S	■	■	■	■		■	■					
Cinnamon Bark Vitality	D	■	■	■	■		■	■					
Cistus	S	■	■					■		■			
Citronella	S	■			■			■		■			■
Citrus Fresh	B				■					■			
Citrus Fresh Vitality	D				■					■			
Citrus Hystrix (Combava)	S				■								
ClaraDerm	P												■
Clarity	B					■							
Clary Sage	S	■					■		■				
Clove	S	■	■		■			■			■	■	
Clove Vitality	D	■	■		■			■			■	■	
Coconut-Lime Replenishing Body Butter	P												■
ComforTone	D		■		■		■						
Common Sense	B					■				■			
Cool Azul	B								■				
Cool Azul Pain Relief Cream	L								■				
Cool Azul Sports Gel	L								■				
Copaiba	S	■	■		■	■		■	■	■		■	■
Copaiba Vanilla Moisturizing Conditioner	P												■
Copaiba Vanilla Moisturizing Shampoo	P												■
Copaiba Vitality	D	■	■		■	■		■	■	■		■	■
Coriander	S	■	■			■	■	■					■
Coriander Vitality	D	■	■			■	■	■					■
CortiStop	D						■						
Cumin	S	■	■		■		■	■					
Cypress	S	■		■			■	■					
Davana	S		■				■						
Deep Relief Roll-On	B		■						■	■			
Detoxzyme	D				■	■							
Digest & Cleanse	D				■								
DiGize	B				■								
DiGize Vitality	D				■								
Dill	S				■			■	■			■	

Essential Oils Complete Home Reference | First Edition

Product Type Key:
- S Essential Oil Single
- B Essential Oil Blend
- D Dietary Supplement
- P Personal Care/Hair and Skin
- L Lotions/Creams/Massage Oils
- G Bath and Shower Gels/Soaps
- A Antiseptic/Sanitizing
- O Oral Care

Product	Product Type	Antiaging	Anti-inflammatory	Cardiovascular System	Digestive / Elimination	Emotional Balance	Glandular / Hormonal	Immune / Anti-infectious	Muscle and Bone	Nervous System	Oral Hygiene	Respiratory System	Skin and Hair
Dill Vitality	D				■			■	■			■	
Dorado Azul	S	■	■				■	■	■			■	
Douglas Fir	S	■							■			■	
Dragon Time	B					■	■						
Dragon Time Bath & Shower Gel	G												■
Dragon Time Massage Oil	L					■							■
Dream Catcher	B					■							
Egyptian Gold	B					■		■		■		■	
Elemi	S		■					■	■				■
EndoFlex	B				■		■						
EndoFlex Vitality	D				■		■						
EndoGize	D						■						
En-R-Gee	B					■							
Envision	B					■							
Essential Beauty Serum (Dry Skin)	P												■
Essentialzyme	D				■								
Essentialzymes-4	D				■								
Eucalyptus Blue	S							■	■			■	
Eucalyptus Citriodora	S							■				■	
Eucalyptus Globulus	S							■	■			■	
Eucalyptus Radiata	S							■				■	■
Eucalyptus Staigeriana	S							■				■	
Evening Peace Bath & Shower Gel	G												■
Exodus II	B							■					
Faith	B					■							
Family	B					■							
FemiGen	D					■	■						
Fennel	S		■		■		■	■	■				
Fennel Vitality	D		■		■		■	■	■				
Field	B					■							
Finance	B					■							
Fitness	B					■							
Forgiveness	B					■							
Frankincense	S	■	■			■		■				■	
Frankincense Vitality	D	■	■			■		■				■	
Freedom	B					■							
Frereana Frankincense	S		■										
Friends	B					■							
Fulfill Your Destiny	B					■							

Appendix

Product Type Key:
- S Essential Oil Single
- B Essential Oil Blend
- D Dietary Supplement
- P Personal Care/Hair and Skin
- L Lotions/Creams/Massage Oils
- G Bath and Shower Gels/Soaps
- A Antiseptic/Sanitizing
- O Oral Care

Product	Product Type	Antiaging	Anti-inflammatory	Cardiovascular System	Digestive / Elimination	Emotional Balance	Glandular / Hormonal	Immune / Anti-infectious	Muscle and Bone	Nervous System	Oral Hygiene	Respiratory System	Skin and Hair
Fun	B					■							
Gary's True Grit Chocolate-Coated Wolfberry Crisp Bars	D				■								
Gary's True Grit Einkorn Berries	D				■								
Gary's True Grit Einkorn Crackers	D				■								
Gary's True Grit Einkorn Flakes Cereal	D				■								
Gary's True Grit Einkorn Flour	D				■								
Gary's True Grit Einkorn Granola	D				■								
Gary's True Grit Einkorn Pancake and Waffle Mix	D				■								
Gary's True Grit Einkorn Rotini Pasta	D				■								
Gary's True Grit Einkorn Spaghetti	D				■								
Gary's True Grit Gluten-Free Pancake and Waffle Mix	D				■								
Gary's True Grit NingXia Berry Syrup	D				■								
Gathering	B					■							
Genesis Hand & Body Lotion	L												■
Gentle Baby	B					■							■
Geranium	S	■	■					■	■				■
German Chamomile	S	■	■		■				■				
German Chamomile Vitality	D	■	■		■				■				
Ginger	S		■		■							■	
Ginger Vitality	D		■		■							■	
GLF	B				■			■					
GLF Vitality	D				■			■					
Goldenrod	S		■										
Grapefruit	S					■							
Grapefruit Lip Balm	P										■		
Grapefruit Vitality	D				■								
Gratitude	B					■							■
Grounding	B					■							
Harmony	B					■							
Helichrysum	S	■							■				
Highest Potential	B					■							
Hinoki	S		■			■		■					■
Hong Kuai	S							■				■	
Hope	B					■							
Ho Wood	S		■			■		■	■				
Humility	B					■							
Hyssop	S		■					■				■	
ICP	D				■								
Idaho Balsam Fir	S		■					■					

First Edition | Essential Oils Complete Home Reference | 967

Essential Oils Complete Home Reference | First Edition

Product Type Key:
- S Essential Oil Single
- B Essential Oil Blend
- D Dietary Supplement
- P Personal Care/Hair and Skin
- L Lotions/Creams/Massage Oils
- G Bath and Shower Gels/Soaps
- A Antiseptic/Sanitizing
- O Oral Care

Product

Product	Product Type	Antiaging	Anti-inflammatory	Cardiovascular System	Digestive / Elimination	Emotional Balance	Glandular / Hormonal	Immune / Anti-infectious	Muscle and Bone	Nervous System	Oral Hygiene	Respiratory System	Skin and Hair
Idaho Blue Spruce	S					■		■		■		■	
Idaho Tansy	S	■						■					■
ImmuPower	B					■		■					
ImmuPro	D	■						■					
Inner Child	B					■							
Inner Defense	D							■				■	
Insect Repellent	P												■
Inspiration	B					■							
InTouch	B					■							
Into the Future	B					■							
Jade Lemon	S					■							
Jade Lemon Vitality	D					■							
Jasmine	S					■	■	■					■
Journey On	B					■							
Joy	B					■							
Juniper	S				■								■
JuvaCleanse	B	■			■								
JuvaCleanse Vitality	D	■			■								
JuvaFlex	B				■	■							
JuvaFlex Vitality	D				■	■							
JuvaPower	D	■			■								
JuvaTone	D	■			■								
K&B	D				■								
KidScents Bath Gel	G												■
KidScents GeneYus	B					■							
KidScents Lotion	L												■
KidScents MightyPro	D				■			■					
KidScents MightyVites	D			■	■		■	■	■	■		■	
KidScents MightyZyme	D				■								
KidScents Owie	B												■
KidScents Shampoo	P												■
KidScents SleepyIze	B					■							
KidScents Slique Toothpaste	O										■		
KidScents SniffleEase	B											■	
KidScents Tender Tush	L												■
KidScents TummyGize	B				■								
Kunzea	S		■										■
Lady Sclareol	B					■	■						
Laurus Nobilis (Bay Laurel)	S							■		■		■	

968 Appendix

Appendix

Product Type Key:

- S Essential Oil Single
- B Essential Oil Blend
- D Dietary Supplement
- P Personal Care/Hair and Skin
- L Lotions/Creams/Massage Oils
- G Bath and Shower Gels/Soaps
- A Antiseptic/Sanitizing
- O Oral Care

Product

Product	Product Type	Antiaging	Anti-inflammatory	Cardiovascular System	Digestive / Elimination	Emotional Balance	Glandular / Hormonal	Immune / Anti-infectious	Muscle and Bone	Nervous System	Oral Hygiene	Respiratory System	Skin and Hair
Laurus Nobilis Vitality	S							■		■		■	
LavaDerm After-Sun Spray	P												■
LavaDerm Cooling Mist	P												■
Lavender	S		■			■		■					■
Lavender Bath & Shower Gel	G												■
Lavender Calming Bath Bombs	G					■							■
Lavender Conditioner	P												■
Lavender Foaming Hand Soap	G												■
Lavender Hand & Body Lotion	L												■
Lavender Lip Balm	P										■		
Lavender Mint Daily Conditioner	P												■
Lavender Mint Daily Shampoo	P												■
Lavender-Oatmeal Bar Soap	G												■
Lavender Shampoo	P												■
Lavender Vitality	D		■			■		■					
Ledum	S		■					■					
Lemon	S				■	■		■					
Lemongrass	S		■	■	■			■				■	
Lemongrass Vitality	D		■	■	■			■				■	
Lemon Myrtle	S		■					■		■			
Lemon-Sandalwood Cleansing Soap	G												■
Lemon Vitality	D		■		■	■		■					
Life 9	D				■			■					
Light the Fire	B					■							
Lime	S							■				■	■
Lime Vitality	D							■				■	■
Live with Passion	B					■							
Live Your Passion	B					■							
Longevity	B	■											
Longevity Softgels	D	■											
Longevity Vitality	D	■				■							
Loyalty	B					■							
Magnify Your Purpose	B					■	■						
Mandarin	S				■			■					■
Manuka	S		■			■		■	■			■	■
Marjoram	S			■		■		■	■				
Marjoram Vitality	D			■		■		■	■				
Master Formula	D	■		■	■		■	■	■	■		■	
Mastrante	S	■						■	■				

Essential Oils Complete Home Reference | **First Edition**

Product Type Key:
- S Essential Oil Single
- B Essential Oil Blend
- D Dietary Supplement
- P Personal Care/Hair and Skin
- L Lotions/Creams/Massage Oils
- G Bath and Shower Gels/Soaps
- A Antiseptic/Sanitizing
- O Oral Care

Product	Product Type	Antiaging	Anti-inflammatory	Cardiovascular System	Digestive / Elimination	Emotional Balance	Glandular / Hormonal	Immune / Anti-infectious	Muscle and Bone	Nervous System	Oral Hygiene	Respiratory System	Skin and Hair
MegaCal	D			■					■				
Melaleuca Ericifolia	S		■					■					
Melaleuca-Geranium Moisturizing Soap	G												■
Melaleuca Quinquenervia (Niaouli)	S		■				■	■				■	
Melissa	S		■			■		■					
Melrose	B		■									■	■
M-Grain	B	■	■							■			
MindWise	D			■						■			
Mineral Essence	D	■						■					
Mineral Sunscreen Lotion - SPF 10 & SPF 50	P												■
Mirah Luminous Cleansing Oil	L												■
Mirah Lustrous Hair Oil	L												■
Mirah Shave Oil	P												■
Mister	B						■						
Morning Start Bath & Shower Gel	G												■
Morning Start Moisturizing Soap	G												■
Motivation	B					■							
Mountain Savory	S	■	■		■			■					
Mountain Savory Vitality	S	■	■		■			■					
MultiGreens	D			■	■			■		■			
Myrrh	S	■	■					■			■		■
Myrtle	S		■							■		■	■
Neroli	S			■	■	■							■
Niaouli (see also Melaleuca Quinquenervia)	S		■				■	■				■	
Ningxia Dried Wolfberries (Organic)	D	■				■							
NingXia Nitro	D	■				■							
NingXia Red	D	■											
NingXia Zyng	D	■		■			■	■		■			
Northern Lights Black Spruce	S		■					■	■			■	
Nutmeg	S		■		■		■		■				
Nutmeg Vitality	D		■		■		■		■				
Ocotea	S		■					■					
OmegaGize^3	D	■											
Oola Balance	B					■							
Oola Grow	B					■							
Orange	S				■	■							■
Orange Blossom Facial Wash	P												■
Orange Blossom Moisturizer	L												■
Orange Vitality	D			■									■

Appendix

Product Type Key:

- S Essential Oil Single
- B Essential Oil Blend
- D Dietary Supplement
- P Personal Care/Hair and Skin
- L Lotions/Creams/Massage Oils
- G Bath and Shower Gels/Soaps
- A Antiseptic/Sanitizing
- O Oral Care

Product

Product	Product Type	Antiaging	Anti-inflammatory	Cardiovascular System	Digestive / Elimination	Emotional Balance	Glandular / Hormonal	Immune / Anti-infectious	Muscle and Bone	Nervous System	Oral Hygiene	Respiratory System	Skin and Hair
Oregano	S	■	■					■					
Oregano Vitality	D	■	■					■					
Ortho Ease Massage Oil	L								■				■
Ortho Sport Massage Oil	L								■				■
Palmarosa	S			■				■					■
Palo Santo	S		■					■				■	
PanAway	B		■	■					■				
ParaFree	D							■					
Patchouli	S		■		■			■					■
PD 80/20	D				■		■						
Peace & Calming	B					■			■	■			
Peace & Calming II	B					■				■			
Peppermint	S		■		■			■	■			■	■
Peppermint-Cedarwood Moisturizing Soap	G												■
Peppermint Vitality	D		■		■			■	■			■	■
Petitgrain	S		■						■	■			
Pine	S				■							■	
Plectranthus Oregano	S	■	■					■					
PowerGize	D								■	■			
Prenolone Plus Body Cream	L	■					■						■
Present Time	B					■							
Progessence Plus	P						■						
Prostate Health	D						■	■					
Protec	B						■						
Pure Protein Complete, Chocolate Deluxe, Vanilla Spice	D	■							■				
Purification	B							■					■
Raven	B							■				■	
Ravintsara	S							■				■	
R.C.	B							■				■	
Reconnect	B					■							
Red Shot	B				■								
Regenolone Moisturizing Cream	L		■				■		■				
Rehemogen	D				■								
Relaxation Massage Oil	L					■							■
Release	B					■	■						
Relieve It	B		■			■			■				
Roman Chamomile	S		■			■			■	■			■
Roman Chamomile Vitality	D		■			■			■	■			■
Rose	S	■				■							

Essential Oils Complete Home Reference, First Edition

Product Type Key:
- S Essential Oil Single
- B Essential Oil Blend
- D Dietary Supplement
- P Personal Care/Hair and Skin
- L Lotions/Creams/Massage Oils
- G Bath and Shower Gels/Soaps
- A Antiseptic/Sanitizing
- O Oral Care

Product	Product Type	Antiaging	Anti-inflammatory	Cardiovascular System	Digestive / Elimination	Emotional Balance	Glandular / Hormonal	Immune / Anti-infectious	Muscle and Bone	Nervous System	Oral Hygiene	Respiratory System	Skin and Hair
Rosemary	S		■	■		■		■					
Rosemary Vitality	D		■	■		■		■					
Rose Ointment	P												■
Royal Hawaiian Sandalwood	S					■							■
Rue	S		■	■	■	■							
RutaVaLa	B					■				■			
RutaVaLa Roll-On	B					■				■			
Sacred Frankincense	S		■			■						■	■
Sacred Mountain	B					■							
Sacred Mountain Moisturizing Soap	G												■
Sacred Sandalwood	S							■					■
Sage	S	■	■	■			■	■					
Sage Vitality	D	■	■	■			■	■					
Sandalwood Moisture Cream	P	■											■
SARA	B					■							
Satin Facial Scrub, Mint	P												■
Savvy Minerals by Young Living - Makeup Line	P												■
SclarEssence	B					■	■						
SclarEssence Vitality	B					■	■						
Seedlings Baby Lotion	L												■
Seedlings Baby Oil	L												■
Seedlings Baby Wash & Shampoo	P												■
Seedlings Baby Wipes	P												■
Seedlings Diaper Cream	P												■
Seedlings Linen Spray	A					■							■
Sensation	B					■							■
Sensation Bath & Shower Gel	G												■
Sensation Hand & Body Lotion	L												■
Sensation Massage Oil	L					■							■
Shutran	B					■							
Shutran 3-in-1 Men's Wash	G												■
Shutran Aftershave Lotion	P												■
Shutran Bar Soap	P												■
Shutran Beard Oil	P												■
Shutran Shave Cream	P												■
SleepEssence	D					■							
Slique Bars	D				■								
Slique Bars - Chocolate-Coated	D				■								
Slique CitraSlim	D				■								

Appendix

Product Type Key:
- S Essential Oil Single
- B Essential Oil Blend
- D Dietary Supplement
- P Personal Care/Hair and Skin
- L Lotions/Creams/Massage Oils
- G Bath and Shower Gels/Soaps
- A Antiseptic/Sanitizing
- O Oral Care

Product	Product Type	Antiaging	Anti-inflammatory	Cardiovascular System	Digestive / Elimination	Emotional Balance	Glandular / Hormonal	Immune / Anti-infectious	Muscle and Bone	Nervous System	Oral Hygiene	Respiratory System	Skin and Hair
Slique Essence	B				■								
Slique Gum	O				■						■		
Slique Shake	D				■								
Slique Tea	D				■								
Spanish Sage	S				■	■			■			■	■
Spearmint	S		■		■			■	■				
Spearmint Vitality	D		■		■			■	■				
Spikenard	S	■	■			■		■					
Stress Away (and Roll-On)	B					■							
Stress Away Relaxing Bath Bombs	G					■							■
Sulfurzyme (Capsules and Powder)	D	■		■	■		■	■	■	■		■	■
Super B	D				■								
Super C (and Chewable)	D	■			■			■					
Super Cal Plus	D					■	■		■				
Surrender	B					■							
Tangerine	S			■	■				■			■	
Tangerine Vitality	D			■	■				■			■	
Tarragon	S		■		■			■	■				
Tarragon Vitality	D		■		■			■	■				
Tea Tree	S		■					■			■	■	■
The Gift	B	■				■		■	■				■
Thieves	B	■						■					
Thieves AromaBright Toothpaste	O							■			■		
Thieves Automatic Dishwasher Powder	A							■					
Thieves Cleansing Soap	A							■					■
Thieves Cough Drops	D							■				■	
Thieves Dental Floss	O										■		
Thieves Dentarome Plus Toothpaste	O										■		
Thieves Dentarome Ultra Toothpaste	O										■		
Thieves Dish Soap	A							■					
Thieves Foaming Hand Soap	A							■					■
Thieves Fresh Essence Plus Mouthwash	O							■			■		
Thieves Fruit & Veggie Soak (and Spray)	A							■					
Thieves Hard Lozenges	O							■			■		
Thieves Household Cleaner	A							■					
Thieves Laundry Soap	A							■					
Thieves Mints	O							■			■		
Thieves Spray	A							■				■	■
Thieves Vitality	D	■			■			■					

Product Type Key:
- **S** Essential Oil Single
- **B** Essential Oil Blend
- **D** Dietary Supplement
- **P** Personal Care/Hair and Skin
- **L** Lotions/Creams/Massage Oils
- **G** Bath and Shower Gels/Soaps
- **A** Antiseptic/Sanitizing
- **O** Oral Care

Product

Product	Product Type	Antiaging	Anti-inflammatory	Cardiovascular System	Digestive / Elimination	Emotional Balance	Glandular / Hormonal	Immune / Anti-infectious	Muscle and Bone	Nervous System	Oral Hygiene	Respiratory System	Skin and Hair
Thieves Waterless Hand Purifier	A							■					■
Thieves Wipes	A							■					
Thyme	S	■	■	■				■	■				
Thyme Vitality	D	■	■	■				■	■				
Thyromin	D						■						
T.R. Care	B					■							
Tranquil Roll-On	B					■							
Transformation	B					■							
Trauma Life	B					■							
Treasure of the Season	B					■							
Tsuga	S											■	
V-6 Vegetable Oil Complex	L								■				■
Valerian	S					■				■			
Valor	B					■							
Valor Moisturizing Soap	P												■
Valor Roll-On	B					■							
Vanilla	S					■							
Vetiver	S				■					■			
Western Red Cedar	S							■					
White Angelica	B					■							
White Fir	S	■											
White Light	B					■							
White Lotus	S		■					■					
Wintergreen	S		■	■					■				
Wolfberry Eye Cream	L	■											■
Xiang Mao	S				■			■					
Yacon Syrup	D	■			■								
Yarrow	S		■				■						
Ylang Ylang	S		■			■			■				■
Yuzu	S		■			■						■	

Index

3 Wise Men: 63, 64, 251, 642, 672, 674-677, 698, 739, 956, 959, 961, 964, 967, 971, 981

25 Years Young (Anniversary Blend): 66

Abscesses: 402, 644

Absolutes: 42

Abundance: 53, 55, 63, 68, 223, 239, 647, 674-679, 739, 956, 957, 959, 960, 964, 965, 971, 978, 981

Acceptance: 63, 68, 70, 71, 642, 674, 676, 678, 739, 955-962, 964, 967, 968, 971, 978, 981

Acne: 23, 37, 39, 144, 150, 153, 165, 173, 236, 254, 334, 338, 361, 362, 391, 398, 405, 412, 443, 444, 457, 458, 473, 486, 504, 514, 556, 566, 596, 597, 755, 959, 962, 963, 966, 968, 981,

Acne Treatment: 596, 959, 962, 963, 966, 968, 981

Acne Treatment, Maximum Strength: 596, 981,

Acupressure: 643, 644, 647

Acupuncture: 650

Addictions: 313

ADHD: 144, 153, 194, 297, 500, 514

Adulterated Oils: 48, 49, 423, 631

Adulteration: 16, 17, 48

Aftershave Lotion: 595, 956, 958, 960-964, 969, 990

Agave: 555, 759, 762

AgilEase: 535, 638, 639, 957, 964, 969, 981

Aging: 38, 114, 125, 354, 514, 542, 548-550, 552, 555, 558, 560, 563, 564, 596, 683, 696, 713, 716, 720, 727-729, 754, 760, 762, 763, 766

Agitation: 96, 121, 278, 674, 740

Agrichemicals: 45

AIDS: 405, 473, 536, 563, 582, 715, 720, 753

Alcohols: 16, 42-44, 236

Aldehydes: 16, 41, 42, 44, 671, 691

AlkaLime: 535, 536, 686, 699, 752, 952, 963, 981

Alkalinity: 535, 685, 686

Alkanes: 41, 42, 596, 597, 599-601

Allergic Rhinitis: 432

Allergies: 39, 90, 216, 369, 411, 517, 536, 684, 685, 697, 711, 714, 715, 717, 718, 722, 755, 756

Allerzyme: 536, 640, 689, 692, 697, 700, 711, 712, 717, 718, 751, 955, 959-961, 963, 965, 968, 981

Alopecia Areata: 144, 444

Aluminum: 12, 45, 575, 576, 613, 723

Aluminum Toxicity: 575, 613

Alzheimer's disease: 23, 135, 182, 443, 454, 473, 482, 493, 563, 576, 613, 722, 759

Amazonian Ylang Ylang: 530, 951, 953, 955, 969, 981

Amino Acids: 536, 543-546, 551, 553, 578, 617, 692, 699, 707, 709, 712-714, 717, 720, 743, 744, 752, 756, 762

AminoWise: 536, 638, 962, 963, 981

Amoressence: 63, 72, 958, 959, 961, 964, 965, 968, 969, 971, 978, 981

Amygdala: 50, 51, 658, 670, 671, 738

Analgesic: 43, 77, 98, 101, 108, 111, 146, 162, 174, 182, 189, 219, 224, 226, 233, 236, 240, 243, 333, 334, 338, 366, 377, 385, 387, 392, 402, 412, 423, 434, 443, 451, 485, 503, 504, 519, 522, 526, 530, 558, 574, 610

Anemia: 576

Angelica: 44, 62, 63, 74, 146, 155, 197, 235, 269, 270, 350, 357, 451, 454, 480, 500, 518, 538, 558, 597, 600, 638, 658, 659, 661, 662, 666, 670, 673-679, 698, 739, 951, 953, 955, 956, 958, 960, 961, 963, 964, 966, 967, 969, 972-977, 979, 981, 992

Anger: 27, 50, 74, 122, 150, 153, 186, 189, 197, 216, 240, 276, 313, 438, 458, 499, 520, 672, 674, 697

Angina: 330, 522, 760

Animals: 19, 165, 341, 547, 549, 550, 559, 561, 577, 582, 602, 608, 617, 629-640, 645, 685, 719, 728-730, 747

Animal Scents Cat Treats: 636, 960, 981

Animal Scents Dental Pet Chews: 636, 955, 967, 981

Animal Scents Essential Oil Blends: 637

Animal Scents Infect Away: 637, 958, 964-966, 981

Animal Scents Mendwell: 637, 959-961, 964, 981

Animal Scents Ointment: 635-638, 640, 642-644, 955, 956, 958, 959, 961, 964, 965, 968, 969, 981

Animal Scents ParaGize: 637, 955, 958-961, 963, 965-967, 981

Animal Scents PuriClean: 637, 957, 961-966, 968, 981

Animal Scents Shampoo: 637, 639, 957, 959, 961, 962, 964, 968, 981

Animal Scents T-Away: 638, 981

Animal Treatment: 638

Anise: 42, 62, 76, 77, 118, 192, 205, 304, 325, 536, 539, 540, 542, 568, 620, 625, 637, 693, 697, 717, 718, 952, 953, 955, 971-973, 976, 977, 981

Antagonism: 674

Anti-infectious: 45, 53, 168, 186, 189, 289, 333, 486, 489, 490, 520, 981, 616

Anti-inflammatory: , 9, 23, 42-45, 64, 67, 68, 71, 72, 77, 79, 80, 83, 84, 86, 89, 90, 93, 95, 96, 98, 103, 104, 107, 111, 112, 114, 117, 118, 122, 126, 130, 133, 135, 146, 153, 155, 156, 158, 161, 162, 165, 168, 170, 174, 177, 178, 181, 182, 185, 189, 191, 194, 197, 199, 202, 205, 206, 209, 211, 215, 219, 220, 223, 224, 226, 230, 233, 235, 236, 239, 240, 243, 244, 247, 251, 252, 254, 257, 259, 260, 263, 266, 269, 270, 273, 275, 276, 278, 281, 283, 284, 286, 289, 293, 294, 297, 299, 304, 307, 310, 313, 314, 319, 320, 322, 325, 327, 328, 330, 334, 337, 341, 342, 348, 350, 353, 354, 357, 358, 362, 369, 370, 373, 374, 377, 379, 380, 382, 385, 387,

388, 392, 395, 398, 401, 402, 405, 406, 409, 412, 414, 417, 419, 420, 423, 431, 432, 434, 438, 441, 443, 444, 447, 448, 451, 452, 454, 458, 461, 465, 466, 469, 474, 477, 479, 480, 485, 486, 489, 490, 493, 495, 496, 499, 500, 503, 508, 513, 514, 519, 522, 525, 526, 529, 530, 533, 537, 538, 547, 583, 588, 608, 638, 645, 657, 669, 688, 735, 736, 981

Antiaging: 125, 174, 220, 401, 493, 525, 550, 606, 754, 981

Antibacterial: 20, 44, 53, 77, 86, 93, 96, 108, 121, 122, 126, 130, 133, 144, 146, 149, 150, 153, 158, 161, 162, 165, 168, 173, 174, 181, 182, 186, 194, 197, 216, 219, 220, 223, 224, 226, 236, 240, 254, 263, 278, 286, 297, 299, 303, 322, 325, 330, 333, 334, 337, 341, 342, 345, 348, 362, 365, 366, 369, 377, 382, 385, 387, 388, 392, 398, 401, 402, 405, 406, 411, 419, 423, 427, 432, 434, 437, 444, 451, 454, 457, 458, 470, 474, 477, 482, 485, 486, 489, 490, 500, 503, 519, 520, 522, 529, 530, 580, 586, 588, 590, 611, 612, 616, 623, 624, 626, 657, 667, 686, 688, 702, 749

Antibiotics: 19, 20, 77, 107, 330, 341, 388, 681, 686, 701,

Anticancer: 23, 96, 135, 150, 168, 174, 182, 243, 264, 337, 341, 348, 365, 370, 387, 388, 444, 447, 458, 477, 482, 547, 548, 550, 560, 570, 633

Anticoagulant: 74, 77, 122, 133, 161, 173, 174, 257, 263, 392, 398, 503, 526

Antidepressant: 42, 67, 74, 96, 135, 168, 197, 239, 264, 278, 297, 303, 366, 377, 385, 392, 405, 420, 434, 444, 451, 477, 503, 513, 519, 530, 736

Antifungal: 43, 44, 67, 86, 96, 98, 101, 111, 125, 126, 130, 133, 144, 161, 165, 173, 174, 182, 185, 194, 197, 200, 216, 219, 220, 233, 236, 239, 254, 257, 273, 278, 281, 299, 322, 327, 333, 334, 338, 341, 342, 361, 362, 365, 366, 369, 377, 382, 385, 388, 395, 401, 405, 406, 411, 412, 419, 420, 423, 434, 444, 447, 454, 470, 477, 482, 486, 490, 493, 500, 503, 520, 526, 529, 530, 608, 609, 616, 686-688

Antimicrobial: 20, 23, 42, 53, 64, 67, 68, 71, 72, 74, 77, 79, 80, 83, 84, 89, 90, 93, 95, 96, 98, 101, 107, 108, 111, 112, 114, 117, 118, 122, 125, 129, 130, 146, 149, 153, 155,

156, 158, 161, 165, 167, 168, 170, 173, 174, 177, 178, 181, 182, 185, 186, 189, 191, 192, 199, 200, 202, 205, 206, 209, 211, 212, 215, 219, 220, 223, 224, 226, 229, 230, 233, 235, 236, 243, 244, 247, 252, 254, 259, 260, 263, 264, 266, 270, 273, 275, 276, 283, 284, 286, 289, 290, 294, 299, 300, 303, 304, 307, 310, 313, 314, 319, 320, 327, 328, 330, 333, 334, 338, 341, 342, 345, 347, 350, 353, 354, 357, 358, 362, 365, 366, 373, 374, 379, 380, 382, 387, 388, 391, 392, 398, 401, 402, 405, 409, 412, 414, 417, 424, 427, 428, 431, 432, 434, 438, 444, 447, 448, 451, 454, 458, 461, 462, 465, 466, 469, 470, 473, 474, 479, 480, 482, 486, 489, 490, 493, 495, 496, 499, 500, 508, 517, 520, 526, 529, 530, 589, 613, 616, 624, 655-657, 667, 686, 687, 741, 747, 764, 766

Antioxidant: 23, 67, 74, 77, 93, 98, 101, 107, 111, 112, 122, 126, 129, 130, 149, 150, 153, 158, 161, 162, 165, 168, 173, 174, 182, 185, 186, 189, 194, 197, 199, 200, 220, 223, 224, 233, 236, 239, 254, 260, 261, 264, 273, 275, 286, 299, 308, 330, 333, 334, 337, 338, 341, 345, 348, 354, 361, 362, 365, 366, 377, 382, 385, 387, 388, 391, 392, 398, 401, 402, 405, 411, 412, 420, 443, 444, 447, 451, 454, 458, 473, 474, 477, 482, 493, 500, 513, 514, 519, 520, 522, 526, 533, 537, 538, 545, 548-553, 558, 561, 566, 584, 596, 608, 609, 617, 696, 699-702, 720, 721, 727-730, 742, 749, 752-754, 762, 763, 766

Antiseptic: 19, 20, 37, 42-44, 103, 104, 130, 161, 174, 181, 185, 199, 209, 220, 223, 233, 263, 264, 286, 289, 300, 303, 308, 327, 333, 334, 338, 342, 369, 373, 392, 411, 420, 423, 428, 434, 473, 474, 486, 490, 500, 504, 514, 517, 522, 981-992, 585, 586, 588, 603, 608, 611, 616, 626, 627, 669, 687, 720

Antispasmodic: 44, 74, 93, 103, 104, 121, 122, 125, 129, 165, 186, 194, 197, 209, 224, 233, 240, 254, 273, 286, 303, 325, 341, 361, 366, 374, 385, 388, 420, 424, 447, 452, 474, 482, 485, 493, 500, 503, 507, 514, 526

Antitumoral: 67, 77, 107, 135, 150, 161, 168, 174, 185, 200, 233, 239, 254, 257, 263, 264, 300, 334, 337, 338, 370, 387, 402, 412, 419, 420, 432, 434, 444, 454, 457, 458, 474, 482, 500, 503, 519, 520, 730

Antiviral: 19, 42, 44, 53, 67, 77, 84, 86, 93, 98, 107, 133, 161, 162, 174, 185, 186, 189, 197, 200, 216, 219, 220, 223, 254, 278, 286, 297, 303, 322, 327, 330, 338, 341, 345, 348, 362, 366, 369, 370, 373, 382, 385, 387, 401, 405, 406, 419, 428, 432, 434, 437, 444, 451, 454, 457, 458, 486, 489, 490, 493, 503, 519, 530, 616, 623, 655, 657, 667, 688

Anxiety: 23, 27, 37-39, 50, 96, 121, 153, 158, 165, 167, 168, 173, 181, 182, 233, 236, 239, 252, 254, 264, 303, 333, 338, 341, 361, 362, 370, 391, 395, 398, 406, 414, 420, 423, 424, 432, 443, 444, 452, 454, 473, 477, 482, 495, 500, 504, 507, 514, 529, 530, 533, 560, 561, 564, 639, 669, 671, 674, 722

Apathy: 674

Appetite, Loss of: 330, 684

Application: 8, 13, 62, 63, 135, 158, 182, 191, 314, 316, 319, 320, 322, 325, 444, 508, 560, 561, 566-568, 570, 580, 582, 584, 597, 607, 619, 620, 629-635, 637, 638, 643, 647, 649-651, 653, 655, 657-663, 665-668, 671, 697, 738

AromaBright Toothpaste, Thieves: 589, 957, 959, 963, 964, 966, 967, 991

AromaEase: 63, 78, 79, 674-679, 956, 959, 960, 965, 967, 981

Aroma Life: 63, 80, 739, 958, 960, 963, 969, 971, 978, 981

Aroma Siez: 63, 82, 83, 645, 658-660, 662, 665, 739, 955, 958, 962, 963, 965, 971, 978, 981

AromaSleep: 971, 978, 981

Aromatherapist: 362

Aromatherapy: 8, 19, 48, 96, 101, 254, 257, 300, 303, 334, 338, 398, 419, 432, 530, 533, 571, 577, 613, 628, 631, 632, 655, 764

ART Beauty Masque: 597, 600, 956, 957, 962-964, 982

ART Chocolate Masque: 597, 959, 967, 969, 982

ART Creme Masque: 597, 600, 958, 959, 964, 966, 968, 969, 982

Arteriosclerosis: 133, 144, 150, 273, 334, 338, 398, 526, 727

ART Gentle Cleanser: 582, 598, 959, 962,

963, 967, 982

Arthritis: 77, 98, 101, 103, 104, 149, 150, 162, 174, 181, 182, 200, 220, 233, 239, 240, 243, 257, 263, 330, 365, 369, 392, 401, 402, 406, 409, 411, 419, 423, 432, 473, 514, 522, 526, 537, 546, 547, 554, 568, 594, 633, 635, 638, 755, 756

Arthritis, Animal Treatment: 638

ART Intensive Moisturizer: 582, 598, 956, 959, 960, 967, 969, 982

ART Light Moisturizer: 582, 599, 959, 967, 982

ART Refreshing Toner: 582, 599, 959, 962, 963, 965, 967, 982

ART Renewal Serum: 582, 597, 599, 955, 958, 959, 961, 969, 982

ART Sheerlumé Brightening Cream: 582, 600, 601, 956-959, 961, 967, 968, 982

Aspartame: 758, 759

Asthma: 149, 189, 199, 200, 263, 286, 377, 473, 522, 533, 642, 722, 755, 756, 766

Athlete's Foot: 477, 486, 609

Attention Deficit Disorder: 722

Australia: 9, 26, 85, 86, 89, 107, 223, 233, 236, 327, 342, 369, 486, 487

Australian Blue: 63, 84, 674-679, 956, 958-962, 964, 966-969, 971, 978, 982

Australian Kuranya: 63, 88, 89, 645, 956, 959, 961, 963, 967, 968, 971, 982

Autism: 731

Automatic Dishwasher Powder: 624, 957, 959, 963, 965, 966, 991

Awaken: 63, 90, 212, 522, 609, 674, 675, 678, 696, 739, 758, 955-969, 971, 978, 982

Backache: 594

Bacteria: 19, 20, 23, 37-39, 108, 122, 165, 168, 182, 200, 220, 230, 273, 341, 362, 388, 398, 402, 419, 432, 444, 474, 486, 490, 529, 547, 559, 575, 576, 584-588, 592, 613, 617, 623-627, 638, 643, 657, 681, 682, 685, 686, 691, 696, 698, 700, 701, 714, 723, 726, 741, 744, 747, 759, 760, 762, 764, 766

Bad Breath: 411, 586, 684, 691

Balance Complete Vanilla Cream Meal Replacement: 552

Balancing Body Energy: 661

Balm of Gilead: 951, 953

Balsam Canada: 568, 581, 951, 953, 961, 971-975

Balsam Copaiba: 178, 180, 191, 244, 304, 375, 479, 568, 572, 580, 594, 604, 951, 953, 957

Balsam Fir: 15, 26, 42, 263, 951, 953, 961, 971-975, 977, 985, 638

Basil: 23, 29, 42, 44, 62, 83, 92, 93, 149, 170, 374, 391, 952, 953, 955, 971, 972, 974, 977, 982, 617, 628, 632, 634, 657-660, 662, 664, 667, 674, 675, 678, 690, 695, 704, 705, 707, 739

Basil Vitality: 92, 628, 952, 953, 955, 977, 982

Bath: 29, 350, 411, 520, 555, 571-573, 583, 608, 615, 752, 955-969, 981-992

Bath & Shower Gel Base: 571, 982

Bay Laurel: 42, 117, 330, 952, 953, 961, 971, 986

Beauty Boost: 602

Beauty Masque: 597, 600, 956, 957, 962-964, 982

Becker, Robert O.: 737, 743

Benign Prostate Hyperplasia (BPH): 564, 568

Bereavement: 672

Bergamot: 23, 26, 43, 44, 62, 71, 90, 95, 96, 118, 146, 155, 170, 197, 205, 223, 235, 252, 266, 270, 284, 293, 304, 307, 314, 320, 328, 358, 417, 434, 465, 466, 500, 519, 951, 953, 955, 971-977, 982, 567-569, 571-574, 580, 584, 600, 604-606, 609, 616, 619-622, 624, 625, 636, 638, 673, 674, 676-679, 695, 697

Bergamot Vitality: 96, 951, 953, 955, 977, 982

Bible: 1, 52, 53, 286, 669

Biblical Sweet Myrrh: 62, 98, 951, 953, 955

Birds: 56, 58, 631, 632, 639, 714

Birthing: 252, 638

Bites: 3, 38, 39, 93, 173, 181, 224, 243, 348, 427, 486, 583, 603, 707

Bitter Orange: 43, 44, 71, 90, 247, 248, 284, 290, 350, 390, 422, 951, 953, 955, 964, 971-974

Black Pepper: 42, 44, 62, 90, 100, 101, 118, 205, 212, 229, 247, 304, 347, 441, 541, 552, 553, 565, 674, 728, 952, 953, 955, 971-975, 977, 982

Black Pepper Vitality: 100, 952, 953, 955, 977, 982

Black Spruce: 14, 26, 62, 64, 68, 102-104, 146, 155, 156, 206, 215, 229, 230, 251, 266, 269, 270, 275, 276, 283, 284, 290, 293, 304, 314, 316, 322, 347, 353, 380, 385, 396, 417, 424, 431, 434, 441, 451, 452, 469, 480, 489, 499, 500, 508, 519, 535, 576, 579, 581, 595, 603, 606, 610-612, 619, 620, 622, 637, 638, 642, 673-679, 698, 751, 952, 953, 955, 956, 964, 971-978, 982, 988

Black Spruce, Northern Lights: 62, 104, 146, 155, 206, 229, 230, 251, 266, 275, 276, 284, 314, 347, 353, 385, 396, 417, 434, 469, 489, 500, 535, 579, 581, 595, 603, 606, 611, 619, 637, 642, 673-679, 698, 751, 952, 953, 956, 964, 972-975, 978, 988

Blanc, Bernard H.: 742

Bleeding: 125, 254, 334, 370, 638, 639, 643, 684

Blends: 23, 62, 64-95, 97-103, 105, 108, 109, 111, 114-533, 971, 978, 15, 538, 568, 569, 584, 594, 596, 615, 616, 619, 624, 627, 628, 631, 637, 639, 642, 658, 662, 671-679, 686, 690-693, 697-699, 701, 738, 739, 741, 747, 748, 750, 752

Blisters: 15, 565, 571, 615, 623

BLM: 537, 638, 639, 957, 961, 969, 982

Blood Cleanse: 691

Blood Pressure, High (Hypertension): 395, 727

BLOOM Brightening Cleanser: 600

BLOOM Brightening Essence: 601

Blue Agave: 555, 759, 762

Blue Cypress: 26, 62, 71, 84, 89, 90, 106, 107, 114, 117, 118, 178, 197, 205, 276, 304, 314, 434, 438, 461, 500, 555, 574, 594, 600, 601, 619, 951, 953, 955, 971-975, 977, 982

Blue Spruce, Idaho: 62, 26, 72, 95, 108, 118, 226, 244, 247, 294, 297, 314, 328, 353, 357, 385, 434, 469, 496, 569, 579, 581, 595, 606, 611, 619, 640, 642, 674-679, 952, 953, 961, 971-975, 977, 986

Blue Tansy: 62, 71, 84, 90, 110, 111, 118, 155, 205, 276, 304, 313, 316, 396, 414, 438, 461, 500, 508, 571, 576, 611, 619, 638, 696, 952, 953, 956, 971-977, 982

Blue Yarrow: 62, 112, 567, 569, 580, 583, 954, 969

Body Systems: 286, 337, 981, 541, 650, 658, 667, 670, 671, 686, 699, 709, 751

Boils: 522

Bone Pain: 537

Bones: 411, 537, 638, 639, 685, 714, 719, 720, 723, 731, 732

Bones, Ligaments, and Muscles: 537

Boredom: 674

Boswellia Wrinkle Cream: 555, 582, 601, 959, 964, 967, 969, 982

Botanical Plant Names: 951

BPH (Benign Prostate Hyperplasia): 564, 568

Brain: 27, 37, 50, 51, 63, 90, 98, 114, 115, 135, 144, 161, 167, 170, 205, 239, 300, 334, 358, 387, 419, 432, 443, 444, 457, 458, 477, 510, 513, 533, 544, 545, 559, 561-563, 569, 596, 618, 631, 666, 669-672, 674-676, 678, 679, 686, 690, 692, 698, 720, 722, 723, 727-729, 736, 738, 739, 747, 752, 753, 759, 762-764, 956, 959, 960, 962, 963, 967, 971, 978, 982

Brain Function: 239, 444, 544, 559, 720, 729

Brain Power: 63, 114, 170, 674-676, 678, 739, 747, 956, 959, 960, 962, 963, 967, 971, 978, 982

Brain Stem Pump: 666

Brazil: 9, 121, 181, 366, 398, 693

Breast Cancer: 86, 122, 150, 174, 240, 243, 254, 257, 365, 398, 411, 423, 447, 477, 558, 560, 561, 564, 566, 569, 736, 764

Breastfeeding: 533, 602

Breathe Again: 63, 116, 639, 690, 698, 956-959, 961, 964, 965, 971, 978, 982

Brigham Young University: 457, 458

Brightening Cleanser, BLOOM: 600

Brightening Cream, ART Sheerlumé: 582, 600, 601, 956-959, 961, 967, 968, 982

Brightening Essence, BLOOM: 601

Bronchitis: 23, 125, 181, 199, 236, 263, 286, 337, 366, 431, 504, 522

Bruising: 38, 39, 520, 638, 640, 684

Brushing Teeth: 586

Build Your Dream: 63, 118, 673-678, 955, 956, 958-963, 967-969, 971, 978, 982

Building Blocks of Health: 709, 711, 713, 715, 717, 719, 721, 723, 725

Burns: 3, 31, 37, 48, 49, 224, 333, 334, 373, 419, 500, 603, 605, 720, 746, 751

Bursitis: 554, 756

Cairo University: 182, 741

Calamus: 53, 55, 57, 59, 62, 120, 121, 230, 951, 953, 956, 972, 977, 982

Calm CBD Roll-On: 142

Camphor: 32, 41, 43, 44, 46, 48, 62, 93, 111, 112, 122, 133, 155, 182, 289, 304, 308, 322, 333, 334, 385, 396, 428, 432, 444, 451, 454, 473, 508, 575, 576, 594, 611, 620, 973, 974, 976

Canada: 9, 14, 26, 103, 104, 112, 125, 260, 263, 337, 423, 504, 517, 522, 568, 575, 581, 655, 746, 750, 761, 764, 951, 953, 961, 971-975

Canadian Fleabane: 15, 62, 124, 229, 347, 539, 541, 565, 951, 953, 956, 974, 977, 982

Cancer: 23, 77, 86, 122, 125, 130, 133, 135, 150, 174, 181, 182, 185, 199, 219, 223, 233, 239, 240, 243, 254, 257, 281, 334, 337, 348, 365, 370, 377, 387, 392, 398, 402, 411, 412, 423, 443, 447, 457, 458, 477, 482, 493, 513, 544, 546-548, 550, 552, 556-558, 560-564, 566, 568-570, 575, 581, 584, 585, 613, 631, 640, 644, 685, 686, 691, 692, 712, 717, 721, 723-725, 730-732, 734-737, 741, 747, 748, 750, 752, 760, 763, 764, 766

Candidiasis: 486

Carbohydrate: 174, 543, 700, 711, 757

Carboxylic Acids: 43

Cardamom: 62, 79, 101, 128, 129, 146, 170, 247, 325, 357, 496, 538, 564, 569, 620, 676-679, 951, 953, 956, 971-977, 982

Cardamom Vitality: 128, 951, 953, 956, 977, 982

CardioGize: 538, 955-958, 960, 962, 966, 982

Carpal Tunnel Syndrome: 150, 568

Carrot Seed: 62, 130, 600, 601, 604, 605, 636, 695, 951, 953, 956, 977, 982

Carrot Seed Vitality: 130, 951, 953, 956, 977, 982

Casabianca, Hervé: 16, 46

Cassia: 42, 43, 53, 59 , 62, 132, 133, 229, 230, 247, 347, 357, 412, 417, 437, 541, 553, 565, 585, 612, 727, 951, 953, 956, 972-975, 977, 982

Cataracts: 133, 174, 546

Cats: 629, 630, 632-638, 647, 715, 726, 766

Cattle: 630, 635

CBD: 63, 134-136, 138, 140, 142, 538, 594, 602

CBD Beauty Boost: 602

CBD Muscle Rub: 594

Cedarwood: 34, 37, 42, 53, 62, 67, 84, 114, 144, 165, 206, 269, 276, 293, 294, 297, 314, 350, 434, 452, 461, 469, 479, 495, 500, 568, 572, 574, 579-581, 583, 595, 597, 599, 606, 610, 611, 619, 639, 674-677, 679, 686, 951, 953, 956, 971-975, 977, 982

Cel-Lite Magic Massage Oil: 583, 956-958, 960, 961, 983

Celery Seed: 43, 62, 148, 158, 259, 310, 951, 643, 684, 692, 696, 953, 956, 973, 977, 982, 983

Celery Seed Vitality: 643, 951, 953, 956, 977, 983

Cellulite: 264, 583

Cervical Cancer: 257

Chakras: 200, 236, 15, 673, 698

Chao, Sue: 490, 555, 596, 657, 741

Charcoal Bar Soap: 609, 962, 965, 966, 983

Chamomile, German: 9, 15, 43, 62, 71, 84, 90, 118, 146, 150, 178, 205, 211, 276, 304,

414, 417, 438, 461, 480, 500, 539, 594, 600, 608, 638, 696, 739, 951-953, 960, 971-975, 977, 985

Chamomile, Vitality German: 150, 952, 953, 960, 985

Chamomile, Roman: 43, 62, 72, 90, 146, 152, 153, 155, 170, 194, 197, 235, 252, 270, 304, 307, 313, 320, 374, 380, 396, 480, 495, 500, 556, 567, 569, 571, 573, 580, 581, 596, 597, 601, 602, 604, 606, 616, 619, 620, 638-640, 674, 676-679, 690, 696, 951, 954, 966, 971-975, 978, 989

Chemistry of Essential Oils: 41, 230

Chemical Structure: 8, 41, 510, 709

Chemotypes: 44, 45, 122, 366, 432

Chernobyl: 701, 748, 750, 752

Chest Rub, Thieves: 574

Children: 31, 38, 54, 62, 63, 144, 153, 156, 178, 224, 230, 252, 290, 297, 314, 316, 319, 320, 322, 325, 342, 373, 398, 409, 412, 428, 444, 465, 479, 507, 514, 526, 533, 15, 539, 552, 559-561, 565, 566, 571, 575, 580, 583, 584, 588-590, 592-594, 602-604, 615-621, 623, 624, 626, 628, 633, 636, 657, 658, 670, 673, 684, 688, 697, 700, 702, 703, 711, 715, 717-720, 723, 726, 731-733, 746, 749-752, 755, 757, 763-765

China: 19, 122, 153, 174, 220, 257, 300, 507, 526, 538, 543, 544, 547, 551, 564, 721, 734, 753, 754, 760, 761

Chlorine: 723-726, 758

Chocolate Coated Wolfberry Crisp Bars: 555, 707

Chocolessence, Ecuadorian Dark: 540, 707

Cholera: 101, 723

Cholesterol, High: 684

Christmas Spirit: 63, 156, 611, 674-679, 739, 956, 957, 965, 971, 978, 983

Chronic Fatigue Syndrome: 722, 759

Chronic Pain: 96, 759

CinnaFresh Deodorant: 576

Cinnamint Lip Balm: 556, 581, 957, 965, 967, 983

Cinnamon Bark: 42, 62, 68, 136, 138, 156, 160, 161, 206, 230, 248, 251, 276, 304,

358, 490, 500, 503, 537, 538, 540, 553, 554, 556, 575, 576, 580, 581, 584, 586, 588-590, 592, 593, 611, 612, 616, 624-628, 741, 750, 951, 953, 956, 957, 971-975, 977, 983

Cinnamon Bark Vitality: 160, 540, 627, 628, 951, 953, 956, 957, 977, 983

Circular Hand Massage: 660, 665

Cistus: 8, 26, 62, 162, 248, 289, 304, 319, 417, 489, 951, 953, 954, 957, 966, 972-975, 977, 983, 604, 616, 619, 637, 639, 674-679, 699

Citronella: 62, 164, 165, 300, 405, 427, 502, 625, 637, 639, 951, 953, 957, 972, 974, 977, 983

Citrus Fresh: 63, 37, 166, 167, 345, 628, 632, 674-677, 679, 700-702, 739, 748, 749, 960, 962, 963, 965, 967, 968, 971, 978, 983

Citrus Fresh Vitality: 166, 960, 628, 962, 963, 965, 967, 968, 971, 978, 983

Citrus Hystrix: 62, 118, 168, 205, 276, 304, 461, 499, 500, 951, 953, 957, 961, 972-975, 983, 638

ClaraDerm: 602, 640, 959, 960, 962, 964, 966, 968, 983

Clarity: 63, 114, 118, 129, 168, 170, 177, 200, 205, 251, 314, 338, 444, 525, 955, 956, 958, 959, 961, 962, 965, 966, 969, 971, 978, 983, 560, 569, 618, 659, 674-676, 678, 688, 699, 717, 739, 747

Clary Sage: 43, 62, 172, 173, 202, 247, 294, 328, 350, 411, 462, 496, 539, 541, 556, 565-569, 571, 578, 580, 583, 674, 677-679, 952, 953, 957, 972-975, 977, 983

Cleaning: 224, 300, 338, 342, 403, 623-627, 638, 644, 720

Cleanse: 43, 53, 58, 219, 254, 259, 334, 338, 373, 406, 411, 504, 537, 540, 555, 572, 578, 583, 598-600, 604, 605, 608-611, 622, 637, 683, 684, 687-697, 716, 722, 751, 753, 955, 959, 960, 962, 965, 983

Cleansing: 42, 43, 96, 111, 149, 153, 158, 182, 185, 233, 236, 248, 264, 299, 301, 310, 330, 401, 427, 432, 486, 537, 539, 540, 556, 571, 572, 578, 589, 592, 596, 599, 602, 604-606, 609, 611, 616, 621, 624, 637, 638, 681-683, 685-697, 699-701, 703-705, 707, 717, 740, 750, 955, 957-963, 965-969, 987, 988, 991

Clove: 8, 10, 20, 23, 42, 43, 62, 68, 174, 191, 212, 289, 304, 319, 354, 373, 385, 409, 490, 510, 951-953, 957, 971-975, 977, 983, 535, 537, 540, 542, 568, 574-576, 580, 584-586, 588-590, 592-594, 600-602, 611, 612, 616, 619, 624-629, 640, 679, 686, 697, 699, 705, 725, 727-730, 741, 750, 763

Clove Vitality: 174, 540, 627, 628, 952, 953, 957, 975, 977, 983

Colds: 37-39, 108, 117, 199, 337, 369, 377, 406, 412, 431, 432, 457, 453, 473, 493, 504, 522, 639, 684, 699

Colic: 224, 233, 639, 640

Colitis: 126, 398, 504, 535, 685

Colon Cleanse: 690, 693

Colorado: 630, 667

ComforTone: 538, 691, 693, 694, 696, 697, 700, 751, 752, 955, 960, 964-966, 968, 983

Common Sense: 63, 176, 177, 632, 635, 647, 674-678, 698, 717, 747, 958-960, 963, 964, 967, 969, 971, 978, 983

Compress: 192, 202, 313, 379, 409, 428, 431, 438, 441, 466, 697

Concentration: 96, 101, 114, 162, 334, 419, 444, 507, 525, 544, 551, 576, 629, 633, 674, 684, 693, 722, 723, 728, 759, 763

Confusion: 112, 290, 420, 630, 675, 684

Constituents: 3, 5, 7, 8, 11, 12, 16, 20, 41-46, 74, 77, 79, 86, 93, 96, 98, 101, 103, 104, 107, 108, 111, 112, 121, 122, 125, 126, 129, 130, 133, 144, 149, 150, 153, 158, 161, 162, 165, 168, 173, 174, 181, 182, 185, 186, 189, 194, 199, 200, 209, 216, 219, 220, 223, 224, 233, 236, 239, 240, 243, 248, 254, 257, 260, 263, 264, 273, 278, 281, 286, 299, 300, 303, 308, 327, 330, 333, 334, 337, 338, 341, 342, 345, 348, 361, 362, 365, 366, 369, 370, 377, 382, 387, 388, 391, 392, 395, 398, 401, 402, 405, 406, 411, 412, 419, 420, 423, 432, 443, 444, 447, 454, 457, 458, 473, 474, 477, 482, 485, 486, 493, 504, 507, 510, 513, 514, 517, 520, 525, 526, 529, 530, 533, 548, 549, 554, 585, 586, 629, 671, 727, 736

Cooking: 10, 12, 45, 101, 125, 185, 338, 342, 402, 403, 473, 513, 533, 553, 627, 628, 704, 705, 707, 709, 711, 718, 741-743, 746, 762, 765

Cool Azul: 63, 178, 594, 640, 956-958, 960, 962, 963, 965-969, 971, 983

Cool Azul Pain Relief Cream: 594, 640, 956-958, 960, 962, 963, 965-968, 983

Cool Azul Sports Gel: 594, 640, 956-958, 960, 962, 963, 965-969, 983

Copaiba: 37, 62, 117, 178, 180, 181, 191, 244, 304, 385, 479, 535, 555, 568, 572, 577, 580, 594, 597, 604, 633, 638-640, 643-645, 675-678, 951, 953, 957, 959, 962, 963, 971-975, 983

Copaiba Vanilla Moisturizing Conditioner: 555, 577, 957, 959, 962, 963, 983

Copaiba Vanilla Moisturizing Shampoo: 555, 577, 957, 959, 962, 963, 983

Copaiba Vitality: 180, 951, 953, 957, 983

Coriander: 42, 62, 71, 90, 95, 118, 146, 155, 158, 170, 182, 235, 252, 266, 270, 284, 293, 307, 314, 328, 358, 434, 451, 465, 466, 469, 500, 519, 569, 571-574, 579, 581, 584, 595, 600, 604-606, 609, 611, 616, 619-622, 636, 638, 705, 951, 953, 957, 958, 971-977, 983

Coriander Vitality: 182, 951, 953, 957, 958, 977, 983

Cortisol: 23, 396, 173, 398, 539, 541, 563, 565, 684

CortiStop: 539, 563, 565, 956, 957, 959, 965, 983

Cosmetics: 129, 162, 401, 473, 520, 533, 596, 623, 681, 746, 754

Coumarins: 43, 44, 74

Cramps: 37, 409, 538, 540, 566, 693

Creme Masque: 597, 600, 958, 959, 964, 966, 968, 969, 982

Croatia: 8, 9, 14, 15, 26, 273, 308, 330, 382

Crohn's Disease: 691

Cumin: 42, 62, 184, 185, 289, 304, 951, 539, 542, 576, 637, 693, 697, 717, 953, 958, 973, 977, 983

Cypress: 11, 26, 62, 71, 80, 83, 84, 89, 90, 106, 107, 114, 117, 118, 178, 186, 187, 197, 205, 276, 278, 281, 304, 314, 322, 385, 431, 434, 438, 461, 500, 538, 555, 574, 583, 594, 600, 601, 607, 619, 620, 632, 634, 643-645, 658-660, 662, 664, 667, 674, 676-679, 951, 953, 954, 956, 958, 968, 971-975, 977, 982, 983

Cystitis: 181, 504

Daily Maintenance: 691, 699, 700

Dandruff: 219, 362, 412, 473, 486

Davana: 62, 71, 72, 84, 90, 118, 188, 189, 205, 276, 304, 417, 438, 461, 469, 499, 500, 555, 572, 573, 579, 581, 595, 597, 600, 601, 606, 611, 638, 674, 676-679, 951, 953, 958, 971-975, 977, 983

Dentarome Plus Toothpaste, Thieves: 957, 959, 963, 966, 969, 991

Dentarome Ultra Toothpaste, Thieves: 644, 957, 963, 966, 969, 991

Deodorants: 575, 623

Depression: 50, 96, 153, 239, 264, 283, 303, 307, 334, 338, 361, 370, 377, 391, 398, 406, 412, 414, 420, 424, 443, 452, 473, 477, 482, 485, 489, 500, 510, 513, 514, 530, 533, 556, 560, 563, 564, 566, 608, 669, 670, 672, 673, 675, 697, 698, 722, 739, 740, 761, 766

Dermatitis (Eczema): 153, 254, 755

Despair: 454, 675, 698

Despondency: 676

Detoxzyme: 955, 958, 959, 983, 539, 640, 689, 692, 696, 697, 700, 701, 711, 712, 717, 751

DeVita, Sabina: 746

DHEA: 539, 541, 556, 559, 561-567, 580

Diabetes: 103, 104, 133, 153, 161, 174, 182, 185, 186, 189, 194, 199, 233, 330, 370, 387, 402, 543, 556, 557, 559, 638, 681-684, 757, 758, 760-762, 765, 766

Diaper Rash: 37, 252, 617, 622, 635, 644

Diarrhea: 19, 125, 135, 341, 377, 419, 504, 536, 539, 631, 643, 684, 685, 689, 694, 695, 711, 715, 717

Diet: 77, 96, 101, 121, 342, 387, 398, 533, 537, 543, 544, 546, 548, 551, 552, 556, 557, 560, 563, 596, 617, 636, 658, 681, 683, 685, 686, 688, 696, 702, 711, 712, 718, 719, 730, 739, 749, 752-754, 757-761

Diffusing: 27, 510, 631, 632, 634, 750

Digest & Cleanse: 540, 695, 697, 751, 955, 959, 960, 962, 965, 983

Digestive Problems: 37, 98, 101, 149, 185, 189, 192, 194, 338, 341, 361, 401, 405, 419, 447, 457, 458, 474, 482, 529, 563, 711

DiGize: 37, 63, 192, 193, 624, 633, 639-641, 643, 693, 695-697, 699, 700, 751, 752, 955, 959-961, 963, 965, 968, 972, 978, 983

DiGize Vitality: 192, 633, 639-641, 643, 751, 955, 959-961, 963, 965, 968, 972, 978, 983

Dill: 62, 146, 194, 951, 953, 958, 977, 983, 984, 636, 679, 704, 716

Dill Vitality: 194, 951, 953, 958, 977, 984

Disappointment: 676

Discouragement: 676

Dish Soap: 624, 644, 955, 957, 959, 963, 967, 991

Dishwasher Powder, Thieves Automatic: 624, 957, 959, 963, 965, 966, 991

Disinfectants: 585, 623, 628

Distillation: 3, 8-16, 25, 42, 45, 107, 122, 264, 345, 443, 510, 513, 530

Divine Release: 63, 196, 197, 955, 956, 959, 960, 962, 963, 966, 967, 972, 978

Dizziness: 149, 447, 566, 722

Dogs: 362, 553, 629, 630, 633-635

Dorado Azul: 62, 177, 178, 198, 199, 216, 248, 289, 304, 322, 385, 431, 594, 620, 637, 640, 677, 678, 951, 953, 958, 971-975, 977, 984

Douglas Fir: 62, 200, 952, 953, 958, 984

Dragon Time: 63, 202, 568, 583, 675, 677, 678, 739, 955-959, 961-963, 965-969, 972, 978, 984

Dragon Time Massage Oil: 583, 957, 959, 961, 962, 967, 969, 984

Dream Catcher: 63, 204, 251, 674-677, 739, 955-961, 966-969, 971, 972, 978, 984

Dysentery: 723

Earache: 93, 503

Ear Infection: 23

Ear problems: 447

Eating Habits: 700

Ecclesiastes: 53

Ecuador: 9, 26, 46, 199, 216, 299, 366, 395,

Index

396, 402, 406, 447, 530, 753, 762, 951, 953

Ecuadorian Dark Chocolessence: 540, 707

Ecuadorian Oregano: 62, 402, 699

Eczema (Dermatitis): 153, 254, 755

Effleurage: 655

Egypt: 44, 150, 158, 185, 186, 194, 254, 303, 365, 493, 525

Egyptian: 63, 129, 133, 182, 206, 233, 239, 387, 493, 669, 674, 676-679, 714, 727, 764, 956, 957, 959, 961, 962, 964, 966, 968, 972, 978, 984

Egyptian Gold: 63, 206, 674, 676-679, 956, 957, 959, 961, 962, 964, 966, 968, 972, 978, 984

Einkorn: 540, 552, 700, 706, 707, 716, 985

Einkorn Flour: 985

Einkorn Grain: 540

Einkorn Granola: 552, 707, 985

Einkorn Pancake and Waffle Mix: 552, 985

Einkorn Rotini Pasta: 985

Einkorn Spaghetti: 985

Einkorn Grain (Wheat): 540

Elemi: 26, 42, 62, 178, 208, 209, 319, 583, 594, 619, 951, 953, 958, 971, 974, 977, 984

Embalming: 107, 144, 209, 493

Emotional: 27, 37, 42, 49-51, 59, 64-77, 103, 104, 108, 133, 186, 189, 199, 205, 215, 226, 235, 236, 248, 251, 270, 278, 290, 294, 370, 414, 423, 438, 451, 461, 474, 499, 514, 517, 533, 981, 569, 582, 638, 647, 648, 655, 658, 661, 666, 669-675, 677, 679, 680, 686, 690, 691, 727, 738, 743

Emotional Challenges: 674

Emotional Health: 569, 670, 672

Emotional Release: 133, 451, 647, 558, 671-673

Emotional Trauma: 51, 186, 499, 514, 658, 670, 671

EndoFlex: 63, 210, 211, 700-702, 739, 748, 749, 751, 959, 960, 964, 967, 972, 978, 984

EndoFlex Vitality: 210, 751, 959, 960, 964, 967, 972, 978, 984

En-R-Gee: 63, 212, 674-679, 739, 955, 957, 961, 963, 964, 966, 972, 978, 984

EndoGize: 541, 565, 956, 957, 960, 964, 984

EndoShield: 701, 702, 748, 749

Energy Centers: 90, 270, 660, 672, 673, 698

Environmental Pollution: 701, 702, 749

Environmental Protection Kits: 701, 702, 748, 749

Envision: 63, 68, 214, 673, 675-678, 739, 959, 962, 965-967, 972, 978, 984

Enzymes: 5, 9, 112, 150, 240, 536, 539, 541, 542, 550, 552, 559, 560, 562, 538, 589, 618, 625, 635, 683, 687-689, 691, 692, 696, 702, 703, 709, 711-722, 730, 733, 736, 741, 742, 744, 749, 754, 757, 760, 764

Epilepsy: 126, 129, 135, 473, 561, 569, 759

Essential Beauty Serum: 555, 574, 956, 957, 962, 964, 967, 984

Essential Brush Set: 582

Essential Oil Chemistry: 40, 41

Essential Oils for Cooking: 627

Essentialzyme: 541, 542, 560, 643, 689, 692, 696, 699-701, 703, 711, 712, 716-718, 751, 955, 957, 959, 965, 968, 984

Essentialzymes-4: 955, 959, 960, 963, 966, 968, 984, 560, 643, 689, 692, 696, 697, 699, 701, 703, 711, 712, 716-718, 751

Esters: 43, 44, 548, 579, 599, 601, 616, 671, 702, 749

Ethers: 42

Eucalyptus Blue: 26, 62, 117, 216, 322, 431, 620, 699, 951, 953, 958, 971, 975, 977, 984

Eucalyptus Citriodora: 62, 216, 218, 219, 322, 385, 431, 620, 951, 953, 958, 974, 975, 977, 984

Eucalyptus Globulus: 62, 117, 142, 216, 220, 223, 322, 385, 423, 431, 583, 586, 612, 620, 627, 639, 677-679, 951, 953, 958, 971, 974, 975, 977, 984

Eucalyptus Radiata: 23, 26, 62, 89, 117, 222, 223, 322, 385, 428, 431, 490, 575, 576, 580, 583, 586, 588-590, 592, 593, 611, 612, 616, 620, 624-627, 640, 657, 667, 951, 953, 959, 971, 974, 975, 977, 984

Eucalyptus Staigeriana: 62, 117, 224, 951, 953, 959, 971, 984

Europe: 12, 19, 77, 101, 126, 150, 153, 161, 194, 206, 209, 224, 333, 365, 454, 457, 458, 473, 485, 493, 561, 583, 761

Evening Peace Bath & Shower Gel: 571, 955-959, 961, 962, 965-967, 969, 984

Evergreen Essence: 63, 226

Exodus II: 63, 230, 239, 638-640, 644, 698, 699, 739, 750, 751, 956, 957, 959, 961, 964, 968, 972, 978, 984

Exotic Pets: 629, 632

Eye Cream: 556, 606, 955, 958-960, 962, 966, 969, 992

Facial Scrub: 582, 606, 965, 966, 990

Facial Wash: 556, 582, 600, 604, 605, 960, 962, 965, 966, 988

Fainting: 168, 734

Farag, Radwan: 728, 741

Fasting: 161, 185, 557, 688, 689, 753, 754

Fat: 101, 161, 257, 334, 345, 387, 544, 557, 559, 560, 563, 583, 607, 636, 681-684, 689, 691, 692, 695, 715, 717, 718, 722, 724, 728, 743, 758, 759, 762

Fatigue: 51, 83, 93, 101, 135, 146, 239, 263, 264, 392, 420, 423, 444, 452, 454, 474, 493, 535, 536, 539, 556, 563, 684, 685, 715, 722, 756, 759

FDA: 20, 575, 657, 583, 708, 721, 734, 746, 758, 759, 761

Fear: 27, 50, 294, 380, 670, 676, 679, 689

Feather Spray: 631

Feathering: 660

FemiGen: 566, 957, 959, 967, 969, 984

Fennel: 42, 43, 62, 79, 89, 192, 202, 232, 233, 313, 325, 379, 462, 951, 953, 959, 971-977, 984, 536, 539, 540, 542, 553, 565-569, 580, 583, 584, 620, 625, 637, 640, 678, 690, 693-697, 704, 707, 717

Fennel Vitality: 232, 951, 953, 959, 977, 984

Fever: 345, 366, 522, 545, 658, 684, 38

Fibromyalgia: 691, 755

Finger Straddle: 660, 664

Fish: 575, 613, 631, 632, 693, 703, 706, 716, 720, 752

Flash Points: 977

Flatulence: 411, 695, 711

Fleas: 39, 423, 639

Flu: 28, 33, 39, 199, 337, 406, 473, 504, 522, 533, 639, 667, 699, 721, 756

Fluoride: 586, 588-590, 613, 723, 731-734, 763, 764

Foaming Hand Soaps: 611

Food Poisoning: 423

Forgetfulness: 37, 454, 676, 684

Forgiveness: 63, 197, 234, 251, 284, 673, 674, 676-678, 739, 955, 958-963, 966, 967, 969, 971, 972, 978, 984

FOS (Fructooligosaccharides): 760

Fractures: 290, 642, 733, 763

France: 9, 11, 16, 26, 46, 47, 112, 130, 153, 173, 186, 273, 286, 333, 334, 342, 370, 454, 586, 657

Franchomme, Pierre: 41, 702, 749

Frankincense: 10, 23, 26, 37, 42, 48, 53, 55-57, 59, 62, 64, 67, 68, 71, 90, 95, 98, 114, 118, 142, 146, 155, 177, 197, 206, 209, 230, 235, 238-244, 247, 248, 251, 254, 266, 270, 275, 276, 284, 289, 293, 294, 304, 314, 316, 320, 353, 354, 357, 361, 385, 387, 396, 406, 434, 457, 458, 489, 496, 499, 500, 503, 508, 535, 539, 553, 555, 556, 565, 568, 569, 576, 580, 591, 596-602, 604, 606, 611, 616, 619, 620, 631, 633, 637-640, 642, 669-679, 695, 697-699, 727, 734-737, 739, 747, 750, 752, 764, 951, 953, 954, 959, 967, 971-978, 984, 990

Frankincense, Frereana: 62, 240, 503, 951, 953, 959, 975, 984, 591, 736, 764

Frankincense, Sacred: 62, 118, 242-244, 248, 275, 314, 320, 357, 434, 489, 496, 568, 569, 580, 600, 619, 620, 640, 642, 669, 670, 672-679, 698, 699, 735, 736, 747, 750, 752, 951, 954, 967, 971-975, 978, 990

Frankincense Vitality: 238, 633, 951, 953, 959, 977, 984

Freedom: 7, 63, 196, 244, 957, 961, 962, 965, 967, 968, 972, 978, 984, 582, 638, 672-679, 697, 744

Frequency: 51, 68, 103, 104, 251, 284, 519, 535, 561, 564, 576, 629, 631, 632, 636, 650, 673, 697, 698, 725, 736-741, 746, 747, 764

Frereana Frankincense: 62, 240, 503, 591, 736, 764, 951, 953, 959, 975, 984

Friedmann, Terry: 144, 514, 596, 656

Fructooligosaccharides (FOS): 760

Fructose: 485, 537, 693, 712, 757-759, 761, 762

Fruit & Veggie Soak: 624, 955, 957, 959-961, 963-968, 991

Fruit & Veggie Spray: 625, 957, 959, 963, 967

Frustration: 27, 276, 677, 697, 740

Fujimoto, Edward: 743

Fulfill Your Destiny: 63, 246, 247, 674, 955-957, 959, 961, 964, 968, 973, 984

Fungal Infections: 98, 101, 103, 104, 133, 165, 219, 236, 254, 281, 362, 365, 387, 405, 419, 486, 609, 631

Furanoids: 44

Galbanum: 53, 951, 953, 739

Gallstones: 561, 684, 695, 718

Gary's Light: 63, 248, 674-679, 690, 698, 699

Gary's True Grit: 540, 552, 555, 707, 962, 965, 985

Gary's True Grit Chocolate Coated Wolfberry Crisp Bars: 707

Gary's True Grit Einkorn Berries: 985

Gary's True Grit Einkorn Flakes Cereal: 985

Gary's True Grit Einkorn Flour: 985

Gary's True Grit Einkorn Granola: 552, 707, 985

Gary's True Grit Einkorn Pancake and Waffle Mix: 552, 985

Gary's True Grit Einkorn Rotini Pasta: 985

Gary's True Grit Einkorn Spaghetti: 985

Gary's True Grit NingXia Berry Syrup: 552, 962, 965, 985

Gas: 10, 16, 37, 38, 46-48, 192, 239, 243, 333, 536, 540, 618, 684, 695, 703, 711, 715, 717, 718, 761, 764

Gas Chromatography: 16, 46-48, 239, 243, 764

Gastritis: 691

Gathering: 63, 250, 251, 673-679, 698, 739, 957, 959, 962, 964, 966-969, 973, 978, 985

Gattefossé, René Maurice: 19

Genesis Hand & Body Lotion: 573, 955, 958, 959, 961, 962, 965, 966, 969, 985

GeneYus, KidScents: 63, 314, 986, 619, 674-679

Gentle Baby: 37, 63, 252, 638, 640, 675, 676, 739, 955, 958, 959, 961, 962, 965, 966, 969, 973, 978, 985

Geranium: 43, 62, 71, 72, 84, 90, 95, 118, 146, 155, 170, 197, 205, 211, 215, 235, 251, 252, 254, 255, 266, 270, 276, 284, 293, 304, 307, 313, 314, 316, 320, 328, 357, 358, 396, 434, 438, 451, 461, 465, 466, 499, 500, 508, 519, 555, 556, 567-569, 571-574, 576, 577, 579, 580, 584, 596, 597, 600-602, 604-606, 609, 611, 616, 619-622, 636-639, 643, 674-679, 695, 696, 702, 749, 952, 953, 959, 960, 971-977, 985

German Chamomile: 9, 15, 43, 62, 71, 84, 90, 118, 146, 150, 178, 205, 211, 276, 304, 414, 417, 438, 461, 480, 500, 539, 594, 600, 608, 638, 696, 739, 951-953, 960, 971-975, 977, 985

German Chamomile Vitality: 150, 952, 953, 960, 985

Germany: 23, 44, 545, 546, 592

Giardia: 726

Gift, The: 63, 68, 251, 488, 489, 642, 673, 674, 676-679, 697-699, 747, 752, 957, 961, 964, 967, 968, 975, 979, 991

Ginger: 42, 43, 62, 68, 79, 192, 256, 257, 325, 350, 358, 536, 539-541, 565, 620, 625, 636, 637, 675-677, 691, 693, 695, 696, 705, 706, 717, 952, 953, 960, 971, 972, 974, 976, 977, 985

Index

Ginger Vitality: 256, 540, 952, 953, 960, 977, 985

Gingivitis and Periodontitis: 588

Glands: 10, 33, 90, 98, 114, 135, 251, 387, 550, 559, 561-563, 698, 702, 749

GLF: 63, 258, 259, 690, 692, 699, 752, 753, 956, 960-962, 967, 973, 979, 985

GLF Vitality: 258, 956, 960-962, 967, 973, 979, 985

Glycemic Index: 548, 549, 553, 700, 759-762

Goldenrod: 15, 26, 62, 177, 260, 952, 953, 960, 971, 977, 985

Good Eating Habits: 700

Gout: 406, 755

Grade B Maple Syrup: 688, 689, 761

Grain: 540, 643, 707, 714, 721

Grand Fir, Idaho: 26, 62, 95, 118, 155, 191, 206, 212, 262, 263, 266, 319, 385, 452, 489, 503, 537, 610, 619, 636, 639, 640, 642, 672, 674, 676-678, 690, 695, 697, 698, 747

Grapefruit: 20, 26, 34, 42, 44, 62, 71, 84, 90, 118, 167, 197, 205, 259, 264, 276, 304, 437, 438, 461, 470, 500, 556, 573, 576, 581, 583, 588, 616, 675, 689, 691, 693, 700, 716, 951, 953, 960, 971-975, 977, 985

Grapefruit Juice Recipe: 691

Grapefruit Lip Balm: 556, 581, 960, 985

Grapefruit Vitality: 34, 264, 951, 953, 960, 973, 977, 985

GRAS: 181, 657, 761

Gratitude: 63, 266, 673, 676-679, 955, 958, 959, 961, 964, 968, 969, 973, 979, 985

Graves' Disease: 752

Grief: 219, 236, 307, 677

Grounding: 63, 103, 104, 108, 133, 186, 200, 209, 233, 240, 263, 268, 269, 276, 283, 366, 423, 447, 451, 452, 457, 458, 507, 514, 620, 639, 642, 672-676, 678, 690, 698, 739, 747, 955, 956, 961, 966, 968, 969, 973, 979, 985

Guilt: 677

Hahn, Scott: 669

Hair Care: 114, 236, 560, 577, 981-992

Hair Loss: 144, 334, 424, 444, 473, 493, 530, 566

Hand Purifier: 957, 959, 963, 966, 967, 992

Hardening of the Arteries: 723

Harmony: 41, 63, 112, 270, 443, 522, 539, 599, 647, 672, 674-679, 697, 698, 739, 740, 747, 955, 956, 958-969, 973, 979, 985

Hawaii: 26, 457, 743

Headache: 150, 168, 200, 419, 443, 447, 507, 545, 629, 689

Health Issues: 135, 666, 724

Healthy Snacks: 707

Heartburn: 37, 192, 686, 696, 711, 715

Heart Health: 135, 158, 538

Heavy Metals: 16, 594, 681, 688, 692, 722, 723, 753

Heavy Metals Cleanse: 692

Hebrew University: 669, 736

Helichrysum: 8, 15, 26, 43, 62, 67, 80, 90, 114, 191, 197, 235, 259, 272, 273, 310, 313, 319, 350, 374, 385, 409, 499, 500, 538, 594, 602-604, 619, 622, 638-640, 642, 643, 674, 678, 684, 692, 696, 739, 751, 951, 953, 960, 971-975, 977, 985

Hemorrhoids: 125, 388, 457, 458

Hepatitis: 125, 149, 150, 174, 254, 260, 303, 310, 337, 387, 392, 432, 444, 474, 493, 526, 530, 547, 681-684, 741

Herb Farming: 9

Herbicides: 9, 13, 45, 559, 681, 715, 724

Herpes Zoster: 107, 419, 457, 458

Hertel, Hans Ulrich: 744

HFCS: 757, 758

Hieroglyphics: 714, 727

Highest Potential: 63, 90, 276, 642, 673-677, 679, 698, 956-962, 964, 966-969, 973, 979, 985

High Fructose Corn Syrup: 758

Highland Flats Tree Farm: 15, 263, 522

Hildegard of Bingen: 93, 174, 194, 233, 365, 387, 392, 401, 444, 493

Hinoki: 62, 197, 229, 278, 279, 281, 469, 579, 581, 595, 599, 606, 611, 674-679, 951, 953, 960, 972, 974, 975, 977, 985

Hippocampus: 51, 392, 670

Hirsch, Alan: 51, 419

Hobble Injury: 640

Home: 1, 15, 27, 29, 36, 64-533, 536, 538, 540, 542, 544, 546, 548, 550, 552, 554, 556, 558, 560, 562-564, 566, 568, 570, 572, 574, 576, 578, 580, 582, 584, 586, 588, 590, 592, 594, 596, 598, 600, 602, 604, 606, 608, 610, 612-614, 616, 618-620, 622-628, 630, 632, 634, 635, 638, 640, 642, 644, 646, 648, 650, 652, 654, 656, 658, 660, 662, 664, 666, 668, 670, 672, 674, 676, 678, 680, 682, 684, 686, 688, 690-692, 694, 696, 698, 700, 702, 704, 706, 708, 710, 712, 714, 716, 718, 720, 722, 724-726, 728, 730, 732, 734, 736, 738-744, 746, 748, 750, 752, 754, 756, 758-760, 762, 764, 766

Hong Kuai: 26, 62, 118, 280, 281, 951, 953, 960, 971, 977, 985

Hope: 1, 63, 95, 254, 282, 283, 496, 647, 673-677, 679, 719, 739, 956, 961, 963, 964, 973, 979, 985

Hormone Balancing: 202, 211, 580

Hormones: 51, 98, 158, 369, 387, 462, 541, 559-564, 566, 583, 681, 682, 714, 717, 720, 727, 733, 754

Horses: 55, 57, 59, 608, 629, 630, 635, 640, 644, 645, 667, 714

Ho Wood: 62, 42, 122, 155, 316, 451, 508, 611, 619, 960, 976, 985

Human Rights: 744

Humility: 63, 284, 674, 677, 678, 739, 955, 958-960, 963, 964, 966, 968, 969, 973, 979, 985

Hunza: 754

Hyperactivity: 38, 144, 273, 507, 514, 608

Hypertension: 23, 185, 260, 273, 338, 341, 369, 377, 391, 392, 395, 398, 412, 443, 452, 477, 479, 486, 526, 530, 557, 684, 722, 727

Hypoglycemia: 557

Hyssop: 43, 53, 54, 58, 62, 90, 146, 155, 206, 230, 248, 259, 270, 286, 287, 289, 304, 314, 434, 441, 451, 500, 519, 619,

637, 638, 752, 951, 953, 961, 972-977, 985

Iceland: 23

ICP: 560, 643, 689, 694-697, 700, 751, 752, 955, 959, 960, 963, 966, 968, 985

Idaho: 13, 26, 62, 72, 95, 108, 118, 155, 191, 200, 206, 212, 226, 244, 247, 262, 263, 266, 294, 297, 314, 319, 328, 353, 357, 385, 434, 452, 469, 489, 496, 503, 517, 522, 537, 569, 579, 581, 595, 606, 610, 611, 619, 636, 638-640, 642, 672, 674-679, 690, 695, 697, 698, 747, 951-953, 961, 971-975, 977, 985, 986

Idaho Blue Spruce: 26, 62, 72, 95, 108, 118, 226, 244, 247, 294, 297, 314, 328, 353, 357, 385, 434, 469, 496, 952, 953, 961, 971-975, 977, 986, 569, 579, 581, 595, 606, 611, 619, 640, 642, 674-679

Idaho Grand Fir: 26, 62, 95, 118, 155, 191, 206, 212, 262, 263, 266, 319, 385, 452, 489, 503, 537, 610, 619, 636, 639, 640, 642, 672, 674, 676-678, 690, 695, 697, 698, 747

Idaho Tansy: 13, 952, 953, 961, 977, 986

Immune System: 42, 109, 126, 158, 162, 173, 174, 200, 206, 236, 337, 432, 482, 489, 520, 533, 537, 552, 554, 563, 631, 648, 657, 658, 670, 672, 684, 698, 699, 702, 709, 712, 721, 743-745, 749, 751-753, 756, 759, 760, 762

ImmuPower: 63, 288, 289, 639, 699, 739, 747, 957-959, 961, 964-966, 973, 979, 986

ImmuPro: 552, 566, 640, 698, 751, 965, 986

Infect Away, Animal Scents: 637, 958, 964-966, 981

Inflammation: 23, 37, 38, 74, 108, 125, 133, 149, 150, 153, 158, 173, 185, 191, 194, 219, 239, 278, 286, 330, 333, 341, 373, 387, 391, 398, 405, 406, 409, 411, 423, 432, 447, 454, 486, 520, 525, 530, 533, 15, 535, 537, 544, 546, 550, 565, 568, 571, 585, 586, 588, 592, 608, 615, 623, 638-640, 656-658, 681, 684, 689, 691, 736, 742, 756, 758, 765

Influenza: 161, 370, 428, 486

Inhalation: 23, 51, 93, 96, 101, 144, 149, 153, 173, 254, 264, 278, 300, 334, 338, 391, 412, 419, 420, 432, 470, 486, 530, 647, 725,

738, 752

Inner Child: 263, 90, 956, 961, 963-965, 967-969, 973, 979, 986, 639, 673, 674, 676-679, 690, 698, 739

Inner Defense: 642, 697, 699, 701, 751, 957, 959, 962, 963, 965, 966, 968, 986

Inner Harmony: 955, 960-969, 973, 979

Insect: 3, 38, 39, 93, 126, 149, 165, 173, 181, 219, 220, 224, 243, 263, 300, 310, 348, 412, 447, 486, 493, 517, 583, 602, 603, 639, 957, 960, 963, 966-968, 986

Insect Repellent: 126, 149, 165, 219, 220, 224, 263, 300, 412, 447, 493, 602, 639, 957, 960, 963, 966-968, 986

Insomnia: 3, 96, 150, 153, 297, 334, 361, 370, 391, 398, 414, 420, 437, 477, 482, 499, 500, 507, 514

Inspiration: 63, 281, 292, 676-679, 698, 739, 955, 956, 958-960, 964, 967-969, 973, 979, 986

Intestinal Fiber Cleanse: 694

Into the Future: 63, 68, 294, 956, 957, 959, 961, 965, 968, 969, 973, 979, 986, 673, 676, 677, 679, 739

InTouch: 63, 296, 676, 679, 698, 956, 961, 963, 967, 968, 973, 979, 986

Iran: 23, 77, 112, 126, 150, 165, 182, 186, 286, 300, 303, 330, 338, 370, 401, 443, 485, 525

Irregular Periods: 202

Irritability: 153, 437, 482, 535, 566, 608, 618, 677, 685, 689

Irritable Bowel Syndrome: 233, 239, 419, 536, 561, 684

Ishpingo: 62, 298, 299, 395, 952, 953, 961

Israel: 26, 54, 55, 377, 764

Itching: 362, 412, 15, 565, 571, 583, 602, 610, 615, 623, 684

Jade Lemon: 26, 62, 229, 300, 624, 625, 674-679, 951, 953, 961, 977, 986

Jade Lemon Vitality: 300, 951, 953, 961, 977, 986

Japan: 122, 278, 533, 657, 681, 735, 761

Jasmine: 62, 42, 43, 62, 71, 72, 84, 90, 118, 146, 155, 170, 202, 205, 235, 252, 270, 275, 276, 290, 294, 302-304, 307, 328, 350, 361, 396, 438, 461, 466, 489, 500, 568,

569, 571-574, 578, 583, 584, 595, 597, 600, 601, 604, 638, 674, 678, 952, 953, 961, 971-975, 977, 986

Jaundice: 525, 684

Jealousy: 57, 677

Journey On: 63, 304, 305, 674-679, 955-962, 964-969, 973, 986

Joy: 27, 50, 63, 68, 122, 156, 248, 249, 306, 307, 365, 391, 396, 496, 569, 603, 642, 647, 673-678, 698, 736, 739, 955, 958, 960-962, 965, 966, 968, 969, 971, 973, 979, 986

Juniper: 26, 42, 43, 62, 64, 118, 192, 205, 212, 269, 283, 294, 304, 308, 952, 953, 961, 971-974, 977, 986, 536, 572, 583, 609, 625, 637, 643, 674-679, 695, 717, 739

JuvaCleanse: 63, 310, 684, 690, 692, 696, 697, 699, 752, 956, 960, 962, 973, 979, 986

JuvaCleanse Vitality: 310, 956, 960, 962, 973, 979, 986

JuvaFlex: 63, 312, 313, 690-693, 696, 699, 739, 956, 959, 960, 966, 973, 974, 979, 986

JuvaFlex Vitality: 312, 956, 959, 960, 966, 974, 979, 986

JuvaPower: 560, 685, 686, 689, 694, 696, 697, 700, 704-706, 751, 752, 955, 959, 986

JuvaTone: 691, 696, 697, 699, 956, 960, 962, 964, 966, 986

K&B: 643, 957, 959-961, 966, 967, 986

Kidney Disorders: 181

Kidney Failure: 643

Kidney Stones: 181, 695

KidPower, KidScents: 63, 316, 619, 674-679

KidScents: 63, 314, 316, 318-320, 322, 324, 325, 552, 586, 588, 615-620, 674-679, 686, 697, 701, 711, 712, 751, 955-960, 962, 964-969, 986

KidScents Bath Gel: 615, 956, 986

KidScents GeneYus: 63, 314, 619, 674-679, 986

KidScents KidPower: 63, 316, 619, 674-

984 | Index

Index

679

KidScents Lotion: 616, 955, 956, 958, 960, 968, 969, 986

KidScents MightyPro: 617, 686, 701, 986

KidScents MightyVites: 552, 617, 751, 986

KidScents MightyZyme: 618, 697, 711, 712, 965, 986

KidScents Oil Collection: 619

KidScents Owie: 63, 318, 986, 619

KidScents Roll-On Collection: 619

KidScents Shampoo: 616, 962, 968, 986

KidScents SleepyIze: 63, 320, 620, 986

KidScents Slique Toothpaste: 588, 957, 959, 960, 962, 964, 966-968, 986

KidScents SniffleEase: 63, 322, 620, 986

KidScents Tender Tush: 616, 955, 957-960, 962, 966, 969, 986

KidScents TummyGize: 63, 324, 986, 620

KidScents Unwind: 618

Kitty Litter: 633

Kitty Raindrop: 632, 634

Korea: 122, 761

Kunzea: 20, 62, 89, 326, 327, 639, 674, 961, 971, 986

Lactones: 43, 44

Lady Sclareol: 63, 328, 569, 677, 678, 955, 957, 958, 960, 961, 965, 967-969, 974, 979, 986

Lakota Indians: 103, 655

Laryngitis: 473

Laundry: 37, 39, 625, 627, 639, 955, 957, 959, 963, 967, 991

Laundry Soap: 625, 639, 955, 957, 959, 963, 967, 991

Laurus Nobilis (Bay Laurel): 117, 952, 953, 961, 971, 986

LavaDerm Cooling Mist: 603, 751, 960, 962, 964, 987

Lavandin: 41-43, 46, 48, 49, 62, 332-334, 427, 438, 625, 637, 952, 953, 961, 974, 975, 977

Lavender: 3, 7, 10, 11, 20, 23, 26, 34, 37, 41, 42, 44, 46-49, 51, 62, 67, 83, 90, 114, 118, 142, 146, 155, 178, 202, 206, 215, 235, 244, 251, 252, 270, 276, 304, 320, 322, 333, 334, 357, 361, 374, 379, 380, 385, 414, 431, 434, 448, 461, 465, 469, 472, 479, 480, 495, 499, 500, 538, 553, 555, 556, 568, 569, 572-574, 576-579, 581, 583, 584, 594-599, 602-607, 609, 611, 612, 616, 619-622, 627, 628, 631, 637-640, 671, 674-679, 690, 698, 739, 751, 952-954, 957, 958, 961, 962, 964, 965, 967, 971-975, 977, 987

Lavender Bath & Shower Gel: 555, 572, 958, 962, 964, 987

Lavender Calming Bath Bombs: 572, 962, 987

Lavender Conditioner: 578, 957, 961, 962, 965, 967, 987

Lavender Foaming Hand Soap: 612, 962, 964, 987

Lavender Hand & Body Lotion: 555, 573, 958, 962, 964, 987

Lavender Lip Balm: 556, 581, 962, 987

Lavender Mint Daily Conditioner: 577, 962, 965, 967, 987

Lavender Mint Daily Shampoo: 578, 962, 965, 967, 987

Lavender Shampoo: 556, 578, 957, 961, 962, 987

Lavender Vitality: 334, 628, 952, 953, 962, 977, 987

Laxative for Foals: 643

Layering: 29, 31

Ledoux, Joseph: 670

Ledum: 15, 62, 197, 259, 310, 336, 337, 640, 684, 690, 692, 695-697, 752, 952, 953, 962, 972, 973, 977, 987

Lee, Lita: 743

Lemon: 20, 23, 26, 34, 38, 42, 44, 62, 71, 84, 89, 90, 118, 146, 155, 167, 170, 191, 205, 224, 229, 235, 252, 270, 275, 276, 300, 304, 307, 338, 341, 342, 344, 345, 347, 366, 370, 385, 396, 428, 438, 461, 469, 470, 480, 490, 496, 500, 507, 536, 540, 552, 553, 555, 569, 571-573, 575, 576, 578-581, 586, 588-590, 592-595, 598, 599, 604-606, 609, 611, 612, 615-617, 624-628, 631, 637, 638, 674-679, 688, 689, 694-696, 699, 700, 702, 703, 707, 718, 725-727, 739, 749, 752, 951, 953, 961-963, 971-975, 977, 986, 987

Lemon Myrtle: 62, 89, 342, 385, 573, 612, 674-676, 951, 953, 963, 971, 972, 974, 977, 987

Lemon Verbena: 20, 62, 344, 345, 699

Lemon Vitality: 34, 300, 538, 627, 628, 951, 953, 961-963, 977, 986, 987

Lemonade Diet: 688

Lemongrass: 20, 26, 38, 42, 43, 62, 90, 192, 212, 248, 264, 290, 340, 341, 405, 427, 529, 536, 572, 583, 602, 609, 624, 625, 637, 639, 643, 644, 657, 695, 700, 707, 717, 741, 752, 951, 953, 963, 972-974, 977, 987

Lemongrass Vitality: 340, 951, 953, 963, 977, 987

Lemon Myrtle: 62, 89, 342, 385, 951, 953, 963, 971, 972, 974, 977, 987, 573, 612, 674-676

Letting Go: 672, 673

Leukemia: 144, 454, 759, 766

Lewis, Roger: 310, 684

Lice: 23, 39, 165, 168, 174, 423, 486, 637

Life 9: 561, 643, 686, 696, 699, 701, 751, 987

Ligaments: 83, 191, 341, 529, 537, 583, 638, 639

Light the Fire: 63, 346, 347, 955, 956, 962-964, 974, 979, 987, 673-679

Limbic System: 27, 28, 50, 51, 98, 387, 670, 672, 673, 686, 698, 738

Lime: 26, 34, 42, 44, 62, 71, 84, 90, 158, 168, 177, 275, 348, 349, 353, 385, 396, 437, 438, 479, 951, 953, 957, 961, 963, 971, 972, 974, 975, 977, 987, 536, 553, 555, 572, 573, 577, 597, 625, 674-679, 752

Lime Vitality: 34, 158, 348, 951, 953, 963, 977, 987

Lin, HK: 23, 239, 243, 457, 458, 764

Linalool: 42-45, 86, 93, 96, 122, 129, 133, 158, 161, 168, 173, 182, 236, 254, 303, 330, 333, 334, 365, 388, 391, 401, 405, 420, 432, 444, 493, 525, 530, 960, 657

Linalyl Acetate: 43, 44, 47, 48, 96, 112, 129, 173, 333, 334, 391, 420, 473

Lip Balm: 556, 581, 957, 960, 962, 965,

967, 983, 985, 987

Lip Balm, Cinnamint: 556, 581, 957, 965, 967, 983

Lip Balm, Grapefruit: 556, 581, 960, 985

Lip Balm, Lavender: 556, 581, 962, 987

Lip Gloss, Savvy Minerals: 965

Lipase: 536, 537, 539, 618, 625, 709, 712, 715, 717

Lipid: 48, 112, 150, 185, 257, 264, 286, 330, 444, 470, 548, 551, 555, 574, 616, 682, 683, 763

Liposomes: 593

Live with Passion: 63, 350, 674-676, 678, 679, 739, 955-957, 960, 961, 963-965, 967, 974, 979, 987

Live Your Passion: 63, 352, 353, 673-676, 678, 679, 959, 961, 963-965, 967, 969, 974, 979, 987

Liver: 32, 37, 44, 77, 93, 112, 125, 130, 149, 150, 153, 161, 182, 185, 186, 194, 199, 211, 219, 233, 254, 257, 259, 260, 264, 273, 308, 310, 313, 330, 337, 388, 391, 392, 401, 402, 419, 438, 443, 444, 454, 474, 482, 525, 526, 539, 540, 543, 546, 547, 553, 560, 562, 563, 575, 596, 608, 629, 644, 666, 672, 681-685, 688, 690-692, 694-697, 707-709, 712, 715, 717, 718, 720, 722, 728, 730, 741, 746, 753, 758, 760-763, 766,

Liver Health: 186, 681, 696, 761

Livestock: 19, 20, 635

Longevity: 63, 51, 354, 365, 473, 688, 699-702, 719, 722, 727-729, 731, 733-735, 737, 739, 741, 743, 745, 747-749, 751-755, 757, 759, 761, 763, 765, 957, 959, 965, 968, 974, 979, 987

Longevity Vitality: 354, 957, 959, 965, 968, 974, 979, 987, 700, 727, 729, 731, 733, 735, 737, 739, 741, 743, 745, 747, 749, 751, 753, 755, 757, 759, 761, 763, 765

Lotion: 555, 573, 595, 601, 604, 616, 620, 955-969, 985-988, 990

Loyalty: 63, 356, 357, 955, 956, 960-963, 965-969, 974, 987

Lung Cancer: 133, 150, 513

Lupus: 756

Lushious Lemon Foaming Hand Soap: 612

Lymphatic Pump: 648, 666

Lymphatic System: 80, 257, 348, 437, 745

Magnify Your Purpose: 63, 68, 358, 673-679, 739, 955, 957, 958, 960, 964, 965, 967, 969, 974, 979, 987

Maintenance Protocol: 700

Malaria: 101, 220, 723

Malaysia: 181

Mandarin: 42, 62, 167, 360, 361, 437, 482, 533, 573, 694, 704, 951, 953, 963, 971, 972, 975, 977, 987

Manuka: 62, 362, 363, 596, 952, 953, 963, 977, 987

Maple Syrup: 354, 688, 689, 691, 696, 703, 704, 706, 761, 762

Marjoram: 29, 62, 80, 83, 202, 322, 364, 365, 374, 385, 431, 493, 568, 583, 620, 632, 634, 645, 657-660, 662, 665, 667, 674, 678, 952, 953, 963, 971, 972, 974, 975, 977, 987

Marjoram Vitality: 364, 952, 953, 963, 977, 987

Mass Spectrometry: 16, 47, 48, 240, 388, 548, 743, 764, 765

Mass Spectroscopy: 48

Massage: 15, 29, 67, 186, 192, 252, 254, 313, 334, 401, 402, 406, 409, 423, 438, 489, 514, 520, 567, 569, 578, 580, 582-584, 594, 598, 600, 604-607, 620, 621, 632, 634, 635, 637-642, 645, 647, 648, 655, 658-660, 665, 673, 697, 698, 955-963, 965, 967-969, 981-992

Massage Oils: 313, 409, 582, 584, 642, 981-992

Master Cleanse: 688, 689, 691, 696, 697

Master Formula: 552, 617, 696, 699, 956, 957, 959, 960, 987

Mastrante: 62, 229, 347, 357, 366, 675-679, 952, 953, 963, 974, 977, 987

Matricaria: 71, 84, 118, 150, 178, 205, 211, 304, 414, 417, 438, 461, 480, 500, 573, 594, 600, 604, 605, 951-953, 960, 971, 972, 974, 975

Meat: 53, 55-57, 59, 608, 628, 696, 707, 713, 715, 716, 718-720, 752

MegaCal: 962, 988, 686

Mein, Carolyn L.: 673

Melaleuca Alternifolia: 23, 338, 486, 952, 954, 968

Melaleuca Ericifolia: 86, 89, 952, 953, 963, 971, 977, 988

Melaleuca Quinquenervia: 62, 178, 368, 369, 373, 952, 594, 701, 953, 963, 964, 971, 974, 977, 988,

Melanoma: 112, 369, 447, 514

Melatonin: 114, 144, 392, 457, 458, 552, 561-563, 566, 569, 570, 698

Melissa: 15, 26, 42, 62, 90, 114, 118, 197, 235, 283, 284, 289, 297, 314, 334, 350, 357, 370, 434, 451, 519, 564, 598-601, 619, 640, 675-679, 695, 697, 699, 707, 739, 752, 952, 953, 963, 971-976, 978, 988

Melrose: 63, 372, 373, 638-640, 642-645, 699-702, 739, 747-752, 957, 963, 966, 968, 974, 979, 988

Memory, Impaired: 444

Mendwell, Animal Scents: 637, 959-961, 964, 981

Menopause: 303, 560, 564, 566, 568-570

Mental: 23, 93, 96, 114, 129, 146, 170, 177, 205, 243, 276, 334, 419, 420, 423, 444, 454, 461, 479, 496, 549, 552, 560, 563, 564, 569, 583, 618, 669-671, 673, 675, 677, 679, 680, 689, 699, 715, 720, 723, 727, 743, 755

Mental Fatigue: 93, 146, 420, 444, 454, 563

Methyl Chavicol: 44, 77, 93, 133, 233, 485

Mexico: 26, 264, 348, 366, 482, 557, 752, 753, 764

M-Grain: 63, 374, 739, 955, 960, 962, 963, 965, 966, 974, 979, 988

Microbes: 19, 20, 220, 585, 586, 657, 687, 707, 712, 737, 741, 742

Micromeria: 62, 376, 377, 952, 953, 963, 978

Microwave: 711, 741-747, 765

Microwave Cooking: 711, 741-743, 746

Microwave Ovens: 741, 743-746, 765

MightyVites, KidScents: 552, 617, 751, 986

MightyZyme, KidScents: 618, 697, 711, 712, 965, 986

MindWise: 955, 959, 962, 963, 965, 988

Mineral Essence: 639, 686, 696, 699, 722, 751, 957, 962, 965, 988

Minerals: 9, 32, 536, 539, 543-546, 551-553, 568, 581, 582, 617, 683, 686-689, 692, 696, 698-700, 702, 709, 716-723, 725, 726, 742, 746, 749, 751, 754, 756, 757, 760-762, 955, 956, 960, 962-968, 990

Mineral Sunscreen Lotion – SPF 50: 604

Mirah Luminous Cleansing Oil: 604, 955, 958, 960-962, 965-969, 988

Mirah Shave Oil: 595, 956, 958, 961, 962, 964, 966, 967, 969, 988

Mister: 63, 378, 569, 678, 679, 739, 959, 962, 964, 965, 967, 969, 974, 979, 988

Mites: 638, 639

Moisture Cream: 556, 605, 955, 958, 960, 962, 964, 966, 967, 969, 990

Moisturizing Bar Soaps: 608

Moles: 38

Monoterpenes: 41, 42, 44, 657, 667

Mood Swings: 202, 535, 563, 564, 566, 678, 685

Morning Sickness: 37

Morning Start Bath & Shower Gel: 572, 961, 963, 965, 966, 988

Morning Start Moisturizing Soap: 609, 961, 963, 965, 966, 988

Motivation: 27, 63, 68, 251, 353, 358, 380, 432, 499, 673-676, 678, 681, 739, 956, 962, 966, 969, 974, 979, 988

Mountain Savory: 42, 62, 289, 304, 382, 480, 637, 638, 645, 667, 699, 741, 750, 952, 953, 964, 973, 975, 978, 988

Mountain Savory Vitality: 382, 952, 953, 964, 978, 988

Moussaieff, Arieh: 669, 736

Mouth Rinse: 586, 593

Mouthwash: 20, 402, 493, 588, 589, 592, 593, 731, 957, 959, 963, 966-968, 991

MSM (methylsulfonylmethane): 537, 755

Mucus: 575, 684, 686, 689

MultiGreens: 696, 699, 751, 752, 962, 963, 966, 988

Muscles: 29, 38, 83, 178, 216, 219, 220, 223, 236, 263, 286, 341, 345, 362, 423, 520, 529, 537, 564, 571, 583, 645, 648, 658, 660, 667, 720

Muscle Rub: 594

My Destiny: 63, 384, 385, 957-969, 974

Myrrh: 10, 26, 42, 44, 53, 55, 57-59, 62, 64, 67, 68, 98, 99, 155, 206, 209, 230, 248, 266, 283, 284, 314, 386, 387, 434, 451, 489, 519, 541, 555, 556, 565, 572-574, 596, 600-602, 604, 605, 612, 619, 636-638, 640, 644, 669, 674, 676-679, 686, 697, 699, 727, 739, 951, 953, 955, 964, 971-976, 978, 988

Myrtle: 23, 55, 56, 59, 62, 89, 117, 211, 293, 322, 342, 379, 385, 388, 389, 427, 431, 564, 568, 569, 573, 612, 620, 625, 637, 640, 674-676, 699, 702, 747, 749, 951-953, 963, 964, 971-975, 977, 978, 987, 988

Natural Soaps: 607

Nature's Ultra: 134, 135, 594, 602

Nausea: 79, 80, 83, 84, 90, 117, 126, 167, 168, 170, 178, 191, 192, 202, 205, 211, 212, 235, 247, 252, 257, 275, 276, 300, 304, 310, 313, 325, 338, 341, 347, 350, 353, 357, 358, 370, 379, 411, 412, 419, 428, 431, 462, 469, 470, 474, 485, 490, 496, 540, 684, 689, 690, 692, 711

Neroli: 44, 62, 71, 90, 247, 284, 290, 350, 390, 424, 951, 953, 955, 964, 971-974, 978, 988

Nervous System: 42, 64, 68, 96, 135, 162, 192, 194, 206, 264, 286, 297, 333, 342, 350, 357, 358, 382, 405, 412, 414, 417, 485, 507, 533, 981, 561, 582, 608, 650, 669, 671, 692, 722, 736, 743, 755, 763

Nervous System, Autonomic: 194, 533

Nervous System, Parasympathetic: 96

Nervous System, Sympathetic: 162, 412, 485

Neuralgia: 254, 369, 522

Neuro Auricular Technique: 647

Neurological Diseases: 575, 669, 692

Neuropathy: 103, 104, 392

Neurotoxin: 613, 731

New Testament: 53, 266, 477, 669

Niaouli: 178, 368, 369, 373, 564, 594, 702, 749, 952, 953, 963, 964, 971, 974, 977, 988

NingXia Berry Syrup: 552, 962, 965, 985

NingXia Nitro: 552, 553, 955, 964, 965, 967, 968, 988

NingXia Red: 354, 437, 553, 635, 640, 696, 697, 699, 701-703, 711, 722, 749, 751, 752, 962, 965, 968, 969, 988

Ningxia Wolfberries (Organic Dried): 552, 553, 706, 707, 988

Ningxia Wolfberry: 536, 537, 543-557, 609, 617, 698, 718, 754, 756, 762

NingXia Zyng: 553, 955, 963, 988

Northern Lights Black Spruce: 62, 104, 146, 155, 206, 229, 230, 251, 266, 275, 276, 284, 314, 347, 353, 385, 396, 417, 434, 469, 489, 500, 535, 579, 581, 595, 603, 606, 611, 619, 637, 642, 673-679, 698, 751, 952, 953, 956, 964, 972-975, 978, 988

Northern Lights Farm: 12

Nutmeg: 10, 42, 62, 211, 212, 229, 247, 347, 353, 358, 385, 392, 540, 552, 628, 676-678, 697, 707, 728, 729, 952, 954, 964, 972-974, 978, 988

Nutmeg Vitality: 392, 540, 628, 952, 954, 964, 978, 988

NutraSweet®: 759

Nutrition: 485, 537, 543-545, 547, 554, 557, 618, 636, 702, 703, 711, 723, 726, 742, 749, 758, 763, 765, 766

Nutritional Support: 354, 617, 698

Obesity: 23, 101, 161, 233, 264, 337, 338, 342, 387, 419, 474, 482, 520, 560, 563, 624, 681-683, 685, 715, 726, 757, 758, 762, 765

Obsessiveness: 678

Ocotea: 26, 62, 71, 72, 84, 90, 118, 177, 205, 229, 276, 298, 299, 304, 347, 394-396, 438, 461, 469, 470, 479, 496, 500, 538, 539, 553, 569, 572, 579, 581, 588-590, 595, 597, 606, 611, 616, 637, 638, 674, 675, 677, 678, 699, 707, 952-954, 961, 964, 971-975, 978, 988

Oil Pulling: 585

Ointment: 53, 59, 252, 373, 574, 605, 616, 635-638, 640, 642-644, 955, 956, 958-961, 964-966, 968, 969, 981, 990

Old Testament: 133, 669

Olive Oil: 28, 31, 32, 34, 53, 230, 438, 573, 575, 578, 583, 584, 595, 603, 609, 610, 622, 635, 641, 685, 694, 704, 705, 972, 975

Oman: 26, 98, 243, 670, 734-736, 747, 764

OmegaGize3: 639, 699

One Heart: 63, 396, 674-679, 698

Onycha: 42, 952, 954

Optical Rotation: 16, 48

ORAC: 549, 754

Oral Health Care: 584, 589

Oral Hygiene: 419, 981, 584-586

Orange: 23, 26, 34, 42-44, 49, 62, 68, 71, 90, 142, 146, 155, 156, 167, 215, 247, 248, 264, 270, 284, 290, 294, 316, 328, 350, 353, 354, 385, 390, 398, 399, 411, 414, 417, 424, 461, 500, 537, 549, 552-554, 556, 564, 566, 569, 573, 578, 579, 581, 582, 590, 596, 601, 604, 605, 609, 611, 612, 616, 617, 619, 624, 627, 628, 631, 638, 674-679, 689, 694, 699, 700, 702, 703, 706, 707, 717, 720, 725, 749, 951, 953-955, 960, 962, 964-966, 971-975, 978, 988

Orange Blossom Facial Wash: 556, 582, 604, 605, 960, 962, 965, 966, 988

Orange Blossom Moisturizer: 605, 962, 965, 966, 988

Orange Vitality: 34, 398, 627, 628, 954, 965, 971, 978, 988

Oregano: 31, 38, 49, 62, 178, 289, 304, 308, 400-403, 568, 581, 583-585, 594, 628, 629, 632, 634, 637, 642, 644, 645, 657-660, 662, 663, 667, 699, 705, 741, 750, 952, 954, 965, 966, 971, 973, 978, 989

Oregano Vitality: 400, 628, 644, 952, 954, 965, 978, 989

Oregano, Ecuadorian: 62, 402, 699

Ortho Ease Massage Oil: 583, 638-640, 659, 958, 959, 961, 963, 965, 968, 969, 989

Ortho Sport Massage Oil: 583, 638-640, 958, 963, 965, 968, 969, 989

OSHA: 746

Osteoarthritis: 257, 474, 756

Osteoporosis: 243, 559, 560, 564, 566, 719

Owie, KidScents: 63, 318, 986, 619

Oxides: 43, 44, 236

Oxygen: 41, 47, 96, 251, 330, 548-550, 608, 650, 671, 687, 702, 709, 716, 717, 720, 722, 749, 754

Pain: 15, 23, 37-39, 48, 68, 71, 72, 79, 83, 84, 89, 90, 95, 96, 98, 101, 104, 108, 117, 118, 121, 125, 133, 135, 144, 146, 149, 150, 155, 156, 165, 167, 168, 170, 174, 178, 181, 191, 192, 199, 200, 202, 209, 212, 215, 226, 229, 233, 236, 251, 252, 254, 263, 266, 270, 275, 278, 284, 289, 290, 293, 297, 303, 304, 307, 313, 319, 327, 328, 333, 338, 347, 354, 357, 362, 365, 370, 373, 374, 379, 385, 392, 398, 402, 409, 414, 417, 419, 423, 428, 431, 434, 438, 441, 447, 461, 462, 465, 466, 469, 470, 474, 477, 479, 480, 489, 490, 496, 499, 508, 520, 522, 526, 537, 539, 563, 565, 568, 571, 592, 594, 608, 610, 615, 618, 623, 638-640, 642, 643, 648, 656-658, 667, 670, 684, 695, 715, 748, 751, 755, 756, 759, 956-958, 960, 962, 963, 965-968, 983

Pain Relief: 104, 108, 149, 181, 362, 594, 640, 667, 956-958, 960, 962, 963, 965-968, 983

Pain Relief Cream: 594, 640, 956-958, 960, 962, 963, 965-968, 983

Pakistan: 753, 754

Palm: 56, 554, 573, 577-582, 595, 597-602, 604-611, 615, 634, 643, 648, 660-662, 665, 698

Palmarosa: 62, 146, 155, 170, 235, 252, 270, 307, 404, 405, 500, 569, 571, 573, 604, 605, 636, 638, 674-679, 951, 954, 965, 971-975, 978, 989

Palm Slide: 660, 665

Palo Santo: 26, 62, 170, 244, 289, 314, 322, 406, 434, 496, 951, 954, 965, 972, 973, 975, 978, 989, 569, 619, 620, 637-639, 642, 645, 674-679, 699, 747, 750

PanAway: 38, 63, 409, 638-640, 739, 957, 960, 965, 969, 974, 979, 989

Pancreatitis: 541

Panic: 678

ParaFree: 639, 640, 690, 697, 955, 957-961, 963-965, 968, 989

ParaGize, Animal Scents: 637, 955, 958-961, 963, 965-967, 981

Parasites, Intestinal: 96, 165, 174, 233

Parasympathetic Nervous System: 96

Parkinson's Disease: 135, 219

Parsley: 62, 410, 411, 636, 705

Parsley Vitality: 410, 411

Patchouli: 42, 62, 68, 192, 350, 357, 358, 412, 414, 417, 477, 500, 513, 952, 536, 604, 605, 609, 625, 636-638, 640, 678, 717, 752, 954, 965, 971, 972, 974, 975, 978, 989

PD 80/20: 989, 566

Peace & Calming: 63, 38, 414, 416, 417, 635, 639, 640, 642, 643, 647, 674, 677, 678, 690, 698, 739, 955-958, 960, 964, 965, 968, 969, 974, 979, 989

Peace & Calming II: 63, 416, 417, 642, 643, 674, 677, 678, 690, 698, 955-958, 960, 964, 965, 968, 969, 974, 989

Pénoël, Daniel: 41, 43, 388, 655, 702, 749, 750

Peppermint: 20, 23, 26, 29, 34, 38, 43, 44, 51, 62, 79, 83, 117, 140, 146, 170, 178, 191, 192, 244, 304, 322, 325, 353, 357, 374, 379, 385, 409, 418, 419, 428, 431, 441, 462, 474, 496, 530, 952, 954, 965, 966, 971-976, 978, 989, 536, 537, 539, 540, 542, 552, 553, 556, 564, 565, 568, 569, 572, 577, 578, 580, 581, 583, 584, 586, 589-594, 599-601, 606, 608-610, 618, 620, 625-628, 631, 632, 634, 637, 639-641, 657-660, 662, 665, 674-678, 693, 695, 706, 707, 717, 718, 725, 739, 741, 750

Peppermint Vitality: 418, 540, 627, 628, 639, 641, 952, 954, 965, 966, 978, 989

Periodontitis: 586, 588

Perry, Bruce D: 670

Personal Care: 555, 571, 577, 582, 596, 615, 656, 981-992

Pert, Candace: 670

Petitgrain: 44, 62, 420, 951, 954, 966, 978, 989

pH Balance: 535, 536, 615, 616, 685, 686, 752

Index

Phenols: 41, 42, 401, 629, 714, 728

Physical Relief: 658

Pigs: 630, 634, 715

Pine: 42, 43, 49, 55, 56, 62, 84, 226, 254, 269, 322, 385, 422, 423, 431, 522, 594, 620, 638-640, 657, 674-679, 951-954, 966, 968, 972-976, 978, 989

Plaque: 20, 526, 585-587, 589, 590, 592, 593, 613

Plectranthus Oregano: 62, 178, 402, 594, 632, 634, 637, 642, 645, 952, 954, 966, 971, 989

Pneumonia: 419, 428, 432, 486, 699

PowerGize: 956, 960, 961, 989

Pregnancy: 37, 111, 177, 233, 252, 255, 300, 320, 338, 560, 564, 694, 726, 731

Pregnenolone: 539, 556, 559, 562, 564-569, 580, 581

Prenolone: 556, 566, 580, 955, 957, 959, 960, 967, 969, 989

Prenolone Plus Body Cream: 556, 566, 580, 955, 957, 959, 960, 967, 969, 989

Present Time: 63, 424, 673-679, 722, 739, 747, 956, 964, 969, 971, 974, 979, 989

Progessence Plus: 567, 580, 955-957, 959, 965, 967, 989

Prostate Cancer: 182, 561, 564, 566, 568

Prostate Health: 568, 959, 960, 962, 964, 965, 989

Prostate Problems: 112, 388, 564

Protec: 958, 959, 964, 967, 989

Protecting Your Home: 623

Protein: 536, 537, 543, 544, 552-556, 563, 567, 568, 577, 578, 580, 581, 591, 605, 606, 635, 636, 638, 643, 644, 681-684, 689, 693, 699, 700, 703, 707, 711-713, 716, 717, 720, 728, 741, 744, 745, 755, 756, 965, 989

Psalms: 58, 59

Psoriasis: 130, 181, 254, 273, 334, 388, 419, 486, 522, 608, 715

Pure Protein Complete Chocolate Deluxe: 989

PuriClean, Animal Scents: 637, 957, 961-966, 968, 981

Purification: 39, 63, 108, 220, 341, 395, 426, 427, 482, 549, 559, 624, 631, 638, 639, 643, 688, 699, 725, 726, 739, 750, 752, 957, 961, 963, 964, 966, 968, 974, 979, 989

Purity: 7, 9, 13, 15-17, 25, 45, 48, 486, 522, 722, 734, 761

QuadShield: 701, 702, 748, 749

Quality Control: 16, 17, 46-48

Radiation: 112, 373, 550, 561, 681, 701, 702, 723, 740, 742, 743, 746-753, 762, 765

Raindrop Technique: 83, 93, 186, 212, 251, 263, 365, 401, 402, 419, 428, 431, 493, 503, 508, 519, 526, 632-635, 638, 642, 644, 645, 648, 655-661, 666, 667

Raindrop Technique for Horses: 644

Raven: 63, 428, 431, 432, 959, 962, 965, 966, 969, 974, 979, 989, 639, 640, 642, 739, 750

Ravintsara: 62, 122, 289, 304, 322, 385, 428, 432, 433, 620, 644, 667, 699, 739, 951, 954, 966, 973-975, 978, 989

R.C.: 39, 63, 117, 430, 431, 639, 640, 642, 667, 739, 741, 956, 958, 959, 962-966, 974, 979, 989

Recipes: 34, 53, 129, 133, 158, 185, 233, 239, 387, 395, 411, 493, 553, 627, 689, 691, 696, 697, 703, 704, 707, 762

Recipes—Delicious and Nutritious: 703

Reconnect: 63, 283, 290, 297, 434, 673-679, 697, 698, 955, 956, 958, 960-969, 975, 979, 989

Red Shot: 436, 437, 956, 960, 963, 967, 968, 975, 979, 989

Refractive Index: 16

Regenolone Moisturizing Cream: 556, 568, 581, 958, 965, 969, 989

Rehemogen: 691, 699, 966, 968, 989

Relaxation Massage Oil: 584, 955, 958, 960, 962, 965, 967-969, 989

Release: 10, 34, 42, 63, 68, 74, 95, 122, 133, 150, 153, 196, 197, 226, 235, 243, 254, 281, 300, 438, 451, 461, 499, 540, 544, 554, 556, 557, 563, 582, 591, 593, 640, 643, 644, 647, 658, 660, 666, 667, 670-674, 676-679, 690, 691, 697, 698, 709, 725, 739, 763, 955, 956, 958-964, 966-969, 972, 975, 978, 979, 989

Relieve It: 63, 440, 955, 956, 961, 965, 975, 979, 989, 640, 739

Research: 1, 15, 19, 20, 23, 27, 46-49, 51, 74, 77, 86, 93, 96, 98, 101, 103, 104, 107, 108, 111, 112, 121, 122, 125, 126, 129, 130, 133, 144, 149, 150, 153, 158, 161, 162, 165, 168, 173, 174, 181, 182, 185, 186, 189, 194, 199, 200, 209, 216, 219, 220, 223, 224, 233, 236, 239, 240, 243, 254, 257, 260, 263, 264, 273, 278, 281, 286, 299, 300, 303, 308, 310, 327, 330, 333, 334, 337, 338, 341, 342, 345, 348, 361, 362, 365, 366, 369, 370, 377, 382, 387, 388, 391, 392, 395, 398, 401, 402, 405, 406, 411, 412, 419, 420, 423, 432, 443, 444, 447, 454, 457, 458, 473, 474, 477, 482, 485, 486, 490, 493, 504, 507, 513, 514, 517, 520, 525, 526, 529, 530, 533, 547, 556, 558-561, 563, 564, 568-570, 577, 585, 586, 613, 647, 655-657, 667, 670, 684, 686, 687, 702, 714-716, 721, 727, 728, 730-732, 734, 736-739, 741-746, 748, 749, 752-755, 753, 761-766

Resentment: 678

Restlessness: 37, 153, 297, 495, 499, 507, 678

Retention: 16, 38, 46, 130, 186, 233, 264, 308, 322, 337, 341, 361, 362, 392, 398, 412, 482, 486, 517, 529, 563, 684, 720, 756

Rheumatoid Arthritis: 243, 330, 369

Rhinitis: 125, 362, 432

Roman Chamomile: 43, 62, 72, 90, 146, 152, 153, 155, 170, 194, 197, 235, 252, 270, 304, 307, 313, 320, 374, 380, 396, 480, 495, 500, 556, 567, 569, 571, 573, 580, 581, 596, 597, 601, 602, 604, 606, 616, 619, 620, 638-640, 674, 676-679, 690, 696, 951, 954, 966, 971-975, 978, 989

Romans: 53, 365, 454, 473

Rose: 15, 42, 43, 59, 62, 67-71, 84, 90, 117, 118, 142, 146, 155, 162, 197, 205, 206, 215, 220, 235, 251, 252, 270, 275, 276, 284, 304, 307, 314, 357, 373, 398, 434, 438, 442, 443, 451, 461, 499, 500, 519, 568, 569, 573, 574, 579, 581, 595, 596, 601, 602, 604-606, 619, 636, 638, 669, 670, 673-678, 694, 697, 737, 739, 951, 952, 954-956, 958, 960, 964-966, 968, 969, 971-976, 978, 989, 950

Rose of Sharon: 162, 951, 954, 966

First Edition | Essential Oils Complete Home Reference | 989

Rose Ointment: 252, 373, 605, 955, 956, 958, 960, 964-966, 968, 969, 990

Rosemary: 23, 43, 44, 53, 62, 146, 170, 212, 257, 308, 313, 373, 427, 444, 445, 473, 490, 538, 539, 556, 572, 573, 575-578, 580, 586, 588, 590, 592, 593, 596, 602, 604, 605, 608-612, 616, 624-628, 636, 637, 639, 657, 674-678, 687, 690, 693, 695, 696, 699, 707, 717, 718, 727, 728, 752, 952, 954, 966, 967, 970-975, 978, 990

Rosemary Vitality: 444, 627, 628, 952, 954, 966, 967, 978, 990

Royal Hawaiian Sandalwood: 62, 64, 71, 90, 118, 197, 235, 251, 276, 290, 293, 297, 328, 350, 353, 434, 438, 456, 457, 496, 499, 500, 555, 569, 571, 574, 595, 598-602, 605, 609, 638, 674, 675, 697, 747, 952, 954, 967, 971-975, 978, 990

Rue: 44, 62, 177, 244, 320, 446-448, 500, 620, 638, 671, 952, 954, 967, 971, 972, 975, 978, 990

Russia: 182, 194

RutaVaLa: 63, 448, 673, 674, 676, 678, 679, 690, 698, 962, 967, 968, 975, 979, 990

Sacred Frankincense: 62, 118, 242-244, 248, 275, 314, 320, 357, 434, 489, 496, 568, 569, 580, 600, 619, 620, 640, 642, 669, 670, 672-679, 698, 699, 735, 736, 747, 750, 752, 951, 954, 967, 971-975, 978, 990

Sacred Mountain: 251, 452, 610, 642, 674-678, 697, 739, 956, 961, 969, 975, 979, 990

Sacred Mountain Moisturizing Soap: 610, 956, 961, 969, 990

Sacred Sandalwood: 62, 67, 89, 114, 146, 155, 205, 270, 275, 304, 314, 357, 358, 385, 451, 458, 500, 519, 952, 967, 971-976, 990, 597, 604, 616, 619, 640, 674, 675, 678, 697, 747

Sage: 20, 26, 43, 62, 146, 155, 172, 173, 178, 202, 211, 215, 247, 270, 294, 308, 328, 350, 358, 379, 411, 454, 462, 472, 473, 496, 500, 539, 541, 556, 565-569, 571, 576, 578-580, 583, 584, 594, 638, 674, 677-679, 728, 952-954, 957, 967, 971-975, 977, 978, 983, 990, 991

Sage Vitality: 454, 967, 978, 990

Sagging Skin: 37, 423

Sandalwood Moisture Cream: 556, 605, 955, 958, 960, 962, 964, 966, 967, 969, 990

Sandalwood, Royal Hawaiian: 62, 64, 71, 90, 118, 197, 235, 251, 276, 290, 293, 297, 328, 350, 353, 434, 438, 456, 457, 496, 499, 500, 555, 569, 571, 574, 595, 598-602, 605, 609, 638, 674, 675, 697, 747, 952, 954, 967, 971-975, 978, 990

Sandalwood, Sacred: 62, 67, 89, 114, 146, 155, 205, 270, 275, 304, 314, 357, 358, 385, 451, 458, 500, 519, 597, 604, 616, 619, 640, 674, 675, 678, 697, 747, 952, 967, 971-976, 990

SARA: 63, 460, 461, 640, 673-679, 690, 698, 739, 956-958, 960-962, 964-969, 975, 979, 990

Satin Facial Scrub Mint: 606, 582, 965, 990

Saunas: 205

Savvy Minerals Accessories: 582

Savvy Minerals Lip Gloss: 965

Scar Tissue: 150, 252, 273, 603, 682, 756

Scarring: 112, 252, 334, 443

Schreuder, Marc: 736

Sciatica: 103, 104, 525, 568, 656, 657, 667

SclarEssence: 63, 462, 569, 957, 959, 965, 967, 975, 979, 990

SclarEssence Vitality: 462, 957, 959, 965, 967, 975, 979, 990

Scleroderma: 756

Scoliosis: 382, 419, 656, 657, 667

Scurvy: 108, 337, 338

Seed to Seal: 8, 9, 15, 17, 25, 27, 31, 46, 135, 263, 396, 510, 582

Seedlings Baby Lotion: 620, 955, 958, 960, 962, 969, 990

Seedlings Baby Oil: 621, 955, 958, 960, 962, 990

Seedlings Baby Wash & Shampoo: 621, 955, 958, 960, 962, 969, 990

Seedlings Baby Wipes: 621, 955, 958, 960, 969, 990

Seedlings Diaper Cream: 956, 960, 962, 990

Seedlings Linen Spray: 622, 955, 958, 960, 962, 969, 990

Seizures: 391, 759

Sensation: 15, 49, 50, 63, 178, 419, 466, 565, 571-573, 583, 584, 594, 600, 615, 623, 739 955, 958, 960, 961, 969, 975, 979, 990

Sensation Bath & Shower Gel: 572, 955, 958, 960, 961, 969, 990

Sensation Hand & Body Lotion: 573, 955, 958, 960, 961, 969, 990

Sensation Massage Oil: 584, 955, 958, 960, 961, 969, 990

Sesquiterpenes: 42, 44, 98, 387, 457, 458, 477, 496, 507, 514, 671, 686, 728, 730, 763

Shampoo: 555, 556, 577, 578, 616, 621, 637, 639, 955, 957-965, 967-969, 981, 983, 986, 987, 990

Shave Cream: 595, 956, 958, 960-964, 968, 969, 990

Shave Oil: 595, 956, 958, 961, 962, 964, 966, 967, 969, 988

Shaving: 548, 594, 595

Sheerlumé Brightening Cream: 582, 600, 601, 956-959, 961, 967, 968, 982

Shock: 678, 722, 763

Shower: 350, 555, 571, 572, 631, 725, 726, 955-969, 981-992

Shutran: 63, 468, 469, 489, 956, 579, 581, 595, 606, 611, 674-679, 958, 960-964, 966, 968, 969, 975, 979, 990

Shutran 3-in-1 Men's Wash: 606, 956, 958, 960-962, 964, 969, 990

Shutran Aftershave Lotion: 595, 956, 958, 960-964, 969, 990

Shutran Bar Soap: 611, 956, 958, 960-964, 966, 969, 990

Shutran Beard Oil: 579, 956, 958, 960-964, 969, 990

Shutran Shave Cream: 595, 956, 958, 960-964, 968, 969, 990

Single Oils: 75, 105, 107, 113, 627, 658, 693, 695, 738, 747, 750, 977

Index

Sinus Congestion: 236

Sinus Infections: 86, 200, 220, 223, 263, 322, 341, 369, 388, 423

Skin Cancer: 546, 640, 748

Skin Candida: 158

Skin Care: 44, 135, 168, 200, 209, 236, 338, 348, 423, 482, 514, 571, 573, 582, 595, 596, 599, 629

Skin Warming: 655

Sleep Disorders: 454

SleepEssence: 962, 967, 968, 990

SleepyIze, KidScents: 63, 320, 986, 620

Slique Bars: 553, 554, 707, 957, 965, 968, 990

Slique Bars—Tropical Berry Crunch: 553

Slique CitraSlim: 956, 959, 961, 963, 964, 967, 990

Slique Essence: 63, 470, 588, 616, 628, 960, 963, 964, 967, 968, 975, 979, 991

Slique Gum: 591, 959, 966, 967, 991

Slique Shake: 554, 696, 699, 703, 707, 960, 963, 964, 967, 968, 991

Slique Tea: 470, 968, 991

Slique Toothpaste: 588, 957, 959, 960, 962, 964, 966-968, 986

Snacks: 707, 754, 757, 762

SniffleEase, KidScents: 63, 322, 620, 986

Snoring: 39

Soaps: 20, 342, 473, 981-992, 571, 607, 608, 611, 612, 623, 624, 714, 746

Sore Muscles: 29, 38, 83, 216, 220, 223, 236, 520

Sore Throat: 39, 181, 545, 592, 593

Sorrow: 489, 679

Spanish Sage: 62, 146, 155, 270, 328, 462, 472, 473, 500, 569, 638, 952, 954, 967, 972-975, 978, 991

Spearmint: 26, 62, 71, 79, 84, 90, 118, 140, 167, 205, 211, 229, 259, 275, 276, 304, 325, 328, 396, 437, 438, 461, 470, 474, 475, 500, 552, 556, 569, 573, 577, 578, 581, 584, 588-591, 593, 600-602, 612, 616, 620, 628, 636, 637, 675, 691, 702, 707, 749, 952, 954, 967, 971-976, 978, 991

Spearmint Vitality: 474, 628, 952, 954, 967, 972, 978, 991

Species: 8, 15, 20, 42, 44, 46, 86, 96, 98, 121, 144, 162, 165, 173, 181, 186, 216, 220, 223, 224, 240, 260, 281, 286, 299, 303, 330, 333, 341, 395, 412, 423, 454, 473, 477, 482, 517, 520, 529, 530, 547, 561, 588, 629, 631, 632, 637, 638, 669, 702, 734-736, 749, 764,

Spikenard: 53, 55, 57, 59, 62, 476, 477, 952, 954, 991

Spinal Tissue Pull: 660, 664

Spiritual: 59, 64, 98, 189, 199, 239, 243, 251, 275, 308, 316, 387, 406, 451, 452, 489, 508, 530, 619, 661, 669, 671-673, 675, 677, 679, 680, 727, 736, 738, 740, 741

Splenda: 724, 758, 759, 766

Sports Gel: 594, 640, 956-958, 960, 962, 963, 965-969, 983

Stanford University: 743

Stanley Burroughs: 650, 688

Steam Distillation: 3, 8, 10, 12, 107, 345

Stevia: 136, 138, 140, 470, 975, 536, 554, 566, 588-593, 616-619, 761, 762, 766

Stings: 489

Stomachache: 522, 718

Stomach Ulcers: 181

Storage: 559, 562, 683, 716, 752

Stress: 3, 27, 34, 37-39, 42, 50, 51, 63, 77, 80, 83, 96, 101, 108, 112, 121, 129, 150, 153, 158, 161, 168, 173, 189, 219, 233, 252, 270, 278, 299, 334, 338, 361, 362, 365, 369, 370, 395, 405, 406, 414, 420, 423, 432, 444, 447, 477-480, 495, 499, 500, 504, 507, 510, 513, 514, 517, 520, 533, 956, 957, 962-964, 968, 975, 979, 991, 539-541, 548, 550, 563, 569, 571, 572, 583, 584, 597, 635, 639, 640, 642, 645, 650, 658, 672, 673, 679, 681-686, 689, 690, 698, 713, 727, 754

Stress Away: 39, 63, 478, 956, 957, 962-964, 968, 975, 979, 991, 571, 572, 597, 635, 639, 640, 642, 673, 679, 690, 698

Stress Away Relaxing Bath Bombs: 572, 964, 991

Stretch Marks: 37, 252, 334, 361, 387, 391, 616

Strokes: 576, 602, 605, 632, 634, 645, 660, 663

Sucralose: 758, 759, 765

Sugar: 158, 189, 194, 264, 273, 395, 405, 473, 536, 540, 544, 546, 548, 549, 552-555, 563, 578, 585, 588, 590, 592, 644, 681, 682, 684-686, 689, 693-696, 700, 711-713, 716, 717, 724, 754, 757-762, 765

Suhail, Mahmoud: 735, 735

Sulfurzyme Capsules and Powder: 554, 991

Sunburn: 37, 38, 362, 525, 603, 747, 748

Super Vitamin B: 699

Super Vitamin C: 699, 751

Super Vitamin C Chewable: 699, 751

Super Vitamin Cal Plus: 700

Super Vitamin D: 699

Surrender: 63, 480, 642, 674, 677, 678, 739, 955, 956, 962-964, 966, 975, 979, 991

Sweeteners: 536, 553, 591, 688, 694, 696, 700, 756-759, 761, 762, 765

Swelling: 37, 38, 68, 71, 72, 79, 83, 84, 89, 90, 108, 117, 118, 146, 153, 156, 167, 170, 178, 191, 192, 212, 215, 229, 251, 252, 266, 270, 275, 284, 289, 290, 293, 304, 307, 313, 319, 328, 347, 354, 357, 373, 374, 379, 409, 414, 417, 428, 431, 438, 441, 461, 462, 465, 466, 469, 470, 479, 480, 489, 490, 496, 499, 508, 515, 565, 571, 615, 623, 642, 644

Switzerland: 726, 744

Sympathetic Nervous System: 162, 412, 485

Synthetic: 1, 5, 7, 8, 12, 16, 25, 43, 45, 47-49, 114, 239, 303, 334, 536, 555, 559, 560, 564, 571, 572, 575, 577, 582, 588, 590, 594, 596, 602-604, 608, 615-617, 622, 623, 631, 636, 656, 700, 711, 722, 743, 746, 754, 757, 758, 761, 762, 765

Syphilis: 181

T-Away, Animal Scents: 638, 981

Taiwan: 8, 26, 122, 278, 281, 300, 529, 551, 761

Tangerine: 34, 42, 62, 71, 84, 90, 118, 155, 167, 205, 229, 247, 276, 290, 304, 307, 320, 325, 414, 417, 437, 438, 461, 470,

482, 500, 539, 540, 553, 569, 573, 584, 588, 604, 615, 616, 620, 627, 628, 638, 675-677, 679, 691, 694, 700, 951, 954, 967, 968, 971-976, 978, 991

Tangerine Vitality: 34, 482, 540, 627, 628, 951, 954, 967, 968, 978, 991

Tarragon: 42, 62, 192, 484, 485, 536, 539, 542, 625, 637, 693, 695, 696, 717, 951, 954, 968, 972, 978, 991

Tarragon Vitality: 484, 951, 954, 968, 972, 978, 991

Tea, Slique: 470, 968, 991

Tea Tree: 20, 23, 26, 39, 62, 74, 89, 236, 319, 327, 362, 373, 411, 427, 486, 487, 952, 576, 594-596, 602, 605, 607, 619, 625, 627, 636, 637, 639, 645, 697, 699, 701, 702, 747, 954, 968, 971, 974, 978, 991,

Techniques for Different Animal Species: 631

Techniques for Essential Oil Application: 647, 649, 651, 653, 655, 657, 659, 661, 663, 665, 667, 668

Tender Tush: 616, 955, 957-960, 962, 966, 969, 986

Tendons: 639

Terpenes: 41-43, 49, 107, 366, 667, 728, 730

Testing: 8, 15, 16, 17, 42, 46-48, 50, 559, 565, 568, 571, 594, 615, 623, 631, 681, 686, 723, 736, 738, 742, 750, 758,

Testing Your pH: 686

Texas: 366, 670, 23

Texas Southern University: 23

The Gift: 63, 68, 251, 488, 489, 642, 673, 674, 676-679, 697-699, 747, 752, 957, 961, 964, 967, 968, 975, 979, 991

Therapeutic: 5-13, 16, 17, 19, 25-27, 34, 41, 42, 44-46, 49, 96, 122, 186, 239, 303, 327, 443, 444, 458, 489, 573, 582, 593, 608, 629, 655, 657, 658, 671, 746, 756

Thieves: 39, 63, 174, 289, 431, 444, 490, 553, 574, 575, 580, 586, 588-590, 592, 593, 611, 612, 616, 623-627, 638-640, 642-644, 698, 699, 739, 750, 752, 955, 957, 959-961, 963-969, 975, 979, 991, 992

Thieves AromaBright Toothpaste: 589, 957, 959, 963, 964, 966, 967, 991

Thieves Automatic Dishwasher Powder: 624, 957, 959, 963, 965, 966, 991

Thieves Chest Rub: 574

Thieves Cleansing Soap: 957, 959, 963, 966, 991, 611

Thieves Cough Drops: 592, 957, 959, 963, 966, 991

Thieves Dental Floss: 590, 957, 959, 963, 966, 991

Thieves Dish Soap: 624, 644, 955, 957, 959, 963, 967, 991

Thieves Foaming Hand Soap: 612, 624, 957, 959, 963, 965, 967, 991

Thieves Fresh Essence Plus Mouthwash: 592, 593, 957, 959, 963, 966-968, 991

Thieves Fruit & Veggie Soak: 624, 955, 957, 959-961, 963-968, 991

Thieves Fruit & Veggie Spray: 625, 957, 959, 963, 967

Thieves Hard Lozenges: 592, 957, 959, 963, 966, 967, 991

Thieves Household Cleaner: 625, 627, 644, 957, 959, 963, 967, 991

Thieves Laundry Soap: 625, 639, 955, 957, 959, 963, 967, 991

Thieves Mints: 592, 957, 959, 963, 966, 967, 991

Thieves Roll-On: 63, 490, 963, 964

Thieves Spray: 626, 627, 957, 959, 963, 967, 991

Thieves Vitality: 490, 644, 957, 959, 963, 967, 968, 975, 979, 991

Thieves Waterless Hand Purifier: 957, 959, 963, 966, 967, 992

Thieves Wipes: 627, 957, 959, 963, 967, 992

Three Mile Island: 701, 748

Throat: 33, 39, 74, 93, 108, 117, 122, 125, 173, 174, 181, 251, 263, 322, 388, 419, 423, 432, 444, 517, 545, 575, 592, 593, 640, 643, 666, 697, 698, 711, 741, 743

Thumb Roll: 660, 665

Thyme: 20, 23, 42, 44, 45, 62, 308, 354, 492, 493, 542, 576, 583-586, 592, 602, 628, 629, 632, 634, 644, 645, 657-660,

662, 664, 667, 674-678, 686, 697, 699, 707, 727-729, 741, 763, 952, 954, 968, 974, 978, 992

Thyme Vitality: 492, 628, 644, 952, 954, 968, 974, 978, 992

Thyroid Problems: 388

Thyromin: 699-702, 748, 749, 751, 964, 966, 967, 992

Ticks: 637, 638, 640

To Disinfect: 444, 642, 643

To Promote Healing: 43, 635, 655, 657

To Reduce Bleeding: 638

Tonsillitis: 181, 362

Tooth Enamel: 586, 587, 593, 732

Toothpaste: 586-590, 616, 644, 731, 732, 957, 959, 960, 962-964, 966-969, 986, 991

Topical Application: 444, 561, 566

Toxic Liver: 684

Transformation: 63, 189, 457, 458, 496, 569, 673, 674, 677-679, 698, 956, 957, 961, 963-967, 975, 979, 992

Trauma, Emotional: 51, 186, 499, 514, 658, 670, 671

Trauma Life: 63, 498, 639, 640, 642, 674, 676-679, 739, 956-960, 962, 966-968, 975, 979, 992

T.R. Care: 63, 500, 955-969, 975, 979, 992

Treasure of the Season: 63, 502, 503, 957, 959, 961, 975, 992

Truman, Karol K: 673

Tsuga: 62, 504, 675-679, 952, 954, 968, 978, 992

Tuberculosis: 20, 93, 149, 181, 391, 401, 419, 428, 525, 657, 667, 760

TummyGize, KidScents: 63, 324, 620, 986

Tumors: 161, 181, 561, 570, 640, 681

Umbilical Cords of Newborn Foals: 644

United Kingdom: 454, 728

University of Delaware: 23

University of Minnesota: 743

University of Oklahoma: 734, 23

Index

Urinary Tract Infection: 233, 423, 485

Usage: 25, 27, 33, 36, 248, 299, 589, 627, 667, 738, 746, 747, 761, 981

USDA: 7, 19, 556, 617, 754, 758, 765

Utah: 26, 46, 173, 308, 310, 457, 517, 568, 586, 625-627, 657, 684, 714, 715, 741, 763, 13, 15,

Unwind, KidScents: 618

V-6 Vegetable Oil Complex: 15, 28, 31, 62, 63, 584, 632, 634, 635, 639-642, 656, 659, 697, 992

Valerian: 43, 62, 244, 320, 448, 499, 500, 506, 507, 620, 638-640, 643, 677, 678, 690, 952, 954, 968, 971, 972, 975, 978, 992

Valnet, Jean: 220, 254, 419, 586, 613, 655

Valor: 34, 39, 63, 68, 251, 396, 508, 576, 611, 632, 634, 635, 639, 640, 642, 644, 658-661, 665, 667, 672-679, 690, 697, 698, 739, 747, 955-961, 967-969, 976, 979, 992

Valor Deodorant: 576

Valor Moisturizing Soap: 611, 955-961, 967-969, 992

Valor Roll-On: 63, 508, 674-679, 690, 956, 959, 960, 976, 979, 992

Vanilla: 62, 72, 316, 479, 510, 512, 513, 952, 954, 957, 959, 962, 963, 965, 968, 971, 975, 983, 989, 992, 552, 554, 555, 572, 577, 597, 599, 619, 706

Varicose Veins: 38, 112, 273, 338, 341, 419, 529

Vegetarian: 536, 545, 618

Vertebrae: 80, 658, 664, 667

Veterinary Medicine: 629

Vetiver: 43, 62, 72, 142, 155, 178, 191, 206, 230, 244, 251, 266, 276, 284, 293, 297, 314, 328, 357, 385, 417, 434, 489, 500, 514, 569, 583, 593, 594, 597, 600, 601, 619, 637, 638, 642, 678, 697, 952, 954, 968, 971-975, 978, 992

Vita Flex: 34, 192, 200, 211, 328, 15, 569, 634, 645, 647, 648, 650, 655, 659, 660, 662, 663, 665, 697

Vita Flex Thumb Roll: 660, 665

Vital Life Juice Recipe: 691, 696

Vitality: 15, 34, 92, 93, 95, 96, 100, 101, 126, 128-130, 149, 150, 158, 160, 161, 166, 167, 170, 174, 180-182, 184, 185, 192, 194, 199, 210-212, 232, 233, 238, 239, 256-259, 264, 300, 310, 312, 313, 330, 334, 338, 340, 341, 348, 354, 364, 365, 382, 392, 393, 400, 401, 410, 411, 418, 419, 444, 454, 462, 474, 482, 484, 485, 490, 492, 493, 499, 503, 537, 540-542, 552, 565, 571, 584, 615, 623, 627, 628, 633, 639-641, 643, 644, 647, 648, 681, 691, 699, 700, 713, 722, 727, 729, 731, 733-735, 737, 739, 741, 743, 745, 747, 749, 751, 753, 755, 757, 759, 761, 763, 765, 951-968, 971-975, 977-979, 982-992

Vitassage: 647

Vitiligo: 254

Water: 9-12, 14, 16, 20, 28, 34, 41, 45, 48, 53, 58, 103, 125, 126, 130, 133, 173, 181, 185, 186, 199, 220, 243, 337, 350, 370, 406, 411, 431, 443, 470, 473, 486, 517, 525, 536-540, 544, 551, 554, 559, 567-569, 571-573, 576-581, 583, 588-590, 592-601, 603-607, 609-612, 615-617, 620-622, 624-628, 631, 632, 635-637, 639, 640, 643, 644, 658, 659, 666, 681, 684, 685, 687-691, 693-696, 698-700, 703-707, 711, 715-719, 722-726, 728, 731-734, 739, 742, 743, 748, 750-752, 754, 756, 763, 765

Water Filtration: 726

Waterless Hand Purifier: 957, 959, 963, 966, 967, 992

Weber State University: 490, 586, 625-627, 657, 741

Western Red Cedar: 62, 226, 516, 952, 954, 968, 992

White Angelica: 63, 518, 658, 659, 661, 662, 666, 673-679, 698, 739, 955, 956, 958, 960, 961, 963, 964, 966, 967, 969, 976, 979, 992

White Fir: 15, 62, 84, 226, 269, 276, 294, 500, 520, 522, 951, 954, 968, 971, 973-976, 978, 992

White Light: 63, 522, 968, 976, 992, 677, 678

White Lotus: 62, 294, 461, 524, 952, 954, 968, 973-975, 992

Whooping Cough: 432

Wintergreen: 43, 62, 178, 191, 385, 409, 428, 526, 535, 537, 556, 568, 581, 583, 586, 592, 594, 596, 632, 634, 638-640, 642, 658-660, 662, 664, 667, 951, 954, 969, 971, 972, 974, 978, 992

Wipes: 575, 621, 627, 955, 957-960, 963, 967, 969, 990, 992

Wolfberry: 26, 536, 537, 540, 543-558, 566-568, 573, 574, 577-581, 596, 601, 605, 606, 609-611, 617, 698, 699, 707, 718, 722, 754, 756, 762, 955, 958-960, 962, 966, 969, 985, 992

Wolfberry Crisp: 552, 555, 707, 985

Wolfberry Crisp Bars, Chocolate Coated: 555, 707

Wolfberry Eye Cream: 556, 606, 955, 958-960, 962, 966, 969, 992

World War II: 742, 744

Worms: 129, 161, 165, 174, 233, 286, 419, 637, 640

Wounds: 108, 112, 209, 216, 219, 220, 224, 286, 377, 411, 419, 504, 520, 530, 575, 594, 602, 619, 635, 636, 638, 640, 643, 720, 721

Wrinkles: 37, 130, 209, 252, 303, 338, 387, 391, 398, 411, 412, 423, 443, 457, 458, 514, 555, 564, 601, 602, 756

Xiang Mao: 26, 62, 66, 528, 951, 954, 969, 972, 978, 992

Yacon: 354, 688, 691, 696, 703, 704, 706, 707, 762, 766, 992

Yacon Syrup: 354, 638, 691, 696, 703, 704, 706, 707, 762, 992

Yarrow: 15, 62, 112, 202, 379, 567-569, 580, 583, 678, 951, 954, 969, 972, 974, 978, 992

Yeast: 17, 20, 200, 419, 493, 535, 539, 636, 685, 686, 691, 714, 715, 720, 721, 741, 760

Yemen: 98, 734

Ylang Ylang: 26, 42, 62, 67, 71, 72, 80, 84, 90, 95, 118, 142, 146, 155, 170, 177, 205, 235, 251, 252, 266, 269, 270, 276, 284, 290, 293, 294, 304, 307, 314, 328, 353, 357, 358, 380, 385, 396, 411, 414, 417, 424, 434, 438, 451, 452, 461, 465, 466, 469, 500, 513, 519, 530, 951, 953-955, 969, 971-976, 978, 981, 992, 555, 556, 566, 567, 569, 571-574, 579-581, 583, 584, 595-597, 599-602, 604-605, 609-612, 616, 619-

622, 636, 638, 673-679

Young: 1, 7-11, 13, 16, 17, 25-28, 31, 34, 36, 41, 42, 44-48, 55-57, 59, 63, 66, 67, 72, 98, 108, 122, 134, 135, 142, 177, 199, 216, 223, 229, 239, 240, 243, 247, 263, 299, 304, 310, 341, 396, 406, 432, 457, 458, 490, 503, 510, 530, 990, 15, 540, 549, 551, 554, 556, 559, 565, 567-569, 571, 572, 575, 577, 582, 583, 594, 599-602, 604, 609, 613, 615, 616, 618, 619, 621, 623, 633, 637, 647, 655, 657, 667, 669, 681, 684, 687, 688, 691, 696, 698, 704, 707, 714-716, 729, 731, 732, 734-737, 741, 747, 750, 753, 754, 763-765.

Young, D. Gary: 177, 199, 229, 240, 243, 396, 554, 559, 567, 569, 647, 655, 657, 681, 691, 696, 704, 707, 715, 736, 741, 750, 753, 754

Young, Gary: 177, 199, 229, 240, 243, 247, 396, 490, 530, 554, 559, 567, 569, 647, 655, 657, 681, 691, 696, 704, 707, 715, 736, 741, 750, 753, 754

Young Living: 1, 7-11, 13, 15, 16, 17, 25-28, 31, 34, 36, 41, 42, 44-48, 67, 72, 98, 108, 122, 134, 135, 142, 177, 216, 243, 263, 299, 304, 396, 432, 503, 510, 530, 540, 549, 565, 571, 572, 575, 577, 582, 594, 599-602, 604, 609, 615, 618, 621, 623, 637, 647, 667, 698, 707, 716, 734-737, 741, 990

Young Living Essential Oils: 1, 8, 13, 25, 27, 31, 34, 41, 46, 47, 108, 142, 177, 510, 540, 549, 594, 637, 647, 734, 736, 741,

Yuzu: 62, 532, 533, 951, 954, 969, 978, 992

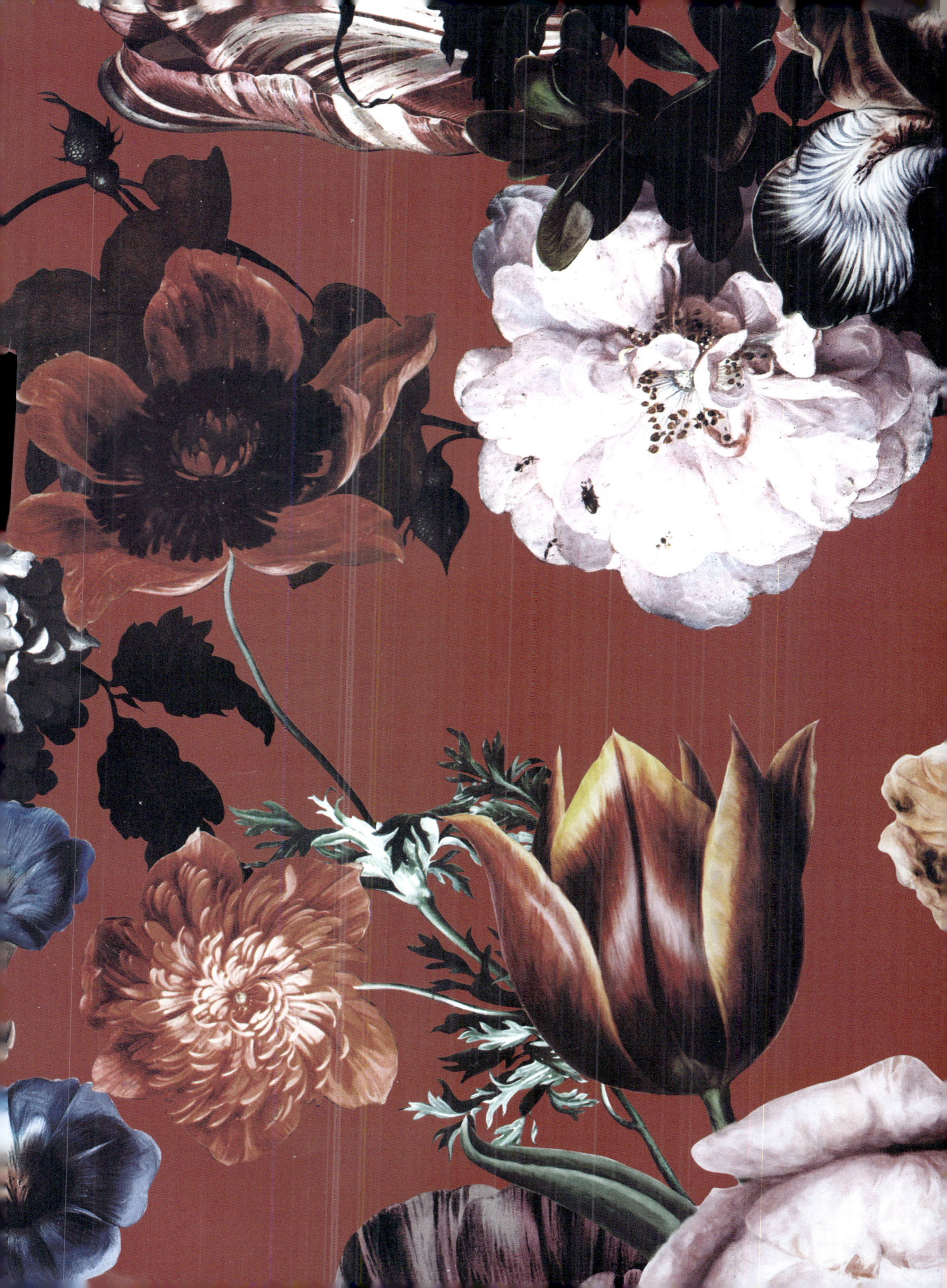

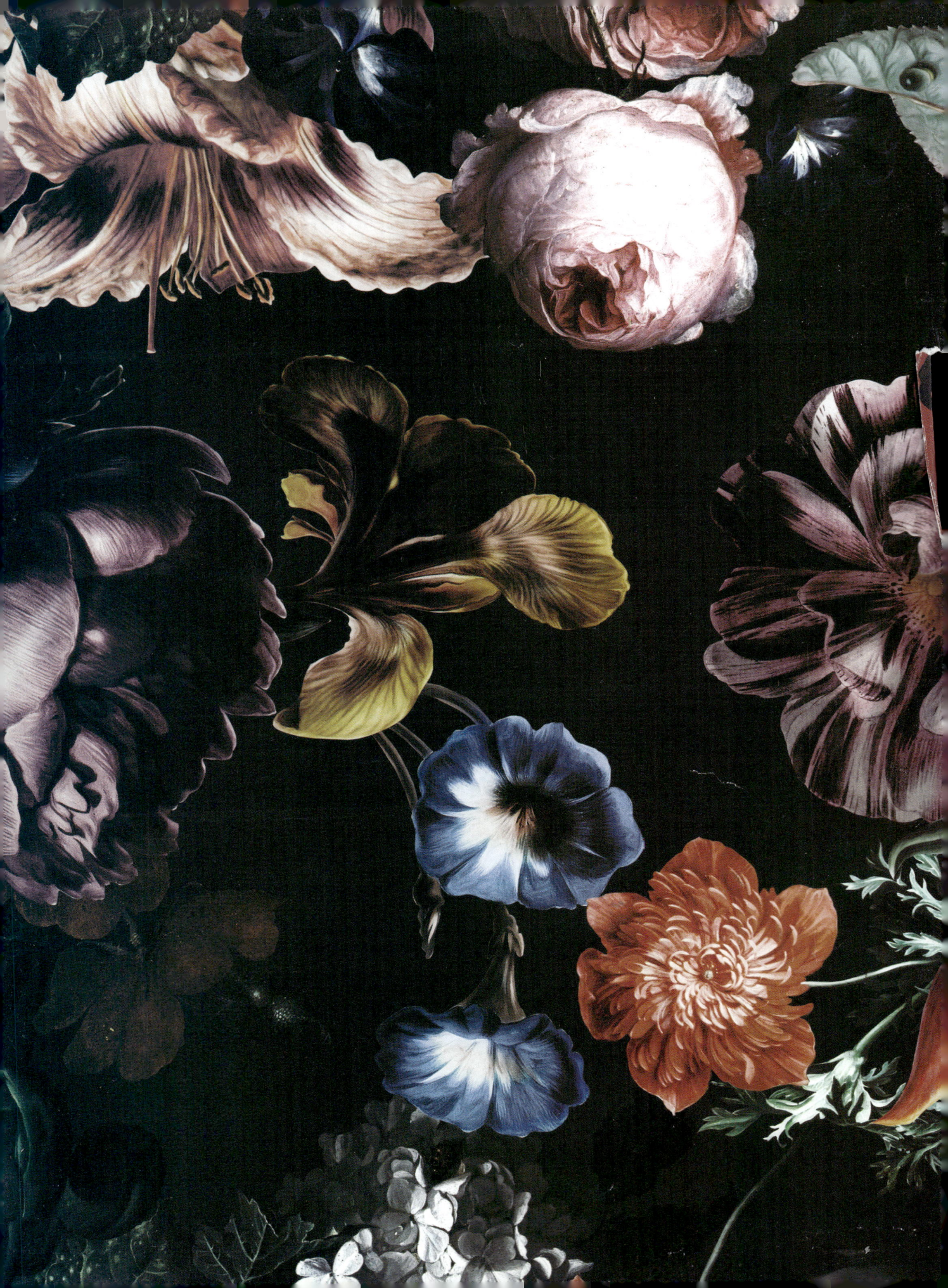